EXPLORE PEARSON mynursingkit™

W9-BMN-784

STEP 1: Register

All you need to get started is a valid email address and the access code below. To register, simply:

1. Go to **www.mynursingkit.com**. Click on the appropriate book cover.
2. In the "First-Time User" column, click "**Register**."
3. Read the **License Agreement** and **Privacy Policy**. If you accept, click "**I Accept**."
4. Under "**Do you have a Pearson account**?" select:
   - "**Yes**" if you have a Pearson account and know your Login Name and Password.
   - "**Not Sure**" if you do not know if you already have an account or do not recall your Login Name and Password.
   - "**No**" if you are sure you do not have a Pearson account.
5. Using a coin, scratch off the silver coating below to reveal your access code. Do not use a knife or other sharp object, which can damage the code.
6. Enter your access code in lowercase or uppercase, without the dashes, then click "**Next**."
7. Follow the on-screen instructions to complete registration.

After completing registration, you will be sent a confirmation email that contains your Login Name and Password. Be sure to save this email for future reference.

Your Access Code is:

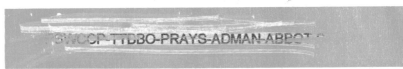

SWOOP-TTDBO-PRAYS-ADMAN-ABBOT

Note: If there is no silver foil covering the access code, it may already have been redeemed, and therefore may no longer be valid. In that case, you can purchase access online using a major credit card. To do so, go to www.mynursingkit.com. Find and click on the cover of your textbook, then click "Get Access," and follow the on-screen instructions.

STEP 2: Log in

1. Go to **www.mynursingkit.com**.
2. Find and click on the appropriate book cover. Cover must match the textbook edition used for your class.
3. Enter the Login Name and Password that you created during registration. If unsure of this information, refer to your registration confirmation email.
4. Click "**Login**."

Got technical questions?

Customer Technical Support: To obtain support, please visit us online anytime at http://247pearsoned.custhelp.com where you can search our knowledgebase for common solutions, view product alerts, and review all options for additional assistance.

SITE REQUIREMENTS
For the latest updates on Site Requirements, go to www.mynursingkit.com. Find and click on the cover of the book you are using. Click on "**Needs help?**" link at bottom of page. Under "**Technical Problems**" select the link "**What do I need on my computer to use this site?**"

Important: Please read the Subscription and End-User License agreement, accessible from the book website's login page, before using the *mynursingkit* website. By using the website, you indicate that you have read, understood, and accepted the terms of this agreement.

0135077591

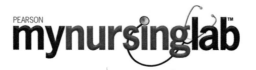
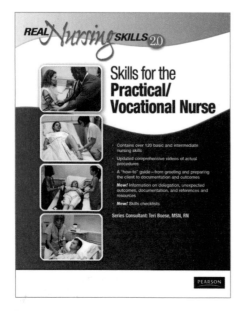

The Nature of Nursing

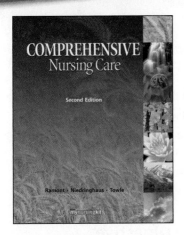

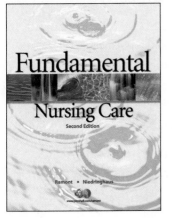

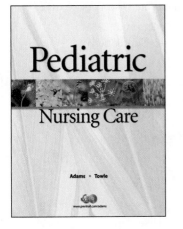

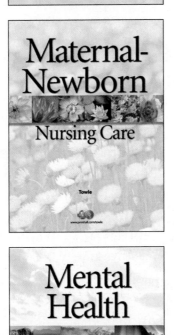

The Nature of Nursing embodies the ever-changing rewards and challenges for today's practical and vocational nursing students. Pearson Nursing addresses these challenges with a series of textbooks written directly for practical and vocational nursing students. Each book in the series shares a similar design and contains similar features to enhance the student's learning experience. It gives students more time to focus on content and less on "learning the book". Books in the series share a consistent reading level and a dedicated focus on what the LPN/LVN needs to know and do and priorities for action.

Shared features include:

- Color-coded boxes for assessment and data collection, client teaching, lifespan and diversity issues
- Clinical Alerts
- Nursing Care sections
- Nursing Process Care Plans
- End of Chapter NCLEX-PN® review questions and test-taking tips
- Clinical Reasoning/Critical Thinking Care Maps
- Extensive Unit Wrap-Ups

The Nature of Nursing— Grow With It!

BRIEF CONTENTS

THIRD EDITION

CORE CONCEPTS IN PHARMACOLOGY

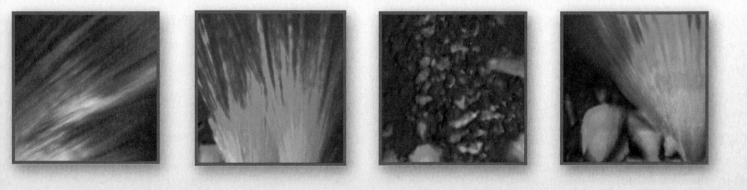

LELAND NORMAN HOLLAND, Jr., PhD

Instructor
Hillsborough Community College, SouthShore Center

MICHAEL PATRICK ADAMS, PhD, RT(R)

Professor, Biological Sciences
Formerly Dean, Health Occupations
Pasco-Hernando Community College

NURSING CONSULTANT

Jeanine Brice, RN, MSN
Pasco-Hernando Community College

Pearson
Boston   Columbus   Indianapolis   New York   San Francisco   Upper Saddle River
Amsterdam   Cape Town   Dubai   London   Madrid   Milan   Munich   Paris   Montreal   Toronto
Delhi   Mexico City   Sao Paulo   Sydney   Hong Kong   Seoul   Singapore   Taipei   Tokyo

Library of Congress Cataloging-in-Publication Data

Holland, Leland Norman, (Date)
   Core concepts in pharmacology / Leland Norman Holland Jr., Michael Patrick Adams.—3rd ed.
     p. ; cm.
   Includes bibliographical references and index.
   ISBN-13: 978-0-13-507759-7
   ISBN-10: 0-13-507759-1
   1. Pharmacology—Outlines, syllabi, etc. I. Adams, Michael, (Date) II. Title.
   [DNLM: 1. Pharmacological Phenomena. 2. Drug Therapy. QV 4 H735c 2011]
   RM301.14.H655 2011
   615'.1—dc22

                                              2010003553

Publisher: Julie Levin Alexander
Assistant to the Publisher: Regina Bruno
Editor-in-Chief: Maura Connor
Senior Acquisitions Editor: Kelly Trakalo
Editorial Assistant: Lauren Sweeney
Development Editor: Michael Giacobbe
Managing Production Editor: Patrick Walsh
Production Liaison: Yagnesh Jani
Production Editor: Mary Tindle, S4Carlisle Publishing Services
Manufacturing Manager: Ilene Sanford
Senior Art Director: Maria Guglielmo
Cover and Interior Designer: Wanda Expaña
Digital Media Product Manager: Travis Moses-Westphal
Media Product Manager: Rachel Collett
Image Interior Permission Coordinator: Richard Rodrigues
Manager, Image Rights and Permissions: Zina Arabia
Manager, Visual Research: Beth Brenzel
Image Cover Permission Coordinator: Rita Wenning
Director of Marketing: David Gesell
Marketing Coordinator: Michael Sirinides
Marketing Assistant: Crystal Gonzalez
Composition: S4Carlisle Publishing Services
Cover Printer: Lehigh Phoenix Color
Printer/Binder: Worldcolor Versailles
Cover Image: Courtesy of Maud S. Bech / Phototake, Inc.

Notice: The authors and the publisher of this volume have taken care to make certain that the doses of drugs and schedules of treatment are correct and compatible with the standards generally accepted at the time of publication. Nevertheless, as new information becomes available, changes in treatment and in the use of drugs become necessary. The reader is advised to carefully consult the instruction and information material included in the package insert of each drug or therapeutic agent before administration. This advice is especially important when using, administering, or recommending new and infrequently used drugs. The authors and publisher disclaim all responsibility for any liability, loss, injury, or damage incurred as a consequence, directly or indirectly, of the use and application of any of the contents of this volume.

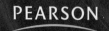

ISBN-13:   978-0-13-507759-7
ISBN-10:   0-13-507759-1

Pharmacology is one of the most challenging subjects for those embarking on careers in the health sciences. By its very nature, pharmacology is an interdisciplinary subject, borrowing concepts from a wide variety of the natural and applied sciences. Prediction of drug action, the ultimate goal in the study of pharmacology, requires a thorough knowledge of anatomy, physiology, chemistry, and pathology as well as the social sciences of psychology and sociology. It is the interdisciplinary nature of pharmacology that makes the subject difficult to learn, but fascinating to study.

This text presents pharmacology from an interdisciplinary perspective. The text draws upon core concepts of anatomy, physiology, and pathology to make drug therapy understandable. The text does not assume that the student comes to the course with a strong background in the natural or applied sciences. Although it is true that many students have prerequisite courses prior to attempting introductory pharmacology, such courses may have been taken many years prior to the current course. The prerequisite science knowledge necessary for understanding drug therapy is reviewed prior to presenting the core concepts in pharmacology.

ORGANIZATION

The authors have created a concise means of communicating the most important pharmacologic information to the student. Through the use of numbered **Core Concepts**, the student is able to quickly identify key ideas. These core concepts are stated at the beginning of each chapter, so that the student can get an overview of what is to be learned. They are repeated at the end of the chapter, with a brief summary of the important concepts.

Disease and Body System Approach

Core Concepts in Pharmacology is organized according to body systems and diseases. This clearly places the drugs in context with how they are used therapeutically. The student is able to easily locate all relevant anatomy, physiology, pathology, and pharmacology in the same chapter in which the drugs are discussed.

Prototype Approach to Drug Therapy

The vast number of drugs taught in a pharmacology course is staggering. To facilitate learning, a prototype approach is used in which the one or two most representative drugs in each classification are introduced in detail. **Drug Profile** boxes are used to clearly indicate these important medications.

Focused Nursing Content

This text provides focused nursing content, which allows students to quickly find the essential content for safe, effective drug therapy. **Nursing Process Focus** charts provide a succinct, easy-to-read view of the most commonly prescribed drug classes. Need-to-know nursing actions are presented in a format that reflects the "flow" of the Nursing Process: nursing assessment, potential nursing diagnoses, planning, interventions, patient education and discharge planning, and evaluation. Rationales for interventions are included in parentheses. The Nursing Process Focus charts identify clearly what nursing actions are most important.

NEW TO THIS EDITION:

- **2 New Chapters!** Chapter 5, The Nursing Process and Chapter, Drugs for Degenerative Diseases and Muscles.

- **New! Safety Alert** feature throughout the text calls attention to medication errors and The Joint Commission safety guidelines.

- **New! Glossary** provided at the end of the book.

- **Updated and Revised!** End of chapter NCLEX-PN® questions completely revised by nurse consultant.

- **Updated and Revised!** All drugs updated and prototypes adjusted to today's drug market.

- **New information** on weight loss surgery and drugs.

- **Drug Profiles** will now include both therapeutic and pharmacological drug classifications.

- **Addition** of off-label uses of drugs and adverse effects to drug tables as appropriate.

- **New information** on the impaired nurse.

DESIGN AND FEATURES

A Focus On Core Information

Through the use of Numbered **Core Concepts**, identify ideas and provide an overview of the chapter.

The **Drug Snapshot** provides an at-a-glance list of the drug classes and related drug profiles covered in each chapter.

Key Terms with page numbers help students review important vocabulary terms.

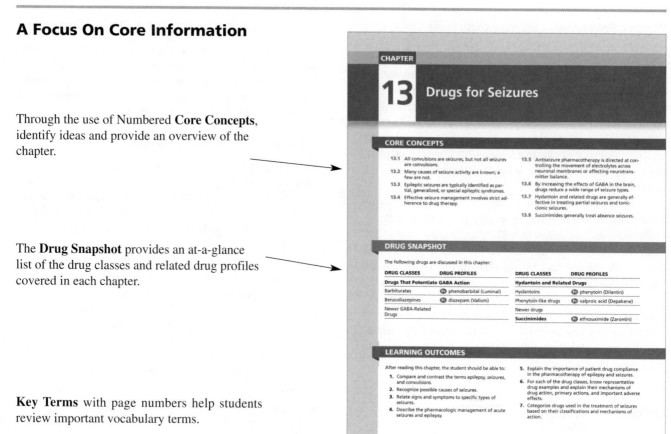

Concept Reviews are questions placed strategically throughout the chapter to stimulate student comprehension and retention as they read.

Concept Review   13.1

■ What is epilepsy? What is the difference between a seizure and a convulsion? Name and identify signs of the more common types of seizures.

Using A Prototype Approach

The prototype approach introduces the one or two most representative drugs in each classification in detail. **Drug Profile** boxes highlight these important drugs. This edition now includes both therapeutic and pharmacologic drug classifications.

DRUG PROFILE: Phenobarbital (Luminal)
Therapeutic Class: Antiseizure drug, sedative, hypnotic
Pharmacologic Class: Barbiturate, GABA_A receptor drug

Actions and Uses:
Phenobarbital is a long-acting barbiturate used for the management of a variety of seizures. It is also used for insomnia. Phenobarbital should not be used for pain relief, because it may increase a patient's sensitivity to pain. Phenobarbital acts biochemically in the brain by enhancing the action of the neurotransmitter GABA, which is responsible for suppressing abnormal neuronal discharges that can cause epilepsy.

Adverse Effects and Interactions:
Phenobarbital is a Schedule IV drug that may cause dependence. Common adverse effects include drowsiness, vitamin deficiencies (vitamin D, folate, B_6, and B_12), and laryngospasms. With overdose, phenobarbital may cause severe respiratory depression, CNS depression, coma, and death. Phenobarbital is a pregnancy category D drug.
Phenobarbital interacts with many other drugs. For example, it should not be taken with alcohol or other CNS depressants. These substances potentiate the action of barbiturates, increasing the risk of life-threatening respiratory depression or cardiac arrest. Phenobarbital increases the metabolism of many other drugs, reducing their effectiveness.

Refer to MyNursingKit for a Nursing Process Focus specific to this drug.

TABLE 13.4	Succinimides	
DRUG	**ROUTE AND ADULT DOSE**	**REMARKS**
ethosuximide (Zarontin)	PO; 250 mg bid, increased every 4–7 days (max: 1.5 g/day)	For absence seizures, myoclonic seizures, and akinetic epilepsy
methsuximide (Celontin)	PO; 300 mg/day, may increase every 4–7 days (max: 1.2 g/day in divided doses)	For absence seizures; may be used in combination with other anticonvulsants in mixed types of seizure activity
phensuximide (Milontin)	PO; 0.5–1 g bid or tid	For absence seizures; similar characteristics to methsuximide

Drug tables provide the most important information for each drug in a user-friendly format. Drugs profiled within that chapter are also identified with a Prototype icon .

HIGHLIGHTS KEY INFORMATION FOR SAFE, EFFECTIVE NURSING CARE

NURSING PROCESS FOCUS

Patients Receiving Drugs for Muscle Spasms or Spasticity

ASSESSMENT

Prior to administration:
- Obtain a complete health history (physical/mental), including allergies, drug history, and possible drug interactions
- Obtain a complete physical examination
- Establish a baseline level of consciousness (LOC) and vital signs

POTENTIAL NURSING DIAGNOSES
- Pain (acute/chronic) related to muscle spasms.
- Impaired Physical Mobility related to acute/chronic pain.
- Risk for Injury related to adverse effects of drug.
- Deficient Knowledge related to information about disease process and drug therapy.

PLANNING: PATIENT GOALS AND EXPECTED OUTCOMES

The patient will:
- Report a decrease in pain, increase in range of motion, and reduction of muscle spasms
- Exhibit no serious adverse effects from the drug therapy
- Demonstrate an understanding of the therapeutic regimen by accurately describing the drug's effects, precautions, and measures to take to minimize adverse effects

IMPLEMENTATION

Interventions and (Rationales)	Patient Education/Discharge Planning
Monitor LOC and vital signs. (Some skeletal muscle relaxants alter the patient's LOC. Others within this class may alter blood pressure and heart rate.)	Instruct the patient to: • Avoid driving and other activities requiring mental alertness until the effects of the medication are known • Report any significant change in sensorium, such as slurred speech, confusion, hallucinations, or extreme lethargy • Report palpitations, chest pain, dyspnea, unusual fatigue, weakness, and visual disturbances • Avoid using other CNS depressants such as alcohol that will intensify sedation
Monitor pain. Determine the location, duration, and precipitating factors of the patient's pain. (Drugs should diminish the patient's pain.)	Instruct the patient: • To report the development of new sites of muscle pain • In relaxation techniques, deep breathing, and meditation methods to facilitate relaxation and reduce pain
Monitor for withdrawal reactions. (Abrupt withdrawal of baclofen may cause visual hallucinations, paranoid ideation, and seizures.)	• Advise the patient to not abruptly discontinue treatment.
Monitor muscle tone, range of motion, and degree of muscle spasm. (This will determine the effectiveness of drug therapy.)	• Instruct the patient to perform gentle range of motion, only to the point of mild physical discomfort, throughout the day.
Provide additional pain relief measures such as positional support, gentle massage, and moist heat or ice packs. (Drugs alone may not be sufficient in providing pain relief.)	• Instruct the patient in complementary pain interventions such as positioning, gentle massage, and the application of heat or cold to the painful area.
Monitor for adverse effects such as drowsiness, dry mouth, dizziness, nausea, vomiting, faintness, headache, nervousness, diplopia, and urinary retention (cyclobenzaprine).	Instruct the patient to: • Report adverse effects • Take medication with food to decrease GI upset • Report signs of urinary retention such as a feeling of urinary bladder fullness, distended abdomen, and discomfort
Monitor for adverse effects such as muscle weakness, dry mouth, dizziness, nausea, diarrhea, tachycardia, erratic blood pressure, photosensitivity, and urinary retention. (These adverse effects occur with certain drugs in this class.)	Instruct the patient: • That frequent mouth rinses, sips of water, and sugarless candy or gum may help with dry mouth • That medication may cause a decrease in muscle strength and dosage may need to be reduced • To use sunscreen and protective clothing when outdoors

EVALUATION OF OUTCOME CRITERIA

Evaluate the effectiveness of drug therapy by confirming that patient goals and expected outcomes have been met (see "Planning").

See Tables 12.6 and 12.7 for lists of drugs to which these nursing actions apply.

Nursing Process Focus charts provide a succinct, easy-to-read view of the most important nursing actions for the commonly prescribed drug classes. Need-to-know nursing actions are presented in the nursing process which also include patient education and discharge planning.

The nursing student needs to learn how to teach drug administration to patients and families. To help the student, each drug chapter contains concise **Patients Need to Know** boxes help students teach patients and families about drug information and administration.

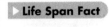

PATIENTS NEED TO KNOW

Patients taking antiseizure medications need to know the following:

In General
1. Never abruptly stop taking antiseizure medication; doing so can cause seizures.
2. Avoid alcohol and other CNS depressants because they can increase sedation.
3. Antiseizure medications may cause drowsiness; avoid driving and the use of machinery that could lead to injury.
4. It may require several dosage adjustments over many months to find the dosage that allows performance of normal daily activities while controlling seizures.
5. It is important to keep laboratory appointments because many antiseizure medications require blood testing to ensure that the drug is at a safe and effective level in the blood.
6. Consult a health care provider before trying to become pregnant; some antiseizure medications are not safe to use during pregnancy.
7. Report excess fatigue, drowsiness, agitation, confusion, or suicidal thoughts to a health care provider.

Regarding Hydantoins and Related Medications
8. Report the following adverse effects to a health care provider: gum overgrowth (gingival hyperplasia) or skin rash, tremors, weight gain, diarrhea, irregular menses, dizziness, nausea, or oversedation.
9. Hydantoins and related medications interact with many other drugs; do not add any other prescription, over-the-counter (OTC) drugs, or herbal supplements until a health care provider is consulted. Do not consume alcohol while taking these medications.

Regarding Succinimides
10. Report the following adverse effects to a health care provider: hiccups or epigastric pain with ethosuximide (Zarontin), drowsiness, or increased bleeding time.

SAFETY ALERT

Interpreting Physician Orders

In many health care facilities, it is the nurse's responsibility to interpret and transcribe doctors' orders for medications. Unfortunately, handwritten orders can be difficult to interpret correctly. For example, an error was made when an order to discontinue "SSRI," intended to mean "sliding scale regular insulin," was misinterpreted as an order to discontinue the "selective serotonin reuptake inhibitor" (Zoloft). It is extremely important for the nurse to know their patients' needs and to clarify with the physician any medication order that is difficult to interpret or is questionable.

Source: SSRI OR SSKI. (2008, May). NurseAdvise-ERR, 6(5), 2–3.

New! Safety Alerts highlight potential medication errors and The Joint Commission Safety Guidelines.

Life Span Facts provide important **pediatric** and **older adult** considerations for drug therapy, so students understand variations in nursing care and drug actions due to age.

▶ Life Span Fact

Onset of epilepsy is most common among the youngest and oldest age groups. About 50% of children have a generalized epilepsy syndrome compared with about 20% of adults. The incidence of epilepsy in elderly adults is greater than among the general population, perhaps because of the greater prevalence of mild strokes and cardiac arrest in this age group.

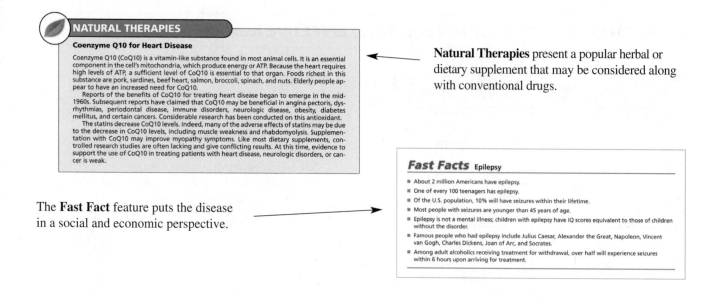

Natural Therapies present a popular herbal or dietary supplement that may be considered along with conventional drugs.

The **Fast Fact** feature puts the disease in a social and economic perspective.

END OF CHAPTER REVIEW RESOURCES

Student practical and vocational nurses from around the country told us that they start their chapter reading from the end of the chapter. So to ensure students' success, in the classroom, on the NCLEX-PN® exam, and in the workplace, we put dynamite review resources at the end of each chapter.

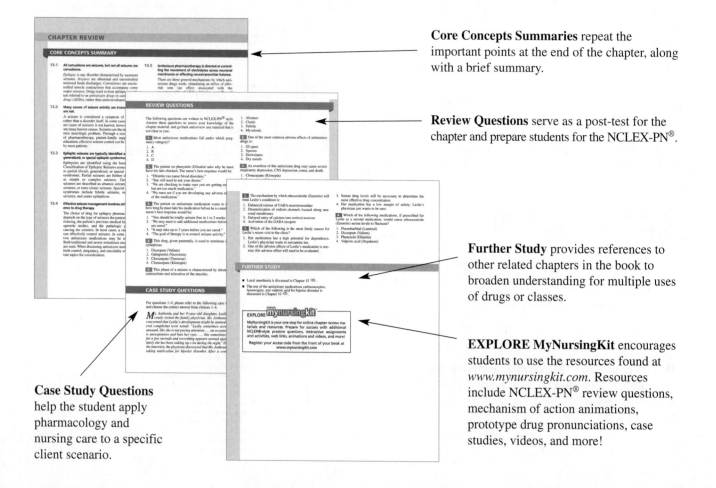

Core Concepts Summaries repeat the important points at the end of the chapter, along with a brief summary.

Review Questions serve as a post-test for the chapter and prepare students for the NCLEX-PN®.

Further Study provides references to other related chapters in the book to broaden understanding for multiple uses of drugs or classes.

EXPLORE MyNursingKit encourages students to use the resources found at *www.mynursingkit.com*. Resources include NCLEX-PN® review questions, mechanism of action animations, prototype drug pronunciations, case studies, videos, and more!

Case Study Questions help the student apply pharmacology and nursing care to a specific client scenario.

ACKNOWLEDGMENTS

We are grateful to all the educators who reviewed the manuscript of this text. Their insights, suggestions, and eye for detail helped us prepare a more relevant and useful book, one that focuses on the essential components of learning in the field of pharmacology. In particular we would like to thank Jeanine Brice, RN, MSN who reviewed and contributed to all nursing material including Nursing Process Focus Charts, Safety Alerts, Patient's Need to Know, Safety Alerts and all of the end of chapter questions. Your nursing experience, expertise, and dedication to the profession is evident in these materials.

Textbook Reviewers

Carol A. Buttz, RN BS CEN
Dakota County Technical College
Rosemount, Minnesota

Charlene M. Chapman, RN BSN
Pennsylvania Institute of Technology
Media, Pennsylvania

Cheryl Puckett, OB-RNC, MSN
Bluegrass Community and Technical College,
Danville Campus
Danville, Kentucky

Christi Blair, MSN, RN
Holmes Community College
Goodman, Mississippi

Gwen Dalida, RN-BC, MSN
South Texas College
McAllen, Texas

Janice C. Hess, M.S., RMT
Metropolitan Community College
Elkhorn, Nebraska

Joan Zarra, RN, BSN, MSN
Dover Business College–School of Practical
Nursing
Dover, New Jersey

Karen Snipe, CPhT, BA, Med
Trident Technical College
Charleston, South Carolina

Kathleen Reilly Dolin, MSN, RN
Northampton Community College
Bethlehem, Pennsylvania

Kristie A. Berkstreser, MSN, RN, CNE, BC
HACC, Central Pennsylvania's Community
College
Lancaster, Pennsylvania

**Mitchell J. Seal, EdD, Med-IT, BSN, AS,
RNBC, CLNC**
Bakersfield College
Bakersfield, California

Shirley Stamford, RN MSN
Brewster Technical Center
Tampa, Florida

Stephanie Justice, RN, BSN
Hondros College School of Nursing
Westerville, Ohio

Vernita A. Smith, MSN, RN
Bohecker College-Cincinnati
Fairfield, Ohio

Supplement Contributors

Sherri Hewlings, RN, BSN
Pennsylvania Institute of Technology
Media, Pennsylvania
*Instructor's Manual and Resource Guide,
PowerPoint Slides*

Stephanie Justice, RN
The Ohio State University College of Nursing
Columbus, Ohio
Test Item File

Supplement Reviewers

Charlene M. Chapman, RN BSN
Pennsylvania Institute of Technology
Media, Pennsylvania

Allison W. McQuirter, RN, MSN, CFNP
Holmes Community College,
Ridgeland Campus
Ridgeland, Mississippi

Michelle Rule, CMT
Metropolitan Community College
Omaha, Nebraska

Karen Snipe, CPhT, BA, Med
Trident Technical College
Charleston, South Carolina

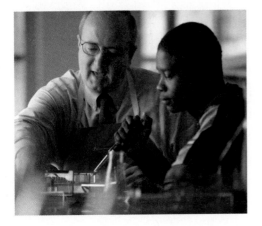

Leland Norman Holland, Jr., PhD (Norm), over twenty years ago started out like many scientists, planning for a career in basic science research. Quickly he was drawn to the field of teaching in higher medical education, where he has spent most of his career since that time. Among the areas where he has been particularly effective are preparatory programs in nursing, medicine, dentistry, pharmacy and allied health. Dr. Holland is both an affiliate and supporter of nursing education nationwide. He brings to the profession a depth of knowledge in biology, chemistry and medically-related subjects such as microbiology, biological chemistry, and pharmacology. Dr. Holland's doctoral degree is in medical pharmacology. He is very much dedicated to the success of students and their preparation for work-life readiness. He continues to motivate students in the life-long pursuit of learning.

I would like to acknowledge the willful encouragement of Farrell and Norma Jean Stalcup. I dedicate this book to my beloved wife, Karen, and my three wonderful children, Alexandria Noelle, my double-deuce daughter; Caleb Jaymes, my number one son; and Joshua Nathaniel, my number three "O"!
—LNH

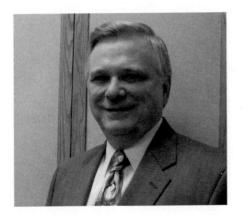

Michael Patrick Adams, PhD, RT(R), is an accomplished educator, author, and national speaker. The National Institute for Staff and Organizational Development in Austin, Texas, named Dr. Adams a Master Teacher. He has published two other textbooks with Pearson Publishing: *Pharmacology and Nursing: A Pathophysiological Approach* and *Pharmacology: Connections to Nursing Practice*.

Dr. Adams obtained his Master's degree in Pharmacology from Michigan State University and his Doctorate in Education at the University of South Florida. Dr. Adams was on the faculty of Lansing Community College and St. Petersburg College, and was Dean of Health Programs at Pasco-Hernando Community College for 15 years. He is currently Professor of Biological Sciences at Pasco-Hernando Community College.

I dedicate this book to nursing educators, who contribute every day to making the world a better and more caring place.
—MPA

CONTENTS

UNIT 7
The Skeletal System, Integumentary System, and Eyes and Ears

593

UNIT 1

Basic Concepts in Pharmacology

UNIT CONTENTS

1 Introduction to Pharmacology: Drug Regulation and Approval

CORE CONCEPTS

1.1 Pharmacology is an expansive and challenging topic.

1.2 For health care providers, the fields of pharmacology and therapeutics are connected.

1.3 Agents may be classified as traditional drugs, biologics, and natural alternatives.

1.4 Drugs are available by prescription or over the counter (OTC).

1.5 Pharmaceutics is the science of pharmacy.

1.6 Drug regulations were created to protect the public from drug misuse.

1.7 U.S. drug standards have become increasingly complex.

1.8 There are four stages of approval for therapeutic and biologic drugs.

1.9 Once criticized for being too slow, governmental agencies face new challenges for ensuring the safety of drugs.

1.10 Similar drug standards protect Canadian consumers.

1.11 Health care providers must be prepared to deal with the threat of biological and chemical attack.

LEARNING OUTCOMES

After reading this chapter, the student should be able to:

1. Explain the interdisciplinary nature of pharmacology and give examples of subject area expertise needed to learn the discipline well.

2. Identify groups of occupations in which a knowledge of pharmacology is important.

3. Explain how the disciplines of therapeutics and pharmacology are interconnected.

4. Distinguish between therapeutic drugs and agents such as foods, household products, and cosmetics.

5. Compare and contrast traditional drugs, biologics, and natural alternative therapies.

6. Identify the advantages and disadvantages of prescription and OTC drugs.

7. Distinguish between pharmaceutics and pharmacology.

8. Discuss the history of U.S. standards, acts, and organizations leading to the requirement that drug safety must be proven before marketing.

9. Discuss the role of the United States Food and Drug Administration (FDA) in determining whether drugs may be used for therapy.

10. Discuss the roles and responsibilities of branches within the FDA in overseeing traditional therapeutic drugs, biologics, and natural alternative therapies.

11. Identify four stages of approval for therapeutic and biologic drugs.

12. Discuss current challenges facing the FDA in approving new drugs for market.

13. Explain the role of Health Canada in the management of Canadian health, drug, and safety issues.

14. Describe the Canadian drug approval process and explain points of similarity to the U.S. approval process.

15. Discuss the challenges facing health care professionals in view of modern-day bioterrorist threats.

KEY TERMS

biologics (beye-oh-LOJ-iks) *4*

clinical pharmacology *8*

formularies (FOR-mew-LEH-reez) *5*

natural alternative therapies *4*

pathophysiology (PATH-oh-fiz-ee-OL-oh-jee) *3*

pharmaceutics (far-mah-SOO-tiks) *5*

pharmacology (far-mah-KOL-oh-jee) *3*

pharmacopoeia (far-mah-KOH-pee-ah) *5*

pharmacotherapeutics (far-mah-koh-THER-ah-PEW-tiks) *4*

therapeutics (ther-ah-PEW-tiks) *4*

D rugs are the most powerful weapon we have against diseases, worldwide epidemics, and bioterrorist activity. More drugs are being administered to consumers than ever before. Because of the number of new drugs becoming available for therapy, some experts are concerned that patients might be harmed if drugs are not thoroughly tested.

The purpose of this chapter is to introduce the subject of pharmacology and to emphasize the role of the government in ensuring that drugs and natural alternatives are safe and effective for public use. The chapter also addresses the role that drug therapy has in fighting disease as governmental regulators, consumers, and health care professionals face new challenges in the years ahead.

Bioterrorist threats have led to widespread changes in emergency preparedness planning. This chapter also briefly introduces the role of pharmacology in the prevention and treatment of diseases or conditions that might develop because of global biological, chemical, or nuclear threat.

Pharmacology is an expansive and challenging topic.

The word **pharmacology** is derived from two Greek words: *pharmakon,* which means "medicine," and *logos,* which means "study." Thus, *pharmacology* is defined as "the study of medicine."

pharmac = *medicine*
ology = *the study of*

Health care providers practice the discipline of pharmacology because it is the study of how drugs improve the health of the human body. If applied properly, drugs can dramatically improve patients' quality of life. If applied improperly, the consequences of drug action can be devastating.

The subject of pharmacology is an expansive topic ranging from a study of how drugs enter and travel throughout the body to the actual responses they produce. To learn the discipline well, students must master concepts from several interrelated areas, including anatomy, physiology, chemistry, and **pathophysiology**. The useful application of drugs depends on knowledge from at least these areas.

patho = *disease*
physio = *the nature of*
ology = *the study of*

More than 10,000 brand and generic varieties of drugs with many different names, interactions, side effects, and complicated mechanisms of action are currently available. Keeping up with the numbers of drugs is a huge challenge. Many drugs may be prescribed for more than one disease, and most produce multiple effects in the body. Further complicating the study of pharmacology is the fact that drugs may cause different responses depending on factors such as gender, age, health status, body mass, and genetics.

For health care providers, the fields of pharmacology and therapeutics are connected.

It is obvious that a thorough knowledge of pharmacology is important to those health professionals who prescribe drugs on a daily basis. This group includes physicians, physician's assistants, dentists, and advanced nurse practitioners. Depending on state or provincial law, members of other groups may also be permitted to prescribe medications. In this textbook, the group of occupations that is allowed to prescribe drugs is referred to as *health care providers.*

A second group of occupations includes nursing, allied health, and community service employees. These occupations have in common direct contact with patients or health care providers. Nurses and some other allied health workers are directly involved with drug administration as well as with issues related to drug education, management, and/or enforcement of drug laws. In this text, these occupations are referred to as *health care providers*.

Some health care providers, such as nurses, may administer drugs on a daily basis, whereas others may administer drugs occasionally. A strong knowledge of pharmacology is necessary to properly educate and advise patients regarding their health care needs. This knowledge is also essential to communicate effectively with health care providers, who rely heavily on nurses and allied health professionals to gather medical data from their patients and to follow up on results of therapy.

For health care providers studying pharmacology, it usually becomes apparent that the fields of pharmacology and therapeutics are connected. **Therapeutics** is the branch of medicine concerned with the treatment of disease and suffering. **Pharmacotherapeutics** is the use of medicine to treat disease.

Agents may be classified as traditional drugs, biologics, and natural alternatives.

CORE CONCEPT 1.3

Drugs are chemical agents that produce biologic responses within the body. From a broader perspective, drugs may be considered a part of the body's normal activities, from the essential gases that people breathe to the foods that they eat. Because drugs are defined so broadly, it is necessary to clearly separate them from other substances such as foods, household products, and cosmetics. Many agents, including antiperspirants, sunscreens, toothpastes, and shampoos, might alter the body's normal activities, but they are not considered to be medically therapeutic, as are drugs taken for a medical disorder.

Therapeutic drugs are sometimes classified on the basis of how they are produced, either chemically or naturally. Most traditional drugs are chemically produced or synthesized in a laboratory. **Biologics** are agents naturally produced in animal cells, in microorganisms, or by the body itself. **Natural alternative therapies** are herbs, natural extracts, vitamins, minerals, or dietary supplements. Table 1.1 shows a summary of characteristics associated with traditional drug therapies, biologics, and natural alternative therapies. Because drugs may be described in many ways, this text limits its focus to agents used for therapy in a clinical or home setting. Traditional drugs and drug classes are discussed more thoroughly in Chapter 2. Natural alternatives are discussed more thoroughly in Chapter 6. In addition, most chapters include a feature called *Natural Alternatives* that highlights a specific herbal therapy or dietary supplement.

Drugs are available by prescription or over the counter (OTC).

CORE CONCEPT 1.4

Legal drugs are obtained either with a prescription or by purchasing them over the counter. There are differences between the two methods of dispensing. To obtain prescription drugs, patients must get a physician's order authorizing them to receive the drugs. The advantages to this are numerous. Practitioners have an opportunity to examine their patients and determine a specific diagnosis. Practitioners can maximize therapy by ordering the proper drug for their patients' conditions and

TABLE 1.1	Characteristics of Traditional Therapeutic Drugs, Biologics, and Natural Alternative Therapies
Traditional Drug Therapies	■ Chemically produced in a laboratory ■ Routinely used by health care providers
Biologics	■ Naturally produced by the body itself, in animal cells, or in microorganisms ■ Include hormones and vaccines ■ Routinely used by health care providers
Natural Alternative Therapies	■ Naturally produced ■ Include herbs, extracts, vitamins, minerals, or dietary supplements

controlling the specific amount and frequency of the drug to be dispensed. Health care providers may give instructions on how to use the drug properly and what side effects to expect.

A drug's safety is related to its effectiveness. The difference between its usual effective dose and a dose that produces severe side effects is called its *margin of safety*. When drugs have been used over long periods and demonstrate "wide" margins of safety—that is, they are very safe and effective—regulators often change them from being prescription drugs to being OTC drugs. Unlike prescription drugs, OTC drugs do not require a physician's order. Patients may treat themselves safely if they carefully follow instructions included with these OTC drugs. If patients do not follow these guidelines, OTC drugs can have serious side effects.

Patients often prefer to take OTC medications for many reasons. They may obtain OTC drugs more easily than prescription drugs. They do not have to make an appointment with a physician, which saves time and money. Without training, however, choosing the proper medication for a specific problem may be challenging. OTC drugs may react with foods, herbal products, and prescription or other OTC drugs. Patients may not be aware that some medications can impair their ability to function safely. Self-treatment is sometimes ineffective, and the potential for injury is much greater if the disease is allowed to progress without proper treatment.

Pharmaceutics is the science of pharmacy.

Pharmaceutics is the science of preparing and dispensing drugs and is a very important part of pharmacotherapy. Often, the general public confuses the science of pharmaceutics with pharmacology. Generally, consumers recognize the root *pharm* and assume that *pharmacology* is the same as *pharmacy*. Correctly, *pharmaceutics* is the science of pharmacy. Speaking simply, pharmaceutics involves dispensing a drug to a patient after he or she has been examined by a licensed health care providers. Pharmacists are experts at cataloguing signs, symptoms, side effects, and drug interactions. They often act as drug advisors to patients, making sure that they receive the proper medication and educating them about undesirable symptoms or interactions.

Concept Review   1.1

■ Explain the meaning of this statement: "Pharmacotherapy involves the science of therapeutics and pharmaceutics."

Drug regulations were created to protect the public from drug misuse.

For many years, there were no standards or guidelines to protect the public from drug misuse. Patients could not be assured that available medicines were not a form of quackery. The archives of drug regulatory agencies are filled with examples of early medicines, including rattlesnake oil for rheumatism; epilepsy treatment for spasms, hysteria, and alcoholism; and fat reducers for a slender, healthy figure. It became quite clear that drug regulations were needed to protect the public.

The first standards commonly used by pharmacists were early **formularies**, or lists of drugs and drug recipes. In 1820, the first comprehensive publication of drug standards, called the *U.S. Pharmacopoeia (USP),* was established. (See the timeline in Figure 1.1 ■.) A **pharmacopoeia** is a medical reference summary indicating standards of drug purity and strength and directions for synthesis. In 1852, a national professional society of pharmacists—the American Pharmaceutical Association (APhA)—was founded. From 1852 until 1975, two major sources maintained drug standards in the United States: the USP and the APhA's *National Formulary (NF)*. All drug substances and products were covered in the USP; the NF focused on pharmaceutic ingredients. In 1975, the two organizations merged and created a single publication named the *U.S. Pharmacopoeia-National Formulary (USP-NF)*. Official updates for the *USP-NF* are published regularly. Today, the USP label can be found on many medication vials verifying the exact ingredients found within the container, as shown in Figure 1.2 ■.

In the early 1900s, to protect the public, the government began to develop and enforce tougher drug legislation. In 1902, the Biologics Control Act was passed to standardize the quality of serums and other blood-related products. The Pure Food and Drug Act of 1906 gave the government power to control the labeling of medicines. In 1912, the Sherley Amendment prohibited the sale of drugs labeled with false therapeutic claims intended to cheat the consumer. In 1938, Congress passed the Food, Drug, and Cosmetic Act. This was the first law preventing the marketing of drugs that had not been thoroughly tested prior to marketing. According to the

FIGURE 1.1	
TIMELINE	**REGULATORY ACTS, STANDARDS, AND ORGANIZATIONS**
1820	A group of physicians established the first comprehensive publication of drug standards called the **U.S. Pharmacopoeia (USP).**
1852	A group of pharmacists founded a national professional society called the **American Pharmaceutical Association (APhA).** The APhA then established the **National Formulary (NF),** a publication listing standardized pharmaceutical ingredients. The USP continued to catalogue all drug-related substances and products.
1862	This was the beginning of the **Federal Bureau of Chemistry,** established by President Lincoln. Over the years, duties were added, and it became the Food and Drug Administration (FDA).
1902	Congress passed the **Biologics Control Act** to control the quality of serums and other blood-related products.
1906	**The Pure Food and Drug Act** gave the government power to control the labeling of medicines.
1912	**The Sherley Amendment** made medicines safer by prohibiting the sale of drugs labeled with false therapeutic claims.
1938	Congress passed the **Food, Drug, and Cosmetic Act.** It was the first law preventing the marketing of drugs not thoroughly tested. This law now requires drug companies to submit a New Drug Application (NDA) to the Food and Drug Administration (FDA) before marketing the drug.
1944	Congress passed the **Public Health Service Act,** covering many health issues including biologic products and the control of communicable diseases.
1975	The U.S. Pharmacopoeia and National Formulary announced their union. The **USP-NF** became a single standardized publication.
1986	Congress passed the **Childhood Vaccine Act.** It authorized the FDA to acquire information about patients taking vaccines, to recall biologics, and to recommend civil penalties if guidelines were not followed.
1988	The **FDA** was officially established as an agency of the **U.S. Department of Health and Human Services.**
1992	Congress passed the **Prescription Drug User Fee Act.** It required that manufacturers of non-generic drugs and biologics pay fees to help improve the drug review process.
1997	**The FDA Modernization Act** was the largest reform effort of the drug review process since 1938.
2003	**Medicare Prescription Drug Improvement and Modernization Act**
2007	**Best Pharmaceuticals for Children's Act**

Historical timeline of regulatory acts, standards, and organizations

provisions of this law, drug companies were required to prove the safety and *efficacy* (that is, effectiveness) of any drug before it could be sold within the United States.

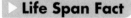

CORE CONCEPT 1.7

U.S. drug standards have become increasingly complex.

Much has changed in the regulation of drugs since 1938. In 1988, the FDA was officially established as an agency of the U.S. Department of Health and Human Services. Today, the Center for Drug Evaluation and Research (CDER), a branch of the FDA, has powerful control over whether prescription drugs and OTC drugs may be used for therapy. The CDER states its mission as "facilitating the availability of safe effective drugs, keeping unsafe or ineffective drugs off the market, improving the health of Americans, and providing clear, easily understandable drug information for safe and effective use." Any pharmaceutical laboratory, whether private, public, or academic, must obtain FDA approval before marketing any drug. Another branch of the FDA, the Center for Biologics Evaluation and Research (CBER), regulates the use of biologics, including serums, vaccines, and products found in the bloodstream.

The FDA also oversees administration of herbal products and dietary supplements, but the Center for Food Safety and Applied Nutrition (CFSAN) regulates use of these substances. Herbal products and dietary supplements are regulated by the Dietary Supplement Health and Education Act of 1994. This act does not provide the same degree of protection as the Food, Drug, and Cos-

▶ **Life Span Fact**

One historical achievement involving biologics is the 1986 Childhood Vaccine Act. This act authorized the FDA to acquire information about patients taking vaccines, to recall biologics, and to recommend civil penalties if guidelines regarding biologics were not followed.

FIGURE 1.2

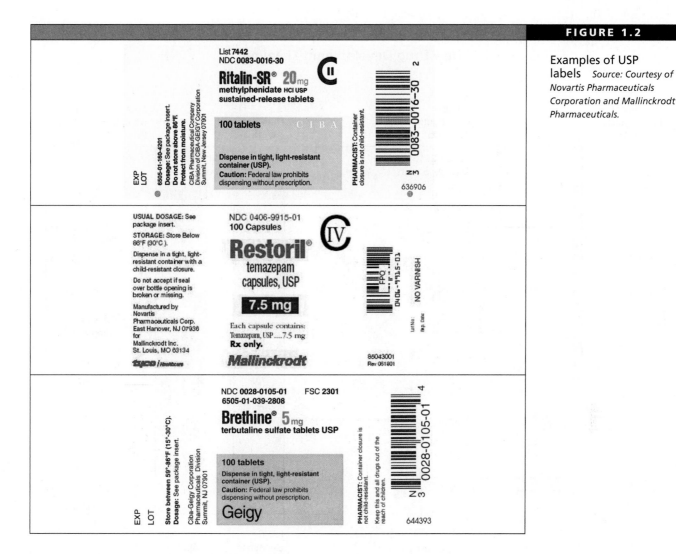

Examples of USP labels   *Source: Courtesy of Novartis Pharmaceuticals Corporation and Mallinckrodt Pharmaceuticals.*

metic Act of 1938. Herbal and dietary supplements may be marketed without prior approval from the FDA. This act is discussed in more detail in Chapter 6.

There are four stages of approval for therapeutic and biologic drugs.

The amount of time spent in the review and approval process for both prescription and OTC drugs depends on several checkpoints in a well-developed and organized plan. Most therapeutic drugs and biologics are reviewed in four stages, which are summarized in Figure 1.3 ■. These stages are (1) preclinical investigation, (2) clinical investigation, (3) submission of a new drug application (NDA) with review, and (4) postmarketing studies.

Preclinical Investigation

Preclinical investigation involves basic science research. Scientists perform many tests on cells grown in the laboratory (a process called *culture*) or on animals to examine the effectiveness of a range of drug doses and to look for any adverse effects. Laboratory tests on cells and animals are important because they assist in predicting whether drugs will cause harm in humans. Because laboratory tests do not always reflect the way a human responds, preclinical investigation results are always inconclusive.

Clinical Investigation

Clinical investigation, the second stage of drug approval, takes place in three different phases, termed *clinical phase trials*. This is the longest part of the drug approval process and involves

FIGURE 1.3

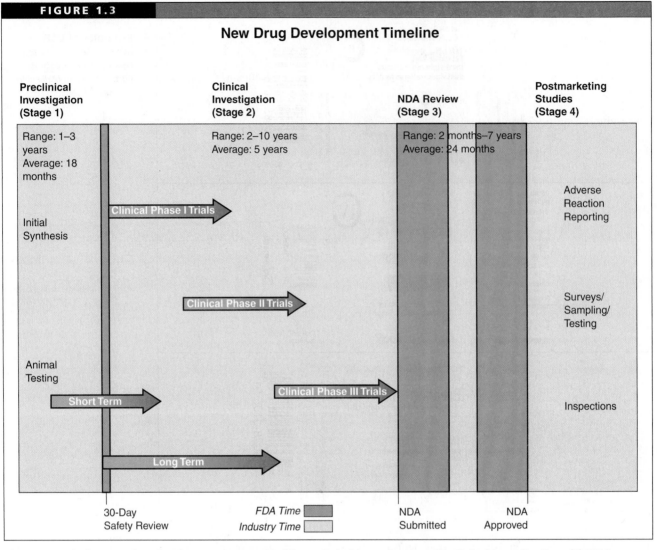

New Drug Development Timeline

The approval of a new drug is a four-stage process: (1) preclinical investigation, (2) clinical investigation, (3) NDA submission and review, and (4) postmarketing studies. Within the second stage (clinical investigation), three phases of trials are conducted over 2 to 10 years. Postmarketing studies, also called *postmarketing surveillance*, continue in large patient groups during the fourth stage of drug development. *Source: Pearson Education/PH College.*

clinical pharmacology, an area of medicine devoted to the evaluation of drugs used for human benefit. During these phases, clinical pharmacologists, researchers, and health care providers examine data from volunteers and large groups of selected patients with certain diseases. Both scientists and health care providers establish drug doses and try to identify adverse effects. Clinical investigators address concerns such as whether the drug worsens other medical conditions, interacts unsafely with existing medications patients are taking, or affects one type of patient more than others.

Clinical Phase Trials. Clinical phase trials are essential because responses among patients vary. If a drug appears to be effective without causing serious side effects, approval for marketing may be accelerated, or the drug may be used for treatment immediately in special cases with careful monitoring. If the drug shows promise but some minor problems are noted, the approval process is delayed until concerns are addressed. In any case, an NDA must be submitted before a drug is allowed to proceed to the next stage of the approval process.

Submission of an NDA with Review

A review of the NDA is the third stage of drug approval. During this stage, clinical Phase III trials and animal testing may continue, depending on the results obtained from preclinical testing.

If the NDA is approved, the process continues to the final stage. If the NDA is rejected, the process stops until concerns are addressed.

Postmarketing Studies

Postmarketing surveillance is the fourth stage of the drug approval process. It takes place after clinical trials and the NDA review process have been completed. Testing in humans is continued to check for any new harmful effects in larger and more diverse populations. Some adverse effects take longer to appear and are not identified until a drug is used by large numbers of patients. One example is the diabetes drug troglitazone (Rezulin), which was placed on the market in 1997. In 1998, Great Britain banned its use after at least one death and several cases of liver failure were reported in patients with diabetes taking the drug. The FDA became aware of a number of cases in the United States in which Rezulin was linked with liver failure. Consumer advocates also claimed that the drug caused several cases of heart failure. Rezulin was recalled in March 2000 after health professionals asked the FDA to reconsider its risks.

The FDA holds annual public meetings to hear comments from patients and professional and pharmaceutical organizations about the effectiveness and safety of new drug therapies. If the FDA discovers a serious problem, it will require that a drug be withdrawn from the market and its use discontinued.

Once criticized for being too slow, governmental agencies face new challenges for ensuring the safety of drugs.

CORE CONCEPT 1.9

The public once criticized the FDA and other regulatory agencies for being too slow in bringing new, potentially lifesaving drugs to the consumer. In the early 1990s, organized consumer groups and drug manufacturers pressured governmental officials to speed up the drug review process. Reasons for delays in the FDA drug approval process were outdated guidelines, poor communication, and agency understaffing.

PEARSON
mynursingkit

U.S. DRUG RECALLS

In 1992, FDA officials, members of Congress, and representatives from pharmaceutical companies negotiated the Prescription Drug User Fee Act on a 5-year trial basis. This act required drug and biologic manufacturers to provide yearly product user fees. With this extra income, the FDA hired more employees and restructured its organization to handle the greater number of drug applications more efficiently. Restructuring was a resounding success. From 1992 to 1996, the FDA approved double the number of drugs while cutting some review times by as much as half. In 1997, the FDA Modernization Act was passed, reauthorizing the Prescription Drug User Fee Act. It allowed drug companies to give health care providers information about *FDA-unapproved* uses of certain drugs. For example, sometimes drugs are approved to treat one condition, but not others; however, physicians may discover that the drug is useful in treating a different problem. When such a benefit is found frequently, a drug company is allowed to share accurate information with other physicians about the drug's "unapproved" but effective use in treating another condition. The act also added nearly 700 employees to the FDA's drug and biologics program, and over $300 million was collected in user fees.

One concern now is that drugs are being developed at a faster rate than risks can be assessed. Officials have been calling for patients, pharmacists, allied health workers, nurses, physicians, hospitals, and pharmaceutical companies to work together to minimize risks. Because of the higher numbers of drugs being approved for therapy, the potential for adverse drug-drug and drug-herbal interactions is greater than ever before.

Concept Review   1.2

■ Can you recall the major U.S. acts, standards, and organizations leading up to the present time? When was the FDA established? What current U.S. laws regulate how drugs are approved for marketing?

Similar drug standards protect Canadian consumers.

CORE CONCEPT 1.10

In Canada as in the United States, drug testing and risk assessment is a major priority (Table 1.2). Governments in both countries have realized a need to monitor very carefully newly developed traditional drugs, as well as natural products, minerals, vitamins, and herbs, because the potential for adverse effects is great.

TABLE 1.2	Steps of Approval for Drugs Marketed Within Canada
Step 1	Preclinical studies or experiments performed in culture, living tissue, and small animals are performed, followed by extensive clinical trials or testing done in humans.
Step 2	A drug company completes a drug submission to Health Canada. This report details important safety and effectiveness information, including testing data, how the drug product will be produced and packaged, expected therapeutic benefits, and adverse reactions.
Step 3	A committee of drug experts, including medical and drug scientists, reviews the drug submission to identify potential benefits and drug risks.
Step 4	Health Canada reviews information about the drug product and passes on important details to health care providers and consumers.
Step 5	Health Canada issues a Notice of Compliance (NOC) and Drug Identification Number (DIN). Both permit the manufacturer to market the drug product.
Step 6	Health Canada monitors the effectiveness of the drug and any concerns after it has been marketed. This is done by regular inspection, notices, newsletters, and feedback from consumers and health care providers.

Health Canada is the federal department working in partnership with provincial and territorial governments. The Health Products and Food Branch (HPFB) of Health Canada is responsible for ensuring that health products and foods approved for sale to Canadians are safe and of high quality. The HPFB regulates the use of therapeutic products through directorates. The Therapeutic Products Directorate (TPD) authorizes marketing of a pharmaceutical drug or medical device once a manufacturer presents sufficient scientific evidence of the product's safety, efficacy, and quality as required by the Canadian Food and Drugs Act and Regulations. The Biologics and Genetic Therapies Directorate (BGTD) regulates biologic drugs (drugs derived from living sources) and radiopharmaceuticals. Products regulated by the BGTD include blood products, vaccines, tissues, organs, and gene therapy products. The Natural Health Products Directorate (NHPD) is the regulating authority for natural health products for sale in Canada.

The Canadian Food and Drugs Act is the important regulatory document specifying that drugs cannot be marketed without a Notice of Compliance (NOC) and Drug Identification Number (DIN) from Health Canada. Foods, drugs, cosmetics, and therapeutic devices must follow established guidelines for approval. Any drug that does not comply with standards established by recognized pharmacopoeias and formularies in the United States, Europe, Great Britain, or France cannot be labeled, packaged, sold, or advertised in Canada. Canadian drugs may share the same names as their counterparts in the United States, or they may have unique names.

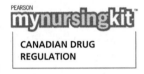

CANADIAN DRUG
REGULATION

CORE CONCEPT 1.11

Health care providers must be prepared to deal with the threat of biological and chemical attack.

Prior to the September 11, 2001, terrorist attacks on the United States, concern about epidemic diseases mainly focused on the possible spread of traditional infectious diseases such as influenza, tuberculosis, cholera, and human immunodeficiency virus (HIV). Health care providers were also concerned about widespread food poisoning and sexually transmitted diseases other than HIV, but because these diseases and conditions produced fewer fatalities, less attention was given to them.

Now, however, the health care community is more aware of the possibility of *bioterrorism*—the intentional use of infectious biological agents, chemical substances, or radiation to cause widespread harm or illness. Such federal agencies as the Centers for Disease Control and Prevention (CDC) and the U.S. Department of Defense have increased efforts to inform, educate, and prepare the public for disease outbreaks caused by bioterrorism. In 2002, the U.S. Department of Homeland Security was organized to provide additional security and defense for the United States in a terrorist attack. The department also prioritized the important issue of citizen preparedness, educating families how best to prepare for natural emergencies and disasters.

Among the goals of a bioterrorist are to create widespread public panic and cause as many casualties as possible. The list of agents that can be used for this purpose is long. Some of these agents are easily obtainable and require little or no specialized knowledge to spread. The most worrisome threats are:

bio = *living microorganisms*
terrorism = *to induce fear*

- Acutely infectious diseases such as anthrax, smallpox, plague, and hemorrhagic viruses

- Incapacitating chemicals such as nerve gas, cyanide, and chlorinated agents
- Nuclear and radiation emergencies

One can easily imagine what devastation would be caused if laboratories and health care professionals were not able to identify, isolate, and treat widespread disease caused by bioterrorism. The following chapters contain important information related to bioterrorism. Chapter 24 reviews the topic of antibiotics for the treatment of anthrax. The treatment of chemical warfare agents is discussed in Chapter 8. Chapter 31 includes a discussion of the treatment of radiation exposure.

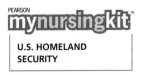

PEARSON
mynursingkit

U.S. HOMELAND
SECURITY

CHAPTER REVIEW

CORE CONCEPTS SUMMARY

1.1 Pharmacology is an expansive and challenging topic.

Pharmacology, the study of medicine, is a subject devoted to proper drug treatment and health of the human body. It is an expansive topic utilizing concepts from human biology, pathophysiology, and chemistry.

1.2 For health care providers, the fields of pharmacology and therapeutics are connected.

Therapeutics is the science associated with the treatment of suffering and the prevention of disease. *Pharmacotherapeutics* is the useful application of drugs for the purpose of fighting disease. The study of pharmacology is important to health professionals from many different fields.

1.3 Agents may be classified as traditional drugs, biologics, and natural alternatives.

Drugs are chemical agents used to treat disease by producing biological responses within the body. Therapeutic drugs are classified as substances produced chemically or naturally. Biologics are natural agents produced by animal cells or microorganisms. Alternative therapies include natural herbs, plant extracts, or dietary supplements.

1.4 Drugs are available by prescription or over the counter (OTC).

There are two major methods of dispensing drugs. Prescription drugs require a physician's order; OTC drugs do not. There are advantages and disadvantages to both dispensing methods.

1.5 Pharmaceutics is the science of pharmacy.

Pharmaceutics involves the successful dispensation of drugs for therapeutic purposes. Dispensing medication safely is a major challenge for health care providers and patients.

1.6 Drug regulations were created to protect the public from drug misuse.

The first drug laws were acts created by Congress to protect patients from wrongful therapeutic claims. These and other standards form the basis of modern drug regulation agencies and organizations such as the Food and Drug Administration and publications such as the *U.S. Pharmacopoeia-National Formulary.*

1.7 U.S. drug standards have become increasingly complex.

The Food and Drug Administration (FDA), a branch of the U.S. Department of Health and Human Services, is the primary agency regulating drug safety. Three branches of the FDA control policies regarding drug therapies: the Center for Drug Evaluation and Research (CDER), the Center for Biologics Evaluation and Research (CBER), and the Center for Food Safety and Applied Nutrition (CFSAN).

1.8 There are four stages of approval for therapeutic and biologic drugs.

Drug approval occurs in four stages: preclinical investigation, clinical investigation, submission of a new drug application (NDA) with review, and post-marketing studies. Clinical phase trials must be completed before drugs are approved for public use.

1.9 Once criticized for being too slow, governmental agencies face new challenges for ensuring the safety of drugs.

FDA officials, members of Congress, and pharmaceutical company representatives negotiated the Prescription Drug User Fee Act and FDA Modernization Act. These acts have sped up the approval process and require drug and biologic manufacturers to provide yearly product user fees. The concern now is that drugs are being approved at a rate faster than risks can be assessed.

1.10 Similar drug standards protect Canadian consumers.

In Canada, the Health Protection Branch of the Department of Health and Welfare enforces regulations concerned with the Canadian Food and Drugs Act. The Health Products and Food Branch of Health Canada regulates the proper use of therapeutic drugs by issuing a Notice of Compliance (NOC) and Drug Identification Number (DIN) before drugs are marketed. Drugs in Canada are regulated in a manner similar to that used in the United States.

1.11 Health care providers must be prepared to deal with the threat of biological and chemical attack.

Drugs are among the most powerful weapons to combat bioterrorism. Federal agencies have taken an active role in educating and preparing the public and the health care community about disease outbreaks caused by bioterrorism.

REVIEW QUESTIONS

The following questions are written in NCLEX-PN® style. Answer these questions to assess your knowledge of the chapter material, and go back and review any material that is not clear to you.

1. Pathophysiology is defined as the study of:
1. How drugs enter and travel throughout the body
2. How drugs improve the health of the human body
3. Drugs and how they elicit different responses
4. Diseases and functional changes occurring as a result of disease

2. Biologics are:
1. Produced in nature and include herbs, natural extracts, vitamins, and minerals
2. Chemically produced in a laboratory
3. Naturally produced in animal cells, microorganisms, or by the body itself
4. Not used routinely by physicians

3. Antiperspirants, sunscreens, toothpaste, and shampoo alter the body's activities. Therefore, they are:
1. Considered to be medically therapeutic
2. Classified as traditional drugs because they are chemically produced and cause biological responses in the body
3. Agents limited to therapy in a clinical or home setting
4. Commonly grouped as cosmetics, which are categorized separately from drugs

4. What are precautions that patients need to know when taking OTC drugs?
1. Self-treatment is sometimes ineffective
2. OTC drugs may react with foods, herbal products, and prescription or other OTC drugs
3. The potential for injury is much greater if the disease is allowed to progress
4. All of the above

5. Dispensing of drugs to patients after they have been examined by a licensed health care providers is:
1. Pharmacology
2. Pharmaceutics
3. Therapeutics
4. Health care

6. The act that provided the reauthorization of drug information to the public regarding unapproved drug use and labeling is the:
1. Pure Food and Drug Act (1906)
2. Food, Drug, and Cosmetics Act (1938)
3. Prescription Drug User Fee Act (1992)
4. FDA Modernization Act (1997)

7. The longest part of the drug approval process is typically:
1. Preclinical investigation
2. Clinical investigation
3. NDA submission and review
4. Postmarketing studies

8. The legislation responsible for cutting new drug application review times as much as 50% is the:
1. Pure Food and Drug Act
2. Sherley Amendment
3. Public Health Services Act
4. Prescription Drug User Fee Act

9. One aspect of health protection standards that is clearly different in Canada compared with in the United States is:
1. Preclinical studies are followed by extensive clinical trials
2. A committee of drug experts reviews the drug submission to identify potential benefits and risks of the drug
3. Drugs cannot be marketed without an NOC and a DIN
4. The effectiveness of and concerns about the drugs are monitored after they have been marketed

10. Which of the following is considered a bioterrorist threat?
1. Anthrax contamination
2. Incapacitating chemicals
3. Radiation exposure
4. All of the above

FURTHER STUDY

- Traditional drugs and drug classes are discussed in Chapter 2.

- Chapter 6 covers natural alternatives and herbal and dietary supplements, including the Dietary Supplement Health and Education Act of 1994.

- Canadian drugs and their U.S. equivalents are listed in Appendix B.

- Chapter 24 reviews antibiotics for the treatment of anthrax.

- The treatment of chemical warfare agents is discussed in Chapter 8.

- Chapter 31 includes a discussion of the treatment of radiation exposure.

EXPLORE PEARSON mynursingkit™

MyNursingKit is your one stop for online chapter review materials and resources. Prepare for success with additional NCLEX®-style practice questions, interactive assignments and activities, web links, animations and videos, and more!

Register your access code from the front of your book at **www.mynursingkit.com**

2 Drug Classes, Schedules, and Categories

CORE CONCEPTS

2.1 Drugs may be organized by their therapeutic and pharmacologic classifications.

2.2 Drugs have more than one name.

2.3 The differences between brand name drugs and their generic equivalents include price, formulations, and, most importantly, bioavailability.

2.4 Drugs with a potential for abuse are categorized into schedules.

2.5 Canadian regulations restrict drugs of abuse.

2.6 In order to protect the unborn, all prescription drugs are classified according to safety in pregnancy categories.

LEARNING OUTCOMES

After reading this chapter, the student should be able to:

1. Discuss the basis for placing drugs into therapeutic and pharmacologic classes.

2. Explain the prototype approach to drug classification.

3. Describe what is meant by a drug's mechanism of action.

4. Distinguish among a drug's chemical name, generic name, and trade name.

5. Explain why generic drug names are preferred to other drug names.

6. Discuss why drugs are sometimes placed on a restrictive list, and the controversy surrounding this issue.

7. Explain the meaning of the term *controlled substance.*

8. Explain the U.S. Controlled Substance Act of 1970 and the role of the U.S. Drug Enforcement Agency (DEA) in controlling drug abuse and misuse.

9. Identify the five drug schedules, and provide examples of drugs at each level.

10. Explain how drugs are scheduled, taking into account Parts III and IV of the Canadian Food and Drugs Act and the Narcotic Control Act.

11. Identify the five pregnancy categories, and explain what each category represents.

KEY TERMS

bioavailability (BEYE-oh-ah-VALE-ah-BILL-ih-TEE) 18
chemical name 16
combination drugs 17
controlled substance 18
generic name (je-NARE-ik) 17
mechanism of action 15
pharmacologic classification (FAR-mah-koh-LOJ-ik) 15
prototype drug (PRO-toh-type) 16
restricted drugs 19
scheduled drugs 18
therapeutic classification (ther-ah-PEW-tik) 15
trade name 17

There are many ways that drugs can be classified, from a strict chemical group name to a trade name provided by the manufacturer. Because of the large number of drugs available, practitioners and consumers must have a system for identifying drugs and determining the limitations of their use. This chapter covers the various methods by which drugs may be organized—by therapeutic or pharmacologic classification. This chapter also discusses drug schedules and pregnancy categories because such information affects the routine uses of drugs.

Drugs may be organized by their therapeutic and pharmacologic classifications.

CORE CONCEPT 2.1

Medications may be classified in two major ways. Drugs may be organized by *therapeutic usefulness*. This is referred to as a **therapeutic classification**. Drugs may also be categorized by *how they work pharmacologically*. This is referred to as a **pharmacologic classification**. Both methods are widely used in studying pharmacology, even though health care providers often do not make the distinction when the primary purpose of drug therapy is to improve the health of their patients.

Table 2.1 shows the method of therapeutic classification, using cardiac care as the example. For instance, the cardiovascular system is concerned with the proper functioning of the heart and blood vessels. Many different types of drugs affect cardiovascular function. Some drugs influence blood clotting, whereas others lower blood cholesterol or prevent the onset of stroke. Drugs may be used to lower blood pressure, treat heart failure, correct abnormal heart rhythm, alleviate chest pain, and treat or prevent circulatory shock. Drugs that affect cardiac disorders may be placed in numerous therapeutic classes. Drugs that influence blood clotting are called *anticoagulants*. Medications that lower blood cholesterol are called *antihyperlipidemics*. Drugs that lower blood pressure are called *antihypertensives*.

A therapeutic classification need not be complicated. For example, it is appropriate to classify a medication simply as "a drug used for stroke" or "a drug used for shock." The key to therapeutic classification is to state clearly what a particular drug does clinically. A few additional examples of therapeutic classification are provided in Table 2.2.

A second way drugs are often grouped is by pharmacologic classification. Pharmacologic classification addresses the drug's **mechanism of action**, or *how* the medication produces its effects within the body.

PEARSON
mynursingkit

THERAPEUTIC DRUG CLASSES

TABLE 2.1	Organizing Drugs by Therapeutic Classification
THERAPEUTIC FOCUS	
Cardiac care / Drugs affecting cardiovascular function	
THERAPEUTIC USEFULNESS	***THERAPEUTIC CLASSIFICATION***
influencing blood clotting	anticoagulants
lowering blood cholesterol	antihyperlipidemics
lowering blood pressure	antihypertensives
treating abnormal heartbeat	antidysrhythmics
treating chest pain (angina)	antianginal drugs

TABLE 2.2	Additional Examples of Therapeutic Classification*
anti-inflammatory drugs	anticoagulants
antiepileptic drugs	drugs for vomiting (emesis)
antipsychotic drugs	antidiarrheal drugs
antianxiety drugs	antacids
antidepressants	antibiotic drugs

Note: Although the names of some therapeutic categories may sound complicated, drug terminology will become more familiar as you begin to study drugs and drug classes. When studying this topic, always refer to a medical dictionary and reference drug guide.

TABLE 2.3	Organizing Drugs by Pharmacologic Classification

FOCUSING ON HOW A THERAPY MAY BE APPLIED
Therapy for high blood pressure may be achieved by:

MECHANISM OF ACTION	PHARMACOLOGIC CLASSIFICATION
lowering plasma volume	diuretics
blocking heart calcium channels	calcium channel blockers
blocking hormonal activity	angiotensin-converting enzyme inhibitors
blocking stress-related activity	adrenergic blockers (drugs that inhibit actions of the sympathetic nervous system)
dilating peripheral blood vessels	vasodilators

Table 2.3 shows various types of pharmacologic classifications using high blood pressure (hypertension) as an example. A *diuretic* is a class of drug used to treat hypertension by lowering plasma volume. Lowering plasma volume is the mechanism of action by which diuretics work. *Calcium channel blockers* treat hypertension by limiting the force of heart contractions. Other drugs, such as angiotensin-converting enzyme inhibitors, block components of the hormonal network called the *renin-angiotensin pathway,* thereby reducing hypertension. Notice that each example describes *how* hypertension may be controlled. Thus, the drug's pharmacologic classification is more specific than its therapeutic classification and requires an understanding of human biochemical and physiologic principles.

When studying a particular drug's mechanism of action, it is recommended that students first become comfortable with the broad drug classes and then gradually move to more specific examples. Prototype drugs are an excellent place to start. A **prototype drug** is the original, well-understood drug model from which other medications in a pharmacologic class have been developed. By learning the prototype drug, students may then predict the actions and adverse effects of other drugs in the same class. For example, by knowing the effects of penicillin V, students can apply this knowledge to the other drugs in the penicillin antibiotic class. *Students should be aware, however, that in many cases the original drug prototype is not the most widely used drug in its class.* As new drugs are developed, features such as antibiotic resistance, fewer side effects, or a more precise site of action might be factors that sway health care providers away from using the older drugs. Therefore, being familiar with the original drug prototypes and keeping up with newer and more popular drugs are essential parts of mastering the subject of pharmacology. For all profiled drugs featured in this book, both pharmacologic and therapeutic classifications are provided to help students organize drug information.

Concept Review 2.1

■ What is the difference between a therapeutic classification and a pharmacologic classification? What is a *prototype drug,* and how is the prototype drug similar and different from other drugs within the same pharmacologic or therapeutic class?

CORE CONCEPT 2.2

Drugs have more than one name.

A major challenge in studying pharmacology is learning the thousands of drug names. Adding to this difficulty is the fact that most drugs have multiple names. The three basic types of drug names are chemical, generic, and trade names.

A **chemical name** is assigned, using standard nomenclature established by the International Union of Pure and Applied Chemistry (IUPAC). A drug has only one chemical name, which is sometimes helpful in predicting its physical and chemical properties. Although chemical names convey a clear and concise meaning about the nature of a drug, they often are very complicated and difficult to pronounce and remember. For example, the chemical name of diazepam is 7-chloro-1, 3-ciphydro-1-methyl-5-phenyl-2H-1,4-benzodiazepin-2-one. In only a few cases, usually when the name is brief and easily remembered, are chemical names useful. Examples of brief (and therefore useful) chemical names include lithium carbonate, calcium gluconate, and sodium chloride.

More practically, drugs are sometimes classified by *a portion* of their chemical structure, known as the chemical group name. Examples are antibiotic drugs such as the fluoroquinolones

TABLE 2.4	Trade Name Products Containing Popular Generic Substances
GENERIC SUBSTANCES	**TRADE NAMES**
aspirin	Acetylsalicylic acid, Acuprin, Anacin, Aspergum, Bayer, Bufferin, Ecotrin, Empirin, Excedrin, Maprin, Norgesic, Salatin, Salocol, Salsprin, Supac, Talwin, Triaphen-10, Vanquish, Verin, Zorprin
diphenhydramine	Allerdryl, Benadryl, Benahist, Bendylate, Caladryl, Compoz, Diahist, Diphenadril, Eldadryl, Fenylhist, Fynex, Hydramine, Hydril, Insomnal, Noradryl, Nordryl, Nytol, Tussat, Wehdryl
ibuprofen	Advil, Amersol, Apsifen, Brufen, Haltran, Medipren, Midol 200, Motrin, Neuvil, Novoprofen, Nuprin, Pamprin-IB, Rufen, Trendar

and cephalosporins. Other common examples include the phenothiazines, thiazides, and benzodiazepines. Although names like these may seem complicated at first, familiarity with chemical group names will grow, and the nomenclature will become more manageable as students continue to communicate with fellow health care providers.

The **generic name** of a drug is assigned by the U.S. Adopted Name Council. With few exceptions, generic names are less complicated and easier to remember than chemical names. Many organizations, including the FDA, the U.S. Pharmacopoeia, and the World Health Organization, routinely describe a medication by its generic name. Because there is only one generic name for each drug, health care providers routinely use this name, and pharmacology students generally must memorize it.

A drug's **trade name** is assigned by the company marketing the drug. The name is usually selected to be snappy and easy to remember. The trade name is also called the *proprietary, product,* or *brand* name. The term *proprietary* relates to ownership. In the United States, a drug developer is given exclusive rights to name and market a drug for 17 years after a new drug application (NDA) is submitted to the FDA. Because it takes several years before a drug can be approved, the amount of time spent in approval is subtracted from the 17 years. For example, if it takes 7 years for a drug to be approved, competing companies will not be allowed to market a generic equivalent drug for another 10 years. The rationale for this is that the developing company must be allowed sufficient time to recoup the millions of dollars spent in research and the time needed to develop the new drug. After 17 years, competing companies may sell a generic equivalent drug, using a different name, which the FDA must approve.

Trade names may be a challenge because of the dozens of product names containing similar ingredients. In addition, some **combination drugs** contain more than one active generic ingredient, making it difficult to match one generic name with one product name. As an example, refer to Table 2.4 and consider the drug diphenhydramine (generic name), also called Benadryl (one of many trade names). Diphenhydramine is an antihistamine. Low doses of diphenhydramine can be purchased over the counter; higher doses require a prescription. When looking for diphenhydramine, health care providers may find it listed under many trade names, such as Allerdryl and Compoz, and provided alone or in combination with other active ingredients. Ibuprofen and aspirin are also examples of drugs with many different trade names. The rule of thumb is that a formulation's active ingredients are described by their generic name. The generic name is usually written in lowercase, whereas the trade name is capitalized.

Concept Review 2.2

■ What are the major differences between a chemical, a generic, and a trade name? Which name is most often used to describe the active ingredients within a drug product?

The differences between brand name drugs and their generic equivalents include price, formulations, and, most importantly, bioavailability.

CORE CONCEPT 2.3

Usually generic drugs are less expensive than brand name drugs. The reason is that a pharmaceutical company determines the price of a proprietary drug during its 17 years of exclusive rights to that new drug. Because there is no competition, the price can be kept quite high. The pharmaceutical company that developed a drug can sometimes use legal tactics to extend its exclusive rights to a drug, which can earn the company hundreds of millions of dollars per year in profits for a popular medicine. Once the exclusive rights end, competing companies market the generic drug for less money, and consumer savings may be considerable. In some states, pharmacists may routinely substitute a generic drug when the prescription calls for a brand name. In other states, the pharmacist must dispense drugs directly as written by a health care providers or obtain approval before providing a generic substitute.

The companies that market brand name drugs often fight aggressively against laws that might restrict the routine use of their products. They claim that significant differences exist between a trade name drug and its generic equivalent, and that switching to the generic drug may be harmful to the patient. Patient advocates, on the other hand, argue that generic substitutions should always be permitted because of the cost savings.

Are there really differences between a brand name drug and its generic equivalent? The answer is unclear. Despite the fact that the dosages may be identical, drug formulations are not always the same. The two drugs may have different *inert* ingredients. For example, in a tablet form, the active ingredients may be more tightly compressed in one of the preparations versus another, and this might affect how well the body can use the drug.

The key to comparing brand name drugs and their generic equivalents lies in measuring the *bioavailability* of the two preparations. **Bioavailability** is the physiologic ability of the drug to reach its target cells and produce its effect. As mentioned, bioavailability can be affected by inert ingredients and tablet compression. Anything that affects absorption of a drug, or its distribution to the target cells, will certainly affect drug action. Measuring how long a drug takes to exert its effect gives pharmacologists a crude measure of bioavailability. For example, if a patient is in circulatory shock and it takes a generic drug 5 minutes longer than the brand name drug to produce its effect, that difference would be significant. However, if a generic medication for arthritis pain relief takes 45 minutes to act, compared with the brand name drug that takes 40 minutes, it probably does not matter which drug is prescribed.

Some states (Florida, Kentucky, Minnesota, and Missouri, for example) have compiled a *negative* formulary list. A negative formulary is a list of trade name drugs that pharmacists may *not* dispense as generic drugs. These drugs must be dispensed exactly as written on the prescription, using the trade name drug the physician prescribed. In some cases, pharmacists must inform or notify patients of substitutions. Pharmaceutical companies and some health care providers have supported this action, claiming that generic drugs—even those that have small differences in bioavailability and bioequivalence—could adversely affect patient outcomes in those with critical conditions or illnesses. However, laws frequently change: In many instances, the efforts of consumer advocacy groups have led to changes in or elimination of negative formulary lists.

bio =*biological effect*
availability =*free to activate cellular targets*

bio =*biological effect*
equivalence =*same*

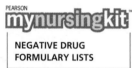

PEARSON
mynursingkit™

NEGATIVE DRUG
FORMULARY LISTS

Drugs with a potential for abuse are categorized into schedules.

Some drugs are frequently abused or have a high potential for becoming addictive. Technically, *addiction* refers to the overwhelming feeling that drives someone to use a drug repeatedly. *Dependence* is a related term, often defined as a physiologic or psychological need for a substance. *Physical dependence* refers to an altered physical condition caused by the nervous system adapting to repeated drug use. In this case, when the drug is no longer available, the individual experiences physical signs of discomfort known as *withdrawal.* In contrast, when an individual is *psychologically dependent,* there are few signs of physical discomfort when the drug is withdrawn; however, the individual feels an intense compelling desire to continue drug use. These concepts are discussed in detail in Chapter 7.

Drugs that cause dependency are restricted to use in situations of medical necessity, that is, if they are allowed at all. According to law, drugs that have a significant potential for abuse are placed into five categories called *schedules.* These **scheduled drugs** are classified according to their potential for abuse: Schedule I drugs have the highest potential for abuse, and Schedule V drugs have the lowest. Schedule I drugs have little or no therapeutic value or are intended for research purposes only. Drugs in the other four schedules may be dispensed only in cases when therapeutic value has been determined. Schedule V is the only category in which some drugs may be dispensed without a prescription because the quantities of the controlled drug are so low that the possibility of causing dependence is extremely remote. Table 2.5 shows the five drug schedules with examples. Not all drugs with an abuse potential are regulated or placed into schedules. Tobacco, alcohol, and caffeine are significant examples.

In the United States, a **controlled substance** is a drug restricted by the Controlled Substances Act of 1970 and later revisions. The Controlled Substances Act is also called the Comprehensive

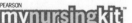
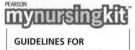

PEARSON
mynursingkit™

GUIDELINES FOR
REFILLING SCHEDULED
DRUGS

TABLE 2.5	Drug Schedule and Examples			
DRUG SCHEDULE	ABUSE POTENTIAL	PHYSICAL DEPENDENCE	PSYCHOLOGICAL DEPENDENCE	THERAPEUTIC USE (EXAMPLES*)
I	Highest	High	High	Limited or no therapeutic use (heroin, LSD, marijuana, and methaqualone)
II	High	High	High	Used therapeutically with prescription; some are no longer used therapeutically (morphine, PCP, cocaine, methadone, and methamphetamine)
III	Moderate	Moderate	High	Used therapeutically with prescription (anabolic steroids, codeine and hydrocodone with aspirin or Tylenol, and some barbiturates)
IV	Lower	Lower	Lower	Used therapeutically with prescription (Darvon, Talwin, Equanil, Valium, and Xanax)
V	Lowest	Lowest	Lowest	Used therapeutically without prescription (OTC cough medicines with codeine)

*All drugs developed for medicinal use in the United States must be approved by the FDA and the DEA. The FDA regulates human testing and the introduction of new drugs into the marketplace, whereas the DEA determines the schedule of and establishes production quotas for drugs with potential for abuse and to prevent their diversion to unlawful channels. The DEA also authorizes health care providers to prescribe controlled substances. The federal legislation that gives the DEA the right to control drugs of abuse (and thus impacts which drugs can be prescribed or not) is the Controlled Substances Act. See http://www.dea.gov.

Drug Abuse Prevention and Control Act. Hospitals and pharmacies must register with the Drug Enforcement Administration (DEA) and use their assigned registration numbers to purchase scheduled drugs. They must maintain complete records of all quantities purchased and sold. Drugs with higher abuse potential have more restrictions. For example, in the hospital a special drug order form must be used to obtain Schedule II drugs, and orders must be written and signed by the health care providers. Telephone orders to a pharmacy are not permitted. Refills for Schedule II drugs are not permitted; patients must visit their health care providers first. Those convicted of unlawful manufacturing, distributing, and dispensing of controlled substances face severe penalties.

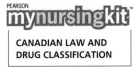

mynursingkit
A–Z INDEX OF U.S. GOVERNMENT DEPARTMENTS AND AGENCIES DEALING WITH DRUGS

Canadian regulations restrict drugs of abuse.

CORE CONCEPT 2.5

In Canada, until 1996, controlled substances were those drugs subject to guidelines outlined in Part III, Schedule G, of the Canadian Food and Drugs Act. According to these guidelines, a health care provider dispensed these medications only to patients suffering from specific diseases or illnesses. Regulated drugs included amphetamines, barbiturates, methaqualone, and anabolic steroids. Controlled drugs were labeled clearly with the letter C on the outside of the container.

Restricted drugs not intended for human use were covered in Part IV, Schedule H, of the Canadian Food and Drugs Act. These were drugs used in the course of a chemical or analytical procedure for medical, laboratory, industrial, educational, or research purposes. They included hallucinogens such as lysergic acid diethylamide (LSD), MDMA, and 2,5-dimethoxy-4-methylamphetamine (DOM; street name STP). Schedule F drugs were those drugs requiring a prescription for their sale. Examples were methylphenidate (Ritalin), diazepam (Valium), and chlordiazepoxide (Librium). Drugs such as morphine, heroin, cocaine, and cannabis were covered under the Canadian Narcotic Control Act and amended schedules. According to Canadian law, narcotic drugs were labeled clearly with the letter N on the outside of the container.

Today Canada's federal drug control statute is the Controlled Drugs and Substances Act. It repeals the Narcotic Control Act and Parts III and IV of the Food and Drugs Act. It further establishes eight schedules of controlled substances; two classes of precursors are covered in one schedule. For a complete listing of drugs, see http://laws.justice.gc.ca/en/C-38.8/. The Controlled Drugs and Substances Act provides broad latitude to the Governor in Council to amend schedules as determined to be in the best interest of Canada's citizens. Drugs and substances covered in the Controlled Drugs and Substances Act correlate with agents named in three United Nations treaties: the Single Convention on Narcotic Drugs, the Convention on Psychotropic Substances, and United Nations Convention Against Illicit Traffic in Narcotic Drugs and Psychotropic Substances.

Throughout Canada, both prescription and nonprescription drugs must meet specific criteria for public distribution and use. Nonprescription drugs are provided according to guidelines and

mynursingkit
CANADIAN LAW AND DRUG CLASSIFICATION

TABLE 2.6	Three-Schedule System for Drugs Sold in Canada
DRUG SCHEDULE	**DRUG TYPE**
I	all prescription drugs
	drugs with no potential for abuse
	controlled drugs
	narcotic drugs
II	all nonprescription drugs monitored for sale by pharmacists
III	all nonprescription drugs not monitored for sale by pharmacists

acts established by the respective Canadian provinces. One recent system establishes three general drug schedules (see Table 2.6). Pharmacies must monitor those drugs used specifically to treat self-limiting discomforts such as colds, flu, and mild gastrointestinal or other symptoms. Other nonprescription drugs may be sold without monitoring.

Concept Review 2.3

- Are controlled drugs described the same way in Canada as in the United States? What about restricted drugs?

TABLE 2.7	Categories of Safety in Pregnancy	
SAFETY CATEGORY	**EXPLANATION**	**EXAMPLES**
A Lowest Risk	Studies HAVE NOT shown a risk to women or to the fetus.	levothyroxine (Synthroid) thyroglobulin (Proloid) potassium chloride (KCl) potassium gluconate (Kaon Tablets) ferrous fumarate (Ferranol)
B	ANIMAL studies HAVE NOT shown a risk to the fetus or, if they have, studies in women have not confirmed this risk.	amoxicillin (Amoxil) insulin (Humulin R) fluoxetine (Prozac) loperamide (Imodium) penicillin V (Pen-Vee-K) ranitidine (Zantac)
C	ANIMAL studies HAVE shown a risk to the fetus, but controlled studies have not been performed in women.	acyclovir (Zovirax) mineral oil (Fleet Mineral Oil) senna (Senokot) hydrochlorothiazide (HydroDIURIL) furosemide (Lasix) iron dextran (K-FeRON) amitriptyline (Elavil)
D	Use of this drug category MAY cause harm to the fetus, but it may provide benefit to the mother in a life-threatening situation or when a safer therapy is not available.	tetracycline (Achromycin) cortisone acetate (Cortistan) warfarin (Coumadin)
X Highest Risk	Studies HAVE shown a significant risk to women and to the fetus.	iodinated glycerol (Organidin) castor oil (Purge) estrogen with progesterone (Ortho Novum) dienestrol (DV) norethindrone (Norlutin) oxymetholone (Anadrol)

In order to protect the unborn, all prescription drugs are classified according to safety in pregnancy categories.

CORE CONCEPT 2.6

Often a major concern of pregnant women is whether a drug will harm their developing baby. Any substance that will harm a developing fetus or embryo is referred to as a *teratogen*. Pregnant patients should never take any prescribed, illegal, or OTC drug or any herbal or dietary supplement without the advice of their health care providers.

terato =*severe deformity*
gen =*something that produces*

To protect the unborn from the teratogenic effects of prescription drugs, the FDA has implemented a category system for classifying drugs based on how safe they are for pregnant women. According to this system, drugs are placed into one of five *pregnancy categories,* labeled as A, B, C, D, and X. These labels appear within package inserts and identify levels of risk to the fetus. The levels are based on degrees to which a drug has been proven to cause birth defects in laboratory animals or in human beings. These categories are summarized in Table 2.7.

Consumers sometimes question whether the testing of laboratory animals is an effective way to predict harm to a developing human fetus or embryo. Results from animal testing are not always transferable to the human body. In fact, results from animal experimentation often vary from species to species. For this reason, consumers should always be cautious, even when there is reasonable assurance that a drug is extremely safe.

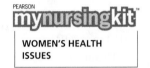

PEARSON
mynursingkit™
WOMEN'S HEALTH ISSUES

CHAPTER REVIEW

CORE CONCEPTS SUMMARY

2.1 Drugs may be organized by their therapeutic and pharmacologic classifications.

Two common ways to classify drugs are by therapeutic classification and pharmacologic classification. Therapeutic classes are based on a drug's clinical usefulness. Pharmacologic classes are based on a drug's mechanism of action. Prototype drugs are used to compare drugs within the same classification.

2.2 Drugs have more than one name.

Drugs may be described by a chemical, generic, or trade name. There are advantages and disadvantages to each type of naming method.

2.3 The differences between brand name drugs and their generic equivalents include price, formulations, and, most importantly, bioavailability.

In most states, generic drugs may be substituted for brand name products if the prescribing practitioner does not object. When generic drugs are substituted, differences in bioavailability may affect the safety and effectiveness of drug therapy.

2.4 Drugs with a potential for abuse are categorized into schedules.

Drugs that have the potential for abuse or dependency are placed into one of five schedules (Schedule I through Schedule V). Schedule I is the most restrictive category. Schedule V is the least restrictive category. The U.S. Drug Enforcement Agency (DEA) handles drug misuse.

2.5 Canadian regulations restrict drugs of abuse.

In Canada, drug use is controlled by eight schedules outlined in the Canadian Controlled Drugs and Substances Act. All prescription drugs, controlled drugs, and narcotic drugs are classified as Schedule I. All nonprescription drugs monitored for sale by pharmacists are classified as Schedule II. Nonprescription drugs not monitored by pharmacists are classified as Schedule III.

2.6 In order to protect the unborn, all prescription drugs are classified according to safety in pregnancy categories.

In the United States, all drugs are placed into one of five pregnancy categories: A, B, C, D, and X. Drugs in category A are the safest; those in category X are the most harmful.

REVIEW QUESTIONS

The following questions are written in NCLEX-PN® style. Answer these questions to assess your knowledge of the chapter material, and go back and review any material that is not clear to you.

1. Which of the following types of drug classification focuses on what a drug does clinically?

1. Therapeutic
2. Pharmacologic
3. Chemical
4. All of the above

2. *How* a medication produces its effects in the body is referred to as a drug's:

1. Therapeutic usefulness
2. Mechanism of action
3. Model for other drugs combating similar diseases
4. Clinical focus

3. In which of the following categories does a drug have only one name?

1. Chemical name
2. Generic name
3. Trade name
4. Both 1 and 2

4. Which of the following statements is correct?

1. Because chemical drug names are often complicated and difficult to remember or pronounce, the chemical structure of a drug is rarely considered in pharmacotherapy.
2. Matching one active ingredient with one trade name product is not a particularly challenging job for the health care provider.
3. When referring to a drug, the generic name is usually capitalized, whereas the trade name is written in lowercase.
4. The drug trade name is sometimes called the *proprietary* name, suggesting ownership.

5. When examining the question, "Are there really differences between brand name drugs and their generic equivalents?" the answer that emerges from reading this chapter is:

1. Unclear.
2. Significant differences exist between a trade name drug and its generic equivalent.
3. Generic drugs are always best because they generally cost less.

4. Brand name drugs are preferred because of differences in bioavailability compared to generic equivalents.

6. An altered physical condition caused by the nervous system adapting to repeated drug use is:

1. Addiction
2. Physical dependence
3. Psychological dependence
4. Withdrawal

7. The Controlled Substances Act of 1970 and later revisions enable the DEA to do which of the following?

1. Introduce drugs into the marketplace
2. Restrict the use of drugs that have a significant potential for abuse
3. Restrict the use of all drugs that have an abuse potential
4. Allow patients to obtain Schedule II drug refills without visiting their health care provider first

8. The drug schedule that allows therapeutic use of a drug with a prescription but contains drugs with relatively lower abuse and dependency potential than other scheduled drugs is:

1. Schedule II
2. Schedule III
3. Schedule IV
4. Schedule V

9. In Canada, nonprescription drugs monitored for sale by pharmacists are classified as:

1. Schedule I
2. Schedule II
3. Schedule III
4. None of the above, because drugs in Canada are not placed into schedules

10. Pregnant patients:

1. Are not at risk if they take drugs placed into pregnancy safety category X
2. Can take herbal or dietary supplements without fear of teratogenic effects to their developing baby
3. Are relatively safe if they take medications within pregnancy safety category B
4. Should never take drugs classified as pregnancy safety category D

FURTHER STUDY

■ Substance abuse is discussed in detail in Chapter 7.

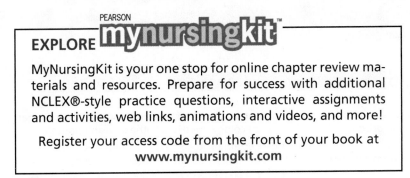

EXPLORE **PEARSON mynursingkit**™

MyNursingKit is your one stop for online chapter review materials and resources. Prepare for success with additional NCLEX®-style practice questions, interactive assignments and activities, web links, animations and videos, and more!

Register your access code from the front of your book at
www.mynursingkit.com

Methods of Drug Administration

CORE CONCEPTS

3.1 A major goal in pharmacotherapy is to limit the number and severity of adverse drug events.

3.2 The rights of drug administration form the basis of proper drug delivery.

3.3 Successful pharmacotherapy depends on patient compliance.

3.4 Health care providers use accepted abbreviations to communicate the directions and times for drug administration.

3.5 Three systems of measurement are used in pharmacology: metric, apothecary, and household.

3.6 Certain protocols and techniques are common to all methods of drug administration.

3.7 Enteral drugs are given orally or via nasogastric or gastrostomy tubes.

3.8 Topical drugs are applied locally to the skin and associated membranes.

3.9 Parenteral administration refers to dispensing medications by routes other than oral or topical.

LEARNING OUTCOMES

After reading this chapter, the student should be able to:

1. Discuss drug administration as a component of safe and effective health care.

2. Describe the roles and responsibilities of nurses, nursing assistants, therapists, and technicians regarding drug administration.

3. Explain how the six rights of drug administration affect patient safety.

4. Give specific examples of how the health care provider can increase patient compliance in taking medications.

5. Interpret abbreviations used in drug administration practices.

6. Compare and contrast the three systems of measurement used in pharmacology.

7. Explain the proper methods to administer enteral, topical, and parenteral drugs.

8. Compare and contrast the advantages and disadvantages of each route of drug administration.

KEY TERMS

allergic reaction 26

anaphylaxis (ANN-ah-fah-LAX-iss) 26

apothecary system (ah-POTH-eh-kare-ee) 29

ASAP order 28

astringent effect (ah-STRIN-jent) 33

buccal route (BUCK-ahl) 32

compliance (kom-PLY-ans) 26

enteral route (EN-tur-ul) 30

enteric-coated (in-TARE-ik) 30

household systems 29

intradermal (ID) route (IN-trah-DERM-ul) 37

intramuscular (IM) route (IN-trah-musk-u-lar) 41

intravenous (IV) route (IN-trah-VEE-nus) 41

metric system 29

parenteral route (pah-REN-tur-ul) 36

prn order 28

routine orders 28

single order 28

six rights of drug administration 26

standing order 28

STAT order 27

subcutaneous (SC or SQ) route (sub-kew-TAY-nee-us) 38

sublingual (SL) route (sub-LIN-gwal) 31

sustained-release 30

three checks of drug administration 26

topical route (TOP-ik-ul) 32

transdermal (trans-DER-mul) 33

transmucosal (trans-mew-KOH-sul) 33

D rug administration is an important part of providing comprehensive care to the patient. During drug administration, members of the health care team collaborate closely with pharmacists, physicians, their patients, and each other to ensure the safe delivery of prescribed medications. The purpose of this chapter is to introduce the roles and responsibilities of nurses and other health care providers, to define the practice of secure and effective distribution of medications, and to provide a basic overview of the major routes of drug administration.

A major goal in pharmacotherapy is to limit the number and severity of adverse drug events.

Whether administering drugs, supervising drug use, or providing assistance, the health care provider is expected to be familiar with the general principles of drug delivery. The large number of different drugs and the potential consequences of medication errors make this an enormous task.

The main responsibilities of the nurse include knowledge and understanding of the following:

- What drug is ordered
- Name (generic and trade) and drug classification
- Intended or proposed use
- Effects on the body
- Contraindications
- Special considerations (for example, the effects of age, weight, body fat distribution, and individual pathophysiological states on pharmacotherapeutic response)
- Side effects
- Why the medication has been prescribed for this particular patient
- What form of the medication is supplied by the pharmacy
- How the medication should be administered, including dosage ranges
- What nursing process considerations related to the medication apply to this patient

Nursing assistants, therapists, and technicians work closely with nurses to provide care to the patients. Members of the health support staff who do not administer medications but who have an equally important role in providing care to the patients have a slightly different list of tasks. These tasks provide opportunity to monitor patients and make sure no unusual reactions or undesirable effects result from the medication. Tasks include:

- Monitoring blood pressure, pulse rate, and respiration rate
- Changing soiled or wet clothing, wraps, or bandages
- Dressing wounds, giving massages, and caring for the skin's surface
- Preparing food trays or helping to feed patients
- Observing patients and reporting significant symptoms, reactions, or changes in condition
- Reporting strange behaviors or habit in patients
- Helping transport patients
- Monitoring special equipment

Before any drug is administered, health care staff must obtain, process, and communicate important information to one another about the patient's medical history, physical assessment, disease processes, learning needs, and capabilities. They must consider growth and developmental factors and remember that many variables can influence how a patient responds to medications. Understanding these variables can increase the success of pharmacotherapy. A major goal of pharmacotherapy is to limit the number and severity of adverse drug events. Many adverse effects are preventable. By applying their experience and knowledge of pharmacotherapeutics to clinical practice, health care providers can avoid many serious adverse drug reactions. Some adverse effects, however, are not preventable. It is vital that the health care team is prepared to recognize and respond to potential adverse medication effects. Allergic and anaphylactic reactions are particularly serious effects that must be carefully monitored and prevented, when possible.

An **allergic reaction** is an acquired hyper-response of body defenses to a foreign substance (allergen). Signs of allergic reactions vary in severity and include skin rash with or without itching, edema, nausea, diarrhea, runny nose, or reddened eyes with tearing. On discovering that a patient is allergic to a product, it is the nurse's responsibility to first alert the charge nurse and patient's physician of the reaction in case it is necessary to give the patient medications to reverse the reaction. Next the nurse should document the allergy in the medical record and apply labels to the chart and medication administration record so that all health care personnel will be aware of the allergy. An agency-approved allergy bracelet should be placed on the patient. The pharmacist should also be told so that the medication can be checked for cross-sensitivity with other pharmacologic products. The pharmacotherapy of allergic reactions is covered in Chapter 24.

Anaphylaxis is a severe type of allergic reaction in which massive amounts of histamine and other chemical mediators of inflammation are released throughout the body. It can lead to life-threatening shock. Symptoms of anaphylaxis are severe shortness of breath, a sudden drop in blood pressure, and tachycardia. These symptoms require immediate attention. The pharmacotherapy of anaphylaxis is covered in Chapter 22.

CORE CONCEPT 3.2

The rights of drug administration form the basis of proper drug delivery.

The traditional **six rights of drug administration** are the basis of safe delivery of medications. The six rights are simple and practical guidelines for nurses to use during drug preparation, delivery, and administration. The six rights are as follows:

- Right patient
- Right medication
- Right dose
- Right route of administration
- Right time of delivery
- Right documentation

Additional rights have been added over the years, depending on particular academic curricula or agency policies. Additions to the original six rights include the right to refuse medication, the right to education, and the right preparation.

The three checks of **drug administration** that nurses use with the six rights help to ensure patient safety and drug effectiveness. Traditionally these checks include the following:

- Checking the drug with the medication administration record (MAR) or medication information system when removing it from the medication drawer, refrigerator, or controlled substance locker
- Checking the drug when preparing it, pouring it, taking it out of the unit dose container, or connecting the IV tubing to the bag
- Checking the drug before administering it to the patient

Despite the use of these checks and rights to provide safe drug delivery, errors still occur, some of them serious and some of them are fatal. Although the nurse is accountable for preparing and administering medications, many individuals—including physicians, pharmacists, and other health care providers—are responsible for safe drug practices.

CORE CONCEPT 3.3

Successful pharmacotherapy depends on patient compliance.

Patient adherence or **compliance** is another major factor affecting the success of pharmacotherapy. Compliance means taking a medication in the way it was prescribed by the practitioner or, in the case of OTC drugs, following the instructions on the label. Patient noncompliance can include not taking the medication at all, taking it at the wrong time, or taking it in the wrong way.

Even when health care providers conscientiously use all the principles of effective drug administration, patients may not agree that the prescribed drug regimen is worthwhile. Before administering the drug, the nurse should use the nursing process to develop a personalized care plan that will allow the patient to be an active participant in his or her care. Support staff can help ensure that the

Fast Facts Potentially Fatal Drug Reactions

Toxic Epidermal Necrolysis (TEN)

- Skin sloughing of 30% or more of the body (caused by skin cell breakdown)
- Severe and deadly allergic reaction caused by the drug
- Occurs when the liver fails to properly break down a drug, which then cannot be excreted normally
- Risk of death decreased if the drug is quickly withdrawn and supportive care is maintained

Stevens-Johnson Syndrome (SJS)

- Skin sloughing of 10% of the body
- Generalized blisterlike lesions following within a few days
- Usually signaled initially by nonspecific upper respiratory infection (URI) with chills, fever, and malaise

care plan works. It is important to remember that a responsible, well-informed adult always has the legal option to refuse any medication. This allows the patient to accept or reject the pharmacotherapy based on accurate information that is presented in a way the patient can understand.

In the plan of care, it is important to address information that the patient must know about the prescribed medications. This includes the name of the drug; why it was ordered; its expected actions; its possible side effects; and its potential interactions with other medications, foods, herbal supplements, or alcohol. Patients need to be reminded that they have an active role in ensuring the effectiveness and safety of their medications.

Many factors influence whether patients comply with pharmacotherapy. The drug may be too expensive or may not be approved by the patient's health insurance plan. Patients sometimes forget doses of medications, especially when they must be taken three or four times per day. Patients often stop using drugs that have annoying side effects or that affect lifestyle. Adverse effects such as headache, dizziness, nausea, diarrhea, or impotence often cause noncompliance. Patients sometimes self-adjust their doses. Some patients believe that if one tablet is good, two must be better. Others believe that they will become dependent on the medication if it is taken as prescribed, and so they take only half the required dose. Patients usually do not want to admit or report noncompliance to the nurse because they are embarrassed or fear being reprimanded. Because there are many reasons for noncompliance, the nurse must carefully question patients about their medications. When pharmacotherapy fails to produce the expected outcomes, noncompliance should be considered as a possible reason.

> ▶ **Life Span Fact**
>
> **Many elderly patients take at least three different drugs each day, with some taking as many as eight. This leads to poor compliance among older patients. Noncompliance can be even greater for elderly patients with dementia or Alzheimer's disease.**

Health care providers use accepted abbreviations to communicate the directions and times for drug administration.

CORE CONCEPT 3.4

Table 3.1 lists common abbreviations that are used to give directions about drug administration. A **STAT order** refers to a medication that should be given immediately and only once. This order is often used with emergency medications that are needed for life-threatening situations. The

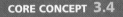

PEARSON
mynursingkit™

ABBREVIATIONS FOR
SAFE MEDICATION
ADMINISTRATION

Fast Facts Grapefruit Juice and Drug Interactions

- Grapefruit juice may not be safe for people who take certain medications.
- Chemicals in grapefruit juice lower the activity of specific enzymes in the intestinal tract that normally break down medications. This allows a larger amount of medication to reach the bloodstream, resulting in increased drug activity.
- Drugs that may be affected by grapefruit juice include certain sedative-hypnotic drugs, antibiotics, drugs that lower blood cholesterol, some antihistamines, and antifungal agents.
- Grapefruit juice should be consumed at least 2 hours before or 5 hours after taking a medication that may interact with it.
- Some drinks that are flavored with fruit juice could contain grapefruit juice, even if grapefruit is not part of the name of the drink. Check the ingredients label.

TABLE 3.1	Drug Administration Abbreviations*		
ABBREVIATION	**MEANING**	**ABBREVIATION**	**MEANING**
ac	before meals	prn	when needed/necessary
ad lib	as desired/as directed	q	every
AM	morning	qh	every hour
ASAP	as soon as possible	qid	four times per day
bid	twice per day	q2h	every 2 hours (even)
cap	capsule	q4h	every 4 hours (even)
/d	per day	q6h	every 6 hours (even)
gtt	drop	q8h	every 8 hours (even)
h or hr	hour	q12h	every 12 hours
hs	hour of sleep/bedtime	Rx	take
no	number	SL	sublingual
pc	after meals; after eating	STAT	immediately; at once
PM	afternoon	tab	tablet
PO	by mouth	tid	three times per day

The Joint Commission (JCAHO) recommends that some previously used abbreviations be spelled out to avoid medication errors: Use "daily" (not qd); use "nightly" (not qhs); use "every other day" (not qod). For other recommendations, see The Joint Commission's official "Do Not Use List": http://www.jointcommission.org/PatientSafety/DoNotUseList.

physician normally notifies the nurse of any STAT order, so it can be obtained from the pharmacy and administered immediately. Although not as urgent, an **ASAP order** (as soon as possible) should be available for administration to the patient within 30 minutes of the written order. (The exact time frame is usually defined by individual facilities.)

A **single order** is for a drug that is to be given only once and at a specific time. An example is a preoperative order. A **prn order** is administered as required by the patient's condition. The nurse makes the judgment, based on patient assessment, as to when the medication should be administered. Orders not written as STAT, ASAP, NOW, or prn are called **routine orders**. These are usually carried out within 2 hours of the time the order is written by the physician, but the exact timing is defined by each facility. A **standing order** is written in advance of a situation and should be carried out under specific circumstances. An example of a standing order is a set of postoperative prn prescriptions that are written for all patients who have undergone a specific surgical procedure. A common standing order for patients who have had a tonsillectomy is "Tylenol elixir 325 mg PO q6h prn sore throat." Because of the legal implications of putting all patients into a single treatment category, standing orders are no longer permitted in some facilities.

Agency policies dictate that drug orders be reviewed by the attending physician within specific time frames, usually at least every 7 days. Prescriptions for narcotics and other scheduled drugs are often automatically stopped after 72 hours, unless specifically reordered by the physician. Automatic stop orders do not generally apply when the number of doses, or an exact period of time, is specified.

Some medications must be taken at specific times. If a drug causes stomach upset, it is usually administered with meals to prevent epigastric pain, nausea, or vomiting. Other medications should be administered between meals because food interferes with absorption. Some CNS drugs and antihypertensives are best administered at bedtime, because they may cause drowsiness. Sildenafil (Viagra) is unique in that it should be taken 30 to 60 minutes prior to expected sexual intercourse to achieve an erection. The nurse must pay careful attention when educating patients about when and how to take their medications to increase compliance and therapeutic success.

Once medications are administered, the nurse must correctly document that the medications have been given to the patient. Depending on the facility, documentation is done on the computer using a special program for medication administration or on a paper copy of the medication administration record (MAR). Either way, it is necessary that the drug name, dosage, time administered, and any assessments data be documented. On the paper copy of the MAR, the nurse must initial and sign his or her name. If a medication is refused or not taken, this fact (along with the patient's reasons) must be recorded on the appropriate form within the medical record. Nursing assistants and health care staff can help verify patient compliance.

Three systems of measurement are used in pharmacology: metric, apothecary, and household.

Dosages are labeled and dispensed according to their weight or volume. The most common system of drug measurement uses the **metric system**. The volume of a drug is expressed in terms of a liter (L) or a milliliter (ml). The abbreviation "cc" for cubic centimeter, a measurement of volume that is equivalent to 1 ml of fluid, is no longer recommended for use in medicine. The metric weight of a drug is stated in terms of kilograms (kg), grams (g), milligrams (mg), or micrograms (mcg). At one time, the abbreviation "µg" was used for micrograms, but this is no longer recommended. It is now recommended that "micrograms" and other small unusual measurements be spelled out.

The **apothecary** and **household systems** are older systems of measurement. Although most physicians and pharmacies use the metric system, these older systems may still be seen. Until the metric system totally replaces the other systems, the health care provider must recognize dosages based on all three systems of measurement. Approximate equivalents among metric, apothecary, and household units of volume and weight are listed in Table 3.2.

Because Americans are familiar with the teaspoon, tablespoon, and cup, it is important for the nurse to be able to convert between the household and metric systems of measurement. In the hospital, a glass of fluid is measured in milliliters—an 8-ounce glass of water is recorded as 240 ml. If a patient being discharged is ordered to drink 2400 ml of fluid per day, the nurse may instruct the patient to drink ten 8-ounce glasses or 10 cups of fluid per day. Likewise, when a child is to be given a drug that is administered in elixir form, the nurse should explain that 5 ml of the drug is the same as 1 teaspoon. The nurse should encourage the use of accurate medical dosing devices at home, such as oral dosing syringes, oral droppers, cylindrical spoons, and medication cups. These are preferred over the traditional household measuring spoon because they are more accurate. Eating utensils that are commonly referred to as teaspoons or tablespoons often do not hold the volume that their names imply.

Certain protocols and techniques are common to all methods of drug administration.

The three general routes of drug administration are enteral, topical, and parenteral, with subcategories among each general route. Each route has both advantages and disadvantages. Although some drugs are formulated to be given by several routes, others are made to be given by only one route. Pharmacokinetic considerations, such as how the route of administration affects drug

TABLE 3.2	Metric, Apothecary, and Household Approximate Measurement Equivalents	
METRIC	**APOTHECARY**	**HOUSEHOLD**
1 ml	15–16 minims	15–16 drops
4–5 ml (cc)	1 fluid dram	1 teaspoon or 60 drops
15 ml	4 fluid drams	1 tablespoon or 3–4 teaspoons
30 ml	8 fluid drams or 1 fluid ounce	2 tablespoons
240 ml	8 fluid ounces (1/2 pint)	1 glass or cup
500 ml	1 pint	2 glasses or 2 cups
1 L	32 fluid ounces or 1 quart	4 glasses or 4 cups or 1 quart
1 mg	1/60 grain	—
60–65 mg	1 grain	—
300–325 mg	5 grains	—
1 g	15–16 grains	—
1 kg	—	2.2 pounds
To convert grains to grams: Divide grains by 15 or 16.		
To convert grams to grains: Multiply grams by 15 or 16.		
To convert minims to milliliters: Divide minims by 15 or 16.		

absorption and distribution, are discussed in Chapter 4. Certain protocols and techniques are common to all methods of drug administration. The student should refer to the drug administration guidelines in the following list before reading about specific routes of administration.

- Review the medication order, and check for drug allergies.
- Wash hands and put on gloves, if indicated.
- Use aseptic technique when preparing and administering parenteral medications.
- Identify the patient by asking the person to state his or her full name (or by asking the parent or guardian if the patient is confused), checking the patient's identification band, and comparing this information with the MAR.
- Ask the patient about known allergies, and check to see if he or she is wearing an allergy identification band.
- Tell the patient what drug you are administering and how you will give it.
- Position the patient for the appropriate route of administration.
- For enteral drugs, assist the patient to a sitting position.
- If the drug is prepackaged as a unit dose, remove it from the packaging at the bedside when possible.
- Unless specifically instructed to do so in the orders, do not leave drugs at the patient's bedside.
- Document the medication administration and any important patient responses on the MAR.

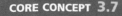

Enteral drugs are given orally or via nasogastric or gastrostomy tubes.

The **enteral route** includes drugs given orally and those administered through nasogastric (NG) or gastrostomy tubes. Oral drug administration (abbreviated PO, which refers to the Latin *per os,* meaning "by mouth") is the most common, most convenient, and usually the least costly of all routes. It is also considered the safest route because the skin's protective barrier is not broken. In cases of overdose, medications remaining in the stomach can be retrieved by causing vomiting. Oral preparations are available in tablet, capsule, caplet, and liquid forms. Medications administered by the enteral route take advantage of the large absorptive surfaces of the oral mucosa, stomach, or small intestine.

Tablets and Capsules

Tablets and capsules are the most common forms of drugs. Patients prefer tablets or capsules over other forms because they are easy to use. In some cases, tablets may be scored so they can easily be broken if the dose needs to be made smaller for a specific patient.

The nurse should always check the manufacturer's instructions for administering the medication to be sure that crushing or opening is allowed. Some tablets and capsules should not be crushed or opened because their ingredients are inactivated by doing so. Other medications can severely irritate the stomach mucosa and cause nausea or vomiting. Occasionally, drugs should not be crushed because they irritate the oral mucosa, are extremely bitter, or contain dyes that stain the teeth. Most drug guides provide lists of drugs that may not be crushed. Guidelines for administering tablets or capsules are given in Table 3.3A.

The strongly acidic contents within the stomach can destroy some medications. To overcome this problem, tablets may have a hard, waxy coating that protects the medicine from acidity. These **enteric-coated** tablets are designed to dissolve in the alkaline environment of the small intestine. It is important that the nurse not crush enteric-coated tablets because the medication would then be directly exposed to the stomach environment.

Studies have clearly shown that patients are less compliant when they must take more than one dose of medicine per day, particularly if the number is three doses or more. With this in mind, pharmacologists have tried to design new drugs that need to be administered only once or twice daily. **Sustained-release** tablets or capsules are designed to dissolve very slowly. They release medication over a longer time, which increases the drug's duration of action (or length of time the medication works). Also called *extended-release (XR), long-acting (LA),* or *slow-release (SR) medications,* these forms allow convenient once or twice daily dosing. These sustained-release medications must not be crushed or opened.

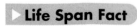

Life Span Fact

For children and elderly patients, as well as those who may have trouble swallowing, the nurse can crush tablets or open capsules and sprinkle the drug over food or mix it with juice to make it easier to swallow and to hide its taste.

TABLE 3.3	Enteral Drug Administration
DRUG FORM	**ADMINISTRATION GUIDELINES**
A. Tablet, capsule, or liquid	1. Check to be sure that the patient is alert and can swallow. 2. Place tablets or capsules into a medication cup. 3. If the medication is liquid, shake the bottle to mix the agent, and measure the dose into the cup at eye level. 4. Hand the patient the medication cup. 5. Offer a glass of water to facilitate swallowing the medication. Milk or juice may be offered (if not contraindicated). 6. Remain with the patient until all medication is swallowed.
B. Sublingual	1. Check that the patient is alert and can hold the medication under the tongue. 2. Instruct the patient not to chew or swallow the tablet, or move it around with the tongue. 3. Instruct the patient to allow the tablet to dissolve completely before swallowing saliva. 4. Place the sublingual tablet under the patient's tongue. 5. Remain with the patient to make sure that all of the medication has dissolved. 6. Offer the patient a glass of water.
C. Buccal	1. Check that the patient is alert and can hold the medication between the gums and the cheek. 2. Instruct the patient to allow the tablet to dissolve completely before swallowing saliva. 3. Instruct the patient not to chew or swallow the tablet or move it around with the tongue. 4. Place the buccal tablet between the gum line and the cheek. 5. Remain with the patient to be sure that all of the medication has dissolved. 6. Offer the patient a glass of water.
D. Nasogastric and gastrostomy	1. Administer liquid forms of the medication when possible to avoid clogging the tube. 2. If the medication is solid, crush it into a fine powder and mix it thoroughly with at least 30 ml of warm water until dissolved. 3. Turn off the feeding tube, if applicable. 4. Verify tube placement and make sure it is clear. 5. Attach a syringe (30 or 60 ml) with plunger. Aspirate the patient's stomach contents and measure the volume. This is termed the *gastric residual volume*. If it is greater than 100 ml (for an adult), check the facility's policy. 6. Attach the syringe without plunger. Return the residual contents by allowing it to flow back into the tube via gravity. Flush the tube with about 10 ml (2 teaspoons) of tap water. 7. Pour the medication into the syringe barrel, also allowing it to flow into the tube by gravity. Give each medication separately, flushing between each with water. 8. Keep the head of the bed elevated 45° for 1 hour to prevent aspiration. 9. Reestablish continual feeding, as scheduled.

Giving medications by the oral route has some disadvantages. The patient must be conscious and able to swallow properly. Certain types of drugs, including proteins, are inactivated by digestive enzymes in the stomach and small intestine. Medications absorbed from the stomach and small intestine first travel to the liver, where they may be inactivated before they ever reach their target organs. This process, called *first-pass metabolism,* is discussed in Chapter 4. The significant variation in the motility of the GI tract among patients and in the tract's ability to absorb medications can create differences in bioavailability. In addition, children and some adults do not like to swallow large tablets and capsules or take oral medications that are distasteful.

Sublingual and Buccal Drug Administration

For sublingual and buccal administration, the patient does not swallow the tablet but instead keeps it in the mouth until it dissolves. The mucosa of the oral cavity contains a rich blood supply that provides an excellent absorptive surface for certain drugs. Medications given by this route are not destroyed by digestive enzymes, nor do they undergo first-pass metabolism in the liver.

For the **sublingual (SL) route,** the medication is placed under the tongue and allowed to dissolve slowly. The rich blood supply under the tongue results in a rapid onset of drug action. Sublingual dosage forms are most often formulated as rapidly disintegrating tablets or as soft gelatin capsules filled with liquid drug.

FIGURE 3.1

(a) Sublingual (under the tongue) drug administration; (b) buccal (between the gums and cheek) drug administration

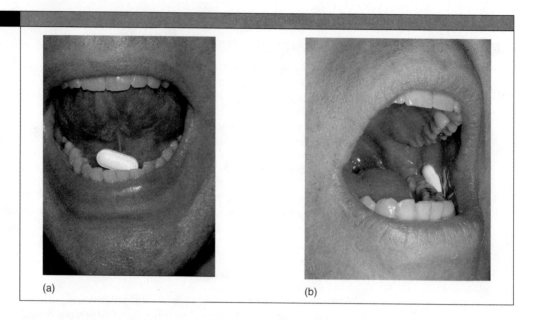

(a)   (b)

When multiple drugs have been ordered, the sublingual preparations should be administered after the oral medications have been swallowed. The patient should be instructed not to move the drug with the tongue, nor to eat or drink anything until the medication has completely dissolved. The sublingual mucosa is not suitable for extended-release formulations because it is a relatively small area and is constantly being bathed by saliva. Table 3.3B and Figure 3.1a ■ present important points about sublingual drug administration.

To administer by the **buccal route**, the tablet, capsule, lozenge, or troche is placed in the oral cavity between the gum and the cheek. The patient must be instructed not to touch the medication with the tongue, because it could get moved to the sublingual area where it would be more rapidly absorbed, or to the back of the throat where it could be swallowed. Medications are absorbed more slowly from the buccal mucosa than from the sublingual area. The buccal route is preferred over the sublingual route for sustained-release delivery because of its greater mucosal surface area. Drugs formulated for buccal administration generally do not cause irritation and are small enough to not cause discomfort to the patient. Table 3.3C and Figure 3.1b ■ provide important guidelines for buccal drug administration.

Nasogastric and Gastrostomy Drug Administration

Patients with a nasogastric (NG) tube or enteral feeding system such as a gastrostomy (G) tube may have their medications administered through these devices. The soft, flexible NG tube is inserted by way of the nasopharynx or oropharynx, with the tip lying in the stomach. A G tube is surgically placed directly into the patient's stomach. Generally, the NG tube is used for short-term treatment, whereas the G tube is inserted for patients who require long-term care. Drugs administered through these tubes are usually in liquid form. Although solid drugs can be crushed or dissolved, they tend to clog the tubes. Sustained-release drugs should not be crushed and administered through NG or G tubes. Drugs administered by this route are exposed to the same physiologic processes as those given orally. Table 3.3D gives important guidelines for administering drugs through NG or G tubes.

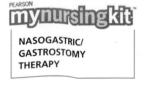

Topical drugs are applied locally to the skin and associated membranes.

CORE CONCEPT 3.8

The **topical route** involves applying drugs locally to the skin or the membranous linings of the eye, ear, nose, respiratory tract, urinary tract, vagina, and rectum. These applications include the following:

- *Dermatologic preparations*   These drugs are applied to the skin using formulations that include creams, lotions, gels, powders, and sprays. The skin is the most common topical route.

- *Instillations and irrigations*   These drugs are applied into body cavities or orifices, including the eyes, ears, nose, urinary bladder, rectum, and vagina.
- *Inhalations*   Inhalers, nebulizers, or positive-pressure breathing apparatuses are used to apply drugs to the respiratory tract. The most common indication for inhaled drugs is bronchoconstriction due to bronchitis or asthma. Many illegal, abused drugs are taken by this route because it provides a very rapid onset of drug action.

Drugs can be applied topically to produce a local or a systemic effect. Many drugs are applied topically to produce a local effect. For example, antibiotics may be applied to the skin to treat skin infections. Antineoplastic agents may be infused into the urinary bladder via catheter to treat tumors of the bladder mucosa. Corticosteroids are sprayed into the nostrils to reduce inflammation of the nasal mucosa due to allergic rhinitis. Local, topical delivery of these drugs produces fewer side effects compared with the same drugs given orally or parenterally. When these drugs are given topically, they are absorbed very slowly, and only small amounts reach the general circulation.

Other drugs are given topically to ensure slow release and absorption of the drug in the general circulation. These agents are given for their systemic (systemwide) effects. For example, a nitroglycerin patch is not applied to the skin to treat a local skin condition, but to treat the systemic condition of coronary artery disease. Likewise, prochlorperazine (Compazine) suppositories are inserted rectally not to treat a disease of the rectum but to alleviate nausea. The distinction between topical drugs given for local effects and those given for systemic effects is an important one for the nurse to know. In the case of local drugs, absorption is undesirable and may cause side effects. For systemic drugs, absorption is necessary for the therapeutic action of the drug. With either type of topical agent, drugs should not be applied to abraded or denuded skin, unless the directions so indicate.

Transdermal Delivery System

Transdermal patches are an effective means of delivering certain medications. Examples include nitroglycerin for angina pectoris and scopolamine (Transderm-Scop) for motion sickness. Although transdermal patches contain a specific amount of drug, the rate of delivery and the actual dose received may vary. Patches are changed on a regular basis, using a site rotation routine, which should be documented in the MAR. Before applying a transdermal patch, the nurse should verify that the previous patch has been removed and disposed of appropriately. Drugs to be administered by this route avoid the first-pass effect in the liver and bypass digestive enzymes. Table 3.4A and Figure 3.2 ■ illustrate the major points of transdermal drug delivery.

Ophthalmic Administration

The ophthalmic route is used to treat local conditions of the eye and surrounding structures. Common indications include excessive dryness, infections, glaucoma, and dilation of the pupil during eye examinations. Ophthalmic drugs are available in the form of eye irrigations, drops, ointments, and medicated disks. Figure 3.3 ■ and Table 3.4B give guidelines for adult administration.

Otic Administration

The otic route is used to treat local conditions of the ear, including infections and soft blockages of the auditory canal. Otic medications include eardrops and irrigations, which are usually ordered for cleaning. Figure 3.4 ■ and Table 3.4C present key points in administering otic medications.

Nasal Administration

The nasal route, a **transmucosal** method of drug delivery, is used for both local and systemic drug administration. The nasal mucosa provides an excellent absorptive surface for certain medications. Advantages of this route include ease of use and avoidance of the first-pass effect in the liver and the digestive enzymes. Nasal spray formulations of corticosteroids have revolutionized the treatment of allergic rhinitis because the medication is very safe when administered by this route.

Although the nasal mucosa provides an excellent surface for drug delivery, there is the potential for damage to the cilia within the nasal cavity, and mucosal irritation is common. In addition, unpredictable mucous secretion in some individuals may affect drug absorption from this site.

Drops or sprays are often used for their local **astringent effect**, which is to shrink swollen mucous membranes or to loosen secretions and facilitate drainage. This brings immediate relief from the nasal congestion caused by the common cold. The nose also provides the route to reach the nasal sinuses and the eustachian tube. Proper positioning of the patient prior to giving nose drops for sinus disorders depends on which sinuses are being treated. The same holds true for

---

▶ Life Span Fact

Although the procedure for administering ophthalmic drugs is the same with a child as with an adult, it is advisable to enlist the help of an adult caregiver. In some cases, the infant or toddler may need to be immobilized, with the arms wrapped to prevent accidental injury to the eye during administration. For the young child, demonstrating the procedure using a doll helps gain the child's cooperation and decreases the level of anxiety.

▶ Life Span Fact

Administration of otic drugs to infants and young children must be performed carefully to avoid injury to sensitive structures of the ear. Otic drops should be at room temperature before adding them to the ear. When giving otic drugs to children, gently pull the pinna down and back. When giving otic drugs to adults, gently pull the pinna down and forward.

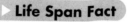

TABLE 3.4	Topical Drug Administration
DRUG FORM	**ADMINISTRATION GUIDELINES**
A. Transdermal	1. Obtain the transdermal patch and read the manufacturer's guidelines. The application site and frequency of changing differ according to medication. 2. Put on gloves before handling the patch to avoid absorbing any medication. 3. Label the patch with the date, time, and your initials. 4. Remove the previous medication or patch, and cleanse the area. 5. If using a transdermal ointment, apply the ordered amount of medication in an even line directly on the premeasured paper that accompanies the medication tube. 6. Press the patch or apply the medicated paper to clean, dry, and hairless skin. 7. Rotate the sites to prevent skin irritation.
B. Ophthalmic	1. Instruct the patient to lie supine or sit with the head slightly tilted back. 2. With your nondominant hand, pull the patient's lower lid down gently to expose the conjunctival sac, creating a pocket. 3. Ask the patient to look upward. 4. Hold the eyedropper 1/4 to 1/8 inch above the conjunctival sac. Do not hold the dropper over the patient's eye because this may stimulate the blink reflex. 5. Instill the prescribed number of drops into the center of the pocket. Avoid touching the eye or conjunctival sac with the tip of the eyedropper. 6. If applying ointment, apply a thin line of ointment evenly along the inner edge of the lower lid margin, from inner to outer canthus. 7. Instruct the patient to gently close the eye. Apply gentle pressure with your finger to the nasolacrimal duct at the inner canthus for 1–2 minutes to avoid overflow drainage into the nose and throat. This minimizes the risk of absorption into the systemic circulation. 8. With a tissue, remove the excess medication from around the patient's eye. 9. Replace the dropper. Do not rinse the eyedropper.
C. Otic	1. Instruct the patient to lie on his or her side or to sit with the head tilted so that the affected ear is facing up. 2. If necessary, use a clean washcloth to clean the pinna of the ear and the meatus to prevent any discharge from being washed into the ear canal during the instillation of the drops. 3. Hold the dropper 1/4 inch above the ear canal, and instill the prescribed number of drops into the side of the ear canal, allowing the drops to flow downward. Avoid placing the drops directly on the tympanic membrane. 4. Gently apply intermittent pressure to the tragus of the ear three or four times. 5. Instruct the patient to remain on his or her side for up to 10 minutes to prevent loss of medication. 6. If cotton ball is ordered, presoak with medication and insert it into the outermost part of ear canal. 7. Wipe off any solution that may have dripped from the ear canal with a tissue.
D. Nasal drops	1. Ask the patient to blow his or her nose to clear the nasal passages. 2. Draw up the correct volume of drug into the dropper. 3. Instruct the patient to open and breathe through the mouth. 4. Hold the tip of the dropper just above the patient's nostril and, without touching the nose with the dropper, direct the solution laterally toward the midline of the superior concha of the ethmoid bone—not at the base of the nasal cavity, where it will run down the throat and into the eustachian tube. 5. Ask the patient to remain in this position for 5 minutes. 6. Discard any remaining solution that is in the dropper.
E. Vaginal	1. Instruct the patient to assume a dorsal recumbent position with her knees bent and separated. 2. Put on gloves; open the suppository and lubricate the rounded end of the suppository and the gloved forefinger of your dominant hand with a water-soluble lubricant. 3. Expose the vaginal orifice by separating the labia with your nondominant hand. 4. Insert the rounded end of the suppository about 8–10 cm along the posterior wall of the vagina, or as far as it will pass. 5. If using a cream, jelly, or foam, gently insert the applicator 5 cm along the posterior vaginal wall and slowly push the plunger until empty. Remove the applicator and place on a paper towel. 6. Ask the patient to lower her legs and remain lying in the dorsal recumbent position for 5–10 minutes following insertion. Offer the patient a perineal pad.

TABLE 3.4	Topical Drug Administration—*Continued*
DRUG FORM	**ADMINISTRATION GUIDELINES**
F. Rectal suppositories	1. Instruct the patient to lie on the left side (Sims' position). 2. Put on gloves; open the suppository and lubricate the rounded end. 3. Lubricate the gloved forefinger of your dominant hand with water-soluble lubricant. 4. Inform the patient when the suppository is to be inserted; instruct the patient to take slow, deep breaths and deeply exhale during insertion to relax the anal sphincter. 5. Gently insert the lubricated end of the suppository into the rectum, beyond the anal-rectal ridge to ensure retention. 6. Instruct the patient to remain in the Sims' position or lie supine to prevent expulsion of the suppository. 7. Instruct the patient to retain the suppository for at least 30 minutes to allow absorption, unless the suppository is administered to stimulate defecation.

FIGURE 3.2

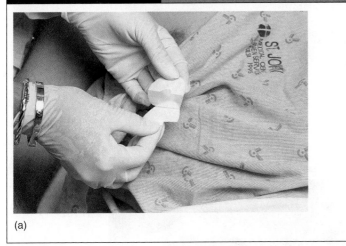
(a)

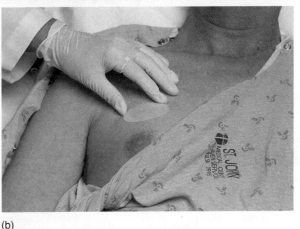
(b)

Transdermal patch administration: Put on gloves before handling the patch and read the manufacturer's directions. Label the patch with the date and time and your initials. Remove any previous medication or patch, and cleanse the area. (a) Remove the protective coating from the patch and (b) apply the patch immediately to clean, dry, hairless skin.   *Source: Pearson Education/PH College*

treatment of the eustachian tube. Table 3.4D and Figure 3.5 ■ illustrate important facts related to nasal drug administration.

Vaginal Administration

The vaginal route is used to deliver medications for treating local infections and to relieve vaginal pain and itching. Vaginal medications are inserted as suppositories, creams, jellies, or foams. It is important that the nurse explains the purpose of treatment and provides privacy for the patient. Before inserting vaginal drugs, the nurse should instruct the patient to empty her bladder. This lessens both discomfort during treatment and the possibility of irritating or injuring the vaginal lining. The patient should be offered a perineal pad following administration. Table 3.4E and Figure 3.6 ■ provide guidelines regarding vaginal drug administration.

Rectal Administration

The rectal route may be used for either local or systemic drug administration. It is a safe and effective means of delivering drugs to patients who are comatose or who are experiencing nausea and vomiting. Rectal drugs are normally in suppository form, although a few laxatives and diagnostic agents are given via enema. Although absorption is slower than by other routes, it is steady and reliable as long as the medication can be retained by the patient. Venous blood from the lower rectum is not transported by way of the liver. Therefore, the first-pass effect is

Ophthalmic administration: (a) Pull the patient's lower lid down gently to expose the conjunctival sac. Have the patient look upward. Apply a thin line of eye ointment into the lower conjunctival sac. (b) Press gently on the nasolacrimal duct.
Source: © Jenny Thomas Photography

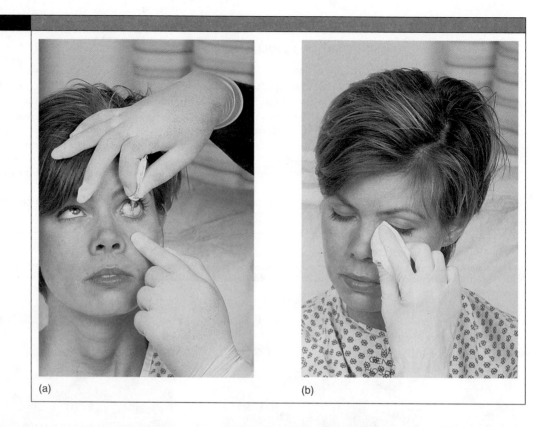

(a)   (b)

Otic drug administration: Instilling eardrops
Source: © Elena Dorfman

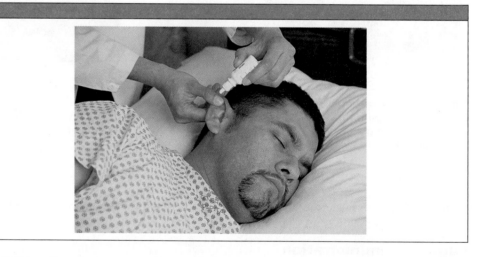

avoided, as are the digestive enzymes of the upper GI tract. Table 3.4F gives details about rectal drug administration.

Parenteral administration refers to dispensing medications by routes other than oral or topical.

CORE CONCEPT 3.9

The **parenteral route** delivers drugs via a needle into the skin layers, subcutaneous tissue, muscles, or veins, with the needle inserted at different degrees, depending on the type of injection, as shown in Figure 3.7 ■. More advanced parenteral delivery includes administration into arteries, body cavities (such as intrathecal), and organs (such as intracardiac). Parenteral drug administration is much more invasive (meaning that the delivery method "invades" the barrier that the skin provides to protect the body) than topical or enteral administration. Because of the possi-

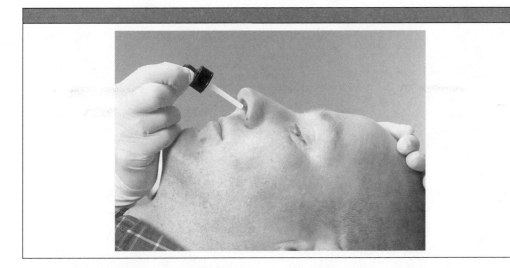

FIGURE 3.5

Nasal drug
administration
*Source: Pearson Education/PH
College*

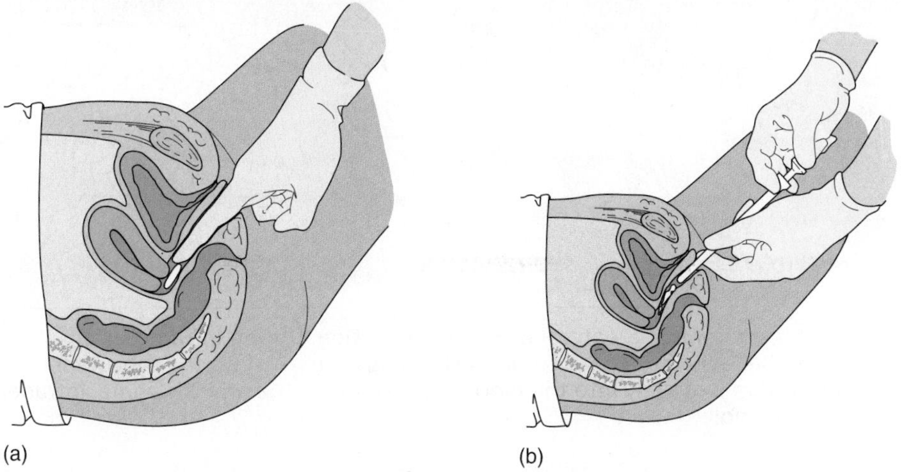

FIGURE 3.6

Vaginal drug
administration:
(a) instilling a vaginal
suppository; (b) using
an applicator to instill a
vaginal cream
*Source: Pearson Education/PH
College*

(a)   (b)

bility of introducing pathogenic microbes directly into the blood or body tissues, aseptic techniques must be strictly used. The nurse is expected to identify and use appropriate materials for parenteral drug delivery, including specialized equipment and techniques involved in the preparation and administration of injectable products. The nurse must know the correct anatomical locations for parenteral administration and safety procedures regarding hazardous equipment disposal.

Intradermal and Subcutaneous Administration

Injection into the skin delivers drugs to the blood vessels that supply the layers of the skin. Drugs may be injected either intradermally or subcutaneously. The major difference between these methods is the depth of injection, which is controlled by the angle of needle placement (see Figure 3.7). An advantage of both methods is that they offer a means of administering drugs to patients who are unable to take them orally. Drugs administered by these routes avoid the first-pass effect in the liver and the digestive enzymes. Disadvantages are that only small volumes can be administered, and injections can cause pain and swelling at the injection site.

An **intradermal (ID) route** injection is administered into the dermis layer of the skin. Because the dermis contains more blood vessels than the deeper subcutaneous layer, drugs are more easily absorbed. This route is usually used for allergy and disease screening or for local anesthetic delivery prior to venous cannulation. Only very small volumes of drug, usually only

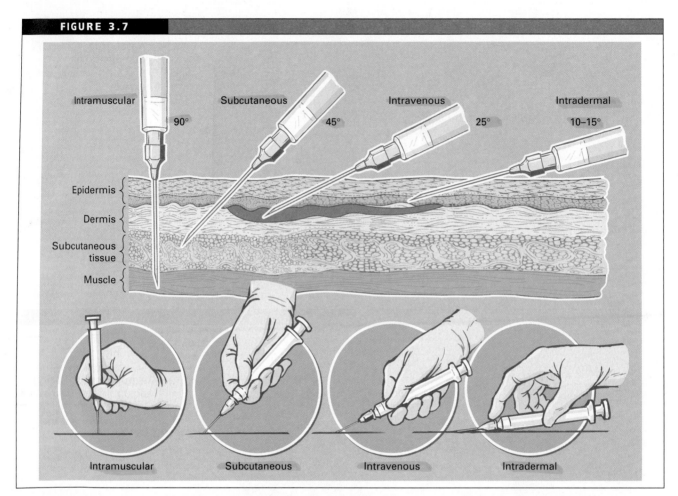

FIGURE 3.7

Intramuscular 90°   Subcutaneous 45°   Intravenous 25°   Intradermal 10–15°

Epidermis
Dermis
Subcutaneous tissue
Muscle

Intramuscular   Subcutaneous   Intravenous   Intradermal

Parenteral drug administration: Gloves are worn for all parenteral drug administration. During intramuscular administration, a drug is injected into muscle at a 90° angle. Subcutaneous administration is into the subcutaneous ~~venous administration~~ ation is directly into the bloodstream and is done at a 25° angle. Intradermal ~~administration is into the dermis~~ 5° angle.   *Source: Pearson Education/PH College.*

Intramuscular   90°
Subcutaneous   45°
Intravenous   25°
Intradermal   10–15°

INJECTIONS

an be given by ID injections. The usual sites for ID injections are the nonhairy ... the upper back, over the scapulae, the high upper chest, and the anterior fore-
... s for intradermal injections are given in Table 3.5A and Figure 3.8 ■.
neous (SC or SQ) route injection is delivered to the deepest layers of the skin.
... vitamins, some vaccines, and other medications are given in this area because

---

ministration

TION GUIDELINES

e medication in a tuberculin or 1 ml syringe, using a 25–27 gauge, 3/8–5/8 inch

ves and cleanse the injection site with an antiseptic swab, using a circular motion.
site to air dry.
humb and index finger of your nondominant hand, spread the patient's skin taut.

4. Insert the needle, with the bevel facing upward, at a 10°–15° angle.
5. Advance the needle until the entire bevel is under the skin; do not aspirate.
6. Slowly inject the medication to form a small wheal or bleb (small raised area).
7. Withdraw the needle quickly, and pat the site gently with a sterile 2 × 2 gauze pad. Do not massage the area.
8. Instruct the patient not to rub or scratch the area.

TABLE 3.5	Parenteral Drug Administration—*Continued*

DRUG FORM	**ADMINISTRATION GUIDELINES**
B. Subcutaneous route	1. Prepare the medication in a 1–3 ml syringe using a 23–25 gauge, 1/2–5/8 inch needle. For heparin, the recommended needle is 3/8 inch and 25–26 gauge.
	2. Choose the site, avoiding bony areas, major nerves, and blood vessels. For heparin, check your facility's policy for the preferred injection sites.
	3. Check the previous rotation sites and select a new area for injection.
	4. Put on gloves and cleanse the injection site with an antiseptic swab using a circular motion.
	5. Allow the site to air dry.
	6. Bunch the skin between the thumb and index finger of your nondominant hand.
	7. Insert the needle at 45° or 90°, depending on the patient's body size and the length of the needle you are using: 90° for obese patients; 45° degrees for average-weight patients.
	8. For nonheparin injections, aspirate by pulling back on the plunger. If blood appears, withdraw the needle, discard the syringe, and prepare a new injection. For heparin, do not aspirate, because aspiration can damage surrounding tissues and cause bruising.
	9. Inject the medication slowly.
	10. Remove the needle quickly. Gently massage the site with an antiseptic swab. *For heparin or insulin, do not massage the size, because bruising or bleeding may occur.*
C. Intramuscular route: ventrogluteal site	1. Prepare the medication using a 20–23 gauge, 1.5 inch needle. (Needle size may vary depending on the site and patient size.)
	2. Put on gloves and cleanse the injection site with an antiseptic swab using a circular motion. Allow the site to air dry.
	3. Locate the site by placing your hand with the heel on the greater trochanter and your thumb pointing toward the umbilicus. Point to the anterior iliac spine with your index finger, spreading your middle finger to point toward the iliac crest (forming a V). Injection of medication is given within the V-shaped area between the index and third finger.
	4. Insert the needle with a smooth, dartlike movement at a 90° angle within the V-shaped area.
	5. Aspirate and observe for blood. If blood appears, withdraw the needle, discard the syringe, and prepare a new injection.
	6. Inject the medication slowly and with smooth, even pressure on the plunger.
	7. Remove the needle quickly.
	8. Apply pressure to the site with a dry, sterile 2 × 2 gauze and gently massage to promote absorption of the medication into the muscle.
D. Intravenous route	1. To add a drug to an IV fluid container:
	a. Verify the order and compatibility of the drug with the IV fluid.
	b. Prepare the medication in a 5–20 ml syringe using a 1–1.5 inch, 19–21 gauge needle.
	c. Put on your gloves and assess the injection site for signs of inflammation or extravasation (oozing of tissue).
	d. Locate the medication port on the IV fluid container and cleanse it with an antiseptic swab.
	e. Carefully insert the needle or access device into the port and inject the medication.
	f. Withdraw the needle and mix the solution by rotating the container end to end.
	g. Hang the container and check the infusion rate.
	2. To add drug to an IV bolus (IV push) using an existing IV line or IV lock (reseal):
	a. Verify the order and compatibility of the drug with the IV fluid.
	b. Determine the correct rate of infusion.
	c. Determine if IV fluids are infusing at the proper rate (IV line) and that the IV site is adequate.
	d. Prepare the drug in a syringe with a 19–21 gauge needle.
	e. Put on your gloves and assess the injection site for signs of inflammation or extravasation (oozing of tissue).
	f. Select an injection port on the tubing that is closest to the insertion site (IV line).
	g. Cleanse the tubing or lock port with an antiseptic swab and insert the needle into the port.
	h. If administering medication through an existing IV line, occlude the tubing by pinching it just above the injection port.
	i. Slowly inject the medication over the designated time (which is not usually faster than 1 ml/min, unless otherwise specified).
	j. Withdraw the syringe. Release the tubing and ensure the proper IV infusion if using an existing IV line.
	k. If using an IV lock, check your facility's policy for use of saline flush before and after injecting medications.

FIGURE 3.8

Intradermal administration: (a) The medication is checked. (b) The medication vial is held nearly vertical at eye level, and the drug is drawn into the syringe. (c) The administration site is prepared. (d) The needle is inserted, bevel up, at 10°–15°. After administration, a 2 × 2 gauze pad is used to gently pat the site dry. *Source: Pearson Education/PH College*

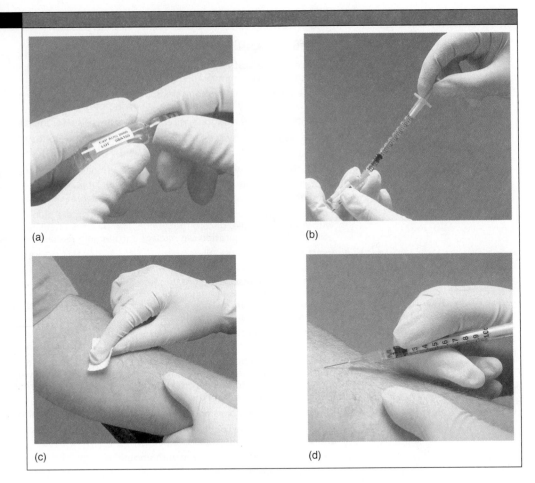

(a) (b) (c) (d)

the sites are easy to reach and provide rapid absorption. Body sites that are ideal for subcutaneous injections include the following:

- Posterior upper arm (above the triceps muscle)
- Middle two thirds of the anterior thigh area
- Subscapular areas of the upper back
- Upper dorsogluteal and ventrogluteal areas
- Abdominal areas, above the iliac crest and below the diaphragm, 2 inches out from the umbilicus

Subcutaneous doses are small in volume, usually ranging from 0.5 to 1 ml, and are given at a 45° (normal weight patient) to 90° angle (obese patient). The needle size varies with the patient's quantity of body fat but is usually 1/2 inch to 5/8 inch. The needle length is usually one-half the size of a pinched/bunched skinfold that can be grasped between the thumb and forefinger. It is important to rotate injection sites in an orderly and documented manner, to promote absorption, minimize tissue damage, and alleviate discomfort. For insulin, however, rotation should be within an anatomical area that promotes reliable absorption and maintains consistent blood glucose levels. When performing subcutaneous injections, it is usually not necessary to aspirate prior to the injection. It depends on what is being injected and the patient's anatomy. Aspiration might prevent inadvertent administration into a vein or artery in a thin person. If the medication should not be administered directly into a vessel, aspiration is recommended. For example, long-acting insulins should not be given IV; therefore, aspiration is justified. Heparin, on the other hand, can be safely administered IV, and so aspiration is not required. Note that tuberculin syringes and insulin syringes are not interchangeable and should not be substituted for each other. Table 3.5B and Figure 3.9 ■ include important information regarding subcutaneous drug administration.

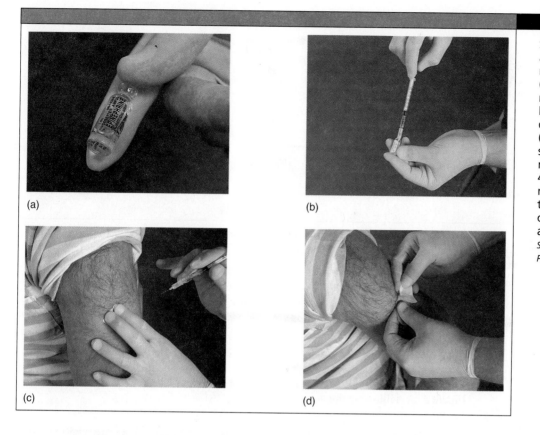

(a)

(b)

(c)

(d)

Subcutaneous administration: (a) The medication is checked. (b) With the vial held nearly vertical at eye level, the medication is drawn into the syringe. (c) The administration site is prepared and the needle is inserted at a 45° angle. (d) The needle is removed, and the puncture site is covered with an adhesive bandage.
Source: Pearson Education/ PH College

FIGURE 3.9

Intramuscular Administration

An **intramuscular (IM) route** injection delivers medication into specific muscles. Because muscle tissue has a rich blood supply, medication moves quickly into blood vessels to produce a more rapid onset of action than with oral, ID, or SC administration. The anatomical structure of muscle permits this tissue to receive a larger volume of medication than the subcutaneous region. An adult with well-developed muscles can safely tolerate up to 5 ml of medication in a large muscle, although only 2 to 3 ml is recommended. The deltoid and triceps muscles should receive a maximum of 1 ml.

A major consideration for the nurse regarding IM drug administration is the selection of an appropriate injection site. Injection sites must be located away from bones, large blood vessels, and nerves. Both the size and length of the needle are determined by body size and muscle mass, the type of drug to be administered, the amount of adipose (fat) tissue overlying the muscle, and the age of the patient. Information regarding IM injections is given in Table 3.5C and Figure 3.10 ■. The four common sites for intramuscular injections are as follows:

- *Ventrogluteal site*   This area provides the greatest thickness of gluteal muscles, contains no large blood vessels or nerves, is sealed off by bone, and contains less fat than the buttock area, thus eliminating the need to determine the depth of subcutaneous fat.
- *Deltoid site*   Used in well-developed teens and adults for volumes of medication not to exceed 1 ml.
- *Dorsogluteal site*   Used for adults and for children who have been walking for at least 6 months. The site is safe as long as the nurse appropriately locates the injection landmarks to avoid puncture or irritation of the sciatic nerve and blood vessels.
- *Vastus lateralis site*   Usually thick and well developed in both adults and children, the middle third of the muscle is the site for IM injections.

Intravenous Administration

The **intravenous (IV) route** enables administration of medications and fluids directly into the bloodstream and allows their immediate availability for use by the body. The IV route is used

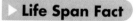

▶ **Life Span Fact**

The ventrogluteal site is a suitable site of IM injection for children and infants over 7 months of age.

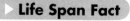

▶ **Life Span Fact**

The vastus lateralis is the site of choice for IM injections in pediatric patients.

FIGURE 3.10

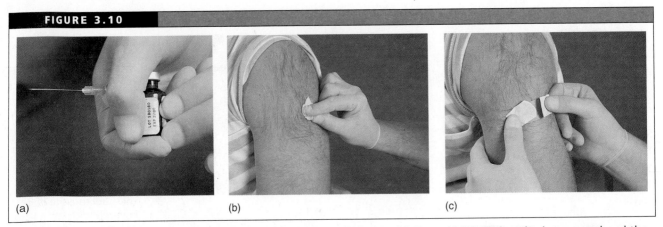

(a) (b) (c)

Intramuscular administration: (a) The medication is checked and drawn. (b) The administration site is prepared and the needle is inserted at a 90° angle. (c) The needle is removed and the puncture site is covered with an adhesive bandage. *Source: Pearson Education/PH College*

when a very rapid onset of action is desired. Like other parenteral routes, IV medications bypass the enzymes of the digestive system and the first-pass effect of the liver. The three basic types of IV administration are as follows:

- *Large-volume infusion* This type of infusion is used for fluid maintenance, replacement, or supplementation. Compatible drugs may be mixed into a large-volume IV container with fluids such as normal saline or Ringer's lactate. Table 3.5D and Figure 3.11 ■ illustrate this technique.

FIGURE 3.11

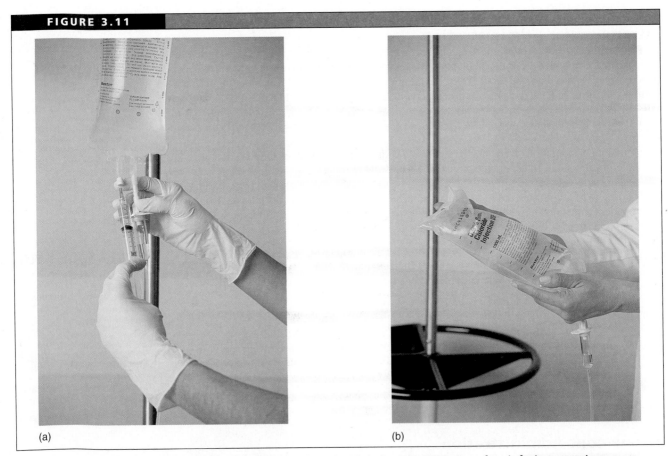

(a) (b)

Adding a drug to an existing infusion: (a) inserting a drug through the injection port of an infusion container; (b) rotating the IV bag to distribute the drug *Source: © Elena Dorfman*

FIGURE 3.12

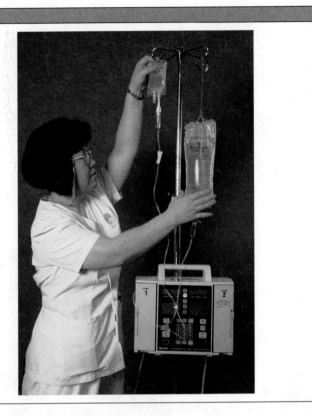

An intermittent IV infusion given piggy-back to the primary infusion   *Source: Pearson Education/PH College*

- *Intermittent infusion*   A small amount of IV solution is "piggy-backed" (added) to the primary large-volume infusion. This type of infusion, illustrated in Figure 3.12 ■, is used to give additional medications such as antibiotics or analgesics over a short time.

- *IV bolus (push) administration*   A concentrated single dose of medication is delivered directly to the circulation via syringe. Bolus injections may be given through an intermittent injection port or by direct IV push. Details on the bolus administration technique are given in Table 3.5D and Figure 3.13 ■.

Although the IV route provides the fastest onset of drug action, it is also the most dangerous. Once injected, the medication cannot be retrieved. If the drug solution or the needle is contaminated, pathogens have a direct route to the bloodstream and body tissues. Patients who are receiving IV injections must be closely monitored for adverse reactions. Some adverse reactions occur immediately after injection; others may take hours or days to appear. Antidotes for drugs that can cause potentially dangerous or fatal reactions must always be readily available. Several types of needleless IV systems are also available and have been shown to greatly reduce the chance of needlestick injuries among health care professionals.

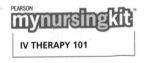

PEARSON
mynursingkit

IV THERAPY 101

SAFETY ALERT

Medication Administration Error – Mistaken Patient Identity

It is the responsibility of the evening nurse on duty to administer medications at 10:00 p.m. When the nurse entered Ms. Brown's room, Ms. Brown was already in bed and had fallen asleep. The nurse gently shook her and said, "I have your 10 p.m. medication, Ms. Brown." Although the patient responded, she was not fully awake. The nurse handed her the medication and a glass of water. Ms. Brown took the medication and quickly returned to sleep. In leaving, the nurse noticed the room number and realized that medication has just been given to Ms. Crown, who is in a room down the hall from Ms. Brown. This situation could have been avoided if the nurse ascertained that the patient receiving the medication was in fact Ms. Brown. Identification needed to be verified by checking the patient's identification band, asking the patient to state her name and date of birth for the nurse, and verifying that these pieces of information matched those listed on the patient's medication administration record.

FIGURE 3.13

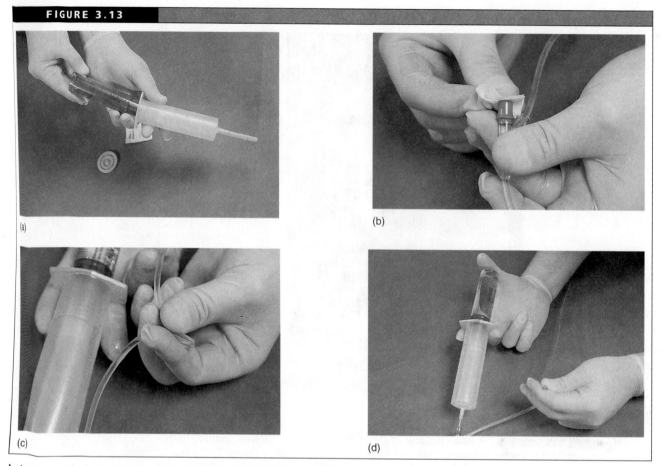

Intravenous bolus administration: (a) The drug is prepared. (b) The administration port is cleaned. (c) The line is pinched. (d) The drug is administered. *Source: Pearson Education/PH College*

PATIENTS NEED TO KNOW

Patients need to know the following:

1. Always ask the health care provider or pharmacist which medications may be taken with food and water to reduce nausea and stomach irritation.
2. Do not crush, cut, or administer enteric-coated tablets with alkaline substances such as antacids.
3. Establish a routine for taking medications by selecting a familiar time of the day, usually on the hour. Special organizers can be obtained to properly store medicines according to times, days, and dosages.
4. Follow the dosing times exactly. If a medication is missed, do not try to "catch up" on the next scheduled dose. If remembered soon after the scheduled time, it is appropriate to take the medicine. Otherwise, wait until the next scheduled dose. An exception would be if the next dose is not scheduled until the next day. For answers to specific questions, consult a health care provider.
5. Store medications in a safe, dry place. Discard them if they become old or outdated.
6. Use the measuring device provided by the drug manufacturer to take medications. Do not rely on kitchen utensils to judge the exact recommended dose.

CHAPTER REVIEW

CORE CONCEPTS SUMMARY

3.1 **A major goal in pharmacotherapy is to limit the number and severity of adverse drug events.**

Health care staff must be familiar with the general principles of drug delivery. The nurse must have a comprehensive knowledge of the actions and side effects of drugs before they are administered to limit the number and severity of adverse drugs events. Allergic and anaphylactic reactions are serious effects that must be carefully monitored and prevented, when possible.

3.2 **The rights of drug administration form the basis of proper drug delivery.**

The six rights and three checks are guidelines to safe drug administration, which involves a collaborative effort among nurses, physicians, and other health care professionals. The six rights are right patient, right medication, right dose, right route of administration, right time of delivery, and right documentation. The three checks are checking the MAR, checking the drug during preparation, and checking the drug before administering it to the patient.

3.3 **Successful pharmacotherapy depends on patient compliance.**

Pharmacologic compliance requires patients to understand and personally accept the value of the prescribed drug regimen. Understanding the reasons for noncompliance can help the health care team increase pharmacotherapeutic success.

3.4 **Health care providers use accepted abbreviations to communicate the directions and times for drug administration.**

There are established orders and time schedules by which medications are routinely administered. The single order (such as a preoperative order) is for a drug that is to be given only once and at a specific time. A prn order is administered as required by the patient's condition. Orders not written as STAT, ASAP, NOW, or prn are called routine orders. A standing order is written in advance of a situation and is to be carried out under specific circumstances. Documenting drug administration and reporting side effects are important responsibilities of the nurse.

3.5 **Three systems of measurement are used in pharmacology: metric, apothecary, and household.**

Health care professionals must recognize dosages based on all three systems of measurement: the metric, apothecary, and household systems. The nurse must be able to convert between household and metric systems of measurement.

3.6 **Certain protocols and techniques are common to all methods of drug administration.**

The student should understand drug administration guidelines before proceeding to a study of specific drug administration routes. The three general routes of drug administration are enteral, topical, and parenteral.

3.7 **Enteral drugs are given orally or via nasogastric or gastrostomy tubes.**

Drugs administered via the enteral route are given orally or through nasogastric (NG) or gastrostomy (G) tubes. The enteral route is the most effective way to administer drugs.

3.8 **Topical drugs are applied locally to the skin and associated membranes.**

Topical drugs are applied locally to the skin or membranous linings of the eye, ear, nose, respiratory tract, urinary tract, vagina, and rectum.

3.9 **Parenteral administration refers to dispensing medications by routes other than oral or topical.**

Parenteral administration is the dispensing of medications via a needle, usually into the skin layers (ID), subcutaneous tissue (SC or SQ), muscles (IM), or veins (IV).

REVIEW QUESTIONS

The following questions are written in NCLEX-PN® style. Answer these questions to assess your knowledge of the chapter material, and go back and review any material that is not clear to you.

1. A nurse enters the patient's room with an intravenous (IV) pole, special tubing, a stethoscope, a fairly large-looking syringe and plunger, and a special container of formula. He explains that in the course of treatment, he will use all of these items. From your understanding of drug administration, which of the following therapies is he likely explaining?

1. Transdermal
2. Intravenous (parenteral)
3. Nasogastric (enteral)
4. Rectal

2. The main reason why extended-release medications must not be crushed is:

1. They are very distasteful, and this reduces patient compliance.
2. Crushing alters the rate of absorption and medication delivery.
3. Multiple drug pieces cause obstructive symptoms.
4. Crushed oral medications have reduced bioavailability.

3. One reason why it is necessary to aspirate the needle during an intramuscular injection is to:

1. Avoid placement of the needle into a blood vessel
2. Produce an air pocket for better drug distribution
3. Avoid nerve puncture
4. Remove air from the syringe

4. Which of the following routes of drug administration has the fastest onset of action?

1. Transdermal
2. Intramuscular
3. Intravenous
4. Ophthalmic

5. Which of the following orders should be carried out immediately?

1. STAT order
2. ASAP order
3. prn order
4. Standing order

6. It is often taught that the nurse should check the label three times during the course of administering a medication: while getting the medication out of the container or drawer, before placing it into the medication cup, and before administering the medication or when placing the stock bottle back on the shelf. Of the "six rights of drug administration," this example mainly refers to which "right"?

1. Right medication
2. Right documentation
3. Right route of administration
4. Right time of delivery

7. When administering medications, the nurse's main responsibilities are to know and understand:

1. The medication being ordered
2. The intended use of the medication
3. Any special considerations such as the patient's age or pathophysiological state
4. All of the above

8. The medication administration record (MAR) contains all of the following information EXCEPT:

1. Date of medication administration
2. Route of drug administration
3. Dose of medication
4. Apothecary system of drug measurement

In questions 9–12, match the abbreviation with the proper meaning in answers 1–4.

9. qh 2

10. qhs 3

11. qid 4

12. qod 1

1. This abbreviation should not be used. Instead write out "every other day."
2. Every hour
3. The abbreviation should not be used. Instead, write out "nightly."
4. Four times per day

FURTHER STUDY

- Chapters 22 and 24 discuss the pharmacotherapy of anaphylaxis and allergic reactions.

- Chapter 4 discusses how pharmacokinetic considerations, such as the route of administration, affect drug absorption and distribution.

- First-pass metabolism is discussed in Chapter 4.

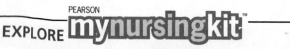

CHAPTER

4

What Happens After a Drug Has Been Administered

CORE CONCEPTS

4.1 Pharmacokinetics focuses on what the body does to the drugs.

4.2 Absorption is the first step in drug transport.

4.3 Distribution refers to how drugs are transported throughout the body.

4.4 Metabolism is a process whereby drugs are made less or more active.

4.5 Excretion processes remove drugs from the body.

4.6 The rate of elimination and half-life characteristics influence drug responsiveness.

4.7 Pharmacodynamics focuses on what the drugs do to the body.

4.8 Drugs activate specific receptors to produce a response.

4.9 *Potency* and *efficacy* are terms often used to describe the success of drug therapy.

LEARNING OUTCOMES

After reading this chapter, the student should be able to:

1. Identify the four major processes of pharmacokinetics.

2. Discuss the factors affecting drug absorption.

3. Describe how plasma proteins affect drug distribution.

4. Explain the significance of the blood-brain barrier, blood-placental barrier, and blood-testicular barrier to drug therapy.

5. Explain the importance of the first-pass effect.

6. Describe how metabolic enzymes differ in younger and in older patients, and explain the significance of this difference to the success of drug therapy.

7. Explain how intermediate products of drug metabolism may produce more intense responses than the original drug.

8. Identify the major processes by which drugs are eliminated from the body.

9. Explain the importance of enterohepatic recirculation to drug therapy.

10. Explain how rate of elimination and plasma half-life ($t_{1/2}$) are related to the duration of drug action.

11. Discuss how successful pharmacotherapy depends on principles of pharmacodynamics.

12. Explain the significance of the receptor theory.

13. Describe how "blockers" of drug action work.

14. Compare and contrast the therapeutic terms *potency* and *efficacy*.

KEY TERMS

absorption (ab-SORP-shun) *49*

agonists (AG-on-ists) *53*

antagonists (an-TAG-oh-nists) *53*

biotransformation (BEYE-oh-trans-for-MAY-shun) *49*

distribution (dis-tree-BU-shun) *49*

efficacy (EFF-ik-ah-see) *53*

enterohepatic recirculation (EN-ter-oh-HEE-pah-tik) *51*

excretion (eks-KREE-shun) *51*

first-pass effect *50*

half-life ($t_{1/2}$) *52*

metabolism (meh-TAHB-oh-liz-ehm) *49*

pharmacodynamics (FAR-mah-koh-deye-NAM-iks) *52*

pharmacokinetics (FAR-mah-koh-kee-NET-iks) *48*

potency (POH-ten-see) *53*

prodrugs *49*

receptor (ree-SEP-tor) *52*

receptor theory *52*

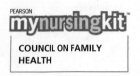

Drugs do not affect all patients the same way. Whether a drug achieves or falls short of achieving a therapeutic response is an important concern to patients and health care providers. Within a population, a dose of medication may produce a dramatic response in one patient while having no effect in another.

Many situations alter a drug's response. Patients sometimes take medications under conditions that interfere with drug activity. This interference is called a *drug interaction.* Well-known examples of food-drug interactions may occur when patients take their medication with food or beverages. Patients often take more than one medication at the same time. After drugs have been absorbed, the effectiveness of drug therapy may be altered by drug-drug interactions in the bloodstream.

To understand the impact that drug interactions have on drug safety and effectiveness, one must understand concepts from two important areas: pharmacokinetics and pharmacodynamics.

CORE CONCEPT 4.1

Pharmacokinetics focuses on what the body does to the drugs.

pharmaco = *drug related*
kinetics = *movement*

As the root words indicate, **pharmacokinetics** focuses on how drugs move within the body. Drug movement involves four processes: absorption, distribution, metabolism, and excretion, as shown in Figure 4.1 ■. A thorough knowledge of pharmacokinetics enables the healthcare provider to understand the therapeutic effects of a drug, as well as to predict potential adverse effects of drug therapy.

FIGURE 4.1

The four processes of pharmacokinetics (drug movement) are absorption, metabolism, distribution, and excretion.

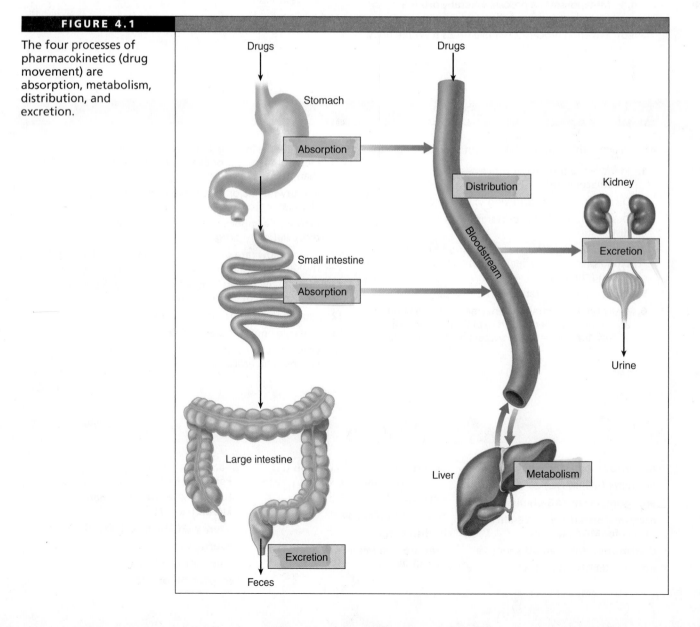

Absorption is the first step in drug transport.

CORE CONCEPT 4.2

Absorption is the first step in how the body handles a drug. Absorption is a process involving the movement of a substance from its site of administration across one or more body membranes. A drug may be absorbed locally and produce a biologic effect at a remote site. Absorption may occur across the skin and associated mucous membranes, or drugs may move across membranes that line blood vessels. Ultimately most drugs move across many membranes to reach their target cells. Many basic science textbooks cover the ways that foods and drugs are absorbed, including passive transport and energy-requiring transport processes. The presence of food in the digestive tract slows the absorption of drugs administered orally.

PEARSON
mynursingkit

FACTORS AFFECTING
DRUG ABSORPTION

Distribution refers to how drugs are transported throughout the body.

CORE CONCEPT 4.3

Distribution is the process by which drugs are transported after they have been absorbed or administered directly into the bloodstream. Between the site of drug administration and the target tissue, many factors affect drug movement. One important example is the *binding* that occurs between drugs and other substances, such as plasma proteins, already present in the bloodstream. When a drug binds with a plasma protein such as albumin, the drug is held by the plasma protein in the bloodstream, where it is unable to reach its target cells. Often, a second drug will interfere with this binding by displacing the first drug from the plasma protein. In this case, the first drug's activity is intensified. The term *bioavailability* is often used to describe how much of a drug will be available after administration to produce a biological effect.

Even if a drug is not bound by plasma proteins, it still may not be able to reach all body tissues. Three important organs contain anatomic barriers that prevent some drugs from gaining access. These are the brain, the placenta, and the testes. Even though these organs have a larger blood supply compared to most other organs in the body, their cellular barriers only allow fat-soluble substances to cross. These special barriers are called the *blood-brain barrier, blood-placental barrier,* and *blood-testicular barrier.*

Some drugs are able to cross the blood-brain barrier without difficulty. These include antianxiety drugs, sedatives (sleep-inducing), and psychoactive (or mind-altering) drugs. Other medications, such as many antibiotics and anticancer medications, are absorbed easily from the intestinal tract, but they do not easily cross into the brain.

The blood-placental barrier serves an important protective function because it regulates which substances pass from the mother's bloodstream to the fetus. However, many potentially damaging agents such as cocaine and alcohol, and even some prescription or OTC medications, are not prevented from crossing this barrier. This is an extremely important issue: All food items and therapeutic drugs should be evaluated to assess their adverse effects on pregnant women and their unborn children, as discussed in Chapter 2. In males, the blood-testicular barrier prevents many drugs from reaching the testes, making it difficult to treat testicular disorders.

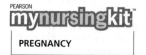

PEARSON
mynursingkit

PREGNANCY

Metabolism is a process whereby drugs are made less or more active.

CORE CONCEPT 4.4

Metabolism is the next step in pharmacokinetics. It is often described as the total of all chemical reactions in the body. Metabolism occurs in almost every cell and organ—including the intestinal tract and kidneys—but the liver is the primary site. The individual chemical reactions of metabolism are called **biotransformation** reactions: They are the chemical conversion of drugs from one form to another that may result in increased or decreased activity. Metabolism is important to drug therapy because these chemical reactions deactivate most drugs. Also, patients with liver disease usually receive much lower doses than normal because their liver is unable to metabolize the drug to a safe, active form.

However, certain drugs called **prodrugs** require metabolism to make them active. In these cases, as the drug is broken down by chemical reactions of metabolism, the products formed by the breakdown produce a more intense response than does the original drug. An example of such a prodrug is sulfasalazine, which is not active in its original form taken by mouth. It is broken down by bacteria in the colon into two products that become active. However, such

bio = *biologic*
transformation =
    changing process
pro =*before*
drug = *medication form*

cases of prodrugs are infrequent. Usually, metabolism is affected by the use of other drugs or the presence of other diseases.

Another important mechanism that affects metabolism and drug action is the **first-pass effect.** Substances absorbed across the intestinal wall enter blood vessels known as the *hepatic portal circulation,* which carries blood directly to the liver (Figure 4.2 ■). Drugs administered orally are absorbed into the hepatic portal circulation and are taken directly to the liver for metabolism. The liver may then metabolize the drug to a less active form before it is distributed to the rest of the body and target organs. In some cases, this first-pass effect can inactivate more than 90% of an orally administered drug before it can reach the general circulation.

Many patients differ in how efficiently their metabolic enzymes work to metabolize drugs. Age, kidney and liver disease, genetics, and other factors can dramatically affect metabolism. Some patients metabolize drugs very slowly; others, very quickly.

FIGURE 4.2

First-pass effect: Drugs given orally are absorbed through the intestinal wall and enter the hepatic portal circulation. Absorbed drugs are taken directly to the liver for metabolism before reaching the heart and circulating throughout the rest of the body.

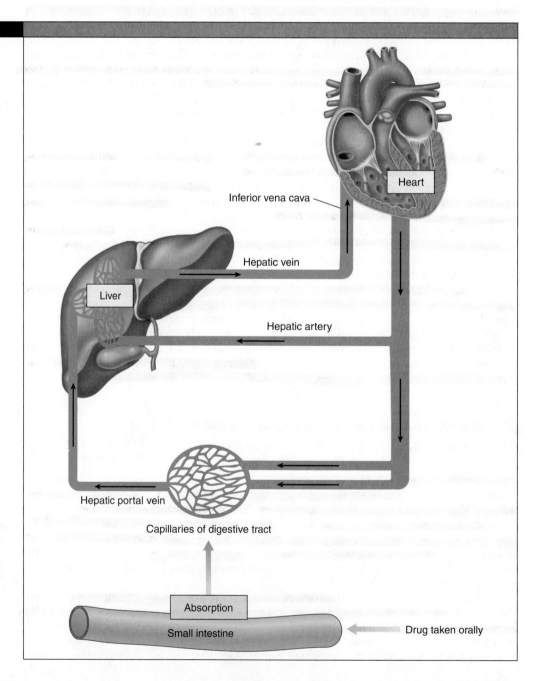

Excretion processes remove drugs from the body.

The last step of pharmacokinetics is **excretion**. Most substances that enter the body are removed by urination, exhalation, defecation, and/or sweating. Drugs are normally removed from the body by the kidneys, the respiratory tract, bile, or glandular activity.

The main organ of excretion is the kidney. The major role of the kidneys is to remove all non-natural and harmful agents in the bloodstream while maintaining a balance of other natural substances. Most drugs are excreted by the kidneys. Therefore, kidney damage can significantly prolong drug action and is a common cause of adverse reactions. Drugs that affect the kidney and its filtration processes are presented in Chapter 23.

Drugs that are easily changed into a gaseous form are especially suited for excretion by the respiratory system. The rate of respiratory excretion is dependent on the many factors that affect gas exchange, including diffusion, gas solubility, and blood flow. The greater the blood flow into lung capillaries, the greater the excretion. In contrast to other methods of excretion, the lungs excrete most drugs in their original unmetabolized form.

Some drugs are excreted through bile. However, most components of bile are circulated back to the liver by a process known as **enterohepatic recirculation**, as shown in Figure 4.3 ■. Recirculating drugs are then metabolized by the liver and excreted by the kidneys. The fraction of drug that is not recirculated continues on its way to the feces. Elimination of drugs through bile may continue for several weeks after therapy has stopped and results in prolonged drug action.

Glands (other than the breast glands) that produce body fluids such as saliva and sweat are less effective at excreting drugs. Most of the substances that are secreted in saliva and perspiration, such as urea or other waste products, are natural products. However, the breast glands can secrete any drug capable of crossing these membranes. Therefore, a breastfeeding mother should always check with her physician before taking any prescription drug, OTC drug, or natural alternative therapy.

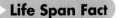

▶ **Life Span Fact**

In general, metabolic enzyme activity is reduced in very young and in elderly patients. Therefore, pediatric and geriatric patients are usually more sensitive to medications than are other patients. Drug doses to the youngest and oldest age groups are often reduced to compensate for these differences.

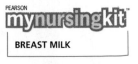

PEARSON
mynursingkit™

BREAST MILK

FIGURE 4.3

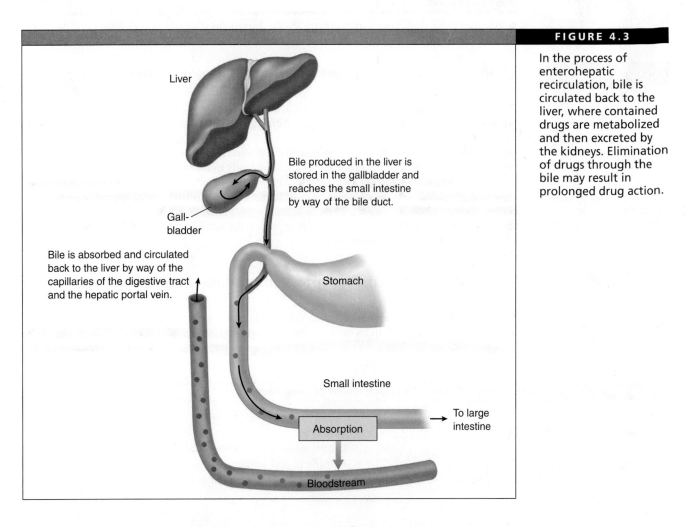

Liver

Bile produced in the liver is stored in the gallbladder and reaches the small intestine by way of the bile duct.

Gall-bladder

Bile is absorbed and circulated back to the liver by way of the capillaries of the digestive tract and the hepatic portal vein.

Stomach

Small intestine

To large intestine

Absorption

Bloodstream

In the process of enterohepatic recirculation, bile is circulated back to the liver, where contained drugs are metabolized and then excreted by the kidneys. Elimination of drugs through the bile may result in prolonged drug action.

Concept Review 4.1

■ What does the term *pharmacokinetics* mean? Describe the four major parts of pharmacokinetics?

CORE CONCEPT 4.6

The rate of elimination and half-life characteristics influence drug responsiveness.

Elimination, which is another term for *excretion,* is often measured so that dosages of drugs can be determined more accurately. The *term rate of elimination* refers to the amount of drug removed per unit of time from the body by normal physiologic processes. The rate of elimination is helpful in determining how long a particular drug will remain in the bloodstream and is thus an indicator of how long a drug will produce its effect.

The **half-life ($t_{1/2}$)** of a drug is a related measurement used to ensure that maximum therapeutic dosages are administered. Half-life is the length of time required for a drug's concentration in the plasma to decrease by one half. It is an indicator of how long a drug will produce its effect in the body. The larger the half-life value, the longer it takes for a drug to be eliminated. For example, a drug with a half-life of 10 hours will take longer to be eliminated from the body than a drug with a half-life of 5 hours. Drugs with longer half-lives may be given less frequently—for example, once per day.

When a patient has a renal or hepatic disease, the plasma half-life of a drug increases. This reflects the important relationship of half-life to metabolism and excretion. Some drugs have a half-life of just a few minutes, whereas others have a half-life of several hours or days.

Concept Review 4.2

■ Why are rate of elimination and half-life ($t_{1/2}$) important to the health care provider?

CORE CONCEPT 4.7

Pharmacodynamics focuses on what the drugs do to the body.

As discussed already, many variables influence the effectiveness of drug therapy, such as rate of administration, frequency of drug dosing, and changing medical condition. Some of these factors are summarized in Table 4.1.

Successful pharmacotherapy depends on these variables as well as how effectively the body responds to drugs at specific target locations. This leads to another important core area of pharmacology: the field of pharmacodynamics. The field of pharmacodynamics is complex and requires extensive knowledge of human physiology and biochemistry. **Pharmacodynamics** deals with the mechanisms of drug action, or how the drug exerts its effects. As the root words suggest, drugs have a powerful influence on body processes. The remaining part of this chapter is devoted to a few basic pharmacodynamic principles.

pharmaco = *drug related*
dynamics = *powerful change*

CORE CONCEPT 4.8

Drugs activate specific receptors to produce a response.

recep = *receiving*
tor = *entity*

Successful pharmacotherapy is based on the principle that to treat a disorder, a drug must interact with specific receptors in its target tissue. The **receptor theory** is a classic theory referring to the cellular mechanism by which most drugs can change body processes. A **receptor** is any struc-

TABLE 4.1	Factors That Influence the Effectiveness of Drug Therapy
Concentration (dose) of administered drug	Metabolic rate (lower in children and elderly patients)
Frequency of drug dosing	Genetics
Food-drug interactions	Excretion rate (rate of elimination)
Drug-drug interactions	Half-life ($t_{1/2}$) of administered drug
Absorption rate (refer to Core Concept 4.1)	Changing medical condition (liver or kidney disease)

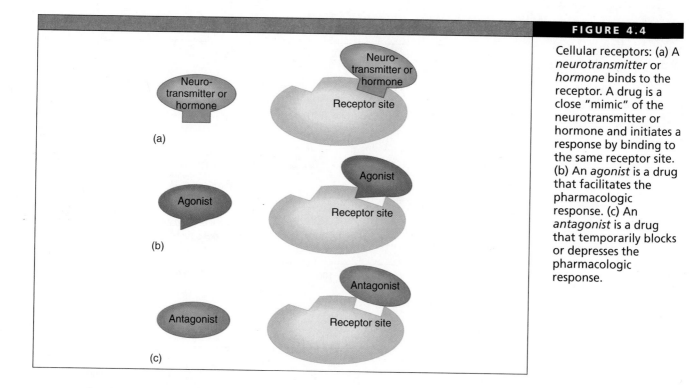

FIGURE 4.4

Cellular receptors: (a) A *neurotransmitter* or *hormone* binds to the receptor. A drug is a close "mimic" of the neurotransmitter or hormone and initiates a response by binding to the same receptor site. (b) An *agonist* is a drug that facilitates the pharmacologic response. (c) An *antagonist* is a drug that temporarily blocks or depresses the pharmacologic response.

tural component of a cell to which a drug binds in a dose-related manner. Receptors can be located on the plasma membrane or in the cytoplasm or nucleus of the cell. The drug or natural body substance attaches to its receptor much like a lock and key (Figure 4.4 ■). Some drug actions are not linked to a receptor but are connected directly with cell function, such as changing the membrane excitability or stability of a nerve or muscle cell.

The terms *agonist* and *antagonist* are often used to describe drug action at the receptor level. **Agonists** are drugs capable of binding with receptors and causing a cellular response; these are *facilitators* of cellular action. When they are present in the bloodstream, agonists cause the tissue to respond, resulting in a therapeutic action. **Antagonists** are drugs that inhibit or block the responses of agonists. Antagonists are called *blockers*.

ant = *against*
agonist = *activator*

Potency and efficacy are terms often used to describe the success of drug therapy.

CORE CONCEPT 4.9

Potency refers to a drug's strength at a certain concentration or dose. As shown in Figure 4.5 ■, *dose-response curves* are used to compare potencies of different drugs. If drug A has a higher potency than drug B, it means that drug A will produce a more intense effect than drug B if both drugs are given at the same dose (Figure 4.5a). A higher potency also means that a much smaller dose of the medication will be needed to produce the same effect as another drug, as shown by the shift to the left of the dose-response curve for drug A in Figure 4.5a.

Another core concept is **efficacy**. Efficacy refers to the ability of a drug to produce a more intense response as its concentration is increased. As an example, consider Figure 4.5b. If the doses of two similarly acting drugs (A and B) are increased, they will both produce a more intense effect, but drug B will have a maximum intensity that is lower than drug A. The drug reaching a lower maximum intensity compared to another drug is said to have a lower efficacy.

efficacy = *effectiveness*

In pharmacotherapeutics, it is generally more important to have a drug with higher efficacy than one with higher potency. For example, at recommended doses ibuprofen (200 mg) and aspirin (650 mg) are equally effective at relieving headache pain; thus, they have the *same efficacy*. The fact that ibuprofen relieves pain at a lower dose indicates that this agent is *more potent* than aspirin. If the patient is experiencing severe pain, however, neither aspirin nor ibuprofen has sufficient efficacy to bring relief. In this instance, morphine has a greater efficacy than aspirin or ibuprofen and can effectively treat this type of pain. In this example, the average dose is unimportant to the patient, but efficacy—the ability of the pain medication to bring essential relief—is crucial.

FIGURE 4.5

Potency and efficacy:
(a) drug A has a higher
potency than drug B;
(b) drug A has a higher
efficacy than drug B.

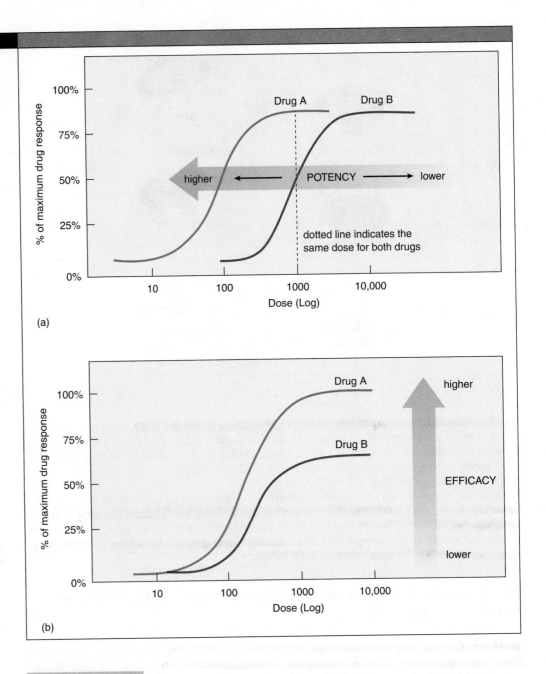

Concept Review 4.3

■ What does the term *pharmacodynamics* mean? Identify the importance of receptors, agonists, and antagonists in influencing drug action. What is the difference between a drug's
potency and its efficacy?

CHAPTER REVIEW

CORE CONCEPTS SUMMARY

4.1 Pharmacokinetics focuses on what the body does to the drugs.

Pharmacokinetics is an area of pharmacology dealing with how drugs move throughout the body. There are four components of drug transport: absorption, distribution, metabolism, and excretion.

4.2 Absorption is the first step in drug transport.

Absorption represents the first step in pharmacokinetics. It involves movement of a drug from its site of administration across body membranes. Drugs cross many membrances before reaching target organs. Drug absorption is affected by many factors.

4.3 Distribution refers to how drugs are transported throughout the body.

Distribution begins after absorption and continues until drug action. Drugs bound to plasma proteins may be isolated in the plasma and prevented from reaching their target cells. The blood-brain barrier, blood-placental barrier, and blood-testicular barrier all represent areas in the body where drug distribution may be limited.

4.4 Metabolism is a process whereby drugs are made less or more active.

Metabolic processes take place in the liver, and to a lesser extent, in organs such as the kidney and cells of the gastrointestinal tract. The first-pass effect is an important phenomenon because many drugs absorbed across intestinal membranes are routed directly to the liver. Metabolic liver enzymes are usually less active in younger and in older patients; therefore, drug effects will most likely be greater in these age groups. Prodrugs are agents converted to a more active form when they are metabolically changed.

4.5 Excretion processes remove drugs from the body.

The kidneys, lungs, sweat glands, mammary glands, and gallbladder are the major structures involved in eliminating drugs from the body. The main organ involved with excretion is the kidney. Enterohepatic recirculation is a unique type of mechanism responsible for recirculating bile back into the bloodstream from the gastrointestinal tract.

4.6 The rate of elimination and half-life characteristics influence drug responsiveness.

The elimination rate of a drug is defined as the amount of drug removed from the body by normal physiologic processes per unit of time. Plasma half-life is the amount of time it takes for the body to remove half of the drug from the general circulation. These factors affect the duration of drug action.

4.7 Pharmacodynamics focuses on what the drugs do to the body.

Pharmacodynamics is an area of pharmacology concerned with how drugs produce responses within the body. Successful drug therapy depends on the effectiveness of these responses.

4.8 Drugs activate specific receptors to produce a response.

Generally, the response of a drug begins when the agent encounters the receptor of its target cell. The receptor theory states that most responses in the body are caused by interactions of drugs with specific receptors. Receptors may be located on the plasma membrane, or they may be found in the cytoplasm or nucleus of the cell.

4.9 *Potency* and *efficacy* are terms often used to describe the success of drug therapy.

Potency relates to the concentration or amount of drug required to produce a maximum response. Efficacy refers to how great the maximal response of a drug will be.

REVIEW QUESTIONS

The following questions are written in NCLEX-PN® style. Answer these questions to assess your knowledge of the chapter material, and go back and review any material that is not clear to you.

1. Patients with liver disorders would most likely have problems with which pharmacokinetic phase?

1. Absorption
2. Distribution
3. Metabolism
4. Excretion

2. The patient asks the nurse why she must take her medication twice a day instead of just once. The nurse's best response would be:

1. "Taking it once a day is fine as long as it is taken at the same time every day."
2. "Taking the medication twice a day ensures that maximum concentrations are maintained within the body."
3. "You will need to speak to your physician about this."
4. "The first dose of the medication is blocked by deactivation and the second dose is metabolized by the body."

3. Which of the following principles is true?

1. For a drug to be effective, it must be potent.
2. For drug efficacy to occur, a lower dose must be administered.
3. Antagonists bind to receptors and produce responses to block agonists.
4. The drug-receptor interaction must occur at its target tissue.

4. Drugs that bind with a receptor to produce a therapeutic response are called:

1. Antagonists
2. Facilitators
3. Agonists
4. Blockers

5. If a patient takes a medication on a full stomach, the nurse is aware that the medication will be:

1. Absorbed more rapidly
2. Absorbed more slowly
3. Neutralized by gastric enzymes
4. Activated by gastric enzymes

6. Which of the following factors does not influence the effectiveness of drug therapy?

1. Temperature
2. Food-drug interactions
3. Route of administration
4. Time of administration within the day

7. An antibiotic has been ordered for the patient with a brain abscess. The nurse understands that:

1. Antibiotics are not effective to treat brain abscesses.
2. Only fat-soluble substances will pass the blood-brain barrier.
3. The half-life of the antibiotic will be decreased.
4. The intestinal tract will prevent absorption from occurring.

8. When orally administered drugs are extensively metabolized by the liver, with only part of the drug dose reaching target organs, this is known as:

1. Half-life
2. Potency
3. First-pass effect
4. Rate of elimination

9. Which of these drugs inhibit cell function by preventing other drugs from binding with receptor sites and blocking cellular response?

1. Agonists
2. Antagonists
3. Facilitators
4. Anesthetics

10. Drug dosing in pediatric and elderly patients is most often decreased due to:

1. Reduced metabolic enzyme activity
2. Enhanced metabolic enzyme activity
3. Decreased metabolic kidney function
4. Increased metabolic kidney function

FURTHER STUDY

■ Pregnant women need to be cautious about the food and medications they take, as discussed in Chapter 2.

■ Drugs that affect the kidney and its filtration processes are discussed in more detail in Chapter 23.

EXPLORE 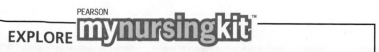 PEARSON **mynursingkit**™

MyNursingKit is your one stop for online chapter review materials and resources. Prepare for success with additional NCLEX®-style practice questions, interactive assignments and activities, web links, animations and videos, and more!

Register your access code from the front of your book at
www.mynursingkit.com

5 Pharmacology and the Nursing Process

CORE CONCEPTS

5.1 The first step of the nursing process is the assessment phase.

5.2 Nursing diagnoses are based on the data gathered in the assessment phase.

5.3 In the planning phase, the nurse creates an individualized plan of care for a patient based on the identified nursing diagnoses and etiologies.

5.4 The implementation phase puts the plan of care into action.

5.5 In the evaluation phase, the nurse obtains data to determine if the goal or outcome has been achieved.

LEARNING OUTCOMES

After reading this chapter, the student should be able to:

1. Compare and contrast the different steps of the nursing process.

2. Describe how the nursing process is used in pharmacology.

3. Identify the purposes of collecting data in the assessment phase of the nursing process.

4. Explain how nursing diagnoses are identified and worded.

5. Describe the steps in the planning phase of the nursing process.

6. Identify specific pharmacology topics employed in the implementation phase of the nursing process.

7. Explain the purpose of the evaluation phase in the nursing process.

8. Explain what actions follow the evaluation phase of the nursing process.

KEY TERMS

assessment *58*

etiologies (e-tee-OL-o-gees) *59*

evaluation criteria *60*

evaluation phase *62*

goal *60*

implementation phase *61*

interventions *59*

nursing diagnosis *59*

nursing process *58*

outcome *60*

planning phase *60*

The **nursing process**, a systematic method of problem solving, forms the foundation of all nursing practice. The use of the nursing process is particularly essential during medication administration. By using the steps of the nursing process, nurses can ensure that the interdisciplinary practice of pharmacology results in safe, effective, and individualized medication administration and outcomes for all patients under their care.

The nursing process is an ongoing activity involving five distinct phases: assessment, diagnosis, planning, implementation, and evaluation. The LPN/LVN contributes to each phase of the process under the direction of the RN. In this chapter, each phase is briefly reviewed, and each phase's use in pharmacology is emphasized. A summary of the phases is shown in Figure 5.1 ■.

CORE CONCEPT 5.1

The first step of the nursing process is the assessment phase.

The **assessment** phase of the nursing process is the systematic collection, organization, validation, and documentation of patient data. The assessment phase serves two purposes. The first is to gather data that will enable the nurse to identify current patient health challenges and problems that the patient is at particular risk for developing. These data are used in developing nursing diagnoses and the plan of care.

The second purpose of the assessment phase is to gather initial *baseline data* on the patient that will be compared to subsequent data during the evaluation phase of the nursing process. These comparisons will indicate to what extent the treatment goals have been achieved. When applying the nursing process to pharmacology, baseline data are necessary for the nurse to be able to evaluate therapeutic drug effects, adverse drug effects, and the capacity for self-care. For example, a common side effect of many antibiotics is the risk for allergic reaction, often identified by a skin rash. To determine whether the rash is due to a particular drug, the nurse must first assess that a rash was not present prior to initiating drug therapy. As another example, if a patient is exhibiting elevated liver enzymes during hospitalization, the nurse will use the baseline assessment data to determine whether the patient had this condition on admission, or whether it is a sign of a recent adverse drug event.

Data collected in the assessment phase can come from many sources. These include the patient, caregivers, medical records, and other health care professionals. *Subjective* data include what the patient says or perceives, such as pain, anxiety, or nausea. Whenever possible, the subjective data are verified by *objective* data that are gathered through physical examination, medical history, laboratory tests, and other diagnostic sources.

FIGURE 5.1

The five overlapping phases of the nursing process. Each phase depends on the accuracy of the other phases. Each phase involves critical thinking.

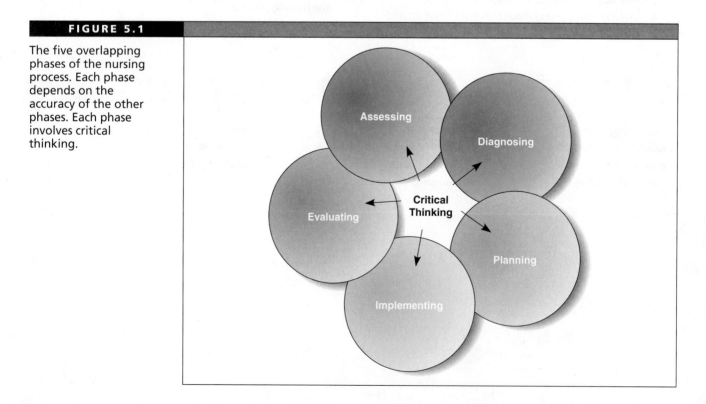

Assessment must always include a comprehensive medical history that includes the patient's use of prescription drugs, OTC agents, dietary supplements, and herbal products. The nurse should inquire about tobacco and alcohol use as well as past or current history of drug abuse because these may influence treatment outcomes. Any allergic or unusual reactions to drugs should be documented, including serious drug events that may have occurred to close family members.

The medical history gathered during the assessment phase is used to determine whether the patient has a contraindication that would present a risk for drug therapy. For example, the nurse may discover during assessment that the patient is pregnant and should not receive isotretinoin (Accutane) for her acne because it is a pregnancy category X drug. The nurse may discover that the patient has a history of allergy to penicillin and, therefore, should not be prescribed ampicillin due to the potential for cross-allergy. A thorough assessment is the best way to prevent adverse drug effects.

Concept Review   5.1

- What types of assessments would be important for patients who will be required to self-administer their medications at home?

Nursing diagnoses are based on the data gathered in the assessment phase.

During the diagnosis phase of the nursing process, the nurse analyzes assessment data, identifies health problems, and formulates diagnostic statements. A **nursing diagnosis** is a clinical judgment of a patient's actual or potential health problem that is within the nurse's scope of practice to address. It is the responsibility of the RN to identify the appropriate diagnosis and develop a plan of care. The LPN/LVN contributes to this phase by collecting data and collaborating with the RN.

dia = *through or complete*
gnosis = *knowledge*

Nursing diagnoses differ from medical diagnoses, which are determined by physicians. Whereas the medical diagnosis remains constant during a patient's hospital stay, nursing diagnoses are in constant flux as the patient responds to treatments. Nursing diagnoses address changes in the patient's condition—for example, alterations in mobility, nutritional intake, urinary elimination, knowledge, ability for self-care, and risk for injury. These nursing diagnoses are used to set goals and plan care.

Nursing diagnoses are often stated as a problem, or the risk for a problem, followed by "related to," which identifies the **etiologies** or those conditions that have caused or contributed to the problem. By altering one or more of these etiologies, nurses are able to effect improvements in the diagnosed problem. This is accomplished by planning and implementing **interventions**, which are actions that the nurse takes to achieve patient goals. The nurse chooses interventions that are patient focused and target the etiologies of the problem. The North American Nursing Diagnosis Association (NANDA) has developed standard wording, known as the nursing diagnosis, for identifying actual and potential patient health problems. For example, a nursing diagnosis may be "*Activity Intolerance* related to acute knee pain." The nurse designs interventions to address the etiology (acute knee pain) that may include the administration of pain medications, heat, or ice packs.

etio = *cause*
ology = *study of*

Nursing diagnoses are prioritized by their level of importance and immediacy to the patient's clinical condition. For example, alterations in breathing would likely take precedence over the potential for skin breakdown. A primary nursing role is to enable patients to become active participants in their own care. Patients need to vocalize, to the extent possible, their priorities for care, which should be considered by the nurse when diagnoses are prioritized. By including patients when identifying needs, the nurse encourages them to take a more active role in working toward meeting the identified goals.

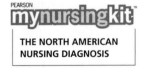

THE NORTH AMERICAN NURSING DIAGNOSIS

When applied to pharmacotherapy, the diagnosis phase of the nursing process addresses three main areas of concern:

- Promoting therapeutic drug effects
- Minimizing adverse drug effects and toxicity
- Maximizing the ability of the patient for self-care, including the knowledge, skills, and resources necessary for safe and effective drug administration

The teaching of patients is one of the basic roles of nursing, and careful attention to drug teaching can promote therapeutic outcomes as well as minimize adverse effects. Examples of nursing diagnoses that intimately involve drug teaching include *Knowledge Deficit* related to new drug therapy and *Noncompliance with Pharmacotherapy* related to side effects. The teaching of patients is discussed further in the planning phase. See Table 5.1 for selected nursing diagnoses for pharmacotherapy. For a complete list, the student should refer to a nursing fundamentals textbook.

In the planning phase the nurse creates an individualized plan of care for a patient based on the identified nursing diagnoses and etiologies.

CORE CONCEPT 5.3

After a nursing diagnosis has been established, the nurse begins to plan ways to assist the patient to return to, or maintain an optimum level of, wellness as defined by that diagnosis. In the **planning phase** of the nursing process, the nurse prioritizes diagnoses, formulates desired goals, and selects nursing interventions.

There are two main steps of the planning phase. The first step is to identify the desired **goal**, or **outcome**, to be achieved, and the specific **evaluation criteria** that will be used to determine if that goal has been met. The outcome may be a short-term or long-term goal, should include the time frame whenever possible, and must be realistic for the patient to achieve. The evaluation criteria should be specific and measurable. These criteria are often indicated by the abbreviation AEB (as evidenced by). The outcome should directly address the problem identified in the nursing diagnosis. For example, if the nursing diagnosis is *Risk for Altered Bowel Elimination* related to opioid analgesic use, a goal might be: the absence of altered bowel elimination, as evidenced by (AEB) regular bowel evacuation, absence of difficulty passing stool, and absence of abdominal bloating or discomfort. Notice how this plan includes a clear goal as well as specific evaluation criteria.

The second step of the planning phase is to develop a list of interventions. The interventions are specific nursing actions designed to help move the patient toward the desired goal.

When planning interventions the nurse should consider the specific health problem and etiologies, current practice guidelines, acceptability to the patient, and the nurse's own capabilities. In addition, the chosen nursing interventions should be safe and appropriate for the patient's age, health, and condition; congruent with the patient's values, beliefs, and culture; and appropriate to the other ordered therapies. The choice of nursing interventions will also depend on what is realistic and practical to the situation in terms of equipment availability, financial status of the patient, and available resources, including staff, agency, family, or community resources.

With respect to pharmacotherapy, the planning phase involves two main issues: drug administration and patient teaching. For the first issue, the nurse must plan how and when to administer the drug. For oral medications, does it need to be given with food or on an empty stomach? Is it more effective if administered at a certain time of day? Can it be crushed or split? For all medications, the nurse will plan interventions to enhance therapeutic outcomes and minimize or prevent adverse drug effects.

TABLE 5.1	Nursing Diagnoses in Pharmacotherapy
Acute Confusion related to drug effects	
Altered Sensory Perception related to drug effects	
Altered Comfort related to drug effects	
Fluid Volume Deficiency related to drug effects	
Fluid Volume Excess related to drug effects	
Noncompliance with Drug Therapy related to lack of knowledge	
Risk for Infection related to adverse drug effects	
Risk for Injury related to drug effects	
Disturbed Sleep Pattern related to drug effects	
Altered Nutrition: Less than body requirements related to drug-induced nausea	
Ineffective Health Maintenance related to knowledge deficit	
Activity Intolerance related to drug effects	
Knowledge Deficiency related to new drug therapy	

TABLE 5.2	Teaching Throughout the Life Span

Patient teaching is an essential component of the nursing process. To be effective, oral and written teaching must be age appropriate. The following are some tips for effective teaching.

CHILDREN

- Use family-centered approaches when providing drug teaching for children and adolescents.
- Engage young children and toddlers by using interactive strategies.
- Use simple, nonthreatening language.
- Provide a developmentally appropriate environment when teaching adolescents.
- Encourage problem solving to help adolescents make choices.

ADULTS

- Adult learners are independent; the nurse should facilitate learning.
- Adults learn best when the topic is of immediate value and when new material is connected to previous experiences.
- Adults vary widely in their learning styles and preferences; learning is enhanced when these things are considered.
- Consider the literacy level of learners; it is recommended that written materials be on a fifth-grade reading level.
- Employ multiple methods of delivering information; a combination of verbal and written material is beneficial.

OLDER ADULTS

- Time needed for learning often increases; plan several short learning sessions; repeat and review material covered.
- Relate new learning to the patient's actual experiences.
- Provide printed material, videotapes, or pictures and diagrams that the patient can refer to at a later time.
- Modify teaching methods to sensory-perceptual deficits or cognitive decline. Ensure that the patient has the necessary aids (glasses, magnifying glass, hearing aid) to maximize the learning experience.
- Offer opportunities for practice of psychomotor skills.

When planning patient drug teaching, the projected length of pharmacotherapy influences the amount and type of teaching provided by the nurse. Is the drug to be given for a short time during an acute care hospitalization, or is pharmacotherapy going to be long term and self-administered following discharge? If a drug is to be given short term, the patient should be told the name of the drug and its basic actions, why the patient is receiving it, and some of the drug's most common and major adverse effects, including any that should be promptly reported to the nurse or health care provider.

For drugs that will be taken after discharge, patient teaching should be more comprehensive and be provided both orally and in writing. This teaching should include the drug name (both generic and trade), the drug class and its major effects, why the drug is being prescribed, the therapeutic effects and when they should occur, how and when to take the drug, the common and major adverse effects and which ones should be reported to the prescriber, the types of follow-up monitoring needed, potential drug interactions, the duration of drug therapy, the activities to avoid while taking the drug, and what to do if a dose is missed or forgotten. Table 5.2 gives tips for effective patient teaching that can be used for patients of all ages.

The implementation phase puts the plan of care into action.

CORE CONCEPT 5.4

The **implementation phase** is when the nurse applies the knowledge, skills, and principles of nursing care to help move the patient toward the desired goal and optimal wellness. Implementation involves *action* on the part of the nurse or patient: administering a drug, providing patient teaching, and initiating other specific actions identified by the nursing diagnoses and plan of care. When applied to pharmacotherapy, the implementation phase involves administering the drug and carrying out the interventions developed in the planning phase to maximize a therapeutic response and prevent adverse events.

It must be remembered that implementation of the plan of care is subject to modification based on the patient's evolving condition. In implementing pharmacotherapy, an important decision that

FIGURE 5.2

Teaching patients about drugs and their effects is an important step in the nursing process.

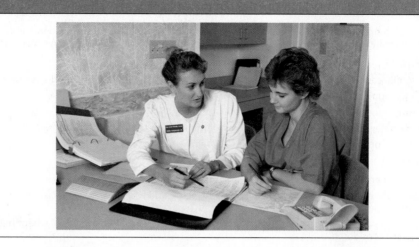

the nurse must make is whether it is appropriate to administer the drug at the planned time. To make this decision, the nurse needs to understand the drug's therapeutic and adverse effects well enough to know the circumstances under which it is appropriate, or not appropriate, to give the drug. After assessing a current vital sign, a laboratory result, a new health problem, or a physical assessment finding, it may be appropriate for the nurse not to administer an ordered drug. For example, if the patient's current serum potassium level is below the normal range, and the nurse has an order to administer furosemide (Lasix), it would be an error for the nurse to administer the drug. Carrying out the order would cause serum potassium to fall, which could trigger cardiac dysrhythmias. Likewise, a patient who has a scheduled dose of morphine for pain relief but currently has a respiratory rate of less than 8 should not receive the drug because it may cause respiratory failure.

As pharmacotherapy progresses, the nurse must be aware of circumstances that might require modification of the implementation phase. The patient may develop new symptoms that contraindicate the use of the drug being administered. For example, the patient may begin to show signs of a developing rash, changes in blood pressure, or alterations in mental status that call for discontinuation of the drug. These examples help illustrate the cyclic nature of the nursing process: the importance of continuous assessment and the revision of the planning and implementation phases.

Implementation also includes providing patient teaching (Figure 5.2 ■). Patient drug teaching should start with what the patient already knows about a drug and build from there. The specific topics to include in this teaching are developed in the planning phase. When preparing to carry out the teaching, other factors that the nurse should consider are the patient's readiness to learn and whether or not it is an appropriate time for teaching. Patients who are in pain, sleepy, anxious, or distracted are less likely to understand instructions. Drug teaching should be tailored to the patient's developmental level, learning capacity, and preferred learning style. Patients may prefer that a family member or caregiver be present for the teaching. This is especially important for pediatric patients, elderly adults with cognitive deficits, and patients with mental illnesses who may be incapable of safe self-administration. Patient teaching is sometimes a collaborative effort, requiring coordination with other medical disciplines as part of the sessions. Often a registered dietician, physical therapist, or diabetes educator collaborates in the patient teaching. When teaching, sufficient time must always be allotted to address any areas of concern for the patient.

Finally, documentation is an essential part of the implementation phase. This includes a thorough reporting of the interventions carried out, the drugs that were given (or withheld), the teaching that took place, and the patient's responses to the interventions.

In the evaluation phase, the nurse obtains data to determine if the goal or outcome has been achieved.

CORE CONCEPT 5.5

The **evaluation phase** compares the patient's current health status with the desired outcome to determine if the plan of care is appropriate or if it needs revision. The evaluation phase is used to determine if the goal or outcome has been met. If it has been met, the plan of care was appropriate, and the problem or risk has been resolved. The next highest priority problem can then be addressed.

If the goal was partially met, the patient is moving toward the goal but the interventions may need to be continued for a longer time or somehow modified to completely resolve the problem.

As it relates to pharmacotherapy, evaluation is used to determine whether the therapeutic effects of the drug have been achieved as well as whether adverse effects have been prevented or kept to acceptable levels. If the evaluation data show no improvement over the baseline data, the interventions may require revision. The drug dose may need to be increased, more time may be needed to achieve therapeutic drug levels, a different or additional drug may be needed, or other changes in nursing interventions may be necessary. The data gathered on the evaluation criteria form part of the assessment data for a continuation of the process as outcomes and interventions are revised or reformulated. These evaluation data need to be documented in the patient's record to ensure proper communication of the patient's response to the nursing interventions.

In an outpatient setting, lack of drug response determined during the evaluation phase may be caused by patient nonadherence to the drug regimen. During the assessment phase, the nurse must determine if the patient is taking the drug as prescribed. If nonadherence is discovered, the nurse must plan and implement strategies for increasing adherence. This always includes addressing the reasons for nonadherence. Additional patient teaching is important to obtaining maximum adherence: The nurse must help the patient to value pharmacotherapy as important to the improvement of the patient's health.

Concept Review 5.2

■ What strategies might the nurse implement to improve adherence to drug therapy for a geriatric patient?

NATURAL THERAPIES

Medication Errors and Dietary Supplements

Herbal and dietary supplements can have powerful effects on the body that can influence the outcomes of prescription drug therapy. In some cases, OTC supplements can enhance the effects of prescription drugs, whereas in other instances supplements may cancel the therapeutic effects of medications. For example, many patients with heart disease take garlic supplements in addition to warfarin (Coumadin) to prevent clots from forming. Because garlic and warfarin are both anticoagulants, taking them together could cause excessive bleeding. As another example, high doses of calcium supplements can cancel the beneficial antihypertensive effects of drugs such as nifedipine (Procardia), a calcium channel blocker.

Life Span Fact

When evaluating the success of chemotherapy in older adults the health care provider should understand that nonadherence may be due to physical limitations. The inability to open childproof containers or to read the instructions on the label are possible causes of nonadherence. Older adults may be depending on caregivers to pick up or administer their medications on a regular basis. In many cases, simply forgetting to take a medication is a cause of lack of drug effect. The health care provider should assist older patients in overcoming these limitations so that pharmacotherapy can be optimized.

CHAPTER REVIEW

CORE CONCEPTS SUMMARY

5.1 The first phase of the nursing process is the assessment phase.

Assessment is the careful, systematic collection of patient data. During this phase, the nurse gathers data in order to identify patient problems and risks for problems.

5.2 Nursing diagnoses are based on the data gathered in the assessment phase.

Nursing diagnoses are clinical judgments on actual or potential patient problems and include the etiologies that are contributing to the health problem. These etiologies are factors that can be addressed by nursing interventions to address the health challenges facing the patient.

5.3 In the planning phase the nurse creates an individualized plan of care for the patient based on the identified nursing diagnoses and etiologies.

The first step of the planning phase is identification of a goal or outcome for the patient, including specified evaluation criteria that will be used to determine the extent to which the goal has been achieved. The second step is the formulation of a list of nursing interventions to be used to help move the patient toward the goal.

5.4 **The implementation phase puts the plan of care into action.**

When applied to pharmacology, the implementation phase involves administering the drug, providing patient drug teaching, and documentation.

5.5 **In the evaluation phase, the nurse obtains data to determine if the goal or outcome has been achieved.**

By comparing the evaluation data to baseline data, the nurse is able to determine if the goal was met, partially met, or unmet. Evaluation data are used to revise goals, plans, or interventions.

REVIEW QUESTIONS

The following questions are written in NCLEX-PN® style. Answer these questions to assess your knowledge of the chapter material, and go back and review any material that is not clear to you.

1. The nurse reviews a patient record for drug allergies, current medications, and disease states that could affect drug responses. These actions are part of which phase of the nursing process?

1. Assessment
2. Planning
3. Implementation
4. Evaluation

2. The implementation phase of the nursing process involves two main activities related to pharmacology. These are:

1. Developing and performing nursing interventions
2. Providing and evaluating patient teaching
3. Administering drugs and providing patient drug teaching
4. Assessing and evaluating adverse drug effects

3. Which of the following would be most important for the nurse to evaluate in the evaluation phase of the nursing process?

1. Patient satisfaction with drug therapy
2. Evidence of therapeutic drug effects
3. Development of minor adverse drug effects
4. The possibility of noncompliance with drug therapy

4. Which of the following is appropriate information to gather in the assessment phase of the nursing process? (Select all that apply.)

1. Drug allergies
2. Therapeutic response to the drug
3. History of renal or hepatic disease
4. Baseline physical assessment data

5. Which of the following is a properly worded nursing diagnosis?

1. Skin breakdown related to diabetes
2. Risk for injury and knowledge deficit related to new medication therapy
3. Pneumonia related to retained secretions
4. Fatigue related to sleep deprivation and physical deconditioning

6. The second phase of the nursing process involves analyzing data and identifying health problems such as *Activity Intolerance* related to pain. This phase is known as:

1. Assessment
2. Implementation
3. Nursing diagnosis
4. Planning

7. The nursing process, as it relates to pharmacology, can be best be described as:

1. A way of determining whether a patient should use a cane or crutches when walking
2. A method of documentation that nurses use in their daily practice
3. A problem-solving method that encourages nurses to rely solely on their textbook knowledge of a patient's condition before determining a course of action
4. A systematic approach to problem solving that ensures the safe and effective administration of medication

8. The role of the LPN/LVN is to:

1. Work independently of the RN and other health care providers when establishing a plan of care for a patient
2. Assist the physician in establishing a patient's plan of care
3. Contribute to each phase of the process under the direction of the RN
4. Rely completely on the RN to utilize the nursing process when caring for patients

6 Herbs and Dietary Supplements

CORE CONCEPTS

6.1 Complementary and alternative therapies are used by a large number of people to prevent and treat disease.

6.2 Natural products from plants have been used as medicines for thousands of years.

6.3 Herbal products are standardized with respect to a specific active ingredient.

6.4 Herbs can have significant pharmacologic actions and can interact with conventional drugs, which may result in adverse effects.

6.5 Specialty supplements are nonherbal products that are widely used to promote wellness.

6.6 Dietary supplements are regulated by the Dietary Supplement Health and Education Act of 1994.

LEARNING OUTCOMES

After reading this chapter, the student should be able to:

1. Explain the role of complementary and alternative medicine in promoting patient wellness.

2. Discuss the reasons why herbal products and dietary supplements have increased in popularity in recent years.

3. Identify the parts of an herb that may contain active ingredients and the types of formulations made from these parts.

4. Describe the strengths and weaknesses of the Dietary Supplement Health and Education Act (DSHEA) of 1994.

5. Describe drug interactions and adverse effects that may be caused by herbal and dietary supplements.

6. Explain how herbal products are sometimes standardized based on specific active ingredients.

7. Discuss the role of the health professional in teaching patients about complementary and alternative therapies.

KEY TERMS

botanicals (boh-TAN-ik-uls) *67*

complementary and alternative medicine (CAM) *66*

dietary supplements *67*

Dietary Supplement and Nonprescription Drug Consumer Protection Act *73*

Dietary Supplement Health and Education Act (DSHEA) of 1994 *72*

herbs *67*

specialty supplements *67*

Herbal and dietary supplements represent a multibillion dollar industry. Sales of these alternative therapies exceed $50 billion annually, with over 158 million consumers using them. Consumers have turned to these treatments for a wide variety of reasons. Many people have the impression that natural substances have more healing power than synthetic medications. The ready availability of OTC herbal supplements at a reasonable cost, combined with effective marketing strategies, has convinced many to try them. This chapter examines the role of herbal and dietary supplements in the prevention and treatment of disease.

CORE CONCEPT 6.1

Complementary and alternative therapies are used by a large number of people to prevent and treat disease.

Complementary and alternative medicine (CAM) comprises an extremely diverse set of therapies and healing systems that are considered to be outside of mainstream health care. CAM systems have the following common characteristics:

- Focus on treating each *individual* person
- Consider the health of the *whole* person
- Emphasize the *integration of mind and body*
- Promote disease *prevention, self-care,* and *self-healing*
- Recognize the role of *spirituality* in health and healing

Because of its popularity, many have focused considerable attention on determining the effectiveness or lack of effectiveness of CAM. Although research into these alternative systems is currently underway, few CAM therapies have been subjected to rigorous clinical and scientific study. It is likely that some of these therapies will become mainstream treatments, whereas others will be found ineffective. The line between what is defined as an alternative therapy and what is considered mainstream is constantly changing. Increasing numbers of practitioners are now accepting CAM therapies and recommending them to their patients. Table 6.1 describes some of these therapies.

Health professionals have long known the value of CAM therapies in preventing and treating disease. For example, prayer, meditation, massage, and yoga have been used for centuries to

TABLE 6.1	Complementary and Alternative Therapies
HEALING METHOD	**EXAMPLES**
Biologic therapies	Herbal therapies Nutritional supplements Special diets
Alternate health care systems	Naturopathy Homeopathy Chiropractic Native American medicine (e.g., sweat lodges, medicine wheel) Chinese traditional medicine (e.g., acupuncture, Chinese herbs)
Manual healing	Massage Pressure-point therapies
Mind-body interventions	Yoga Meditation Hypnotherapy Guided imagery Biofeedback Movement-oriented therapies (e.g., music, dance)
Spiritual	Shamans Faith and prayer

Fast Facts Alternative Therapies in America

Possibly the largest nonscientific study of attitudes toward alternative therapies surveyed 45,000 people and was reported in *Consumer's Reports,* May 2000. Findings of this study include the following:

- Of those surveyed, 55% did not use alternative therapies, primarily because they were satisfied with standard medical treatments.
- Of those surveyed, 35% used alternative therapies to relieve symptoms that were not successfully treated with conventional therapies.
- The people most likely to try alternatives were those in severe pain or under stress.
- For almost all medical conditions, respondents stated that prescription drugs were more effective than herbal therapies.
- For back pain and fibromyalgia, deep muscle massage was rated more effective than prescription drugs.
- Of those who tried alternatives, 25% did so at the recommendation of a doctor or nurse. Only 5% of doctors disapproved of alternative therapies.

treat both body and mind. From a therapeutic perspective, much of the value of CAM therapies is their ability to reduce the need for medications. If a patient can find anxiety relief through massage or biofeedback therapy, for example, the use of anxiolytic drugs may be reduced or eliminated. Reduction of drug dose leads to fewer adverse effects and better compliance with drug therapy. Two of the CAM therapies are covered in detail here: **herbs** and **specialty supplements** (including vitamins and minerals), and their use as **dietary supplements.**

Concept Review 6.1

- How does the healing philosophy of complementary and alternative medicine differ from that of conventional mainstream medicine?

HERBAL PRODUCTS

In the past two decades, the number of people seeking herbal alternatives to conventional medical therapies has greatly increased. Many herbs are extensively used by patients as supplements to traditional pharmacotherapy.

Natural products from plants have been used as medicines for thousands of years.

CORE CONCEPT 6.2

Technically, an herb is a plant that lacks woody stems or bark. Over time, the terms *botanical* and *herb* have come to be used interchangeably to refer to any plant product with a useful application, either as a food enhancer (such as a flavoring) or as a medicine.

The use of **botanicals** in the treatment of disease has been recorded for thousands of years. One of the earliest recorded uses of plant products was a prescription for garlic in 3000 B.C. Eastern and Western medicine have recorded thousands of herbs and herb combinations claimed to have therapeutic value. Some of the most popular herbs and their primary uses are shown in Table 6.2.

The public's interest in herbal medicine began to decline when the pharmaceutical industry was born in the late 1800s. Drugs could be standardized and produced more cheaply than natural herbal products. In the early 1900s, regulatory agencies required that medicines be safe and effective. The focus of health care shifted to treating specific diseases, rather than promoting wellness and holistic care. Information about most herbal and alternative therapies was no longer taught in medical schools; these healing techniques were criticized as being unscientific relics of the past.

Beginning in the 1970s and continuing to the present day, herbal medicine has experienced a remarkable comeback. The majority of adult Americans are either currently taking herbal products on a regular basis or have taken them in the past. This increase in popularity has been due to a number of factors, including increased availability of herbal products, aggressive marketing by

TABLE 6.2		Popular Medicinal Herbs
COMMON NAME	**MEDICINAL PART**	**PRIMARY USE(S)**
Aloe	Juice from the leaves	Treat skin ailments (topical), constipation (oral)
Bilberry	Berries/leaf	Terminate diarrhea, improve and protect vision
Black cohosh	Roots	Relieve menopause symptoms
Cranberry	Berries/juice	Prevent urinary tract infection
Echinacea	Entire plant	Enhance immune system, as an anti-inflammatory
Evening primrose	Seeds/oil	Relieve pain and inflammation
Garlic	Bulbs	Reduce blood cholesterol and blood pressure, as an anticoagulant
Ginger	Root	Relieve GI upset and motion sickness, as an anti-inflammatory
Ginkgo biloba	Leaves and seeds	Improve memory, reduce dizziness
Ginseng	Root	Relieve stress, enhance immune system, decrease fatigue
Horny goat weed	Leaves and roots	Enhance sexual function
Milk thistle	Seeds	As an antitoxin, protect against liver disease
Saw palmetto	Ripe fruit/berries	Relieve urinary problems related to prostate enlargement
Soy	Beans	Source of protein, vitamins, and minerals; relieve menopausal symptoms; prevent cardiovascular disease; as an anticancer agent
St. John's wort	Flowers, leaves, stems	Reduce depression, reduce anxiety, as an anti-inflammatory
Valerian	Roots	Relieve stress, promote sleep

▶ **Life Span Fact**

Dietary supplements such as herbs and other specialty products have the ability to positively influence the health of older patients. Nutritional deficiencies greatly increase with age, and supplements help to prevent or eliminate these deficiencies in seniors. The health care provider should assess the need for such supplements in all elderly patients. Herbal remedies and specialty supplements have been successfully used to enhance the immune systems of older patients, reduce short-term memory loss, and improve overall health.

the herbal industry, increased attention to natural alternatives, and renewed interest in preventive medicine. The gradual aging of the population has led to more patients seeking therapeutic alternatives for chronic conditions such as pain, arthritis, prostate difficulties, and the need for hormone replacement. In addition, the high cost of prescription medicines has driven many people to seek less expensive alternatives.

CORE CONCEPT 6.3

Herbal products are standardized with respect to a specific active ingredient.

The active ingredients in an herbal product may be present in only one specific part of the plant or in all parts. For example, the active chemicals in chamomile are in the aboveground portion, such as the leaves, stems, berries, or flowers. For other herbs, such as ginger, the underground rhizomes and roots are used for their healing properties. When collecting or purchasing herbs for home use, it is important to know which portion of the plant contains the active chemicals.

Most modern drugs contain only one active ingredient. This chemical is standardized, accurately measured, and delivered to the patient in precise amounts. It is a common misconception that herbs also contain one active ingredient, which can be extracted and delivered to patients in exact amounts, like drugs. Each herb, however, may contain dozens of active chemicals, many of which have not yet been isolated, studied, or even identified. It is possible that some of these substances work together and may not have the same activity if isolated. Furthermore, the strength of an herbal preparation may vary depending on where the herb was grown and how it was collected, prepared, and stored.

Recent attempts have been made to standardize herbal products, using such measurements as the percent of flavones in ginkgo or the percent of lactones in kava kava. Some of these standardizations are shown in Table 6.3. Until science can better characterize these substances, however, it is best to view the active ingredient of an herb as being the entire herb. An example of lack of standardization—the ingredients of ginkgo biloba—is shown in Figure 6.1 ■.

The two basic formulations of herbal products are solid and liquid. Solid products include pills, tablets, and capsules made from dried herbs. Other solid products are salves and ointments that are administered topically. Liquid formulations are made by extracting the active chemicals from the plant using solvents such as water, alcohol, or glycerol. The liquids are then

TABLE 6.3	Standardization of Selected Herb Extracts	
HERB	**STANDARDIZATION**	**PERCENT**
Black cohosh	Triterpene glycosides	2.5
Echinacea	Phenolics	4
Ginger	Pungent compounds	>10
Ginkgo	Flavonglycosides	24–25
	Lactones	5
Ginseng root	Ginseosides	20–30
Kava kava	Kavalactones	40–45
St. John's wort	Hypericins	0.3–0.5
	Hyperforin	3–5
Saw palmetto fruit	Total fatty acids	80–90

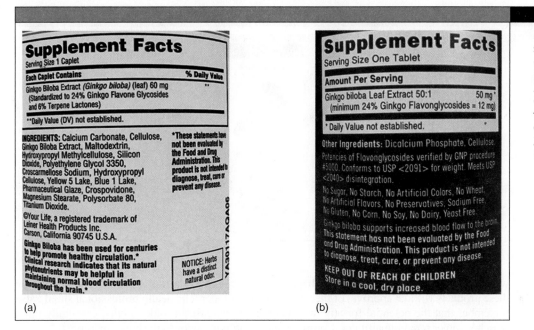

(a)   (b)

FIGURE 6.1

Note the lack of standardization of two ginkgo biloba labels: (a) 60 mg of extract, 24% Ginkgo Flavone Glycosides, and 6% terpenes; and (b) 50:1 Ginkgo Leaf Extract, 24% Ginkgo Flavonglycosides.

concentrated in various strengths. Liquid formulations of herbal preparations are described in Table 6.4. Some formulations of ginkgo biloba, one of the most popular herbals, are illustrated in Figure 6.2 ■.

Herbs can have significant pharmacologic actions and can interact with conventional drugs, which may result in adverse effects.

CORE CONCEPT 6.4

A key concept to remember when dealing with alternative therapies is that natural does not always mean better or safe. There is no question that some botanicals contain active chemicals as powerful as and perhaps more effective than currently approved medications. Thousands of years of experience, combined with current scientific research, have shown that some of these herbal remedies have therapeutic actions. Because a substance comes from a natural product, however, does not make it either safe or effective. For example, poison ivy is natural, but it certainly is not safe or therapeutic. Natural products may not offer an improvement over conventional therapy in treating certain disorders and, indeed, may be of no value whatsoever. Most importantly, a patient who substitutes an unproven alternative therapy for an established, effective medical treatment may delay healing, suffer harmful effects, and endanger his or her health.

Some herbal products contain ingredients that may interact with prescription drugs. For example, patients taking medications with potentially serious adverse effects, such as insulin, warfarin (Coumadin), or digoxin (Lanoxin), should be warned never to take any dietary supplement

TABLE 6.4	Liquid Formulations of Herbal Products
PRODUCT	**DESCRIPTION**
Tea	Fresh or dried herbs are soaked in hot water for 5–10 minutes before ingestion; convenient.
Infusion	Fresh or dried herbs are soaked in hot water for long periods, at least 15 minutes; stronger than teas.
Decoction	Fresh or dried herbs are boiled in water for 30–50 minutes until much of the liquid has boiled off; very concentrated.
Tincture	Active ingredients are extracted by soaking the herb in alcohol; alcohol remains as part of the liquid.
Extract	Active ingredients are extracted using organic solvents to form a highly concentrated liquid or solid form; solvent may be removed or be part of the final product.

FIGURE 6.2

Three different ginkgo formulations: tablets, tea bags, and liquid extract.

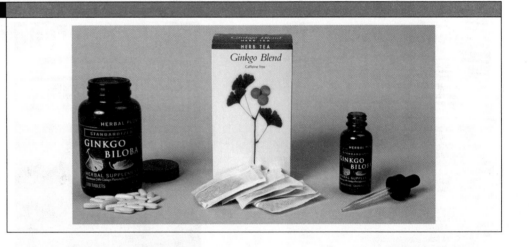

PEARSON mynursingkit

MEDLINE FOR HERBAL PRODUCTS

without first discussing their needs with a physician. Pregnant or lactating women should not take these products without approval of their health care provider. The health professional should also remember that the potential for any drug interaction increases in older adults, especially those with hepatic or renal impairment. Common herb-drug interactions are shown in Table 6.5.

Another warning that must be heeded with natural products is to beware of allergic reactions. Most herbal products contain a mixture of ingredients, and it is not unusual to find dozens of different chemicals in teas and infusions made from the flowers, leaves, or roots of a plant. Patients who have known allergies to certain foods or medicines should seek medical advice before taking an herbal product. It is always wise to take the smallest amount possible—less than the recommended dose—when starting herbal therapy to see if allergies or other adverse effects occur.

Health care providers have an obligation to seek the latest medical information on herbal products, because there is a good possibility that their patients are using them to supplement traditional medicines. Patients should be advised to be skeptical of claims on the labels of dietary supplements and to seek their health information from reputable sources. Health professionals must never condemn patients' use of alternative therapies, but instead be supportive and seek to understand their goals for taking the supplements. The health care provider will often need to educate patients on the role of alternative therapies in the treatment of their disorders and discuss which treatments or combination of treatments will best meet their health goals.

SPECIALTY SUPPLEMENTS

Specialty supplements are *nonherbal* dietary supplements that can come from plant and animal sources. Like herbal therapies, they are widely used to enhance wellness.

TABLE 6.5 — Common Herb-Drug Interactions

COMMON NAME	INTERACTS WITH	COMMENTS
Echinacea	Amiodarone, anabolic steroids, ketoconazole, methotrexate	Possible increased hepatotoxicity
Garlic	Aspirin and other NSAIDs, warfarin (Coumadin)	Increased bleeding risk
	Insulin, oral hypoglycemic agents	Additive hypoglycemic effects
Ginger	Aspirin and other NSAIDs, heparin, warfarin	Increased bleeding risk
Ginkgo biloba	Anticonvulsants	Possible decreased anticonvulsant effectiveness
	Aspirin and NSAIDs	Increased bleeding potential
	Heparin and warfarin	Increased bleeding potential
	Tricyclic antidepressants	Possible decreased seizure threshold
Ginseng	CNS depressants	Increased sedation
	Digoxin (Lanoxin)	Increased toxicity
	Diuretics	Possible weakened diuretic effects
	Insulin and oral hypoglycemic agents	Increased hypoglycemic effects
	Warfarin	Decreased anticoagulant effects
St. John's wort	CNS depressants and opiates	Increased sedation
	Cyclosporine (Sandimmune)	Possible decreased cyclosporine levels
	Oral contraceptives	Decreased drug effectiveness
	Selective serotonin reuptake inhibitors (SSRIs), tricyclic antidepressants	Possible serotonin syndrome (headache, dizziness, sweating, agitation)
	Warfarin (Coumadin)	Decreased anticoagulant effects
Valerian	Barbiturates, benzodiazepines, and other CNS depressants	Increased sedation

Specialty supplements are nonherbal products that are widely used to promote wellness.

CORE CONCEPT 6.5

Specialty supplements are used to enhance a wide variety of body functions. Their actions are more specific than those of herbal products, and they are generally targeted for one or a small number of conditions. The most popular specialty supplements are listed in Table 6.6.

In general, the reasons for using specialty supplements is rational. For example, chondroitin and glucosamine are natural substances in the body necessary for cartilage growth and maintenance.

TABLE 6.6 — Popular Specialty Supplements

NAME	COMMON USES
Amino acids	Build protein, muscle strength, and endurance
Carnitine	Enhance energy and sports performance, heart health, memory, immune function, and male fertility
Coenzyme Q10	Treat heart disease, as an antioxidant
Dehydroepiandrosterone (DHEA)	Boost immune functions and memory
Fish oil	Reduce cholesterol, enhance brain function, increase visual acuity (due to presence of omega-3 fatty acids)
Flaxseed oil	Reduce cholesterol, enhance brain function, increase visual acuity (due to presence of omega-3 fatty acids)
Glucosamine and chondroitin	Treat arthritis and other joint problems
Lactobacillus acidophilus	Maintain intestinal health
Methyl sulfonyl methane (MSM)	Reduce allergic reactions to pollen and foods, relieve pain and inflammation of arthritis and similar conditions
Selenium	Reduce the risk of certain types of cancer

Amino acids are natural building blocks of muscle protein. Flaxseed and fish oils contain omega fatty acids that have been shown to reduce the risk of heart disease in certain patients.

Unfortunately, the link between most specialty supplements and their benefits is unclear. In some cases, the body already has sufficient quantities of the substance; therefore, taking additional amounts may be of no benefit. In other cases, the supplement is marketed for conditions for which it has no proven effect. The good news is that these substances are generally not harmful unless taken in large amounts. The bad news, however, is that they can give patients false hopes of an easy cure for a chronic condition such as heart disease or the pain of arthritis. As with herbal products, the health professional should advise patients to be skeptical about the health claims regarding the use of these supplements.

PEARSON
mynursingkit™

COMPLEMENTARY
MEDICINES AND
ALTERNATIVE THERAPIES

Concept Review 6.2

■ Explain the difference between an herb and a specialty dietary supplement.

CORE CONCEPT 6.6

Dietary supplements are regulated by the Dietary Supplement Health and Education Act of 1994.

Since the passage of the Food, Drug, and Cosmetic Act of 1935, Americans have come to expect that all prescription and OTC drugs have passed rigid standards of safety prior to being marketed. Furthermore, it is assumed that the effectiveness of these drugs has been tested, and that they truly provide the therapeutic benefits claimed by the manufacturer. Indeed, most people would be outraged if they found out that the drug they purchased for pain relief or to cure an infectious disease was totally ineffective. Unfortunately, dietary supplements are regulated by a far less restrictive law, the **Dietary Supplement Health and Education Act (DSHEA) of 1994,** than are drugs. Therefore, Americans must be cautious.

According to the DSHEA, "dietary supplements" are exempted from the Food, Drug, and Cosmetic Act and are defined as products intended to enhance or supplement the diet. They are not approved as drugs by the FDA. The DSHEA also requires these products to be clearly labeled as dietary supplements. Figure 6.3 ■ shows the labels for the herbal supplement black cohosh.

One strength of the DSHEA is that it gives the FDA the power to remove from the market any product that poses a "significant or unreasonable" risk to the public. The FDA used this legislative guideline for the first time in 2004, when the dietary supplement ephedra was removed from the market because of reported serious side effects in some patients. It took 7 years from the time the FDA first warned consumers of the dangers of ephedra (1997) until it was removed in 2004.

FIGURE 6.3

Labeling of black cohosh: (a) front label with general health claim; and (b) back label with more health claims and FDA disclaimer.

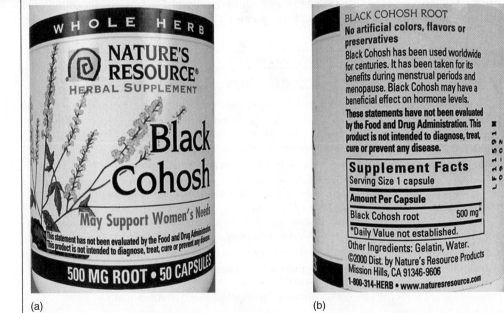

(a)   (b)

Unfortunately, the DSHEA has significant weaknesses that allow a lack of standardization in the dietary supplement industry and lowered protection of the consumer. The following list describes these weaknesses:

- Dietary supplements do not have to be *tested* prior to marketing.
- The *effectiveness* of a dietary supplement does not have to be demonstrated by the manufacturer.
- The manufacturer does not have to prove the *safety* of the dietary supplement. It is the government's job to prove that the dietary supplement is *unsafe* and to take the necessary steps to remove it from the market.
- The label of a dietary supplement is not permitted to state that the product is intended to diagnose, treat, cure, or prevent any disease. However, claims about a product's effect on body structure and function are allowed, including the following:
  - Helps promote healthy immune systems
  - Reduces anxiety and stress
  - Helps to maintain cardiovascular function
  - May reduce pain and inflammation
- The DSHEA does not regulate the *accuracy* of the label; the product may or may not contain the product listed in the amounts claimed.

Several steps have been taken to address the lack of purity and mislabeling of herbal and dietary supplements. In an attempt to protect consumers, Congress passed the **Dietary Supplement and Nonprescription Drug Consumer Protection Act,** which took effect in 2007. Companies marketing herbal and dietary supplements are now required to include contact information (address and phone number) on the product labels for consumers to use in reporting adverse events. Companies must notify the FDA of any serious adverse event reports within 15 days of receiving such reports.

Also in 2007, the FDA announced a final rule that requires the manufacturers of dietary supplements to evaluate the identity, purity, potency, and composition of their products. The labels must accurately reflect what is in the product, which must be free of contaminants such as pesticides, toxins, glass, or heavy metals.

Concept Review 6.3

- How does the federal regulation of an herb by the DSHEA differ from the federal regulation of a prescription drug?

CHAPTER REVIEW

CORE CONCEPTS SUMMARY

6.1 Complementary and alternative therapies are used by a large number of people to prevent and treat disease.

Complementary and alternative medicine (CAM) is a set of different therapies and healing systems used by many patients for disease prevention and self-healing. Complementary therapies offer nonpharmacologic alternatives to promote health and healing. They focus on the holistic treatment of each patient, integrate mind and body, and are often used in conjunction with conventional medical therapies.

6.2 Natural products from plants have been used as medicines for thousands of years.

Thousands of herbal therapies are recorded in Eastern and Western history. The popularity of alternative herbal remedies has increased in recent years.

6.3 Herbal products are standardized with respect to a specific active ingredient.

Herbal products are marketed in a number of different formulations, some consisting of standardized extracts of specific chemicals, others containing whole herbs. Unlike drugs, herbs contain a large number of chemicals that may act in a coordinated manner, or *synergistically,* to produce a therapeutic effect. The active ingredients may be in the flowers, leaves, stems, or roots of an herb. Formulations include tablets, capsules, teas, or extracts.

6.4 Herbs can have significant pharmacologic actions and can interact with conventional drugs, which may result in adverse effects.

Just because a substance comes from a natural product does not make it safe or effective. Although botanicals may have therapeutic applications, they may not be the best product for treating the disease and may interact with prescription medicines.

6.5 Specialty supplements are nonherbal products that are widely used to promote wellness.

Specialty supplements include nonherbal therapies that are used to promote a specific aspect of well-

ness. These products usually have a rational basis for therapy, although their benefits have not always been proven.

6.6 Dietary supplements are regulated by the Dietary Supplement Health and Education Act of 1994.

The DSHEA loosely regulates herbal and dietary supplements. Dietary supplements and herbal products can be marketed without any proof that they are safe or effective. They do not have to be tested prior to marketing. The labels list ingredients but may contain statements that are inaccurate or unproven.

REVIEW QUESTIONS

The following questions are written in NCLEX-PN® style. Answer these questions to assess your knowledge of the chapter material, and go back and review any material that is not clear to you.

1. The patient is to be started on warfarin (Coumadin) therapy. It is important for the nurse to assess for the use of which herbs? (Select all that apply.)

1. Ginseng
2. Ginger
3. St. John's wort
4. Valerian

2. Patients often use herbal therapies for which of the following reasons?

1. To prevent overuse of prescription medications
2. To increase feelings of wellness and promote holistic treatment
3. Because herbal therapies are much more regulated than prescription drugs
4. Because herbal therapies are so much safer than man-made drugs

3. It is important that patients receive education regarding herbal products because:

1. Herbal products are approved under strict FDA regulations.
2. Labeling is not always reliable and herbal products should be used with caution.
3. There are so few side effects, and they can be purchased without a prescription.
4. The manufacturer has repeatedly demonstrated effectiveness.

4. An example of a specialty supplement is:

1. *Lactobacillus acidophilus*
2. Ginseng
3. Garlic
4. Ginkgo biloba

5. It is important for the nurse to assess for the use of complementary and alternative medicine (CAM) because:

1. Patients must be warned that most CAM therapies are dangerous.
2. Additional treatment may not be needed.
3. CAM therapies could interact with prescription and OTC medications.
4. Most CAM therapies are totally ineffective.

6. The nurse understands that specialty supplements are used:

1. For a diverse range of disease conditions
2. For treatment of a targeted condition
3. When prescriptive medications are no longer effective
4. When the body no longer makes sufficient quantities of the substance

7. The Dietary Supplement Health and Education Act (DHSEA) is responsible for:

1. Strict herbal product testing
2. Ensuring that herbal products are labeled as "dietary supplements"
3. Sending the herbal product to the FDA for evaluation
4. Ensuring safety of the product

8. The patient is admitted with digoxin (Lanoxin) toxicity. The nurse assesses for which of the following herbal products?

1. St. John's wort
2. Valerian
3. Fish oil
4. Ginseng

9. The patient requests information on alternative treatments for her arthritis. The nurse identifies which of the following supplements?

1. Garlic and soy
2. Fish oil
3. Chondroitin and glucosamine
4. DHEA

10. Which of the following herbal products is commonly used to enhance the immune system?

1. Soy
2. Saw palmetto
3. Cranberry
4. Echinacea

PEARSON
EXPLORE mynursingkit™

MyNursingKit is your one stop for online chapter review materials and resources. Prepare for success with additional NCLEX®-style practice questions, interactive assignments and activities, web links, animations and videos, and more!

Register your access code from the front of your book at
www.mynursingkit.com

7 Substance Abuse

CORE CONCEPTS

7.1 Abused substances belong to many different chemical classes.

7.2 Addiction depends on multiple, complex, and interacting variables.

7.3 Substance dependence is classified as physical dependence or psychological dependence.

7.4 Withdrawal results when an abused substance is no longer available.

7.5 Tolerance occurs when higher and higher doses of a drug are needed to achieve the initial response.

7.6 Central nervous system (CNS) depressants decrease the activity of the central nervous system.

7.7 Marijuana produces little physical dependence or tolerance.

7.8 Hallucinogens cause an altered state of thought and perception similar to that found in dreams.

7.9 CNS stimulants increase the activity of the central nervous system.

7.10 Nicotine is powerful and highly addictive.

7.11 Health care providers strive to remain free of impairment due to alcohol and drug addiction.

LEARNING OUTCOMES

After reading this chapter, the student should be able to:

1. Discuss the underlying causes of addiction.
2. Compare and contrast psychological and physical dependence.
3. Compare and contrast classic and conditioned withdrawal.
4. Explain the significance of drug tolerance to pharmacotherapy.
5. Explain the major characteristics of abuse, dependence, and tolerance resulting from the following substances:
   a. Alcohol
   b. Nicotine
   c. Marijuana
   d. Hallucinogens
   e. CNS stimulants
   f. Sedatives
   g. Opioids
6. List reasons why health care providers may have problems with alcohol or substance abuse.
7. Identify signs of substance abuse exhibited by the health care provider.

KEY TERMS

addiction (ah-DIK-shun) 78
alcohol intoxication (AL-ku-hol in-tak-su-KA-shun) 82
attention deficit disorder (ADD) 85
cross-tolerance (krause TOL-er-ans) 80
designer drugs (de-ZEYE-ner drugs) 77

narcolepsy (NAR-koh-lep-see) 85
opioids (OH-pee-oyd) 77
physical dependence (FI-zi-kul dee-PEN-dens) 79
psychedelics (seye-keh-DEL-iks) 83
psychological dependence (seye-koh-LOJ-i-kul dee-PEN-dens) 79

tetrahydrocannabinol (THC) (TEH-trah-HEYE-droh-cah-NAB-in-ol) 83
tolerance (TOL-er-ans) 80
withdrawal syndrome (with-DRAW-ul SIN-drom) 79

*S*ubstance abuse is the self-administration of a drug in a way that one's culture or society views as abnormal and not acceptable. Throughout history, individuals have consumed both natural and prescription drugs to increase physical or mental performance, cause a relaxed feeling, change a psychological state, or simply fit in with the crowd. Substance abuse has a tremendous economic, social, and public health impact on society.

Abused substances belong to many different chemical classes.

CORE CONCEPT 7.1

Substances from a wide variety of chemical classes are abused and can be taken by many different routes. Abused substances have in common an ability to affect the nervous system, particularly the brain. Some agents, such as opium, marijuana, cocaine, nicotine, caffeine, and alcohol, are obtained from natural sources. Others agents are synthetic or **designer drugs** that are created in illegal laboratories solely for making money in illegal drug trafficking.

Although the public often connects substance abuse with illegal drugs, this is not necessarily the case: Alcohol and nicotine are the two most commonly abused drugs. Legal prescription medications such as methylphenidate (Ritalin) and meperidine (Demerol) are sometimes abused. Volatile inhalants, found in common household products such as aerosols and paint thinners, are often abused as with "huffing." Frequently abused illegal substances include marijuana, **opioids** (which are *narcotic analgesics*), sedatives, and hallucinogens such as lysergic acid diethylamide (LSD) and methamphetamines. Phencyclidine (PCP), although once used more widely, is less prevalent in today's culture.

Several drugs once used therapeutically are now illegal because of their high potential for abuse. Cocaine was once widely used as a local anesthetic, but today nearly all cocaine use and purchase is illegal. LSD is now illegal, although in the 1940s and 1950s it was used in psychotherapy. Phencyclidine was popular in the early 1960s as an anesthetic but was taken off the market in 1965 because patients reported hallucinations, delusions, and anxiety after recovering from anesthesia. Many of

Fast Facts   Substance Abuse in the United States

- Twenty-eight million Americans have used illicit drugs at least once.
- Twenty-five percent of high school students use an illegal drug monthly.
- An estimated 2.4 million Americans have used heroin during their lives.
- About one in five Americans has lived with an alcoholic while growing up. Children of alcoholic parents are four times more likely to become alcoholics than children of nonalcoholic parents.
- Alcohol is an important factor in 68% of manslaughters, 54% of murders, 48% of robberies, and 44% of burglaries.
- Among youth between the ages of 12 and 17, approximately 7.2 million have drunk alcohol at least are. Girls are as likely as boys to drink alcohol.
- Barbiturate overdose is a factor in almost one third of all drug-related deaths.
- Thirty-six percent of 10th graders and 46% of 12th graders have reported using marijuana and hashish.
- Almost 8% of high school seniors have reported using cocaine.
- Two million Americans have used cocaine on a monthly basis; about 567,000 have used crack cocaine.
- Approximately 70% of the cocaine entering the United States comes from Colombia and passes through south Florida.
- Sixteen percent of 8th graders and 11% of 12th graders have reported using volatile inhalants.
- Thirty percent of all Americans are cigarette smokers, including 25% who are between the ages of 12 and 25.
- Forty-three percent of 10th graders and 54% of 12th graders have reported smoking cigarettes. Eight percent of 12th graders consume half a pack or more each day.
- Eight percent of 12th graders have reported using Ecstasy (MDMA).
- LSD is one of the most potent drugs known, with only 25–150 mcg constituting a dose. Almost 9% of 12th graders have reported using LSD.

TABLE 7.1	Commonly Abused Substances	NATURAL SUBSTANCES	MEDICATIONS
LEGAL SUBSTANCES WITHOUT PRESCRIPTION			
Ethyl alcohol		✓ Drinking alcohol	✓ OTC drugs
Methanol		✓ Solvents, varnishes	
Caffeine		✓ Coffee	✓ OTC drugs
Nicotine		✓ Tobacco	✓ Smoking cessation
LEGAL SUBSTANCES WITH PRESCRIPTION			
Barbiturates			✓ Sedative; CNS depressant
Benzodiazepines			✓ Sedative; CNS depressant
Opioids			✓ Pain therapy
Ketamine			✓ Anesthetic
Gamma hydroxybutyrate (GHB)			✓ Anesthetic
Amphetamines, methamphetamines, and methylphenidate (Ritalin)			✓ CNS stimulants
Anabolic steroids			✓ Weight gain; other uses
ILLEGAL SUBSTANCES OR DISCONTINUED IN TRADITIONAL THERAPIES			
Opioids		✓ Opium	✓ Heroin
Cannabinoids (THC)*		✓ Marijuana	✓ Glaucoma therapy
LSD		✓ Rye/grain fungus	✓ Psychiatric therapy
Psilocybin		✓ Mushrooms	
Mescaline		✓ Peyote	
Phencyclidine (PCP)			✓ Anesthetic
MDA*—designer drug—synthetic—no medicinal use			
MMDA* (Ecstasy)—designer drug—synthetic—no medicinal use			
DOM* (STP)—designer drug—synthetic—no medicinal use			
Cocaine		✓ Coca plant	✓ Local anesthetic

Chemical names are complicated and extensive; see Core Concepts 7.7 and 7.8 for more information.

the amphetamines, once prescribed for bronchodilation, were stopped in the 1980s after psychotic episodes were reported. Some commonly abused substances are summarized in Table 7.1.

CORE CONCEPT 7.2	**Addiction depends on multiple, complex, and interacting variables.**

addict = *given over*

Addiction, the progressive and chronic abuse of a substance, is an overwhelming feeling that drives someone to use a drug repeatedly despite serious health and social consequences. It is impossible to predict accurately whether a person will become an addict. Scientists have used psychological profiles and investigated genetic links to attempt to predict a person's addictive tendency, but no firm connections have been found. Addiction depends on multiple, complex, and interacting variables. These variables fall into the following categories:

- *Agent or drug of abuse* Cost, availability, dose, method of administration (e.g., oral, IV, inhalation), speed of onset/duration of effect, and length of drug use
- *User factors* Genetic factors (e.g., metabolic enzymes, natural tolerance), tendency toward risk-taking behavior, prior experiences with drugs, disease that may require a scheduled drug
- *Environment* Social/community *norms* (behavior accepted within a community), role models, peer influences, educational opportunities

Addiction may begin with a real need for pharmacotherapy. For example, narcotic analgesics may be prescribed for pain, or sedatives for a sleep disorder. A favorable experience of pain relief or being able to fall asleep may cause a patient to want to repeat these positive experiences.

It is a common misunderstanding, even among some health professionals, that the therapeutic use of scheduled drugs creates large numbers of patients with addiction. In fact, prescription drugs rarely cause addiction when used as prescribed. The risk of addiction for prescription medications is mostly a function of the dose and the length of therapy. For this reason, medications having a potential for abuse are usually prescribed at the lowest effective dose for the shortest time necessary to treat the medical problems (see Chapter 14 ⚭ for more information on pain management). As mentioned in Chapters 1 ⚭ and 2, numerous laws have been passed in an attempt to limit drug abuse and addiction.

Substance dependence is classified as physical dependence or psychological dependence.

CORE CONCEPT **7.3**

Whether a substance is addictive relates to how easily an individual can stop taking it repeatedly. When a person has an overwhelming desire to take a drug and cannot stop, it is referred to as *substance dependence*. Substance dependence is classified into two categories: physical dependence and psychological dependence.

Physical dependence is an altered physical condition caused by the nervous system adapting to repeated substance use. Over time, the body's cells are tricked into believing that it is normal for the substance to continually be present. With physical dependence, uncomfortable symptoms, known as **withdrawal syndrome**, occur when the agent is stopped. Opioids, such as morphine and heroin, may produce physical dependence rather quickly with repeated doses, particularly when taken intravenously. Alcohol, sedatives, some stimulants, and nicotine are other examples of substances that may easily produce physical dependence with repeated use.

In contrast to physical dependence, **psychological dependence** causes no apparent signs of physical discomfort after the agent is stopped. The person, however, will have an intense craving and display an overwhelming desire to continue using the substance even if there are obvious negative economic, physical, or social consequences. The intense craving may be associated with the individual's home environment or social contacts. Strong psychological cravings for a substance may continue for months or even years and is often responsible for relapses (return to the original drug-seeking behavior) during substance abuse therapy. Psychological dependence usually occurs only after relatively high doses of the substance have been used for a long time, such as with marijuana and antianxiety drugs. However, psychological dependence may develop quickly, perhaps after only one use, as with crack cocaine—a potent, inexpensive form of the drug.

Withdrawal results when an abused substance is no longer available.

CORE CONCEPT **7.4**

Once an individual becomes physically dependent and the substance is stopped, withdrawal syndrome will occur. Symptoms of withdrawal syndrome may be severe for patients who are physically dependent on alcohol and sedatives. Helping a patient withdraw from these agents is best done in a substance abuse treatment facility. Examples of withdrawal syndromes related to different abused substances are listed in Table 7.2.

Prescription drugs may be used to reduce the severity of withdrawal symptoms. For example, alcohol withdrawal can be treated with a benzodiazepine such as diazepam (Valium), and opioid withdrawal can be treated with methadone. Symptoms of nicotine withdrawal may be relieved by nicotine replacement therapy in the form of patches or chewing gum and the use of bupropion (Wellbutrin). No specific pharmacologic treatments are indicated for withdrawal from CNS stimulants, hallucinogens, marijuana, or inhalants.

With chronic substance abuse, patients will often associate their conditions and surroundings—including social contacts with other users—with use of the drug. Users tend to return to drug-seeking behavior when they interact with other substance abusers. Counselors often encourage patients to stop associating with past social contacts or having relationships with other substance abusers to lessen the possibility of relapse. With the assistance of self-help groups such as Alcoholics Anonymous, some patients are able to move to a drug-free lifestyle by making friends with new people who are drug free and alcohol free.

TABLE 7.2	Withdrawal Symptoms of Selected Drugs of Abuse
DRUG	**SYMPTOMS**
Alcohol	Tremors, fatigue, anxiety, abdominal cramping, hallucinations, confusion, seizures, delirium
Barbiturates and other sedative-hypnotics	Insomnia, anxiety, weakness, abdominal cramps, tremor, anorexia, seizures, hallucinations, delirium
Benzodiazepines	Insomnia, restlessness, abdominal pain, nausea, sensitivity to light and sound, headache, fatigue, muscle twitches
Cocaine and amphetamines	Mental depression, anxiety, extreme fatigue, hunger
Hallucinogens	Rarely observed; dependent on specific drug
Marijuana	Irritability, restlessness, insomnia, tremor, chills, weight loss
Nicotine	Irritability, anxiety, restlessness, headaches, increased appetite, insomnia, inability to concentrate, decreased heart rate and blood pressure
Opioids	Excessive sweating, restlessness, dilated pupils, agitation, goosebumps, tremor, violent yawning, increased heart rate and blood pressure, nausea/vomiting, abdominal cramps and pain, muscle spasms with kicking movements, weight loss

CORE CONCEPT 7.5

Tolerance occurs when higher and higher doses of a drug are needed to achieve the initial response.

Tolerance is a biological condition that occurs when the body adapts to a substance after it is repeatedly administered. Over time, higher doses of the agent are needed to produce the initial effect. For example, at the start of pharmacotherapy, a patient may find that 2 mg of a sedative is effective for causing sleep. After taking the medication for several months, the patient notices that it takes 4 mg or perhaps 6 mg to fall asleep. Development of drug tolerance is common for substances that affect the nervous system. Tolerance should be thought of as a natural consequence of continued drug use and not be considered evidence of addiction or substance abuse.

Tolerance does not develop at the same rate for all actions of a drug. For example, patients usually develop tolerance to the nausea and vomiting produced by narcotic analgesics after only a few doses. Tolerance to the mood-altering effects of these drugs and to their ability to reduce pain develops more slowly but eventually may be complete. Tolerance never develops to the drug's ability to constrict the pupils. Patients will often put up with annoying side effects of drugs, such as the sleepiness caused by antihistamines, if they know that tolerance to these effects will develop quickly.

Once tolerance develops to one substance, it often also occurs with use of closely related drugs. This reaction is known as **cross-tolerance**. For example, a heroin addict will be tolerant to the analgesic effects of other opioids such as morphine or meperidine. Patients who have developed tolerance to alcohol will show tolerance to other CNS depressants such as barbiturates, benzodiazepines, and some general anesthetics. This is important to know because doses of related medications may need to be adjusted so that the patient receives maximum therapeutic benefit.

PEARSON
mynursingkit

THE TEMPTATION OF ANABOLIC STEROIDS

NATURAL THERAPIES

Milk Thistle for Liver Damage

Milk thistle is a plant found growing in North America, from Mexico to Canada, that has been used as an herbal medicine for centuries. The active ingredient in the milk thistle plant (*Silybum marianum*), silymarin, has been confirmed to protect the liver against injury. Studies have shown that silymarin is able to neutralize the effects of alcohol and actually stimulate liver regrowth. It acts as an antioxidant and free-radical scavenger. It is typically taken for liver cirrhosis, chronic hepatitis, and gallbladder disorders. The herb has few side effects other than mild diarrhea, bloating, and upset stomach.

Anti-inflammatory and anticarcinogenic properties of milk thistle have also been documented. Milk thistle has been claimed to reduce the growth of cancer cells, but this has not been confirmed by controlled research studies. The nurse should urge patients to report the use of this herb to their health care provider.

The terms *immunity* and *resistance* are often confused with *tolerance*. These terms more correctly refer to the immune system and infections, and they should not be used to mean tolerance. For example, microorganisms become *resistant* to the effects of an antibiotic; they do not become *tolerant*. Patients become *tolerant* to the effects of pain relievers; they do not become *resistant*. It is not acceptable to say that patients are *immune* to drug therapy.

Concept Review   7.1

■ What is the difference between physical dependence and psychological dependence? How do patients know when they are physically dependent on a substance?

Central nervous system (CNS) depressants decrease the activity of the central nervous system.

CORE CONCEPT 7.6

CNS depressants form a group of drugs that cause patients to feel sedated or relaxed. Drugs in this group include barbiturates, nonbarbiturate sedative-hypnotics, benzodiazepines, alcohol, and opioids. Although the majority of these substances are legal, they are controlled because of their abuse potential.

Sedatives and Sedative-Hypnotics

Sedatives, sometimes referred to as *tranquilizers,* are prescribed mostly for sleep disorders and some forms of epilepsy. The two primary classes of sedatives are the barbiturates (see Chapter 9 ⬭ for their use in treating sleep disorders, and Chapter 13 ⬭ for their use in treating epilepsy) and the nonbarbiturate sedative-hypnotics. Their actions, indications, safety profiles, and addictive potential are roughly the same. Physical dependence, psychological dependence, and tolerance develop when these agents are taken for long periods at high doses. Patients sometimes abuse these drugs by taking more doses than prescribed or by sharing their medication with friends. These drugs are frequently combined with other drugs of abuse such as CNS stimulants or alcohol. People with addiction often alternate between amphetamines, which keep them awake for several days, and barbiturates, which help them relax and fall asleep.

Many sedatives have a long duration of action. Effects may last an entire day, depending on the specific drug. Patients may appear dull or apathetic, with slurred speech and lack of motor coordination. Four commonly abused barbiturates are pentobarbital (Nembutal), amobarbital (Amytal), secobarbital (Seconal), and a combination of secobarbital and amobarbital (Tuinal). The medical use of barbiturates and nonbarbiturate sedative-hypnotics has noticeably declined over the past 20 years.

Overdoses of barbiturates and nonbarbiturate sedative-hynotics are extremely dangerous. These drugs suppress the respiratory centers in the brain, and the user may stop breathing or enter a coma. Death may result from barbiturate overdose. Withdrawal symptoms from these drugs are similar to those of alcohol withdrawal and may be life threatening.

Benzodiazepines

Benzodiazepines are another group of CNS depressants that have a potential for abuse. They are one of the most widely prescribed classes of drugs and have largely replaced the barbiturates for certain disorders. Their primary indication is anxiety; thus they are called *anxiolytic* drugs (see Chapter 9 ⬭). They are also used for short-term treatment of seizures (see Chapter 13 ⬭) and as muscle relaxants (see Chapter 12 ⬭). Popular benzodiazepines include alprazolam (Xanax), diazepam (Valium), temazepam (Restoril), triazolam (Halcion), and midazolam (Versed).

anxio = *anxiety/restlessness*
lytic = *destruction*

Although benzodiazepines are the most frequently prescribed drug class, benzodiazepine abuse is varied. Those individuals who do abuse benzodiazepines may appear carefree, detached, sleepy, or disoriented. Death due to overdose is rare, even with high doses, unless benzodiazepines are used in combination with other CNS depressants. Abusers may combine these agents with alcohol, cocaine, or heroin to increase their drug experience. If combined with other agents, death due to overdose is very likely. Benzodiazepine withdrawal syndrome by itself is less severe than barbiturate withdrawal or alcohol withdrawal.

Opioids

Opioids are prescribed for severe pain, persistent cough, and diarrhea. The opioid class includes opium, morphine, and codeine, which are processed from natural substances found in the unripe seeds of the poppy plant, and synthetic drugs, such as propoxyphene (Darvon), hydromorphone

(Dilauded), oxycodone (OxyContin), fentanyl (Duragesic, Sublimaze), methadone (Dolophine), and heroin. The therapeutic effects of the opioids are discussed in detail in Chapter 14 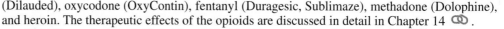 .

eu = *healthy or well*
phoria = *bearing*

The effects of *oral* opioids begin within 30 minutes and may last over a day. *Parenteral* forms produce immediate effects, including the brief, intense rush of *euphoria* (pleasure) sought by heroin addicts. Individuals experience a range of CNS effects, from extreme pleasure to slowed body activities and extreme sedation. Signs include constricted pupils, an increase in the ability to withstand pain, and respiratory depression.

Addiction to opioids can occur rapidly, and withdrawal can produce intense symptoms. Although extremely unpleasant, withdrawal from opioids is not necessarily life threatening. Methadone is a narcotic sometimes used to treat opioid addiction. Although methadone has addictive properties of its own, it does not produce the same degree of euphoria as other opioids, and its effects are longer lasting. Heroin addicts may be switched to methadone to prevent unpleasant withdrawal symptoms. Because methadone is taken orally, the serious risks associated with intravenous drug use, such as hepatitis and AIDS, are eliminated. Patients sometimes remain on methadone maintenance for their lifetimes. Withdrawal from methadone is more prolonged than from heroin or morphine, but the symptoms are less intense.

Ethyl Alcohol

Ethyl alcohol, commonly known as alcohol, is one of the most widely abused drugs. Alcohol is a legal substance for adults and is available as beer, wine, and liquor. The economic, social, and health consequences of alcohol abuse are staggering. In contrast to the many negative consequences associated with long-term abuse of alcohol, drinking small quantities of alcohol on a daily basis has been found to reduce the risk of stroke and heart attack.

Alcohol is classified as a CNS depressant, because it slows the actions of the region of the brain responsible for alertness and wakefulness. Alcohol easily crosses the blood-brain barrier, and its effects can be noticed within 5 to 30 minutes. Effects of alcohol are directly related to the amount consumed within a certain time frame and include relaxation, sedation, memory impairment, loss of motor coordination, reduced judgment, and decreased inhibition. **Alcohol intoxication** occurs when muscle coordination is lost and mental function is affected. It results in a characteristic odor to the breath and increased blood flow in certain areas of the skin, causing a flushed face, pink cheeks, or red nose. Although these symptoms are easily recognized, the nurse must be aware that other substances and disorders may cause similar effects. For example, many antianxiety agents, sedatives, and antidepressants can cause drowsiness, memory difficulties, and loss of motor coordination. Certain mouthwashes, medicines, and other substances containing alcohol can give the breath an "alcoholic" smell.

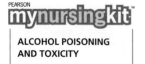

ALCOHOL POISONING
AND TOXICITY

The presence of food in the stomach will slow the absorption of alcohol, thus delaying the onset of drug action. *Metabolism,* or detoxification of alcohol by the liver, occurs at a slow, constant rate, which is not affected by the presence of food. The average rate is about 15 ml per hour—equal to one alcoholic beverage per hour. If consumed at a higher rate, alcohol will accumulate in the blood and produce greater effects on the brain. An overdose of alcohol produces vomiting, severe hypotension, respiratory failure, and coma. Death due to alcohol poisoning is common.

Chronic alcohol consumption produces both psychological and physiological dependence and results in a large number of adverse health effects. The organ most affected by chronic alcohol abuse is the liver. Alcoholism is a common cause of *cirrhosis,* a harmful and often fatal failure of the liver to perform its vital functions. Liver failure causes abnormalities in blood clotting and nutritional deficiencies and sensitizes the patient to the effects of all medications metabolized by the liver.

cirr = *orange/yellow*
osis = *condition*

Alcohol withdrawal syndrome is severe and may be life threatening. The use of antiseizure medications for treating severe alcohol withdrawal symptoms is discussed in Chapter 13 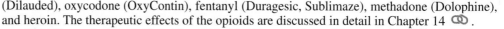 . Long-term treatment for alcohol abuse includes behavioral counseling and participation in self-help groups such as Alcoholics Anonymous. Disulfiram (Antabuse) may be given to discourage relapses. Disulfiram inhibits acetaldehyde dehydrogenase, the enzyme that metabolizes alcohol. If alcohol is consumed while taking disulfiram, the patient becomes violently ill within 5 to 10 minutes, with headache, shortness of breath, nausea/vomiting, and other unpleasant symptoms. Disulfiram is only effective in highly motivated patients, because the success of pharmacotherapy is entirely dependent on patient compliance. Alcohol sensitivity can continue for up to 2 weeks after disulfiram has been discontinued. As a pregnancy category X drug, disulfiram should never be taken during pregnancy.

In addition to disulfiram, acamprosate calcium (Campral, Forest) is an FDA-approved drug for maintaining alcohol abstinence in patients with alcohol dependence. Additional studies comparing the therapeutic benefit of disulfiram with acamprosate are needed. Adverse reactions to acamprosate include diarrhea, flatulence, and nausea. The drug is not recommended for patients who have impaired kidney functioning.

■ Compare the potential to cause coma or death of barbiturates and benzodiazepines.

Marijuana produces little physical dependence or tolerance.

Cannabinoids are substances obtained from the hemp plant *Cannabis sativa,* which grows in tropical climates. Cannabinoid agents are usually smoked and include marijuana, hashish, and hash oil. Although more than 61 cannabinoid chemicals have been identified, the ingredient responsible for most of the psychoactive properties is delta-9-**tetrahydrocannabinol (THC)**.

Marijuana (street names "grass," "pot," "weed," "reefer," or "dope") is a natural product obtained from *C. sativa.* It is the most commonly used illegal drug in the United States. Use of marijuana slows motor activity, decreases coordination, and causes disconnected thoughts, paranoia, and euphoria. It increases thirst and craving for food, particularly chocolate and other candies. One hallmark symptom of marijuana use is red or bloodshot eyes, caused by dilation of blood vessels. THC accumulates in the gonads.

para = *beside*
noia = *mind*

When inhaled, marijuana produces effects that occur within minutes and last up to 24 hours. Because marijuana smoke is inhaled more deeply and held within the lungs for a longer time than cigarette smoke, marijuana smoke introduces four times more tar into the lungs than tobacco smoke. Smoking marijuana on a daily basis may increase the risk of lung cancer and other respiratory disorders. Chronic use is associated with lack of motivation and loss of productivity.

Unlike many abused substances, marijuana produces little physical dependence or tolerance. Withdrawal symptoms are mild, if they are experienced at all. Metabolites of THC, however, remain in the body for months to years, allowing laboratory specialists to determine easily whether someone has used marijuana. For several days after use, THC can also be detected in the urine. Despite numerous attempts by scientists and clinicians to demonstrate therapeutic applications for marijuana, results have been controversial and the medical value of the drug remains to be proven.

■ Name three legal substances that are both used in traditional therapies and frequently abused. Are these substances natural or synthetic? Compare ethyl alcohol and marijuana in terms of common use.

Hallucinogens cause an altered state of thought and perception similar to that found in dreams.

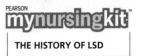

Hallucinogens consist of an assorted class of chemicals that have in common the ability to produce an altered, dreamlike state of consciousness. Sometimes called **psychedelics**, the prototype substance for this class is LSD. All hallucinogens are Schedule I drugs and have no medical use.

For nearly all drugs of abuse, predictable symptoms occur in every user. Effects from hallucinogens, however, are highly variable and depend on the mood and expectations of the user and the surrounding environment in which the substance is used. Two patients taking the same agent will report completely different symptoms, and the same patient may report different symptoms with each use. Users who take LSD or *psilocybin* (Figure 7.1 ■) may experience symptoms such as laughter, visions, religious revelations, or deep personal insights. Common occurrences are hallucinations and afterimages (images that are projected onto people as they move). Users also report unusually bright lights and vivid colors. Some users hear voices; others report smells. Many experience a profound sense of truth and deep-directed thoughts. Unpleasant experiences can be terrifying and may include anxiety, panic attacks, confusion, severe depression, or paranoia.

LSD (street names "acid," "the beast," "blotter acid," "California sunshine") is made from a fungus that grows on rye and other grains. LSD is almost always used in an oral form. It can be manufactured in capsules, tablets, or liquids. A common and inexpensive method for distributing LSD is to place drops of the drug on small pieces of paper that often contain images of cartoon characters or graphics related to the drug culture. After drying, the paper containing the LSD is swallowed to produce the drug's effects.

LSD is distributed throughout the body immediately after use. Effects are experienced within an hour and may last 6 to 12 hours. It affects the central and autonomic nervous systems, increasing

FIGURE 7.1

Comparison of the chemical structures of psilocybin and LSD. Psilocybin is derived from a mushroom, shown in (a); an LSD "blot" is shown in (b).
Source: Pearson Education/ PH College

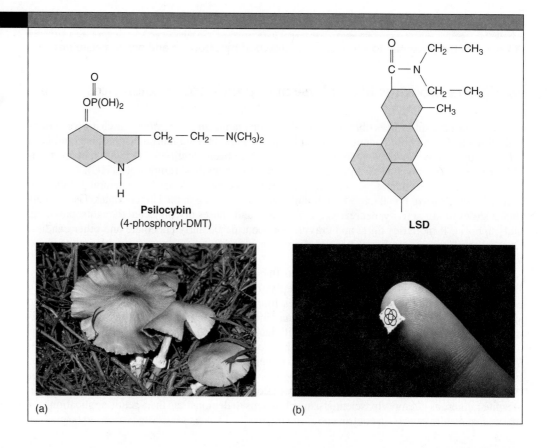

Psilocybin
(4-phosphoryl-DMT)

LSD

(a)

(b)

blood pressure, elevating body temperature, dilating pupils, and increasing heart rate. Repeated use may cause memory loss and inability to reason. In extreme cases, patients may develop psychoses. One unusual adverse effect is flashbacks, in which the user experiences the effects of the drug again—sometimes weeks, months, or years after the drug was initially taken. Although users may experience tolerance, they have little or no dependence with hallucinogens.

Other hallucinogenic drugs that are abused include the following:

- *Mescaline* found in the peyote cactus of Mexico and Central America (Figure 7.2 ■)
- *MDMA (3,4-methylenedioxymethamphetamine, "XTC," or "Ecstasy")* an amphetamine originally created for research purposes but now extremely popular as a drug of abuse
- *DOM (2,5 dimethoxy-4-methylamphetamine, "STP")* a recreational drug often linked with rave parties
- *MDA (3,4-methylenedioxyamphetamine)* called the "love drug" because of a belief that it enhances sexual desires

FIGURE 7.2

The chemical structure of mescaline, derived from the peyote plant (shown in photo)
Source: Pearson Education/ PH College

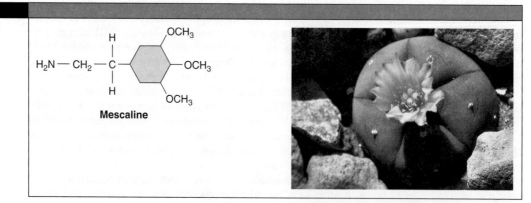

Mescaline

- *PCP (chemical name phenylcyclohexylpiperadine; also called phencyclidine; street name "angel dust")* produces a trancelike state that may last for days and results in severe brain damage; used as an animal tranquilizer

- *Ketamine ("date rape" drug or "special coke")* produces unconsciousness and amnesia; primary legal use is as an anesthetic

Concept Review 7.4

- In examining and interviewing a patient, how could you determine whether he or she is under the influence of marijuana or hallucinogens?

CNS stimulants increase the activity of the central nervous system.

narco = *numbness or stupor*
lepsy = *seizure*

Stimulants include a varied family of drugs with the ability to increase the activity of the CNS. Some are available by prescription for use in the treatment of **narcolepsy** (a sleep disorder in which people fall asleep unexpectedly), obesity, and **attention deficit disorder (ADD)** (or attention deficit hyperactivity disorder [ADHD]). As drugs of abuse, CNS stimulants are taken to produce a sense of exhilaration, improve mental and physical performance, reduce appetite, prolong wakefulness, or simply "get high." Stimulants include amphetamines, cocaine, methylphenidate, and caffeine.

CNS stimulants have effects similar to the neurotransmitter norepinephrine, which is discussed in Chapter 8 ⟳. Norepinephrine activates neurons in a part of the brain that affects awareness and wakefulness, called the *reticular formation* (see Chapter 9 ⟳ for an in-depth discussion). High doses of amphetamines give the user a feeling of self-confidence, euphoria, alertness, and empowerment. Long-term use, however, often causes feelings of restlessness, anxiety, and fits of rage, especially when the user is coming down from a drug high.

Most CNS stimulants affect cardiovascular and respiratory activity, raising blood pressure and increasing respiration rate. Other symptoms include dilated pupils, sweating, and tremors. Overdoses of some stimulants lead to seizures and cardiac arrest.

Amphetamines and dextroamphetamines were once widely prescribed for depression, obesity, drowsiness, and congestion. In the 1960s, the health care profession realized that the risk for amphetamine dependence outweighed the drug's therapeutic usefulness. Because of the development of safer medications, the current therapeutic uses of these drugs are extremely limited. Most substance abusers get these agents from illegal laboratories, which can easily produce amphetamines and make tremendous profits.

Dextroamphetamine (Dexedrine) may be used to treat narcolepsy and for short-term weight loss when all other attempts to lose weight have been exhausted. Methamphetamine (street name "ice" or "crank") is often used as a recreational drug for those who like the "rush" that it provides. It usually is administered in powder or crystal form, but it also may be smoked. Methamphetamine is a Schedule II drug marketed under the trade name Desoxyn, although most abusers obtain it from illegal methamphetamine laboratories. A drug related to methamphetamine, called methcathinone (street name "cat"), is made illegally and snorted, taken orally, or injected intravenously. Methcathinone is a Schedule I agent.

Methylphenidate (Ritalin) is a CNS stimulant (Schedule II drug) that is widely prescribed for children diagnosed with ADD/ADHD (see Chapter 10 ⟳). Ritalin has a calming effect on children who are inattentive or hyperactive. It stimulates the alertness center in the brain and allows the child to focus on tasks for longer periods.

In adults, Ritalin usually produces the same effects as cocaine and amphetamines and is sometimes abused by adolescents and adults seeking euphoria. The tablets are crushed and used intranasally or dissolved in liquid and injected intravenously. Ritalin is also sometimes mixed with heroin (street name "speedball").

Cocaine is a natural substance obtained from leaves of the coca plant, which grows in the Andes Mountain region of South America. The plant has been used by Andean cultures since 2500 B.C. Natives of this region chew the coca leaves or make teas of the dried leaves. Because it is taken orally, its absorption is slow, and the leaves contain only 1% cocaine, users do not have the ill effects caused by chemically pure extracts from the plant. In the Andean culture, use of coca leaves is not considered substance abuse because it is part of that society's culture.

Cocaine is a Schedule II drug that produces actions similar to those of the amphetamines, although its effects are usually more rapid and intense. It is the second most commonly abused illegal drug in the United States. Routes of administration include snorting, smoking, and injecting. In smaller doses, cocaine produces feelings of intense euphoria, a decrease in hunger, analgesia, illusions of physical strength, and increased sensory perception. Larger doses will magnify these effects and also cause rapid heartbeat, sweating, dilation of the pupils, and elevated body temperature. After euphoria diminishes, the user often feels irritable, depressed, and distrustful and usually has insomnia. Some users report the sensation that insects are crawling under their skin. Users who snort cocaine develop a chronic runny nose, a crusty redness around the nostrils, and deterioration of the nasal cartilage. Overdose can cause dysrhythmias, convulsions, stroke, or death due to respiratory arrest. The withdrawal syndrome for amphetamines and cocaine is much less intense than that from alcohol or barbiturates.

Caffeine is a natural substance found in the seeds, leaves, or fruits of more than 63 plant species throughout the world. Significant amounts of caffeine are consumed in chocolate, coffee, tea, and soft drinks (Table 7.3). Sometimes caffeine is added to OTC pain relievers to help relieve migraines and other conditions. Caffeine travels to almost all parts of the body after ingestion, and several hours are needed for the body to metabolize and eliminate the drug. Caffeine has a pronounced diuretic effect.

Caffeine is considered a CNS stimulant because it produces increased mental alertness, restlessness, nervousness, irritability, and insomnia. The physical effects of caffeine include bronchodilation, increased blood pressure, increased production of stomach acid, and changes in blood glucose levels. Repeated use of caffeine may result in physical dependence and tolerance.

Concept Review 7.5

■ Identify three groups of stimulants discussed in this section, and give examples for each group. Identify major systems in the body affected by these stimulants.

TABLE 7.3	Caffeine Content of Common Drugs, Foods, and Beverages	
	SERVING SIZE	**CAFFEINE (MG)**
OTC DRUGS		
NoDoz, maximum strength; Vivarin	1 tablet	200
Excedrin	2 tablets	130
NoDoz, regular strength	1 tablet	100
Anacin (also available in caffeine-free formulation)	2 tablets	64
COFFEES		
Coffee, brewed and instant	8 ounces	95–135
Coffee, decaffeinated	8 ounces	5
TEAS		
Tea, leaf or bag	8 ounces	50
Tea, green	8 ounces	30
Tea, instant	8 ounces	15
SOFT DRINKS		
Mountain Dew	12 ounces	55.5
Diet Coke	12 ounces	46.5
Coca-Cola Classic	12 ounces	34.5
Pepsi-Cola	12 ounces	37.5
CHOCOLATES AND CANDIES		
Hershey's Special Dark chocolate bar	1 bar (1.5 ounces)	31
Hershey Bar (milk chocolate)	1 bar (1.5 ounces)	10
Cocoa or hot chocolate	8 ounces	85

Nicotine is powerful and highly addictive.

Nicotine is sometimes considered a CNS stimulant because of its ability to increase alertness. However, its actions and long-term consequences place it into a class by itself. Nicotine is unique among abused substances in that it is legal, strongly addictive, and highly carcinogenic. Furthermore, use of tobacco can cause harmful effects from secondhand smoke to those in the immediate area of the smoker. Patients often do not consider tobacco use to be substance abuse.

The most common method by which nicotine enters the body is through the inhalation of cigarette, pipe, or cigar smoke. Tobacco smoke contains more than 1000 chemicals, many of which are carcinogens. The primary addictive substance in cigarette smoke is nicotine. Effects of inhaled nicotine may last from 30 minutes to several hours.

Nicotine affects many body systems, including the nervous, cardiovascular, and endocrine systems. Nicotine stimulates the CNS directly, causing increased alertness and ability to focus, feelings of relaxation, and lightheadedness. The cardiovascular effects of nicotine include accelerated heart rate and increased blood pressure, caused by activation of nicotinic receptors located within the autonomic nervous system (see Chapter 8 ∞). These cardiovascular effects can be serious in patients taking oral contraceptives. The risk of a fatal heart attack is five times greater in smokers than in nonsmokers. Muscular tremors may occur with moderate doses of nicotine, and convulsions may result from very high doses. Nicotine affects the endocrine system by increasing the basal metabolic rate, leading to weight loss. Nicotine also reduces appetite. Chronic use may lead to bronchitis, emphysema, and lung cancer.

Both psychological and physical dependence occur relatively quickly with nicotine. Once started on tobacco, patients tend to continue their drug use for many years, despite overwhelming medical evidence that their quality of life may be adversely affected and their life span shortened. Discontinuation results in agitation, weight gain, anxiety, headache, and an extreme craving for the drug. Although nicotine replacement therapy, such as patches, gum, and buproprion, assists patients in dealing with the unpleasant withdrawal symptoms, only 25% of patients who attempt to stop smoking remain tobacco-free 1 year later.

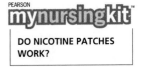

DO NICOTINE PATCHES WORK?

PATIENTS NEED TO KNOW

Patients taking medications with abuse potential need to know the following regarding:

Alcohol

1. Limit alcoholic beverage intake to two drinks per day for men or one drink per day for women.
2. Avoid alcohol use entirely if liver disease, gastric reflux, peptic ulcers, or pregnancy exists.
3. Check with your health care provider when combining alcohol and medications (prescription or over the counter). Alcohol is considered a CNS depressant, so never combine it with other CNS depressants.
4. Consuming more than one alcoholic drink per hour will usually result in blood alcohol levels above the legal limit for operating a vehicle.

CNS Stimulants

5. Avoid sources of caffeine such as OTC drugs with caffeine, chocolate, coffee, and tea if taking methylphenidate.
6. Always take methylphenidate (Ritalin) at least 6 hours prior to sleep to avoid insomnia.

CNS Depressants

7. Never take more CNS depressant medication than prescribed. If the prescribed dose is not providing sufficient relief, a health care provider should be notified due to the possibility of a developed tolerance.
8. Never combine CNS depressants (including alcohol) unless advised to do so by a health care provider.

Tobacco

9. Nicotine is a major contributor to cancer, heart disease, and stroke.
10. Secondhand smoke is dangerous, particularly to children and pregnant women.
11. If using nicotine replacement therapy (NRT), discontinue smoking immediately and follow the instruction sheet provided with the NRT of choice.

CORE CONCEPT 7.11

Health care providers strive to remain free of impairment due to alcohol and drug addiction.

Most healthcare providers report that they have encountered coworkers with perceived alcohol or substance abuse problems. For example, as compared to nurses in other specialties, critical care nurses are especially likely to use cocaine and marijuana. Generally among nurses, alcohol is the most commonly abused substance; prescription drugs are abused secondly.

Reasons for these problems seem to be increasing tension due to the demands of the health care profession; social environments among medical professionals that promote self-reliance and independence; difficulty sleeping, in particular among workers with rotating shifts; and in general, fatigue. Warning signs of substance abuse are overworking habits (e.g., arriving early and staying late for many days on end), high performance following by deteriorating performance, isolation from other working staff, and unexplained or complicated variables related to the nurse's professional or social life.

Obvious signs may be frequent mood swings, irritability or tearful outbursts followed by depression. Signs of substance abuse may be smell of alcohol on the breath covered up by mints or mouthwash, frequent absence from the unit to visit the restroom, or patients complaining of not receiving medications. Patients may complain about feeling pain despite having received seemingly adequate or repeated dosing of medication.

There are organizations and groups of organizations that focus chiefly on addiction and the nursing profession as well as psychiatric disorders among nurses and health care workers. The focus need not be just on disciplinary action but also on monitoring and support services. Agencies have adopted alternative disciplinary and peer assistance programs to make sure that both patients and health care providers receive proper assistance.

CHAPTER REVIEW

CORE CONCEPTS SUMMARY

7.1 **Abused substances belong to many different chemical classes.**

Abused substances come from many different chemical classes. Some abused substances, such as alcohol and nicotine, are available without a prescription. Others, such as barbiturates, benzodiazepines, and most opioids, have legitimate medical uses. Still others, such as LSD and heroin, are illegal, having no current medical applications.

7.2 **Addiction depends on multiple, complex, and interacting variables.**

Addiction is an overwhelming feeling that causes someone to continue taking drugs. Although ideas have changed about addiction over the years, health care providers now recognize it as being related to on drug factors, genetic factors, and environmental factors.

7.3 **Substance dependence is classified as physical dependence or psychological dependence.**

Dependence is an overwhelming need to take a drug on a continual basis. Physical dependence occurs when the patient exhibits signs of withdrawal after

the drug is discontinued. Psychological dependence is an intense craving for the drug.

7.4 **Withdrawal results when an abused substance is no longer available.**

When an abused drug is discontinued, patients may experience uncomfortable physical symptoms known as withdrawal syndrome. Symptoms vary depending on the specific drug of abuse and range from mild to life threatening.

7.5 **Tolerance occurs when higher and higher doses of a drug are needed to achieve the initial response.**

Tolerance occurs over time when patients adapt to continued drug use and require higher doses to produce the same effect. Cross-tolerance or tolerance resulting from prior exposure to a related drug also results in higher doses needed to produce the same effect.

7.6 **Central nervous system (CNS) depressants decrease the activity of the central nervous system.**

Substances that make patients feel relaxed and sleepy, and work by generally slowing neuronal activity in the brain, include sedatives, opioids, and ethyl alcohol. Examples of sedatives are barbiturates and benzodiazepines. Because of their abuse potential, many of these substances are controlled. Ethyl alcohol is a legal substance.

7.7 Marijuana produces little physical dependence or tolerance.

The most commonly abused illegal substance is marijuana. Marijuana produces less physical dependence than most other drugs and produces less tolerance. The medical value of this drug remains controversial and unproven. The risks of using this substance are lung cancer, respiratory problems, and lack of motivation.

7.8 Hallucinogens cause an altered state of thought and perception similar to that found in dreams.

Hallucinogens, also called psychedelics, have the ability to produce altered states of consciousness and dreams. They include LSD, mescaline, MDMA (Ecstacy), DOM (STP), MDA (love drug), and ketamine (an anesthetic).

7.9 CNS stimulants increase the activity of the central nervous system.

Amphetamines, methylphenidate, cocaine, and caffeine increase alertness by stimulating the central nervous system. Some substances are available by prescription and are used for narcolepsy, obesity, and attention deficit disorder. Caffeine is available in many consumer products, including chocolate, coffee, tea, soft drinks, and coffee ice cream. Cocaine is among the most commonly abused substances in America.

7.10 Nicotine is powerful and highly addictive.

Nicotine is a unique, legal, carcinogenic, highly addictive substance. The most common method of entry into the body is by inhalation of cigarette, pipe, or cigar smoke. Important effects of inhaled nicotine include stimulation of the CNS and increased cardiovascular effects.

7.11 Health care providers strive to remain free of impairment due to alcohol and drug addiction.

Reasons why health care providers have problems with alcohol or drug abuse seem to be related to demands in the health profession, including self-reliant social and professional environments, rotating working shifts, and fatigue. Signs of impairment are frequent mood swings, irritability or depressive symptoms, smell of alcohol on the breath, frequent absences from the unit, or patients not receiving proper medications. Support groups and organizations assist with these related issues.

REVIEW QUESTIONS

The following questions are written in NCLEX-PN® style. Answer these questions to assess your knowledge of the chapter material, and go back and review any material that is not clear to you.

1. The two most commonly abused drugs are:
1. Methylphenidate (Ritalin) and meperidine (Demerol)
2. Lysergic acid diethylamide (LSD) and phencyclidine (PCP)
3. Alcohol and nicotine
4. Opioids and inhalants

2. The patient has been diagnosed with a narcotic analgesic overdose. Which of the following symptoms are most likely associated with a narcotic analgesic overdose?
1. Irritability, restlessness, abdominal cramping
2. Excessive sweating, agitation, goosebump chills, increased heart rate
3. Insomnia, hallucinations, tremors
4. Delirium, extreme fatigue, hunger, headaches

3. When the patient requires a higher dose of the substance to produce the initial effect, this is known as:
1. Toxicity
2. Resistance
3. Immunity
4. Tolerance

4. The patient has developed an opioid addiction. The nurse anticipates that which of the following medications will be used for opioid withdrawal?
1. Methadone
2. Heroin
3. Diazepam (Valium)
4. Alprazolam (Xanax)

5. The nurse understands that which of the following substances produces little physical dependence or tolerance?
1. Heroin
2. Marijuana
3. Alcohol
4. Cocaine

6. The nurse recognizes that methylphenidate (Ritalin) is classified as a:
1. Schedule I drug
2. Schedule II drug
3. Schedule III drug
4. Schedule IV drug

7. The nurse assesses the patient and finds the following: increased heart rate, dilated pupils, elevated body temperature, and sweating. The nurse suspects:
1. Marijuana use
2. Heroin use

3. Cocaine use
4. Amphetamine use

8. Which of the following would the nurse find when assessing the patient for use of barbiturates?

1. Slurred speech, lack of muscle coordination, decreased respirations
2. Euphoria and irritability
3. Increased pain threshold and hallucinations
4. Increased blood pressure and respirations

9. Physical dependence differs from psychological dependence in that with physical dependence:

1. There is an intense craving for the drug.
2. There is an overwhelming need to take the drug.

3. The patient exhibits signs of withdrawal after the drug is discontinued.
4. Higher doses are required to produce the initial effect of the drug.

10. The nurse educates the patient on disulfiram (Antabuse), saying that:

1. Only small amounts of alcohol may be ingested while on this drug.
2. If alcohol is ingested, the patient may experience shortness of breath, nausea and vomiting, and headache.
3. It is safe for use in pregnancy.
4. It enhances alcohol metabolism within the body.

FURTHER STUDY

- The use of barbiturates is discussed in Chapter 9 ⚄ (for treating sleep disorders) and in Chapter 13 ⚄ (for treating epilepsy).

- Benzodiazepines are discussed in Chapter 9 ⚄ (for treating anxiety), in Chapter 13 ⚄ (for short-term control of seizures), and in Chapter 12 ⚄ (for muscle relaxation).

- The therapeutic effects of opioids in managing pain are covered in detail in Chapter 14 ⚄ .

- The use of antiseizure drugs as they relate to alcohol withdrawal symptoms is discussed in Chapter 13 ⚄ .

- Similarities between CNS stimulants and the neurotransmitter norepinephrine are covered in Chapter 8 ⚄ .

- An in-depth discussion of the reticular formation in wakefulness and anxiety is in Chapter 9 ⚄ .

- The therapeutic applications of methylphenidate are discussed in Chapter 10 ⚄ .

- The cardiovascular effects of nicotine are discussed in Chapter 8 ⚄ .

8 Drugs Affecting Functions of the Autonomic Nervous System

CORE CONCEPTS

8.1 The nervous system is divided into central and peripheral components.

8.2 The autonomic nervous system has sympathetic and parasympathetic branches.

8.3 Synapses are common sites of drug action.

8.4 Acetylcholine and norepinephrine are the two primary neurotransmitters in the autonomic nervous system.

8.5 Autonomic drugs are classified according to the receptors they stimulate or block.

8.6 Parasympathomimetics have few therapeutic uses because of their numerous adverse effects.

8.7 Anticholinergics are mainly used to dry secretions and to treat asthma.

8.8 Sympathomimetics are primarily used for their effects on the heart, bronchial tree, and nasal passages.

8.9 Adrenergic blockers are primarily used to treat hypertension and are the most widely prescribed class of autonomic drugs.

DRUG SNAPSHOT

The following drugs are discussed in this chapter:

DRUG CLASSES	DRUG PROFILES
Parasympathomimetics	**Pr** bethanechol (Urecholine)
Anticholinergics	**Pr** atropine (Atro-Pen, Atropain, Atropisol)
Sympathomimetics	**Pr** phenylephrine (Neo-Synephrine)
Adrenergic blockers	**Pr** prazosin (Minipress)

LEARNING OUTCOMES

After reading this chapter, the student should be able to:

1. Identify the two primary divisions of the nervous system.

2. Identify the three primary functions of the nervous system.

3. Compare and contrast the actions of the sympathetic and parasympathetic nervous systems.

4. Describe the three parts of a synapse.

5. Identify the neurotransmitters important to the autonomic nervous system and the types of nerves with which they are associated.

6. Compare and contrast nicotinic and muscarinic receptors.

7. Compare and contrast the types of effects when a drug stimulates $alpha_1$, $alpha_2$, $beta_1$, or $beta_2$-adrenergic receptors.

8. For each of the classes in the Drug Snapshot, explain the mechanism of drug action, primary actions, and important adverse effects.

acetylcholine (Ach) (ah-SEET-ul-
KOH-leen) 96

adrenergic (add-rah-NUR-jik) 96

adrenergic blockers 97

adrenergic drugs 97

alpha receptor 96

anticholinergics 97

beta receptor 96

cholinergic (kol-in-UR-jik) 96

cholinergic blockers 97

cholinergic drugs 97

ganglia (GANG-lee-ah) 96

muscarinic (MUS-kah-RIN-ik) 96

nicotinic (NIK-oh-TIN-ik) 96

norepinephrine (nor-EH-pin-NEF-
rin) 96

parasympathetic nervous system
(PAIR-ah-SIM-pah-THET-ik) 93

parasympathomimetics (PAIR-ah-
SIM-path-oh-mah-MET-iks) 97

sympathetic nervous system
(SIM-pah-THET-ik) 93

sympatholytics (SIM-path-oh-LIT-
ik) 97

sympathomimetics (SIM-path-oh-
mih-MET-ik) 97

N euEuropharmacology represents one of the largest, most complicated, and least understood branches of pharmacology. Nervous system medications are used to treat a large and diverse set of conditions, including pain, anxiety, depression, schizophrenia, insomnia, and convulsions. Through their effects on nerves, medications are also used to treat many disorders that are considered diseases of other organ systems. Examples include abnormalities in heart rate and rhythm, high and low blood pressure, pressure within the eyeball, asthma, and even a runny nose.

The next seven chapters of this text cover topics in nervous system pharmacology. Traditionally, the study of neuropharmacology begins with the autonomic nervous system. A firm grasp of autonomic pharmacology is necessary to understand the pharmacology of other systems in the body.

The nervous system is divided into central and peripheral components.

CORE CONCEPT 8.1

The nervous system has two major divisions: the *central nervous system (CNS)* and the *peripheral nervous system*. The CNS is made up of the brain and spinal cord. The peripheral nervous system consists of all nervous tissue outside the CNS. The basic functions of the nervous system are to:

- Recognize changes in the internal and external environments
- Process and integrate these environmental changes
- React to the environmental changes by producing an action or response

Figure 8.1 ■ shows the fundamental functional divisions of the peripheral nervous system. Nerves in the peripheral nervous system either recognize changes to the environment (sensory division) or respond to these changes by moving muscles or secreting chemicals (motor division). The *somatic nervous system* consists of nerves that provide voluntary control over skeletal muscle. Nerves of the *autonomic nervous system*, on the other hand, give involuntary control over smooth muscle, cardiac muscle, and glands. Organs and tissues regulated by nerves from the autonomic nervous system include the heart, digestive tract, respiratory tract, reproductive tracts, arteries, salivary glands, and portions of the eye.

auto = *self*
ic = *relating to*
soma = *body*

The autonomic nervous system has sympathetic and parasympathetic branches.

CORE CONCEPT 8.2

The autonomic nervous system has two subsystems called the **sympathetic nervous system** and the **parasympathetic nervous system**. Almost all organs and glands receive nerves from both branches of the autonomic nervous system.

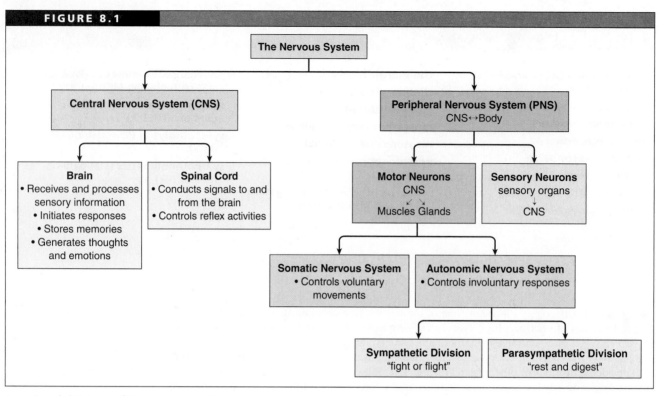

FIGURE 8.1

Functional divisions of the nervous system

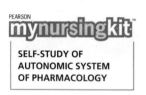

**SELF-STUDY OF
AUTONOMIC SYSTEM
OF PHARMACOLOGY**

The sympathetic nervous system is activated under conditions of stress and produces a set of actions called the *fight-or-flight response*. On the other hand, the parasympathetic nervous system is activated under nonstressful conditions and produces symptoms called the *rest-and-digest response*. Most of the actions of the sympathetic branch are opposite to those of the parasympathetic branch. For example, activation of sympathetic nerves increases heart rate, whereas activation of parasympathetic nerves decreases heart rate. The major actions of the two branches are shown in Figure 8.2 ■. It is essential to learn these actions early in the study of pharmacology because knowledge of autonomic effects is used to predict the actions and adverse effects of many drugs.

Concept Review   8.1

■ How would a person who is engaging in stressful or energetic activity benefit from the sympathetic effects of bronchodilation, slowed GI motility, and pupil dilation?

CORE CONCEPT 8.3   **Synapses are common sites of drug action.**

pre = *before*
post = *after*
synaptic = *relating to
    the synapse*

The basic functional cell of the nervous system is the *neuron*. For information to be transmitted throughout the nervous system, neurons must communicate with each other and with muscles and glands. A nerve impulse travels along a neuron to an area at the end of the neuron called a *synapse*. The synapse contains a space called the *synaptic cleft*, which must be crossed for the impulse to reach the next neuron. The neuron generating the original impulse is called the *presynaptic neuron*. The nerve on the other side of the synapse, waiting to receive the impulse, is called the *postsynaptic neuron*. The basic structure of a synapse is shown in Figure 8.3 ■.

Chemicals called *neurotransmitters* allow nerve impulses to cross the synaptic cleft. Neurotransmitters are released into the synaptic cleft when a nerve impulse reaches the end of a presynaptic neuron. The neurotransmitter travels across the synaptic cleft to reach receptors on the postsynaptic neuron, which then regenerates the impulse. Many different types of neurotransmitters are located throughout the nervous system, each related to particular functions. *Many drugs are identical to or have the same general structure as neurotransmitters.* These drugs are used to affect autonomic functions by either blocking or enhancing the activity of these neurotransmitters.

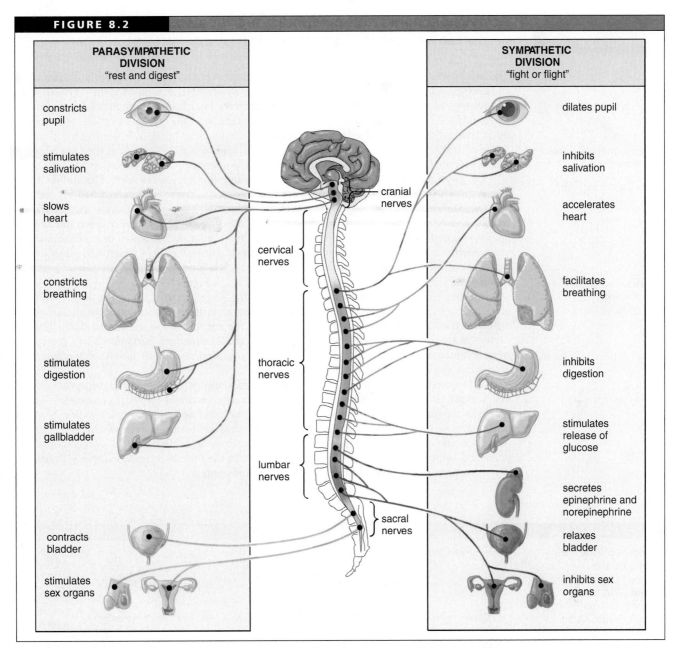

FIGURE 8.2

PARASYMPATHETIC DIVISION "rest and digest"

constricts pupil

stimulates salivation

slows heart

constricts breathing

stimulates digestion

stimulates gallbladder

contracts bladder

stimulates sex organs

cranial nerves

cervical nerves

thoracic nerves

lumbar nerves

sacral nerves

SYMPATHETIC DIVISION "fight or flight"

dilates pupil

inhibits salivation

accelerates heart

facilitates breathing

inhibits digestion

stimulates release of glucose

secretes epinephrine and norepinephrine

relaxes bladder

inhibits sex organs

Effects of the sympathetic and parasympathetic nervous systems   *Source: Pearson Education/PH College*

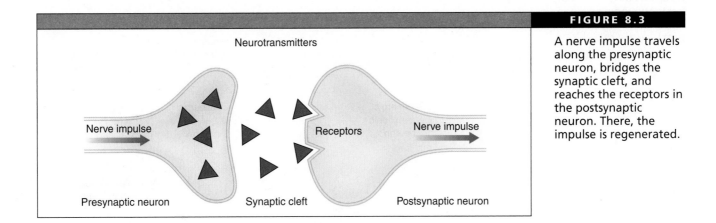

Neurotransmitters

Nerve impulse

Presynaptic neuron

Synaptic cleft

Receptors

Nerve impulse

Postsynaptic neuron

FIGURE 8.3

A nerve impulse travels along the presynaptic neuron, bridges the synaptic cleft, and reaches the receptors in the postsynaptic neuron. There, the impulse is regenerated.

Acetylcholine and norepinephrine are the two primary neurotransmitters in the autonomic nervous system.

The two primary neurotransmitters of the autonomic nervous system are **norepinephrine (NE)** and **acetylcholine (Ach)**. In the sympathetic nervous system, NE is released at the junction of the postsynaptic neuron and the organ or gland to be acted on. For example, sympathetic nerves in the heart release NE on cardiac muscle, which stimulates the heart to contract faster and with greater force. Sympathetic nerves also release NE in the smooth muscle lining the digestive tract, and its action is to slow contractions, or motility. Sympathetic nerves are sometimes called **adrenergic**. This term comes from the word *adrenaline,* which is a chemical closely related to NE.

adren = *adrenal gland (adrenaline)*

The physiology of Ach is more complicated because it is released in several locations. When released at the ends of parasympathetic neurons, it produces the opposite effects of NE, such as slowing the heart and increasing the motility of the digestive tract. Ach is also the neurotransmitter released at the end of all presynaptic neurons at sites called **ganglia**, which are collections of neuron cell bodies located outside the spinal cord. In addition, Ach is also a neurotransmitter of sympathetic neurons that activate sweat glands—this is a unique case in which Ach is associated with sympathetic rather than parasympathetic activity. Neurons that release Ach are often called **cholinergic**. The sites of Ach and NE action are shown in Figure 8.4 ■.

cholin = *acetylcholine*
erg = *work*
ic = *relating to*

Because Ach can stimulate receptors both in the ganglia and at the organ level, different names are assigned to these receptors. Ach receptors in the ganglia and in skeletal muscle are called **nicotinic** receptors, named after nicotine, the agent found in tobacco products. Ach receptors at the end of postsynaptic neurons in the parasympathetic nervous system are called **muscarinic** receptors, named after an extract of the mushroom *Amanita muscaria.* Nicotinic and muscarinic receptors are indicated in Figure 8.4.

Norepinephrine receptors are of two basic subtypes, **alpha (α)** and **beta (β) receptors**. *Alpha* and *beta* are Greek letters commonly used in naming chemical and scientific compounds. These receptors are further subdivided into beta$_1$, beta$_2$, alpha$_1$, and alpha$_2$. Drugs may be selective and affect only one type of NE receptor, or they may affect all of them. The type of response depends on the specific type of receptor that is activated. Drugs may also affect one type of receptor at low doses and begin to affect other receptor subtypes when the dose is increased. Table 8.1 contains a list of receptors and expected responses to neurotransmitters.

FIGURE 8:4

Norepinephrine (NE) receptors are adrenergic receptors (α and β) in the sympathetic pathway. Acetylcholine (Ach) receptors in the ganglia and skeletal muscles (not shown here) are called *nicotinic*. Ach receptors at the ends of postganglionic neurons in the parasympathetic pathway are called *muscarinic*.

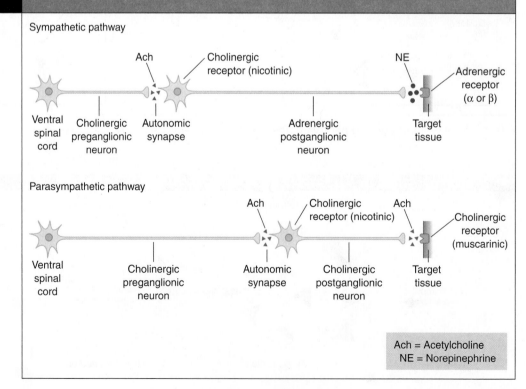

TABLE 8.1	Types of Autonomic Receptors		
NEUROTRANSMITTER	**RECEPTOR**	**PRIMARY LOCATIONS**	**RESPONSES**
Acetylcholine (cholinergic)	Muscarinic	Parasympathetic target: organs other than the heart	Stimulation of smooth muscle contractions and gland secretions
		Heart	Decrease in heart rate and force of contraction
	Nicotinic	Cell bodies of postganglionic neurons (sympathetic and parasympathetic pathways)	Stimulation of smooth muscle contractions and gland secretions
Norepinephrine (adrenergic)	Alpha$_1$	All sympathetic target organs except the heart	Constriction of blood vessels, dilation of pupils
	Alpha$_2$	Presynaptic adrenergic neuron terminals	Inhibition of norepinephrine release
	Beta$_1$	Heart and kidneys	Increase in heart rate and force of contraction; release of renin
	Beta$_2$	All sympathetic target organs except the heart	Inhibition of smooth muscle contractions

Autonomic drugs are classified according to the receptors they stimulate or block.

Because they can block or stimulate either the sympathetic or parasympathetic nervous systems, autonomic drugs are classified based on one of four possible actions:

1. *Stimulation of the sympathetic nervous system.* These drugs are called **sympathomimetics** or **adrenergic drugs** and produce the classic symptoms of the fight-or-flight response.
2. *Stimulation of the parasympathetic nervous system.* These drugs are called **parasympathomimetics** or **cholinergic drugs** and produce the classic symptoms of the rest-and-digest response.
3. *Inhibition of the sympathetic nervous system.* These drugs are called **adrenergic blockers** or **sympatholytics** and produce actions opposite to those of the sympathomimetics.
4. *Inhibition of the parasympathetic nervous system.* These drugs are called **anticholinergics** or **cholinergic blockers** and produce actions opposite to those of the parasympathomimetics.

sympatho = *sympathetic*
parasympatho = *parasympathetic*
mimetic = *to mimic*
lytic = *to undo*

Students beginning their study of pharmacology often have difficulty understanding the terminology and actions of autonomic drugs. It is only necessary to learn one group well because the others are logical extensions of the first. If the fight-or-flight symptoms of the sympathomimetics are learned, the actions of the other three groups can be remembered as being either the same or opposite. For example, both the sympathomimetics and the cholinergic blockers increase heart rate and dilate the pupils. The other two groups, the parasympathomimetics and the adrenergic blockers, have the opposite effects of slowing heart rate and constricting the pupils. Mastering the actions and terminology of autonomic drugs early in the study of pharmacology will reap rewards later in the course when these drugs are applied to various systems. See Table 8.2 for a quick review of the autonomic drugs.

TABLE 8.2	Review of Autonomic Drug Classes	
	STIMULATION	**INHIBITION**
Parasympathetic Nervous System	Parasympathomimetics (cholinergic drugs)	Anticholinergics (cholinergic blockers)
Sympathetic Nervous System	Sympathomimetics (adrenergic drugs)	Sympatholytics (adrenergic blockers)

CORE CONCEPT 8.6

Parasympathomimetics have few therapeutic uses because of their numerous adverse effects.

Parasympathomimetics are drugs that mimic actions of the parasympathetic nervous system. These drugs are associated with rest-and-digest responses. Because of their high potential for serious adverse effects, direct-acting parasympathomimetics are used only in a clinical setting. For instance, in ophthalmology, they are used to reduce intraocular pressure in patients with glaucoma (see Chapter 35 ⊂⊃). Others are used after anesthesia to stimulate the smooth muscles of the bowel or urinary tract.

Indirect-acting parasympathomimetic drugs, or drugs that inhibit the important enzyme acetylcholinesterase, have the same effect as direct-acting drugs. These acetylcholinesterase inhibitors facilitate the effects of the natural neurotransmitter Ach. Therefore, neostigmine (Prostigmin) and physostigmine (Antilirium) can induce actions in the body associated with rest and digestion. (Refer back to Figure 8.2.)

Several drugs in this class are used for their effects on Ach receptors *in skeletal muscle* rather than for their parasympathetic action. For example, myasthenia gravis is an autoimmune disorder characterized by destruction of cholinergic receptors found in skeletal muscles. Administration of pyridostigmine (Mestinon), neostigmine (Prostigmin), and other drugs (Table 8.3) will stimulate skeletal muscle contraction and diagnose or temporarily help to restore the severe muscle weakness found in this disease. Because several drugs structurally similar to myasthenia drugs are useful in treating Alzheimer's disease, drugs such as donepezil (Aricept, Aricept ODT), galantamine hydrobromide (Reminyl, Razadyne), rivastigmine (Exelon), and tacrine (Cognex) are included in the table. These drugs increase the amount of Ach binding to receptors located *within the CNS* (see Chapter 10 ⊂⊃).

Nerve agents (see Chapter 1 ⊂⊃) such as Sarin and organophosphate insecticides are chemicals that inhibit acetylcholinesterase in the synaptic cleft throughout the entire nervous system. These agents can cause widespread and toxic parasympathomimetic effects. Symptoms are severe salivation, increased sweating, muscle twitching, involuntary urination and defecation, confusion, convulsions, and death. In an emergency, if nerve agents are released, Mark I injector kits containing the anticholinergic drug atropine or related medications are used to counteract toxic effects. Atropine blocks the attachment of Ach to receptor sites and prevents overstimulation caused by harmful nerve agents. In instances in which too much anticholinergic activity occurs, as with atropine overdose or ingestion of poisonous substances, physostigmine (Antilirium) can be used as an antidote to counter adverse CNS effects resulting from intense cholinergic blockade.

TABLE 8.3	Selected Parasympathomimetics
DRUG	**CLINICAL USE**
ⓟ bethanechol (Urecholine)	To contract bladder muscles (for treating urinary retention)
cevimeline HCl (Evoxac)	To increase salivation (for treating dry mouth)
ambenonium (Mytelase)	Treatment of myasthenia gravis
donepezil (Aricept, Aricept ODT) (see page 178 for the Drug Profile box)	Treatment of Alzheimer's disease
edrophonium (Tensilon)	Diagnosis of myasthenia gravis
galantamine hydrobromide (Reminyl, Razadyne)	Treatment of Alzheimer's disease
neostigmine (Prostigmin)	Treatment of myasthenia gravis
physostigmine (Antilirium)	To counteract anticholinergic (atropine-related) drug overdose
pilocarpine (Isopto Carpine; Salagen)	To decrease intraocular pressure (for treating glaucoma)
pyridostigmine (Mestinon)	Treatment of myasthenia gravis
rivastigmine (Exelon)	Treatment of Alzheimer's disease
tacrine (Cognex)	Treatment of Alzheimer's disease

DRUG PROFILE: Ⓟ *Bethanechol (Urecholine)*

Therapeutic Class: Urinary retention (incomplete bladder emptying) treatment
Pharmacologic Class: Parasympathomimetic, cholinergic receptor drug

Actions and Uses:

Bethanechol is a direct-acting parasympathomimetic that interacts with Ach receptors to cause actions typical of parasympathetic stimulation. It affects mostly the digestive and urinary tracts, where it stimulates smooth muscle contraction. These actions are particularly useful in stimulating the return of normal gastrointestinal (GI) and urinary tract function following general anesthesia.

Adverse Effects and Interactions:

The adverse effects of bethanechol are parasympathetic actions: increased salivation, sweating, abdominal cramping, and hypotension that can lead to fainting. It should not be given to patients with suspected urinary or intestinal obstruction or those with active asthma.

Do not use with ambenonium, neostigmine, and other cholinergic drugs; mecamylamine (blocker of Ach at the ganglia) may cause abdominal symptoms and hypotension. Procainamide, quinidine, atropine, and epinephrine reduce the effects of bethanechol.

 Refer to MyNursingKit for a Nursing Process Focus specific to this drug.

NURSING PROCESS FOCUS

Patients Receiving Direct- and Indirect-Acting Parasympathomimetic Therapy

ASSESSMENT

Prior to administration:
- Obtain complete health history, including vital signs, allergies, blood chemistry and liver function panel, and drug history for possible drug interactions
- Assess reason for drug administration
- Assess for contraindications of drug administration
- Assess for urinary retention, urinary patterns initially and throughout therapy (direct acting)
- Assess muscle strength and neuromuscular status, ptosis, diplopia, and chewing

POTENTIAL NURSING DIAGNOSES

- Urinary Incontinence related to the adverse effects of direct-acting drugs.
- Impaired Urinary Elimination related to adverse effects of direct-acting drugs.
- Impaired Physical Mobility related to adverse effects of indirect-acting drugs.
- Deficient Knowledge related to information about administration and adverse effects of drug therapy.
- Risk for Injury related to adverse effects of medication.

PLANNING: PATIENT GOALS AND EXPECTED OUTCOMES

The patient will:
- Exhibit increased bowel and bladder function and tone by regaining normal pattern of elimination (direct acting)
- Exhibit a decrease in myasthenia gravis symptoms such as muscle weakness, ptosis, and diplopia (indirect acting)
- Demonstrate understanding of the drug's action by accurately describing drug adverse effects and precautions

IMPLEMENTATION

Interventions and (Rationales)

All Parasympathomimetics

- Monitor for adverse effects such as abdominal cramping, diarrhea, excessive salivation, increased sweating, difficulty breathing, muscle cramping, and hypotension. (These may indicate cholinergic crisis that requires atropine.)

Patient Education/Discharge Planning

- Instruct the patient to report nausea, vomiting, diarrhea, rash, jaundice, or change in color of stool, feeling faint, or any other adverse reactions to the drug.

continued . . .

NURSING PROCESS FOCUS *(continued)*

Interventions and (Rationales)	Patient Education/Discharge Planning
■ Monitor liver enzymes at the start of therapy and weekly for 6 weeks (for possible liver toxocity).	■ Instruct the patient to adhere to laboratory testing regimen for serum blood level tests of liver enzymes as directed.
■ Assess and monitor for appropriate self-care administration to prevent complications.	Instruct the patient to: ■ Take the drug as directed on regular schedule to maintain serum levels and control symptoms ■ Not chew or crush sustained-release tablets ■ Take oral parasympathomimetics on empty stomach to lessen incidence of nausea and vomiting and to increase absorption

Direct Acting

■ Monitor intake and output ratio. Palpate the abdomen for bladder distention. (These drugs have an onset of action within 60 minutes, stimulating the smooth muscle of the bladder to contract and causing urination.)	■ Advise the patient to be near bathroom facilities after taking these drugs.
■ Monitor for blurred vision (a cholinergic effect).	■ Advise the patient that blurred vision is a possible adverse effect and to take appropriate precautions. ■ Instruct the patient not to drive or engage in potentially hazardous activities until the drug's effects are known.
■ Monitor for orthostatic hypotension.	■ Instruct the patient to avoid abrupt position changes. Avoid prolonged standing in one place.

Indirect Acting

■ Monitor muscle strength and neuromuscular status, ptosis, diplopia, and chewing to determine if the therapeutic effect is achieved.	■ Instruct the patient to report difficulty with vision or swallowing.
■ Schedule the medication around mealtimes. (This will achieve therapeutic effect and aid in chewing and swallowing.)	■ Instruct the patient to take the medication about 30 minutes before a meal.
■ Schedule activities to avoid fatigue.	Instruct the patient to: ■ Plan activities according to muscle strength and fatigue ■ Take frequent rest periods to avoid fatigue
■ Monitor for muscle weakness. (This symptom, depending on time onset, indicates cholinergic crisis—overdose—OR myasthenic crisis—underdose.)	Instruct the patient to: ■ Report any severe muscle weakness that occurs 1 hour after administration of medication ■ Report any muscle weakness that occurs 3 or more hours after medication administration because this is a major symptom of myasthenic crisis

EVALUATION OF OUTCOME CRITERIA

Evaluate the effectiveness of drug therapy by confirming that patient goals and expected outcomes have been met (see "Planning").

See Table 8.3 for a list of drugs to which these nursing actions apply.

Anticholinergics are mainly used to dry secretions and to treat asthma.

Anticholinergics are drugs that have actions opposite those of the parasympathetic branch. They mimic the fight-or-flight response. Although the term *anticholinergic* is commonly used, a better term for this class of drugs would be *muscarinic blockers,* which more accurately describes the nature of their action. Most therapeutic uses of the anticholinergics relate to their autonomic actions: dilation of pupils, increase in heart rate, drying of secretions, and dilation of the bronchi. Anticholinergics have been widely used in medicine for many disorders. A relatively high incidence of adverse effects and the development of safer, and sometimes more effective, medications has limited the current use of anticholinergics. For example, anticholinergics were once drugs of choice in treating peptic ulcers, but they have been replaced by proton-pump inhibitors and H_2-receptor blockers (see Chapter 29 ⊙). Two important adverse effects that limit their usefulness include tachycardia (fast heart rate) and the tendency to cause urinary retention in men with prostate disorders.

Some of the anticholinergics are used for their effects *in the CNS,* rather than their autonomic actions. Scopolamine (Hyoscine, Transderm-Scop) is used to produce sedation and prevent motion sickness (see Chapter 6 ⊙); benztropine (Cogentin) and trihexyphenidyl (Artane) are prescribed to reduce the muscular tremor and rigidity associated with Parkinson's disease (see Chapter 10 ⊙).

Some of the more common anticholinergics and their clinical uses are listed in Table 8.4.

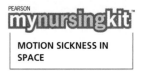

Sympathomimetics are primarily used for their effects on the heart, bronchial tree, and nasal passages.

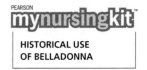

Sympathomimetics, or adrenergic drugs, have actions similar to activation of the sympathetic nervous system. They will produce responses characteristic of the fight-or-flight response. The sympathomimetics produce many of the same symptoms as the anticholinergics. However, because the sympathetic nervous system has alpha- and beta-subreceptors, the actions of many of the sympathomimetics are more specific and have wider therapeutic application.

Although most effects of sympathomimetics are predictable based on their autonomic actions, their primary effects depend on which adrenergic subreceptors are stimulated. Drugs such as phenylephrine (Neo-Synephrine) stimulate alpha$_1$-receptors and are often used to dry nasal secretions. Because beta$_1$-receptors are predominant in the heart, beta$_1$-drugs such as dobutamine (Dobutrex) are used to stimulate the heart rate and increase its strength of contraction. Beta$_2$-drugs such as albuterol (Proventil) cause bronchodilation and are useful in the treatment of asthma.

TABLE 8.4	Selected Anticholinergics
DRUG	**CLINICAL USE**
℗ atropine (Atro-Pen, Atropair, Atropisol)	To dry secretions prior to anesthesia, increase heart rate, dilate pupils
benztropine (Cogentin) (see page 175 for the Drug Profile box)	Parkinson's disease, neuroleptic adverse effects
cyclopentolate (Cyclogyl)	To dilate pupils
dicyclomine (Bentyl)	Irritable bowel syndrome
glycopyrrolate (Robinul)	To dry secretions prior to anesthesia, peptic ulcers
ipratropium (Atrovent)	Asthma
oxybutynin (Ditropan)	Urinary bladder urgency and incontinence
propantheline (Pro-banthine)	Irritable bowel syndrome, peptic ulcers
scopolamine (Hyoscine, Transderm-Scop)	Irritable bowel syndrome, motion sickness
tiotropium (Spiriva)	Asthma
tolterodine (Detrol)	Overactive bladder with symptoms of urinary incontinence, urgency, and frequency
trihexyphenidyl (Artane, others)	Parkinson's disease

DRUG PROFILE: **⊕** *Atropine (Atro-Pen, Atropair, Atropisol)*

Therapeutic Class: Antidote for anticholinerase poisoning, antidysrhythmic, mydriatic (pupil dilating drug)
Pharmacologic Class: Anticholinergic, cholinergic receptor blocker

Actions and Uses:

Atropine is a natural product found in the deadly nightshade plant, or Atropa belladonna. By blocking Ach (muscarinic) receptors, atropine causes symptoms of the fight-or-flight response, such as increased heart rate, bronchodilation, decreased motility in the GI tract, mydriasis (pupil dilation), and decreased secretions from glands. Throughout history, atropine has been used for a variety of purposes, although its use has declined because of the development of safer, more effective medications. Atropine is used to treat hypermotility diseases of the GI tract such as irritable bowel syndrome, to suppress secretions during surgical procedures, to increase the heart rate in patients with a slow heart beat bradycardia), to dilate the pupil during eye examinations, and to cause bronchodilation in patients with asthma. Atropine is an antidote for poisoning with nerve gas agents and organophosphate insecticides.

Adverse Effects and Interactions:

The adverse effects of atropine limit its therapeutic usefulness. Adverse effects include dry mouth, constipation, urinary retention, and an increased heart rate. Atropine is usually contraindicated in patients with glaucoma because the drug may increase pressure within the eyeball.

Use of amantadine, antihistamines, tricyclic antidepressants, quinidine, disopyramide, and procainamide can increase the anticholinergic effects of atropine. Use with levodopa may decrease the effects of the latter. Use with methotrimeprazine may cause extrapyramidal effects. The antipsychotic effects of phenothiazines are generally decreased.

Refer to MyNursingKit for a Nursing Process Focus specific to this drug.

NURSING PROCESS FOCUS

Patients Receiving Anticholinergic Therapy

ASSESSMENT

Prior to administration:
- Obtain a complete health history, including drug history, to determine possible drug interactions and allergies
- Assess the reason for drug administration
- Assess for heart rate, blood pressure, temperature, and elimination patterns (initially and throughout therapy)

POTENTIAL NURSING DIAGNOSES

- Deficient Knowledge related to information about administration and adverse effects of drug therapy.
- Decreased Cardiac Output related to adverse effects of drug therapy.
- Risk for Imbalanced Body Temperature related to inhibited sweat gland secretions.
- Impaired Oral Mucous Membranes related to decrease in exocrine secretions.
- Constipation related to adverse effect of drug therapy.
- Urinary Retention related to adverse effects of drug therapy.

PLANNING: PATIENT GOALS AND EXPECTED OUTCOMES

The patient will:
- Exhibit a decrease in symptoms for which the medication is prescribed
- Demonstrate an understanding of the drug's action by accurately describing drug adverse effects and precautions
- Verbalize techniques to avoid hazardous adverse effects associated with anticholinergic therapy

continued . . .

NURSING PROCESS FOCUS (continued)

IMPLEMENTATION

Interventions and (Rationales)	Patient Education/Discharge Planning
■ Monitor for signs of anticholinergic crisis resulting from overdosage: fever, tachycardia, difficulty swallowing, ataxia, reduced urine output, psychomotor agitation, confusion, hallucinations.	■ Instruct patients to report adverse effects related to therapy, such as shortness of breath, cough, dysphagia, syncope, fever, anxiety, right upper quadrant pain, extreme lethargy, or dizziness.
■ Report significant changes in heart rate or blood pressure, or development of dysrhythmias.	■ Instruct the patient to monitor vital signs, ensuring proper use of home equipment.
■ Observe for adverse effects such as drowsiness, blurred vision, tachycardia, dry mouth, urinary hesitancy, and decreased sweating.	Instruct the patient to: ■ Report adverse effects ■ Avoid driving and hazardous activities until effects of drugs are known ■ Wear sunglasses to decrease sensitivity to bright light
■ Provide comfort measures for dryness of mucous membranes, such as apply lubricant to moisten lips and oral mucosa, assist in rinsing mouth. Use artificial tears for dry eyes, as needed.	Instruct the patient to: ■ Use oral rinses, sugarless gum or candy, and frequent oral hygiene to help relieve dry mouth ■ Avoid alcohol-containing mouthwashes that can further dry oral tissue
■ Minimize exposure to heat or cold and strenuous exercise. (Anticholinergics can inhibit sweat gland secretions due to direct blockade of the muscarinic receptors on the sweat glands. Sweating is necessary for patients to cool down, so this inhibition of sweating can increase their risk for hyperthermia.)	■ Advise the patient to limit activity outside when the temperature is hot. Strenuous activity in a hot environment may cause heat stroke.
■ Monitor intake and output ratio. Palpate the abdomen for bladder distention.	■ Instruct the patient to notify the health care provider if difficulty in voiding occurs.
■ Monitor patients routinely for abdominal distention, and auscultate for bowel sounds.	■ Advise the patient to increase fluid intake and add bulk to the diet, if constipation becomes a problem.

EVALUATION OF OUTCOME CRITERIA

Evaluate the effectiveness of drug therapy by confirming that patient goals and expected outcomes have been met (see "Planning").

See Table 8.4 for a list of drugs to which these nursing actions apply.

Some sympathomimetics are nonselective, stimulating more than one type of adrenergic receptor. For example, epinephrine stimulates all four types of adrenergic receptors and is used for cardiac arrest and asthma. Pseudoephedrine (Sudafed and others) stimulates both alpha$_1$- and beta$_2$-receptors and is used orally as a nasal decongestant. Isoproterenol (Isuprel) stimulates both beta$_1$- and beta$_2$-receptors and is used to increase the rate, force, and conduction speed of the heart and, occasionally, to treat asthma. The nonselective drugs generally cause more autonomic-related adverse effects.

Some of the more commonly used sympathomimetics are shown in Table 8.5. Most drugs in this class are presented in other chapters of this text. For profiles of drugs in this class, see epinephrine (Adrenalin) and norepinephrine (Levophed) in Chapter 19 ⬤, oxymetazoline (Afrin, others) in Chapter 23 ⬤, and salmeterol (Serevent) in Chapter 27 ⬤.

Concept Review 8.2

■ Why do the sympathomimetics produce many of the same symptoms as the anticholinergics?

TABLE 8.5   Selected Sympathomimetics

DRUG	PRIMARY RECEPTOR SUBTYPE	CLINICAL USE
albuterol (Proventil, Ventolin)	Beta$_2$	Asthma
clonidine (Catapres)	Alpha$_2$ in CNS	Hypertension
dexmedetomidine HCl (Precedex)	Alpha$_2$ in CNS	Sedation
dobutamine (Dobutrex)	Beta$_1$	To stimulate the heart
dopamine (Dopastat, Intropin) (see page 361 for the Drug Profile box)	Alpha$_1$ and beta$_1$	Shock
epinephrine (Adrenalin) (see page 362 for the Drug Profile box)	Alpha and beta	Hypertension, asthma, cardiac arrest
formoterol (Foradil)	Beta$_2$	Asthma, chronic obstructive pulmonary disease (COPD)
isoproterenol (Isuprel)	Beta$_1$ and beta$_2$	Asthma, dysrhythmias, heart failure
metaproterenol (Alupent)	Beta$_2$	Asthma
metaraminol (Aramine)	Alpha$_1$ and beta$_1$	Shock
methyldopa (Aldomet)	Alpha$_2$ in CNS	Hypertension
norepinephrine (Levophed) (see page 361 for the Drug Profile box)	Alpha and beta$_1$	Shock
oxymetazoline (Afrin, others) (see page 492 for the Drug Profile box)	Alpha	Nasal congestion
(Pr) phenylephrine (Neo-Synephrine)	Alpha	Nasal congestion
pseudoephedrine (Sudafed, Afrin, and others)	Alpha and beta	Nasal congestion
ritodrine (Yutopar)	Beta$_2$	To slow uterine contractions
salmeterol (Serevent) (see page 497 for the Drug Profile box)	Beta$_2$	Nasal congestion
terbutaline (Brethine and others)	Beta$_2$	Asthma

DRUG PROFILE: (Pr) *Phenylephrine (Neo-Synephrine)*

Therapeutic Class: Nasal decongestant, mydriatic agent, antihypotensive

Pharmacologic Class: Sympathomimetic, alpha$_1$-adrenergic drug

Actions and Uses:

Phenylephrine is a selective alpha-adrenergic drug that is available in several formulations, including intranasal, ophthalmic, IM, SC, and IV. All of its actions and indications result from sympathetic stimulation. When applied intranasally by spray or drops, it reduces nasal congestion by constricting small blood vessels in the nasal mucosa. Applied topically to the eye during ophthalmic examinations, phenylephrine can dilate the pupil without causing significant paralysis of the eye muscles (cycloplegia). The parenteral administration of phenylephrine can reverse acute hypotension caused by spinal anesthesia or vascular shock. Because it lacks beta-adrenergic activity, it produces relatively few cardiac adverse effects at therapeutic doses. Its longer duration of activity and lack of significant cardiac effects gives phenylephrine some advantages over epinephrine or norepinephrine in treating acute hypotension.

Adverse Effects and Interactions:

When used topically or intranasally, adverse effects are uncommon. Prolonged intranasal use can cause burning of the mucosa and rebound congestion (see Chapter 35 ∞). Ophthalmic preparations can cause narrow-angle glaucoma because of their mydriatic effect. High doses can cause reflex bradycardia due to the elevation of blood pressure caused by stimulation of alpha$_1$-receptors. When given parenterally, the drug should be used with caution in patients with advanced coronary artery disease or hypertension. Anxiety, restlessness, and tremor may occur due to the drug's stimulatory effect on the CNS. Patients with hyperthyroidism may experience a severe increase in basal metabolic rate, resulting in increased blood pressure and tachycardia. Drug interactions may occur with monoamine oxidase (MAO) inhibitors, causing a hypertensive crisis. Increased effects may also occur with tricyclic antidepressants. This drug is incompatible with iron preparations (ferric salts).

Refer to MyNursingKit for a Nursing Process Focus specific to this drug.

NURSING PROCESS FOCUS

Patients Receiving Sympathomimetic Therapy

ASSESSMENT

Prior to administration:
- Determine the reason for drug administration
- Monitor vital signs, urinary output, and cardiac output (initially and throughout therapy)
- For treatment of nasal congestion, assess the nasal mucosa for changes such as excoriation or bleeding
- Obtain a complete health history, including allergies, drug history, and possible drug interactions

POTENTIAL NURSING DIAGNOSES

- Deficient Knowledge related to information about administration and adverse effects of drug therapy.
- Decreased Cardiac Output related to bradycardia (disorder).
- Ineffective Cardiopulmonary Tissue Perfusion related to bronchoconstriction (disorder).
- Risk for Injury related to adverse effects of drug therapy.
- Ineffective Breathing Pattern related to nasal congestion.
- Disturbed Sleep Pattern related to adrenergic stimulation and drug-induced excitation.

PLANNING: PATIENT GOALS AND EXPECTED OUTCOMES

The patient will:
- Exhibit a decrease in symptoms for which the drug is being given
- Demonstrate understanding of the drug's action by accurately describing drug adverse effects and precautions
- Demonstrate proper nasal/ophthalmic medication instillation technique

IMPLEMENTATION

Interventions and (Rationales)	Patient Education/Discharge Planning
<ul><li>Closely monitor IV insertion sites for extravasation with IV administration. Use an infusion pump to deliver medication.</li><li>Use a tuberculin syringe when administering SC doses that are extremely small.</li><li>For metered-dose inhalation, shake the container well, and wait at least 2 minutes between medications.</li><li>Instill only the prescribed number of drops when using ophthalmic solutions.</li></ul>	Instruct the patient to:<ul><li>Use the drug as prescribed and not "double up" on doses</li><li>Take the medication early in the day to avoid insomnia</li></ul>
<ul><li>Monitor the patient for adverse effects. (Adverse effects of sympathomimetics may be serious and limit therapy.)</li></ul>	Instruct the patient to:<ul><li>Immediately report shortness of breath, palpitations, dizziness, chest/arm pain or pressure, or other angina-like symptoms</li><li>Consult the health care provider before attempting to use sympathomimetics to treat nasal congestion or eye irritation</li><li>Monitor blood pressure, pulse, and temperature to ensure proper use of home equipment</li></ul>
<ul><li>Monitor breathing patterns and observe for shortness of breath and/or audible wheezing.</li><li>Observe the patient's responsiveness to light. (Some sympathomimetics cause photosensitivity by affecting the pupillary light accommodation/response.)</li><li>Provide eye comfort by reducing exposure to direct bright light in the environment; shield the eyes with a rolled washcloth or eye bandages for severe photosensitivity.</li></ul>	<ul><li>Instruct the patient to immediately report any difficulty breathing. Instruct the patient with a history of asthma to consult a health care provider before using over-the-counter (OTC) drugs to treat nasal stuffiness.</li><li>Instruct patients using ophthalmic sympathomimetics that transient stinging and blurred vision on instillation is normal. Headache and/or brow pain may also occur.</li><li>Instruct the patient to avoid driving and other activities requiring visual acuity until blurring subsides.</li></ul>
<ul><li>For patients receiving nasal sympathomimetics, observe the nasal cavity. Monitor for rhinorrhea and epistaxis.</li></ul>	Instruct the patient to:<ul><li>Observe the nasal cavity for signs of excoriation or bleeding before instilling nasal spray or drops; review procedure for safe instillation of nasal sprays or eyedrops</li><li>Limit usage of OTC sympathomimetics; inform the patient about rebound nasal congestion</li></ul>

EVALUATION OF OUTCOME CRITERIA

Evaluate the effectiveness of drug therapy by confirming that patient goals and expected outcomes have been met (see "Planning").

See Table 8.5 for a list of drugs to which these nursing actions apply.

Adrenergic blockers are primarily used to treat hypertension and are the most widely prescribed class of autonomic drugs.

Adrenergic blockers inhibit the actions of the sympathetic nervous system. These drugs produce many of the same responses as the parasympathomimetics, but they are more widely used. Because the sympathetic nervous system has alpha- and beta-subreceptors, the actions of adrenergic blockers are specific and have wide therapeutic application. In fact, they are the most widely prescribed class of autonomic drugs. Some of the adrenergic blockers are shown in Table 8.6.

Alpha-adrenergic blockers, or simply *alpha blockers*, are primarily used for their effects on vascular smooth muscle. By relaxing vascular smooth muscle in small arteries, alpha$_1$-blockers such as doxazosin (Cardura) cause vasodilation, which results in decreased blood pressure. Their primary use is in the treatment of hypertension, either alone or in combination with other drugs.

Some drugs in this class selectively block beta$_1$-receptors. Because beta$_1$-receptors are only present in the heart, the effects of drugs such as atenolol (Tenormin) are often called *cardioselective*. By slowing the heart rate, they lower blood pressure, which is their primary use.

Some beta blockers, such as propranolol (Inderal, InnoPran XL), are nonselective, blocking both beta$_1$- and beta$_2$-receptors. The nonselective beta blockers are used to treat hypertension, angina, and cardiac rhythm abnormalities. Their nonselective actions generally result in more adverse effects than the selective beta blockers. Profiles of adrenergic blockers can be found for doxazosin (Cardura) in Chapter 17 ⬤, propranolol (Inderal, InnoPran XL) in Chapter 19 ⬤, and atenolol (Tenormin) and metoprolol (Lopressor) in Chapter 20 ⬤.

Concept Review   8.3

■ Both parasympathomimetics and adrenergic blockers produce similar actions. Why are adrenergic blockers used to treat hypertension, but parasympathomimetics are not used for this purpose?

TABLE 8.6	**Selected Adrenergic Blockers (Sympatholytics)**	
DRUG	**PRIMARY RECEPTOR SUBTYPE**	**CLINICAL USE**
acebutolol (Sectral)	Beta$_1$	Hypertension, dysrhythmias, angina
atenolol (Tenormin) (see page 345 for the Drug Profile box)	Beta$_1$	Hypertension and angina
carteolol (Cartrol)	Beta$_1$ and beta$_2$	Hypertension and glaucoma
carvedilol (Coreg) (see page 300 for the Drug Profile box)	Alpha$_1$, beta$_1$, and beta$_2$	Hypertension
doxazocin (Cardura)	Alpha$_1$	Hypertension
esmolol (Brevibloc)	Beta$_1$	Hypertension and dysrhythmias
metoprolol (Lopressor)	Beta$_1$	Hypertension, heart failure, myocardial infarction (MI)
nadolol (Corgard)	Beta$_1$ and beta$_2$	Hypertension
phentolamine (Regitine)	Alpha	Severe hypertension
Pr prazosin (Minipress)	Alpha$_1$	Hypertension
propranolol (Inderal, InnoPran XL) (see page 314 for the Drug Profile box)	Beta$_1$ and beta$_2$	Dysrhythmias, hypertension, migraines, angina
sotalol (Betapace)	Beta$_1$ and beta$_2$	Dysrhythmias
tamsulosin (Flomax)	Alpha$_1$	Benign prostatic hypertrophy
terazosin (Hytrin)	Alpha$_1$	Hypertension
timolol (Blocadren, Timoptic XE) (see page 637 for the Drug Profile box)	Beta$_1$ and beta$_2$	Hypertension, angina, glaucoma

DRUG PROFILE: Pr *Prazosin (Minipress)*

Therapeutic Class: Antihypertensive

Pharmacologic Class: Sympatholytic, alpha$_1$-adrenergic blocker

Actions and Uses:

Prazosin is a selective alpha$_1$-adrenergic blocker that competes with NE at its receptors on vascular smooth muscle in arterioles and veins. Its major action is a rapid decrease in peripheral resistance that reduces blood pressure. It has little effect on cardiac output or heart rate, and it causes less reflex tachycardia than some other drugs in this class. Tolerance may occur to its antihypertensive effect. Its most common use is in combination with other drugs, such as beta blockers or diuretics, in the pharmacotherapy of hypertension. Prazosin has a short half-life and is often taken two or three times per day.

Adverse Effects and Interactions:

Like other alpha blockers, prazosin has a tendency to cause orthostatic hypotension due to alpha$_1$-inhibition in vascular smooth muscle. In rare cases, this hypotension can be so severe as to cause unconsciousness about 30 minutes after the first dose. This is called the *first-dose phenomenon*. To avoid this situation, the first dose should be very low and given at bedtime. Dizziness, drowsiness, or lightheadedness may occur as a result of decreased blood flow to the brain due to the drug's hypotensive action. Reflex tachycardia may occur due to the rapid falls in blood pressure. The alpha blockade may also result in nasal congestion or inhibition of ejaculation.

Drug interactions include increased hypotensive effects with concurrent use of antihypertensives and diuretics.

Refer to MyNursingKit for a Nursing Process Focus specific to this drug.

NURSING PROCESS FOCUS

Patients Receiving Adrenergic Blocker Therapy

ASSESSMENT

Prior to administration:
- Assess vital signs, urinary output, and cardiac output (initially and throughout therapy)
- Assess the reason for drug administration
- Obtain a complete health history, including allergies, drug history, and possible drug interactions

POTENTIAL NURSING DIAGNOSES

- Deficient Knowledge related to information about drug therapy.
- Disturbed Sensory Perception related to hypotensive action of drug.
- Risk for Injury related to dizziness, syncope.
- Impaired Urinary Elimination (frequency) related to adverse effects of drug therapy.
- Sexual Dysfunction related to adverse effects of drug therapy.

PLANNING: PATIENT GOALS AND EXPECTED OUTCOMES

The patient will:
- Exhibit a decrease in blood pressure with fewer adverse effects
- Report a decrease in urinary symptoms such as hesitancy and difficulty voiding
- Demonstrate an understanding of the drug's action by accurately describing drug adverse effects and precautions and importance of follow-up care

continued . . .

NURSING PROCESS FOCUS *(continued)*

IMPLEMENTATION

Interventions and (Rationales)	Patient Education/Discharge Planning
■ In patients with prostatic hypertrophy, monitor for urinary hesitancy/feeling of incomplete bladder emptying, and interrupted urinary stream.	■ Instruct the patient to report increased difficulty with urination to a health care provider.
■ Monitor for syncope. (Alpha-adrenergic blockers produce first-dose syncope phenomenon and may cause loss of consciousness.)	Instruct the patient to: ■ Take this medication at bedtime, and to take the first dose *immediately* before getting into bed ■ Avoid abrupt changes in position; warn the patient about first-dose phenomenon and reassure that this effect diminishes with continued therapy
■ Monitor vital signs (especially blood pressure), level of consciousness, and mood. (Adrenergic blockers can exacerbate existing mental depression.)	■ Instruct the patient to immediately report any feelings of dysphoria. ■ Interview the patient regarding suicide potential; obtain a "no-self harm" verbal contract from the patient.
■ Monitor carefully for dizziness, drowsiness, or lightheadedness. (These are signs of decreased blood flow to the brain due to the drug's hypotensive action.)	Instruct the patient: ■ To monitor vitals signs, especially blood pressure, ensuring proper use of home equipment ■ Regarding the normotensive range of blood pressure; instruct the patient to consult the nurse regarding "reportable" blood pressure readings ■ To report dizziness or syncope that persists beyond the first dose, as well as paresthesia and other neurologic changes
■ Observe for adverse effects that may include blurred vision, tinnitus, epistaxis, and edema.	Inform the patient: ■ That nasal congestion may be an adverse effect ■ To report any adverse reactions to the health care provider ■ About the potential danger of concomitant use of OTC nasal decongestants
Interventions and (Rationales)	**Patient Education/Discharge Planning**
■ Monitor liver function (because of increased risk for liver toxicity).	Instruct the patient: ■ To adhere to a regular schedule of laboratory testing for liver function as ordered by the health care provider ■ To report signs and symptoms of liver toxicity: nausea, vomiting, diarrhea, rash, jaundice, abdominal pain, tenderness or distention, or change in color of stool ■ About importance of ongoing medication compliance and follow-up

EVALUATION OF OUTCOME CRITERIA

Evaluate the effectiveness of drug therapy by confirming that patient goals and expected outcomes have been met (see "Planning").

See Table 8.6 for a list of drugs to which these nursing actions apply.

PATIENTS NEED TO KNOW

Patients treated with autonomic medications need to know the following:

In General

1. Do not take any OTC cold, cough, or sinus drugs without seeking medical advice because these likely contain autonomic drugs.
2. Report any palpitations, shortness of breath, chest pain, or large changes in blood pressure immediately to a health care provider. Some of the most significant adverse effects of autonomic drugs relate to the cardiovascular system.
3. Notify a health care provider before taking autonomic drugs if the following conditions are present: thyroid disease, diabetes mellitus, dysrhythmias, or hypertension. Such medications have the potential to cause serious adverse effects in individuals with these conditions.
4. Move slowly when changing from a supine to an upright position to avoid dizziness and perhaps fainting. Many of the autonomic medications affect blood pressure.
5. Notify a health care provider if any significant change in bowel habits or abdominal cramping/constipation occurs after taking autonomic drugs.
6. Inform a health care provider before taking anticholinergic drugs if urinating difficulty is present or if the diagnosis of benign prostatic hypertrophy (BPH) has been made.
7. Chew gum or suck on hard candies if dry mouth is experienced when taking autonomic drugs. Proper oral hygiene is important to avoid dental caries.

Regarding Adrenergic Blockers

8. Do not discontinue the use of beta blockers abruptly because doing so can result in chest pain or rebound hypertension.
9. Alpha blockers can sometimes cause impotence as an adverse effect. If there are difficulties with ejaculation, notify a health care provider so that other drug options can be explored.

CHAPTER REVIEW

CORE CONCEPTS SUMMARY

8.1 **The nervous system is divided into central and peripheral components.**

The central nervous system consists of the brain and spinal cord. The peripheral nervous system consists of a sensory portion and a motor portion. Outgoing motor signals are characterized as voluntary (somatic) or involuntary (autonomic).

8.2 **The autonomic nervous system has sympathetic and parasympathetic branches.**

Stimulation of sympathetic nerves causes symptoms of the fight-or-flight response. Stimulation of parasympathetic nerves induces the rest-and-digest response. With few exceptions, the actions of the two divisions oppose each other.

8.3 **Synapses are common sites of drug action.**

Synapses consist of a presynaptic nerve and a postsynaptic nerve with a space between them called the synaptic cleft. Neurotransmitters cross this synaptic cleft to regenerate the nerve impulse.

8.4 **Acetylcholine and norepinephrine are the two primary neurotransmitters in the autonomic nervous system.**

Acetylcholine is the neurotransmitter at the end of all presynaptic nerves (ganglia), at sweat glands, and in skeletal muscle. Acetylcholine receptors may be nicotinic or muscarinic. Norepinephrine is the neurotransmitter at the organ level in the sympathetic nervous system. Norepinephrine receptors may be alpha or beta subtypes.

8.5 **Autonomic drugs are classified according to the receptors they stimulate or block.**

Sympathomimetics stimulate sympathetic nerves, and parasympathomimetics primarily stimulate parasympathetic nerves. Adrenergic blockers inhibit the sympathetic division, whereas cholinergic blockers mostly inhibit the parasympathetic branch.

8.6 **Parasympathomimetics have few therapeutic uses because of their numerous adverse effects.**

Parasympathomimetics are used to treat glaucoma and to stimulate the urinary or digestive tracts following general anesthesia. Toxic nerve agents are parasympathomimetics, producing harmful effects in the body.

8.7 **Anticholinergics are mainly used to dry secretions and to treat asthma.**

The use of cholinergic blockers has declined due to their numerous adverse effects. They are used to dry secretions, dilate the bronchi, and dilate the pupils.

8.8 **Sympathomimetics are primarily used for their effects on the heart, bronchial tree, and nasal passages.**

Sympathomimetics may stimulate one or several subtypes of adrenergic receptors. Uses include increasing the heart rate, dilating the bronchi, and drying excess secretions caused by colds.

8.9 **Adrenergic blockers are primarily used to treat hypertension and are the most widely prescribed class of autonomic drugs.**

Adrenergic blockers are the most commonly prescribed autonomic medications. They may be selective for only one receptor subtype, such as the $beta_1$-blockers, or inhibit several subtypes. Hypertension is their primary indication.

REVIEW QUESTIONS

The following questions are written in NCLEX-PN® style. Answer these questions to assess your knowledge of the chapter material, and go back and review any material that is not clear to you.

1. The nurse recognizes that which of the following drugs is contraindicated in patients with glaucoma?

1. Sotalol (Betapace)
2. Betaxolol HCl (Betoptic)
3. Timolol (Timoptic)
4. Atropine

2. The patient diagnosed with glaucoma would most likely be prescribed which of the following drugs?

1. Adrenergic drugs
2. Cholinergic drugs
3. Adrenergic blockers
4. Cholinergic blockers

3. The nurse teaches the patient that rebound congestion can occur with long-term use of this sympathomimetic.

1. Albuterol (Proventil)
2. Ritodrine (Yutopar)
3. Salmeterol (Serevent)
4. Phenylephrine (Neo-Synephrine)

4. The patient is diagnosed with urinary bladder urgency and incontinence. The nurse recognizes which of the following anticholinergics as being appropriate for this condition?

1. Dicyclomine (Bentyl)
2. Ipratropium (Atrovent)
3. Oxybutynin (Ditropan)
4. Scopolamine (Transderm-Scop)

5. Alpha$_1$-adrenergic blockers cause what to occur in the body?

1. Vasoconstriction and increased blood pressure
2. Vasodilation and decreased blood pressure

3. Bronchodilation
4. Increased heart rate and cardiac output

6. Metoprolol (Lopressor) is classified as a(n):

1. Alpha blocker
2. Beta blocker
3. Cholinergic
4. Anticholinergic

7. Prior to administering atenolol (Tenormin), the nurse should assess:

1. Respirations and blood pressure
2. Respirations and heart rate
3. Heart rate and blood pressure
4. Temperature and blood pressure

8. The body's response to stimulation of this autonomic receptor is increased heart rate and force of contraction and release of renin.

1. Muscarinic
2. Beta$_1$
3. Alpha$_1$
4. Beta$_2$

9. The patient given bethanechol (Urecholine) must be assessed for:

1. Increased heart rate
2. Hypertension
3. Fluid overload
4. Dehydration

10. Anticholinergic drugs would be suspected for which of the following patient complaints?

1. Diaphoresis
2. Confusion
3. Dry mouth
4. Increased urination

CASE STUDY QUESTIONS

For questions 1–4, please refer to the following case studies, and choose the correct answer from choices 1–4.

*M*rs. Wheaton, a 74-year-old woman, has been having problems with nonobstructive urinary retention following surgery, a retropubic urethral suspension. She required a Foley catheter for 4 days but was unable to void after removal of the catheter. The physician ordered bethanechol (Urecholine) for Mrs. Wheaton.

1. Why would the physician order this medication for Mrs. Wheaton?

1. It causes the kidneys to produce more urine, which increases the pressure within the bladder, forcing her to urinate.
2. It inhibits smooth muscle contractions, causing the bladder to relax.
3. It stimulates smooth muscle contractions, causing the bladder to function normally.
4. It decreases the amount of urine produced in the kidneys so as not to put as much pressure on the bladder.

2. What should Mrs. Wheaton be aware of when taking bethanechol? (Select all that apply.)

1. No adverse effects are significant to report when taking this medication.
2. To avoid abrupt position changes.
3. That vision may become blurred.
4. To be near a bathroom after taking this medication.

Mrs. Lopez has been diagnosed with severe hypertension.

3. Which of the following drugs might she be prescribed?

1. Ipratropium (Atrovent)
2. Salmeterol (Serevent)
3. Prazosin (Minipress)
4. Phenylephrine (Neo-Synephrine)

4. Which class(es) of drugs effectively reverse Mrs. Lopez's hypertension?

1. Parasympathomimetics and anticholinergics
2. Sympathomimetics
3. Sympathomimetics and cholinergics
4. Adrenergic blockers

FURTHER STUDY

- Direct-acting parasympathomimetics that are used in ophthalmology are discussed in Chapter 35 ⚭ .

- See Chapter 29 ⚭ for information on proton-pump inhibitors and H_2-receptor blockers.

- Additional information about several sympathomimetics is provided in Chapter 22 ⚭ (epinephrine and norepinephrine), Chapter 28 ⚭ (oxymetazoline), and Chapter 28 ⚭ (salmeterol).

- Certain adrenergic blockers are also featured in Chapter 17 ⚭ (doxazosin), Chapter 19 ⚭ (propranolol), and Chapter 21 ⚭ (atenolol and metoprolol).

9 Drugs for Anxiety and Insomnia

CORE CONCEPTS

9.1 Anxiety disorders fall into several categories.

9.2 Specific regions of the brain are responsible for anxiety and wakefulness.

9.3 Anxiety is managed with both pharmacologic and nonpharmacologic strategies.

9.4 An inability to sleep is linked with anxiety.

9.5 Anxiety and insomnia are treated with many types of central nervous system (CNS) agents.

9.6 When taken properly, antidepressants reduce symptoms of panic and anxiety.

9.7 Benzodiazepines are useful for the short-term treatment of anxiety and insomnia.

9.8 Barbiturates depress CNS function and cause drowsiness.

9.9 Additional drugs provide therapy for anxiety-related symptoms and sleep disorders.

DRUG SNAPSHOT

The following drugs are discussed in this chapter:

DRUG CLASSES	DRUG PROFILES
Antidepressants	
Benzodiazepines	(Pr) lorazepam (Ativan)
Barbiturates	
Nonbenzodiazepine, Nonbarbiturate CNS Agents	(Pr) zolpidem (Ambien)

LEARNING OUTCOMES

After reading this chapter, the student should be able to:

1. Identify the major categories of anxiety disorders.

2. Discuss factors contributing to anxiety, and explain some nonpharmacologic therapies used to cope with this disorder.

3. Identify the four categories of CNS agents used to treat anxiety and sleep disorders.

4. Explain the pharmacologic management of anxiety and insomnia.

5. Categorize drugs used for anxiety and insomnia based on their classification and mechanism of action.

6. For each of the classes listed in the Drug Snapshot, know representative drugs and explain their related clinical uses.

KEY TERMS

Patients experience nervousness and tension more often than any other symptoms. Seeking relief from these symptoms, patients often turn to a variety of pharmacologic and alternative therapies. Most health care providers agree that even though drugs do not cure the underlying problem, they can provide short-term help to calm patients who are experiencing acute anxiety or who have simple sleep disorders. This chapter discusses drugs that treat anxiety, cause sedation, or help patients sleep.

ANXIETY

According to the *International Classification of Diseases,* 10th edition (ICD-10), **anxiety** is a state of "apprehension, tension, or uneasiness that stems from the anticipation of danger, the source of which is largely unknown or unrecognized." Based on actual events or circumstances, people admit that feelings of anxiety are greater than what they should experience. Anxious individuals often have trouble dealing with the factors that bring on their symptoms.

Anxiety disorders fall into several categories.

CORE CONCEPT 9.1

The anxiety experienced by people faced with a stressful environment or situations is called *situational anxiety.* To a certain degree, situational anxiety is beneficial because it motivates people to accomplish tasks in a prompt manner—if for no other reason than to end the source of nervousness. Situational stress may be intense, but many people often learn to cope with this kind of stress without seeking conventional medical intervention.

Generalized anxiety disorder (GAD) is difficult-to-control, excessive anxiety that lasts 6 months or more. It occurs in response to a variety of life events or activities, and it interferes with normal, day-to-day functions. It is by far the most common type of stress disorder routinely observed by health care providers. Symptoms include restlessness, fatigue, muscle tension, nervousness, inability to focus or concentrate, an overwhelming sense of dread, and sleep disturbances. Autonomic signs of sympathetic nervous system activation involve sweating, blood pressure elevation, heart palpitations, varying degrees of respiratory change, and dry mouth. Parasympathetic responses may involve abdominal cramping, diarrhea, and urinary urgency. Additional motor symptoms experienced by the patient may include increased reflexes and numbness and tingling of the extremities. Females are slightly more likely to experience GAD, and its prevalence is highest in those ages 20 to 35.

A second category of anxiety, called **panic disorder**, is characterized by intense feelings of immediate apprehension, fearfulness, terror, or impending doom, accompanied by increased autonomic nervous system activity. Although panic attacks usually last less than 10 minutes, patients

Fast Facts Anxiety Disorders

- Millions of Americans experience anxiety every year.
- Other illnesses commonly coexist with anxiety, including depression, eating disorders, and substance abuse.
- The top five causes of anxiety affecting people between the ages of 18 and 54 are:
  - Phobias
    - Over 19.2 million Americans have some type of specific phobia.
    - Specific phobias usually begin in childhood and lasts for many years.
    - Over 15 million Americans have *social phobia*.
    - Over 1.8 million Americans have *agoraphobia*, an intense fear of crowds.
  - Post-traumatic stress disorder (PTSD)
    - Over 7.7 million Americans have PTSD.
    - PTSD can develop at any age.
  - Generalized anxiety disorder (GAD)
    - Over 6.8 million Americans are diagnosed with GAD in a given year.
    - Generalized anxiety symptoms usually begin in an individual's early 30s.
  - Panic
    - Over 6 million Americans have panic disorder.
    - About one third of Americans with panic disorder have phobic tendencies.
  - Obsessive-compulsive disorder (OCD)
    - Over 2.2 million Americans have OCD.
    - The first symptoms of OCD usually begin in the late teenage years.
- For details, see the National Institutes of Mental Health Web site: http://www.nimh.nih.gov/.

may describe them as seemingly endless. As many as 5% of the population will experience one or more panic attacks during their lifetimes, and women are affected about twice as often as men.

phobia = *fear*

Other categories of anxiety disorders include phobias, post-traumatic stress disorder, and obsessive-compulsive disorder. **Phobias** are fearful feelings attached to specific objects or situations. Examples include elevators, heights, and crowds. Attacks may occur when a person feels trapped, embarrassed, or unable to escape. Fear of crowds or *agoraphobia* is a form of *social anxiety*. Feeling nervous before a recital, an athletic event, or sexual intimacy is a form of *performance anxiety*. Experiencing signs of anxiety in a crowd or feeling anxious just before an event may be normal, but feeling *extreme* fear to the point at which the person avoids the situation altogether is not normal.

Post-traumatic stress disorder (PTSD) is a type of anxiety that develops in response to reexperiencing a previous traumatic life event such as combat experience, physical or sexual abuse, a natural disaster, or a murder. The person may dream about the event or be constantly reminded of the event by common everyday occurrences. This reexperiencing of the trauma leads to feelings of helplessness and anxiety that affect the person's ability to function normally.

Obsessive-compulsive disorder (OCD) describes recurrent, disturbing thoughts or repetitive behaviors that interfere with a person's normal activities or relationships. For example, a person may have a fear of being exposed to germs. This fear may eventually lead the person to wash his or her hands over and over. After some time, this handwashing may be done so frequently that the person is unable to perform regular activities of life.

Specific regions of the brain are responsible for anxiety and wakefulness.

CORE CONCEPT 9.2

Anxiety and restlessness are associated with the limbic system and the reticular activating system. The **limbic system** is an area of the brain that is responsible for emotional expression, learning, and memory. Signals routed through the limbic system connect with the hypothalamus. Emotional states associated with this connection include anxiety, fear, anger, aggression, remorse, depression, appetite, sexual drive, and euphoria.

The hypothalamus is an important center that triggers unconscious responses to extreme stress, such as increased blood pressure, elevated breathing rate, and dilated pupils. These are responses associated with the fight-or-flight response of the autonomic nervous system (see Chapter 8 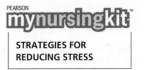). The endocrine functions of the hypothalamus are discussed in Chapter 31 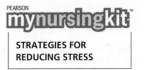 .

The hypothalamus also connects with the **reticular formation**, a network of neurons found along the entire length of the brainstem. Stimulation of the reticular formation causes increased alertness and arousal; inhibition causes drowsiness and sleep.

The larger area in which the reticular formation is found is called the **reticular activating system (RAS)**. The RAS controls sleeping and wakefulness and performs an alerting function for the cerebral cortex. It also helps a person focus attention on individual tasks by transmitting information to higher brain centers. The RAS is the neural mechanism thought to be responsible for emotions such as anxiety and fear. It is also the mechanism associated with restlessness and an interrupted sleeping pattern.

Anxiety is managed with both pharmacologic and nonpharmacologic strategies.

CORE CONCEPT 9.3

Although stress itself may be incapacitating, it is often only a symptom of an underlying disorder. Uncovering and addressing the cause of the anxiety is more productive than merely treating the symptoms with medications. Patients should be encouraged to explore and develop nonpharmacologic coping strategies to deal with the underlying causes. Such strategies may include behavioral therapy, biofeedback techniques, meditation, and other complementary therapies. One model for anxiety management is shown in Figure 9.1 ■.

When anxiety becomes severe enough to significantly interfere with daily activities of life, pharmacotherapy is indicated. In most types of stress, **anxiolytics**, or drugs having the ability to relieve anxiety, are quite effective. These include medications in a number of therapeutic categories, involving drugs for depression (see Chapter 10 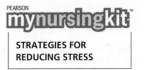), seizures (see Chapter 13 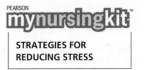), and cardiovascular disorders (see Chapter 17 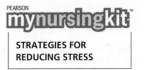). Anxiolytics provide treatment for GAD, panic disorder, phobias, PTSD, and OCD.

PEARSON
mynursingkit

STRATEGIES FOR
REDUCING STRESS

anxio = *anxiety*
lytic = *to dissolve away; break*

Concept Review   9.1

■ What does the term *anxiolytic* mean? What disorders do anxiolytic drugs treat?

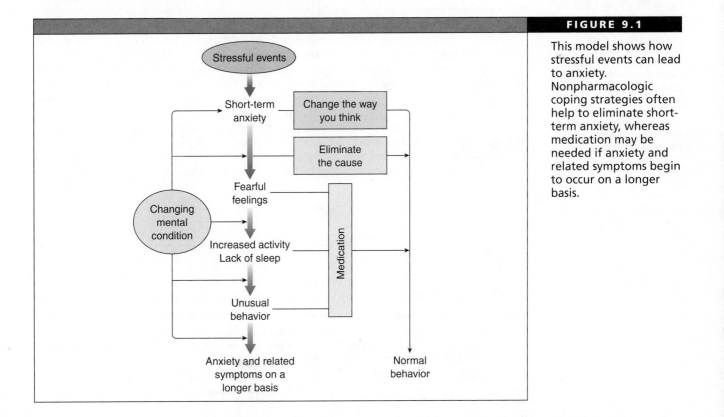

FIGURE 9.1

This model shows how stressful events can lead to anxiety. Nonpharmacologic coping strategies often help to eliminate short-term anxiety, whereas medication may be needed if anxiety and related symptoms begin to occur on a longer basis.

INSOMNIA

Insomnia is a condition characterized by a patient's inability to fall asleep or remain asleep. Pharmacotherapy may be needed if the sleeplessness interferes with normal daily activities.

CORE CONCEPT 9.4

An inability to sleep is linked with anxiety.

PEARSON
mynursingkit

STAGES OF SLEEP

PEARSON
mynursingkit

NATIONAL CENTER ON
SLEEP DISORDERS
RESEARCH

Why is it that we need sleep? During an average lifetime, about 33% of our time is spent sleeping or trying to sleep. Insufficient sleep is associated with increased workplace and driving accidents. Although it is well established that sleep is essential for wellness, scientists are unsure of its function or how much is needed. Following are some theories:

- Inactivity during sleep gives the body time to repair itself.
- Sleep is a function that evolved as a protective mechanism. Throughout history, nighttime was the safest time of day.
- Sleep deals with "electrical" charging and discharging of the brain. The brain needs time for processing and filing new information collected throughout the day. When this is done without interference from the environment, these vast amounts of data can later be retrieved through memory.

The acts of sleeping and waking are synchronized with many different bodily functions. Body temperature, blood pressure, hormone levels, and respiration fluctuate cyclically throughout the 24-hour day. When this cycle is impaired, pharmacologic and other interventions may be needed to readjust it. Increased levels of the neurotransmitter serotonin help initiate the various processes of sleep.

Insomnia, or sleeplessness, is a disorder associated with anxiety. There are several major types of insomnia. *Short-term* or *behavioral insomnia* may be attributed to stress caused by a hectic lifestyle or the inability to resolve day-to-day conflicts within the home or workplace. Worries about work, marriage, children, and health are common reasons for short-term sleep loss. When stress interrupts normal sleeping patterns, patients cannot sleep because their minds are too active. *Long-term insomnia* may be caused by more intense emotional and mood-related illnesses such as depression, manic disorders, or chronic pain.

Foods or beverages containing stimulants such as caffeine may interrupt sleep. Patients may also find that using tobacco products makes them restless and edgy. Alcohol, although often enabling a person to fall asleep, may produce vivid dreams and frequent awakening that prevent restful sleep. Eating a large meal—especially one high in protein and fat—close to bedtime may interfere with sleep because metabolism increases to digest the food. Certain medications cause CNS stimulation, and these should not be taken immediately before bedtime. Stressful conditions—for example, too much light, an uncomfortable room temperature (especially one that is too warm), snoring, sleep apnea, and recurring nightmares—also interfere with sleep.

Nonpharmacologic means of relieving insomnia are usually tried before drug therapy, because long-term use of sleep medications will likely worsen insomnia and may cause physical or

▶ **Life Span Fact**

Older patients are more likely to experience medication-related sleep problems. For the first night or two, drugs may seem to help the insomnia of an elderly patient, but as the medication accumulates in the system, it produces generalized brain dysfunction. The agitated patient may then be mistakenly overdosed with further medication.

Fast Facts Insomnia

- One third of the world's population has trouble sleeping during part of the year.
- Insomnia is more common in women than in men.
- Patients older than 65 years old sleep less than patients in any other age group.
- Only about 70% of people with insomnia ever report this problem to their health care provider.
- People buy over-the-counter (OTC) sleep medications and combination drugs with sleep additives more than any other drug category. Trade name products include Anacin P.M., Exedrin P.M., Nytol, Quiet World, Sleep-Fez, Sominex, Tylenol P.M., and Unisom.
- As a natural alternative for sleep, some people take melatonin, kava kava, or valerian.

psychological dependence. Some patients experience a phenomenon called **rebound insomnia**. This effect occurs when a sedative drug is stopped abruptly or when it has been taken for a long time and drug dependence occurs. Alcohol abuse can also cause rebound insomnia.

Concept Review	9.2

■ Why might a patient not be able to enjoy normal sleep? Why is long-term drug therapy for lack of sleep not a good idea?

Anxiety and insomnia are treated with many types of central nervous system (CNS) agents.

CORE CONCEPT 9.5

CNS agents are used to alter brain activity in patients with anxiety or sleep disorders. These medications are grouped into four major classes: (1) antidepressants, (2) benzodiazepines, (3) barbiturates, and (4) nonbarbiturate and nonbenzodiazepine CNS agents.

Antidepressants have an ability to enhance mood by altering the levels of two important neurotransmitters in the brain—norepinephrine and serotonin. By restoring the balance of these neurotransmitters, antidepressants can reduce the symptoms associated with depression, panic, obsessive-compulsive behavior, and phobia. Antidepressants used to treat anxiety and insomnia include selective serotonin reuptake inhibitors (SSRIs), serotonin–norepinephrine reuptake inhibitors (SNRIs), atypical antidepressants, tricyclic antidepressants (TCAs), and monoamine oxidase inhibitors (MAOIs). Use of the latter two types of drugs has declined in recent years. The mechanisms of action and important considerations of these drugs are covered in Chapter 10 ⊂⊃ .

Another approach to relieving anxiety is the use of **CNS depressants** that slow neuronal activity in the brain. These drugs range from those that relax to those that sedate to those that cause sleep and anesthesia. Coma and death are the end stages of CNS depression. Some drug classes can produce the full range of CNS depression from relaxation to full anesthesia, whereas others are less effective across this range. Medications that depress the CNS are sometimes called **sedatives** because of their ability to sedate or relax a patient. At higher doses, many of the same drugs can cause sleep and therefore are called *hypnotics*. The term **sedative-hypnotic** is often used to describe a drug with the ability to produce a calming effect at lower doses and sleep at higher doses. *Tranquilizer* is an older term used to describe a drug that produces a calm or tranquil feeling.

CNS depressants used for anxiety and sleep disorders are categorized into two major classes: benzodiazepines and barbiturates. An additional category consists of miscellaneous drugs chemically unrelated to the other drug groups. These have additional therapeutic usefulness in the treatment of anxiety-related symptoms and insomnia:

- Buspirone (BuSpar), a mild tranquilizer
- Valproate (Depakote), an antiseizure medication
- Atenolol (Tenormin) and propranolol (Inderal, InnoPran XL), beta blockers to reduce stress
- Eszopiclone (Lunesta), zolpidem (Ambien), and zaleplon (Sonata), sleep disorder medications that directly activate benzodiazepine receptors in the brain
- Ramelteon (Rozerem), medication that activates melatonin receptors in the brain
- Diphenhydramine (Nytol and Sominex) and doxylamine (Unisom), OTC antihistamine sleep aids

As discussed in Chapter 7 ⊂⊃ , long-term use of many CNS depressants can lead to physical or psychological dependence. The withdrawal syndrome for some CNS depressants can cause life-threatening neurologic reactions, including fever, psychosis, and seizures. Other withdrawal symptoms include increased heart rate and lowered blood pressure; loss of appetite; muscle cramps; impaired memory, concentration, and orientation; abnormal sounds in the ears and blurred vision; and insomnia, agitation, anxiety, and panic. Noticeable withdrawal symptoms typically last 2 to 4 weeks. Subtle ones can last months.

Concept Review	9.3

■ Describe what each of the following terms means in relation to anxiety and alertness: *CNS depressants, sedatives, hypnotics, sedative-hypnotics,* and *tranquilizers.*

PEARSON
mynursingkit™
ANXIETY SELF-HELP WEB SITE

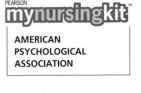

PEARSON
mynursingkit™
AMERICAN PSYCHOLOGICAL ASSOCIATION

CORE CONCEPT 9.6

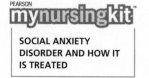

NATIONAL INSTITUTE OF MENTAL HEALTH

When taken properly, antidepressants reduce symptoms of panic and anxiety.

In the 1960s, antidepressants were mainly used for the treatment of depression or depression that occurred with anxiety. Today, antidepressants are used not only to treat major depressive disorder (see Chapter 10 ⬤), but also symptoms of anxiety associated with panic disorder, OCD, social phobia, and PTSD. Because many of the features observed in patients with depressive disorder overlap with anxiety disorders, methods of intervention are often the same.

For most patients, panic symptoms come in two stages. The first stage is called *anticipatory anxiety,* when the patient begins to think about an upcoming challenge and starts to feel dread. The second stage is when physical symptoms such as shortness of breath, rapid heart rate, and muscle tension begin. Many of the stressful symptoms are associated with activation of the autonomic nervous system. The strategy in treating panic attacks is to help the patient face the fear and suppress symptoms during one or more of these stages. Drugs can lessen the negative thoughts associated with anticipating the panic, thereby reducing the stress. Drugs also decrease neuronal activity and suppress functions of the autonomic nervous system, helping the patient to remain calm. The patient can then use self-help skills to control behavior.

Antidepressants are often used to reduce symptoms of panic and anxiety. These medications are summarized in Table 9.1. SSRIs, SNRIs, and atypical antidepressants not only treat panic symptoms but also treat symptoms of PTSD, OCD, and phobias. SSRIs and SNRIs produce fewer major adverse effects than the TCAs or MAOIs.

As with all CNS agents, precautions must be taken to make sure that medications are effective. Because of adverse reactions, some patients might find antidepressant treatment unacceptable. In 2004, the Food and Drug Administration issued an advisory warning (**black box warning**) pointing out the potential warning signs of suicide in adults and children when doses are changed and at the beginning of antidepressant therapy. In the course of treatment, it is possible that several signs that are the focus of anxiety therapy—for example, irritability, panic attacks, agitation, insomnia, and hostility—may emerge. See Chapter 10 ⬤ for more detailed primary actions and adverse effects of these drugs. Following is a brief introduction of important considerations for each type of antidepressant:

- *TCAs* These are not recommended in patients with a history of heart attack, heart block, or abnormal heart rhythm. Patients often have annoying anticholinergic effects (see Chapter 8 ⬤). Most TCAs are pregnancy category C or D. These drugs should not be used with alcohol or other CNS depressants. Patients with asthma, gastrointestinal disorders, alcoholism, schizophrenia, or bipolar disorder should use these drugs with extreme caution.

- *MAOIs* Patients should strictly avoid foods containing tyramine (a form of the amino acid tyrosine) and caffeine. MAOIs intensify the effects of insulin and other diabetes drugs. Common adverse effects include orthostatic hypotension, headache, and diarrhea. MAOIs are prescribed less often due to food interactions and serious adverse effects.

- *SSRIs and SNRIs* These drugs are safer than the other classes of antidepressants and result in fewer occurrences of unfavorable sympathomimetic effects and anticholinergic effects (see Chapter 8 ⬤). SNRIs inhibit the reuptake of both serotonin and norepinephrine. Because both neurotransmitters are thought to play a role in mood, these medications have received more attention in recent years. SSRIs and SNRIs can cause weight gain and sexual dysfunction. Excessive doses of these medications can cause confusion, anxiety, restlessness, hypertension, tremors, sweating, fever, blurred vision, constipation, and muscle incoordination. SSRIs are often drugs of choice for anxiety.

- *Atypical antidepressants* These are chemically unrelated to the other antidepressants. Their adverse effects are generally similar to those of SSRIs and SNRIs. Atypical antidepressants were the first effective alternatives to TCAs because of their more tolerable adverse effects. Common adverse effects are headache, insomnia, nervousness, dry mouth, dizziness, weight loss, sexual dysfunction, and chills.

SOCIAL ANXIETY DISORDER AND HOW IT IS TREATED

TABLE 9.1	Antidepressants for Anxiety Disorders	
DRUG	**ROUTE AND ADULT DOSE**	**CLINICAL USES**
TRICYCLIC ANTIDEPRESSANTS (TCAs)		
amitriptyline (Elavil)	PO; 75–100 mg/day, may gradually increase to 150–300 mg/day (use lower doses in outpatients)	Depression
clomipramine (Anafranil)	PO; 75–100 mg/day in divided doses	OCD, depression
desipramine (Norpramin, Pertofrane, and others)	PO; 75–100 mg/day at bedtime or in divided doses, may gradually increase to 150–300 mg/day (use lower doses in older adults)	Depression
doxepin (Sinequan or Adapin)	PO; 30–150 mg/day at bedtime or in divided doses, may gradually increase to 300 mg/day (use lower doses in older adults)	Depression
imipramine (Tofranil) (see page 137 for the Drug Profile box)	PO; 75–100 mg/day in divided doses (max: 300 mg/day)	Depression, GAD
nortriptyline (Aventyl or Pamelor)	PO; 25 mg three times/day or four times/day, gradually increased to 100–150 mg/day	Depression
trimipramine (Surmontil)	PO; 75-100 mg/day (max: 300 mg/day) in divided doses	Depression
MONOAMINE OXIDASE INHIBITORS (MAOIs)		
phenelzine (Nardil) (see page 142 for the Drug Profile box	PO; 15 mg three times/day, rapidly increase to at least 60 mg/day, may need up to 90 mg/day	Social anxiety, depression
tranylcypromine (Parnate)	PO; 30 mg/day in two divided doses (20 mg in a.m., 10 mg in p.m.), may increase by 10 mg/day at 3-week intervals (max: 60 mg/day)	Depression
SELECTIVE SEROTONIN REUPTAKE INHIBITORS (SSRIs)		
citalopram (Celexa)	PO; start at 20 mg/day, may increase to 40 mg/day if needed	Depression
escitalopram oxalate (Lexapro)	PO; 10 mg/day, may increase to 20 mg/day if needed after 1 week	Depression, GAD, social anxiety
fluoxetine (Prozac) (see page 141 for the Drug Profile box)	20 mg/day in a.m., may increase by 20 mg/day at weekly intervals (max: 80 mg/day); 20 mg/day in a.m.; when stable may switch to 90 mg sustained-release capsule every week (max: 90 mg/week)	Depression, social anxiety, OCD
fluvoxamine (Luvox)	PO; start with 50 mg/day, may increase slowly up to 300 mg/day given at bedtime or divided two times/day	Depression, social anxiety, OCD
paroxetine (Paxil)	PO; 20–60 mg/day	Depression, GAD, social anxiety, panic disorder, OCD, PTSD
sertraline (Zoloft)	PO; begin with 50 mg/day, gradually increase every few weeks according to response (max: 200 mg)	Depression, social anxiety, panic disorder, OCD, PTSD
SEROTONIN-NOREPINEPHRINE REUPTAKE INHIBITORS (SNRIs)		
desvenlafaxine (Pristiq)	PO; 50 mg/day	Depression
duloxetine (Cymbalta)	PO; 40–60 mg/day in one or two divided doses	Depression, GAD, neuropathic pain, chronic fatigue syndrome, stress urinary continence, fibromyalgia
venlafaxine (Effexor)	Start with 37.5 mg sustained release every day and increase to 75–225 mg sustained release per day	Depression, social anxiety, GAD, neuropathic pain, migraines
ATYPICAL ANTIDEPRESSANTS		
trazodone (Desyrel)	PO; 150 mg/day in divided doses, may increase by 50 mg/day every 3–4 days (max: 400–600 mg/day)	Depression, GAD

Benzodiazepines are useful for the short-term treatment of anxiety and insomnia.

CORE CONCEPT 9.7

benzo = *aromatic or ring structure*
di = *two*
azepine = *nitrogen containing*

The **benzodiazepines** are one of the most widely prescribed drug classes. The root word *benzo* refers to an aromatic compound, one having a carbon ring structure attached to different atoms or another carbon ring. Two nitrogen atoms incorporated into the ring structure are the reason for the *diazepine* portion of the name.

The benzodiazepines are used for panic disorder, generalized anxiety, phobias, and insomnia (Table 9.2). Since the introduction of the first benzodiazepines—chlordiazepoxide (Librium) and diazepam (Valium)—in the 1960s, the class has become one of the most widely prescribed in medicine. Although about 15 benzodiazepines are available, all have the same actions and adverse effects. They differ primarily in their onset and duration of action. Some, such as midazolam (Versed), have a rapid onset time of 15 to 30 minutes; others, such as oxazepam (Serax), take 2 to 3 hours to reach peak blood levels. In cases in which the benzodiazepines are used for insomnia therapy, this is important because *time of onset* translates to *time until sleep* for the patient. *Duration of action* translates to *time of anticipated sleep* or *drowsiness*. The benzodiazepines are categorized as Schedule IV drugs, although they produce considerably less physical dependence and result in less tolerance than the barbiturates.

Benzodiazepines act by binding to the gamma-aminobutyric acid (GABA) receptor–chloride channel molecule (see Chapter 10). These drugs intensify the effect of GABA, which is a natural inhibitory neurotransmitter found throughout the brain. Most are metabolized in the liver to active metabolites and excreted primarily in urine. One major advantage of the benzodiazepines is that they do not produce life-threatening respiratory depression or coma if taken in excessive amounts. Death is unlikely, unless the benzodiazepines are taken in large quantities in combination with other CNS depressants, or the patient suffers from sleep apnea.

TABLE 9.2 Benzodiazepines for Anxiety and Insomnia

DRUG	ROUTE AND ADULT DOSE	RELATED CLINICAL USES
ANXIETY		
alprazolam (Xanax)	For panic: PO; 1–2 mg three times/day For anxiety: PO; 0.25–0.5 mg three times/day	GAD, phobias, social anxiety
clonazepam (Klonopin)	PO; 1–2 mg/day in divided doses (max: 4 mg/day)	Phobias, social anxiety, seizures
chlordiazepoxide (Librium)	Mild anxiety: PO; 5–10 mg three or four times/day Severe anxiety: PO; 20–25 mg three or four times/day	Phobias, alcohol withdrawal
clorazepate (Tranxene)	PO; 15 mg/day at bedtime (max: 4 mg/day)	Alcohol withdrawal, seizures
diazepam (Valium) (see page 199 for the Drug Profile box)	PO; 2–10 mg two times/day	Alcohol withdrawal, seizures, muscle spasms, induction of anesthesia
Pr lorazepam (Ativan)	For anxiety: PO; 2–6 mg/day in divided doses (max: 10 mg/day)	Panic disorder, phobias, alcohol withdrawal, seizures, induction of anesthesia
oxazepam (Serax)	PO; 10–30 mg three or four times/day	Phobias, alcohol withdrawal
INSOMNIA		
estazolam (ProSom)	PO; 1 mg at bedtime, may increase to 2 mg if necessary	Insomnia: 15–60 min onset and medium duration
flurazepam (Dalmane)	PO; 15–30 mg at bedtime	Insomnia: 30–60 min onset and long duration
quazepam (Doral)	PO; 7.5–15 mg at bedtime	Insomnia: 20–45 min onset and long duration
temazepam (Restoril)	PO; 7.5–30 mg at bedtime	Insomnia: 45–60 min onset and medium duration
triazolam (Halcion)	PO; 0.125–0.25 mg at bedtime (max: 0.5 mg/day)	Insomnia: 15–30 min onset and short duration

NURSING PROCESS FOCUS

Patients Receiving Antianxiety Therapy

ASSESSMENT

Prior to administration:
- Obtain a complete health history (both physical/mental), including allergies and drug history for possible drug interactions
- Identify factors that precipitate anxiety or insomnia
- Identify actions that have been previously tried to decrease anxiety or insomnia
- Assess likelihood of drug abuse and dependence
- Establish baseline vital signs and level of consciousness

POTENTIAL NURSING DIAGNOSES

- Risk for Injury related to adverse effects of drug therapy.
- Anxiety related to patient specific cause.
- Deficient Knowledge related to administration and information about adverse effects of drug.
- Ineffective Individual Coping related to anxiety.
- Risk for Activity Intolerance related to sedative effect of drug.
- Sleep Deprivation related to anxiety or adverse effects of drug therapy.

PLANNING: PATIENT GOALS AND EXPECTED OUTCOMES

The patient will:
- Experience an increase in psychological comfort
- Report absence of physical and behavioral manifestations of anxiety
- Demonstrate an understanding of the drug's action by accurately describing drug adverse effects and precautions

IMPLEMENTATION

Interventions and (Rationales)	Patient Education/Discharge Planning
■ Monitor vital signs. Observe respiratory patterns, especially during sleep, for evidence of apnea or shallow breathing. (Benzodiazepines can reduce the respiratory drive in susceptible patients.)	Instruct the patient: ■ To consult a health care provider before taking this drug if snoring is a problem (Snoring may indicate an obstruction in the upper respiratory tract, resulting in hypoxia.) ■ Regarding methods to monitor vital signs at home, especially respirations
■ Monitor neurologic status, especially level of consciousness. (Confusion or lack of response may indicate overmedication.)	■ Instruct the patient to report extreme lethargy, slurred speech, disorientation, or ataxia.
■ Ensure patient safety. (Drug may cause excessive drowsiness.)	Instruct the patient to: ■ *Not* drive or perform hazardous activities until the effects of the drug are known ■ Request assistance when getting out of bed and walking until the effect of the medication is known
■ Monitor the patient's intake of stimulants, including caffeine (in beverages such as coffee, tea, cola, and other soft drinks and in OTC analgesics such as Excedrin) and nicotine from tobacco products and nicotine patches. (These products can reduce the drug's effectiveness.)	Instruct the patient to: ■ Avoid taking OTC sleep-inducing antihistamines such as diphenhydramine ■ Consult a health care provider before self-medicating with any OTC preparation
■ Monitor effect and emotional status. (Drug may increase risk of mental depression, especially in patients with suicidal tendencies.)	Instruct the patient to: ■ Report significant mood changes, especially depression ■ Avoid consuming alcohol or taking other CNS depressants while on benzodiazepines because these increase depressant effect
■ Avoid abrupt discontinuation of therapy. (Withdrawal symptoms, including rebound anxiety and sleeplessness, are possible with abrupt discontinuation after long-term use.)	Instruct the patient: ■ To take the drug exactly as prescribed ■ To keep all follow-up appointments as directed by the health care provider to monitor response to medication ■ About nonpharmacologic methods for reestablishing sleep regimen

EVALUATION OF OUTCOME CRITERIA

Evaluate effectiveness of drug therapy by confirming that patient goals and expected outcomes have been met (see "Planning").

See Table 9.2 for a list of drugs to which these nursing actions apply.

DRUG PROFILE: Ⓟ *Lorazepam (Ativan)*

Therapeutic Class: Sedative-hypnotic, anxiolytic, anesthetic adjunct
Pharmacologic Class: Benzodiazepines, GABA receptor agent

Actions and Uses:

Lorazepam is a benzodiazepine that acts by increasing the effects of GABA, an inhibitory neurotransmitter, in the thalamic, hypothalamic, and limbic levels of the CNS. It is one of the most potent benzodiazepines. It has an extended half-life of 10 to 20 hours that allows for once or twice a day oral dosing. In addition to its use as an anxiolytic, lorazepam is used as a preanesthetic medication to provide sedation and for the management of status epilepticus.

Adverse Effects and Interactions:

The most common adverse effects of lorazepam are drowsiness and sedation, which may decrease with time. When given in higher doses or by the intravenous (IV) route, more severe effects may be observed, such as amnesia, weakness, disorientation, ataxia, sleep disturbance, blood pressure changes, blurred vision, double vision, nausea, and vomiting.

Lorazepam interacts with multiple drugs; for example, concurrent use of CNS depressants, including alcohol, increases sedation effects and the risk of respiratory depression and death. Lorazepam may contribute to digoxin toxicity by increasing the serum digoxin level. Symptoms include visual changes, nausea, vomiting, dizziness, and confusion.

Lorazepam should be used with caution with herbal supplements. For example, sedation-producing herbs such as kava, valerian, chamomil or hops may have an additive effect with medication. Stimulant herbs such as gotu-kola and ma huang may reduce the drug's effectiveness.

 Refer to MyNursingKit for a Nursing Process Focus specific to this drug.

Most benzodiazepines are given orally. Those that can be given parenterally, such as diazepam (Valium) and lorazepam (Ativan), should be monitored carefully because of their rapid onset of CNS effects and possible respiratory depression.

Because of their greater safety, the benzodiazepines are preferred over the barbiturates for the short-term treatment of insomnia caused by anxiety. Benzodiazepines shorten the length of time it takes to fall asleep and reduce the frequency of interrupted sleep. Although most benzodiazepines increase total sleep time, some reduce Stage IV sleep, and some affect REM sleep. In general, the benzodiazepines used to treat short-term insomnia are different from those used to treat GAD (see Table 9.2).

Benzodiazepines have a number of other important indications. Diazepam (Valium) is featured as a profile drug in Chapter 13 ⬭ for its use in treating seizure disorders. Other uses include treatment of alcohol withdrawal symptoms (see Chapter 7 ⬭), central muscle relaxation (see Chapter 12 ⬭), and as induction agents in general anesthesia (see Chapter 15 ⬭).

CORE CONCEPT 9.8

Barbiturates depress CNS function and cause drowsiness.

Barbiturates are drugs derived from barbituric acid. They are powerful CNS depressants that have been used in pharmacotherapy since the early 1900s for their sedative, hypnotic, and antiseizure effects.

Until the discovery of the benzodiazepines, barbiturates were the drug of choice for treating anxiety and insomnia (Table 9.3). Although barbiturates are still indicated for several conditions, they are rarely, if ever, prescribed for treating anxiety or insomnia because of their significant adverse effects and the availability of more effective medications. The risk of psychological and physical dependence is high—several are Schedule II drugs. The withdrawal syndrome from barbiturates is extremely severe and can be fatal. Overdose results in profound respiratory depression, hypotension, and shock. People have used barbiturates to commit suicide, and death due to overdose is not uncommon.

TABLE 9.3	Barbiturates for Sedation and Insomnia
DRUG	**ROUTE AND ADULT DOSE**
SHORT ACTING	
pentobarbital sodium (Nembutal)	Sedative: PO; 20–30 mg two or three times/day Hypnotic: PO; 120–200 mg
secobarbital (Seconal)	Sedative: PO; 100–300 mg/day in three divided doses Hypnotic: PO; 100–200 mg
INTERMEDIATE ACTING	
amobarbital (Amytal)	Sedative: PO; 30–50 mg two or three times/day Hypnotic: PO; 65–200 mg (max: 500 mg)
aprobarbital (Alurate)	Sedative: PO; 40 mg three times/day Hypnotic: PO; 40–160 mg
butabarbital sodium (Butisol)	Sedative: PO; 15–30 mg three or four times/day Hypnotic: PO; 50–100 mg at bedtime
LONG ACTING	
mephobarbital (Mebaral)	Sedative: PO; 32–100 mg three times/day
phenobarbital (Luminal) (see page 199 for the Drug Profile box)	Sedative: PO; 30–120 mg/day

Barbiturates are capable of depressing CNS function at all levels. Like benzodiazepines, barbiturates act by binding to GABA receptor–chloride channel molecules, intensifying the effect of GABA throughout the brain. At low doses, they reduce anxiety and cause drowsiness. At moderate doses, they inhibit seizure activity (see Chapter 10 ⬤) and promote sleep, probably by inhibiting brain impulses traveling through the limbic system and the reticular activating system. At higher doses, some barbiturates can produce anesthesia (see Chapter 15 ⬤).

When taken for prolonged periods, barbiturates stimulate the microsomal enzymes in the liver that metabolize medications. This means that barbiturates can stimulate their own metabolism as well as that of hundreds of other drugs that use these enzymes for their breakdown. With repeated use, tolerance develops to the sedative effects of these drugs, and cross-tolerance to other CNS depressants such as the opioids occurs. Tolerance does not develop, however, to the respiratory depressant effects.

Concept Review 9.4

■ Identify the major drug classes used for sedation and insomnia. Why are CNS depressants especially dangerous if administered in high doses?

Additional drugs provide therapy for anxiety-related symptoms and sleep disorders.

CORE CONCEPT 9.9

The final group of CNS agents used for anxiety and sleep disorders consists of miscellaneous drugs that are chemically unrelated to either benzodiazepines or barbiturates.

Additional drugs for anxiety include the mild tranquilizer buspirone (BuSpar), the antiseizure medication valproate (Depakene/Depakote), and the beta blockers atenolol (Tenormin) and propranolol (Inderal, InnoPran XL). Drugs for insomnia therapy include nonbenzodiazepine CNS depressants, eszopiclone (Lunesta), zaleplon (Sonata), and zolpidem (Ambien); the melatonin receptor agent ramelteon (Rozerem); and OTC antihistamines, diphenhydramine (Nytol and Sominex) and doxylamine (Unisom) (Table 9.4).

The mechanism of action for buspirone (BuSpar) is unclear but appears to be related to serotonin and dopamine receptors in the brain. Buspirone is less likely than benzodiazepines to affect cognitive and motor performance and rarely interacts with other CNS depressants. Common adverse effects include dizziness, headache, and drowsiness. Its main use is for anxiety symptoms.

TABLE 9.4	Nonbenzodiazepine, Nonbarbiturate CNS Agents for Anxiety and Insomnia	
DRUG	**ROUTE AND ADULT DOSE**	**CLINICAL USES**
ANXIETY THERAPY		
CNS Depressant (Mild Tranquilizer)		
buspirone (BuSpar)	PO; 7.5–15 mg in divided doses, may increase by 5 mg/day every 2–3 days if needed (max: 60 mg/day)	GAD, OCD
Antiseizure Medication		
valproate (Depakote)	For mania: PO; 250 mg three times/day (max: 60 mg/kg/day)	Panic disorder, seizures, smoking, bipolar disorder, prevention of migraines
Beta Blockers		
atenolol (Tenormin) (see page 345 for the Drug Profile box)	PO; 25–100 mg once/day	Performance anxiety, social anxiety
propranolol (Inderal, InnoPran XL) (see page 314 for the Drug Profile box)	For trembling: PO; 40 mg two times/day (max: up to 320 mg/day)	Performance anxiety, social anxiety
INSOMNIA THERAPY		
Nonbenzodiazepines		
eszopiclone (Lunesta)	PO; 2 mg at bedtime; depending on the age, clinical response, and tolerance of the patient, dose may be lowered to 1 mg PO	60 min onset and medium duration
zaleplon (Sonata)	PO; 10 mg at bedtime (max: 20 mg at bedtime)	15–30 min onset and short duration
(Pr) zolpidem (Ambien), zolpidem CR (Ambien CR)	PO; 5–10 mg at bedtime	30 min onset and short (medium CR) duration
Melatonin Receptor Agent		
ramelteon (Rozerem)	PO; 8 mg at bedtime	30 min onset and short duration
Antihistamines		
diphenhydramine (Nytol and Sominex)	OTC medication	60–180 min onset and long duration
doxylamine (Unisom)	OTC medication	60–120 min onset and long duration

Therapy may take several weeks to achieve optimal results. Dependence and withdrawal problems are not major concerns.

The antiseizure medication valproic acid (Depakene) is an important drug used to treat a variety of seizure types. Common uses include treatment for all partial and generalized seizures (see Chapter 13), control of symptoms in patients with bipolar disorder (see Chapter 10), and prevention of migraine headaches (see Chapter 14). For these reasons, valproic acid is listed as one medication that might be helpful in reducing anxiety symptoms among patients predisposed to panic disorders, mood swings, or migraine headaches. Adverse gastrointestinal effects such as nausea and vomiting are common. Rare life-threatening hepatotoxicity and pancreatitis are a concern.

Beta blockers were covered in Chapter 8 and are covered more thoroughly as they pertain to management of hypertension (see Chapter 17), angina (see Chapter 20), and cardiac dysrhythmias (see Chapter 19). Sweating, heart palpitations, and shaking are expected signs of situational, social, and performance anxiety. Low doses of beta blockers reduce symptoms connected with panic, tension, and excitement.

Zolpidem (Ambien) is a Schedule IV controlled substance limited to the short-term treatment of insomnia. It is highly specific to the GABA receptor and produces muscle relaxation (see Chapter 12) and antiseizure effects (see Chapter 13) only at doses much higher than the hypnotic dose. As with other CNS depressants, zolpidem should be used cautiously in patients with respiratory impairment, in elderly persons, and when used along with other CNS depressants. Lower

DRUG PROFILE: ℞ *Zolpidem (Ambien)*

Therapeutic Class: Sedative-hypnotic

Pharmacologic Class: Nonbenzodiazepine, nonbarbiturate CNS depressant, GABA receptor agent

Actions and Uses:

Although it is a nonbenzodiazepine, zolpidem acts in a similar fashion to facilitate GABA-mediated CNS depression in the limbic, thalamic, and hypothalamic regions. The only indication for zolpidem is short-term insomnia management (7–10 days). Zolpidem is pregnancy category B.

Adverse Effects and Interactions:

Adverse effects include daytime sedation, confusion, amnesia, dizziness, depression, nausea, and vomiting.

Drug interactions with zolpidem include an increase in sedation when used concurrently with other CNS depressants, including alcohol. When taken with food, absorption is slowed significantly and the onset of action may be delayed.

Refer to MyNursingKit for a Nursing Process Focus specific to this drug.

NATURAL THERAPIES

Valerian for Anxiety and Insomnia

Valerian (*Valeriana officinalis*) is a perennial plant that grows in Europe, Asia, and North America. Valerian has several substances in its roots that affect the CNS; the exact active chemical has yet to be identified. This herb has been used to treat nervousness, anxiety, and insomnia for thousands of years and is one of the most widely used herbal CNS depressants. The drug appears to have effects similar to benzodiazepines such as diazepam (Valium). The major side effects of valerian are extensions of its therapeutic effects: drowsiness and decreased alertness. Valerian should not be combined with alcohol or other drugs that cause sedation or drowsiness because excessive drowsiness may occur.

---

dosages may be necessary. Also, because of the rapid onset of this drug (within 30 minutes), it should be taken just prior to expected sleep. Adverse reactions are usually minimal (mild nausea, dizziness, diarrhea, daytime drowsiness). Rebound insomnia may occur when the drug is discontinued.

Although structurally unrelated to other drugs used to treat insomnia, eszopiclone (Lunesta) has properties similar to those of zolpidem (Ambien). The effectiveness of eszopiclone has been shown in outpatient and sleep laboratory studies, but the drug has not been directly compared with zolpidem or other hypnotics. However, eszopiclone's longer elimination half-life, about twice as long as that of zolpidem, may give it an advantage in maintaining sleep and decreasing early-morning awakening. On the other hand, eszopiclone is more likely to cause daytime sedation.

Zaleplon (Sonata) may be useful for people who desire to fall asleep but need to awake early in the morning. It is sometimes used for travel purposes and has been advertised by pharmaceutical companies for this purpose.

In 2005, remelteon (Rozerem) was approved by the Food and Drug Administration (FDA) in a single 8-mg dose. Ramelteon is a melatonin receptor agent, which has been shown to mainly improve sleep induction. It has a relatively short onset of action (30 minutes), and its duration is comparable to the noncontrolled release form of zolpidem. The FDA indications for remelteon or zolpidem are not limited to short-term use because they do not appear to produce dependence or tolerance to dose.

Drugs included in Table 9.4 without dosing information are diphenhydramine (Nytol and Sominex) and doxylamine (Unisom). These are OTC sleep aids. Antihistamines produce drowsiness and are beneficial in calming patients. They offer the advantage of not causing dependence, although their use is often limited by anticholinergic adverse effects. Diphenhydramine is a common component of antihistamine combinations available OTC for allergic rhinitis and cough and for allergic reactions in general (see Chapter 28).

Concept Review 9.5

- What are the major drug classes used to treat GAD and panic disorder?
- Name popular drugs within these classes.

PATIENTS NEED TO KNOW

Patients taking anxiolytics and CNS depressants need to know the following:

1. Stimulants such as coffee, tea, and chocolate should be avoided because they counteract anxiolytics and sedatives and increase the symptoms of anxiety.
2. Exercise, progressive muscle relaxation, and slow, deep breathing can assist with anxiety relief.
3. Alcohol, antihistamines, and other CNS depressants can increase the effects of anxiolytics. They should be avoided to decrease the risk of accidental depressant overdose and death.
4. Anxiolytics can cause drowsiness. Until effects of these drugs have been established, assistance with getting out of bed or avoidance of driving may be necessary.
5. Anxiolytics and sedatives should be stored in a secure place to avoid accidental ingestion by children and animals.
6. Avoid abrupt discontinuation of medication because withdrawal symptoms are possible after long-term use.
7. Report any significant changes in mood to the health care provider.
8. Do not take any OTC medications without first consulting the health care provider.

SAFETY ALERT

Interpreting Physician Orders

In many health care facilities, it is the nurse's responsibility to interpret and transcribe doctors' orders for medications. Unfortunately, handwritten orders can be difficult to interpret correctly. For example, an error was made when an order to discontinue "SSRI," intended to mean "sliding scale regular insulin," was misinterpreted as an order to discontinue the "selective serotonin reuptake inhibitor" (Zoloft). It is extremely important for the nurse to know their patients' needs and to clarify with the physician any medication order that is difficult to interpret or is questionable.

Source: SSRI OR SSKI. (2008, May). NurseAdvise-ERR, 6(5), 2–3.

CHAPTER REVIEW

CORE CONCEPTS SUMMARY

9.1 Anxiety disorders fall into several categories.

There are at least five major types of anxiety disorders: generalized anxiety, panic disorder, phobias, obsessive-compulsive disorder, and post-traumatic stress disorder.

9.2 Specific regions of the brain are responsible for anxiety and wakefulness.

The limbic system and the reticular activating system control anxiety and wakefulness. Neural signals passing between these two brain regions are responsible for anxiety, fear, restlessness, and an interrupted sleep pattern.

9.3 Anxiety is managed with both pharmacologic and nonpharmacologic strategies.

Patients should be encouraged to explore and develop coping strategies for dealing with stress. In cases when anxiety becomes too severe, anxiolytics are an effective treatment.

9.4 An inability to sleep is linked with anxiety.

There are many reasons why a patient might experience sleeplessness. Stress is one factor in short-term insomnia. Others include caffeine, nicotine, room temperature, light, snoring, and sleep apnea.

In long-term insomnia, psychological and physiological factors may be involved.

9.5   Anxiety and insomnia are treated with many types of central nervous system (CNS) agents.

Antidepressants treat stress and related symptoms by altering levels of norepinephrine and serotonin in the brain. *Sedatives, sedative-hypnotics,* and *CNS depressants* are terms used to describe benzodiazepines, barbiturates, and other drugs. These agents suppress impulses traveling through the limbic and reticular activating systems, thereby reducing symptoms of stress, producing drowsiness, and promoting sleep.

9.6   When taken properly, antidepressants reduce symptoms of panic and anxiety.

Several classes of antidepressants treat panic and anxiety symptoms: tricyclic antidepressants (TCAs), monoamine oxidase inhibitors (MAOIs), selective serotonin reuptake inhibitors (SSRIs), serotonin-norepinephrine reuptake inhibitors (SNRIs), and atypical antidepressants. The new SSRIs are preferred because they produce fewer sympathomimetic and anticholinergic effects.

9.7   Benzodiazepines are useful for the short-term treatment of anxiety and insomnia.

Benzodiazepines are commonly prescribed for insomnia. Several drugs are used; in general, they differ from the ones used to treat anxiety. Onset and duration of action help determine therapeutic application.

9.8   Barbiturates depress CNS function and cause drowsiness.

Barbiturates are rarely, if ever, prescribed for insomnia. The primary role of this class of drugs is sedation. They depress CNS function by binding to GABA receptors and causing drowsiness.

9.9   Additional drugs provide therapy for anxiety-related symptoms and sleep disorders.

Miscellaneous drugs provide relief from anxiety and anxiety-related symptoms. These include CNS depressants, antiseizure medications, and beta blockers. Additional drugs employed for insomnia therapy involve nonbenzodiazepines, melatonin receptor agents, and antihistamines. Antihistamines are often found in OTC medications.

REVIEW QUESTIONS

The following questions are written in NCLEX-PN® style. Answer these questions to assess your knowledge of the chapter material, and go back and review any material that is not clear to you.

1. After 8 months of use, the patient abruptly discontinues his zaleplon (Sonata). The patient is now complaining of anxiety and inability to sleep. The nurse suspects:

1. A panic disorder
2. Long-term insomnia
3. Behavioral insomnia
4. Rebound insomnia

2. Your patient was started on buspirone (BuSpar) for his anxiety disorder 3 days ago. The patient now calls the physician's office stating that it "just isn't working." The nurse's best response would be:

1. "BuSpar should give you immediate relief. I will notify the physician that this medication is not effective."
2. "It will take 3 to 4 weeks for BuSpar to be fully effective."
3. "You may need an increased dose of BuSpar for it to work."
4. "You will need additional medications to ease your anxiety."

3. The patient is sleeping at the time the next sedative is ordered. The nurse should:

1. Wake the patient and administer the next dose of sedative
2. Notify the physician
3. Hold the dose and document the reason
4. Hold this dose and administer it with the next dose

4. The nurse educates the patient on zolpidem (Ambien) that it:

1. Will take a week for the medication to be effective
2. May be taken 2 to 3 hours before bedtime
3. Should be taken just prior to going to bed
4. Must be used long term to be effective

5. The patient has been taking barbiturates for the last few months for difficulty sleeping. The nurse's main concern for the patient who stopped taking the barbiturate would be:

1. Respiratory depression
2. Severe withdrawal
3. Hypotension
4. Shock

6. Which of the following nursing interventions would be most appropriate for a patient who has just been administered a sedative?

1. Orient to surroundings.
2. Assess for respiratory dysfunction.
3. Shut off the lights and close the door.
4. Make sure the call light is within the patient's reach.

7. The patient has been diagnosed with a panic disorder. The nurse recognizes that symptoms of a panic disorder include:

1. Fatigue, muscle tension, nervousness
2. Dry mouth, diarrhea, restlessness
3. Feelings of immediate apprehension, terror, impending doom
4. Chronic insomnia, terror, nervousness

8. It is important to teach the patient to avoid _____, which can increase the effects of sedatives.

1. Nicotine
2. Alcohol
3. Chocolate
4. Tea

9. Which of the following is not used in the treatment of panic disorders?

1. alprazolam (Xanax)
2. estazolam (ProSom)
3. clonazepam (Klonopin)
4. lorazepam (Ativan)

10. The nurse should monitor the patient taking lorazepam (Ativan) for which of the following adverse effects?

1. Ataxia
2. Euphoria
3. Astigmatism
4. Tachypnea

CASE STUDY QUESTIONS

For questions 1 and 2, please refer to the following case study and choose the correct answer from choices 1–4.

Ms. Reynolds is a 34-year-old interior designer who witnessed and was nearly involved in a fatal car accident on her way to a patient house about 6 months ago. Since that time she has been having dreams about the accident, and during the day she often thinks about the events and the injured people she saw. She is fearful of driving and does all she can to avoid leaving her home-based office. When she hears a siren, she feels immediate anxiety and terror.

1. The disorder Ms. Reynolds is likely experiencing is called:

1. Obsessive-compulsive disorder (OCD)
2. Panic disorder

3. Phobia
4. Post-traumatic stress disorder (PTSD)

2. Not recognizing that she is experiencing a type of anxiety, Ms. Reynolds does not seek help. Instead, she finds that more and more she is compelled to perform a series of actions prior to driving anywhere in her car. She gets into the car, puts on her seat belt and pulls it tight, checks all her mirrors, and then takes her seat belt back off and refastens it. Sometimes it takes her 20 to 30 minutes to repeatedly perform these actions before she leaves her driveway. Which of the following disorders might she also be experiencing?

1. Obsessive-compulsive disorder (OCD)
2. Panic disorder
3. Phobia
4. Generalized anxiety disorder

FURTHER STUDY

- Benzodiazepines are also discussed in Chapter 12 ∞ (for skeletal muscle spasms).

- Phenobarbital for the treatment of seizures is discussed in Chapter 13 ∞.

- Barbiturates can cause physical and psychological dependence, as discussed in Chapter 7 ∞.

- Valproic acid (Depakene) is also used to treat bipolar disorder, as discussed in Chapter 10 ∞.

- Phenytoin's antidysrhythmic properties are discussed in Chapter 19 ∞.

- Drugs for depression and hallucinations are also covered in Chapter 10 ∞.

- Drugs for alcohol abuse are discussed in Chapter 7 ∞.

- Drugs for seizure disorders are covered in Chapter 13 ∞.

10 Drugs for Emotional and Mood Disorders

CORE CONCEPTS

10.1 People suffer from depression for many reasons.

10.2 Treatment of severe depression requires both medication and psychotherapy for the best results.

10.3 Antidepressants enhance mood by boosting the actions of neurotransmitters, including norepinephrine and serotonin.

10.4 Patients with bipolar disorder may experience emotions ranging from depression to extreme agitation.

10.5 Mood stabilization in patients with bipolar disorder is accomplished with lithium and other drugs.

10.6 Attention deficit–hyperactivity disorder (ADHD) presents challenges for children and adults.

10.7 Central nervous system (CNS) stimulants have been the main course of treatment for ADHD.

DRUG SNAPSHOT

The following drugs are discussed in this chapter:

DRUG CLASSES	DRUG PROFILES
Antidepressants	
Tricyclic antidepressants (TCAs)	**Pr** imipramine (Tofranil)
Selective serotonin reuptake inhibitors (SSRIs)	**Pr** fluoxetine (Prozac)
Serotonin-norepinephrine reuptake inhibitors (SNRIs)	
Monoamine oxidase inhibitors (MAOIs)	**Pr** phenelzine (Nardil)
Atypical antidepressants	

DRUG CLASSES	DRUG PROFILES
Drugs for Bipolar Disorder	
Mood stabilizers	**Pr** lithium (Eskalith)
Antiseizure drugs	
Atypical antipsychotic drugs	
Drugs for Attention Deficit–Hyperactivity Disorder (ADHD)	
CNS stimulants	**Pr** methylphenidate (Ritalin)
Nonstimulant drugs for ADHD	

LEARNING OUTCOMES

After reading this chapter, the student should be able to:

1. Identify the two major categories of mood disorders and their symptoms.

2. Explain the causes of major depressive disorder.

3. Discuss the pharmacologic management of patients with depression, bipolar disorder, and attention deficit–hyperactivity disorder (ADHD).

4. Identify symptoms of ADHD.

5. Know representative drug examples, and explain the mechanism of action, primary actions, and important adverse effects for each of the drug classes covered in this chapter.

6. Categorize drugs used for mood and emotional disorders based on their classes and drug actions.

antidepressants (AN-tee-dee-PRESS-ahnts) 132

attention deficit–hyperactivity disorder (ADHD) 145

bipolar disorder (bi-PO-ler) 142

dysthymic disorder (dis-THEYE-mick) 131

major depressive disorder 131

monoamine oxidase inhibitors (MAOIs) (mon-oh-AHM-een OK-se-daze) 140

mood disorder 130

mood stabilizers 143

selective serotonin-reuptake inhibitors (SSRIs) (sir-eh-TO-nin) 135

serotonin-norepinephrine reuptake inhibitors (SNRIs) 136

serotonin syndrome (SES) 136

tricyclic antidepressants (TCAs) (treye-SICK-lick) 132

nappropriate or unusually intense emotions are among the leading causes of mental health disorders. Although mood changes are a normal part of life, when those changes become severe and impair functioning within the family, work environment, or interpersonal relationships, an individual may be diagnosed as having a **mood disorder**. The two major categories of mood disorders are depression and bipolar disorder. A third emotional disorder, ADHD, is also included in this chapter.

DEPRESSION

Depression is a disorder characterized by many symptoms, some of which are depressed mood, lack of energy, sleep disturbances, abnormal eating patterns, and feelings of despair, guilt, and misery (Table 10.1).

CORE CONCEPT 10.1

People suffer from depression for many reasons.

▶ **Life Span Fact**

Depression is the most common mental health disorder of elderly patients, encompassing a variety of physical, emotional, cognitive, and social considerations.

In some cases, depression may be situational or reactive, meaning that it results from challenging circumstances such as severe physical illness, loss of a job, death of a loved one, divorce, or financial difficulties coupled with inadequate psychosocial support. In other cases, the depression

TABLE 10.1	Situational and Biological Causes of Depression

SITUATIONAL CAUSES OF DEPRESSION

- Unpleasant life circumstances—grief from a lost loved one, divorce, loss of or dissatisfaction with a job, financial difficulty, excessive stress or responsibilities
- Negative thinking patterns—an environment that is likely to cause an individual to feel as if any attempts to escape or correct a situation are hopeless; poor self-image or lack of support from family or friends
- Substance abuse—substances that produce unpleasant adverse effects or withdrawal symptoms, such as opiates, alcohol, or other CNS depressants
- Medication intended for therapeutic use—unfavorable adverse effects from medication intended to treat a medical disorder (for example, some antihypertensive drugs and oral contraceptives)

BIOLOGICAL (PHYSIOLOGICAL) CAUSES OF DEPRESSION

- Genetic—history of depression in one's family
- Hormonal changes in the body—fluctuations of reproductive or metabolic hormones
- Neurobiological dysfunction—chemical disturbances in the brain; usually related to abnormal functioning or release of neurotransmitters (for example, dopamine, norepinephrine, serotonin, or melatonin)
- Symptoms from a second disorder—almost any debilitating disorder, including head trauma, dementia, brain stroke or tumors, chronic pain, or thyroid dysfunction

may be biological or organic in origin, associated with dysfunction of neurologic processes leading to an imbalance of neurotransmitters. Family history of depression increases the risk of biological depression.

Most depressed patients are not found in psychiatric hospitals but in mainstream everyday settings. **Dysthymic disorder** is a condition characterized by less severe depressive symptoms that may prevent a person from feeling well or functioning normally. Recognizing depression to properly diagnose and treat patients is a collaborative effort among health care providers, who should all be alert for signs and symptoms of depression in patients they treat. Often it is the pharmacist, working in a neighborhood pharmacy or supermarket, who recognizes that a person is depressed when the individual is self-medicating with remedies that enhance mood or using over-the-counter (OTC) sleep aids.

Some women experience intense mood shifts associated with hormonal changes during the menstrual cycle, pregnancy, childbirth, and menopause. For example, up to 80% of women experience depression 2 weeks to 6 months after the birth of a baby. Many women face additional stresses such as responsibilities both at work and home, single parenthood, and caring for children and aging parents. If mood is severely depressed and persists long enough, many women, including women with premenstrual distress disorder, postpartum depression, or menopausal distress, may benefit from medical treatment.

During the dark winter months, some patients experience a type of depression known as *seasonal affective disorder (SAD)*. This type of depression is associated with a reduced release of the brain neurohormone melatonin. Exposing patients on a regular basis to specific wavelengths of light may relieve SAD depression and prevent future episodes.

Psychotic depression is another condition characterized by the expression of mood shifts and unusual behaviors. Intense behaviors include hallucinations, combativeness, and disorganized speech patterns. For patients with psychosis and for patients with extreme mood swings, unusual behaviors are often treatable with antipsychotic drugs (see Chapter 11 ⊕).

Treatment of severe depression requires both medication and psychotherapy for the best results.

The first step to treating depression is a complete health examination. Drugs such as glucocorticoids, levodopa, and oral contraceptives can cause the same symptoms as depression, and the health care provider should rule out this possibility. Medical and neurologic disorders, ranging from vitamin B deficiencies to thyroid gland problems to early Alzheimer's disease, can mimic depression. If physical causes for depression are ruled out, a psychological evaluation is often performed by a psychiatrist or psychologist to confirm the diagnosis.

During the health examination, inquiries should be made about alcohol and drug use, and whether the patient has had thoughts about death or suicide. Further, a history should include questions about whether other family members have had a depressive illness and, if treated, what therapies they received and which of them were effective.

To determine a course of treatment, health care providers assess for well-accepted symptoms of depression. Patients diagnosed with **major depressive disorder** must show at least five of the following symptoms:

- Difficulty sleeping or sleeping too much
- Extreme fatigue; lack of energy
- Abnormal eating patterns (eating too much or not enough)
- Vague physical symptoms (gastrointestinal [GI] pain, joint/muscle pain, or headaches)
- Inability to concentrate or make decisions
- Feelings of despair, lack of self-worth, guiltiness, and misery
- Obsession with death (a wish to die or to commit suicide)
- Avoidance of psychosocial and interpersonal interactions
- Lack of interest in personal appearance or sex
- Delusions or hallucinations

In general, severe depressive illness, particularly that which reoccurs, requires treatment with both medication and psychotherapy to achieve the best response. Counseling therapies help patients gain insight into and resolve their problems through verbal give-and-take with the therapist. Behavioral therapies help patients learn how to obtain more satisfaction and rewards through their own actions and how to unlearn the behavioral patterns that contribute to or result from their depression.

Two short-term psychotherapies that are helpful for some forms of depression are interpersonal and cognitive-behavioral therapies. *Interpersonal therapy* focuses on the patient's disturbed personal relationships that both cause and worsen the depression. *Cognitive-behavioral therapy* helps the patient change the negative style of thought and behavior that are often associated with depression. *Psychodynamic therapies,* often postponed until the depressive symptoms are significantly improved, focus on resolving the patient's internal conflicts.

In patients with serious and life-threatening mood disorders that are unresponsive to pharmacotherapy, *electroconvulsive therapy (ECT)* has been the traditional treatment. Although ECT has been found to be safe, there may be serious complications related to the anesthesia that is used and to seizure activity caused by ECT. Studies suggest that *repetitive transcranial magnetic stimulation (rTMS)* may improve mood in major depressive disorder. In contrast to ECT, it has minimal effects on memory, does not require general anesthesia, and produces its effects without a generalized seizure.

CORE CONCEPT 10.3
Antidepressants enhance mood by boosting the actions of neurotransmitters, including norepinephrine and serotonin.

Antidepressants are medications that combat depression by enhancing mood. Depression is associated with an imbalance of neurotransmitters in certain regions of the brain. Although medication does not completely restore these chemical imbalances, it does help to reduce depressive symptoms while the patient develops effective means of coping.

Antidepressants work by increasing the action of certain neurotransmitters in the brain, including norepinephrine and serotonin (chemical name, 5-hydroxytryptamine, or 5-HT). There are two main ways in which most antidepressants work: (1) by blocking the enzymatic breakdown of norepinephrine, and (2) by slowing the reuptake of serotonin and/or norepinephrine. The primary classes of antidepressant drugs, also shown in Table 10.2, are as follows:

- Tricyclic antidepressants (TCAs)
- Selective serotonin-reuptake inhibitors (SSRIs)
- Serotonin-norepinephrine reuptake inhibitors (SNRIs)
- Monoamine oxidase inhibitors (MAOIs)
- Atypical antidepressants

The atypical antidepressants consist of agents that do not conveniently fit into the first four drug categories. The *atypical* label here refers to the unique chemical nature of the group. Drugs such as bupropion (Wellbutrin) not only inhibit the reuptake of serotonin, but may also affect the activity of norepinephrine and dopamine. Catecholamine (relating to nonreprinephrine- and dopamine-like) neurotransmitters may play a more active role in stability of mood than once thought. Additional examples of atypical antidepressants are mirtazapine (Remeron), nefazodone (Serzone), and trazodone (Desyrel).

Desvenlafaxine (Pristiq), duloxetine (Cymbalta), and venlafaxine (Effexor) are SNRIs. Sometimes these drugs have been grouped with the atypical antidepressants. Because of their unique physiologic significance, SNRIs are being separated out and placed into their own subgroup.

Concept Review 10.1

- What are the major causes of depression? Identify symptoms of major depressive disorder. What is the name used to describe drugs that treat depression?

Tricyclic Antidepressants
Tricyclic antidepressants (TCAs) are drugs named for their three-ring chemical structure. They were the mainstay of depression pharmacotherapy from the early 1960s until the 1980s and are still widely used.

TABLE 10.2	Antidepressants	
DRUG	**ROUTE AND ADULT DOSE**	**REMARKS**

TRICYCLIC ANTIDEPRESSANTS (TCAs)

amitriptyline (Elavil)	Adult: PO; 75–100 mg/day (may gradually increase to 150–300 mg/day); geriatric: PO; 10–25 mg at bedtime (may gradually increase to 25–150 mg/day)	For biological depression; inhibits gastric acid secretion by blocking histamine-2 receptors in the body
amoxapine (Asendin)	Adult: PO; begin with 100 mg/day, may increase on day 3 to 300 mg/day; geriatric: PO; 25 mg at bedtime, may increase every 3–7 days to 50–150 mg/day (max: 300 mg/day)	For situational and biological depression; not associated with cardiotoxicity; mild sedative
clomipramine (Anafranil)	PO; 75–300 mg/day in divided doses	For depression accompanying obsessive-compulsive disorder
desipramine (Norpramin)	PO; 75–100 mg/day, may increase to 150–300 mg/day	Active metabolite of imipramine
doxepin (Sinequan)	PO; 30–150 mg/day at bedtime, may gradually increase to 300 mg/day	For depression accompanying anxiety or alcohol dependence
Pr imipramine (Tofranil)	PO; 75–100 mg/day (max: 300 mg/day)	For biological depression or alcohol or cocaine dependence; may cause cardiac dysfunction and abnormal blood cell count; available IM; may control bed-wetting in children
maprotiline (Ludiomil)	Mild to moderate depression: PO; start at 75 mg/day and gradually increase every 2 weeks to 150 mg/day; severe depression: PO; start at 100–150 mg/day and gradually increase to 300 mg/day	For a broad range of depression from mild to severe
nortriptyline (Aventyl, Pamelor)	PO; 25 mg tid or qid; may increase to 100–150 mg/day	For biological depression; interactions similar to imipramine
protriptyline (Vivactil)	PO; 15–40 mg/day in three to four divided doses (max: 60 mg/day)	For symptoms of depression; few sedative qualities; causes increased heart rate
trimipramine (Surmontil)	PO; 75–100 mg/day (max: 300 mg/day)	For depression accompanied by a sleep disorder (has strong sedative effects)

SELECTIVE SEROTONIN REUPTAKE INHIBITORS (SSRIs)

citalopram (Celexa)	PO; start at 20 mg/day (max: 40 mg/day)	Does not mimic the sympathetic response; has no acetylcholine blocking properties; does not inhibit MAOIs
escitalopram oxalate (Lexapro)	PO; 10 mg daily, may increase to 20 mg after 1 week	May be used for generalized anxiety disorder; does not inhibit MAOIs
Pr fluoxetine (Prozac)	PO; 20 mg/day in the a.m. (max: 80 mg/day)	May be used for obsessive-compulsive disorder and eating disorders
fluvoxamine (Luvox)	PO; start with 50 mg/day (max: 300 mg/day)	May be used for obsessive-compulsive disorder; no severe adverse cardiovascular effects; fewer acetylcholine blocking effects
paroxetine (Paxil)	Depression: PO; 10–50 mg/day (max: 80 mg/day); obsessive-compulsive disorder: PO; 20–60 mg/day; panic attacks: PO; 40 mg/day	May be used for obsessive-compulsive disorder and panic attacks
sertraline (Zoloft)	Adult: PO; start with 50 mg/day, gradually increase every few weeks to a range of 50–200 mg; geriatric: start with 25 mg/day	Does not mimic sympathetic response; has no acetylcholine blocking properties; does not inhibit MAOIs

SEROTONIN-NOREPINEPHRINE REUPTAKE INHIBITORS (SNRIs)

desvenlafaxine (Pristiq)	PO; 50 mg/day	For major depression; active metabolite of venlafaxine; available in once-daily extended release form

continued . . .

TABLE 10.2	Antidepressants—*Continued*	
DRUG	**ROUTE AND ADULT DOSE**	**REMARKS**
duloxetine (Cymbalta)	PO; 40–60 mg/day in one or two divided doses	For major depression, generalized anxiety disorder, neuropathic pain, chronic fatigue syndrome, stress urinary continence, and fibromyalgia (some uses are being reviewed by the Food and Drug Administration [FDA])
venlafaxine (Effexor)	Start with 37.5 mg sustained release every day and increase to 75–225 mg sustained release per day	For major depression, situational depression, generalized anxiety disorder, neuropathic pain, and migraines (some uses are being reviewed by the FDA)
MONOAMINE OXIDASE INHIBITORS (MAOIs)		
isocarboxazid (Marplan)	PO; 10–30 mg/day (max: 30 mg/day)	May cause peripheral edema and high blood pressure; used in cases in which other approaches for treatment of depression are not successful
Pp phenelzine (Nardil)	PO; 15 mg tid (max: 90 mg/day)	May cause a hypertensive crisis or respiratory depression; use cautiously in patients with epilepsy or diabetes, or who are likely to abuse drugs and alcohol
tranylcypromine (Parnate)	PO; 30 mg/day (give 20 mg in a.m. and 10 mg in p.m.), may increase by 10 mg/day at 3-week intervals up to 60 mg/day	For severe depression in cases in which patients have not responded to other medications
ATYPICAL ANTIDEPRESSANTS		
bupropion (Wellbutrin)	PO; 75–100 mg tid (greater than 450 mg/day increases risk for adverse reactions)	For changing moods, schizoaffective disorders, and to quit smoking; increased risk for seizures; weaker blocker of serotonin and norepinephrine uptake
mirtazapine (Remeron)	PO; 15 mg/day in a single dose at bedtime, may increase every 1–2 weeks (max: 45 mg/day)	Potent blocker of 5-HT$_2$ and 5-HT$_3$ receptor subtypes; blocks presynaptic alpha$_2$-receptors, enhancing norepinephrine release; use caution in cases in which patients have kidney or liver dysfunction
nefazodone	PO; 50–100 mg bid, may increase up to 300–600 mg/day	Minimal cardiovascular effects; fewer effects in blocking acetylcholine; less sedation; less sexual dysfunction compared to other antidepressants
trazodone (Desyrel)	PO; 150 mg/day, may increase by 50 mg/day every 3–4 days up to 400–600 mg/day	Increases total sleep time; reduces night awakenings; has anxiolytic effects

pre = *before*
post = *after*
synaptic = *the synapse*

TCAs act by inhibiting the reuptake of both norepinephrine and serotonin into presynaptic nerve terminals, as shown in Figure 10.1 ■. TCAs are used mainly for major depressive disorder and occasionally for milder situational depression. Clomipramine (Anafranil) is approved for treatment of obsessive-compulsive disorder, and other TCAs are sometimes used as offlabel treatments for panic attacks (see Chapter 9 ⬬). One use for TCAs, not related to psychopharmacology, is to treat childhood enuresis (bed-wetting).

Although TCAs work well in depression, they have some unpleasant and serious adverse effects. The most common adverse effect is *orthostatic hypotension* (feeling dizzy when changing to an upright or standing position), which occurs due to vasoconstriction of blood vessels. Sedation is a frequently reported complaint at the beginning of therapy, but patients usually become tolerant to this effect after several weeks of treatment. Most TCAs have a long half-life, which increases the risk of adverse effects for patients with delayed excretion (see Chapter 4 ⬬). Anticholinergic effects, such as dry mouth, constipation, urinary retention, blurred vision, and tachycardia, are common (see Chapter 4 ⬬). Significant drug interactions can occur with CNS depressants, sympathomimetics, anticholinergics, and MAOIs. Now that newer antidepressants

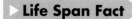

▶ Life Span Fact

TCAs can cause heart block and other adverse cardiac effects. They must be used cautiously in elderly patients or those with cardiac disease.

FIGURE 10.1

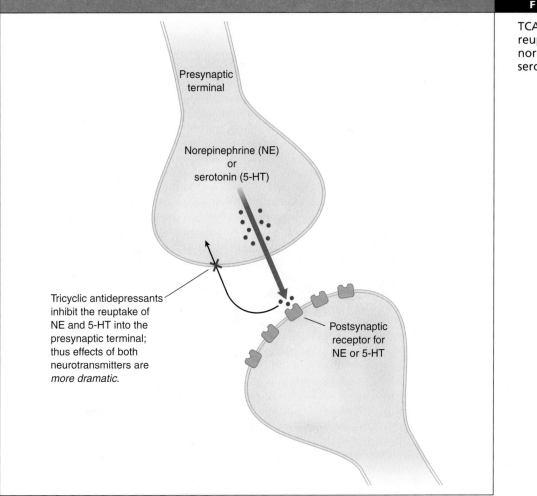

Presynaptic
terminal

Norepinephrine (NE)
or
serotonin (5-HT)

Tricyclic antidepressants
inhibit the reuptake of
NE and 5-HT into the
presynaptic terminal;
thus effects of both
neurotransmitters are
more dramatic.

Postsynaptic
receptor for
NE or 5-HT

TCAs inhibit the
reuptake of both
norepinephrine and
serotonin.

with fewer adverse effects are available, TCAs are less likely to be used as first-choice drugs in the treatment of depression.

Selective Serotonin Reuptake Inhibitors

Selective serotonin-reuptake inhibitors (SSRIs) are drugs that slow the reuptake of serotonin into presynaptic nerve terminals. They have become drugs of choice in the treatment of depression.

In the 1970s, it became increasingly clear that serotonin had a more substantial role in depression than once thought. Clinicians knew that the TCAs altered the sensitivity of serotonin to certain receptors in the brain, but they did not know how this was connected with depression. Ongoing efforts to find antidepressants with fewer adverse effects led to the development of the SSRIs.

Serotonin (5-HT) is a natural neurotransmitter in the CNS and is found in high concentrations in neurons of the hypothalamus, limbic system, medulla oblongata, and spinal cord. Serotonin is important to several body activities, including the cycling between NREM and REM sleep, pain perception, and emotional states (see Chapter 9 ⬤⬤). Lack of adequate serotonin in the CNS can lead to depression. Serotonin is metabolized to a less active substance by an enzyme located in presynaptic terminals called *monoamine oxidase (MAO).* A second enzyme, *catecholamine O-methyl transferase (COMT),* metabolizes serotonin in the synaptic cleft.

The TCAs inhibit the reuptake of both norepinephrine and serotonin into presynaptic nerve terminals, whereas the SSRIs are selective for just serotonin. Increased levels of serotonin in the synaptic gap cause complex neurotransmitter changes in presynaptic and postsynaptic neurons in the brain. Presynaptic receptors become less sensitive, whereas postsynaptic receptors become more sensitive. This concept is illustrated in Figure 10.2 ■.

SSRIs are about as effective as the TCAs for relieving depression. The major advantage of the SSRIs, and the one that makes them drugs of choice, is their greater safety. Sympathomimetic effects (increased heart rate and hypertension) and anticholinergic effects (dry mouth, blurred

FIGURE 10.2

SSRIs selectively inhibit the reuptake of serotonin, causing complex changes in the presynaptic and postsynaptic neurons.

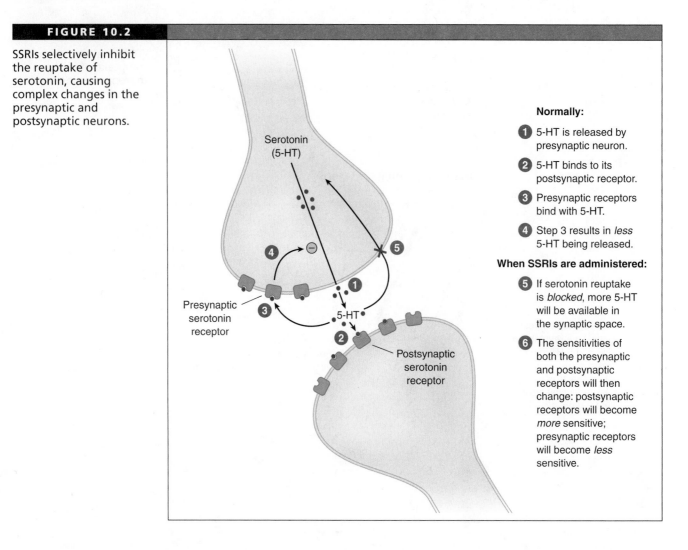

Normally:

1. 5-HT is released by presynaptic neuron.

2. 5-HT binds to its postsynaptic receptor.

3. Presynaptic receptors bind with 5-HT.

4. Step 3 results in *less* 5-HT being released.

When SSRIs are administered:

5. If serotonin reuptake is *blocked*, more 5-HT will be available in the synaptic space.

6. The sensitivities of both the presynaptic and postsynaptic receptors will then change: postsynaptic receptors will become *more* sensitive; presynaptic receptors will become *less* sensitive.

vision, urinary retention, and constipation) are less common with this drug class. Sedation is also experienced less frequently, and heart toxicity is not observed. All drugs in the SSRI class are equally effective and have similar adverse effects.

The most common adverse effects of SSRIs relate to sexual dysfunction. Up to 70% of both men and women may experience decreased libido and lack of ability to reach orgasm. In men, delayed ejaculation and impotence may occur. For patients who are sexually active, these adverse effects may result in noncompliance with pharmacotherapy. Other common adverse effects of SSRIs include nausea, headache, anxiety, and insomnia.

Serotonin syndrome (SES) is an adverse event that may occur when a patient is taking an SSRI and an additional medication that affects the metabolism, synthesis, or reuptake of serotonin. The result is that serotonin accumulates in the body. Symptoms can begin as early as 2 hours or as late as several weeks after taking the first dose. SES can be produced by the administration of an SSRI with an MAOI, a TCA, lithium, or a number of other medications. Symptoms of SES include mental status changes (confusion, anxiety, restlessness), hypertension, tremors, sweating, fever, and lack of muscular coordination. Conservative treatment is to discontinue the SSRI and provide supportive care. In severe cases, mechanical ventilation and muscle relaxants may be necessary. If left untreated, death may occur.

Serotonin-Norepinephrine Reuptake Inhibitors

Serotonin-norepinephrine reuptake inhibitors (SNRIs) inhibit both the reuptake of serotonin and norepinephrine with minimal effects on other neurotransmitters or their receptor subtypes. SNRIs affect the same neurotransmitters as the TCAs shown in Figure 10.1; therefore, this figure also depicts the drug mechanism for the SNRIs. With the SNRIs, adverse effects are less of a concern than for the TCAs; however, a few more important adverse effects are observed compared to the SSRIs. Higher doses of SRNIs are likely to produce liver toxicity, and they lower the patient's

DRUG PROFILE: ℞ *Imipramine (Tofranil)*

Therapeutic Class: Antidepressant, treatment of nocturnal enuresis (bed-wetting) in children
Pharmacologic Class: Tricyclic antidepressant (TCA), serotonin and norepinephrine reuptake inhibitor (SNRI)

Actions and Uses:

Imipramine blocks the reupake of serotonin and norepinephrine into nerve terminals. It is mainly used for major depressive disorder, although it is occasionally used for the treatment of nocturnal enuresis in children. The nurse may find imipramine prescribed for a number of offlabel uses, including intractable pain, anxiety disorders, and withdrawal syndromes from alcohol and cocaine.

Adverse Effects and Interactions:

Adverse effects include sedation, drowsiness, blurred vision, dry mouth, and cardiovascular symptoms such as dysrhythmias, heart block, and extreme hypertension. Agents that mimic the action of norepinephrine or serotonin should be avoided because imipramine inhibits their metabolism and may produce toxicity. Some patients may experience photosensitivity. Concurrent use of other CNS depressants, including alcohol, may cause sedation. Cimetidine (Tagamet) may inhibit the metabolism of imipramine, leading to increased serum levels and possible toxicity. Clonidine may decrease its antihypertensive effects and increase risk for CNS depression. Use of oral contraceptives may increase or decrease imipramine levels. Disulfiram may lead to delirium and tachycardia.

Imipramine should be used with caution with herbal supplements, such as evening primrose oil or ginkgo biloba, which may lower the seizure threshold. St. John's wort used with imipramine may cause serotonin syndrome.

Refer to MyNursingKit for a Nursing Process Focus specific to this drug.

NURSING PROCESS FOCUS

Patients Receiving Antidepressant Therapy

ASSESSMENT

Prior to drug administration:
- Obtain a complete health history (both physical/mental), including allergies, drug history, and possible drug interactions
- Obtain history of cardiac (including recent myocardial infarction [MI]), renal, biliary, liver, and mental disorders, including electrocardiogram (ECG) and blood studies: complete blood count (CBC), platelets, glucose, blood urea nitrogen (BUN), creatinine, electrolytes, liver function tests and enzymes, and urinalysis
- Assess neurologic status, including seizure activity, level of consciousness (LOC), and identification of recent mood and behavior patterns
- Identify factors that may have precipitated the depressive episode

POTENTIAL NURSING DIAGNOSES

- Ineffective Coping related to inadequate level of confidence in ability to cope.
- Risk for injury related to adverse effects of medications and depressive state.
- Disturbed Thought Processes related to adverse effects of drug and lack of positive coping skills.
- Deficient Knowledge related to information about disorder and drug therapy.
- Urinary Retention related to adverse anticholinergic effects of drug.

continued . . .

NURSING PROCESS FOCUS (continued)

PLANNING: PATIENT GOALS AND EXPECTED OUTCOMES

The patient will:
- Report mood elevation and effectively engage in activities of daily living
- Report an absence of suicidal ideations and improvement in thought processes
- Demonstrate a decrease in anxiety (e.g., ritual behaviors)
- Demonstrate an understanding of the drug's action by accurately describing drug effects and precautions

IMPLEMENTATION

Interventions and (Rationales)	Patient Teaching/Discharge Planning
■ Monitor vital signs, especially pulse and blood pressure. (Imipramine may cause orthostatic hypotension.)	Instruct the patient to: ■ Report any change in sensorium, particularly impending syncope ■ Avoid abrupt changes in position ■ Monitor vital signs (especially blood pressure), ensuring proper use of home equipment ■ Consult the health care provider regarding "reportable" blood pressure readings (e.g., lower than 80/50 mmHg)
■ Observe for serotonin syndrome in SSRI use: confusion, mania, headache, respiratory problems, kidney failure, and possibly death (usually occurs with concurrent use of St. John's wort or MAOIs). If suspected, discontinue the drug and initiate supportive care. Respond according to intensive care unit (ICU)/emergency department protocols. ■ Monitor for paradoxical diaphoresis, which must be considered a significant sign and is especially serious when coupled with nausea/vomiting or chest pain. ■ Monitor cardiovascular status. Observe for hypertension and signs of impending stroke or MI and heart failure.	■ Inform the patient that overdosage may result in serotonin syndrome, which can be life threatening. ■ Instruct the patient to seek immediate medical attention for dizziness, headache, tremor, nausea/vomiting, anxiety, disorientation, hyperreflexia, diaphoresis, and fever. ■ Instruct the patient to immediately report severe headache, dizziness, paresthesias, bradycardia, chest pain, tachycardia, nausea/vomiting, or diaphoresis.
■ Monitor neurologic status. Observe for somnolence and seizures. (TCAs may cause somnolence related to CNS depression; may reduce the seizure threshold.)	Instruct the patient to: ■ Report significant changes in neurologic status, such as seizures, extreme lethargy, slurred speech, disorientation, or ataxia, and to discontinue the drug ■ Take the dose at bedtime to avoid daytime sedation
■ Monitor mental and emotional status. Observe for suicidal ideation. (Therapeutic benefits may be delayed. Outpatients should have no more than a 7-day medication supply.) Also monitor for underlying or concomitant psychoses such as schizophrenia or bipolar disorders (may trigger manic states).	Instruct the patient: ■ To immediately report dysphoria or suicidal impulses ■ To commit to a "no-self harm" verbal contract ■ That it may take 10–14 days before improvement is noticed, and about 1 month to achieve full therapeutic effect
■ Monitor sleep–wake cycle. Observe for insomnia and/or daytime somnolence.	Instruct the patient to: ■ Take the drug very early in the morning to promote normal timing of sleep onset ■ Avoid driving or potentially hazardous activities until the effects of the drug are known ■ Take at bedtime if daytime drowsiness persists
■ Monitor renal status and urinary output. (This drug may cause urinary retention due to muscle relaxation in urinary tract. Imipramine is excreted through the kidneys. Fluoxetine is slowly metabolized and excreted, increasing the risk of organ damage. Urinary retention may exacerbate existing symptoms of prostatic hypertrophy.)	Instruct the patient to: ■ Monitor fluid intake and output ■ Notify the health care provider of edema, dysuria (hesitancy, pain, diminished stream), changes in urine quantity or quality (e.g., cloudy, with sediment) ■ Report fever or flank pain that may be indicative of a urinary tract infection related to urine retention

continued . . .

NURSING PROCESS FOCUS *(continued)*

Interventions and (Rationales)

- Use cautiously with elderly or young patients. (Diminished kidney and liver function related to aging can result in higher serum drug levels and may require lower doses. Children, due to an immature CNS, respond paradoxically to CNS-active drugs.)

- Monitor gastrointestinal status. Observe for abdominal distention. (Muscarinic blockade reduces tone and motility of intestinal smooth muscle and may cause paralytic ileus.)

- Monitor liver function. Observe for signs and symptoms of hepatotoxicity.
- Monitor blood studies, including CBC, differential, platelets, prothrombin time (PT), partial thromboplastin time (PTT), and liver enzymes.

- Monitor hematologic status. Observe for signs of bleeding. (Imipramine may cause blood dyscrasias. Use with warfarin may increase bleeding time.)

- Monitor immune/metabolic status. Use with caution in patients with diabetes mellitus or hyperthyroidism. (If given in hyperthyroidism, this drug can cause agranulocytosis. Imipramine may either increase or decrease serum glucose. Fluoxetine may cause initial anorexia and weight loss, but prolonged therapy may result in weight gain of up to 20 pounds.)

- Observe for extrapyramidal and anticholinergic effects. In overdosage, 12 hours of anticholinergic activity is followed by CNS depression. Do not treat overdosage with quinidine, procainamide, atropine, or barbiturates. (Quinidine and procainamide can increase the possibility of dysrhythmia; atropine can lead to severe anticholinergic effects; and barbiturates can lead to excess sedation.)

- Monitor visual acuity. Use with caution in narrow-angle glaucoma. (Imipramine may cause an increase in intraocular pressure. Anticholinergic effects may produce blurred vision.)

- Ensure patient safety. (Dizziness caused by postural hypotension increases the risk of fall injuries.)

Patient Teaching/Discharge Planning

Instruct the patient that:
- Elderly patients may be more prone to adverse effects such as hypertension and dysrhythmias
- Children on imipramine for nocturnal enuresis may experience mood alterations

Instruct the patient to:
- Exercise, drink adequate amounts of fluids, and add dietary fiber to promote stool passage
- Consult the nurse regarding a bulk laxative or stool softener if constipation becomes a problem

Instruct the patient to:
- Report nausea, vomiting, diarrhea, rash, jaundice, epigastric or abdominal pain, tenderness, or change in color of stool
- Adhere to laboratory testing regimen for blood tests and urinalysis as directed

- Instruct the patient to report excessive bruising, fatigue, pallor, shortness of breath, frank bleeding, and/or tarry stools.
- Conduct guaiac testing on stool for occult blood.

Instruct the patient:
- With diabetes to monitor glucose level daily and to consult the nurse regarding reportable serum glucose levels.
- To monitor weight. Possible anorexia and weight loss will diminish with continued therapy.

Instruct the patient to:
- Immediately report involuntary muscle movement of the face or upper body (e.g., tongue spasms), fever, anuria, lower abdominal pain, anxiety, hallucinations, psychomotor agitation, visual changes, dry mouth, and difficulty swallowing
- Relieve dry mouth with (sugar-free) hard candies, by chewing gum, and by drinking fluids
- Avoid alcohol-containing mouthwashes, which can further dry oral mucous membranes

Instruct the patient to:
- Report visual changes, headache, or eye pain
- Inform an eye care professional of imipramine therapy

Instruct the patient to:
- Call for assistance before getting out of bed or attempting to ambulate alone
- Avoid driving or performing hazardous activities until blood pressure is stabilized and effects of the drug are known

EVALUATION OF OUTCOME CRITERIA

Evaluate the effectiveness of drug therapy by confirming that patient goals and expected outcomes have been met (see "Planning").
See Table 10.2 for a list of drugs to which these nursing actions apply.

threshold for seizures. Also, as seen with the TCAs and owing to the effects of norepinephrine, SNRIs may result in heart toxicity and sexual dysfunction in some patients.

From 2004 until the present, a number of FDA alerts about SNRIs were issued, including the *black box warning* cautioning patients to avoid taking these drugs with other antidepressants and with other medications (e.g., migraine drugs). Taking multiple antidepressant drugs or similar chemically based drugs might produce SES or cause patients to commit suicide (see Chapter 9 ∞).

In 2004, duloxetine (Cymbalta) was approved by the FDA for the treatment of neuropathic pain. Other clinical uses since that time have been conditionally supported and then rescinded. Venlafaxine (Effexor) has been approved for the treatment of major depression, neuropathic pain, and migraines. Effexor is available in an intermediate-release form that requires two or three doses a day. In 2008, the FDA granted one drug manufacturer permission to market desvenlafaxine (Pristiq), an active metabolite of venlafaxine, in once-daily extended-release tablets. Pristiq has been approved for the treatment of major depressive disorder.

Monoamine Oxidase Inhibitors

As discussed, the action of norepinephrine at adrenergic synapses is terminated through two means: (1) reuptake into the presynaptic nerve and (2) enzymatic destruction by the enzyme monoamine oxidase (MAO). By decreasing the effectiveness of the enzyme MAO, **monoamine oxidase inhibitors (MAOIs)** limit the breakdown of norepinephrine, dopamine, and serotonin in the CNS. This creates higher levels of these neurotransmitters in the brain to facilitate neurotransmission and to alleviate the symptoms of depression (Figure 10.3 ■).

In the 1950s, the MAOIs were the first drugs approved to treat depression. They are just as effective as the TCAs and SSRIs in treating depression. However, because of drug–drug and food–drug interactions, hepatotoxicity, and the development of safer antidepressants, MAOIs are now reserved for patients who are not responsive to the other antidepressant classes.

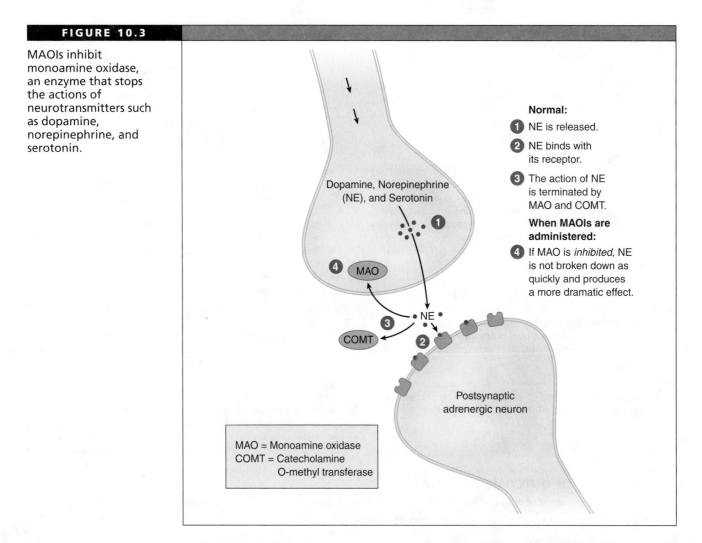

FIGURE 10.3

MAOIs inhibit monoamine oxidase, an enzyme that stops the actions of neurotransmitters such as dopamine, norepinephrine, and serotonin.

Dopamine, Norepinephrine (NE), and Serotonin

MAO

4

NE

3

COMT

2

Postsynaptic adrenergic neuron

MAO = Monoamine oxidase
COMT = Catecholamine O-methyl transferase

Normal:

1 NE is released.

2 NE binds with its receptor.

3 The action of NE is terminated by MAO and COMT.

When MAOIs are administered:

4 If MAO is *inhibited*, NE is not broken down as quickly and produces a more dramatic effect.

DRUG PROFILE: ℞ *Fluoxetine (Prozac)*

Therapeutic Class: Antidepressant

Pharmacologic Class: Selective serotonin reuptake inhibitor (SSRI)

Actions and Uses:

Fluoxetine acts by selectively inhibiting serotonin reuptake into presynaptic nerve terminals. Its main use is in major depressive disorder, although it may be prescribed for obsessive-compulsive and eating disorders. Therapeutic actions include improved affect, mood enhancement, and increased appetite, with maximum effects observed after several days to weeks. Fluoxetine is pregnancy category B.

Adverse Effects and Interactions:

Fluoxetine may cause headaches, nervousness, insomnia, nausea, and diarrhea. Foods high in the amino acid tryptophan should be avoided. Coadministration with selegiline may increase the risk of a hypertensive crisis. TCAs administered with fluoxetine may produce SES. Symptoms of fluoxetine overdose include fever, confusion, shivering, sweating, and muscle spasms. Fluoxetine cannot be used if the patient took an MAOI within 14 days. Use with benzodiazepines may cause increased adverse CNS effects. Use with beta blockers can cause their decreased elimination, leading to hypotension or bradycardia. Use with phenytoin, clozapine, or theophylline may lead to decreased elimination of these drugs and toxicity. Use with warfarin may lead to increased risk of bleeding due to competitive protein binding.

Fluoxetine should be used with caution with herbal supplements such as St. John's wort or L-tryptophan, which may cause SES, and kava, which may increase the effects of fluoxetine.

Mechanism in Action:

Fluoxetine (Prozac) is an SSRI. It acts by blocking the recycling of the brain neurotransmitter serotonin into presynaptic nerve terminals. At the synaptic cleft, serotonin continually binds with postsynaptic receptors and activates excitatory postsynaptic potentials (EPSPs). This is thought to restore the mental state of a patient with depression to normal.

Refer to MyNursingKit for a Nursing Process Focus specific to this drug.

Common adverse effects of the MAOIs include orthostatic hypotension, headache, insomnia, and diarrhea. A primary concern is that these agents interact with a large number of foods and other medications, sometimes with serious effects. A hypertensive crisis can occur when a MAOI is used together with other antidepressants or sympathomimetic drugs. Combining an MAOI with an SSRI can produce SES. If given with antihypertensives, the patient can experience excessive hypotension. MAOIs also increase the hypoglycemic effects of insulin and oral antidiabetic drugs. Extreme fever is known to occur in patients taking MAOIs with meperidine (Demerol), dextromethorphan (Pedia Care and others), and TCAs.

A hypertensive crisis can also result from an interaction between MAOIs and foods containing tyramine, a form of the amino acid tyrosine. In fact, tyrosine is a presursor to norepinephrine in the nervous system. In many respects, tyramine resembles norepinephrine. Tyramine is usually degraded by MAO in the intestines. If a patient is taking MAOIs, however, tyramine enters the bloodstream in high amounts and displaces norepinephrine in presynaptic nerve terminals. The result is a sudden increase in norepinephrine, causing acute hypertension. Symptoms usually occur within minutes of ingesting the food and include occipital headache, stiff neck, flushing, palpitations, profuse sweating, and nausea. Calcium channel blockers may be given as an antidote to increased cardiovasular effects. Examples of foods containing tyramine are listed in Table 10.3.

Concept Review   **10.2**

■ Name the major classes of antidepressants. Name representative drugs within each class, and describe how each drug works pharmacologically.

TABLE 10.3	Foods Containing Tyramine		
FRUITS	**DAIRY PRODUCTS**	**ALCOHOL**	**MEATS**
Avocados	Cheese (except cottage cheese)	Beer	Beef or chicken liver
Bananas	Sour cream	Wines (especially red wines and Chianti)	Pate
Raisins	Yogurt		Meat extracts
Papaya products, including meat tenderizers			Pickled or kippered herring
Canned figs			Pepperoni
			Salami
			Sausage
			Bologna/hot dogs
VEGETABLES	**SAUCES**	**YEASTS**	**OTHER**
Pods of broad beans (fava beans)	Soy sauce	All yeasts or yeast extracts	Chocolate

DRUG PROFILE: Ⓟ *Phenelzine (Nardil)*

Therapeutic Class: Antidepressant

Pharmacologic Class: Monoamine oxidase inhibitor (MAOI)

Actions and Uses:

Phenelzine produces its effects by irreversible inhibition of MAO; therefore, it intensifies the effects of norepinephrine in adrenergic synapses. It is used to manage symptoms of depression not responsive to other types of pharmacotherapy, and it is occasionally used for panic disorder. Drug effects may continue for 2 to 3 weeks after therapy is discontinued.

Adverse Effects and Interactions:

Common adverse effects are constipation, dry mouth, orthostatic hypotension, insomnia, nausea, and loss of appetite. It may increase heart rate and neural activity, leading to delirium, mania, anxiety, and convulsions. Severe hypertension may occur when ingesting foods containing tyramine. Seizures, respiratory depression, circulatory collapse, and coma may occur in cases of severe overdose. Many other drugs affect the action of phenelzine. Use with TCAs and SSRIs should be avoided, because the combination can cause temperature elevation and seizures. Opiates, including meperidine, should be avoided due to increased risk of respiratory failure or hypertensive crisis.

Phenelzine should be used with caution with herbal supplements such as ginseng, which could cause headache, tremors, mania, insomnia, irritability, and visual hallucinations. Concurrent use of ephedra could cause hypertensive crisis.

Refer to MyNursingKit for a Nursing Process Focus specific to this drug.

BIPOLAR DISORDER

bi = *two*
polar = *extremes*

Bipolar disorder is characterized by extreme and opposite moods. Patients may display signs of euphoria and depression or feelings of excitement and calm.

NATURAL THERAPIES

St. John's Wort for Depression

One of the most popular herbs in the United States, St. John's wort (*Hypericum perforatum*) grows throughout Asia, Europe, and North America. Its modern use is as an antidepressant. It gets its name from a legend that red spots once appeared on its leaves on the anniversary of the beheading of St. John the Baptist. The word *wort* is a British term for "plant."

Research suggests that substances found in St. John's wort selectively inhibit serotonin re-uptake in certain brain neurons. A number of clinical studies suggest that St. John's wort is an effective treatment for mild to moderate depression, and that it may be just as effective as TCAs and SSRIs. Recent analyses also suggest that the herb may be effective for major depression and that it causes fewer adverse effects than traditional drugs. St. John's wort may interact with many medications, including oral contraceptives, warfarin, digoxin, and cyclosporine. It should not be taken concurrently with antidepressant medications.

St. John's wort is well tolerated, producing mild adverse effects such as gastrointestinal (GI) distress, fatigue, and allergic skin reactions. The herb contains compounds that photosensitize the skin; thus patients should be advised to apply sunscreen or to wear protective clothing when outdoors.

Patients with bipolar disorder may experience emotions ranging from depression to extreme agitation.

CORE CONCEPT 10.4

Once known as *manic depression*, bipolar disorder is characterized by extreme and opposite moods, such as euphoria and depression. Although the moods of patients may shift between extremes, usually patients will remain in one state for awhile, or they may remain in a normal state for prolonged times.

Depressed and slightly depressed *(dysphoric)* signs and symptoms are the same as those described earlier in this chapter. Patients with bipolar disorder also display signs of *mania,* an emotional state characterized by high psychomotor activity and irritability. Symptoms of mania are shown in the following list; these are generally the opposite of depressive symptoms.

dys = *difficulty (as in illness)*
phoric = *bearing*

- Insomnia
- Activity for days without rest and without appearing tired
- Easy agitation and aggression
- Feelings of exaggerated confidence
- Making choices without regard for a long-term plan or consequences of action
- Attention seeking
- Unusual interest in sex
- Drug abuse, including alcohol, cocaine, or sleeping medications
- Denial that the behavior is a problem

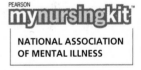

NATIONAL ASSOCIATION OF MENTAL ILLNESS

Concept Review 10.3

- Identify the symptoms of mania. How do manic symptoms generally compare with depressive symptoms?

Mood stabilization in patients with bipolar disorder is accomplished with lithium and other drugs.

CORE CONCEPT 10.5

Drugs for bipolar disorder are called **mood stabilizers** because they have the ability to moderate extreme shifts in emotions between mania and depression. Currently, lithium, antiseizure drugs, and atypical antipsychotic drugs are the choices used for mood stabilization in patients with bipolar disorder. Table 10.4 and Table 11.4 (see page 162) list selected drugs used to treat bipolar disorder.

For years, the traditional treatment of bipolar disorder has been lithium (Eskalith), which was used as monotherapy or in combination with other drugs. Lithium was approved in the United States in 1970. With lithium, serum levels must be checked every 1 to 3 days when beginning

TABLE 10.4	Drugs for Bipolar Disorder: Mood Stabilizers	
DRUG	**ROUTE AND ADULT DOSE**	**REMARKS**
Pr lithium (Eskalith)	PO; initial 600 mg tid, maintenance 300 mg tid (max: 2.4 g/day)	For treatment of mania and depressive symptoms; must be used cautiously in epilepsy and in psychosis
ANTISEIZURE DRUGS		
carbamazepine (Tegretol)	PO; 200 mg bid, gradually increased to 800–1200 mg/day in three to four divided doses	For treatment of manic depressive and schizoaffective symptoms; used as antiseizure medication
iamotrigine (Lamictal)	PO; 50 mg/day for 2 weeks, then 50 mg bid for 2 weeks; may increase gradually up to 300–500 mg/day in two divided doses (max: 700 mg/day)	Used as antiseizure medication; fatal rash has been reported in children less than 16 years old
valproic acid (Depakene) (see page 203 for the Drug Profile box)	PO; 250 mg tid (max: 60 mg/kg/day)	For treatment of mania and prevention of migraine headache; used as antiseizure medication

DRUG PROFILE: **Pr** *Lithium (Eskalith)*

Therapeutic Class: Bipolar affective disorder drug, antimanic, antidepressant

Pharmacologic Class: Serotonin receptor blocker, glutamate inhibiting agent, inhibitor of glycogen synthase kinase-3 beta

Actions and Uses:

Although the exact mechanism of action is not clear, lithium has been thought to alter the activity of neurons containing dopamine, norepinephrine, and serotonin by influencing their release, synthesis, and reuptake. More recent studies suggest that lithium may inhibit the action of glutamate, an excitatory neurotransmitter in the synapse. Other promising information indicates that serotonin at the receptor may be blocked and that glycogen synthase kinase-3 beta may be inhibited within the neuron. These actions tend to stabilize a wider range of cellular activation pathways. Therapeutic actions are stabilization of mood during periods of mania, and antidepressant effects during periods of depression. Lithium has neither antimanic nor antidepressant effects in individuals without bipolar disorder. After taking lithium for 2 to 3 weeks, patients are able to better concentrate and function in self-care.

Adverse Effects and Interactions:

Lithium may cause dizziness, fatigue, short-term memory loss, increased urination, nausea, vomiting, loss of appetite, abdominal pain, diarrhea, dry mouth, muscular weakness, and slight tremors. Some drugs, including diuretics, sodium bicarbonate, and potassium citrate, increase the rate at which the kidneys remove lithium from the bloodstream. Other drugs, such as methyldopa and probenecid, inhibit the rate of lithium excretion. Patients should not have a salt-free diet when taking this drug, because such a diet reduces lithium excretion. Diuretics enhance excretion of sodium and increase the risk of lithium toxicity. Use with anticholinergic drugs can cause urinary retention that, coupled with the polyuria effect of lithium, may cause a medical emergency. Alcohol can increase drug action.

Refer to MyNursingKit for a Nursing Process Focus specific to this drug.

therapy, and every 2 to 3 months thereafter. To ensure therapeutic action, concentrations of lithium in the blood must remain within the range of 0.6 to 1.5 mEq/L. Close monitoring encourages compliance and helps to avoid toxicity. Lithium acts like sodium in the body, so conditions in which sodium is lost (e.g., excessive sweating or dehydration) can cause lithium toxicity. Lithium overdose may be treated with hemodialysis and supportive care.

For the most complete control of bipolar disorder, it is not unusual for other drugs to be used in combination with lithium. During the depressed stage, a TCA or an atypical antidepressant such as bupropion (Wellbutrin) may be necessary. During manic phases, a benzodiazepine will moderate manic symptoms (see Chapter 9 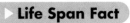). In cases of extreme agitation, delusions, or hallucinations, an antipsychotic agent may be indicated (see Chapter 11 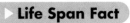). Continued patient compliance is essential to achieving successful pharmacotherapy because some patients do not perceive their condition as abnormal.

Today, antiseizure drugs (see Chapter 13 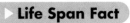) and antipsychotic drugs (see Chapter 11 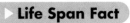) have emerged as probably the most effective agents for mood stabilization. For example, valproic acid (Depakene), carbamazepine (Tegretol), and lamotrigine (Lamictal) are the antiseizure drugs most often used in the treatment of rapidly cycling and mixed states of bipolar disorder. Lithium has remained effective for purely manic or purely depressive states. Atypical antipsychotics have been very effective for the treatment of extreme mania. Clozapine (Clozaril) was the first atypical antipsychotic. Newer agents with less risk for agranulocytosis have replaced the older drugs. The newer antipsychotic drugs are aripiprazole (Abilify), olanzapine (Zyprexa), quetiapine (Seroquel), risperidone (Risperdal, Risperdal Consta), and ziprasidone (Zeldox). Longer term stabilization of extreme and unusual behaviors with atypical antipsychotics is covered in Chapter 11 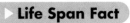.

Concept Review   10.4

- Give the general name of drugs used to treat bipolar disorder. What has been the main drug used to treat bipolar disorder, and how does it work pharmacologically? What other drugs treat bipolar disorder?

ATTENTION DEFICIT–HYPERACTIVITY DISORDER

Attention deficit–hyperactivity disorder (ADHD) is a condition characterized by poor attention span, behavior control issues, and/or hyperactivity. Although usually diagnosed in childhood, symptoms of ADHD may extend into adulthood.

Attention deficit–hyperactivity disorder presents challenges for children and adults.

CORE CONCEPT 10.6

ADHD is characterized by developmentally inappropriate behaviors involving difficulty in paying attention or focusing on tasks. ADHD may be diagnosed when a child's hyperactive behaviors significantly interfere with normal play, sleep, or learning activities. Hyperactive children usually have increased motor activity shown by a tendency to be fidgety and impulsive and to interrupt and talk excessively during their developmental years; therefore, they may not be able to interact with others appropriately at home or school. In boys, the activity levels are usually more overt. Girls show less aggression and impulsiveness but may show more anxiety, mood swings, social withdrawal, and cognitive and language delays. Girls also tend to be older at the time of diagnosis, so problems and setbacks related to the disorder exist for a longer time before treatment interventions are undertaken. Symptoms of ADHD are shown in the following list:

▶ **Life Span Fact**

ADHD affects as many as 5% of all children. Most children diagnosed with this condition are between the ages of 3 and 7 years, and boys are four to eight times more likely to be diagnosed than girls.

- Easy distractability
- Failure to receive or follow instructions properly
- Inability to focus on one task at a time and tendency to jump from one activity to another
- Difficulty remembering
- Frequent loss or misplacing of personal items
- Excessive talking and interrupting other children in a group
- Inability to sit still when asked repeatedly
- Impulsiveness
- Sleep disturbances

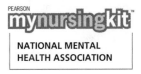

NATIONAL MENTAL HEALTH ASSOCIATION

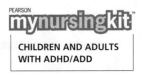

CHILDREN AND ADULTS WITH ADHD/ADD

Most children with ADHD have associated challenges. Many find it difficult to concentrate on tasks assigned in school. Even if they are gifted, their grades may suffer because they have difficulty following a conventional routine; discipline may also be a problem. Teachers are often the first to suggest that a child should be examined for ADHD and receive medication when

Fast Facts ADHD

- ADHD is the major reason why children are referred for mental health treatment.
- About 50% of children are also diagnosed with oppositional defiant or conduct disorder.
- Anxiety disorder is diagnosed in 25% of children.
- About one third are also diagnosed with depression.
- Learning disabilities are present in about 20% of children.

behaviors in the classroom escalate to the point of interfering with learning. A diagnosis is based on psychological and medical evaluations.

The cause of ADHD is not clear. Recent evidence suggests that hyperactivity may be related to a deficit or dysfunction of dopamine, norepinephrine, and serotonin in the reticular activating system of the brain (see Chapter 9 ⊙). ADHD was once thought to be caused by sugar, chocolate, high-carbohydrate foods and beverages, and certain food additives, but these have been disproved as causing or aggravating ADHD.

One third to one half of children diagnosed with ADHD also experience symptoms of attention dysfunction in their adult years. Symptoms of *attention deficit disorder (ADD)* in adults appear similar to those of mood disorders and include anxiety, mania, restlessness, and depression, which can also cause difficulties in interpersonal relationships. Attention dysfunction in adults is often linked with poor self-esteem, diminished social success, and introverted behaviors. Patients may have mood swings similar to bipolar disorder.

CNS Stimulants

Traditional medications used to treat ADHD are CNS stimulants. These drugs activate specific areas of the brain.

DRUG PROFILE: ⊕ *Methylphenidate (Ritalin)*

Therapeutic Class: Drug for attention-deficit-hyperactivity disorder, narcolepsy drug
Pharmacologic Class: Central nervous system stimulant, norepinephrine and dopamine releasing agent

Actions and Uses:

Methylphenidate activates the reticular activating system, causing heightened alertness in various regions of the brain, particularly those centers associated with focus and attention. Activation is partially achieved by the release of neurotransmitters such as norepinephrine, dopamine, and serotonin. Impulsiveness, hyperactivity, and disruptive behavior are usually reduced within a few weeks. These changes promote improved psychosocial interactions and academic performance.

Adverse Effects and Interactions:

In a patient with no ADHD, methylphenidate causes nervousness and insomnia. All patients are at risk for irregular heartbeat, high blood pressure, and liver toxicity. Methylphenidate is a Schedule II drug, indicating its potential to cause dependence when used for extended periods. Periodic drug-free "holidays" are recommended to reduce drug dependence and to assess the patient's condition.

Methylphenidate interacts with many drugs. For example, it may decrease the effectiveness of anticonvulsants, anticoagulants, and guanethidine. Use with clonidine may increase adverse effects. Antihypertensives or other CNS stimulants could increase the vasoconstrictive action of methylphenidate. MAOIs may produce hypertensive crisis.

Mechanism in Action:

Methylphenidate (Ritalin) is a medication used for the treatment of ADHD in children and narcolepsy in adults. Methylphenidate increases norepinephrine (NE) release in ascending pathways of the reticular activating system (RAS), which maintains arousal and alertness. Methylphenidate also directly stimulates dopamine release in areas of the brain responsible for concentration.

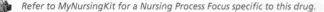 *Refer to MyNursingKit for a Nursing Process Focus specific to this drug.*

Central nervous system (CNS) stimulants have been the main course of treatment for ADHD.

These drugs stimulate specific areas of the CNS that heighten alertness and increase focus. Recently, a non-CNS stimulant was approved to treat ADHD. Agents for treating ADHD are listed in Table 10.5.

Stimulants reverse many of the symptoms and help patients to focus on tasks. The most widely prescribed drug for ADHD is methylphenidate (Ritalin). Other CNS stimulants less prescribed include d- and 1-amphetamine racemic mixture (Adderall), dextroamphetamine (Dexedrine), or methamphetamine (Desoxyn). More recently, extended release forms have been made available: dextroamphetamine mixture (Adderall XR), dexmethylphenidate (Focalin XR), and slow-releasing methylphenidate (Ritalin, LA/SR).

Patients taking CNS stimulants must be carefully monitored because the drugs may cause paradoxical hyperactivity. Adverse reactions include insomnia, nervousness, anorexia, and weight loss. Occasionally, a patient may suffer from dizziness, depression, irritability, nausea, or abdominal pain. These drugs are Schedule II controlled substances and pregnancy category C.

Non-CNS Stimulants

Non-CNS stimulants have been tried for ADHD; however, they are less effective. Clonidine (Catapres) is sometimes prescribed when patients are extremely aggressive or active or have difficulty falling asleep. Atypical antidepressants such as bupropion (Wellbutrin) and TCAs such as desipramine

TABLE 10.5	Drugs for Attention Deficit-Hyperactivity Disorder	
DRUG	**ROUTE AND ADULT DOSE**	**REMARKS**
CNS STIMULANTS		
d- and l-amphetamine racemic mixture (Adderall)	>6 years old: PO; 5 mg daily to bid, may increase by 5 mg at weekly intervals (max: 40 mg/day); 3–5 years old: PO; 2.5 mg one to two times/day, may increase by 2.5 mg at weekly intervals	May be used for daytime sleep disorder (narcolepsy); high potential for abuse; also called amphetamine sulfate
dextroamphetamine mixture (Adderall XR)	3–5 years old: PO; 2.5 mg daily to bid, may increase by 2.5 mg at weekly intervals; 6 years old: PO; 5 mg daily to bid, increase by 5 mg at weekly intervals (max: 40 mg/day)	Potent appetite suppressant; should only be used for short-term treatment of ADHD; safety in children less than 3 years old has not been established
methamphetamine (Desoxyn)	≤6 years old: PO; 2.5–5 mg daily to bid, may increase by 5 mg at weekly intervals (max: 20–25 mg/day)	Abuse potential high in adults
(Pr) methylphenidate (Ritalin)	PO; 5–10 mg before breakfast and lunch, with gradual increase of 5–10 mg/week as needed (max: 60 mg/day)	Most widely used drug for patients with ADHD; more dramatic effect on attention deficit than for hyperactivity
benzphetamine (Didrex)	PO; 25–50 mg one to three times per day (max: 150 mg/day)	Drug for patients with ADHD
dexmethylphenidate (Focalin XR)	Child older than 6 years: PO: 2.5 mg bid may increase by 2.5–5 mg/week (max: 20 mg/day); 5 mg/day extended release may increase by 5 mg/week. Adult: PO: 2.5 mg bid; may increase by 2.5–5 mg/day at weekly intervals (max: 20 mg/day)	Drug for patients with ADHD
lisdexamfetamine (Vyvanse)	PO: 30 mg once daily in the a.m. (max: 70 mg/day)	Drug for patients with ADHD
NONSTIMULANTS		
atomoxetine (Strattera)	PO; start with 40 mg in a.m., may increase after 3 days to target dose of 80 mg/day given either once in the morning, divided morning, or late afternoon/early evening; may increase to max of 100 mg/day if needed	Inhibits reuptake of norepinephrine; safety and efficacy in children less than 6 years old has not been established
clonidine (Catapres)	PO; 5 mcg/kg/day in four divided doses, average dose is 0.15–0.2 mg/day	Sometimes prescribed when patients are extremely aggressive, active, or have difficulty sleeping; stimulates alpha$_2$-receptors in the brain; available in transdermal patch

PATIENTS NEED TO KNOW

Patients taking antidepressants need to know the following:

In General

1. Avoid driving or operating machinery until response to the medication is known. Its sedating effects can increase the risk for accidental injury.
2. Do not stop taking the medication without consulting a health care provider.
3. Antidepressants may take 1–4 weeks to become fully effective.

Regarding Tricyclics

4. Tricyclics may increase appetite, cause dizziness upon rapid change of position, and be sedating. Report dry mouth, constipation, urinary retention, increase in heart rate and palpitations, or blurred vision if they occur.
5. Avoid the use of alcohol; it increases sedative effects.

Regarding MAOIs

6. MAOIs may cause problems with sleep, agitation, dizziness when rapidly changing position, and dangerous interactions with other medications. Eating foods high in tyramine can cause a hypertensive crisis. Such foods include aged cheeses, wine, luncheon meats, and sausages.
7. Report any of the following adverse effects to a health care provider: increased heart rate or lightheadedness when changing positions.
8. Monitor weight; an increase or a decrease may occur.
9. A decrease in sexual interest or performance may occur. If this does, discuss a change in medication with a health care provider.

Regarding SSRIs

10. SSRIs may cause GI upset, dizziness, skin rash, and headache. Report these signs and symptoms to a health care provider.
11. Avoid foods containing large amounts of tryptophan, such as cottage cheese, poultry, peanuts, and sesame seeds.
12. Do not combine MAOIs and SSRIs. Do not take St. John's wort with any antidepressant. These combinations, such as confusion, mania, headache, respiratory problems, kidney failure, and possibly death, can cause serious adverse effects, termed SES.
13. If insomnia is a problem, take the medication in the morning.
14. If nausea is a problem, take the medication with food, unless otherwise instructed.

For Attention Deficit–Hyperactivity Disorder (ADHD)

15. Many drugs used for the treatment of ADHD are controlled substances.
16. Dependence may occur due to the high abuse potential of CNS stimulants.
17. CNS stimulants often increase blood pressure. Monitor blood pressure closely.
18. Take drugs at least 6 hours before bedtime to avoid insomnia.
19. Avoid giving drinks containing caffeine to children who are seizure prone and those with diabetes. (CNS stimulants lower the threshold in patients with seizure disorders and alter insulin needs in patients with diabetes.)
20. Monitor height and weight in children with prolonged therapy.
21. Administer drugs after meals to reduce appetite-suppressive effects.
22. Do not take medication used to combat fatigue.
23. Even though atomoxetine (Strattera) is a nonstimulant ADHD medication, it still has many of the adverse effects of the other ADHD medications.

(Norpramin) and imipramine (Tofranil) are considered second-choice drugs for use when CNS stimulants fail to work or are contraindicated.

A recent addition to the treatment of ADHD in children and adults is atomoxetine (Strattera). Although its exact mechanism is not known, it is classified as a norepinephrine reuptake inhibitor. Patients on atomoxetine showed improved ability to focus on tasks and reduced hyperactivity. Efficacy appears to be equivalent to methylphenidate (Ritalin), although the drug is too new for long-term comparisons. Common adverse effects include headache, insomnia, upper abdominal pain, decreased appetite, and cough. Unlike methylphenidate, it is not a scheduled drug; thus, parents who are hesitant to place their child on stimulants now have a reasonable alternative.

Concept Review 10.5

■ What are the symptoms experienced by patients with ADHD? Which drug is most often used in the treatment of these symptoms? What are the common symptoms experienced by adults with ADD?

10.1 People suffer from depression for many reasons.

The two major categories of mood disorders are depression and bipolar disorder. Depression may involve both situational and biological causes. The recognition of depression is a collaborative effort among health care providers. A third emotional disorder is attention deficit–hyperactivity disorder.

10.2 Treatment of severe depression requires both medication and psychotherapy for the best results.

After a health examination is performed to rule out physical causes of depression, a psychological evaluation may be performed. Patients diagnosed with a major depressive disorder have at least five symptoms of recognized depression. Treatment may include medication in addition to a number of other approaches, including counseling and behavioral therapy, short-term psychotherapies, interpersonal therapy, psychodynamic therapies, and in extreme cases, electroconvulsive therapy (ECT) and repetitive transcranial magnetic stimulation (rTMS). Most therapeutic approaches involve a long-term commitment from patients, health care providers, and family.

10.3 Antidepressants enhance mood by boosting the actions of neurotransmitters, including norepinephrine and serotonin.

Drugs for depression are called antidepressants. The major classes of antidepressants are tricyclic antidepressants (TCAs), selective serotonin reuptake inhibitors (SSRIs), serotonin-norepinephrine reuptake inhibitors (SNRIs), and monoamine oxidase inhibitors (MAOIs). All drug classes work mainly by increasing the amount of norepinephrine, serotonin, and possibly other neurotransmitters in the nerve synapse and thereby intensifying neurotransmitter action and enhancing mood. Atypical antidepressants are a fifth class of drugs grouped mainly based on their similar actions but different chemical structures.

10.4 Patients with bipolar disorder may experience emotions ranging from depression to extreme agitation.

Bipolar disorder is characterized by sometimes extreme and opposite moods, such as depression and euphoria. During the depressive stages, patients express signs of major depression. Patients may then change to signs of mania or high psychomotor activity and irritability.

10.5 Mood stabilization in patients with bipolar disorder is accomplished with lithium and other drugs.

Drugs for bipolar disorder are called mood stabilizers. Lithium (Eskalith) may be used alone or in combination with other drugs, including antidepressants and antianxiety agents. Antiseizure drugs and atypical antipsychotic drugs have emerged as more effective drug treatments for bipolar disorder. Drugs are selective for extreme mania, extreme depression, or cycling of mood that occurs between the extremes.

10.6 Attention deficit–hyperactivity disorder (ADHD) presents challenges for children and adults.

ADHD is a condition characterized by poor attention span, behavior control issues, and/or hyperactivity. ADHD is normally diagnosed in childhood, although one third to one half of children with symptoms of attention deficit experience them into adulthood. As adults, patients with ADD have symptoms similar to mood disorders.

10.7 Central nervous system (CNS) stimulants have been the main course of treatment for ADHD.

The traditional drugs used to treat attention deficit in children have been the CNS stimulants. Patients taking CNS stimulants must be carefully monitored to avoid adverse reactions. Recently, non-CNS stimulants, including the new drug atomoxetine (Strattera), have been used as a reasonable alternative to existing Schedule II controlled substances.

REVIEW QUESTIONS

The following questions are written in NCLEX-PN® style. Answer these questions to assess your knowledge of the chapter material, and go back and review any material that is not clear to you.

1. Patient education for the patient started on antidepressants would include:

1. The avoidance of tyramine-containing foods
2. The signs and symptoms of hypertension
3. That drowsiness is a common adverse effect
4. That it may take a combination of antidepressants for effectiveness to occur

2. If a patient taking MAOIs experiences a hypertensive crisis, what may be given as an antidote?

1. Meperidine (Demerol)
2. Dextromethorphan
3. Calcium channel blockers
4. Carbamazepine (Tegretol)

3. When the patient on lithium is dehydrated, this could lead to:

1. Lower serum lithium levels
2. Increased effectiveness
3. The need to increase the lithium dosage
4. Lithium toxicity

4. The patient on methylphenidate (Ritalin) should be assessed for:

1. Signs of weight loss
2. Hypotension
3. Renal toxicity
4. Extreme euphoria and insomnia

5. Which of the following symptoms would indicate to the nurse that a patient is experiencing lithium toxicity?

1. Increased urination, diarrhea, tremors
2. Dry mouth, vomiting, hypotension
3. Constipation, blurred vision, hypertension
4. Increased appetite, increased energy, memory loss

6. Imipramine (Tofranil) has been ordered in a patient experiencing depression. Patient teaching would include which of the following?

1. The use of alcohol is permitted with this drug.
2. Avoid standing up too quickly.
3. Effectiveness occurs within a few hours of administration.
4. If a dose is missed, double up on the next dose.

7. The patient is taking phenelzine (Nardil). The nurse teaches her to avoid eating:

1. Eggs
2. Aged cheeses
3. Onions
4. Apples

8. Which of the following antiseizure mediations may be used as a mood stabilizer?

1. Diazepam (Valium)
2. Phenytoin (Dilantin)
3. Valproic acid (Depakene)
4. Lorazepam (Ativan)

9. The patient has been started on an MAOI for depression and is now asking if she can add St. John's wort to increase the effectiveness of the antidepressant. The nurse's best response would be:

1. "St. John's wort is highly effective for depression. Adding it to your current medication will increase its effectiveness."
2. "Although St. John's wort has been found to be effective for depression, you should consult with your physician before adding it to your current medication routine."
3. "St. John's wort cannot be mixed with MAOIs because of drug interactions."
4. "Because St. John's wort is effective for depression, you will no longer need your medication."

10. Antidepressants improve mood by increasing levels of:

1. Epinephrine and norepinephrine
2. Reticular formation within the hypothalamus
3. Norepinephrine and serotonin
4. GABA and serotonin

CASE STUDY QUESTIONS

For questions 1–4, please refer to the following case study, and choose the correct answer from choices 1–4.

Mr. Coxilean, a 38-year-old man, visits his family doctor and explains that lately he has been experiencing frequent headaches, disinterest in eating and sex, and a hard time "keeping focused." For the past 2 years, he has been taking OTC medication to help him sleep. Two times within the last year, he missed work because of extreme fatigue. Mr. Coxilean does not drink alcohol but admits, "The pressure is almost overwhelming sometimes." Mr. Coxilean is diagnosed with major depressive disorder.

1. The main reason why Mr. Coxilean would not be treated with mood stabilizers is the lack of:

1. Complaints from the patient, suggesting attention deficit disorder
2. Toxicity concerns for this class of drug
3. Evidence that the patient feels his condition is normal
4. Extreme shifts between mania and depression

2. If the lab values for Mr. Coxilean were normal, which of the following medications would be considered the drug of choice for his condition?

1. Doxepin (Sinequan)
2. Tranylcypromine (Parnate)
3. Sertraline (Zoloft)
4. Bupropion (Wellbutrin)

3. If phenelzine (Nardil) were prescribed for Mr. Coxilean, the health care provider would most likley tell him:

1. "Avoid reducing your salt intake. It increases excretion of this medication."
2. "Avoid chocolate and some other foods when taking this medication."
3. "You can take herbals, but avoid the use of St. John's wort."
4. "You can continue to take OTC medication for sleep, but monitor the frequency."

4. If SSRIs were prescribed for Mr. Coxilean, which of the following effects might still remain a problem?

1. Headaches
2. Loss of appetite
3. Poor sexual activity
4. Both 1 and 3

FURTHER STUDY

- Tricyclic antidepressants for panic attacks are covered in Chapter 9 ⚇ .

- Antiseizure drugs are discussed in Chapter 13 ⚇ .

- Benzodiazepines for treating anxiety are covered in Chapter 9 ⚇ .

- Antipsychotic agents are discussed in Chapter 11 ⚇ .

- The reticular activating system of the brain is further discussed in Chapter 9 ⚇ .

EXPLORE PEARSON **mynursingkit**™

MyNursingKit is your one stop for online chapter review materials and resources. Prepare for success with additional NCLEX®-style practice questions, interactive assignments and activities, web links, animations and videos, and more!

Register your access code from the front of your book at www.mynursingkit.com

11 Drugs for Psychoses

CORE CONCEPTS

11.1 Most psychoses have no identifiable cause and require long-term drug therapy.

11.2 Patients with schizophrenia experience many different symptoms that may change over time.

11.3 The experience and skills of the health care provider are critical to the pharmacologic management of psychoses.

11.4 Conventional antipsychotic drugs include the phenothiazines, phenothiazine-like drugs, and nonphenothiazines.

11.5 Atypical antipsychotic drugs and a newer drug class have been developed to better meet the needs of patients with psychoses.

DRUG SNAPSHOT

The following drugs are discussed in this chapter:

DRUG CLASSES	DRUG PROFILES
Conventional Antipsychotics	
Phenothiazines	**Pr** chlorpromazine (Thorazine)
Nonphenothiazines	**Pr** haloperidol (Haldol)

DRUG CLASSES	DRUG PROFILES
Atypical Antipsychotics	
	Pr risperidone (Risperdal, Risperdal Consta)
Dopamine System Stabilizers (DSSs)	

LEARNING OUTCOMES

After reading this chapter, the student should be able to:

1. Identify signs characteristic of psychosis.

2. Compare and contrast the positive and negative symptoms of schizophrenia.

3. Describe theories for the cause of schizophrenia.

4. Explain the importance of patient drug compliance in the pharmacotherapy of schizophrenia.

5. Explain the symptoms associated with extrapyramidal adverse effects of antipsychotic drugs.

6. For each of the drug classes, identify representative drug examples and explain their mechanism of action, primary actions, and important adverse effects.

7. Explain the goals of pharmacotherapy and categorize antipsychotic drugs based on their classification and drug action.

KEY TERMS

akathisia (ACK-ah-THEE-shea) *157*

extrapyramidal symptoms (EPS) (peh-RAM-ed-el) *157*

negative symptoms *154*

neuroleptic malignant syndrome (NMS) (noo-roh-LEP-tik) *158*

neuroleptics (noo-roh-LEP-ticks) *156*

parkinsonism *157*

positive symptoms *154*

schizoaffective disorder (SKIT-soh-ah-FEK-tiv) *154*

schizophrenia (SKIT-soh-FREN-ee-uh) *154*

tardive dyskinesia (TAR-div dis-ki-NEE-zee-uh) *157*

S evere mental illness can be incapacitating for the patient and intensely frustrating for family members dealing with the patient on a regular basis. Before the 1950s, patients with acute mental dysfunction were institutionalized, often for their entire lives. With the introduction of chlorpromazine (Thorazine) in the 1950s and the development of newer drugs, antipsychotic drugs have revolutionized the treatment of mental illness.

Most psychoses have no identifiable cause and require long-term drug therapy.

CORE CONCEPT 11.1

Patients with psychoses often are unable to distinguish what is real from what is illusion. Because of this, patients may be viewed as medically and legally incompetent. The following signs are characteristic of psychosis:

- *Delusions*   (strong beliefs in something that is false or not based on reality); for example, the patient may believe that someone is planting thoughts in his or her head.
- *Hallucinations*   (seeing, hearing, or feeling something that is not there); for example, the patient may hear voices or see spiders crawling on walls that others around the patient do not hear or see.
- *Illusions*   (distorted or misleading perceptions of something that is actually real); for example, the patient may see a shadow and believe it is really a person.
- *Disorganized behavior*   For example, the patient may wear clothes in an entirely inappropriate manner and for no apparent reason, such as dressing up with layers of clothes including a hat, sunglasses, and several pairs of socks over the hands and feet.
- *Difficulty relating to others*   For example, the patient may become withdrawn from other people in the room, showing signs of distress, maybe even turning combative if confronted or questioned. Behavior may range from total inactivity to extreme agitation.
- *Paranoia*   For example the patient may have an extreme suspicion that he or she is being followed, or that someone is trying to kill him or her.

In many cases, the condition of psychosis is devastating. Psychosis may be classified as *acute* or *chronic*. Acute psychotic episodes occur over hours or days, whereas chronic psychoses develop over months or years. Sometimes a cause may be attributed to the psychosis, such as brain damage, overdoses of certain medications, extreme depression, chronic alcoholism, or drug addiction. Genetic factors are known to play a role in some psychoses. Unfortunately, the vast majority of psychoses have no identifiable cause.

People with psychosis are usually unable to function in society without long-term drug therapy. Patients must see their health care provider periodically, and medication must be taken for life. Family members and social support groups are important sources of help for patients who cannot function without continuous drug therapy.

Fast Facts Psychosis

- Symptoms of psychosis are often associated with other mental health problems, including substance abuse, depression, and dementia.
- Psychotic disorders are among the most misunderstood mental health disorders in North America.
- Approximately 3 million Americans have schizophrenia.
- Patients with psychosis often develop symptoms between the ages of 13 and the early 20s.
- As many as 50% of homeless people in America have schizophrenia.
- The probability of developing schizophrenia is 1 in 100 for the general population, 1 in 10 if one parent has the disorder, and 1 in 4 if both parents are schizophrenic.

Source: National Mental Health Association (http://www.nmha.org/)

SCHIZOPHRENIA

schizo = *split*
phrenia = *mind*

Schizophrenia is a type of psychosis characterized by abnormal thoughts and thought processes, disordered communication, withdrawal from other people and the outside environment, and a high risk for suicide. Several subtypes of schizophrenic disorders are based on clinical presentation.

CORE CONCEPT 11.2

Patients with schizophrenia experience many different symptoms that may change over time.

PEARSON
mynursingkit™

NATIONAL ASSOCIATION OF MENTAL ILLNESS

Schizophrenia is the most common psychotic disorder, affecting 1% to 2% of the population. Symptoms generally begin to appear in early adulthood, with a peak incidence in men 15 to 24 years of age and in women 25 to 34 years of age. Patients experience a variety of symptoms that may change over time.

When observing patients with schizophrenia, health care workers should look for both positive and negative symptoms. **Positive symptoms** are those that *add on* to normal behavior. These include hallucinations, delusions, and disorganized thoughts or speech. **Negative symptoms** are those that *subtract from* normal behavior. These include lack of interest, motivation, responsiveness, or pleasure in daily activities. Proper diagnosis of positive and negative symptoms is important for selecting the most appropriate antipsychotic drug for treatment. The following symptoms may appear quickly or take several months or years to develop:

POSITIVE SYMPTOMS

- Hallucinations, delusions, or paranoia
- Strange behavior, such as talking in rambling statements or making up words
- Strange or irrational actions
- Changes from stupor to extreme hyperactivity

NEGATIVE SYMPTOMS

- Attitude of indifference toward or detachment from life activities
- Neglect of personal hygiene, job, and school
- Noticeable withdrawal from social activities and relationships
- Changes from extreme hyperactivity to stupor

Concept Review 11.1

- What are the characteristic signs of schizophrenia? What distinguishes a positive symptom from a negative symptom?

schizo = *schizophrenia*
affective = *mood*

Schizoaffective disorder is a related condition in which the patient exhibits symptoms of both schizophrenia and mood disorder. For example, an acute schizoaffective reaction may include distorted perceptions, hallucinations, and delusions, followed by extreme depression. Over time, both positive and negative psychotic symptoms appear.

Many conditions can cause bizarre behavior, and these should be distinguished from schizophrenia. Chronic use of amphetamines or cocaine can create a paranoid syndrome. Certain complex partial seizures (see Chapter 13 ⊂⊃) can cause unusual symptoms that are sometimes mistaken for psychoses. Brain neoplasms, infections, or hemorrhage can also cause bizarre, psychotic-like symptoms.

The causes of schizophrenia have not been determined, although several theories have been proposed. There appears to be a genetic component to schizophrenia, because many patients suffering from it have family members who have been afflicted with the same disorder. Another theory suggests that the disorder is caused by imbalances in neurotransmitters in specific brain areas. This theory suggests the possibility of overactive dopaminergic pathways found in the basal nuclei, an area of the brain that controls motor activity. The basal ganglia with associated nuclei are responsible for starting and stopping synchronized motor activity, such as leg and arm motions during walking.

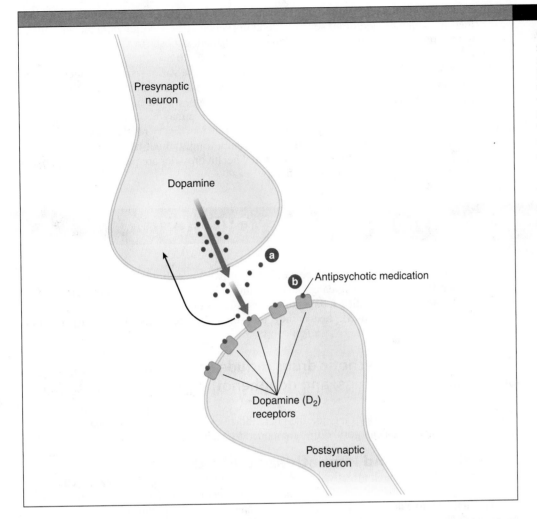

FIGURE 11.1

One theory of schizophrenia is that (a) too much dopamine is produced by neurons within basal ganglia of the brain. The extra dopamine overexcites the receptors. (b) Antipsychotic drugs act by attaching to D_2 receptors and preventing the extra dopamine from overstimulating of the postsynaptic neuron.

Synchronized motor activity seems to be associated with dopamine receptors. The basal nuclei are particularly rich in D_2 receptors, whereas the cerebrum contains very few. All antipsychotic drugs act by entering dopaminergic synapses and competing with dopamine. By blocking a majority of the D_2-type receptors, antipsychotic drugs reduce the symptoms of schizophrenia (Figure 11.1 ■).

Concept Review   11.2

■ What are the major types of psychoses, and how are they differentiated? How are the symptoms of schizophrenia reduced?

The experience and skills of the health care provider are critical to the pharmacologic management of psychoses.

CORE CONCEPT 11.3

Management of severe mental illness is difficult. Many patients do not see their behavior as abnormal and have difficulty understanding the need for medication. When that medication produces undesirable adverse effects, such as severe twitching or loss of sexual function, compliance diminishes and patients experience symptoms of their pretreatment illness. Agitation, distrust, and extreme frustration are common, because patients cannot comprehend why others are unable to think and see the same as they do.

The primary goal of pharmacotherapy for patients with schizophrenia is to reduce psychotic symptoms to a level that allows the patient to maintain normal social relationships, including self-care and keeping a job. From a pharmacologic perspective, therapy has both a positive and a negative side. Although many symptoms of psychoses can be controlled with current drugs, adverse effects are common and often severe. The antipsychotic drugs do not cure mental illness, and symptoms remain in remission only as long as the patient chooses to take the drug. The relapse rate for patients who discontinue their medication is 60% to 80%.

In terms of effectiveness, there is little difference among the various antipsychotic drugs; in other words, there is no single drug of choice for schizophrenia. Selection of a specific drug is based on clinician experience, the occurrence of adverse effects, and the needs of the patient. For example, patients with psychosis due to a degenerative disease may need an antipsychotic with minimal extrapyramidal adverse effects. Those who operate machinery need a drug that does not cause sedation. Men who are sexually active may want a drug without negative sexual effects. The experience and skills of the physician and mental health provider are particularly valuable in achieving successful psychiatric pharmacotherapy.

CONVENTIONAL ANTIPSYCHOTICS

neuro = *nervous*
leptic = *state of mind*

Because of the common neurologic adverse effects, antipsychotic drugs are sometimes referred to as **neuroleptics**. The two basic categories of antipsychotic drugs are conventional antipsychotics and atypical antipsychotics. Conventional or typical antipsychotic drugs were the first category of drugs to be developed; hence they are sometimes referred to as first-generation antipsychotics.

CORE CONCEPT 11.4

Conventional antipsychotic drugs include the phenothiazines, phenothiazine-like drugs, and nonphenothiazines.

The conventional antipsychotics include the phenothiazines and phenothiazine-like drugs listed in Table 11.1. Within each category, drugs are named by their chemical structure.

Phenothiazines and Phenothiazine-like Drugs

The phenothiazines are most effective at treating the positive symptoms of schizophrenia, such as hallucinations and delusions, and have been the treatment of choice for psychoses for 50 years.

The first effective drug used to treat schizophrenia was the low-potency phenothiazine chlorpromazine (Thorazine), approved by the Food and Drug Administration (FDA) in 1954. A number of other phenothiazines are now available to treat mental illness. All block the excitement associated with the positive symptoms of schizophrenia, although they differ in their potency and adverse effect profiles. Hallucinations and delusions often begin to diminish within days. Other symptoms, however, may require as long as 7 to 8 weeks of pharmacotherapy to improve. Be-

TABLE 11.1	Conventional Antipsychotics: Phenothiazines and Phenothiazine-like Drugs	
DRUG	**ROUTE AND ADULT DOSE**	**REMARKS**
Pr chlorpromazine (Thorazine)	PO; 25–100 mg tid or qid (max: 1000 mg/day) IM/IV; 25–50 mg (max: 600 mg every 4–6 hours)	Strong sedative properties; controls nausea and vomiting, dementia, and hiccups not treated by any other means; for agitated patients
fluphenazine (Permitil, Prolixin)	PO; 0.5–10 mg/day (max: 20 mg/day)	Also for dementia; available in IM or subcutaneous forms
perphenazine (Phenazine, Trilafon)	PO; 4–16 mg bid to qid (max: 64 mg/day)	Also for dementia and nausea; available in IM and IV forms
prochlorperazine (Compazine) (see page 522 for the Drug Profile box	PO; 0.5–10 mg/day (max: 20 mg/day)	Antiemetic drug used to treat nausea and vomiting
thioridazine (Mellaril)	PO; 50–100 mg tid (max: 800 mg/day)	Strong sedative properties; for moderate to severe depression and dementia
trifluoperazine (Stelazine)	PO; 1–2 mg bid (max: 20 mg/day)	Also for dementia; use cautiously in patients with seizure disorders; available in IM form

cause of the high rate of recurrence of psychotic episodes, pharmacotherapy should be considered long term, often for the life of the patient. Phenothiazines are thought to act by preventing both dopamine and serotonin from occupying critical neurologic receptor sites.

Although the phenothiazines once revolutionized treatment of severe mental illness, they continue to exhibit numerous adverse effects that can limit pharmacotherapy. General adverse effects are listed in Table 11.2. Anticholinergic effects such as dry mouth, postural hypotension, and urinary retention are common. Ejaculation disorders occur in a high percentage of patients; delay in achieving orgasm (in both men and women) is a common cause for noncompliance. Menstrual disorders are common. Each phenothiazine has a slightly different spectrum of adverse effects.

Unlike many other drugs whose primary action is on the central nervous system (CNS) (e.g., amphetamines, barbiturates, anxiolytics, alcohol), antipsychotic drugs do not cause physical or psychological dependence. They also have a wide safety margin between a therapeutic dose and a lethal dose; deaths due to overdoses of antipsychotic drugs are uncommon.

Extrapyramidal symptoms (EPS) are a particularly serious set of adverse reactions to antipsychotic drugs. EPS include acute dystonia, akathisia, parkinsonism, and tardive dyskinesia. Acute *dystonias* (see Chapter 12 🔗) occur early in the course of pharmacotherapy and involve severe muscle spasms, particularly of the back, neck, tongue, and face. **Akathisia**, the most common EPS, is an inability to rest or relax. The patient paces, has trouble sitting or remaining still, and has difficulty sleeping. Symptoms of phenothiazine-induced **parkinsonism** include tremor, muscle rigidity, stooped posture, and a shuffling gait. Parkinsonism results from abnormal neuronal activity in areas of the corpus striatum and substantia nigra. Long-term use of phenothiazines may lead to **tardive dyskinesia**, which is characterized by unusual tongue and face movements such as lip smacking and wormlike motions of the tongue. If extrapyramidal effects are reported early and the drug is withdrawn or the dosage is reduced, the adverse effects can be reversible. With higher doses given for prolonged periods, the EPS may become permanent.

With the conventional antipsychotics, it is not always possible to control the disabling symptoms of schizophrenia without producing some degree of extrapyramidal effects. In these patients, drug therapy may be warranted to treat EPS. Concurrent pharmacotherapy with an anticholinergic drug may prevent some of the extrapyramidal signs (see Chapter 12 🔗). For acute dystonia, benztropine (Cogentin) may be given parenterally. Levodopa (Larodopa) is usually avoided, because its ability to increase dopamine function antagonizes the action of the phenothiazines. Beta-adrenergic blockers and benzodiazepines are sometimes given to reduce signs of akathisia.

Nonphenothiazine Drugs

The nonphenothiazine antipsychotic medications and the phenothiazines have equal effectiveness. Although the incidence of sedation and anticholinergic adverse effects is less, extrapyramidal effects may be common, particularly in elderly patients.

The nonphenothiazine antipsychotic class consists of drugs whose chemical structures are dissimilar to the phenothiazines (Table 11.3). Introduced shortly after the phenothiazines, the nonphenothiazines were initially expected to produce fewer adverse effects. Unfortunately, this appears not to be the case. The spectrum of adverse effects for the nonphenothiazines is identical

substantia = *substance*
nigra = *black*

corpus = *body*
striatum = *striped*

tardive = *late*
dyskinesia = *abnormal movement*

TABLE 11.2	**Adverse Effects of the Conventional Antipsychotics**
EFFECT	**DESCRIPTION**
Acute dystonia	Severe spasms, particularly the back muscles, tongue, and facial muscles; twitching movements
Akathisia	Constant pacing with repetitive, compulsive movements
Anticholinergic effects	Dry mouth, tachycardia, blurred vision
Hypotension	Particularly severe when quickly moving from a recumbent position to an upright position
Neuroleptic malignant syndrome	High fever, confusion, muscle rigidity, and elevated serum creatine kinase levels; can be fatal
Parkinsonism	Tremor, muscle rigidity, stooped posture, and shuffling gait
Sedation	Usually diminishes with continued therapy
Sexual dysfunction	Impotence and diminished libido
Tardive dyskinesia	Bizarre tongue and face movements such as lip smacking and wormlike motions of the tongue; puffing of cheeks, uncontrolled chewing movements

TABLE 11.3	Conventional Antipsychotics: Nonphenothiazines	
DRUG	**ROUTE AND ADULT DOSE**	**REMARKS**
chlorprothixene (Taractan)	PO; 75–150 mg/day (max: 600 mg/day)	Prominent sedative effects; less hypotensive than phenothiazines; available in IV form
(Pr) haloperidol (Haldol)	PO; 0.2–5 mg bid or tid	For severe psychosis, dementia, and Tourette's syndrome; available in IM form
loxapine succinate (Loxitane)	PO; start with 20 mg/day and rapidly increase to 60–100 mg/day in divided doses (max: 250 mg/day)	Also for dementia
molindone HCl (Moban)	PO; 50–75 mg/day in three to four divided doses, may increase to 100 mg/day in 3–4 days (max: 225 mg/day)	May produce insomnia and drowsiness
pimozide (Orap)	PO; 1–2 mg/day in divided doses; gradually increase every other day to 7–16 mg/day, whichever is less (max: 10 mg/day)	For Tourette's syndrome; use cautiously in patients with seizure disorders
thiothixene HCl (Navane)	PO; 2 mg tid; may increase up to 15 mg/day (max: 60 mg/day)	Also for dementia; offlabel use as an antidepressant

to that for the phenothiazines, although the degree to which a particular effect occurs depends on the specific drug. In general, the nonphenothiazine drugs cause less sedation and fewer anticholinergic adverse effects than chlorpromazine (Thorazine) but exhibit an equal or even greater incidence of extrapyramidal signs. Concurrent therapy with other CNS depressants must be carefully monitored because of the potential additive effects.

DRUG PROFILE: (Pr) *Chlorpromazine (Thorazine)*

Therapeutic Class: Conventional antipsychotic, schizophrenia agent
Pharmacologic Class: Phenothiazine, D_2 dopamine receptor blocker

Actions and Uses:

Chlorpromazine provides symptomatic relief of positive symptoms of schizophrenia and controls manic symptoms in patients with schizoaffective disorder. Many patients must take chlorpromazine for 7 or 8 weeks before they experience improvement. Extreme agitation may be treated with IM or IV injections, which begin to act within minutes. Chlorpromazine can also control severe nausea and vomiting.

Adverse Effects and Interactions:

Strong blockade of alpha$_2$-adrenergic receptors and weak blockade of cholinergic receptors explain some of chlorpromazine's adverse effects. Common adverse effects are dizziness, drowsiness, and orthostatic hypotension.

EPS occur mostly in elderly patients, women, and pediatric patients who are dehydrated. **Neuroleptic malignant syndrome (NMS)** may also occur. Patients taking chlorpromazine and exposed to warmer temperatures should be monitored more closely for symptoms of NMS.

Chlorpromazine interacts with several drugs. For example, use with sedative medications such as phenobarbital should be avoided. Taking chlorpromazine with tricyclic antidepressants can elevate blood pressure. Use of chlorpromazine with antiseizure medication can lower the seizure threshold.

Use with caution with herbal supplements, such as kava and St. John's wort, which may increase the risk and severity of dystonia.

 Refer to MyNursingKit for a Nursing Process Focus specific to this drug.

DRUG PROFILE: 🅟 *Haloperidol (Haldol)*
Therapeutic Class: Conventional antipsychotic, schizophrenia agent
Pharmacologic Class: Nonphenothiazine, D_2 dopamine receptor blocker

Actions and Uses:

Haloperidol is classified chemically as a butyrophenone. Its primary use is for the management of acute and chronic psychotic disorders. It may be used to treat patients with Tourette's syndrome and children with severe behavior problems such as unprovoked aggressiveness and explosive hyperexcitability. It is approximately 50 times more potent than chlorpromazine but has equal efficacy in relieving symptoms of schizophrenia. Haldol LA is a long-acting preparation that lasts for approximately 3 weeks following IM or SC administration. This is particularly beneficial for patients who are uncooperative or unable to take oral medications.

Adverse Effects and Interaction:

Haloperidol produces less sedation and hypotension than chlorpromazine, but the incidence of EPS is high. Elderly patients are more likely to experience adverse effects and often are prescribed half the adult dose until the adverse effects of therapy can be determined. Although NMS is rare, it can occur.

Haloperidol interacts with many drugs. For example, the following drugs decrease the effects/absorption of haloperidol: aluminum- and magnesium-containing antacids, levodopa (also increases chances of levodopa toxicity), lithium (increases chance of severe neurologic toxicity), phenobarbital, phenytoin (also increases chances of phenytoin toxicity), rifampin, and beta blockers (may increase blood levels of haloperidol, thus leading to possible toxicity). Haloperidol inhibits the action of centrally acting antihypertensives.

Use with caution with herbal supplements such as kava, which may increase the effect of haloperidol.

Refer to MyNursingKit for a Nursing Process Focus specific to this drug.

Drugs in the nonphenothiazine class have the same therapeutic effects and effectiveness as the phenothiazines. They are also believed to act by the same mechanism as the phenothiazines—that is, by blocking postsynaptic D_2 dopamine receptors. As a class, they offer no significant advantages over the phenothiazines in the treatment of schizophrenia.

ATYPICAL ANTIPSYCHOTICS

Atypical antipsychotics treat both positive and negative symptoms of schizophrenia. They have become drugs of choice for treating psychoses.

Atypical antipsychotic drugs and a newer drug class have been developed to better meet the needs of patients with psychoses.

CORE CONCEPT 11.5

The approval of clozapine (Clozaril), the first atypical antipsychotic, marked the first major advance in the pharmacotherapy of psychoses since the discovery of chlorpromazine decades earlier. Clozapine and the other drugs in this class are called second generation or *atypical*, because they have a broader spectrum of action than the conventional antipsychotics, controlling both the positive and negative symptoms of schizophrenia (Table 11.4). Furthermore, at therapeutic doses they exhibit their antipsychotic actions without producing the EPS effects of the conventional drugs. Some drugs, such as clozapine, are especially useful for patients in whom other drugs have proved unsuccessful.

The mechanism of action of the atypical drugs is largely unknown, but they are thought to act by blocking several receptor types in the brain. Like the phenothiazines, the atypical drugs block dopamine D_2 receptors. However, the atypicals also block serotonin (5-HT) and

NURSING PROCESS FOCUS

Patients Receiving Phenothiazines and Conventional Nonphenothiazine Therapy

ASSESSMENT

Prior to administration:
- Obtain a complete health history (physical/mental), including allergies, drug history, and possible drug interactions
- Obtain baseline laboratory studies (electrolytes, complete blood count [CBC], blood urea nitrogen [BUN], creatinine, white blood cells [WBCs], liver enzymes, drug screens)
- Assess for hallucinations, level of consciousness, and mental status
- Assess patient support system(s)

POTENTIAL NURSING DIAGNOSES

- Ineffective Therapeutic Regimen Management related to noncompliance with medication regimen, presence of adverse effects, and need for long-term medication use.
- Anxiety related to symptoms of psychosis.
- Risk for Injury related to adverse effects of drug therapy and thought processes.
- Noncompliance related to length of time before medication reaches therapeutic levels, desire to use alcohol or illegal drugs.
- Deficient Knowledge related to information about disease process and drug therapy.

PLANNING: PATIENT GOALS AND EXPECTED OUTCOMES

The patient will:
- Report a reduction of psychotic symptoms, including delusions, paranoia, irrational behavior, hallucinations
- Demonstrate an understanding of the drug's action by accurately describing drug effects, precautions, and measures to take to decrease any adverse effects
- Immediately report adverse effects or adverse reactions
- Adhere to recommended treatment regimen

IMPLEMENTATION

Interventions and (Rationales)	Patient Education/Discharge Planning
■ Monitor for decreased psychotic symptoms. (If the patient continues to exhibit symptoms of psychosis, he or she may not be taking the drug as ordered, may be taking an inadequate dose, or may not be affected by the drug; it may need to be discontinued and another antipsychotic begun.)	Instruct the patient to: ■ Notice increases or decreases of symptoms of psychosis, including hallucinations, abnormal sleep patterns, social withdrawal, delusions, or paranoia ■ Contact the physician if no decrease of symptoms occurs over a 6-week period
■ Monitor for adverse effects such as drowsiness, dizziness, lethargy, headaches, blurred vision, skin rash, diaphoresis, nausea/vomiting, anorexia, diarrhea, menstrual irregularities, depression, hypotension, or hypertension.	Instruct the patient: ■ To report adverse effects ■ That impotence, gynecomastia, amenorrhea, and anuresis may occur
■ Monitor for anticholinergic adverse effects such as orthostatic hypotension, constipation, anorexia, genitourinary problems, respiratory changes, and visual disturbances.	Instruct the patient to: ■ Avoid abrupt changes in position ■ Not drive or perform hazardous activities until the effects of the drug are known ■ Report vision changes ■ Comply with required laboratory tests ■ Increase dietary fiber, fluids, and exercise to prevent constipation ■ Relieve symptoms of dry mouth with sugarless hard candy or gum and frequent drinks of water ■ Notify the physician immediately if urinary retention occurs
■ Monitor for extrapyramidal effects such as the development of tremors, involuntary repetitive movements, decreased muscle tone, or increased restlessness. (Presence of EPS may be sufficient reason for the patient to discontinue the antipsychotic. Monitor for NMS, which is life threatening and must be reported and treated immediately.)	Instruct the patient to: ■ Recognize tardive dyskinesia, dystonia, akathisia, pseudoparkinsonism ■ Immediately seek treatment for elevated temperature, unstable blood pressure, profuse sweating, dyspnea, muscle rigidity, incontinence

NURSING PROCESS FOCUS (continued)

Interventions and (Rationales)

- Monitor for alcohol/illegal drug use. (Patient may decide to use alcohol or illegal drugs as a means of coping with symptoms of psychosis, so he or she may stop taking the antipsychotic. Concurrent use will cause increased CNS depressant effect.)

- Monitor caffeine use. (Use of caffeine-containing substances will negate effects of antipsychotics.)

- Monitor for cardiovascular changes, including hypotension, tachycardia, and electrocardiogram (ECG) changes. (Haloperidol has fewer cardiotoxic effects than other antipsychotics and may be preferred for patients with existing cardiovascular problems.)

- Monitor for smoking. (Heavy smoking may decrease metabolism of haloperidol, leading to decreased effectiveness.)

- Monitor elderly patients closely. (Elderly patients may need lower doses and a more gradual dosage increase. Elderly women are at greater risk for developing tardive dyskinesia.)

- Monitor laboratory results, including red blood cell (RBC) counts, white blood cell (WBC) counts, and drug levels.

- Monitor for use of medication. (All antipsychotics must be taken as ordered for therapeutic results to occur.)

- Monitor for seizures. (Drug may lower seizure threshold.)

- Monitor the patient's environment. (Drug may cause the patient to perceive a brownish discoloration of objects or experience photophobia. Drug may also interfere with the ability to regulate body temperature.)

Patient Education/Discharge Planning

- Instruct the patient to refrain from alcohol and illegal drug use. Refer the patient to community support groups such as Alcoholics Anonymous (AA) or Narcotics Anonymous (NA) as appropriate.

Instruct the patient to:
- Avoid caffeine
- Recognize common caffeine-containing products and assist in finding acceptable substitutes, such as decaffeinated coffee and tea, caffeine-free colas

- Instruct the patient that dizziness and falls, especially on sudden position changes, may indicate cardiovascular changes. Teach safety measures.

- Instruct the patient to stop or decrease smoking. Refer to smoking cessation programs, if indicated.

Instruct the patient:
- To look for unusual reactions such as confusion, depression, and hallucinations and for symptoms of tardive dyskinesia, and to report them immediately
- On ways to counteract anticholinergic effects of medication while taking into account any other existing medical problems

- Advise the patient of the necessity of having regular laboratory studies done.

- Instruct the patient that medication must be continued as ordered, even if no therapeutic benefits are felt, because it may take several months for full therapeutic benefits to take effect.

- Instruct the patient that seizures may occur and review appropriate safety precautions.

Instruct the patient to:
- Wear dark glasses to avoid discomfort from photophobia
- Avoid temperature extremes
- Be aware that perception of brownish discoloration of objects may appear, but that it is not harmful

EVALUATION OF OUTCOME CRITERIA

Evaluate the effectiveness of drug therapy by confirming that patient goals and expected outcomes have been met (see "Planning").

See Tables 11.1 and 11.3 for lists of the drugs to which these nursing actions apply.

TABLE 11.4 | Atypical Antipsychotic Drugs

DRUG	ROUTE AND ADULT DOSE	REMARKS
aripiprazole (Abilify)	PO; 10–15 mg daily (max: 30 mg/day)	For schizophrenia; may cause loss of glycemic control in patients with diabetes
clozapine (Clozaril)	PO; start at 25–50 mg/day and titrate to a target dose of 50–450 mg/day in 3 days, may increase further (max: 900 mg/day)	For schizophrenia (adults older than 16 years)
olanzapine (Zyprexa)	PO adult: start with 5–10 mg/day, may increase by 2.5–5 mg every week (range 10–15 mg/day, max: 20 mg/day); geriatric: start with 5 mg/day	Blocks alpha receptors and acetylcholine
quetiapine fumarate (Seroquel)	PO; start with 25 mg bid, may increase to a target dose of 300–400 mg/day in divided doses	Patients may experience hypotension when changing positions; use cautiously in elderly patients; also used for depression
Pr risperidone (Risperdal, Risperdal Consta)	PO; 1–6 mg bid, increase by 2 mg daily to an initial target dose of 6 mg/day	Offlabel use in behavioral disturbances (patients with mental retardation)
ziprasidone (Geodon)	PO; 20 mg bid (max: 80 mg bid)	Offlabel use for Tourette's syndrome; patients may experience hypotension when changing positions

DRUG PROFILE: Pr *Risperidone (Risperdal, Risperdal Consta)*

Therapeutic Class: Atypical antipsychotic, schizophrenia agent, psychotic depression agent
Pharmacologic Class: Serotonin (5-HT) receptor antagonist, D_2 dopamine receptor antagonist (weaker affinity)

Actions and Uses:

Therapeutic effects of risperidone include treatment and prevention of schizophrenia relapse and expression of bipolar mania symptoms. Risperidone also treats symptoms of irritability in children with autism. Expected results are a reduction of excitement, paranoia, or negative behaviors associated with psychosis. Effects result from blockade of dopamine type 2, serotonin type 2, and alpha$_2$-adrenergic receptors located within the CNS. For a full range of effectiveness, the drug is sometimes combined with lithium (Eskalith) or valproic acid (Depakene). Risperidone is a long-acting preparation, which, following IM administration, releases only a small amount. After a 3-week lag, the rest of the drug releases and lasts for approximately 4 to 6 weeks. PO preparations release sooner and have a 1- to 2-week onset of action.

Adverse Effects and Interactions:

If elderly patients with dementia-related psychoses are given risperidone, they are at an increased risk for heart failure, pneumonia, or sudden death. Patients with underlying cardiovascular disease may be especially prone to dysrhythmias and hypotension. Risperidone should be avoided in patients with a history of seizures, suicidal ideations, or kidney/liver disease. This medication may cause hyperglycemia and worsen glucose control in patients with diabetes. It is not known whether risperidone passes into breast milk or if it could harm a nursing baby. Due to its category C classification, safety in pregnancy has not been established.

Common adverse effects are extrapyramidal reactions (involuntary shaking of the head, neck, and arms), hyperactivity, fatigue, nausea, dizziness, visual disturbances, fever, and orthostatic hypotension. Risperidone may cause weight gain.

Patients taking risperidone should avoid CNS depressants such as alcohol, antihistamines, sedative-hypnotics, or opioid analgesics. These can increase some of the adverse effects of risperidone. Due to inhibition of liver enzymes, other drugs that increase the adverse effects of risperidone include the selective serotonin reuptake inhibitors (SSRIs) such as paroxetine, sertraline, and fluoxetine (Prozac), and antifungal drugs such as fluconazole, itraconazole, and ketoconazole. Risperidone may interfere with elimination by the kidneys of clozapine, also increasing the risk of adverse reactions.

Kava, valerian, or chamomile may increase risperidone's CNS depressive effects.

Refer to MyNursingKit for a Nursing Process Focus specific to this drug.

alpha$_2$-adrenergic receptors, which is thought to account for some of their properties. Because the atypical drugs are only loosely bound to D$_2$ receptors, they produce fewer extrapyramidal adverse effects than the conventional antipsychotics.

Although there are fewer adverse effects with atypical antipsychotics, adverse effects are still significant, and patients must be carefully monitored. Although most antipsychotics cause weight gain, the atypical drugs are associated with obesity and its risk factors. Risperidone (Risperdal, Risperdal Consta) and some of the other antipsychotic drugs increase prolactin levels, which can lead to menstrual disorders, decreased libido, and osteoporosis in women. In men, high prolactin levels can cause lack of libido and impotence. There is also concern that some atypical drugs alter glucose metabolism, which can lead to type II diabetes.

Risperidone (Risperdal, Risperdal Consta) is the first atypical antipsychotic available as a long-acting IM formulation for the treatment of schizophrenia. The licensed indications of Risperdal and Consta are in line with oral formulations of risperidone. Other advances in the "extended release" treatment of psychosis include the antipsychotic medications, paliperidone (Invega) and quetiapine XR (Seroquel). Intramuscular and extended-release (XR) formulations have advantages of greater dosing flexibility among patients.

Concept Review 11.3

■ What is a neuroleptic drug? What are the two general classes of drugs used to treat psychoses? How does each drug category generally affect positive and/or negative symptoms of schizophrenia?

DOPAMINE SYSTEM STABILIZERS

Owing to adverse effects caused by conventional and atypical antipsychotic medications, a newer drug class was developed to better meet the needs of patients with psychoses. The newer class is called *dopamine system stabilizers (DSSs)* or dopamine partial agonists. Aripiprazole (Abilify) received FDA approval in November 2002 for the treatment of schizophrenia and schizoaffective disorder. Because aripiprazole controls both the positive and negative symptoms of schizophrenia, it is grouped in Table 17.4 with the atypical antipsychotic drugs.

Patients treated with aripiprazole appear to exhibit fewer EPS than patients treated with haloperidol (Haldol). Anticholinergic adverse effects are virtually nonexistent. In fact, the incidence of adverse effects generally compared to the other atypical antipsychotic drugs is very low. Notable adverse effects, however, include bradykinesia, headache, nausea/vomiting, fever, constipation, and anxiety.

brady = *slow*
kinesia = *movement*

NURSING PROCESS FOCUS

Patients Receiving Atypical Antipsychotic Therapy

ASSESSMENT

Prior to administration:
■ Obtain a complete health history (physical/mental, including allergies, drug history, and possible drug interactions
■ Obtain baseline laboratory studies, especially RBC and WBC counts
■ Assess for hallucinations, mental status, and level of consciousness
■ Assess patient support system(s)

POTENTIAL NURSING DIAGNOSES

■ Injury, Risk for, related to adverse effects of drug therapy, and thought processes.
■ Ineffective Therapeutic Regimen Management related to noncompliance with medication regimen, presence of adverse effects, and need for long-term medication use.
■ Anxiety related to symptoms of psychosis.
■ Noncompliance related to length of time before drug reaches therapeutic levels, desire to use alcohol or illegal drugs.
■ Deficient Knowledge related to information about disease process and treatment.

continued . . .

NURSING PROCESS FOCUS (continued)

PLANNING: PATIENT GOALS AND EXPECTED OUTCOMES

The patient will:
- Adhere to recommended treatment regimen
- Report a reduction of psychotic symptoms, including delusions, paranoia, irrational behavior, and hallucinations
- Demonstrate an understanding of the drug's actions by accurately describing drug effects and precautions

IMPLEMENTATION

Interventions and (Rationales)	Patient Education/Discharge Planning
■ Monitor RBC and WBC counts. (Agranulocytosis [WBCs below 3,500] can be a life-threatening adverse effect of these medications, which may also suppress bone marrow and lower infection-fighting ability.)	Instruct the patient to: ■ Keep appointments for laboratory testing ■ Report any sore throat, signs of infection, fatigue without apparent cause, or bruising
■ Observe for adverse effects. (These drugs may affect blood pressure, heart rate, and other autonomic functions.)	■ Instruct the patient to report adverse effects, such as drowsiness, dizziness, depression, anxiety, tachycardia, hypotension, nausea/vomiting, excessive salivation, changes in urinary frequency or urgency, incontinence, weight gain, muscle pain or weakness, rash, and fever.
■ Monitor for anticholinergic adverse effects. (These medications may cause mouth dryness, constipation, or urinary retention.)	Instruct the patient to: ■ Increase dietary fiber, fluids, and exercise to prevent constipation ■ Relieve symptoms of dry mouth with sugar-free hard candy or chewing gum and frequent drinks of water ■ Immediately notify the health care provider if urinary retention occurs. Possible catheter placement may be necessary
■ Monitor for decrease of psychotic symptoms. (Decreased symptoms indicate an effective dose and type of medication.)	Instruct the patient to: ■ Notice increases or decreases of symptoms of psychosis, including hallucinations, abnormal sleep patterns, social withdrawal, delusions, or paranoia ■ Contact the health care provider if symptoms do not decrease over a 6-week period
■ Monitor for alcohol or illegal drug use. (Used concurrently, these will cause increased CNS depression. The patient may decide to use alcohol or illegal drugs as a means of coping with symptoms of psychosis and may stop taking the drug.)	■ Instruct the patient to avoid alcohol or illegal drug use. Refer the patient to AA, NA, or other support group as appropriate.
■ Monitor caffeine use. (Use of caffeine-containing substances inhibits the effects of antipsychotics.)	Instruct the patient about: ■ Common caffeine-containing products ■ Acceptable substitutes, including decaffeinated coffee and tea, and caffeine-free soda
■ Monitor for smoking. (Heavy smoking may decrease blood levels of the drug.)	■ Instruct the patient to stop or decrease smoking. Refer to smoking cessation programs if indicated.
■ Monitor elderly patients closely. (Older patients may be more sensitive to anticholinergic adverse effects.)	■ Instruct elderly patients on ways to counteract anticholinergic effects of the medication while taking into account any other existing medical problems.

EVALUATION OF OUTCOME CRITERIA

Evaluate the effectiveness of drug therapy by confirming that patient goals and expected outcomes have been met (see "Planning").

See Table 11.4 for a list of drugs to which these nursing actions apply.

PATIENTS NEED TO KNOW

Patients being treated for psychoses of the nervous system need to know the following:

1. It is important to report the development of tremors, muscle spasms, involuntary repetitive movements, decreased muscle tone, or increased restlessness to the health care provider. These symptoms may indicate serious adverse effects that can be reversed if medication is changed soon after they start.
2. Consult a health care provider if dry mouth, rapid heart rate, constipation, or urinary retention occurs. An additional medication may be prescribed to relieve these signs and symptoms.
3. Avoid taking antacids with antipsychotics because they delay or decrease antipsychotic absorption.
4. Avoid alcohol or other sedatives while taking antipsychotics; it increases the depressant effects.
5. Extra protection from the sun is necessary; wear a hat and sunscreen.
6. Avoid driving or operating machinery until response to the medication is known. Its sedating effects can increase the risk for accidental injury.
7. Contact a health care provider for guidance if symptoms get worse or are not relieved by the medication. Do not stop the medication unless directed to do so.

CHAPTER REVIEW

CORE CONCEPTS SUMMARY

11.1 Most psychoses have no identifiable cause and require long-term drug therapy.

Psychosis is characterized by delusions, hallucinations, illusions, disorganized behavior, difficulty relating to others, and paranoia. Psychoses may be classified as acute or chronic. Sometimes a cause can be found for the psychosis, but the vast majority of cases have no identifiable cause. Most patients with psychoses are not able to function normally in society without long-term drug therapy.

11.2 Patients with schizophrenia experience many different symptoms that may change over time.

Schizophrenia is the most common psychiatric disorder; it is characterized by abnormal thoughts, disordered communication, withdrawal, and suicidal risk. Patients with schizophrenia exhibit positive (adding) or negative (subtracting) symptoms. Proper diagnosis of these symptoms is important for selecting the appropriate antipsychotic drug. The cause of schizophrenia has not been determined. Symptoms seem to be associated with neural *dopamine type 2 (D_2) receptors* found in the basal ganglia. Schizoaffective disorders are characterized by symptoms of both schizophrenia and mood disorder.

11.3 The experience and skills of the health care provider are critical to the pharmacologic management of psychoses.

Management of severe mental illness is difficult. Many patients do not see themselves as abnormal and have difficulty understanding the need for medication. Although many symptoms of psychosis can be controlled with current drug therapy, adverse effects are common and often severe. Skills of the health care team are particularly valuable to achieving successful psychiatric drug treatment.

11.4 Conventional antipsychotic drugs include the phenothiazines, phenothiazine-like drugs, and nonphenothiazines.

Antipsychotic drugs are sometimes called *neuroleptics.* The two basic categories of drugs for psychosis are conventional antipsychotics and atypical antipsychotics. With conventional antipsychotics, it is not always possible to control *extrapyramidal symptoms (EPS)* which include muscle spasms (*dystonia*), inability to sit down (*akathisia*), and unusual tongue and facial movements (*tardive dyskinesia*). Phenothiazines, phenothiazine-like drugs, and nonphenothiazines treat positive signs of schizophrenia, but all have unpleasant adverse effects.

11.5 **Atypical antipsychotic drugs and a newer drug class have been developed to better meet the needs of patients with psychoses.**

Atypical antipsychotic drugs treat both positive and negative signs of schizophrenia and have become drugs of choice for treating psychoses. Like the phenothiazine drugs, atypical drugs block D_2 recep-

tors. Although there are fewer adverse effects with atypical drugs, adverse effects are still significant, and patients must be carefully monitored. Dopamine system stabilizers (DSSs) represent a newer drug category developed to better meet the needs of patients with psychoses.

REVIEW QUESTIONS

The following questions are written in NCLEX-PN® style. Answer these questions to assess your knowledge of the chapter material, and go back and review any material that is not clear to you.

1. Which of the following statements is true?
1. Antipsychotic medications cure mental illnesses.
2. The severe adverse effects of antipsychotic drugs can lead to noncompliance.
3. Antipsychotic medications are only administered when the patient is symptomatic.
4. Antipsychotic drugs improve symptoms within hours of administration.

2. Family members of a patient diagnosed with schizophrenia are educated on the adverse effects of phenothiazines. Which of the following should be included?
1. The patient may experience withdrawal and slowed activity.
2. Severe muscle spasms may occur early in therapy.
3. Tardive dyskinesia is likely early in therapy.
4. Medications should be taken as prescribed to prevent adverse effects.

3. Which of the following symptoms does the nurse recognize as an anticholinergic effect of chlorpromazine (Thorazine)?
1. Hallucinations, illusions, paranoia
2. Hypertension, polyuria, increased salivation
3. Dry mouth, postural hypotension, urinary retention
4. Fever, flulike symptoms, decreased WBC count

4. The patient is on thioridazine (Mellaril) and has developed muscle spasms, difficulty sleeping, and a shuffling gait. The nurse recognizes this as:
1. Anticholinergic effects
2. Cholinergic effects
3. Extrapyramidal adverse effects
4. Serotonin syndrome

5. The patient states that he has not taken his antipsychotic drug for the past 2 weeks because it was causing sexual dysfunction. The name *antipsychotic* explains that continuing the medication as prescribed is important because:
1. Hypertensive crisis may occur with abrupt withdrawal.
2. Muscle twitching may occur.

3. Noncompliance may bring on parkinsonism.
4. Symptoms of psychosis are likely to return.

6. Neuroleptic malignant syndrome (NMS) is most likely to occur with use of which of the following drugs?
1. Chlorpromazine (Thorazine)
2. Thiothixene HCl (Navane)
3. Haloperidol (Haldol)
4. Clozapine (Clozaril)

7. For which of the following conditions would haloperidol (Haldol) be indicated?
1. Seizures
2. Combativeness
3. Severe mental depression
4. Alcoholism

8. Which of the following drug groups can lead to type II diabetes?
1. Phenothiazines
2. Nonphenothiazines
3. Atypical antipsychotics
4. Dopamine system stabilizers (DSSs)

9. Which of the following patients should be monitored for dehydration symptoms?
1. A 15-year-old girl who is taking chlorpromazine (Thorazine)
2. A 67-year-old woman who is taking aripiprazole (Abilify)
3. A 57-year-old man who is taking benztropine (Cogentin)
4. A 73-year-old woman who is taking haloperidol (Haldol)

10. Which of the following drugs can cause bone marrow suppression?
1. Clozapine (Clozaril)
2. Risperidone (Risperdal)
3. Benztropine (Cogentin)
4. Chlorpromazine (Thorazine)

CASE STUDY QUESTIONS

For questions 1–4, please read the following case study, and then choose the correct answer from choices 1–4.

Mr. Wayne, age 38, has been diagnosed with a psychosis characterized by the following symptoms: reports of seeing people who are not there, talking about government agents who are trying to kill him, and communicating with "double agents" about suspicious behavior. This patient has been in and out of the hospital for the last 4 weeks. Mr. Wayne's family reports difficulty in controlling him because he has not been taking his medication. Members in the community have seen Mr. Wayne pacing up and down the highway for several weeks. It becomes necessary to temporarily confine Mr. Wayne for medical treatment. He has had this disorder for 10 years and has a strong, supportive family (mother and father).

1. The symptoms described for Mr. Wayne are called _____ symptoms and respond best to treatment with which class of antipsychotic medication?

1. Positive; conventional or typical antipsychotics
2. Negative; conventional or typical antipsychotics
3. Positive; atypical antipsychotics
4. Negative; atypical antipsychotics

2. Assume that Mr. Wayne has been taking chlorpromazine (Thorazine) for most of the 10 years he has been experiencing psychotic episodes. Identify the effects that Thorazine may have on Mr. Wayne. (Choose all that apply.)

1. Drowsiness
2. Muscle spasms
3. Difficulty sleeping
4. Fever

3. Which of the following medications would have been given to him to reduce the incidence of extrapyramidal adverse effects—particularly dystonia?

1. Levodopa (Larodopa)
2. Benztropine (Cogentin)
3. Thioridazine (Mellaril)
4. Trifluoperazine (Stelazine)

4. Extrapyramidal adverse effects develop for the same neurochemical reasons as for which of the following disorders?

1. Schizoaffective disorder
2. Parkinson's disease
3. Alzheimer's disease
4. Multiple sclerosis

FURTHER STUDY

- A discussion of complex partial seizures, some of which are mistaken for psychosis, is included in Chapter 13 ⚭.

- Chapter 8 ⚭ includes more information on acetylcholinesterase inhibitors and their effects on the parasympathetic nervous system.

- More information on anxiolytics can be found in Chapter 9 ⚭.

- Mood stabilizers are discussed in greater detail in Chapter 10 ⚭.

- Parkinsonism and other extrapyramidal-related symptoms are discussed in more detail in Chapter 12 ⚭.

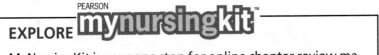
EXPLORE **PEARSON mynursingkit**™

MyNursingKit is your one stop for online chapter review materials and resources. Prepare for success with additional NCLEX®-style practice questions, interactive assignments and activities, web links, animations and videos, and more!

Register your access code from the front of your book at
www.mynursingkit.com

CORE CONCEPTS

12.1 Medications are unable to cure most degenerative diseases of the CNS.

12.2 Parkinson's disease is progressive, with the occurrence of full symptoms taking many years.

12.3 Parkinsonism drugs focus on the brain by restoring the balance between dopamine and acetylcholine.

12.4 Patients with Alzheimer's disease experience a dramatic loss of ability to perform tasks that require acetylcholine as the CNS neurotransmitter.

12.5 Alzheimer's disease is treated with acetylcholinesterase inhibitors.

12.6 Symptoms of multiple sclerosis result from demyelination of CNS nerve fibers.

12.7 Drugs for multiple sclerosis reduce immune attacks in the brain and treat unfavorable symptoms.

12.8 Muscle spasms are caused by injury, overmedication, hypocalcemia, and debilitating neurologic disorders.

12.9 Muscle spasms may be treated with nonpharmacologic or pharmacologic therapies.

12.10 Many muscle relaxants treat muscle spasms by inhibiting upper motor neuron activity, causing sedation, or altering simple reflexes.

12.11 Effective treatment for spasticity includes both physical therapy and medications.

12.12 Some drugs for spasticity provide relief by acting directly on muscle tissue, interfering with the release of calcium ions.

12.13 Neuromuscular blocking agents block the effect of acetylcholine at the receptor.

DRUG SNAPSHOT

The following drugs are discussed in this chapter:

DRUG CLASSES	DRUG PROFILES
Drugs for Parkinson's Disease	
Dopaminergic agents	(Pr) levodopa (Larodopa)
Cholinergic blockers (anticholinergics)	(Pr) benztropine (Cogentin)
Drugs for Alzheimer's Disease	
Acetylcholine sterase inhibitors	(Pr) donepezil (Aricept, Aricept ODT)
Combination NMDA drug therapy	
Drugs for Multiple Sclerosis	
Immune system modulating drugs	
Immunosuppressants	

DRUG CLASSES	DRUG PROFILES
Drugs for Muscle Spasms	
Centrally acting muscle relaxants	(Pr) cyclobenzaprine (Cycoflex, Flexeril)
Drugs for Spasticity	
Direct-acting antispasmodics	(Pr) dantrolene sodium (Dantrium)
Neuromuscular Blocking Agents	
Nondepolarizing blockers	
Depolarizing blockers	

After reading this chapter, the student should be able to:

1. Identify the most common degenerative diseases of the CNS.

2. Describe symptoms of Parkinson's disease, Alzheimer's disease, multiple sclerosis, and spasticity.

3. Explain the neurochemical bases of central degenerative diseases and muscle spasms.

4. Explain the goals of pharmacotherapy, and categorize drugs used in the treatment of degenerative diseases based on their class and drug action.

5. Describe the pharmacologic management of muscle spasms.

6. Discuss nonpharmacologic therapies used to treat muscle spasms and spasticity.

7. Discuss the pharmacology of neuromuscular blocking agents.

8. Compare and contrast the roles of the following drug categories in treating muscle spasms and spasticity: centrally acting skeletal muscle relaxants and direct-acting antispasmodics.

9. For each of the drug classes, identity representative drugs, and explain their mechanisms of action, primary actions, and important adverse effects.

KEY TERMS

acetylcholinesterase (AchE) (AS-ee-til-KOH-lin-ES-ter-ays) *176*

Alzheimer's disease (AD) (ALLZ-heye-mers) *174*

dementia (dee-MEN-she-ah) *175*

dystonia (diss-TONE-ee-ah) *184*

multiple sclerosis (MS) (skle-ROH-sis) *178*

neuromuscular blocking agents (NEWR-oh-musc-you-lahr) *186*

parkinsonism *171*

spasticity (spas-TISS-ih-tee) *182*

Central degenerative diseases and muscle disorders affect a patient's ability to perform daily activities and most often lead to immobility. Appropriate body movement depends on intact neural pathways and proper muscle functioning. Without medical intervention, major sensory, cognitive, and/or motor problems occur. Parkinson's disease, Alzheimer's disease, and multiple sclerosis are three common debilitating and progressive neurologic disorders. Although medications are unable to stop or reverse the progressive nature of these diseases, therapy can often slow down the disorders and offer symptomatic relief. Common muscle disorders are muscle spasms and spasticity. This chapter focuses on the pharmacotherapy of neurodegenerative diseases, muscle disorders, and treatments involving the neuromuscular junction.

Medications are unable to cure most degenerative diseases of the CNS.

CORE CONCEPT 12.1

Degenerative diseases of the CNS include a variety of disorders with different causes and outcomes. Some, such as Huntington's disease, are quite rare, affect younger patients, and are caused by chromosomal defects. Others, such as Alzheimer's disease, affect millions of people, mostly elderly patients, and have a devastating economic and social impact. Table 12.1 lists major degenerative diseases of the CNS.

The cause of most neurologic degenerative diseases is unknown. Most progress from hardly noticeable signs and symptoms early in the disease to serious neurologic and cognitive deficits. In their early stages, disorders may be difficult to diagnose. With the exception of Parkinson's disease, pharmacotherapy provides only minimal benefit. Currently, medication is unable to cure any of the major neurodegenerative diseases.

TABLE 12.1	Degenerative Diseases of the Central Nervous System
DISEASE	**DESCRIPTION**
Alzheimer's disease	Progressive loss of brain function characterized by memory loss, confusion, and dementia
Amyotrophic lateral sclerosis (ALS)	Progressive weakness and wasting of muscles caused by destruction of motor neurons
Huntington's chorea	Autosomal dominant genetic disorder resulting in progressive dementia and involuntary, spasmodic movements of limb and facial muscles
Multiple sclerosis (MS)	Demyelination of neurons in the central nervous system (CNS), resulting in progressive weakness, visual disturbances, mood alterations, and cognitive deficits
Parkinson's disease	Progressive loss of dopamine in the CNS, causing tremor, muscle rigidity, and abnormal movement and posture

Fast Facts Neurodegenerative Diseases

Parkinson's Disease

- Approximately 1.5 million Americans have Parkinson's disease.
- Most patients with Parkinson's disease are above the age of 50.
- Greater than 50% of patients with Parkinson's disease who have difficulty with voluntary movement are less than 60 years of age.
- More men than women develop this disorder.

Dementia

- Of all patients with dementia, 60% to 70% have Alzheimer's disease.
- Approximately 4 million Americans have Alzheimer's disease.
- Alzheimer's disease mainly affects patients over the age of 65.

Multiple Sclerosis

- About 1.1 million people worldwide have MS.
- Onset of symptoms typically occurs between ages 15 and 40.
- Women are affected twice as often as men.
- MS occurs most often in Caucasian people of northern European origin.
- MS is about five times more prevalent in temperate climates than in tropical climates.

Source: The National Parkinson's Foundation and the National Mental Health Association.

PARKINSON'S DISEASE

Parkinson's disease is a degenerative disorder of the CNS caused by death of neurons that produce the brain neurotransmitter dopamine. It is the second most common degenerative disease of the nervous system, affecting many Americans. Pharmacotherapy is often successful in reducing some of the distressing symptoms of this disorder.

CORE CONCEPT 12.2

Parkinson's disease is progressive with the occurrence of full symptoms taking many years.

Parkinson's disease primarily affects patients older than 50 years of age; however, even teenagers can develop the disorder. Men are affected slightly more often than women. The disease is progressive. The appearance of full symptoms often takes many years. The symptoms of Parkinson's disease, described as **parkinsonism**, are summarized as follows:

- *Tremors*   The hands and head develop a palsy-like motion or shakiness when at rest; *pill-rolling* is a common behavior in progressive states, in which patients rub the thumb and forefinger together as if a pill were between them.

- *Muscle rigidity*   Stiffness may resemble symptoms of arthritis. Patients often have difficulty bending over or moving limbs. Some patients develop a rigid *masked face*. These symptoms may not be noticeable at first but become more obvious as the disease progresses.

- *Bradykinesia*   This is the most noticeable of all symptoms. Patients may have difficulty chewing, swallowing, or speaking. Patients with Parkinson's disease have difficulties initiating movement and controlling fine muscle movements. Walking often becomes difficult, and patients shuffle their feet without taking normal strides.

- *Postural instability*   Patients may be humped over slightly and may easily lose their balance. Stumbling results in frequent falls and injuries.

brady = *slow*
kinesia = *movement*

Although Parkinson's disease is a progressive neurologic disorder primarily affecting muscle movement, other health problems often develop in these patients, including anxiety, depression, sleep disturbances, dementia, and disturbances of the autonomic nervous system (difficulty urinating and performing sexually). Several theories have been proposed to explain the development of parkinsonism. Because some patients with Parkinson's symptoms have a family history of this disorder, a genetic link is highly probable. Numerous environmental toxins, such as carbon monoxide, cyanide, manganese, chlorine, and pesticides, also have been suggested as a cause, but results of studies have not proven the cause-effect link. Viral infections, head trauma, and stroke have also been proposed as causes of parkinsonism.

Symptoms of parkinsonism develop due to the degeneration and destruction of dopamine-producing neurons found within an area of the brain known as the *substantia nigra*. When not enough dopamine is released, this neurotransmitter cannot make contact with other critical areas of the brain.

substantia = *substance*
nigra = *black*

The most critical area for dopamine contact is the *corpus striatum*, an area responsible for controlling unconscious muscle movement. Patients with Parkinson's disease have a problem initiating and controlling movements. Balance, posture, muscle tone, and involuntary muscle movements depend on the proper balance between dopamine (inhibitory) and acetylcholine (stimulatory). If dopamine is absent, acetylcholine is able to overstimulate the corpus striatum. For this reason, drug therapy for parkinsonism focuses not only on restoring dopamine function, but also on blocking the effect of acetylcholine within this sensitive area of the brain.

corpus = *body*
striatum = *striped*

Extrapyramidal symptoms (EPS) develop in response to the same neurochemical actions that cause Parkinson's disease. Recall that antipsychotic drugs act by blocking dopamine receptors. Treatment with some antipsychotic drugs may cause parkinsonism-like symptoms by interfering with the same neural pathway and functions affected by the lack of dopamine.

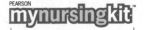

EPS may occur suddenly and become a medical emergency. With acute EPS, patients' muscles may spasm or lock up. Fever and confusion are other signs or symptoms of this reaction. If acute EPS occur in a health care facility, short-term medical treatment may be provided by administering diphenhydramine (Benadryl). When symptoms are recognized outside a health care facility, the patient should be immediately taken to the emergency department. Untreated acute episodes of EPS can be fatal.

THE NATIONAL PARKINSON FOUNDATION

THE AMERICAN PARKINSON DISEASE ASSOCIATION

PARKINSON SOCIETY OF CANADA

Concept Review   12.1

- Parkinson's disease primarily affects which body functions? What are the four major symptoms of this disorder?

Parkinsonism drugs focus on the brain by restoring the balance between dopamine and acetylcholine.

CORE CONCEPT 12.3

The goal of pharmacotherapy for Parkinson's disease is to increase the ability of the patient to perform normal daily activities such as eating, walking, dressing, and bathing. Although pharmacotherapy does not cure this disorder, it can dramatically reduce symptoms in some patients.

As mentioned, antiparkinsonism drugs are given to restore the balance of dopamine and acetylcholine within the corpus striatum of the brain. These drugs include dopaminergic agents and anticholinergics (cholinergic blockers).

TABLE 12.2	Dopaminergic Drugs Used for Parkinsonism	
DRUG	**ROUTE AND ADULT DOSE**	**REMARKS**
amantadine (Symmetrel)	PO; 100 mg daily or bid	Also for infection with influenza A virus; for relief of drug-induced EPS; may cause release of dopamine from nerve terminals
apomorphine	SC; 2 mg for the first dose; every few days, doses may be increased by 1 mg (max: 6 mg); if more than 1 week passes between doses, titration should be restarted at 2 mg	Activates dopamine receptors; may improve ability to walk, talk, and move
bromocriptine (Parlodel)	PO; 1.25–2.5 mg/day up to 100 mg/day in divided doses	Also for suppression of lactation, female infertility, and overproduction of growth hormone; activates the dopamine receptor directly
carbidopa-levodopa (Sinemet)	PO; 1 tablet containing 10 mg carbidopa/ 100 mg levodopa or 25 mg carbidopa/100 mg levodopa tid (max: 6 tablets/day)	Prevents metabolism of levodopa, enhancing dopamine action
entacapone (Comtan)	PO; 200 mg given with levodopa/carbidopa up to eight times/day	Blocks synaptic enzyme (catecholamine O-methyl transferase [COMT]) responsible for metabolizing dopamine
(Pr) levodopa (Larodopa)	PO; 500 mg–1 g/day, may be increased by 750 mg every 3–7 days	Chemical precursor to dopamine; dosage can be reduced by 70–80% if administered with carbidopa
pramipexole (Mirapex)	PO; start with 0.125 mg tid for 1 week, double this dose for the next week, continue to increase by 0.25 mg/dose tid every week to a target dose of 1.5 mg tid	Activates dopamine receptors
ropinirole (Requip)	PO; start with 0.25 mg tid, may increase by 0.25 mg/dose tid every week to a target dose of 1 mg tid	Activates dopamine receptors
selegiline (L-Deprenyl, Eldepryl)	PO; 5 mg/dose bid; doses greater than 10 mg/day are potentially toxic	Blocks monoamine oxidase (MAO) type B, the enzyme that degrades dopamine within brain nerve terminals
tolcapone (Tasmar)	PO; 100 mg tid (max: 600 mg/day)	Blocks synaptic enzyme (COMT) responsible for metabolizing dopamine

Dopaminergic Agents

Dopaminergic drugs, shown in Table 12.2, are used to increase dopamine levels within critical areas of the corpus striatum. The drug of choice for parkinsonism is levodopa (Larodopa), a dopaminergic drug that has been used more often than any other medication for this disorder. As shown in Figure 12.1 ■, levodopa is a precursor of (an agent that stimulates) dopamine synthesis. Supplying it directly with drug therapy leads to increased synthesis of dopamine within the nerve terminals. Levodopa can cross the blood-brain barrier, but dopamine cannot. Therefore, dopamine by itself is not used for therapy. The effectiveness of levodopa can be "boosted" by combining it with carbidopa. A combination, marketed as Sinemet, makes more levodopa available to enter the CNS.

Several approaches to enhancing dopamine may be used in treating parkinsonism. Tolcapone (Tasmar), entacapone (Comtan), and selegiline (L-Deprenyl, Eldepryl) inhibit enzymes that normally destroy levodopa and dopamine. Apomorphine (Apokyn), bromocriptine (Parlodel), pramipexole (Mirapex), and ropinirole (Requip) directly activate the dopamine receptor. Amantadine (Symmetrel), an antiviral agent, causes the release of dopamine from its nerve terminals. All of these drugs, because they are not as effective as levodopa, are considered adjuncts (or additions) to the pharmacotherapy of parkinsonism.

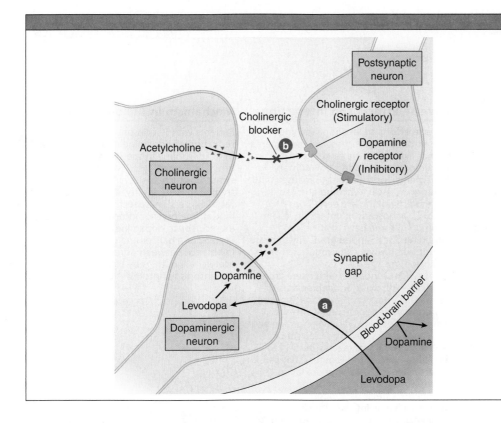

FIGURE 12.1

Dopamine cannot cross the blood-brain barrier. Levodopa, its precursor, can. Once levodopa crosses the blood-brain barrier and enters neurons, it is converted into dopamine, which normally inhibits firing of the next neuron. Natural acetylcholine in the brain stimulates the same postsynaptic neuron. Thus, to restore normal neuronal activity, drug therapy attempts to either (a) restore dopamine inhibitory action, or (b) block acetylcholine (cholinergic) stimulatory activity.

Cholinergic Blockers (Anticholinergics)

A second approach to changing the balance between dopamine and acetylcholine in the brain is to give cholinergic blockers, or anticholinergics. Again, by blocking the effect of acetylcholine, anticholinergics inhibit the overactivity of this neurotransmitter within the corpus striatum. These agents are listed in Table 12.3.

Anticholinergics such as atropine were the first drugs used to treat parkinsonism. The large number of adverse effects has limited use of these drugs. The anticholinergics used now for parkinsonism act within the CNS and produce fewer adverse effects. However, they continue to cause adverse autonomic effects such as dry mouth, blurred vision, tachycardia, urinary retention, and constipation (very troublesome). The centrally acting anticholinergics are not as effective as levodopa in relieving severe symptoms of parkinsonism. They are used early in the courses of the

TABLE 12.3	Anticholinergic Drugs Used for Parkinsonism	
DRUG	**ROUTE AND ADULT DOSE**	**REMARKS**
(Pr) benztropine (Cogentin)	PO; 0.5–1 mg/day, gradually increase as needed (max: 6 mg/day)	Also used to relieve EPS from neuroleptic drugs; does not lighten tardive dyskinesia
biperiden (Akineton)	PO; 2 mg daily to qid	Blocks acetylcholine receptors; thus, actions associated with muscarinic blockade are observed (e.g., blurred vision, dry mouth); available in IM/IV forms.
diphenhydramine (Benadryl) (see page 487 for the Drug Profile box)	PO; 25–50 mg tid or qid (max: 300 mg/day)	Also for allergic reactions, motion sickness, sedation, and coughing; blocks cholinergic function even though it is an antihistamine; available in IM/IV forms.
procyclidine (Kemadrin)	PO; 2.5 mg tid pc; may be increased to 5 mg tid if tolerated, with an additional 5 mg at bedtime (max: 45–60 mg/day)	Blocks acetylcholine receptors in the brain
trihexyphenidyl (Artane)	PO; 1 mg for day 1; double this for day 2; then increase by 2 mg every 3–5 days up to 6–10 mg/day (max: 15 mg/day)	Also used to relieve EPS; offlabeled use for Huntington's chorea and spasmodic torticollis

---

DRUG PROFILE: ℗ *Levodopa (Larodopa)*

Therapeutic Class: Antiparkinson agent
Pharmacologic Class: Dopamine precursor

Actions and Uses:

Levodopa restores the neurotransmitter dopamine in extrapyramidal areas of the brain, thus relieving some Parkinson's symptoms. To increase its effect, levodopa is often combined with other medications, such as carbidopa, that prevent its enzymatic breakdown. As long as 6 months may be needed to achieve the maximum therapeutic effect of levodopa.

Adverse Effects and Interactions:

Adverse effects of levodopa include uncontrolled and purposeless movements such as extending the fingers and shrugging the shoulders, involuntary movements, loss of appetite, nausea, and vomiting. Muscle twitching and spasmodic winking are early signs of toxicity. Orthostatic hypotension is common in some patients. The drug should be discontinued gradually because abrupt withdrawal can produce acute parkinsonism.

Levodopa interacts with many drugs. For example, tricyclic antidepressants decrease the effects of levodopa, increase postural hypotension, or may increase sympathetic activity with hypertension and sinus tachycardia. Levodopa cannot be used if an MAOI was taken within 14 to 28 days because their use together may cause hypertensive crisis. Haloperidol taken concurrently may antagonize the therapeutic effects of levodopa. Methyldopa may increase toxicity. Antihypertensives may cause increased hypotensive effects. Anticonvulsants may decrease the therapeutic effects of levodopa. Antacids containing magnesium, calcium, or sodium bicarbonate may increase levodopa absorption, which could lead to toxicity. Pyridoxine reverses the antiparkinsonian effects of levodopa.

Levodopa should be used with caution with herbal supplements, such as kava, because symptoms of Parkinson's may worsen.

Mechanism in Action:

Patients with Parkinson's disease have a reduction of dopamine and an elevation of acetylcholine in specific regions of the brain. This imbalance is responsible for symptoms such as slow movements, tremor, muscle rigidity, shuffling gait, flat facial expression, speech impairment, and lack of fine psychomotor skills. Levodopa, a precursor to dopamine, crosses the blood-brain barrier and restores the imbalance between dopamine and acetylcholine, thereby treating Parkinson's symptoms.

Refer to MyNursingKit for a Nursing Process Focus specific to this drug.

---

disease when symptoms are less severe, in patients who cannot tolerate levodopa, and in combination therapy with older antiparkinsonism drugs.

Concept Review 12.2

■ Antiparkinson's drugs attempt to restore the balance of which two major CNS neurotransmitters?

ALZHEIMER'S DISEASE

Alzheimer's disease (AD) is a devastating, progressive, degenerative disease that generally begins after age 60. As many as 50% of people are affected with this disease by the age of 85. A patient generally lives 5 to 10 years after being diagnosed with AD. This kind of dementia is the seventh leading cause of death in the United States. Pharmacotherapy has limited success in improving cognitive function in patients with this disorder.

DRUG PROFILE: 🆁 *Benztropine (Cogentin)*

Therapeutic Class: Antiparkinson agent
Pharmacologic Class: Centrally acting cholinergic receptor blocker

Actions and Uses:

Benztropine acts by blocking excess cholinergic stimulation of neurons in the corpus striatum. It is used for relief of parkinsonism symptoms and for the treatment of EPS brought on by antipsychotic pharmacotherapy. This medication suppresses tremors but does not affect tardive dyskinesia.

Adverse Effects and Interactions:

As expected from its autonomic action, benztropine can cause typical anticholinergic adverse effects such as sedation, dry mouth, constipation, and tachycardia.

Benztropine interacts with many drugs. For example, benztropine should not be taken with alcohol, tricyclic antidepressants, MAOIs, phenothiazines, procainamide, or quinidine because of combined sedative effects. Over-the-counter (OTC) cold medicines and alcohol should be avoided. Other drugs that enhance dopamine release or activation of the dopamine receptor may produce additive effects. Haloperidol will cause decreased effectiveness.

Antihistamines, phenothiazines, tricyclics, and disopyramide quinidine may increase anticholinergic effects, and antidiarrheals may decrease absorption.

Refer to MyNursingKit for a Nursing Process Focus specific to this drug.

AD is responsible for most of the cases of dementia. **Dementia** is a degenerative disorder characterized by progressive memory loss, confusion, and inability to think or communicate effectively. Consciousness and perception are usually unaffected. Most causes of dementia are unknown, but atrophy (wasting away) or other structural changes within the brain are common. Some of the known (but less frequent) causes of dementia include multiple strokes, severe infections, and toxins.

Despite extensive, ongoing research, the cause of AD remains unknown. The early-onset form of AD that runs in families accounts for about 10% of cases and is caused by gene defects on chromosome 1, 14, or 21. Environmental, immunologic, and nutritional factors, as well as viruses, may be possible causes of brain damage seen in patients with AD. Chronic inflammation and damage to cells from pollutants, radiation, drugs, or the body's own immune response may decrease the number and function of neurons within the brain.

Although the cause may be unknown, structural damage within the brain of patients with AD has been well documented. *Amyloid plaques* and *neurofibrillary tangles*, found at autopsy, are present in nearly all patients with AD. It is suspected that these structural changes are caused by chronic inflammatory or oxidative cellular damage to surrounding neurons. There is a loss in both the number and function of neurons in patients with AD.

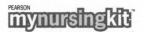

PEARSON
mynursingkit

ALZHEIMER'S DISEASE
INFORMATION PAGE
ALZHEIMER SOCIETY
OF CANADA

Patients with Alzheimer's disease experience a dramatic loss of ability to perform tasks that require acetylcholine as the CNS neurotransmitter.

CORE CONCEPT 12.4

Patients with AD experience a dramatic loss of ability to perform tasks that require acetylcholine as the neurotransmitter. Because acetylcholine is a major neurotransmitter within the *hippocampus* (an area of the brain responsible for learning and memory) and other parts of the cerebral cortex, neuronal function within these brain areas is especially affected. Thus, an inability to remember and to recall information is among the early symptoms of AD. Symptoms of AD include the following:

- Impaired memory and judgment
- Confusion or disorientation

- Inability to recognize family or friends
- Aggressive behavior
- Depression
- Psychoses, including paranoia and delusions
- Anxiety

Alzheimer's disease is treated with acetylcholinesterase inhibitors.

Drugs are used to slow memory loss and other progressive symptoms of dementia. Some drugs are given to treat associated symptoms such as depression, anxiety, or psychoses. The acetylcholinesterase inhibitors are the most widely used class of drugs for treating AD. Representative cholinesterase inhibitors are listed in Table 12.4.

Acetylcholinesterase Inhibitors

The Food and Drug Administration (FDA) has approved only a few drugs for AD. The most effective of these medications acts by intensifying the effect of acetylcholine at the cholinergic receptor, as shown in Figure 12.2 ■. Acetylcholine is naturally degraded in the synapse by the enzyme **acetylcholinesterase (AchE)**. When AchE is inhibited, acetylcholine levels increase and greatly affect the receptors. As described in Chapter 8 ∞ , the AchE inhibitors *indirectly* stimulate the receptors for acetylcholine.

When treating AD, the goal of pharmacotherapy is to improve function in activities of daily living, behavior, and cognition. Although the AchE inhibitors improve all three functions, their effectiveness is limited at best. These agents do not cure AD—they only slow its progression. Therapy is begun as soon as the diagnosis of AD is established. These agents are ineffective in treating the severe stages of this disorder, probably because so many neurons have died. Increasing the levels of acetylcholine is only effective if there are functioning neurons present. Therefore, as the disease progresses, the AchE inhibitors are often discontinued. Their therapeutic benefit is not great enough to outweigh their expense or the adverse effects they may cause.

All AchE inhibitors used to treat AD are equally effective. Their adverse effects are those expected of drugs that enhance the parasympathetic nervous system (see Chapter 8 ∞). These include nausea, vomiting, and diarrhea. Of the agents available for AD, tacrine (Cognex) is associated with liver toxicity. Rivastigmine (Exelon) is associated with weight loss, a potentially serious adverse effect in some elderly patients. When discontinuing therapy, doses of the AchE inhibitors should be lowered gradually.

Although AchE inhibitors are the mainstay of treatment for AD dementia, several other agents are being investigated for their possible benefit in delaying the progression of this disease. Because at least some of the neuronal changes in AD are caused by oxidative cellular damage, antioxidants such as vitamin E are being examined for their effects in affected patients. Other agents currently being examined are anti-inflammatory agents, estrogen, and ginkgo biloba.

TABLE 12.4	Acetylcholinesterase Inhibitors Used for Alzheimer's Disease	
DRUG	**ROUTE AND ADULT DOSE**	**REMARKS**
Pr donepezil (Aricept, Aricept ODT)	PO; 5–10 mg at bedtime	For mild to moderate dementia; may cause nausea, diarrhea, muscle cramps, and weight loss
galantamine (Reminyl)	PO; start with 4 mg bid at least 4 weeks; if tolerated, may increase by 4 mg bid every 4 weeks to target a dose of 12 mg bid (max: 8–16 mg bid)	For mild to moderate dementia; may cause weight loss, dizziness, nausea, vomiting, and hypotension when changing positions
rivastigmine tartrate (Exelon)	PO; start with 1.5 mg bid with food, may increase by 1.5 mg bid every 2 weeks if tolerated; target dose is 3–6 mg bid (max: 12 mg bid)	For mild to moderate dementia; may cause flulike symptoms, dizziness, and weight loss
tacrine (Cognex)	PO; 10 mg qid, increase in 40 mg/day increments not sooner than every 6 weeks (max: 160 mg/day)	For mild to moderate dementia; offlabeled used for severe dementia in patients with HIV infection; may cause nausea, vomiting, and liver toxicity

FIGURE 12.2

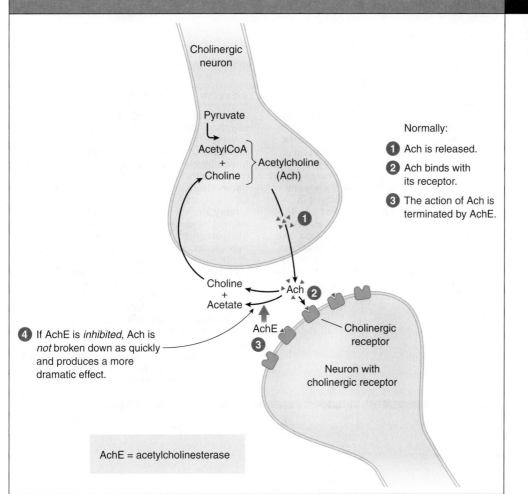

Alzheimer's medications work by intensifying the effect of acetylcholine at the receptor.

Cholinergic neuron

Pyruvate

AcetylCoA
+
Choline
} Acetylcholine (Ach)

Normally:

1 Ach is released.

2 Ach binds with its receptor.

3 The action of Ach is terminated by AchE.

1

Choline
+
Acetate

→ Ach **2**

AchE **3**

Cholinergic receptor

4 If AchE is *inhibited*, Ach is *not* broken down as quickly and produces a more dramatic effect.

Neuron with cholinergic receptor

AchE = acetylcholinesterase

In 2003, memantine (Namenda) was approved by the FDA for combination treatment of moderate to severe AD. Its mechanism of action differs from that of the cholinesterase inhibitors. Unlike cholinesterase inhibitors that address the cholinergic defect in the brains of patients with AD, memantine reduces the abnormally high levels of glutamate. Glutamate exerts its neural effects through interaction with the *N*-methyl-D-aspartate (NMDA) receptor. When bound to the receptor, glutamate causes calcium to enter neurons, producing an excitatory effect. Too much glutamate in the brain may be responsible for brain cell death. Memantine, along with cholinesterase inhibitors such as donepezil, may have a protective function in reducing neuronal calcium overload.

Agitation occurs in most patients with AD. This may be accompanied by delusion, paranoia, hallucinations, or other psychotic symptoms. Atypical antipsychotic agents such as risperidone (Risperdal, Risperdal Consta) and olanzapine (Zyprexa) may be used to control these episodes. Conventional antipsychotics such as haloperidol (Haldol) are occasionally prescribed, although EPS often limit their use.

Although not as common as agitation, anxiety and depression may also occur in patients with AD. Anxiolytics such as buspirone (BuSpar) or some of the benzodiazepines are used to control excessive anxiety (see Chapter 9 ⚭). Mood stabilizers such as sertraline (Zoloft), citalopram (Celexa), or fluoxetine (Prozac) are given when major depression interferes with daily activities (see Chapter 10 ⚭).

Concept Review   12.3

■ Alzheimer's disease is a dysfunction of which brain neurotransmitters? How do drugs for Alzheimer's disease restore neurotransmitter function and improve symptoms of dementia?

DRUG PROFILE: 🔵 *Donepezil (Aricept, Aricept ODT)*

Therapeutic Class: Alzheimer's disease agent
Pharmacologic Class: Acetylcholinerase inhibitor

Actions and Uses:

Donepezil is an AchE inhibitor that improves memory in cases of mild to moderate Alzheimer's dementia by enhancing the effects of acetylcholine in neurons in the cerebral cortex that have not yet been damaged. Patients should receive pharmacotherapy for at least 6 months prior to assessing the maximum benefits of drug therapy. Improvement in memory may be observed as early as 1 to 4 weeks following medication. The therapeutic effects of donepezil are often short-lived, and the degree of improvement is modest at best. An advantage of donepezil over other drugs in its class is that its long half-life permits it to be given once daily.

Adverse Effects and Interactions:

Common adverse effects of donepezil are vomiting, diarrhea, and darkened urine. CNS adverse effects include insomnia, syncope, depression, headache, and irritability. Musculoskeletal adverse effects include muscle cramps, arthritis, and bone fractures. Generalized adverse effects include headache, fatigue, chest pain, increased libido, hot flashes, urinary incontinence, dehydration, and blurred vision. Unlike tacrine, hepatotoxicity has not been observed. Patients with bradycardia, hypotension, asthma, hyperthyroidism, or active peptic ulcer disease should be monitored carefully. Anticholinergics will be less effective. Donepezil interacts with several other drugs. For example, bethanechol causes a synergistic effect. Phenobarbital, phenytoin, dexamethasone, and rifampin may speed elimination of donepezil. Quinidine or ketoconazole may inhibit metabolism of donepezil. Because donepezil acts by increasing cholinergic activity, two parasympathomimetics should not be administered at the same time.

Refer to MyNursingKit for a Nursing Process Focus specific to this drug.

NATURAL THERAPIES

Ginkgo Biloba for Dementia

The seeds and leaves of ginkgo biloba have been used in traditional Chinese medicine for thousands of years. The tree is planted throughout the world, including the United States. In Western medicine, the focus has been on treating depression and memory loss. In Germany, an extract of ginkgo biloba is approved for the treatment of dementia.

Ginkgo has been shown to improve mental functioning and stabilize AD. The mechanism of action seems to be related to increasing the blood supply to the brain by dilating blood vessels, decreasing the viscosity of the blood, and modifying the neurotransmitter system. The exact benefit of ginkgo remains unclear because some studies concluded that cognitive performance improved, whereas others have shown no improvement in the symptoms or progress of AD. Ginkgo is considered safe; however, it may increase the risk of bleeding in patients taking anticoagulants. Other potential uses for ginkgo being investigated include asthma, multiple sclerosis, intermittent claudication, sexual dysfunction due to antidepressants, and insulin resistance (Birks, 2007).

MULTIPLE SCLEROSIS

Multiple sclerosis (MS) is an autoimmune disorder of the CNS. This is a condition in which antibodies target and slowly destroy tissues in the brain and spinal cord.

Symptoms of multiple sclerosis result from demyelination of CNS nerve fibers.

As tissues are damaged, inflammation of nervous tissue causes *demyelination*, or the loss of myelin, a fatty material that acts as a protective insulator of nerve fibers. The loss of myelin leaves multiple areas of hard scarred tissue (plaques) along the covering of nerve cells. Axons are gradually destroyed, disrupting the ability of the nerves to conduct electrical impulses to and from the brain.

Over time, as demyelination continues, various symptoms of MS occur. Some of the more common symptoms include fatigue, heat sensitivity, pain, spasticity (muscle cramps and spasms), cognitive problems, balance and coordination problems, and bowel and bladder symptoms. The course of MS is unpredictable, and each patient will experience a variety of symptoms.

Drugs for multiple sclerosis reduce immune attacks in the brain and treat unfavorable symptoms.

The two basic strategies for treating MS are shown in Table 12.5. One approach attempts to reduce inflammation and prevent attacks on the nervous system. The other strategy emphasizes treatments to relieve symptoms.

The most treatable form of this disorder is *relapsing-remitting MS (RRMS)*. This condition involves unpredictable relapses (attacks) during which time new symptoms appear or existing symptoms become more severe. These symptoms can last for varying periods (days or months), followed by partial or total remission (recovery). In RRMS, the disease may be inactive for months or years. On average, people with RRMS have one or two attacks a year.

Immune system modulating drugs (also described later in the text as *immunostimulants* [see Chapter 24 ∞]) are clinically proven drugs for treating the underlying causes of MS and for decreasing the overall relapse rate. Interferon beta 1a (Avonex, Rebif) is available as an IM or SC medication; interferon beta 1b (Betaseron) is available only as an SC medication. Although generally well tolerated, the interferons have unfavorable adverse effects, including flulike symptoms (e.g., headaches, fever, chills, muscle aches), anxiety, discomfort experienced at the injection site, and liver toxicity. Due to toxicity concerns and additive effects, caution should be exercised when taking these drugs in combination with chemotherapeutic agents or bone marrow-suppressing drugs.

Another drug treatment, glatiramer acetate (Copaxone), formerly known as *copolymer-1*, is an immunomodulating synthetic protein that resembles myelin basic protein, an essential part of the nerve's myelin coating. Because glatiramer acetate resembles myelin, it is thought to curb the body's attack on the myelin covering and reduce the creation of new brain lesions. Copaxone is available in prefilled syringes that can be kept at room temperature for several days. However, patients often complain of adverse effects and having to inject themselves. Adverse effects include redness, pain, swelling, itching, or a lump at the site of injection. Flushing, chest pain, weakness, infection, pain, nausea, joint pain, anxiety, and muscle stiffness are common adverse effects.

TABLE 12.5	Drugs Used for Multiple Sclerosis	
DRUG	**DRUG CLASSIFICATION**	**ADMINISTERED**
FOR IMMUNE ATTACKS AGAINST THE CNS		
interferon beta-1a (Avonex, Rebif)	Immune system modulating drug	IM and SC
interferon beta-1b (Betaseron)	Immune system modulating drug	SC
glatiramer acetate (Copaxone, Copolymer-1)	Immune system modulating drug, myelin protein protectant	IV
mitoxantrone (Novantrone)	Immunosuppressant	IV
FOR THE RELIEF OF MS SYMPTOMS		**Symptoms**
modafinil (Provigil)	Alpha-adrenergic stimulant	Fatigue, memory loss, weakness
amantadine (Symmetrel)	Dopaminergic drug	Fatigue, memory loss, weakness
gabapentin (Neurontin)	Antiseizure drug	Anxiety, insomnia, neuropathic pain
methylprednisolone (Solu-Medrol)	Glucocorticoid	Myelin swelling and inflammation

Mitoxantrone (Novantrone) is an FDA-drug approved for patients with MS who have not responded to interferon or Copaxone therapy. Primarily a chemotherapeutic drug, mitoxantrone is substantially more toxic than the immune system modulating drugs. Toxicity is a concern due to irreversible cardiac injury and potential harm to the fetus. Notable adverse effects are reversible hair loss, gastrointestinal (GI) discomfort (nausea and vomiting), and allergic symptoms (itching, rash, hypotension). Some patients experience a blue-green tint to their urine, which is harmless.

Miscellaneous drugs used for MS include modafinil (Provigil) and amantadine (Symmetrel) for treating fatigue, memory loss, and progressive weakness symptoms. Modafinil is an alpha$_1$-adrenergic agent thought to activate receptors that respond to the brain neurotransmitter norepinephrine. This agent increases alertness and energy and improves memory. Gabapentin (Neurontin) is an antiseizure drug that is used for treating mood disturbances, including depression and sensitivity to pain (see Chapter 13 ⌾). Methylprednisolone (Solu-Medrol), a steroidal anti-inflammatory agent, may be administered IV to treat symptoms of swelling and inflammation in the brain.

MUSCLE SPASMS

Muscle spasms are involuntary contractions of a muscle or groups of muscles. The muscles tighten, develop a fixed pattern of resistance, and lose functioning ability.

CORE CONCEPT 12.8

Muscle spasms are caused by injury, overmedication, hypocalcemia, and debilitating neurologic disorders.

Muscle spasms are a common condition usually associated with overuse of and local injury to the skeletal muscle. Other causes of muscle spasms include overmedication with antipsychotic drugs (see Chapter 11 ⌾), epilepsy, hypocalcemia, pain, and debilitating neurologic disorders. Patients with muscle spasms may experience inflammation, edema, and pain at the affected muscle; loss of coordination; and reduced mobility. When a muscle goes into spasm, it freezes in a contracted state. A single, prolonged contraction is called a *tonic spasm*, whereas multiple, rapidly repeated contractions are called *clonic spasms*. Treatment of muscle spasms includes use of both nonpharmacologic and pharmacologic therapies.

CORE CONCEPT 12.9

Muscle spasms may be treated with nonpharmacologic or pharmacologic therapies.

Identifying the etiology of muscle spasms requires a careful history and a physical exam. After a determination has been made, nonpharmacologic therapies are normally used in conjunction with medications. Nonpharmacologic measures may be immobilization of the affected muscle, application of heat or cold, hydrotherapy, ultrasound, supervised exercises, massage, or manipulation.

Pharmacotherapy for muscle spasms may include combinations of analgesics, anti-inflammatory agents, and centrally acting skeletal muscle relaxants. Most skeletal muscle re-

Fast Facts Muscle Spasms

- More than 12 million people worldwide have muscle spasms.
- Muscle spasms severe enough to warrant drug therapy are often found in patients who have had other debilitating disorders, such as neurodegenerative diseases, stroke, injury or cerebral palsy.
- Cerebral palsy is usually associated with events that occur before or during birth, but it may be caused by head trauma or infection during the first few months or years of life.
- Dystonia affects about 250,000 people in the United States; it is the third most common movement disorder after Parkinson's disease and essential tremor.
- Researchers have recognized multiple forms of inheritable dystonia and identified at least 10 genes or chromosomal locations responsible for the various manifestations.

laxants relieve symptoms of muscular stiffness and rigidity that result from muscular injury. Agents also help improve mobility. Therapeutic goals are to minimize pain and discomfort, increase range of motion, and improve the patient's ability to function independently.

Concept Review **12.4**

■ Give several reasons why muscle spasms develop. What is the main goal of therapy for muscle spasms?

Many muscle relaxants treat muscle spasms by inhibiting upper motor neuron activity, causing sedation, or altering simple reflexes.

CORE CONCEPT 12.10

Antispasmodic drugs relieve symptoms of muscular stiffness and rigidity. They improve mobility in cases in which patients have restricted movements.

Many antispasmodic drugs treat muscle spasms at the level of the CNS. The exact mechanisms of action are not fully known, but it is believed that these agents affect the brain and/or spinal cord by inhibiting upper motor neuron activity, causing sedation, or altering simple reflexes.

Skeletal muscle relaxants are used to treat local spasms resulting from muscular injury and may be prescribed alone or in combination with other medications to reduce pain and increase range of motion. Commonly used centrally acting medications are baclofen (Lioresal), cyclobenzaprine (Cycoflex, Flexeril), tizanidine (Zanaflex), and benzodiazepines such as diazepam (Valium), clonazepam (Klonopin), and lorazepam (Ativan) (Table 12.6). All of the centrally acting agents can cause sedation.

TABLE 12.6	Centrally Acting Antispasmodic Drugs	
DRUG	**ROUTE AND ADULT DOSE**	**REMARKS**
baclofen (Lioresal)	PO; 5 mg tid (max: 80 mg/day)	May be administered orally or by an implantable pump, which infuses medication directly into the subarachnoid space
carisoprodol (Soma)	PO; 350 mg tid	CNS depressant; does not inhibit motor activity like other conventional muscle relaxers; muscle relaxation seems to be related to sedation
chlorzoxazone (Paraflex, Parafon Forte, Remular-S)	PO; 250–500 mg tid–qid (max: 3 g/day)	Depresses nerve transmission in the brain and spinal cord, possibly by sedation; not effective for cerebral palsy
clonazepam (Klonopin)	PO; 0.5 mg tid (max: 20 mg/day)	Benzodiazepine usually taken in combination with other drugs; used for the relief of skeletal muscle spasms; primarily for seizure disorders
(Pr) cyclobenzaprine (Cycoflex, Flexeril)	PO; 10–20 mg bid–qid (max: 60 mg/day)	Short-term relief of muscle spasms associated with acute musculoskeletal conditions; not for cerebral palsy or central nervous system diseases
diazepam (Valium) (see page 199 for the Drug Profile box)	PO; 4–10 mg bid–qid; IM/IV 2–10 mg, repeat if needed in 3–4 hours; IV pump; administer emulsion at 5 mg/min	Benzodiazepine used for the relief of skeletal muscle spasms associated with cerebral palsy, partial paralysis
lorazepam (Ativan) (see page 122 for the Drug Profile box)	PO; 1–2 mg bid–tid (max: 10 mg/day)	Benzodiazepine used for extreme muscle tension
metaxalone (Skelaxin)	PO; 800 mg tid–qid for maximum of 10 days	For acute musculoskeletal conditions; causes its effect through sedation
methocarbamol (Robaxin)	PO; 1.5 g qid for 2–3 days, then reduce to 1 g qid	Adjunct to physical therapy for acute musculoskeletal disorders and tetanus
orphenadrine citrate (Banflex, Flexon, Myolin, Norflex)	PO; 100 mg bid	IM/IV forms available
tizanidine (Zanaflex)	PO; 4–8 mg tid–qid (max: 36 mg/day)	To relax muscle tone associated with spasticity

Baclofen (Lioresal) is structurally similar to the inhibitory neurotransmitter gamma amino butyric acid (GABA) and produces its effect by a mechanism that is not fully known. It inhibits neuronal activity within the brain and, possibly, the spinal cord, although there is some uncertainty about whether the spinal effects of baclofen are associated with GABA. Baclofen may be used to reduce muscle spasms in patients with multiple sclerosis, cerebral palsy, or spinal cord injury. Common adverse effects of baclofen are drowsiness, dizziness, weakness, and fatigue. Baclofen is often the drug of first choice because of its wide safety margin.

Tizanidine (Zanaflex) is a centrally acting alpha$_2$-adrenergic agonist that inhibits motor neurons, mainly at the spinal cord level. Patients receiving high doses report drowsiness; thus, it also affects some neural activity in the brain. Though uncommon, one adverse effect of tizanidine is hallucinations. The drug's most frequent adverse effects are dry mouth, fatigue, dizziness, and sleepiness. Tizanidine is as effective as baclofen and is considered by some to be the drug of first choice.

As discussed in Chapter 13 ⬭ , benzodiazepines inhibit both sensory and motor neuron activity by enhancing the effects of GABA. Common adverse effects include drowsiness and ataxia (loss of coordination). Benzodiazepines are usually prescribed for muscle relaxation when baclofen and tizanidine fail to produce adequate relief.

SPASTICITY

Spasticity is a condition in which muscle groups remain in a continuous state of contraction, usually as a result of damage to the CNS. The contracting muscles become stiff with increased muscle tone. Signs and symptoms may include mild to severe pain, exaggerated deep tendon reflexes, muscle spasms, scissoring (involuntary crossing of the legs), and fixed joints.

CORE CONCEPT 12.11

Effective treatment for spasticity includes both physical therapy and medications.

Spasticity usually results from damage to the motor area of the cerebral cortex, which controls muscle movement. Etiologies most commonly associated with this condition include neurologic

---

DRUG PROFILE: ℗ℳ *Cyclobenzaprine (Cycloflex, Flexeril)*

Therapeutic Class: Skeletal muscle relaxant, central-acting
Pharmacologic Class: Catecholamine reuptake inhibitor

Actions and Uses:

Cyclobenzaprine relieves muscle spasms of local origin without interfering with general muscle function. This drug acts by depressing motor activity, primarily in the brainstem, with limited effects also occurring in the spinal cord. It increases circulating levels of norepinephrine, blocking presynaptic uptake. Its mechanism of action is similar to that of tricyclic antidepressants (see Chapter 10 ⬭). It causes muscle relaxation in acute muscle spasticity, but it is not effective in cases of cerebral palsy or diseases of the brain and spinal cord. This medication is meant to provide therapy for only 2 to 3 weeks.

Adverse Effects and Interactions:

Adverse reactions to cyclobenzaprine include drowsiness, blurred vision, dizziness, dry mouth, rash, and tachycardia. It should be used with caution in patients with myocardial infarction (MI), dysrhythmias, or severe cardiovascular disease. One reaction, although rare, is swelling of the tongue.

Alcohol, phenothiazines, and other CNS depressants may cause additive sedation. Cyclobenzaprine should not be used within 2 weeks of an MAOI because hyperpyretic crisis and convulsions may occur.

Mechanism in Action:

Cyclobenzaprine relaxes skeletal muscle and prevents local muscle spasms to alleviate pain. These effects are produced by depression of motor activity originating at the level of the brainstem and spinal motor neurons. Cyclobenzaprine also increases circulating levels of norepinephrine in the bloodstream and causes intense anticholinergic activity throughout the nervous system.

 Refer to MyNursingKit for a Nursing Process Focus specific to this drug.

NURSING PROCESS FOCUS

Patients Receiving Drugs for Muscle Spasms or Spasticity

ASSESSMENT

Prior to administration:
- Obtain a complete health history (physical/mental), including allergies, drug history, and possible drug interactions
- Obtain a complete physical examination
- Establish a baseline level of consciousness (LOC) and vital signs

POTENTIAL NURSING DIAGNOSES

- Pain (acute/chronic) related to muscle spasms.
- Impaired Physical Mobility related to acute/chronic pain.
- Risk for Injury related to adverse effects of drug.
- Deficient Knowledge related to information about disease process and drug therapy.

PLANNING: PATIENT GOALS AND EXPECTED OUTCOMES

The patient will:
- Report a decrease in pain, increase in range of motion, and reduction of muscle spasms
- Exhibit no serious adverse effects from the drug therapy
- Demonstrate an understanding of the therapeutic regimen by accurately describing the drug's effects, precautions, and measures to take to minimize adverse effects

IMPLEMENTATION

Interventions and (Rationales)	Patient Education/Discharge Planning
■ Monitor LOC and vital signs. (Some skeletal muscle relaxants alter the patient's LOC. Others within this class may alter blood pressure and heart rate.)	Instruct the patient to: ■ Avoid driving and other activities requiring mental alertness until the effects of the medication are known ■ Report any significant change in sensorium, such as slurred speech, confusion, hallucinations, or extreme lethargy ■ Report palpitations, chest pain, dyspnea, unusual fatigue, weakness, and visual disturbances ■ Avoid using other CNS depressants such as alcohol that will intensify sedation
■ Monitor pain. Determine the location, duration, and precipitating factors of the patient's pain. (Drugs should diminish the patient's pain.)	Instruct the patient: ■ To report the development of new sites of muscle pain ■ In relaxation techniques, deep breathing, and meditation methods to facilitate relaxation and reduce pain
■ Monitor for withdrawal reactions. (Abrupt withdrawal of baclofen may cause visual hallucinations, paranoid ideation, and seizures.)	■ Advise the patient to not abruptly discontinue treatment.
■ Monitor muscle tone, range of motion, and degree of muscle spasm. (This will determine the effectiveness of drug therapy.)	■ Instruct the patient to perform gentle range of motion, only to the point of mild physical discomfort, throughout the day.
■ Provide additional pain relief measures such as positional support, gentle massage, and moist heat or ice packs. (Drugs alone may not be sufficient in providing pain relief.)	■ Instruct the patient in complementary pain interventions such as positioning, gentle massage, and the application of heat or cold to the painful area.
■ Monitor for adverse effects such as drowsiness, dry mouth, dizziness, nausea, vomiting, faintness, headache, nervousness, diplopia, and urinary retention (cyclobenzaprine).	Instruct the patient to: ■ Report adverse effects ■ Take medication with food to decrease GI upset ■ Report signs of urinary retention such as a feeling of urinary bladder fullness, distended abdomen, and discomfort
■ Monitor for adverse effects such as muscle weakness, dry mouth, dizziness, nausea, diarrhea, tachycardia, erratic blood pressure, photosensitivity, and urinary retention. (These adverse effects occur with certain drugs in this class.)	Instruct the patient: ■ That frequent mouth rinses, sips of water, and sugarless candy or gum may help with dry mouth ■ That medication may cause a decrease in muscle strength and dosage may need to be reduced ■ To use sunscreen and protective clothing when outdoors

EVALUATION OF OUTCOME CRITERIA

Evaluate the effectiveness of drug therapy by confirming that patient goals and expected outcomes have been met (see "Planning").

See Tables 12.6 and 12.7 for lists of drugs to which these nursing actions apply.

dys = *abnormal*
tonia = *tension*

disorders such as cerebral palsy, severe head injury, spinal cord injury or lesions, and stroke. **Dystonia**, a chronic neurologic disorder, is characterized by involuntary muscle contraction that forces body parts into abnormal, occasionally painful movements or postures. It affects the muscle tone of the arms, legs, trunk, neck, eyelids, face, or vocal cords. Spasticity, whether short-term or long term, can be distressing and greatly impacts an individual's quality of life. In addition to causing pain, it also impairs physical mobility, thereby influencing the person's ability to perform activities of daily living (ADL) and diminishing his or her sense of independence.

Effective treatment for spasticity includes both physical therapy and medications. Medications alone are not adequate to reduce the complications of spasticity, but regular and consistent physical therapy exercises have been shown to be effective in decreasing the severity of symptoms. Types of treatment include muscle stretching to help prevent contractures, muscle group strengthening exercises, and repetitive motion exercises for improvement of accuracy. In extreme cases, surgery for tendon release or to sever the nerve-muscle pathway has been used.

CORE CONCEPT 12.12

Some drugs for spasticity provide relief by acting directly on muscle tissue, interfering with the release of calcium ions.

Drugs that are effective in the treatment of spasticity include two centrally acting drugs, baclofen (Lioresal) and diazepam (Valium), and a direct-acting drug, dantrolene (Dantrium). The direct-acting drugs produce an antispasmodic effect at the level of the neuromuscular junction, as shown in Figure 12.3 ■.

Dantrolene relieves spasticity by interfering with the release of calcium ions in skeletal muscle. Other direct-acting drugs include botulinum toxin type A (Botox, Dysport) and botulinum toxin type B (Myobloc). Although botulinum toxins are generally known for their use in cosmetic procedures, in some instances they may offer temporary relief of dystonia symptoms.

Botulinum toxin is an unusual drug because, in high doses, it acts as a poison. *Clostridium botulinum* is the bacterium responsible for food poisoning or botulism. At lower doses, however, this drug is safe and effective as a muscle relaxant. It produces its effect by blocking the release of acetylcholine from cholinergic nerve terminals (see Chapter 8 ⬡). Botulinum can cause extreme weakness, so its use may require the addition of other therapies to improve muscle strength. To prevent major problems with mobility or posture, botulinum toxin is often applied to small muscle groups. Sometimes this drug is administered together with centrally acting oral medications to further increase the functional use of a range of muscle groups.

Drawbacks to botulinum therapy are its delayed and limited effects. The treatment is mostly effective within 6 weeks of administration, and its effects last for only 3 to 6 months. Another drawback is the pain of injecting botulinum directly into the muscle. Local anesthetics are usually given to block this pain.

Quinine sulfate (Quinamm, Quiphile) has been used to treat nocturnal leg cramps, but in 2006 the FDA issued a warning that quinidine sulfate produces serious adverse effects such as cardiac dysrhythmias, severe hypersensitivity reactions, and an abnormal platelet count. Labelling of the drug was modified to restrict the use of quinine sulfate for malaria only and not for leg cramps. Direct-acting antispasmotic drugs are summarized in Table 12.7.

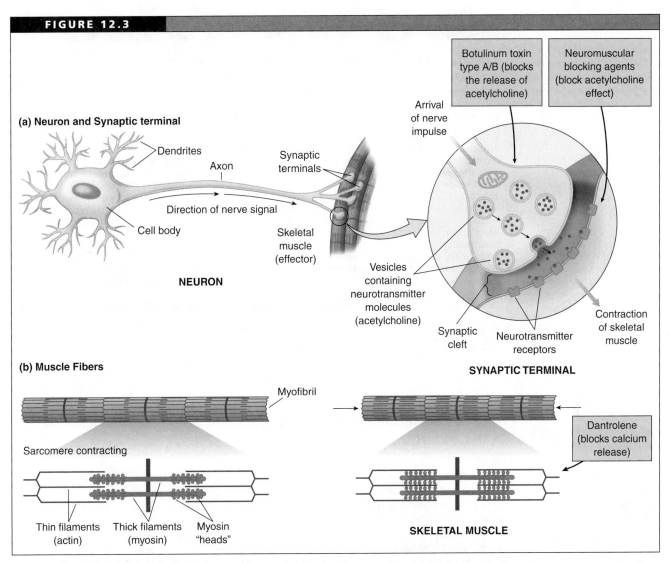

FIGURE 12.3

(a) Drugs affecting the neuromuscular junction may block either the release of acetylcholine at the synaptic terminal or the action of acetylcholine at its receptor (located on the surface of muscle fibers). (b) Drugs also block the release of calcium ions from muscle tissue, preventing the muscle fibers from contracting.

TABLE 12.7	Direct-Acting Antispasmodic Drugs	
DRUG	**ROUTE AND ADULT DOSE**	**REMARKS**
botulinum toxin type A (Botox, Dysport)	25 units injected directly into target muscle (max: 30-day dose should not exceed 200 units)	Mainly used for cosmetic procedures, this drug has been used to treat excessive sweating and wrinkles; relaxes facial muscles around the eye and forehead
botulinum toxin type B (Myobloc)	2500–5000 units/dose injected directly into target muscle; doses should be divided among muscle groups	May be used in cases of cervical dystonia
Pr dantrolene sodium (Dantrium)	PO; 25 mg daily; increase to 25 mg bid–qid; may increase every 4–7 days up to 100 mg bid–tid	Hydantoin-like medication; also for the treatment of malignant hyperthermia; IV form available

DRUG PROFILE: *Dantrolene Sodium (Dantrium)*

Therapeutic Class: Skeletal muscle relaxant, peripheral-acting
Pharmacologic Class: Skeletal muscle calcium release blocker

Actions and Uses:

Dantrolene is often used for spasticity, especially for spasms of the head and neck. It directly relaxes muscle spasms by interfering with the release of calcium ions from storage areas inside skeletal muscle cells. It does not affect cardiac or smooth muscle. Dantrolene is especially useful for muscle spasms when they occur after spinal cord injury or stroke and in cases of cerebral palsy, multiple sclerosis, and occasionally for the treatment of muscle pain after heavy exercise. It is also used for the treatment of malignant hyperthermia.

Adverse Effects and Interactions:

Adverse effects include muscle weakness, drowsiness, dry mouth, dizziness, nausea, diarrhea, tachycardia, erratic blood pressure, photosensitivity, and urinary retention. Dantrolene interacts with many other drugs. For example, it should not be taken with OTC cough preparations and antihistamines, alcohol, or other CNS depressants. Verapamil and other calcium channel blockers taken with dantrolene increase the risk of ventricular fibrillation and cardiovascular collapse. Patients with impaired cardiac or pulmonary function or hepatic disease should not take this drug.

Refer to MyNursingKit for a Nursing Process Focus specific to this drug.

CORE CONCEPT 12.13

Neuromuscular blocking agents block the effect of acetylcholine at the receptor.

nicotin = *nicotine*
ic = *related to*

cholin = *acetycholine*
erg = *work (action)*
ic = *related to*

fascicu = *muscle fascicle (bundle)*
lation = *movement*

Neuromuscular blocking agents bind to nicotinic receptors located on the surface of skeletal muscle fibers. For pharmacotherapy drugs called *nicotinic blocking agents* interfere with the binding of acetylcholine, thereby preventing voluntary muscle contraction. Nicotinic blocking agents are *cholinergic* (see Chapter 8 ⬡).

Neuromuscular blocking agents are classified into two major categories: nondepolarizing blockers and depolarizing blockers. *Nondepolarizing blockers* compete with acetylcholine for the receptor. As long as agents interfere with the binding of acetylcholine, muscles remain relaxed. By a related mechanism, *depolarizing blockers* bind to the acetylcholine receptor and produce a state of continuous depolarization. This action first results in small *fasciculations* or a time of brief repeated muscle movements, followed by relaxation of muscle fibers. Relaxation is short-lived until charges across the muscle membrane are restored (repolarization). Importantly, patients treated with neuromuscular blockers are able to feel pain. Thus, for surgical procedures, concomitant use of anesthetic agents is essential (see Chapter 15 ⬡).

It is important to note that neuromuscular blocking agents are different from *ganglionic blocking agents* that target the autonomic nervous system. In this instance, acetylcholine does indeed bind to nicotinic receptors, but the resulting actions of these agents are involuntary and do not involve skeletal muscle (see Chapter 8 ⬡). Ganglionic blockers dampen parasympathetic tone and produce effects such as increased heart rate, dry mouth, urinary retention, and reduced GI activity. They also dampen sympathetic tone, resulting in reduced sweating and less norepinephrine being released from postsynaptic nerve terminals. As an example, mecamylamine (Inversine) is a ganglionic blocker primarily used to treat patients with essential hypertension (see Chapter 17 ⬡).

The classic example of a nondepolarizing blocker is tubocurarine. Tubocurarine and related blocking agents are used to relax the muscles of patients being prepared for longer surgical procedures (Table 12.8). Although not preferred for mechanical ventilation or endotracheal intubation, small doses of these agents may be used for intermediate surgical procedures. Concerns of tubocurarine-like treatment include over-relaxation of muscles. For example, normal breathing activity (involving the diaphragm, glottic, and intercostal muscles) and swallowing activity (involving the neck and certain esophageal muscles) require skeletal muscle contraction.

Depolarizing agents are used primarily to relax the muscles of patients receiving electroconvulsive therapy (ECT) (see Chapter 13 ⬡) and for brief surgical procedures (see Chapter 15 ⬡).

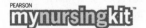

THE NATIONAL
INSTITUTE OF ARTHRITIS
AND MUSCULOSKELETAL
AND SKIN DISEASES

TABLE 12.8   Neuromuscular Blocking Agents

DRUG	DURATION	ADMINISTRATION ROUTE
NONDEPOLARIZING BLOCKERS		
atracurium (Tracrium)	Long duration	IV
cisatracurium (Nimbex)	Long duration	IV
doxacurium ((Nuromax)	Longest duration	IV
metocurine (Metubine)	Longest duration	IV
mivacurium (Mivacron)	Shorter duration	IV
pancuronium	Long duration	IV
pipecuronium (Arduan)	Longest duration	IV
rocuronium (Zemuron)	Long duration	IV
tubocurarine	Longest duration; oldest of the nondepolarizing agents	IV and IM
vecuronium (Norcuron)	Long duration	IV
DEPOLARIZING BLOCKERS		
succinylcholine (Anectine) (see page 244 for the Drug Profile box)	Shortest duration	IV and IM

Short surgical procedures involve mechanical ventilation and endotracheal intubation. Succinylcholine (Anectine) is the prototype example of a depolarizing blocker. Adverse effects include elevated blood levels of potassium, malignant hyperthermia, and postoperative muscle pain and persistent paralysis in some patients. As a specific antidote for persistent paralysis, patients are often given cholinesterase inhibitors.

PATIENTS NEED TO KNOW

Patients being treated for degenerative diseases and disorders of the neuromuscular system need to know the following:

Regarding Drugs for Parkinson's Disease or Dementia

1. Do not eat high-protein foods or foods high in vitamin B_6 (such as wheat germ, liver, green leafy vegetables, bananas, and fish) if you are taking levodopa. These foods interfere with drug effectiveness.
2. Be extremely careful about getting up quickly from a seated position. Many dementia drugs cause dizziness, lightheadedness, blurred vision, and difficulty in concentrating.
3. Do not skip taking the medications, and do not take OTC preparations (especially cold or cough medicines) without checking with a health care provider.
4. Be aware that urine may become a little dark. This is a normal side effect of dopamine-like drugs.
5. Do not drink alcoholic beverages or take sedatives. Combined effects may be harmful.
6. Be familiar with adverse effects specific for the drugs being taken. Drugs used for Parkinson's may produce nausea, dry mouth, and diminished sweating in some cases. Drugs used for dementia may cause nausea, diarrhea, muscle cramps, weight loss, and change in urine color.

Regarding Drugs for Muscle Spasms and Spasticity

7. When receiving treatment for problems with mobility, it often takes several weeks for effectiveness to begin. Follow the advice of a health care provider in order to achieve full therapeutic effect.
8. Most antispasmodic drugs produce adverse effects such as drowsiness and dizziness. Therefore, avoid CNS depressants and alcohol.

Regarding Neuromuscular Blockers

9. Some patients react adversely to neuromuscular blockers. Inform the health care provider about any important family history, such as malignant hyperthermia, myasthenia gravis, cardiovascular disease, and any other unusual problems.
10. Be aware that unpleasant muscle pain may be associated with surgical procedures.

CHAPTER REVIEW

CORE CONCEPTS SUMMARY

12.1 Medications are unable to cure most degenerative diseases of the CNS.

Degenerative diseases of the CNS include Alzheimer's disease, multiple sclerosis, and Parkinson's disease. The cause of most neurologic degenerative disorders is unknown. With the exception of Parkinson's disease, drug therapy provides only minimal benefit.

12.2 Parkinson's disease is progressive, with the occurrence of full symptoms taking many years.

Parkinson's disease, or *parkinsonism*, is a degenerative disorder caused by death of neurons that produce the brain neurotransmitter dopamine. Dopamine-producing neurons in the substantia nigra supply nerve signals to the corpus striatum. When dopamine is depleted, symptoms of parkinsonism, including tremors, muscle rigidity, bradykinesia (slow movement), and postural instability, occur. These symptoms are the same EPS effects caused by prolonged antipsychotic drug treatment.

12.3 Parkinsonism drugs focus on the brain by restoring the balance between dopamine and acetylcholine.

Balance, posture, muscle tone, and involuntary muscle movement depend on the proper balance between the neurotransmitter dopamine (inhibitory) and acetylcholine (stimulatory) in the corpus striatum. Drug therapy for parkinsonism focuses on restoring dopamine function (dopaminergic agents) and blocking the effect of acetylcholine overactivity (cholinergic blockers).

12.4 Patients with Alzheimer's disease experience a dramatic loss of ability to perform tasks that require acetylcholine as the CNS neurotransmitter.

Alzheimer's disease (AD) is a devastating, progressive, degenerative disease characterized by impaired memory, confusion or disorientation, inability to recognize family or friends, aggressive behavior, depression, psychoses, and anxiety. AD is responsible for 70% of all *dementia*. Although the cause of AD is unknown, structural brain damage and a dramatic loss of ability to perform tasks that require acetycholine as the neurotransmitter have been documented.

12.5 Alzheimer's disease is treated with acetylcholinesterase inhibitors.

Only a few drugs for AD have been approved. Most drugs act by intensifying the effect of acetylcholine at the cholinergic receptor. Acetylcholine is naturally degraded in the synapse by the enzyme acetyl-cholinesterase. When acetylcholinesterase is inhibited, acetylcholine levels increase and produce a greater effect on the receptor. This treatment improves function in activities of daily living, behavior, and cognition.

12.6 Symptoms of multiple sclerosis result from demyelination of CNS nerve fibers.

Multiple sclerosis is an autoimmune disorder of the CNS. Antibodies slowly destroy myelin in the brain and spinal cord, disrupting the ability of nerves to conduct electrical impulses. Over time, debilitating symptoms appear, including fatigue, heat sensitivity, pain, muscle cramps and spasms, impaired ability to think and reason, balance and coordination problems, and bowel and bladder symptoms.

12.7 Drugs for multiple sclerosis reduce immune attacks in the brain and treat unfavorable symptoms.

Two strategies for treating MS are reducing the immune response and relieving the symptoms. The most treatable form of MS is *relapsing-remitting MS (RRMS)*, in which unpredictable relapses occur. Drug treatments include immune system modulating drugs, immunosuppressants, and miscellaneous drugs used for treatment of MS symptoms such as inflammation, pain, fatigue, memory loss, and progressive weakness.

12.8 Muscle spasms are caused by injury, overmedication, hypocalcemia, and debilitating neurologic disorders.

Muscle spasms, or involuntary contractions of a muscle or group of muscles, occur for many reasons, including overmedication with antipsychotic drugs, epilepsy, hypocalcemia, pain, and incapacitating neurologic disorders. Two types of muscle spasms are tonic spasms and clonic spasms.

12.9 Muscle spasms may be treated with nonpharmacologic or pharmacologic therapies.

After a thorough medical exam, nonpharmacologic therapies such as immobilization, heat or cold, hydrotherapy, ultrasound, supervised exercises, massage, and manipulation may be used along with medications. Medications include analgesics, anti-inflammatory agents, and centrally acting skeletal muscle relaxants.

12.10 Many muscle relaxants treat muscle spasms by inhibiting upper motor neuron activity, causing sedation, or altering simple reflexes.

Skeletal muscle relaxants treat local spasms resulting from muscular injury and may be prescribed alone or in combination with medications that reduce pain and increase range of motion. These include centrally acting agents (affecting the brain and/or spinal cord) that have the potential to cause sedation and alter reflex activity.

12.11 Effective treatment for spasticity includes both physical therapy and medications.

Spasticity is a condition in which certain muscle groups remain in a state of contraction. Symptoms associated with spasticity include pain, exaggerated deep tendon reflexes, muscle spasms, scissoring, and fixed joints. Medications alone are not adequate in reducing the complications of spasticity.

12.12 Some drugs for spasticity provide relief by acting directly on muscle tissue, interfering with the release of calcium ions.

Direct-acting drugs produce an antispasmodic effect at the level of the neuromuscular junction. Drugs affect either calcium release from the muscle, or they interfere with the release of acetylcholine.

12.13 Neuromuscular blocking agents block the effect of acetylcholine at the receptor.

Neuromuscular blocking agents are classified as nondepolarizing blockers and depolarizing blockers. Both agents bind to acetylcholine receptors, relaxing muscles by slightly different mechanisms and durations of action.

REVIEW QUESTIONS

The following questions are written in NCLEX-PN® style. Answer these questions to assess your knowledge of the chapter material, and go back and review any material that is not clear to you.

1. The patient taking levodopa must avoid foods high in:

1. Vitamin A
2. Vitamin B_{12}
3. Folic acid
4. Vitamin B_6

2. The patient has developed which of the following degenerative CNS diseases that is characterized by progressive dementia and involuntary muscle spasms?

1. Parkinson's disease
2. Huntington's chorea
3. Multiple sclerosis
4. Alzheimer's disease

3. Drug therapy for the patient with Parkinson's disease focuses on:

1. Increasing cholinergic stimulation within the brain
2. Restoring acetylcholine and blocking dopamine within the brain
3. Restoring dopamine function and blocking acetylcholine within the brain
4. Destroying dopamine receptors within the brain

4. The patient on haloperidol (Haldol) is experiencing tardive dyskinesia. Which of the following drugs would the nurse anticipate being ordered?

1. Levodopa
2. Risperidone (Risperdal)
3. Benztropine (Cogentin)
4. Chlorpromazine (Thorazine)

5. The patient with Alzheimer's disease has been started on rivastigmine (Exelon). The nurse assesses the patient for:

1. Liver toxicity
2. Weight loss
3. Renal failure
4. Extrapyramidal adverse effects

6. The patient taking gingko biloba must be assessed for use of which of the following drugs?

1. Lanoxin
2. Coumadin
3. Lasix
4. Dilantin

7. Which of the following patients would be most likely to experience advanced memory loss?

1. A 45-year-old man who is taking glatiramer acetate (Copaxone)
2. A 67-year-old woman who is taking levodopa
3. A 57-year-old man who is taking benztropine (Cogentin)
4. A 53-year-old woman who is taking cyclobenzaprine (Cycloflex, Flexeril)

8. An interferon is prescribed for a patient with MS. The nurse should include which of the following points when teaching the patient about drug therapy?

1. Report flulike symptoms to the health care provider.
2. Expect urine to be orange.
3. Report the development of diarrhea.
4. The symptoms will get better over a period of a year.

CASE STUDY QUESTIONS

For questions 1–4, please read the following case study, and choose the correct answer from choices 1–4.

Mr. Wing, a 35-year-old man with MS, has persistent pain in his right hip and comes in for treatment. He explains that he has been taking enteric-coated aspirin for several weeks. He explains that he has been experiencing severe headaches. He has also been experiencing muscle twitches (multiple, rapidly repeating contractions) in his right hamstring. The muscle twitches have not been severe, but he is concerned that they may be related to his condition. Lately he has been experiencing quite a bit of fatigue, and his vision is sometimes "blurry." Laboratory values show slight hypocalcemia. The patient explains that he hasn't had any trouble with his diet. No abnormalities in bone structure or peripheral inflammatory symptoms are observed on examination.

1. Mr. Wing will probably be a candidate for which of the following medications?

1. Amantadine (Symmetrel)
2. Interferon Beta-1b (Betaseron)
3. Memantine (Namenda)
4. Choices 1 and 2 are correct

2. Mr. Wing's disorder is most correctly classified as:
1. Tonic spasms
2. Clonic spasms
3. Spasticity
4. Dystonia

3. Treatment with multiple types of antispasmodic therapy in this case would:
1. Improve Mr. Wing's symptoms for the long term
2. Improve Mr. Wing's symptoms for the short term
3. Make Mr. Wing's symptoms worse
4. Cause Mr. Wing to be sedated

4. Which of the following medications would likely be indicated if Mr. Wing's condition and symptoms were to progress significantly?
1. Selegiline (L-Deprenyl, Eldepryl)
2. Gabapentin (Neurontin)
3. Mitoxantrone (Novantrone)
4. Donepezil (Aricept)

FURTHER STUDY

- Chapter 8 ⊙⊙ includes more information on acetylcholinesterase inhibitors and their effects on the parasympathetic nervous system.

- More information on anxiolytics can be found in Chapter 9 ⊙⊙ .

- Chapter 24 ⊙⊙ discusses immunostimulants.

- In addition to its use in parkinsonism, diphenhydramine is a drug profile for allergies in Chapter 24 ⊙⊙ .

- Amantadine is also an antiviral drug and is discussed in Chapter 26 ⊙⊙ .

- Other causes of muscle spasms can include overmedication with antipsychotic drugs, which are discussed in Chapter 11 ⊙⊙ .

- As discussed in Chapter 13 ⊙⊙ , benzodiazepines inhibit both sensory and motor neuron activity by enhancing the effects of GABA.

- Acetylcholine is discussed in detail in Chapter 8 ⊙⊙ .

- Drugs for relieving pain are discussed in Chapter 14 ⊙⊙ .

- Adjunctive agents for surgery are covered in Chapter 15 ⊙⊙ .

- Depolarization and repolarization concepts are mentioned in Chapters 13 and 15 ⊙⊙ .

- Nicotinic receptors and the neuromuscular junction are presented in Chapters 8 and 15 ⊙⊙ .

13 Drugs for Seizures

CORE CONCEPTS

13.1 All convulsions are seizures, but not all seizures are convulsions.

13.2 Many causes of seizure activity are known; a few are not.

13.3 Epileptic seizures are typically identified as partial, generalized, or special epileptic syndromes.

13.4 Effective seizure management involves strict adherence to drug therapy.

13.5 Antiseizure pharmacotherapy is directed at controlling the movement of electrolytes across neuronal membranes or affecting neurotransmitter balance.

13.6 By increasing the effects of GABA in the brain, drugs reduce a wide range of seizure types.

13.7 Hydantoin and related drugs are generally effective in treating partial seizures and tonic-clonic seizures.

13.8 Succinimides generally treat absence seizures.

DRUG SNAPSHOT

The following drugs are discussed in this chapter:

DRUG CLASSES	DRUG PROFILES
Drugs That Potentiate GABA Action	
Barbiturates	**℞** phenobarbital (Luminal)
Benzodiazepines	**℞** diazepam (Valium)
Newer GABA-Related Drugs	

DRUG CLASSES	DRUG PROFILES
Hydantoin and Related Drugs	
Hydantoins	**℞** phenytoin (Dilantin)
Phenytoin-like drugs	**℞** valproic acid (Depakene)
Newer drugs	
Succinimides	**℞** ethosuximide (Zarontin)

LEARNING OUTCOMES

After reading this chapter, the student should be able to:

1. Compare and contrast the terms *epilepsy, seizures,* and *convulsions.*

2. Recognize possible causes of seizures.

3. Relate signs and symptoms to specific types of seizures.

4. Describe the pharmacologic management of acute seizures and epilepsy.

5. Explain the importance of patient drug compliance in the pharmacotherapy of epilepsy and seizures.

6. For each of the drug classes, know representative drug examples and explain their mechanisms of drug action, primary actions, and important adverse effects.

7. Categorize drugs used in the treatment of seizures based on their classifications and mechanisms of action.

action potential (poh-TEN-shial)
  200

convulsions (kon-VULL-shuns) 192

eclampsia (ee-KLAMP-see-uh) 194

epilepsy (EPP-ih-lepp-see) 192

febrile seizures 193

generalized seizures 194

partial (focal) seizures 194

pre-eclampsia (pree-ee-KLAMP-
  see-uh) 194

seizure (SEE-zhurr) 192

status epilepticus (ep-ih-LEP-tih-
  kus) 195

epilepsy = *taking hold or to seize*

A s the most common neurologic disorder, epilepsy affects more than 2 million Americans. By definition, **epilepsy** is any condition characterized by recurrent seizures. Symptoms of epilepsy depend on the type of seizure and may include signs such as blackout, fainting spells, sensory disturbances, jerking body movements, and temporary loss of memory. This chapter examines the drug therapies used to treat different kinds of seizures and epilepsy.

SEIZURES

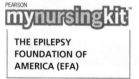

THE EPILEPSY FOUNDATION OF AMERICA (EFA)

A **seizure** is a disturbance of electrical activity in the brain that may affect consciousness, motor activity, and sensation. Seizures are caused by abnormal or uncontrolled neuronal discharges. Uncontrolled charges start in one area of the brain and may propagate to other areas. As a valuable tool in measuring uncontrolled neuronal activity, the electroencephalogram (EEG) is useful in diagnosing seizure disorders. Figure 13.1 ■ compares normal and abnormal neuronal tracings.

CORE CONCEPT 13.1

All convulsions are seizures, but not all seizures are convulsions.

The terms *seizure* and *convulsion* are not synonymous. **Convulsions** specifically refer to involuntary, violent spasms of the large skeletal muscles of the face, neck, arms, and legs. Although

---

FIGURE 13.1

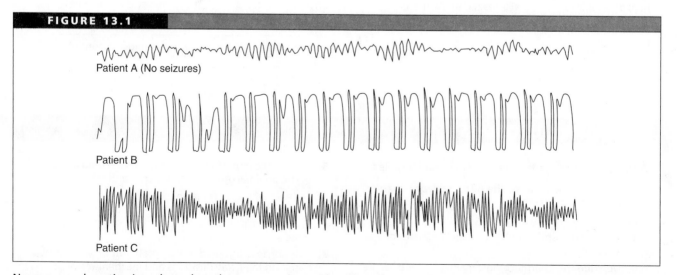

Neurons produce tiny impulses when they communicate. These impulses may be detected by an electroencephalogram (EEG), a device that captures brain-wave activity. Brain waves have characteristic patterns termed *alpha, beta, delta*, and *theta*. Although interpretation of brain waves is a complex art, you can see from these examples that the EEG tracings of patients B and C are dramatically different from those of patient A, who has no seizures. Alpha waves are the predominant waveform observed in patients with normal brain activity.

Fast Facts Epilepsy

- About 2 million Americans have epilepsy.
- One of every 100 teenagers has epilepsy.
- Of the U.S. population, 10% will have seizures within their lifetime.
- Most people with seizures are younger than 45 years of age.
- Epilepsy is not a mental illness; children with epilepsy have IQ scores equivalent to those of children without the disorder.
- Famous people who had epilepsy include Julius Caesar, Alexander the Great, Napoleon, Vincent van Gogh, Charles Dickens, Joan of Arc, and Socrates.
- Among adult alcoholics receiving treatment for withdrawal, over half will experience seizures within 6 hours upon arriving for treatment.

some types of seizures involve convulsions, other seizures do not. Thus, it may be stated that all convulsions are seizures, but not all seizures are convulsions.

Drugs described in this chapter are generally referred to as *antiseizure drugs* rather than *anticonvulsants*. Recognizing also that antiseizure drugs are commonly called *antiepileptic drugs* (AEDs), the term *antiseizure* in this chapter applies to the treatment of all seizure-related symptoms, including signs of epilepsy.

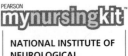

NATIONAL INSTITUTE OF NEUROLOGICAL DISORDERS AND STROKE (NINDS)

Many causes of seizure activity are known; a few are not.

CORE CONCEPT **13.2**

A seizure is considered symptomatic of an underlying disorder, rather than the disease itself. Triggers include exposure to strobe or flickering lights or the occurrence of small fluid and electrolyte imbalances. Patients appear to have a lower tolerance to environmental triggers, and seizures often occur when patients are sleep deprived.

There are many different causes of seizure activity. In some cases, the cause of seizure activity may be clear, but not in all situations. Seizures represent the most common serious neurologic problem affecting children, with an overall incidence approaching 2% for **febrile seizures** and 1% for idiopathic epilepsy. Certain medications for mood disorders, psychoses, and local anesthesia may cause seizures when given in high doses, possibly because of increased levels of stimulatory neurotransmitters or toxicity. Seizures may also occur from drug abuse, as with cocaine, or during withdrawal from alcohol or sedative–hypnotic drugs.

Seizures may present as an acute situation, or they may occur on a chronic basis. Seizures resulting from an acute complication are generally not recurrent after the situation has been resolved. On the other hand, if a *brain abnormality* exists following an acute complication, recurrent seizures are likely. The following are known causes of seizures:

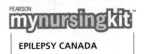

EPILEPSY CANADA

idio = *one's unknown arising*
pathic = *abnormal state*

- *Infectious diseases*   Acute infections such as meningitis and encephalitis can cause inflammation in the brain.
- *Trauma*   Physical trauma such as direct blows to the skull may increase intracranial pressure; chemical trauma such as the presence of toxic substances or the ingestion of poisons may cause brain injury.
- *Metabolic disorders*   Changes in fluid and electrolytes such as hypoglycemia, hyponatremia, and water intoxication may cause seizures by altering electrical impulse transmission at the cellular level.
- *Vascular diseases*   Changes in oxygenation such as those caused by respiratory hypoxia and carbon monoxide poisoning, and changes in perfusion such as those caused by hypotension, cerebral vascular accidents, shock, and cardiac dysrhythmias may be causes.
- *Pediatric disorders*   Rapid increase in body temperature may result in a febrile seizure.
- *Neoplastic disease*   Tumors, especially rapidly growing ones, may occupy space, increase intracranial pressure, and damage brain tissue by disrupting blood flow.

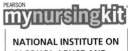

NATIONAL INSTITUTE ON ALCOHOL ABUSE AND ALCOHOLISM (NIAAA)

An important topic when discussing epilepsy and seizure treatment is birth control. Because several antiseizure drugs decrease the effectiveness of oral contraceptives, additional barrier methods of birth control should be practiced to avoid unintended pregnancy. Prior to pregnancy and considering the serious nature of epilepsy, patients should consult with their health care provider to determine the most appropriate plan of action for seizure control.

If patients become pregnant, extreme caution is necessary. Most antiseizure drugs are pregnancy category D. Some antiseizure drugs may cause folate deficiency, a condition correlated with fetal neural tube defects. Vitamin supplements may be necessary. **Pre-eclampsia** and **eclampsia** are severe hypertensive disorders of pregnancy, characterized by seizures, coma, and perinatal mortality. Eclampsia is likely to occur from around the 20th week of gestation to at least one week following delivery of the baby. Roughly one-fourth of patients with eclampsia experience seizures within 72 hours postpartum.

Seizures can have a significant impact on the quality of life. They may cause serious injury if they occur when a person is driving a vehicle or performing a dangerous activity. Without successful pharmacotherapy, epilepsy can severely limit participation in school, employment, or social activities and can affect self-esteem. Chronic depression may accompany poorly controlled seizures. Important considerations in health care include identifying patients at risk for seizures, documenting the pattern and type of seizure activity, and implementing safety precautions. In collaboration with the patient, the health care provider, pharmacist, and all clinical staff are instrumental in achieving positive therapeutic outcomes. Through a combination of pharmacotherapy, patient–family support, and education, effective seizure control can be achieved in the majority of patients.

Epileptic seizures are typically identified as partial, generalized, or special epileptic syndromes.

CORE CONCEPT 13.3

Seizure symptoms vary depending on the areas of the brain affected by the abnormal electrical activity. These symptoms range from sudden, violent shaking and total loss of consciousness to muscle twitching or slight tremor (shaking) of a limb. Staring into space, altered vision, and difficult speech are other behaviors a person may exhibit during a seizure. It is important to determine the cause of recurrent seizures in order to plan for appropriate treatment options.

Methods of classifying epilepsy have changed over time. For example, the terms *grand mal* and *petit mal* epilepsy have been replaced by more descriptive and detailed categorization. Epilepsies are typically identified using the International Classification of Epileptic Seizures. Example nomenclatures are *partial* (less used term *focal*), *generalized*, and *special epileptic syndromes*. Types of partial or generalized seizures may be recognized based on symptoms observed during a seizure episode. Some symptoms are hard to notice and reflect the simple nature of neuronal misfiring in specific areas of the brain; others are more complex.

Partial Seizures
Partial (focal) seizures involve a limited portion of the brain. Abnormal electrical activity starts on one side and travels only a short distance before it stops. The area where the abnormal electrical activity starts is known as the abnormal *focus* (plural, *foci*).

Simple partial seizures have an onset from a small, limited focus. Patients may feel for a brief moment that their precise location is vague, and they may hear and see things that are not there. Some patients smell and taste things that are not present, or have an upset stomach. Others may become emotional and experience a sense of joy, sorrow, or grief. The arms, legs, or face may twitch.

Complex partial seizures (formerly known as *psychomotor* or *temporal lobe seizures*) have sensory, motor, or autonomic symptoms with some degree of altered or impaired consciousness. Total loss of consciousness may not occur during a complex partial seizure, but a period of brief confusion and somnolence may follow the seizure. Such seizures are often preceded by an *aura*, sometimes described as an unpleasant odor or taste. Seizures may start with a blank stare, and patients may begin to chew or swallow repetitively. Some patients fumble with clothing; others try to take off their clothes. Most patients will not pay attention to verbal commands and will act as if they are having a psychotic episode. After a seizure, patients do not remember the seizure incident.

Generalized Seizures
As the name suggests, **generalized seizures** are not localized to one area but travel throughout the entire brain on both sides. The seizure is thought to originate bilaterally and symmetrically within the brain.

---

pre = *before*
ec = *out*

lamp(s) = *to shine*
ia = *sudden condition of*

post = *after*
partum = *delivery*

▶ **Life Span Fact**

Onset of epilepsy is most common among the youngest and oldest age groups. About 50% of children have a generalized epilepsy syndrome compared with about 20% of adults. The incidence of epilepsy in elderly adults is greater than among the general population, perhaps because of the greater prevalence of mild strokes and cardiac arrest in this age group.

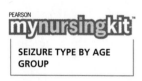

PEARSON
mynursingkit

SEIZURE TYPE BY AGE GROUP

somno = *sleepiness*
lence = *filled with*

bi = *two*
lateral = *sides*

sym = *same*
metrically = *measurement*

Absence seizures (formerly known as *petit mal seizures*) most often occur in children and last for only a few seconds. Because episodes are short-lived, they are difficult to detect. Absence epilepsy often goes unrecognized, or this disorder may be mistaken for daydreaming/signs of attention deficit disorder. Staring and temporary loss of responsiveness are the most common signs. There may be slight motor activity with eyelid fluttering or myoclonic jerks.

Atonic seizures are sometimes called *drop attacks*. Patients often stumble and fall for no apparent reason. Lasting for only a matter of seconds, episodes are very short.

Tonic-clonic seizures (formerly known as *grand mal seizures*) are the most common type of seizure. This applies to all age groups. Seizures may be preceded by an aura (e.g., spiritual feeling, flash of light, special noise). Intense muscle contractions indicate the *tonic phase*. Due to air being forced out of the lungs, a hoarse cry may occur at the onset of the seizure. Patients may temporarily lose bladder or bowel control. Breathing may become shallow and even stop momentarily. The *clonic phase* is characterized by alternating contraction and relaxation of muscles. The seizure usually lasts 1 to 2 minutes, after which the patient becomes drowsy, disoriented, and sleeps deeply.

Special Epileptic Syndromes

Special epileptic seizures include the febrile seizures of infancy, reflex epilepsies, and other forms of myoclonic epilepsies. Myoclonic epilepsies often go along with other neurologic abnormalities or progressively debilitating symptoms.

Febrile seizures typically cause tonic-clonic motor activity lasting for 1 to 2 minutes, with rapid return of consciousness. These occur together with a rapid rise in body temperature and usually occur only once during any given illness. Febrile seizures are most likely to occur within the 3-month to 5-year-old age group.

Myoclonic seizures are characterized by large, jerking body movements. Major muscle groups contract quickly, and patients appear unsteady and clumsy. They may fall from a sitting position or drop whatever they are holding. *Infantile spasms* are an example of a type of *generalized, myoclonic seizure* and are distinguished by short-lasting muscle spasms in the trunk and extremities. Such spasms are often not identified as seizures by parents or health care providers because the movements are much like the normal infantile startle reflex.

Status epilepticus is a medical emergency caused by the repeated occurrence of a seizure. This state could result with any type of seizure, but usually generalized tonic-clonic seizures are observed. When generalized tonic-clonic seizures are long and continuous, hypoxia may develop. Continuous muscle contractions also lead to hypoglycemia, acidosis, and hyperthermia (due to increased metabolic needs, lactic acid production, and heat loss during muscle movement). Carbon dioxide retention also leads to acidosis. If not treated, status epilepticus can cause brain damage and, ultimately, death. Medical treatment involves the IV administration of antiseizure medications. During seizure activity, steps must be taken to make sure that the airway remains open.

a = *without*
tonic = *tension*

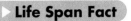 **Life Span Fact**

Preventing the onset of high fever is the best way to control febrile seizures in children.

febrile = *fever*

myo = *muscle*
clonic = *agitation*

status = *state of*
epilepticus = *seizure activity*

Concept Review   13.1

■ What is epilepsy? What is the difference between a seizure and a convulsion? Name and identify signs of the more common types of seizures.

Effective seizure management involves strict adherence to drug therapy.

CORE CONCEPT 13.4

The choice of drug for antiseizure pharmacotherapy depends on signs presented by the patient, the patient's previous medical history, and associated pathologies. Once a medication is selected, the patient is placed on a low initial dose. The amount is gradually increased until seizure control is achieved, or until drug adverse effects prevent additional increases in dose. Serum drug levels may be obtained to assist the health care provider in determining the most effective drug concentration. If seizure activity continues, a different medication is added in small-dose increments while the dose of the first drug is slowly reduced. Because seizures are likely to occur if antiseizure drugs are abruptly withdrawn, the medication is usually discontinued over a period of 6 to 12 weeks.

Traditional and newer antiseizure drugs with indications are shown in Table 13.1. The newer antiseizure drugs offer advantages over the older traditional drugs, mainly due to fewer troublesome adverse effects. Owing to the limited induction of drug-metabolizing enzymes, the pharmacokinetic profiles of the newer antiseizure drugs are less complicated. In addition, the newer antiseizure drugs are generally better tolerated and pose less of a health risk in pregnancy.

TABLE 13.1	Drugs Used for the Management of Specific Types of Seizures			
		GENERALIZED SEIZURES		**SPECIAL**
	PARTIAL SEIZURES	**ABSENCE**	**TONIC–CLONIC**	**MYOCLONIC**
DRUGS THAT POTENTIATE GABA				
diazepam (Valium)		✓	✓	✓
gabapentin (Neurontin)	✓			
lorazepam (Ativan)			✓	
phenobarbital (Luminal)	✓		✓	
pregabalin (Lyrica)	✓			
primidone (Mysoline)	✓		✓	
tiagabine (Gabitril)	✓			
topiramate (Topamax)	✓		✓	✓
HYDANTOIN AND RELATED DRUGS				
carbamazepine (Tegretol)	✓		✓	
lamotrigine (Lamictal)	✓	✓	✓	✓
levetiracetam (Keppra)	✓			
oxcarbazepine (Trileptal)	✓		✓	
phenytoin (Dilantin)	✓		✓	
valproic acid (Depakene)	✓	✓	✓	✓
zonisamide (Zonegran)	✓	✓	✓	✓
SUCCINIMIDES				
ethosuximide (Zarontin)		✓		

One issue of antiseizure drug therapy relates to recent warnings issued by the Food and Drug Administration (FDA). In 2008, the FDA analyzed reports from clinical studies involving patients taking a variety of antiseizure medications, mostly newer nontraditional drugs. Epilepsy, bipolar disorder, psychoses, migraines, and neuropathic pain were among the disorders included in the study. Compared to placebo trials, 11 popular antiseizure examples were found to almost double the risk of suicidal behavior and ideation among patients. In a warning issued by the FDA, health care professionals were admonished to carefully *balance clinical need for antiseizure drugs with risk for suicidality*. Patients and caregivers were encouraged to play close attention to changes in mood and *not to make changes in antiseizure regimen* without consulting with their health care provider. The summary of this review indicated that although the older antiseizure drugs have serious clinical drawbacks, so do the newer antiseizure drugs.

Many of the newer antiseizure medications are used in adjunctive therapy. Some drugs are being evaluated for their potential use in monotherapy. In most cases, effective seizure management can be obtained using only a single drug. For some patients, two antiseizure medications may be needed, although unwanted adverse effects may appear. Some antiseizure drug combinations may actually increase the incidence of seizures.

Once seizures are controlled, treatment is continued indefinitely. After several years of being seizure free, patients may question the need for their medication. In general, withdrawal of antiseizure drugs should be attempted only after at least 3 years of seizure-free activity and only under close direction from the health care provider. Doses of medications are reduced slowly, one at a time, over a period of several months. If seizures recur during the withdrawal process, pharmacotherapy is resumed, usually with the original stabilizing drug.

adjunctive = *joined or added*

mono = *only*
therapy = *treatment*

Concept Review 13.2

■ Give the names of traditional and newer drugs used for the management of specific seizure types. Match the drugs with the types of seizures they best control. Which drugs are generally used for a broader range of seizures?

Antiseizure pharmacotherapy is directed at controlling the movement of electrolytes across neuronal membranes or affecting neurotransmitter balance.

In a resting state, neurons are normally surrounded by a higher concentration of sodium ions, calcium ions, and chloride ions. Potassium ion levels are higher inside the cell. An influx of sodium or calcium ions into the neuron *enhances* neuronal activity, whereas an influx of chloride ions *suppresses* neuronal activity.

The goal of antiseizure pharmacotherapy is to suppress neuronal activity just enough to prevent abnormal or repetitive firing. To this end, there are three general mechanisms by which antiseizure drugs work:

- Stimulating an influx of chloride ions, an effect associated with the neurotransmitter gamma-aminobutyric acid (GABA)
- Delaying an influx of sodium ions
- Delaying an influx of calcium ions

Some drugs act by more than one mechanism. This has prompted drug researchers to try to understand more clearly various drug mechanisms and to develop newer, better-controlled drugs. Recently a fourth mechanism has been studied: blocking of the primary excitatory neurotransmitter glutamate. Glutamate works in concert with the cell's Na^+-K^+ ATPase pump, which helps to restore ion balances across neuronal membranes after firing. Any drug that blocks glutamate activity prevents an influx of positive ions into the cell, so this is consistent with the last two mechanisms.

By increasing the effects of GABA in the brain, drugs reduce a wide range of seizure types.

Several important antiseizure drugs act by changing the action of GABA, the primary inhibitory neurotransmitter in the brain. These drugs mimic the effects of GABA by stimulating an influx of chloride ions that interact with the GABA receptor–chloride channel molecule. A model of this receptor is shown in Figure 13.2 ■. When the receptor is stimulated, chloride ions move into the cell and suppress the firing of neurons. A number of drugs have GABA-related potentiation. Drugs may bind directly to the GABA receptor through specific binding sites designated as $GABA_A$ or $GABA_B$. Most antiseizure drugs bind to the $GABA_A$ site. Drugs may enhance GABA

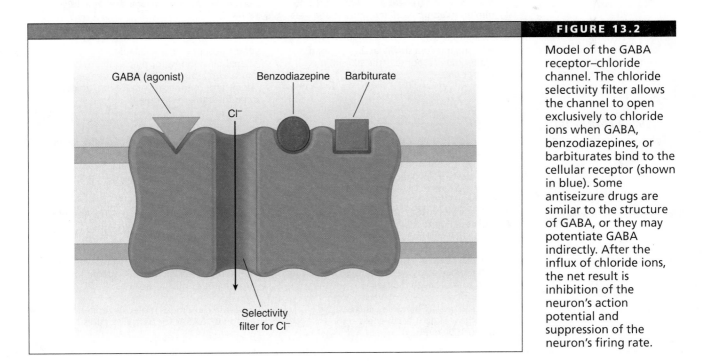

FIGURE 13.2

Model of the GABA receptor–chloride channel. The chloride selectivity filter allows the channel to open exclusively to chloride ions when GABA, benzodiazepines, or barbiturates bind to the cellular receptor (shown in blue). Some antiseizure drugs are similar to the structure of GABA, or they may potentiate GABA indirectly. After the influx of chloride ions, the net result is inhibition of the neuron's action potential and suppression of the neuron's firing rate.

release, or drugs may block the reuptake of GABA into nerve cells and glia. Newer drugs have been developed that inhibit GABA degrading enzymes.

Barbiturates, benzodiazepines, and several newer drugs reduce seizure activity by intensifying GABA action. These drugs are listed in Table 13.2. The predominate effect of GABA potentiation is central nervous system (CNS) depression.

The antiseizure properties of phenobarbital were discovered in 1912, and this drug is still commonly prescribed for seizures. As a class, barbiturates generally have a low margin for safety, a high potential for dependence, and cause profound CNS depression. Phenobarbital, however, is able to suppress abnormal neuronal discharges without causing sedation. It is inexpensive, long acting, and produces a low incidence of adverse effects. When the drug is given orally, several

TABLE 13.2	**Antiseizure Drugs That Potentiate GABA Action**	
DRUG	**ROUTE AND ADULT DOSE**	**REMARKS**
BARBITURATES		
amobarbital (Amytal)	IV; 65–500 mg (max: 1 g)	For control of status epilepticus or acute convulsive episodes; Schedule IV drug
mephobarbital (Mebaral)	PO; 400–600 mg/day	Rarely used in the management of seizures; converted to phenobarbital by the liver
🅟🅻 phenobarbital (Luminal)	For seizures: PO; 100–300 mg/day, IV/IM; 200–600 mg up to 20 mg/kg For status epilepticus: IV; 15–18 mg/kg in single or divided doses (max: 20 mg/kg)	For the management of tonic-clonic seizures, partial seizures, status epilepticus, and eclampsia; Schedule IV drug
primidone (Mysoline)	PO; 250 mg/day, increased by 250 mg/wk up to a maximum of 2 g in two to four divided doses	Similar treatment profile to phenobarbital
BENZODIAZEPINES		
clonazepam (Klonopin)	PO; 1.5 mg/day in three divided doses, increased by 0.5–1 mg every 3 days until seizures are controlled	For absence seizures and minor motor seizures; also for panic disorder; Schedule IV drug
clorazepate dipotassium (Tranxene)	PO; 7.5 mg tid	For partial seizures; also for anxiety; Schedule IV drug
🅟🅻 diazepam (Valium)	IV push, administer emulsion at 5 mg/min; IM/IV 5–10 mg (repeat as needed at 10–15 min intervals up to 30 mg; repeat again as needed every 2–4 hr)	Treatment for status epilepticus; also for anxiety-related symptoms and muscle spasms
lorazepam (Ativan) (see page 122 for the Profile Drug box)	IV; 4 mg injected slowly at 2 mg/min; if inadequate response after 10 min, may repeat once	Most potent of the available benzodiazepines; for management of status epilepticus; also for nausea and vomiting, preoperative sedation, anxiety, and insomnia; Schedule IV drug
NEWER GABA-RELATED DRUGS		
gabapentin (Neurontin)	For additional therapy: PO; start with 300 mg on day 1, 300 mg bid on day 2, 300 mg tid on day 3, continue to increase over 1 week to a dose of 1200 mg/day (400 mg tid); may increase to 1800–2400 mg/day	Chemical structure similar to GABA; speeds up the release of GABA from brain neurons; used for partial seizures or seizures that could become generalized
pregabalin (Lyrica)	PO; start with 150 mg/day; may be increased up to 300 mg/day within 1 week, (max: 600 mg/day)	Chemical structure similar to GABA; used in the treatment of partial seizures
tiagabine (Gabitril)	PO; start with 4 mg/day, may increase by 4–8 mg/day every week up to 56 mg/day in two to four divided doses	Inhibits uptake of GABA into presynaptic neurons, prolonging GABA action; for the treatment of partial seizures
topiramate (Topamax)	PO; start with 50 mg/day, increase by 50 mg/week to effectiveness (max: 1600 mg/day)	Sugar-like chemical molecule; enhances the action of GABA; for partial seizures

DRUG PROFILE: ℗ *Phenobarbital (Luminal)*

Therapeutic Class: Antiseizure drug, sedative, hypnotic
Pharmacologic Class: Barbiturate, GABA$_A$ receptor drug

Actions and Uses:

Phenobarbital is a long-acting barbiturate used for the management of a variety of seizures. It is also used for insomnia. Phenobarbital should not be used for pain relief, because it may increase a patient's sensitivity to pain.

Phenobarbital acts biochemically in the brain by enhancing the action of the neurotransmitter GABA, which is responsible for suppressing abnormal neuronal discharges that can cause epilepsy.

Adverse Effects and Interactions:

Phenobarbital is a Schedule IV drug that may cause dependence. Common adverse effects include drowsiness, vitamin deficiencies (vitamin D, folate, B$_9$, and B$_{12}$), and laryngospasms. With overdose, phenobarbital may cause severe respiratory depression, CNS depression, coma, and death. Phenobarbital is a pregnancy category D drug.

Phenobarbital interacts with many other drugs. For example, it should not be taken with alcohol or other CNS depressants. These substances potentiate the action of barbiturates, increasing the risk of life-threatening respiratory depression or cardiac arrest. Phenobarbital increases the metabolism of many other drugs, reducing their effectiveness.

Refer to MyNursingKit for a Nursing Process Focus specific to this drug.

DRUG PROFILE: ℗ *Diazepam (Valium)*

Therapeutic Class: Antiseizure drug, sedative-hypnotic, anxiolytic, anesthetic adjunct, skeletal muscle relaxant (centrally acting)
Pharmacologic Class: Benzodiazepine, GABA$_A$ receptor drug

Actions and Uses:

Diazepam binds to GABA receptors located throughout the CNS. It produces its effects by suppressing neuronal activity in the limbic system and subsequent impulses that might be transmitted to the reticular activating system. Effects of this drug are suppression of abnormal neuronal foci that may cause seizures, calming without strong sedation, and skeletal muscle relaxation. When used orally, maximum therapeutic effects may take from 1 to 2 weeks. Tolerance may develop after about 4 weeks. When given IV, effects occur within minutes, and its anticonvulsant effects last for about 20 minutes.

Adverse Effects and Interactions:

Diazepam should not be taken with alcohol or other CNS depressants because of combined sedation effects. Other drug interactions include cimetidine, oral contraceptives, valproic acid, and metoprolol, which potentiate diazepam's action, and levodopa and barbiturates, which decrease diazepam's action. Diazepam increases the levels of phenytoin in the bloodstream and may cause phenytoin toxicity. When given IV, hypotension, muscular weakness, tachycardia, and respiratory depression are common. Because of tolerance and dependency, use of diazepam is reserved for short-term seizure control or for status epilepticus.

Diazepam should be used with caution with herbal supplements, such as kava and chamomile, which may cause an increased effect.

Refer to MyNursingKit for a Nursing Process Focus specific to this drug.

NATURAL THERAPIES

The Ketogenic Diet for Epilepsy

The ketogenic diet may be used when seizures cannot be controlled through pharmacotherapy or when there are unacceptable adverse effects to medications. Before antiepileptic drugs were developed, this diet was a primary treatment for epilepsy.

The ketogenic diet is a strict diet that is high in fat and low in carbohydrates and protein. It limits water intake and carefully controls caloric intake. Each meal has the same ketogenic ratio of 4 g of fat to 1 g of protein and carbohydrate. Extra fat is usually given in the form of cream.

Research suggests that the diet produces a high success rate for certain patients. The diet appears to be equally effective for every seizure type. The most frequently reported adverse effects include vomiting, fatigue, constipation, diarrhea, and hunger. Kidney stones, acidosis, and slower growth rates are possible risks. Those interested in trying the diet must consult with their health care provider; this is not a do-it-yourself diet and may be harmful if not carefully monitored by skilled professionals.

weeks may be necessary to achieve optimum effects. Phenobarbital is the drug of choice in the pharmacotherapy of neonatal seizures.

Other than phenobarbital, mephobarbital is occasionally used for epilepsy treatment. Mephobarbital (Mebaral) is converted to phenobarbital in the liver and offers no significant advantages over phenobarbital. Primidone (Mysoline) has a pharmacologic profile similar to phenobarbital and is among the drugs used effectively to potentiate GABA action.

Amobarbital (Amytal) is an intermediate-acting barbiturate given IV or IM to terminate status epilepticus. Unlike phenobarbital, which is a Schedule IV drug, amobarbital is a Schedule II drug and has a higher risk for dependence. As an antiseizure medication, amobarbital is not given orally.

Like barbiturates, benzodiazepines and newer drugs intensify the effect of GABA in the brain. The benzodiazepines bind directly to the GABA receptor, suppressing abnormal neuronal foci. Benzodiazepines used in treating epilepsy include clonazepam (Klonopin), clorazepate (Tranxene), lorazepam (Ativan), and diazepam (Valium). Parenteral diazepam is used to terminate status epilepticus. Other short-term indications of benzodiazepines include *absence seizures* and *myoclonic seizures*. Because tolerance may begin to develop after only a few months of therapy, seizures may recur unless doses are periodically adjusted. Benzodiazepines and other GABA-related drugs are generally not used alone in seizure pharmacotherapy, but instead serve as adjuncts to other antiseizure medications.

CORE CONCEPT 13.7

Hydantoin and related drugs are generally effective in treating partial seizures and tonic-clonic seizures.

Hydantoins and related drugs dampen CNS activity by delaying an influx of sodium ions across neuronal membranes. Sodium movement is the major factor that determines whether a neuron will undergo an **action potential**. Sodium channels guide the movement of sodium ions into the cell. If sodium channels are temporarily inactivated, neuronal activity will be suppressed. If sodium channels are blocked, neuronal activity completely stops, as occurs with local anesthetic drugs (see Chapter 15 ⬭). With hydantoin and related drugs, sodium channels are not blocked completely; they are just made to be less sensitive.

Several drugs in this group may not only desensitize sodium channels but also affect the threshold of neuronal firing, or they may interfere with transduction of the excitatory neurotransmitter glutamate. These actions may be slightly removed from the direct desensitization of sodium channels; however, the result (delayed depolarization of the neuron) is the same. Hydantoin and related drugs are listed in Table 13.3.

The oldest and most commonly prescribed antiseizure medication is phenytoin (Dilantin). Approved in the 1930s, phenytoin is a broad-spectrum hydantoin drug, useful in treatment of all kinds of epilepsy except absence seizures. It provides effective seizure suppression without the potential for abuse or extreme sedative effects. Patients vary significantly in their ability to metabolize phenytoin; therefore, dosages are highly individualized. Because of the very narrow range between therapeutic dose and toxic dose, patients must be carefully monitored. Phenytoin and fosphenytoin are first-line drugs in the treatment of status epilepticus.

Some phenytoin-related drugs are used less frequently; others are more widely used. Most drugs share a mechanism similar to the hydantoins, including carbamazepine (Tegretol), oxcar-

TABLE 13.3	Hydantoins and Related Drugs	
DRUG	**ROUTE AND ADULT DOSE**	**REMARKS**
HYDANTOINS		
fosphenytoin sodium (Cerebyx)	IV; initial dose 15–20 mg PE/kg at 100–150 mg PE/min followed by 4–6 mg PE/kg/day (PE = phenytoin equivalents)	Converted to phenytoin in the body; for control of status epilepticus; short-term substitute for oral phenytoin
℗ phenytoin (Dilantin)	PO; 15–18 mg/kg or 1 g initial dose, then 300 mg/day in one to three divided doses; may be gradually increased 100 mg/week	For tonic-clonic seizures, complex partial seizures, and seizures after head trauma
PHENYTOIN-LIKE DRUGS		
carbamazepine (Tegretol)	PO; 200 mg bid, gradually increased to 800–1200 mg/day in three to four divided doses	For tonic-clonic and complex partial seizures; useful in trigeminal neuralgia (condition characterized by intense pain along the angle of the jaw); also for bipolar disorder
felbamate (Felbatol)	Partial seizures: PO; start with 1200 mg/day in three to four divided doses; may increase by 600 mg/day every 2 weeks (max: 3600 mg/day) Lennox-Gastaut syndrome: PO; start at 15 mg/kg/day in three to four divided doses; may increase 15 mg/kg at weekly intervals to max of 45 mg/kg/day	For use in Lennox-Gastaut syndrome and partial seizures; may cause anemia and liver toxicity in some patients
lamotrigine (Lamictal)	PO; 50 mg/day for 2 weeks, then 50 mg bid for 2 weeks; may increase gradually up to 300–500 mg/day in two divided doses (max: 700 mg/day)	For partial seizures, generalized tonic-clonic seizures, myoclonic seizures; also for bipolar disorder
levetiracetam (Keppra)	PO; 500 mg twice daily (max: 3000 mg total per day)	For use in partial seizures
oxcarbazepine (Trileptal)	PO; initiation of monotherapy, 300 mg twice daily, increase 300 mg/day every third day up to 1200 mg/day	Derivative of carbamazepine with similar treatment profile; may cause serious skin and organ hypersensitivity reactions in some patients
℗ valproic acid (Depakene)	PO/IV; 15 mg/kg/day in divided doses when total daily dose is greater than 250 mg; increase 5–10 mg every week until seizures are controlled (max: 60 mg/kg/day)	Broad-spectrum medication; for absence seizures, mixed generalized types of seizures; also for bipolar disorder
zonisamide (Zonegran)	PO; 100–400 mg/day	Broad-spectrum medication; for partial seizures; it is a sulfonamide, which means that it may cause an allergic reaction in some patients

bazepine (Trileptal), and valproic acid (Depakene), which is also available as valproate and divalproex sodium. Because carbamazepine produces fewer adverse effects than phenytoin or phenobarbital, it is the drug of choice for tonic-clonic and partial seizures. Oxcarbazepine is a derivative of carbamazepine, so its treatment profile is similar. Oxcarbazepine is slightly better tolerated than carbamazepine, although serious skin and organ hypersensitivity reactions have been noted. Valproic acid is the drug of choice for absence seizures and is used in combination with other drugs for partial seizures. Both carbamazepine and valproic acid are used in the treatment of bipolar disorder (see Chapter 10 ⬥).

Newer antiseizure drugs show promise in treatment for a range of disorders, including absence seizures, partial seizures, myoclonic seizures, generalized tonic-clonic seizures, and mood disorders. The most common adverse effects of the newer antiseizure drugs are drowsiness, dizziness, and blurred vision. Lamotrigine (Lamictal) has a broad spectrum of antiseizure activity, and is FDA approved for longer term maintenance of bipolar disorder. This drug's duration of action is greatly affected by other drugs that inhibit or enhance hepatic metabolizing enzymes. Levetiracetam (Keppra) and zonisamide (Zonegram) are approved for adjunctive therapy of partial seizures in adults. Among the newer antiseizure drugs, levetiracetam has been generally less reactive than the other antiseizure medications. Conversely, zonisamide (a sulfonamide) has triggered hypersensitivity reactions in some patients. In addition, felbamate (Felbatol) has induced potentially harmful reactions, including liver toxicity and aplastic anemia.

TABLE 13.4	Succinimides	
DRUG	**ROUTE AND ADULT DOSE**	**REMARKS**
(Pr) ethosuximide (Zarontin)	PO; 250 mg bid, increased every 4–7 days (max: 1.5 g/day)	For absence seizures, myoclonic seizures, and akinetic epilepsy
methsuximide (Celontin)	PO; 300 mg/day, may increase every 4–7 days (max: 1.2 g/day in divided doses)	For absence seizures; may be used in combination with other anticonvulsants in mixed types of seizure activity
phensuximide (Milontin)	PO; 0.5–1 g bid or tid	For absence seizures; similar characteristics to methsuximide

---

CORE CONCEPT 13.8

Succinimides generally treat absence seizures.

succin = *chemical related to succinic acid*
imide = *having an NH functional group*

Neurotransmitters, hormones, and some medications bind to neuronal membranes, stimulating the entry of calcium. Without calcium influx, neuronal transmission would not be possible. Succinimides delay entry of calcium into neurons by blocking low-threshold calcium channels, increasing the electrical threshold of the neuron, and reducing the likelihood of an action potential. By raising the seizure threshold, succinimides keep neurons from firing too quickly, thus suppressing abnormal foci. The succinimides are generally effective only against absence seizures. These drugs are listed in Table 13.4.

DRUG PROFILE: (Pr) *Phenytoin (Dilantin)*

Therapeutic Class: Antiseizure drug, antidysrhythmic
Pharmacologic Class: Hydantoin, sodium influx suppressing drug

Actions and Uses:

Phenytoin acts by desensitizing sodium channels in the CNS responsible for neuronal responsivity. Desensitization prevents the spread of disruptive electrical charges in the brain that produce seizures. It is effective against most types of seizures except absence seizures. Phenytoin has antidysrhythmic activity similar to lidocaine (Class IB). An offlabeled use is for digitalis-induced dysrhythmias.

Adverse Effects and Interactions:

Phenytoin may cause dysrhythmias such as bradycardia or ventricular fibrillation, severe hypotension, and hyperglycemia. Severe CNS reactions include headache, nystagmus, ataxia, confusion and slurred speech, paradoxical nervousness, twitching, and insomnia. Peripheral neuropathy may occur with long-term use. Phenytoin can cause multiple blood dyscrasias, including agranulocytosis and aplastic anemia. It may cause severe skin reactions, such as rashes, including exfoliative dermatitis, and Stevens-Johnson syndrome. Connective tissue reactions include lupus erythematosa, hypertrichosis, hirsutism, and gingival hypertrophy.

Phenytoin interacts with many other drugs, including oral anticoagulants, glucocorticoids, H_2 antagonists, antituberculin drugs, and food supplements such as folic acid, calcium, and vitamin D. It impairs the effectiveness of drugs such as digitoxin, doxycycline, furosemide, estrogens and oral contraceptives, and theophylline. Phenytoin, when combined with tricyclic antidepressants, can trigger seizures.

Phenytoin should be used with caution with herbal supplements such as herbal laxatives (buckthorn, cascara sagrada, and senna), which may increase potassium loss.

Refer to MyNursingKit for a Nursing Process Focus specific to this drug.

DRUG PROFILE: ℞ *Valproic Acid (Depakene)*

Therapeutic Class: Antiseizure drug, bipolar disorder drug, migraine prophylaxis

Pharmacologic Class: Valproate, sodium influx suppressing drug, calcium influx suppressing drug, GABA potentiating drug

Actions and Uses:

The mechanism of action of valproic acid is the same as phenytoin, although effects on GABA and calcium channels may cause some additional actions. It is useful for a wide range of seizure types, including absence seizures and mixed types of seizures. Other uses include treatment of bipolar disorder and prevention of migraine headaches.

Adverse Effects and Interactions:

Adverse effects include sedation, drowsiness, gastrointestinal (GI) upset, and prolonged bleeding time. Other effects include visual disturbances, muscle weakness, tremor, psychomotor agitation, bone marrow suppression, weight gain, abdominal cramps, rash, alopecia, pruritus, photosensitivity, erythema multiforme, and fatal hepatotoxicity.

Valproic acid interacts with many drugs. For example, aspirin, cimetidine, chlorpromazine, erythromycin, and felbamate may increase valproic acid toxicity. Concomitant warfarin, aspirin, or alcohol use can cause severe bleeding. Alcohol, benzodiazepines, and other CNS depressants potentiate CNS depressant action. Lamotrigine, phenytoin, and rifampin lower valproic acid levels. Valproic acid increases serum phenobarbital and phenytoin levels. Use of clonazepam concurrently with valproic acid may induce absence seizures.

Refer to MyNursingKit for a Nursing Process Focus specific to this drug.

DRUG PROFILE: ℞ *Ethosuximide (Zarontin)*

Therapeutic Class: Antiseizure drug

Pharmacologic Class: Succinimide, low-threshold calcium channel blocking drug

Actions and Uses:

Ethosuximide is a drug of choice for absence (petit mal) seizures. It depresses the activity of neurons in the motor cortex by elevating the neuronal threshold. It is usually ineffective against psychomotor or tonic-clonic seizures; however, it may be given in combination with other medications that better treat these conditions. It is available in tablet and flavored syrup formulations.

Adverse Effects and Interactions:

Ethosuximide may impair mental and physical abilities. Psychosis or extreme mood swings, including depression with suicidal intent, can occur. Behavioral changes are more prominent in patients with a history of psychiatric illness. CNS effects include dizziness, headache, lethargy, fatigue, ataxia, sleep pattern disturbances, attention difficulty, and hiccups. Bone marrow suppression and blood dyscrasias are possible, as is systemic lupus erythematosus.

Other reactions include gingival hypertrophy and tongue swelling. Common adverse effects are abdominal distress and weight loss.

Drug interactions include ethosuximide, which increases phenytoin serum levels. Valproic acid causes ethosuximide serum levels to fluctuate (increase or decrease).

Refer to MyNursingKit for a Nursing Process Focus specific to this drug.

NURSING PROCESS FOCUS

Patients Receiving Antiseizure Drug Therapy

ASSESSMENT

Prior to administration:
- Obtain a complete health history (physical/mental), including allergies and drug history, to determine possible drug interactions
- Assess neurologic status, including identification of recent seizure activity
- Assess growth and development

POTENTIAL NURSING DIAGNOSES

- Risk for Injury related to effects of seizure and adverse effects of drug therapy.
- Deficient Knowledge related to information about disorder and drug therapy.
- Noncompliance related to maintenance of drug therapy.

PLANNING: PATIENT GOALS AND OUTCOMES

The patient will:
- Experience the absence of seizures, or a reduction in the number or severity of seizures
- Avoid physical injury related to seizure activity or medication-induced sensory changes
- Demonstrate an understanding of the drug's action by accurately describing drug effects and precautions

IMPLEMENTATION

Interventions and (Rationales)	Patient Education/Discharge Planning
Monitor neurologic status, especially changes in level of consciousness and/or mental status. (Sedation may indicate impending toxicity.)	Instruct the patient to: - Report any significant change in sensorium, such as slurred speech, confusion, hallucinations, or lethargy - Report any changes in seizure quality or unexpected involuntary muscle movement such as twitching, tremor, or unusual eye movement - Be aware of the risk for suicidality when not following proper medication regimen
Protect the patient from injury during seizure events until the therapeutic effects of the drugs are achieved.	Instruct the patient to avoid driving and other hazardous activities until the effects of the drug are known.
Monitor effectiveness of drug therapy. Observe for developmental changes, which may indicate a need for dose adjustment.	Instruct the patient to: - Keep a seizure diary to chronicle events during symptoms phase or during dose adjustment - Take the medication exactly as ordered, including the same manufacturer's drug, each time the prescription is refilled (Switching brands may result in alterations in seizure control.) - Take a missed dose as soon as remembered, but do not take double doses (Doubling doses could result in toxic serum level.)
Monitor for adverse effects. Observe for hypersensitivity, nephrotoxicity, and hepatotoxicity.	Instruct the patient to report adverse effects specific to the drug regimen.
Monitor oral health. Observe for signs of gingival hypertrophy, bleeding, or inflammation (phenytoin specific).	Instruct the patient to: - Use a soft toothbrush and oral rinses as prescribed by a dentist - Avoid mouthwashes containing alcohol - Report changes in oral health such as excessive bleeding or inflammation of the gums - Maintain a regular schedule of dental visits
Monitor gastrointestinal status. (Valproic acid is a GI irritant and anticoagulant.) Conduct guaiac stool testing for occult blood. (Phenytoin's CNS depressant effects decrease GI motility, producing constipation.)	Instruct the patient to: - Take the drug with food to reduce GI upset - Immediately report any severe or persistent heartburn, upper GI pain, nausea, or vomiting - Increase exercise, fluid intake, and fiber intake to facilitate stool passage

continued . . .

NURSING PROCESS FOCUS *(continued)*

Interventions and (Rationales)	Patient Education/Discharge Planning
■ Monitor nutritional status. (Phenytoin's action on electrolytes may cause decreased absorption of folic acid, vitamin D, magnesium, and calcium. Deficiencies in these vitamins and minerals lead to anemia and osteoporosis. Valproic acid may cause an increase in appetite and weight.)	Instruct the patient: ■ In dietary or drug administration techniques specific to prescribed medications ■ To report significant changes in appetite or weight gain
■ Obtain information and monitor use of other medications. Antiseizure medications should not be used with CNS depressants or alcohol.	■ Instruct the patient to report use of any medication to the health care provider. ■ Inform the patient not to drink alcohol while taking these medications.

EVALUATION OF OUTCOME CRITERIA

Evaluate effectiveness of drug therapy by confirming that patient goals and expected outcomes have been met (see "Planning").

See Tables 13.2, 13.3, and 13.4 for a list of drugs to which these nursing actions apply.

Ethosuximide (Zarontin) is the most commonly prescribed drug in this class. It remains the drug of choice for absence seizures. It joins the other positive ion suppressing drugs that successfully treat absence seizures: valproic acid (Depakene), lamotrigine (Lamictal), and zonisamide (Zonegran).

Concept Review   13.3

■ Name three general drug classes introduced by the Drug Snapshot feature at the beginning of this chapter. Identify the various stated chemical categories of antiseizure medications. Based on pharmacologic mechanisms, which of the drug examples do not conveniently fit into only one drug class? Which of the drugs control a wide range of seizure types? Which of the drugs have therapeutic applications other than seizure management?

PATIENTS NEED TO KNOW

Patients taking antiseizure medications need to know the following:

In General

1. Never abruptly stop taking antiseizure medication; doing so can cause seizures.
2. Avoid alcohol and other CNS depressants because they can increase sedation.
3. Antiseizure medications may cause drowsiness; avoid driving and the use of machinery that could lead to injury.
4. It may require several dosage adjustments over many months to find the dosage that allows performance of normal daily activities while controlling seizures.
5. It is important to keep laboratory appointments because many antiseizure medications require blood testing to ensure that the drug is at a safe and effective level in the blood.
6. Consult a health care provider before trying to become pregnant; some antiseizure medications are not safe to use during pregnancy.
7. Report excess fatigue, drowsiness, agitation, confusion, or suicidal thoughts to a health care provider.

Regarding Hydantoins and Related Medications

8. Report the following adverse effects to a health care provider: gum overgrowth (gingival hyperplasia) or skin rash, tremors, weight gain, diarrhea, irregular menses, dizziness, nausea, or oversedation.
9. Hydantoins and related medications interact with many other drugs; do not add any other prescription, over-the-counter (OTC) drugs, or herbal supplements until a health care provider is consulted. Do not consume alcohol while taking these medications.

Regarding Succinimides

10. Report the following adverse effects to a health care provider: hiccups or epigastric pain with ethosuximide (Zarontin), drowsiness, or increased bleeding time.

CHAPTER REVIEW

CORE CONCEPTS SUMMARY

13.1 All convulsions are seizures, but not all seizures are convulsions.

Epilepsy is any disorder characterized by recurrent seizures. *Seizures* are abnormal and uncontrolled neuronal brain discharges. *Convulsions* are uncontrolled muscle contractions that accompany some major seizures. Drugs used to treat epilepsy are often referred to as *antiseizure drugs* or *antiepileptic drugs* (AEDs), rather than anticonvulsants.

13.2 Many causes of seizure activity are known; a few are not.

A seizure is considered a symptom of epilepsy rather than a disorder itself. In some cases, the exact cause of seizures is not known; however, there are many known causes. Seizures are the most common neurologic problem. Through a combination of pharmacotherapy, patient-family support, and education, effective seizure control can be achieved by most patients.

13.3 Epileptic seizures are typically identified as partial, generalized, or special epileptic syndromes.

Epilepsies are identified using the International Classification of Epileptic Seizures nomenclature, as partial (focal), generalized, or special epileptic syndromes. Partial seizures are further described as simple or complex seizures. Generalized seizures are described as absence seizures, atonic seizures, or tonic-clonic seizures. Special epileptic syndromes include febrile seizures, myoclonic seizures, and status epilepticus.

13.4 Effective seizure management involves strict adherence to drug therapy.

The choice of drug for epilepsy pharmacotherapy depends on the type of seizures the patient is experiencing, the patient's previous medical history, diagnostic studies, and the pathologic processes causing the seizures. In most cases, a single drug can effectively control seizures. In some patients, two antiseizure medications may be necessary. Both traditional and newer antiseizure medications are used. When discussing antiseizure medications, birth control, pregnancy, and suicidality are important topics for consideration.

13.5 Antiseizure pharmacotherapy is directed at controlling the movement of electrolytes across neuronal membranes or affecting neurotransmitter balance.

There are three general mechanisms by which antiseizure drugs work: stimulating an influx of chloride ions (an effect associated with the neurotransmitter GABA), delaying an influx of sodium, and delaying an influx of calcium. Antiseizure drugs are represented by these and possibly one additional mechanism: blocking of the excitatory neurotransmitter, glutamate.

13.6 By increasing the effects of GABA in the brain, drugs reduce a wide range of seizure types.

Some antiseizure drugs mimic the effects of GABA by stimulating an influx of chloride ions. Drugs may bind directly to the GABA receptor, enhance GABA release, block the reuptake of GABA into nerve cells and glia, or inhibit GABA degrading enzymes. Barbiturates, benzodiazepines, and several newer GABA-related drugs reduce seizure activity by potentiating GABA action.

13.7 Hydantoin and related drugs are generally effective in treating partial seizures and tonic-clonic seizures.

This class of drugs depresses CNS activity by desensitizing sodium channels and also by affecting the threshold of neuronal firing. Several widely used drugs, including phenytoin (Dilantin), carbamazepine (Tegretol), and valproic acid (Depakene), work by this mechanism. Some drugs act by more than one mechanism. Additional newer antiseizure drugs have been added to the regimen and may be used alone in therapy or as adjunctive drugs.

13.8 Succinimides generally treat absence seizures.

Succinimides delay entry of calcium into neurons by blocking calcium channels, increasing the electrical threshold, and reducing the likelihood that an action potential will be generated. Ethosuximide (Zarontin) is the most commonly prescribed drug in this class.

REVIEW QUESTIONS

The following questions are written in NCLEX-PN® style. Answer these questions to assess your knowledge of the chapter material, and go back and review any material that is not clear to you.

1. Most antiseizure medications fall under which pregnancy category?

1. A
2. B
3. C
4. D

2. The patient on phenytoin (Dilantin) asks why he must have his labs checked. The nurse's best response would be:

1. "Dilantin can cause blood disorders."
2. "You will need to ask your doctor."
3. "We are checking to make sure you are getting enough but not too much medication."
4. "We must see if you are developing any adverse effects of the medication."

3. The patient on antiseizure medication wants to know how long he must take his medication before he is cured. The nurse's best response would be:

1. "You should be totally seizure free in 1 to 3 weeks."
2. "We may need to add additional medications before you are cured."
3. "It may take up to 3 years before you are cured."
4. "The goal of therapy is to control seizure activity."

4. This drug, given parentally, is used to terminate status epilepticus.

1. Diazepam (Valium)
2. Gabapentin (Neurontin)
3. Clorazepate (Tranxene)
4. Clonazepam (Klonopin)

5. This phase of a seizure is characterized by alternating contractions and relaxation of the muscles.

1. Absence
2. Clonic
3. Febrile
4. Myoclonic

6. One of the most common adverse effects of antiseizure drugs is:

1. GI upset
2. Spasms
3. Drowsiness
4. Dry mouth

7. An overdose of this antiseizure drug may cause severe respiratory depression, CNS depression, coma, and death.

1. Clonazepam (Klonopin)
2. Lorazepam (Ativan)
3. Diazepam (Valium)
4. Phenobarbital (Luminal)

8. The nurse should assess the patient on ethosuximide (Zarontin) for which of the following?

1. Urinary dysfunction
2. Gingival hyperplasia
3. Tremors
4. Depression

9. The nurse must assess for gingival hyperplasia with this antiseizure medication.

1. Valproic acid (Depakene)
2. Carbamazepine (Tegretol)
3. Phenytoin (Dilantin)
4. Primidone (Mysoline)

10. This antiseizure medication increases phenytoin serum levels.

1. Ethosuximide (Zarontin)
2. Phenobarbital (Luminal)
3. Carbamazepine (Tegretol)
4. Valproic acid (Depakene)

CASE STUDY QUESTIONS

For questions 1–4, please refer to the following case study, and choose the correct answer from choices 1–4.

*M*s. Anthonia and her 9-year-old daughter, Leslie, recently visited the family physician. Ms. Anthonia was concerned that Leslie's development might be stunted. Several complaints were noted: "Leslie sometimes acts very unusual, like she is not paying attention . . . on occasion she is unresponsive and bats her eyes . . . this sometimes lasts for a few seconds and everything appears normal again . . . lately she has been waking up a lot during the night." During the interview, the physician discovered that Ms. Anthonia was taking medication for bipolar disorder. After a complete

neurologic exam and set of laboratory tests, the family physician prescribed ethosuximide (Zarontin) for Leslie to be taken in gradually increased doses over 7 days and then for a sustained period at the same dose. The physician then scheduled a return visit to the clinic in 7 days.

1. Which of the following is the most likely diagnosis for Leslie?

1. Bipolar disorder
2. Partial seizures
3. Absence seizures
4. Tonic-clonic seizures

2. The mechanism by which ethosuximide (Zarontin) will treat Leslie's condition is:

1. Enhanced release of GABA neurotransmitter
2. Desensitization of sodium channels located along neuronal membranes
3. Delayed entry of calcium into cortical neurons
4. Activation of the GABA receptor

3. Which of the following is the most likely reason for Leslie's return visit to the clinic?

1. Her medication has a high potential for dependence; Leslie's physician wants to reexamine her.
2. One of the adverse effects of Leslie's medication is anemia; this adverse effect will need to be evaluated.

3. Serum drug levels will be necessary to determine the most effective drug concentration.
4. Her medication has a low margin of safety; Leslie's physician just wants to be sure.

4. Which of the following medications, if prescribed for Leslie as a second medication, would cause ethosuximide (Zarontin) serum levels to fluctuate?

1. Phenobarbital (Luminal)
2. Diazepam (Valium)
3. Phenytoin (Dilantin)
4. Valproic acid (Depakene)

FURTHER STUDY

- Local anesthesia is discussed in Chapter 15 ⚭ .

- The use of the antiseizure medications carbamazepine, lamotrigine, and valproic acid for bipolar disorder is discussed in Chapter 10 ⚭ .

- Phenytoin as an antidysrhythmic is discussed in Chapter 19 ⚭ .

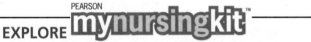

EXPLORE PEARSON **mynursingkit**™

MyNursingKit is your one stop for online chapter review materials and resources. Prepare for success with additional NCLEX®-style practice questions, interactive assignments and activities, web links, animations and videos, and more!

Register your access code from the front of your book at
www.mynursingkit.com

14 Drugs for Pain Control

CORE CONCEPTS

14.1 Pain assessment is the first step to pain management.

14.2 Nonpharmacologic techniques assist patients in obtaining adequate pain relief.

14.3 Pain transmission processes allow several targets for pharmacologic intervention.

14.4 Opioid analgesic medications exert their effects by interacting with specific receptors.

14.5 Narcotic opioids have multiple therapeutic effects, including relief of severe pain.

14.6 Nonsteroidal anti-inflammatory drugs are the drugs of choice for pain due to inflammatory.

14.7 Headaches can be effectively treated with a variety of drug classes.

DRUG SNAPSHOT

The following drugs are discussed in this chapter:

DRUG CLASSES	DRUG PROFILES
Opioid (Narcotic) Analgesics	
Opioid agonists	**Pr** morphine (Astramorph PF, Duramorph, others)
Opioid antagonists	**Pr** naloxone (Narcan)
Opioids with mixed agonist–antagonist activity	
Nonopioid Analgesics	
Nonsteroidal anti-inflammatory drugs (NSAIDs)	
Aspirin and other salicylates	**Pr** aspirin (Acetylsalicylic acid, ASA)

DRUG CLASSES	DRUG PROFILES
Ibuprofen and ibuprofen-like drugs	
Selective COX-2 inhibitors	
	Pr acetaminophen (Tylenol)
Centrally acting drugs	
Antimigraine Drugs	
Triptans	**Pr** sumatriptan (Imitrex)
Ergot alkaloids	
Other antimigraine drugs	

LEARNING OUTCOMES

After reading this chapter, the student should be able to:

1. Relate the importance of pain assessment to effective pharmacotherapy.

2. Explain the neural mechanism for pain at the level of the spinal cord.

3. Explain how pain can be controlled by inhibiting the release of spinal neurotransmitters.

4. Describe the role of nonpharmacologic therapies in pain management.

5. Compare and contrast the types of opioid receptors and their importance to pharmacology.

6. Explain the role of opioid antagonists in the diagnosis and treatment of acute opioid toxicity.

7. Describe the long-term treatment of opioid dependence.

8. Compare the pharmacotherapeutic approaches of preventing migraines to those of aborting migraines.

9. For each of the major drug classes, indentify representative drug examples, and explain the

mechanisms of drug action, primary actions, and important adverse effects for each.

10. Categorize drugs used in the treatment of pain based on their classifications and mechanisms of action.

KEY TERMS

Aδ fibers 212

analgesic (an-ul-JEE-zik) 212

aura (AUR-uh) 225

bradykinin (bray-dee-KYE-nin) 223

C fibers 212

cyclooxygenase (cox) (sye-klo-OK-sah-jen-ays) 220

endogenous opioids (en-DAHJ-en-nuss O-pee-oyds) 212

migraine (MYE-grayne) 225

narcotic (nar-KOT-ik) 212

nociceptor (no-si-SEPP-ter) 210

opiate (OH-pee-aht) 212

opioid (OH-pee-oyd) 212

patient-controlled analgesia (PCA) (patient-controlled an-ul-JEE-ziah 216

prostaglandins (pros-tah-GLAN-dins) 223

substance P 212

tension headache 225

Pain is a physiological and emotional experience characterized by unpleasant feelings, usually associated with trauma and disease. On a simple level, pain may be viewed as a defense mechanism that helps people to avoid potentially damaging situations and encourages them to seek medical help. Although the neural and chemical mechanisms for pain are fairly straightforward, many psychological and emotional processes modify this sensation. Anxiety, fatigue, and depression can increase the perception of pain. Positive attitudes and support from caregivers may reduce the perception of pain. Patients are more likely to tolerate their pain if they know the source of the sensation and the medical course of treatment designed to manage the pain.

ACUTE OR CHRONIC PAIN

The purpose of classifying pain is to guide appropriate treatment measures. Pain can be classified as either acute or chronic. Acute pain is an intense pain occurring over a brief time, usually from injury to recovery. Chronic pain persisting longer than 6 months can interfere with daily activities and is associated with feelings of helplessness or hopelessness.

CORE CONCEPT 14.1

Pain assessment is the first step to pain management.

The psychological reaction to pain is a subjective experience. The same degree and type of pain may be described as excruciating and unbearable by one patient, whereas not be mentioned by another. Several numerical scales and survey instruments are available to help health care providers standardize pain assessment and measure the progress of drug therapy. Successful pain management depends on an accurate assessment of both the degree of pain experienced by the patient and the potential disorders that may be causing the pain. Selection of the correct therapy is dependent on the nature and character of the pain.

Although pain is termed *acute* or *chronic*, it can also be classified by its source. Injury to *tissues* produces *nociceptor pain*. This type of pain may be further subdivided into *somatic pain*, which produces sharp, localized sensations, or *visceral pain*, which is described as a generalized dull, throbbing, or aching pain. The term **nociceptor** refers to activation of receptor nerve endings that receive and transmit pain signals to the spinal cord and brain. In contrast, *neuropathic pain* is caused by direct injury to the *nerves* and typically is described as burning, shooting, or

noci = *pain or injury*
ceptor = *receiver*

210

Fast Facts Pain

- Pain is a common symptom.
  - Approximately 16 million people experience chronic arthritic pain.
  - At least 31 million adults report low back pain, with 19 million people experiencing this on a chronic basis.
  - Currently, 50 million people are fully or partially disabled as a result of pain.
  - Over 50% of adults experience muscle pain each year.
  - Up to 40% of people with cancer report moderate to severe pain.
- About 28 million Americans suffer from headaches and migraines.
  - Use of drug therapy and other measures controls 95% of migraines.
  - After puberty, women have four to eight times more migraines than men.
  - Before puberty, more boys have migraines than do girls.
  - Headaches and migraines appear mostly among people ages 20 to 40.
  - Persons with a family history of headache or migraine have a greater chance of developing these disorders.

numb pain. Whereas nociceptor pain responds quite well to conventional pain relief medications, neuropathic pain responds less successfully.

Concept Review 14.1

- What questions would you ask to identify a patient's type of pain? How would you distinguish between acute pain and chronic pain? Which is the more difficult type of pain to treat?

Nonpharmacologic techniques assist patients in obtaining adequate pain relief.

CORE CONCEPT 14.2

Although drugs are quite effective at relieving pain in most patients, they can have significant adverse effects. For example, at high doses, aspirin causes gastrointestinal (GI) bleeding, and opioids cause significant drowsiness and have the potential for inducing dependence.

To help patients obtain adequate pain relief, nonpharmacologic techniques may be used in place of drugs or in addition to pharmacotherapy. When used together with medication, nonpharmacologic techniques often allow medication doses to be lowered. Lower doses typically mean fewer drug-related adverse effects. Some nonpharmacologic techniques used for reducing pain include the following:

- Acupuncture
- Biofeedback therapy
- Massage
- Heat or cold packs
- Meditation
- Relaxation therapy
- Art or music therapy
- Imagery
- Chiropractic manipulation
- Hypnosis
- Therapeutic touch
- Transcutaneous electrical nerve stimulation (TENS)
- Energy therapies such as reiki and qi gong

Patients with *intractable* (meaning "not easy to relieve") cancer pain sometimes require more *invasive* techniques if rapidly growing tumors press on vital tissues and nerves. In addition, chemotherapy and surgical treatments for cancer can cause severe pain. Radiation therapy may

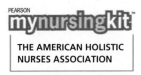

THE AMERICAN HOLISTIC NURSES ASSOCIATION

in = *opposite of*
tractable = *control*
invasive = *tending to spread*

provide pain relief by shrinking solid tumors that may be pressing on nerves. Surgery may be used to reduce pain by removing part of or the entire tumor. Injection of alcohol or other neurotoxic substance into neuronal tissue is occasionally performed to create nerve blocks. Nerve blocks irreversibly stop impulse transmission along treated nerves and have the potential to provide total pain relief.

Pain transmission processes allow several targets for pharmacologic intervention.

CORE CONCEPT 14.3

The process of pain transmission begins when nociceptors are stimulated. These receptors are free nerve endings located throughout the entire body. The nerve impulse signaling the pain is sent to the spinal cord along two types of sensory neurons, called Aδ and C fibers. **Aδ fibers** are wrapped thinly in myelin, a fatty substance that speeds nerve transmission. **C fibers** are *unmyelinated;* thus, they carry nerve transmissions more slowly. The Aδ fibers signal sharp, well-defined pain, whereas the C fibers conduct dull, poorly localized pain.

Once pain impulses reach the spinal cord, neurotransmitters pass the message along to the next neuron. Here, a neurotransmitter called **substance P** is thought to be responsible for continuing the pain message, although other neurotransmitter candidates have been proposed. Spinal substance P is critical because it controls whether pain signals will continue to the brain. The activity of substance P may be affected by other neurotransmitters released from neurons in the central nervous system (CNS). One group of neurotransmitters, called **endogenous opioids**, includes endorphins, dynorphins, and enkephalins. Figure 14.1 ■ shows one point of contact where endogenous opioids modify, or change, sensory information at the level of the spinal cord. If the pain impulse reaches the brain, it may respond with many possible actions. For instance, the brain may signal the skeletal muscles to jerk away from a sharp object. In other instances, such as in those suffering from chronic pain, the impulses reaching the brain may result in mental depression brought on by thoughts of death or disability.

endo = *within*
genous = *coming from*

Because pain signals begin at nociceptors located within peripheral body tissues and then proceed through the CNS, there are several targets where medications can work to stop pain transmission. In general, the two main classes of pain medications act at different locations: The nonsteroidal anti-inflammatory drugs (NSAIDs) act at the peripheral level, whereas the opioids act within the CNS.

Concept Review 14.2

■ What is a nociceptor? Consider substance P and endogenous opioids, and describe how pain can be regulated.

Opioid analgesic medications exert their effects by interacting with specific receptors.

CORE CONCEPT 14.4

an = *without*
algesia = *pain*

opi = *opium*
oid = *shape or form*

Analgesics are medications used to relieve pain. The two basic categories of analgesics are the opioids and the nonopioids. An **opioid** analgesic is a natural or synthetic morphine-like substance responsible for reducing severe pain. Opioids are *narcotic* substances, meaning that they produce numbness or stuporlike symptoms.

Terminology associated with the narcotic analgesic medications is often confusing. Several of these drugs are obtained from opium, a milky extract from the unripe seeds of the poppy plant containing over 20 different chemicals having pharmacologic activity. Opium consists of 9% to 14% morphine and 0.8% to 2.5% codeine. These natural substances are called **opiates**. In a search for safer analgesics, chemists have created several dozen synthetic drugs with activity similar to that of the opiates. *Opioid* is a general term referring to any of these substances, natural or synthetic, and is often used interchangeably with the term *opiate*.

narc = *numbness or stupor*
otic = *like*

Narcotic is a general term used to refer to the stupor associated with morphine-like drugs that produce analgesia and CNS depression. In the context of drug enforcement, the term *narcotic* may be used to describe a much broader range of abused illegal drugs such as hallucinogens, heroin, amphetamines, and marijuana. Opioid narcotics may be natural, such as morphine, or synthetic such as meperidine (Demerol).

FIGURE 14.1

Neural pathways for pain

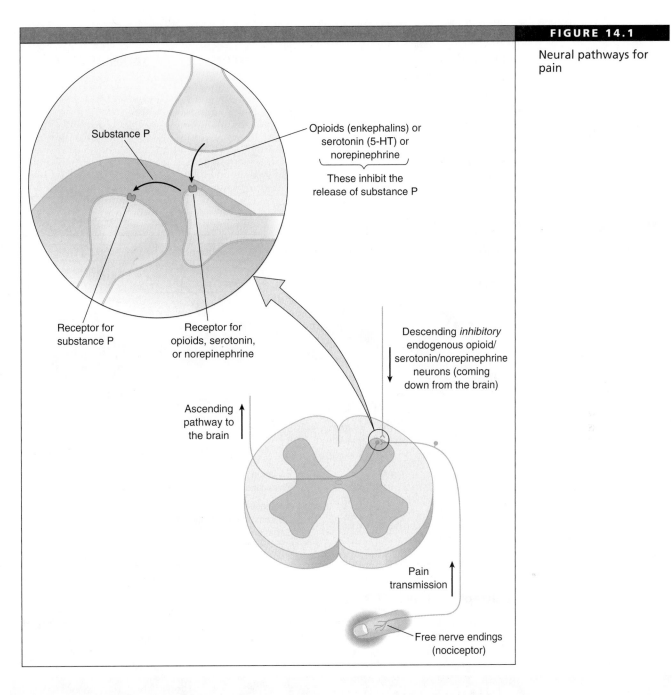

Opioids interact with at least six types of receptors: mu (types one and two), kappa, sigma, delta, and epsilon. From the perspective of pain management, the *mu* and *kappa receptors* are the most important. Some opioids stimulate a particular receptor; others block a receptor. The types of actions produced by activating mu and kappa receptors are listed in Table 14.1.

Some opioids, such as morphine, activate both mu and kappa receptors. Other opioids such as pentazocine (Talwin) exert mixed opioid stimulating-blocking effects by activating the kappa receptor but blocking the mu receptor. Opioid blockers such as naloxone (Narcan) inhibit both the mu and kappa receptors. This is the body's natural way of providing the mechanism for different body responses from one substance. Figure 14.2 ■ illustrates opioid actions on the mu and kappa receptors.

Opioids are drugs of choice for moderate to severe pain that cannot be controlled with other classes of analgesics. More than 20 different opioids are available as medications, and they can be classified by similarities in their chemical structures, by their mechanisms of action, or by their effectiveness. The most useful method is by effectiveness, which places opiates into categories of high or moderate narcotic activity (Table 14.2).

TABLE 14.1	Responses Produced by Activation of Specific Opioid Receptors	
RESPONSE	MU RECEPTOR	KAPPA RECEPTOR
Analgesia	✓	✓
Decreased GI motility	✓	✓
Euphoria	✓	
Miosis (constricted pupils)		✓
Physical dependence	✓	
Respiratory depression	✓	
Sedation	✓	✓

FIGURE 14.2

Opioid receptors

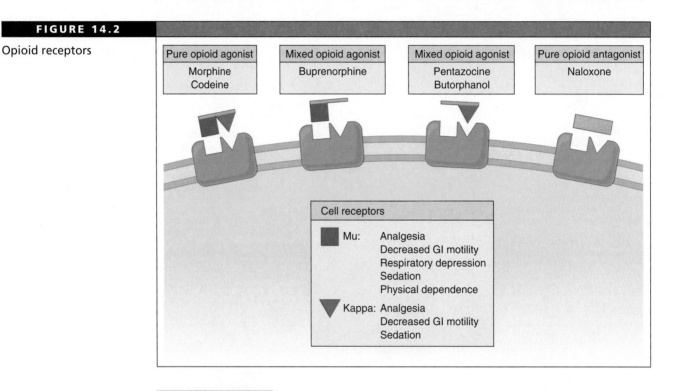

Pure opioid agonist	Mixed opioid agonist	Mixed opioid agonist	Pure opioid antagonist
Morphine Codeine	Buprenorphine	Pentazocine Butorphanol	Naloxone

Cell receptors

Mu: Analgesia
      Decreased GI motility
      Respiratory depression
      Sedation
      Physical dependence

Kappa: Analgesia
       Decreased GI motility
       Sedation

Concept Review   **14.3**

■ Distinguish between the following terms: *opioid, opiate,* and *narcotic*. Name six classes of opioid receptors, and identify those that are connected with analgesia.

OPIOID AGONISTS

Narcotic opioid agonists bind to opioid receptors and produce multiple responses throughout the body. Morphine is the "representative" drug used to treat severe pain. It is usually the standard by which the effectiveness of other opioids is compared.

Narcotic opioids have multiple therapeutic effects, including relief of severe pain.

CORE CONCEPT 14.5

Opiates produce many important effects other than analgesia. They are effective at suppressing the cough reflex and at slowing the *motility*, or movement, of the GI tract for cases of severe diarrhea. As powerful CNS depressants, opioids can cause sedation, which may be a therapeutic effect or an adverse effect, depending on the patient's disease state. Some patients experience

TABLE 14.2	Opioids for Pain Management	
DRUG	**ROUTE AND ADULT DOSE**	**REMARKS**
OPIOID AGONISTS WITH MODERATE EFFECTIVENESS		
codeine	PO; 15–60 mg qid	Also for cough; available in IM and subcutaneous forms; combination drug with aspirin is called Empirin with codeine and with acetaminophen, Tylenol with codeine
hydrocodone bitartrate (Hycodan)	PO; 5–10 mg every 4–6 hours prn (max: 15 mg/dose)	Also for cough; combination drug with acetaminophen is called Amacodone C, Co-Gesic, Vicodin, Dolacet, Norcet, and Norco
oxycodone hydrochloride (OxyContin) oxycodone terephthalate (Percocet-5, Roxicet, others)	PO; 5–10 mg qid prn	Combination drug with acetaminophen is called Percocet or Tylox; with aspirin is called Percodan or Roxiprin
propoxyphene hydrochloride (Darvon) propoxyphene napsylate (Darvon-N)	PO; 65 mg (HCl form) or 100 mg (napsylate form) every 4 hours prn (max: 390 HCl/day; max: 600 mg napsylate/day)	Combination drug with acetaminophen is called Darvocet or Propacet; with aspirin and caffeine is called Darvon or Dolene
OPIOID AGONISTS WITH HIGH EFFECTIVENESS		
fentanyl (Sublimaze)	IM; 0.05-0.1 mg Transdermal 25–100 mcg every 72 hours	Used with anesthesia for surgery and other procedures
hydromorphone hydrochloride (Dilaudid)	PO; 1–4 mg every 4–6 hours prn	Also for cough; available in IM, IV, subcutaneous, and rectal forms
levorphanol tartrate (Levo-Dromoran)	PO; 2–3 mg tid to qid prn	Also available in subcutaneous form
meperidine hydrochloride (Demerol)	PO; 50–150 mg every 3–4 hours prn	For preoperative medication or obstetric analgesia; available in IM, IV, and subcutaneous forms
methadone hydrochloride (Dolophine)	PO; 2.5–10 mg every 3–4 hours prn	For detoxification treatment of opioid dependency; available in IM and IV forms
Pr morphine sulfate (Astramorph PF, Duramorph, others)	PO; 10–30 mg every 4 hours prn	Available in IM, IV, subcutaneous, intrathecal, epidural, and rectal forms
oxymorphone hydrochloride (Numorphan)	Subcutaneous/IM; 1–1.5 mg every 4–6 hours prn; 5 mg every 4–6 hours prn	Also available in IV and rectal forms
OPIOID ANTAGONISTS		
nalmefene hydrochloride (Revex)	Subcutaneous/IM/IV; use 1 mg/ml concentration; nonopioid dependent: 0.5 mg/70 kg; opioid dependent: 0.1 mg/70 kg	For opioid overdose and postoperative opioid depression
Pr naloxone (Narcan)	IV; 0.4–2 mg, may be repeated every 2–3 min up to 10 mg if necessary	For opioid overdose and postoperative opioid depression
naltrexone hydrochloride (Trexan, ReVia)	PO; 25 mg followed by another 25 mg in 1 hour if no withdrawal response (max: 800 mg/day)	For management of opiate or alcohol dependence; longer lasting effect than naloxone
OPIOIDS WITH MIXED AGONIST–ANTAGONIST EFFECTS		
buprenorphine hydrochloride (Buprenex)	IM/IV; 0.3 mg every 6 hours (max: 0.6 mg every 4 hours)	For moderate to severe pain; also available in subcutaneous, epidural, and rectal forms
butorphanol tartrate (Stadol)	IM; 1–4 mg every 3–4 hours prn (max: 4 mg/dose)	For obstetrical analgesia during labor, cancer pain, renal colic, and burns; available in IV and intranasal forms
dezocine (Dalgan)	IV; 2.5–10 mg (usually 5 mg) every 2–4 hours; IM; 5–10 mg (usually 10 mg) every 3–4 hours	Causes less respiratory depression than morphine sulfate

continued . . .

TABLE 14.2	Opioids for Pain Management—*Continued*	
DRUG	**ROUTE AND ADULT DOSE**	**REMARKS**
nalbuphine hydrochloride (Nubain)	Subcutaneous/IM/IV; 10–20 mg every 3–6 hours prn (max: 160 mg/day)	For moderate to severe pain
pentazocine hydrochloride (Talwin)	PO; 50–100 mg every 3–4 hours (max: 600 mg/day); subcutaneous/IM/IV; 30 mg every 3–4 hours (max: 360 mg/day)	For moderate to severe pain (much lower dose for women in labor)

DRUG PROFILE: ⓟ *Morphine (Astramorph PF, Duramorph, Others)*

Therapeutic Class: Opioid analgesic
Pharmacologic Class: Opioid receptor drug

Actions and Uses:

Morphine binds with both mu and kappa receptor sites to produce strong analgesia. It causes euphoria, constriction of the pupils, and stimulation of cardiac muscle. It is used for relief of serious acute and chronic pain after nonnarcotic analgesics have failed, as preanesthetic medication, to relieve shortness of breath associated with heart failure and pulmonary edema, and for acute chest pain connected with myocardial infarction (MI).

Adverse Effects and Interactions:

Morphine may cause dysphoria (restlessness, depression, and anxiety), hallucinations, nausea, constipation, dizziness, and an itching sensation. Overdose may result in severe respiratory depression or cardiac arrest. Tolerance develops to the analgesic, sedative, and euphoric effects of the drug. Cross-tolerance also develops between morphine and other opioids such as heroin, methadone, and meperidine. Physical and psychological dependence develop when high doses are taken for prolonged periods. Morphine may intensify or mask the pain of gallbladder disease due to biliary tract spasms.

Morphine interacts with several drugs. For example, use with CNS depressants, such as alcohol, other opioids, general anesthetics, sedatives, and antidepressants such as monoamine oxidase (MAO) inhibitors and tricyclics, increases the action of opiates and thereby raises the risk of severe respiratory depression and death.

Use with caution with herbal supplements, such as yohimbe, which may increase the effect of morphine.

Mechanism in Action:

Morphine is an opioid that produces many actions throughout the CNS. One important action occurs at the level of the dorsal horn of the spinal cord. Here, morphine binds presynaptically to primary afferent neurons, reducing the amount of neurotransmitter released. Simultaneously, morphine binds postsynaptically to second-order neurons responsible for transmitting ascending pain impulses to the brain.

Refer to MyNursingKit for a Nursing Process Focus specific to this drug.

euphoria and intense relaxation, which are reasons why opiates are sometimes abused. There are many adverse effects, including respiratory depression, sedation, nausea, and vomiting.

All of the narcotic analgesics have the potential to cause physical and psychological dependence, as discussed in Chapter 7 ⚛. Over the years, health care providers and nurses have hesitated to administer the proper amount of opioid analgesics for fear of causing patient dependence or of producing serious adverse effects such as sedation or respiratory depression. Because of this tendency, some patients have not received complete pain relief.

When used according to accepted medical practice, patients can, and indeed should, receive the pain relief they need without fear of addiction or adverse effects. One method available to accomplish this is **patient-controlled analgesia (PCA)**. In this instance patients are allowed to self-medicate with opiate medication by pressing a button. Safe levels of pain medication are delivered with an infusion pump.

In the pharmacologic management of pain, it is common practice to combine opioids and nonnarcotic analgesics into a single tablet or capsule. The two classes of analgesics work *synergistically* to relieve pain, and the dose of narcotic can be kept small to avoid dependence and opioid-related adverse effects. Popular combination analgesics include:

syn = *together*
erg = *work*
istically = *ability to*

- Vicodin (hydrocodone, 5 mg; acetaminophen, 500 mg)
- Percocet (oxycodone HCl, 5 mg; acetaminophen, 325 mg)
- Percodan (oxycodone HCl, 4.5 mg; oxycodone terephthalate, 0.38 mg; aspirin, 325 mg)
- Darvocet-N 50 (propoxyphene napsylate, 50 mg; acetaminophen, 325 mg)
- Empirin with Codeine No. 2 (codeine phosphate, 15 mg; aspirin, 325 mg)
- Tylenol with Codeine (single dose may contain from 15 to 60 mg of codeine phosphate and from 300 to 1000 mg of acetaminophen)

Some opioids are used primarily for conditions other than general complaints of pain. For example, alfentanil (Alfenta), fentanyl (Sublimaze), remifentanil (Ultiva), and sufentanil (Sufenta) are used for general anesthesia; these are discussed further in Chapter 15 ⬢. Codeine is most often prescribed as a cough suppressant and is covered in Chapter 27 ⬢. Opiates used in treating diarrhea are presented in Chapter 28 ⬢.

Opioid Antagonists

Opioid antagonists are substances that prevent the effects of opioid agonists. These drugs are sometimes called "competitive antagonists" because they compete with opioid agonists for access to the opioid receptor site.

Opioid overdose can occur as a result of overly aggressive pain therapy or as a result of substance abuse. Any opioid may be abused for its psychoactive effects; however, morphine, meperidine, and heroin are preferred because of their potency. Although heroin is currently available as a legal analgesic in many countries, it is considered by the Food and Drug Administration (FDA) to be too dangerous for therapeutic use. It is a major drug of abuse. Once injected or inhaled, heroin rapidly crosses the blood-brain barrier to enter the brain, where it is metabolized to morphine. Thus, the effects and symptoms of heroin administration are actually caused by the activation of mu and kappa receptors by morphine. The initial effect is an intense euphoria, called a *rush*, followed by several hours of deep relaxation.

Acute opioid intoxication is a medical emergency. Respiratory depression is the most serious problem. The opioid antagonist naloxone (Narcan) may be infused to reverse respiratory

---

DRUG PROFILE: ℞ *Naloxone (Narcan)*

Therapeutic Class: Drug for treatment of acute opioid overdose and misuse
Pharmacologic Class: Opioid receptor blocker

Actions and Uses:

Naloxone is a pure opioid antagonist, blocking both mu and kappa receptors. It is used for complete or partial reversal of opioid effects in emergency situations when acute opioid overdose is suspected. Given intravenously, it begins to reverse opioid-initiated CNS and respiratory depression within minutes. It will immediately cause opioid withdrawal symptoms in patients physically dependent on opioids. It is also used to treat postoperative opioid depression. It is occasionally given as adjunctive therapy to reverse hypotension caused by septic shock. Naloxone is pregnancy category B.

Adverse Effects and Interactions:

Naloxone itself has minimal toxicity. However, in reversing the effects of opioids, the patient may experience rapid loss of analgesia, increased blood pressure, tremors, hyperventilation, nausea/vomiting, and drowsiness. It should not be used for respiratory depression caused by nonopioid medications.

Drug interactions include a reversal of the analgesic effects of narcotic agonists and agonist–antagonists.

Refer to MyNursingKit for a Nursing Process Focus specific to this drug.

depression and other acute symptoms. In cases in which the patient is unconscious and the health care provider is unclear what drug has been taken, opioid antagonists may be given to diagnose the overdose. If the opioid antagonist fails to quickly reverse the acute symptoms, the overdose was likely due to a nonopioid substance.

Opioids With Mixed Agonist–Antagonist Activity

Narcotic opioids that have mixed agonist–antagonist activity stimulate the opioid receptor; thus, they cause analgesia. However, the withdrawal symptoms or adverse effects are not as intense due to partial activity of receptor subtypes.

Although effective at relieving pain, the opioids have a greater risk for dependence than almost any other class of medications. Tolerance develops relatively quickly to the euphoric effects of opioids, causing users to increase their doses and take the drug more frequently. The higher and more frequent doses rapidly cause physical dependence in opioid abusers.

When physically dependent patients attempt to discontinue drug use, they experience extremely uncomfortable symptoms that may lead them to continue their drug-taking behavior. As long as the drug is continued, they feel "normal" and continue to work and engage in social activities. If a person abruptly discontinues the drug, however, he or she experiences withdrawal symptoms for about 7 days before overcoming the physical dependence.

The intense craving that characterizes psychological dependence may occur for many months, and even years, following discontinuation of opioids. This often results in a return to drug-seeking behavior unless significant support is available.

One method of treating opioid dependence has been to switch the patient from IV and inhalation forms of illegal drugs to methadone (Dolophine). Although oral methadone is an opioid, it does not cause the euphoria of the injectable opioids. Methadone also does not cure the dependence, and the patient must continue taking the drug to avoid withdrawal symptoms. This therapy, called *methadone maintenance*, may continue for many months or years until the patient decides to enter a total withdrawal treatment program. Methadone maintenance allows patients to return to productive work and social relationships without the physical, emotional, and criminal risks of illegal drug use.

A newer treatment option is to administer buprenorphine (Subutex), a mixed opioid agonist–antagonist, by the sublingual route. Subutex is used early in opioid abuse therapy to prevent opioid withdrawal symptoms. Another combination drug, Suboxone, contains both buprenorphine and naloxone and is used later in the maintenance of opioid addiction.

Practitioners must be aware when administering opioids with mixed agonist–antagonist activity that in some ways they act similarly to pure opioid agonists; however, when mixed drugs are administered in combination with opioid agonists, their pain-blocking properties are reduced. Thus, there is a tendency to overprescribe mixed opioids, thereby promoting drug misuse. This is true even though the potential for causing opioid addiction in most cases with mixed agonist–antagonists is lower than with the pure opioid agonists.

NURSING PROCESS FOCUS

Patients Receiving Opioids

ASSESSMENT

Prior to administration:
- Obtain a complete health history (physical/mental), including allergies, drug history, and possible drug interactions
- Assess pain (quality, intensity, location, duration)
- Assess respiratory function
- Assess level of consciousness before and after administration
- Obtain vital signs

POTENTIAL NURSING DIAGNOSES

- Deficient Knowledge related to information about drug therapy.
- Acute Pain related to injury, disease, or surgical procedure.
- Ineffective Breathing Pattern related to action of drug.
- Constipation related to adverse effect of drug.
- Disturbed Sleep Pattern related to pain.

continued . . .

NURSING PROCESS FOCUS *(continued)*

PLANNING: PATIENT GOALS AND EXPECTED OUTCOMES

The patient will:
- Report pain relief or a reduction in pain intensity
- Demonstrate an understanding of the drug's action by accurately describing adverse effects and precautions
- Immediately report effects such as untoward or rebound pain, restlessness, anxiety, depression, hallucination, nausea, dizziness, and itching

IMPLEMENTATION

Interventions and (Rationales)	Patient Education/Discharge Planning
■ Monitor the use of opioids. Opioids are Schedule II controlled substances and can produce both physical and psychological dependence. Administer the drug using the correct route. They may be administered PO, subcutaneously, IM, IV, or PR.	Instruct the patient: ■ To take necessary steps to safeguard drug supply; avoid sharing medications with others ■ That oral *capsules* may be opened and mixed with cool foods; extended-release *tablets*, however, may not be chewed, crushed, or broken ■ That the oral solution for taking sublingually, may be more concentrated than the solution for swallowing
■ Monitor liver function via laboratory tests. (Opioids are metabolized in the liver. Hepatic disease can increase blood levels of opioids to toxic levels.)	Instruct the patient to: ■ Report nausea, vomiting, diarrhea, rash, jaundice, abdominal pain, tenderness or distention, or change in color of stool ■ Adhere to laboratory testing regimen for liver function as ordered by the health care provider
■ Monitor vital signs, especially depth and rate of respirations/pulse oximetry. Withhold the drug if the patient's respiratory rate is below 12, and notify the health care provider. Keep resuscitative equipment and a narcotic antagonist such as naloxone (Narcan) accessible. (Opioid antagonists may reverse respiratory depression, decrease level of consciousness, and initiate other symptoms of narcotic overdose.)	Instruct the patient to: ■ Monitor vital signs regularly, particularly respirations ■ Withhold medication for any difficulty in breathing or respirations below 12 breaths per minute; report symptoms to the health care provider
■ Monitor neurologic status; perform neuro checks regularly. Especially monitor for changes in level of consciousness (LOC) or seizure activity. Decreased LOC and sluggish pupillary response may occur with high doses, and the drug may increase intracranial pressure.	Instruct the patient to: ■ Report headache or any significant change in sensorium, such as an aura or other visual effects that may indicate an impending seizure ■ Recognize seizures and methods to ensure personal safety during a seizure ■ Report any seizure activity immediately
■ If ordered prn, administer the medication upon patient's request or when nursing observations indicate patient detect expressions of pain by the patient.	Instruct the patient to: ■ Alert the nurse immediately upon the return or increase of pain ■ Notify the nurse regarding the drug's effectiveness
■ Monitor renal status and urinary output (may cause urinary retention, which may exacerbate existing symptoms of prostatic hypertrophy).	Instruct the patient to: ■ Measure and monitor fluid intake and output ■ Report symptoms of dysuria (hesitancy, pain, diminished stream), changes in urine quality, or scanty urine output ■ Report fever or flank pain that may be indicative of a urinary tract infection

continued . . .

NURSING PROCESS FOCUS (continued)

Interventions and (Rationales)	Patient Education/Discharge Planning
■ Monitor for other adverse effects such as restlessness, dizziness, anxiety, depression, hallucinations, nausea, and vomiting. (Hives or itching may indicate an allergic reaction due to the production of histamine.)	Instruct the patient to: ■ Recognize adverse effects and symptoms of an allergic or anaphylactic reaction ■ Immediately report any shortness of breath, tight feeling in the throat, itching, hives or other rash, feelings of dysphoria, nausea, or vomiting ■ Avoid the use of sleep-inducing over-the-counter (OTC) antihistamines without first consulting the health care provider
■ Monitor for constipation. (Drug slows peristalsis.)	Instruct the patient to: ■ Maintain adequate fluid and fiber intake to facilitate stool passage ■ Use a stool softener or laxative as recommended by the health care provider
■ Ensure patient safety. Monitor ambulation until response to the drug is known. (Drug can cause sedation and dizziness.)	Instruct the patient to: ■ Request assistance when getting out of bed ■ Avoid driving or performing hazardous activities until effect of the drug is known
■ Monitor frequency of requests and stated effectiveness of narcotic administered. (Opioids cause tolerance and dependence.)	Instruct the patient: ■ Regarding cross-tolerance issues ■ To monitor medication supply to observe for hoarding, which may signal an impending suicide attempt ■ Who is suffering from a terminal illness about the issue of drug dependence from the perspective of reduced life expectancy.

EVALUATION OF OUTCOME CRITERIA

Evaluate the effectiveness of drug therapy by confirming that patient goals and expected outcomes have been met (see "Planning").

See Table 14.2 for a list of drugs to which these nursing actions apply.

CORE CONCEPT 14.6

Nonsteroidal anti-inflammatory drugs are the drugs of choice for pain due to inflammation.

The NSAIDs have antipyretic (antifever) and anti-inflammatory activity, as well as analgesic (pain-reducing) properties. Some of the NSAIDs, such as the selective COX-2 inhibitors, are used primarily for their anti-inflammatory properties. Celecoxib (Celebrex) and rofecoxib (Vioxx), once top-selling arthritis medications, have been linked to the risk of heart attack and stroke. Vioxx was removed from the market on September 30, 2004, after a study revealed that this drug was linked to heart attacks, strokes, blood clots, and cardiovascular injuries. NSAIDs are also used in the treatment of fever (see Chapter 23 ⬤). Table 14.3 highlights the common nonopioid analgesics.

Nonsteroidal Anti-inflammatory Drugs

The nonopioid analgesics include the NSAIDs, acetaminophen, and a few centrally acting drugs. The NSAIDs inhibit **cyclooxygenase (COX)**, an enzyme responsible for the formation of prostaglandins. When cyclooxygenase is inhibited, inflammation and pain are reduced.

NSAIDs are the drugs of choice for mild to moderate pain, especially for pain associated with inflammation. These drugs have many advantages over the opioids. Aspirin and ibuprofen are available as OTC drugs and are inexpensive. Ibuprofen is available in many different formulations, including those designed for children. Many are safe and produce adverse effects only at high doses. Other NSAIDs, such as the COX-2 inhibitors, have been carefully scrutinized for possible adverse effects.

PEARSON
mynursingkit

THE OXFORD PAIN
INTERNET SITE

mediators = *middle drugs*
brady = *slow*
kinin = *movement*
syn = *together*
thesis = *put*

TABLE 14.3   Nonopioid Analgesics

DRUG	ROUTE AND ADULT DOSE	REMARKS
Pr acetaminophen (Tylenol)	PO; 325–650 mg every 4–6 hours	Also for fever; available in rectal form

NSAIDS
Selective COX-2 Inhibitor

celecoxib (Celebrex)	PO; 100–200 mg bid or 200 mg/daily	Also for inflammation

Ibuprofen and Ibuprofen-like: Nonsalicylates

diclofenac (Cataflam, Voltaren)	PO; 50 mg bid to qid (max: 200 mg/day)	Also for inflammation
diflunisal (Dolobid)	PO; 1000 mg followed by 500 mg bid to tid	Also for inflammation
etodolac (Lodine)	PO; 200–400 mg tid to qid	Also for inflammation
fenoprofen calcium (Nalfon)	PO; 200 mg tid to qid	Also for inflammation
flurbiprofen (Ansaid)	PO; 50–100 mg tid to qid (max: 300 mg/day)	Similar to ibuprofen
ibuprofen (Advil, Motrin)	PO; 400 mg tid to qid (max: 1200 mg/day)	Also for fever and inflammation
indomethacin (Indocin)	PO; 25–50 mg bid or tid (max: 200 mg/day) or 75 mg sustained release one to two times/day	Also used for moderate to severe rheumatoid arthritis and acute gouty arthritis
ketoprofen (Actron, Orudis)	PO; 12.5–50 mg tid to qid	Also for inflammation
ketorolac tromethamine (Toradol)	PO; 10 mg qid prn (max: 40 mg/day)	Also for allergic conjunctivitis, available in IM/IV forms
mefenamic acid (Ponstel)	PO; loading dose 500 mg, maintenance dose 250 mg every 6 hours prn	Used for short-term relief of mild to moderate pain, including menstrual cramps
meloxicam (Mobic)	PO; 7.5 mg daily (max: 15 mg/day)	Used for osteoarthritis
nabumetone (Relafen)	PO; 1000 mg daily (max: 2000 mg/day)	Inhibits COX-2 more than COX-1
naproxen (Naprosyn) (see page 391 for the Drug Profile box)	PO; 500 mg followed by 200–250 mg tid to qid (max: 1000 mg/day)	Also for inflammation
naproxen sodium (Aleve, Anaprox) (see page 391 for the Drug Profile box)	PO; 250–500 mg bid (max: 1000 mg/day naproxen)	Also for dysmenorrhea
oxaprozin (Daypro)	PO; 600–1200 mg daily (max: 1800 mg/day)	Similar to naproxen; once-a-day dosage
piroxicam (Feldene)	PO; 10–20 mg daily to bid (max: 20 mg/day)	Has prolonged half-life
sulindac (Clinoril)	PO; 150–200 mg bid (max: 400 mg/day)	Also for inflammation
tolmetin (Tolectin)	PO; 400 mg tid (max: 2 g/day)	Also for inflammation

Salicylates

Pr aspirin (Acetylsalicylic acid, ASA)	PO; 350–650 mg every 4 hours (max: 4 g/day)	Also for fever, inflammation, and thromboembolic disorders, prevention of transient ischemic attacks and heart attacks; rectal form available
choline salicylate (Arthropan)	PO; 435–870 mg (2.5–5 ml) every 4 hours	Also for inflammation; may be indicated for patients who have difficulty swallowing tablets or capsules
salsalate (Disalcid)	PO; 325–3000 mg daily in divided doses (max: 4 g/day)	Also for fever, inflammation

CENTRALLY ACTING DRUGS

clonidine (Catapres)	PO; 0.1 mg bid to tid (max: 0.8 mg/day)	Also used for hypertension
tramadol (Ultram)	PO; 50–100 mg every 4–6 hours prn (max: 400 mg/day), may start with 25 mg/day and increase by 25 mg every 3 days up to 200 mg/day	Causes less respiratory depression than morphine
ziconotide (Prialt)	Intrathecal; 0.1 mcg/hr via infusion, may increase by 0.1 mcg/hr every 2–3 days (max: 0.8 mcg/hr)	Also used for muscle spasticity

DRUG PROFILE: ℗ *Aspirin (Acetylsalicylic Acid, ASA)*

Therapeutic Class: Nonopioid analgesic, nonsteroidal anti-inflammatory drug (NSAID), antipyretic; drug for myocardial infarction prophylaxis and transient ischemia

Pharmacologic Class: Salicylate, cyclooxygenase (COX) inhibitor, prostaglandin synthesis inhibitor, platelet aggregation inhibitor

Actions and Uses:

Aspirin inhibits prostaglandin synthesis involved in the processes of pain and inflammation and produces mild to moderate relief of fever. It has limited effects on peripheral blood vessels, causing vasodilation and sweating. Aspirin has significant anticoagulant activity, and this property is responsible for its ability to reduce the risk of mortality following MI and to reduce the incidence of strokes. Aspirin has also been found to reduce the risk of colorectal cancer, although the mechanism by which it affords this protective effect is unknown.

Adverse Effects and Interactions:

At high doses, such as those used to treat severe inflammatory disorders, aspirin may cause gastric discomfort and bleeding because of its antiplatelet effects. Enteric-coated tablets and buffered preparations are available for patients who experience GI adverse effects.

Because aspirin increases bleeding time, it should not be given to patients receiving anticoagulant therapy such as warfarin, heparin, and plicamycin. ASA may increase the action of oral hypoglycemic drugs. Effects of NSAIDs, uricosuric drugs such as probenecid, beta blockers, spironolactone, and sulfa drugs may be decreased when combined with ASA.

Use with phenobarbital, antacids, and glucocorticoids may decrease ASA effects. Insulin, methotrexate, phenytoin, sulfonamides, and penicillin may increase effects. When taken with alcohol, pyrazolone derivatives, steroids, or other NSAIDs, there is an increased risk for gastric ulcers.

Use with caution with herbal supplements, such as feverfew, which may increase the risk of bleeding.

Refer to MyNursingKit for a Nursing Process Focus specific to this drug.

DRUG PROFILE: ℗ *Acetaminophen (Tylenol)*

Therapeutic Class: Antipyretic, nonopioid analgesic

Pharmacologic Class: Central noninflammatory-type prostaglandin inhibitor

Actions and Uses:

Acetaminophen reduces fever by direct action at the level of the hypothalamus and causes dilation of peripheral blood vessels, enabling sweating and dissipation of heat. Acetaminophen and aspirin have equal efficacy in relieving pain and reducing fever.

Acetaminophen has no peripheral anti-inflammatory action; therefore, it is not effective in treating arthritis or pain caused by tissue swelling following injury. Acetaminophen's pain and fever reducing qualities relate to its ability to reduce the formation of prostaglandin-type chemicals in the brain. The primary therapeutic usefulness of acetaminophen is for the treatment of fever in children and for relief of mild to moderate pain when aspirin is contraindicated. Acetaminophen is pregnancy category B.

Adverse Effects and Interactions:

Acetaminophen is quite safe, and adverse effects are uncommon at therapeutic doses. Unlike aspirin, acetaminophen has no direct anti-inflammatory effect and does not affect blood coagulation or cause gastric irritation. It is not recommended in patients who are malnourished. In such cases, acute toxicity may result, leading to renal failure, which can be fatal. Other signs of acute toxicity include nausea, vomiting, chills, and abdominal discomfort.

Acetaminophen inhibits warfarin metabolism, causing warfarin to accumulate to toxic levels. High-dose or long-term acetaminophen usage may result in elevated warfarin levels and bleeding. Ingestion of this drug with alcohol is not recommended due to the possibility of liver failure from hepatic necrosis.

The patient should avoid taking herbs that have the potential for liver toxicity, including comfrey, coltsfoot, and chaparral.

Refer to MyNursingKit for a Nursing Process Focus specific to this drug.

NSAIDs act by inhibiting pain mediators at the nociceptor level. When tissue is damaged, chemical mediators are released locally, including histamine, potassium ions, hydrogen ions, bradykinin, and prostaglandins. **Bradykinin** is associated with the sensory impulse of pain. **Prostaglandins** can cause pain through the formation of proinflammatory substances.

Prostaglandins are formed with the help of two enzymes: cyclooxygenase type one (COX-1) and cyclooxygenase type two (COX-2). Aspirin inhibits both COX-1 and COX-2. Because the COX-2 enzyme is more specific for the *synthesis* of those prostaglandins that cause pain and inflammation, the selective COX-2 inhibitors were developed to provide more specific pain relief. Figure 14.3 ■ illustrates the mechanisms involved in pain at the nociceptor level.

Acetaminophen
Several important nonopioid analgesics are not classified as NSAIDs. Acetaminophen is a nonopioid analgesic that is as equally effective as aspirin and ibuprofen for relieving pain. Acetaminophen is featured as a representative medication also used to reduce fever.

Centrally Acting Drugs
Clonidine (Catapres), tramadol (Ultram), and ziconotide (Prialt) are centrally acting analgesics. Tramadol has weak opioid activity, although it is not thought to relieve pain by this mechanism.

FIGURE 14.3

Mechanisms of pain at the nociceptor level

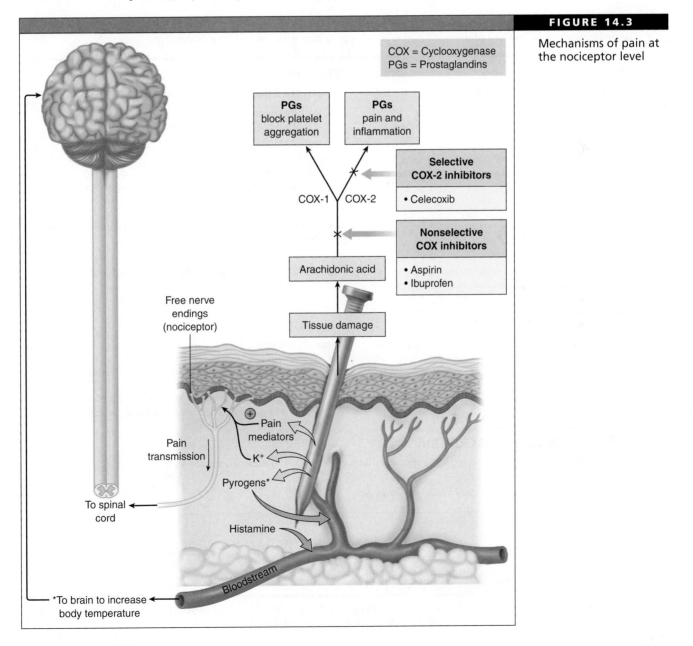

NURSING PROCESS FOCUS

Patients Receiving Antipyretic Therapy

ASSESSMENT

Prior to administration:
- Obtain a complete health history (physical/mental), including data on the origin of the fever, recent surgeries, or trauma
- Obtain vital signs; assess in context of the patient's baseline values
- Obtain the patient's complete medication history, including nicotine and alcohol consumption, to determine possible drug allergies and/or interactions

POTENTIAL NURSING DIAGNOSES

- Hyperthermia related to side effect of illness or dehydration.
- Risk for Injury (hepatic toxicity) related to pain and side effects of hyperthermia.
- Risk Deficient Knowledge related to information about disorder and drug therapy.

PLANNING: PATIENT GOALS AND EXPECTED OUTCOMES

The patient will:
- Experience a reduction in body temperature
- Demonstrate an understanding of the drug's action by accurately describing adverse effects and precautions

IMPLEMENTATION

Interventions and (Rationales)	Patient Education/Discharge Planning
■ Assess for intolerance to ASA for possible cross-hypersensitivity to other NSAIDs or acetaminophen.	■ Inform the patient to immediately report any difficulty breathing, itching, or skin rash.
■ Monitor hepatic and renal function. (Antipyretics are metabolized in the liver and excreted by the kidneys.)	Instruct the patient: ■ To report signs of liver toxicity: nausea, vomiting, anorexia, bleeding, severe upper or lower abdominal pain, heartburn, jaundice, or a change in the color or character of stools ■ To adhere to laboratory testing regimen for serum blood tests, as directed
■ Use with caution in patients with a history of excessive alcohol consumption. (Alcohol increases the risk of liver damage associated with acetaminophen or NSAID administration.)	■ Advise the patient to abstain from alcohol while taking this medication.
■ Use with caution in patients with diabetes. Observe for signs of hypoglycemia, which may occur with acetaminophen usage.	Instruct the patient: ■ To immediately report excessive thirst ■ To immediately report large increases or decreases in urine output ■ With diabetes mellitus that acetaminophen may cause low blood sugar and require insulin dose adjustments.

EVALUATION OF OUTCOME CRITERIA

Evaluate the effectiveness of drug therapy by confirming that patient goals and expected outcomes have been met (see "Planning").

See Table 14.3 for a list of drugs to which these nursing actions apply.

Concept Review 14.4

- Think about cyclooxygenase inhibitors (NSAIDs) and prostaglandins, and then describe how pain might be regulated at the nociceptor.

TENSION HEADACHE AND MIGRAINE

Headache is one of the most common complaints of patients. Living with headaches can interfere with activities of daily life and can cause great distress. Pain and difficulty may result in work-related absences and neglect of home and family life. When headaches are persistent, or as migraines occur, drug therapy is needed.

Of the many types of headaches, the most common is the **tension headache**. It occurs when muscles of the head and neck tighten in response to stress. The tightness causes a steady and lingering pain. Although quite painful, tension headaches usually end when the stress is resolved. They are generally considered an annoyance rather than a medical emergency. Tension headaches are effectively treated with OTC analgesics such as aspirin, acetaminophen, or ibuprofen.

The most painful type of headache is the **migraine**, which is characterized by throbbing or pulsating pain, sometimes preceded by an aura similar to those that warn of a seizure (see Chapter 13 ⬭). The **auras** of migraines are sensory cues, such as seeing jagged lines or flashing lights, smelling, tasting, or hearing something strange. They let the patient know that a migraine attack is coming soon. Most patients with migraines also have nausea and vomiting. Triggers for migraines include nitrates and monosodium glutamate (MSG) found in many Asian foods, red wine, perfumes, food additives, caffeine, chocolate, and aspartame (a sugar substitute). By avoiding these substances, some patients can prevent the onset of a migraine attack.

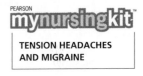

TENSION HEADACHES AND MIGRAINE

Headaches can be effectively treated with a variety of drug classes.

CORE CONCEPT 14.7

There are two primary goals for the pharmacologic management of migraines (Table 14.4). The first is to stop migraines in progress, and the second is to prevent migraines from occurring (*prophylaxis*). For the most part, the drugs used to stop migraines are different than those used for prophylaxis. Drug therapy is most effective if begun before a migraine has reached a severe level.

pro = *before*
phylaxis = *guarding*

The two major drug classes used as antimigraine drugs, the triptans and the ergot alkaloids, both stimulate serotonin (5-HT). Serotonin receptors are found throughout the CNS and in the cardiovascular and GI systems. At least five receptor subtypes have been identified. In addition to the triptans, other drugs acting on serotonin receptors include the popular antianxiety drugs fluoxetine (Prozac) and buspirone (BuSpar).

Triptans

Pharmacotherapy to stop migraines usually begins with acetaminophen or NSAIDs. If OTC analgesics are unable to stop the migraine, the drugs of choice are most often the triptans. The first of the triptans, sumatriptan (Imitrex), was marketed in the United States in 1993. These drugs are selective for the 5-HT$_1$ receptor subtype, and they are thought to act by constricting certain vessels within the brain. They are effective in stopping migraines with or without auras. Although oral forms of the triptans are the most convenient, patients who experience nausea and vomiting during a migraine may require an alternate dosage form. Intranasal formulation and prefilled syringes of triptans are available for patients who are able to self-administer the medication.

TABLE 14.4	Antimigraine Drugs	
DRUG	**ROUTE AND ADULT DOSE**	**REMARKS**
DRUGS FOR TERMINATING MIGRAINES		
Ergot Alkaloids		
dihydroergotamine mesylate (D.H.E. 45, Migranal)	IM; 1 mg, may be repeated at 1-hour intervals to a total of 3 mg (max: 6 mg/week)	Also available as nasal spray; pregnancy category X; for migraine termination; may be used in combination with low-dose heparin to prevent postop deep vein thrombosis
ergotamine tartrate (Ergostat)	PO; 1–2 mg followed by 1–2 mg every 30 minutes until headache stops (max: 6 mg/day or 10 mg/week)	Also available in sublingual, inhalant, or rectal forms; may cause physical dependence; pregnancy category X; for migraine termination
Triptans		
almotriptan (Axert)	PO; 6.25–12.5 mg, may repeat in 2 hours if necessary (max: two tablets/day)	May cause heart palpitations and rapid heartbeat
eletriptan (Relpax)	PO; 20–40 mg, may repeat in 2 hours if necessary (max: 80 mg/day)	May cause hypotension in elderly patients
frovatriptan (Frova)	PO; 2.5 mg, may repeat in 2 hours if necessary (max: 7.5 mg/day)	May cause chest pains and heart palpitations
naratriptan (Amerge)	PO; 1–2.5 mg, may repeat in 4 hours if necessary (max: 5 mg/day)	Serotonin stimulator; for migraine termination
rizatriptan (Maxalt)	PO; 5–10 mg, may repeat in 2 hours if necessary (max: 30 mg/day); 5 mg with concurrent propranolol (max: 15 mg/day)	May cause myocardial infarction
Pr sumatriptan (Imitrex)	PO; 25 mg for one dose (max: 100 mg)	Serotonin stimulator; subcutaneous and intranasal forms available; for termination of migraine
zolmitriptan (Zomig)	PO; 2.5–5 mg, may repeat in 2 hours if necessary (max: 10 mg/day)	Serotonin stimulator; for termination of migraine
DRUGS FOR PREVENTING MIGRAINES		
Antiseizure Drugs		
topiramate (Topamax)	PO; start with 50 mg/day, increase by 50 mg/week to effectiveness (max: 1600 mg/day)	Sugar-like chemical molecule; enhances the action of GABA; also for partial seizures
valproic acid (Depakene) (see page 203 for the Drug Profile box)	PO; 250 mg bid (max: 100 mg/day)	Also for absence seizures and mixed generalized types of seizures and mania
Beta-Adrenergic Blockers		
atenolol (Tenormin) (see page 345 for the Drug Profile box)	PO; 25–50 mg daily (max: 100 mg/day)	Also used for hypertension and angina
metoprolol (Lopressor)	PO; 50–100 mg daily bid (max: 450 mg/day)	Also for angina and MI; sustained-release and IV forms available
propranolol (Inderal, InnoPran XL) (see page 314 for the Drug Profile box)	PO; 80–240 mg/day in divided doses, may need 160–240 mg/day	Beta-adrenergic blocker for migraine prevention
timolol (Blocadren)	PO; 10 mg bid, may increase to 60 mg/day in two divided doses	Also for hypertension, angina, and glaucoma
Calcium Channel Blockers		
nifedipine (Adalat, Procardia) (see page 277 for the Drug Profile box)	PO; 10–20 mg tid (max: 180 mg/day)	Selective for calcium channels in blood vessels; decreases peripheral vascular resistance and increases cardiac output; also for hypertension and angina; sustained-release form available
nimodipine (Nimotop)	PO; 60 mg every 4 hours for 21 days; start therapy within 96 hours of subarachnoid hemorrhage	Offlabeled use for migraines; primary use is for improvement of neurologic symptoms following a stroke

continued . . .

TABLE 14.4	Antimigraine Drugs—*Continued*	
DRUG	**ROUTE AND ADULT DOSE**	**REMARKS**
verapamil (Calan, Isoptin, others) (see page 316 for the Drug Profile box)	PO; 40–80 mg tid	Offlabeled use for migraine prevention
Tricyclic Antidepressants amitriptyline hydrochloride (Elavil)	PO; 75–100 mg/day	Offlabeled use for migraine prevention
imipramine (Tofranil) (see page 137 for the Drug Profile box)	PO; 75–100 mg/day (max: 300 mg/day)	May cause cardiac dysfunction and abnormal blood cell count; also for alcohol or cocaine dependence; may control bedwetting in children; available IM
protriptyline (Vivactil)	PO; 15–40 mg/day in three to four divided doses (max: 60 mg/day)	For symptoms of depression; few sedative qualities; causes increased heart rate
Miscellaneous Drugs methysergide (Sansert)	PO; 4–8 mg/day in divided doses	Similar to ergotamine; for migraine prevention
riboflavin (vitamin B_2)	PO; as a supplement: 5–10 mg/day; for deficiency: 5–30 mg/day in divided doses	Deficiency caused by chronic diarrhea, liver disease, alcoholism, or inadequate consumption of milk or animal products

Ergot Alkaloids

For patients who are unresponsive to triptans, the ergot alkaloids may be used to stop migraines. The actions of the ergot alkaloids have been known for thousands of years. The first purified alkaloid, ergotamine (Ergostat), was isolated from the ergot fungus in 1920. Ergotamine is an inexpensive drug that is available in oral, sublingual, and suppository forms. Modification of the original molecule has produced a number of other useful drugs, such as dihydroergotamine (Migranal). Dihydroergotamine is given parenterally and as a nasal spray. Because the ergot alkaloids interact with adrenergic and dopaminergic receptors as well as serotonin receptors, they produce multiple actions and adverse effects. Many ergot alkaloids are pregnancy category X drugs.

DRUG PROFILE: ℗ *Sumatriptan (Imitrex)*

Therapeutic Class: Antimigraine drug
Pharmacologic Class: Triptan, 5-HT (serotonin) receptor drug, vasoconstrictor of intracranial arteries

Actions and Uses:

Sumatriptan belongs to a relatively new group of antimigraine drugs known as the triptans. The triptans act by causing vasoconstriction of cranial arteries; this vasoconstriction is moderately selective and does not usually affect overall blood pressure. This medication is available in oral, intranasal, and subcutaneous forms. Subcutaneous administration ends migraine attacks in 10 to 20 minutes; the dose may be repeated 60 minutes after the first injection to a maximum of two doses per day. If taken orally, sumatriptan should be administered as soon as possible after the migraine is suspected or has begun.

Adverse Effects and Interactions:

Some dizziness, drowsiness, or a warming sensation may be experienced after taking sumatriptan; however, these effects are not normally severe enough to warrant stopping therapy. Because of its vasoconstricting action, the drug should be used cautiously, if at all, in patients with recent MI, or with a history of angina pectoris, hypertension, or diabetes.

Sumatriptan interacts with several drugs. For example, an increased effect may occur when taken with MAOIs and selective serotonin reuptake inhibitors (SSRIs). Further vasoconstriction can occur when taken with ergot alkaloids and other triptans.

Refer to MyNursingKit for a Nursing Process Focus specific to this drug.

Other Antimigraine Drugs

Drugs for migraine prophylaxis include many classes of drugs discussed throughout this text-book. These include beta-adrenergic blockers (see Chapter 19 ⬮), calcium channel blockers (see Chapter 17 ⬮), antidepressants (see Chapter 10 ⬮), and antiseizure drugs (see Chapter 13 ⬮). Because these drugs have the potential to produce adverse effects, prophylaxis is started only if the number of migraines is high and the patient does not respond to the drugs used to stop migraines. Of the various drugs, propranolol (Inderal, InnoPran XL) is one of the most commonly prescribed. Amitriptyline (Elavil) is an example of a mood disorder drug for patients suffering from anxiety symptoms and insomnia in addition to migraines.

PATIENTS NEED TO KNOW

Patients taking pain medication need to know the following facts and recommendations:

In General

1. Carefully describe pain to your health care provider so that the analgesic medication being taken is suited to the complaint.
2. Report any OTC medication taken for pain to your health care provider to minimize adverse effects and interactions.
3. Aspirin has many undesirable adverse effects mainly related to gastric upset and bleeding.
4. Follow instructions carefully and watch for drug interactions or contraindications.

Regarding Opiates

5. Avoid combining pain medications with alcohol and other CNS depressants (especially opioids).
6. Vital signs will be monitored with all opioid medications because of their CNS depressant effects.
7. Get up slowly from seated positions because certain pain medications cause lightheadedness.
8. Avoid operating machinery or driving a car if taking opiates because dizziness, blurred vision, and drowsiness can occur.
9. Do not abruptly stop taking opioids; this could result in withdrawal. Signs include chills, abdominal and muscle cramps, severe itching, sweating, restlessness, anxiety, yawning, and drug-seeking behavior.

CHAPTER REVIEW

CORE CONCEPTS SUMMARY

14.1 **Pain assessment is the first step to pain management.**

Pain is a subjective experience in which many patients describe discomfort differently. Pain may be classified as acute (from injury to recovery) or chronic (longer than 6 months). Pain may be classified as nociceptor pain and further divided into somatic or visceral pain and neuropathic pain.

14.2 **Nonpharmacologic techniques assist patients in obtaining adequate pain relief.**

Nonpharmacologic techniques may be used in place of drugs or as an adjunct to drug therapy. When used along with medication, nonpharmaco-

logic techniques may allow lower doses to be given with possibly fewer drug-related adverse effects. More invasive techniques in patients with intractable pain may include chemotherapy, surgery, radiation therapy, and injection of alcohol or neurotoxic substances for nerve blocks.

14.3 **Pain transmission processes allow several targets for pharmocologic intervention.**

Pain signals involve nerve impulses along two types of sensory neurons, Aδ and C fibers. Once impulses reach the spinal cord, substance P is thought to transmit pain at the spinal level. The release of substance P is controlled by descending neurons that release neurotransmitters called *endogenous opioids*. If not blocked, the impulse travels to the brain, where pain information is sensed and a response to the sensation is initiated. Opioids act at the level of the central nervous system (CNS); nonsteroidal anti-inflammatory drugs (NSAIDs) act at the level of the peripheral nervous system (PNS).

14.4 Opioid analgesic medications exert their effects by interacting with specific receptors.

Two types of receptors mediate analgesia (pain relief)—mu receptors and kappa receptors. Both are opioid receptors that respond to natural or synthetic morphine-like substances. Natural substances extracted from unripe seeds of the poppy plant are called *opiates*. *Narcotic* is a general term referring to morphine-like drugs. In the context of drug enforcement, the term *narcotic* includes a much broader classification of abused illegal drugs.

14.5 Narcotic opioids have multiple therapeutic effects, including relief of severe pain.

Opioids produce many effects, including analgesia for intense pain, cough suppression, suppression of GI motility in diarrhea treatment, sedation, and euphoria. It is common practice to place opioids and nonnarcotic analgesics in a single tablet or capsule. Acute opioid intoxication is treated with the opioid antagonist naloxone. All of the narcotic analgesics have the potential to cause physical and psychological dependence. The opioids have a greater risk of dependency than most any of the other classes of medications. In treating opioid dependence, medication is often switched to another narcotic drug with less intense withdrawal symptoms.

14.6 Nonsteroidal anti-inflammatory drugs are the drugs of choice for inflammatory pain.

NSAIDs are used to treat less severe pain associated with inflammation. NSAIDs have antifever as well as pain-reducing properties. These effects are achieved by inhibition of enzymes called cyclooxygenase type one (COX-1) and cyclooxygenase type two (COX-2). When cyclooxygenase (COX) is inhibited, prostaglandin synthesis is prevented. Some medications are selective for the COX-2 receptor. Other antifever and pain-reducing medications, including acetaminophen and centrally acting drugs, do not have anti-inflammatory or COX-inhibiting properties.

14.7 Headaches can be effectively treated with a variety of drug classes.

Headaches in two categories—tension headaches and migraines—are the most common complaints of patients. The two primary goals of migraine therapy are migraine termination and migraine prevention. The two major classes of antimigraine drugs are ergot alkaloids and triptans. Drugs for migraine prophylaxis include beta-adrenergic blockers, calcium channel blockers, antidepressants, and antiseizure drugs.

REVIEW QUESTIONS

The following questions are written in NCLEX-PN® style. Answer these questions to assess your knowledge of the chapter material, and go back and review any material that is not clear to you.

1. The patient has osteoarthritis. Which of the following drugs would the nurse anticipate being ordered?

1. Sumatriptan (Imitrex)
2. Acetaminophen (Tylenol)
3. Fentanyl (Sublimaze)
4. Etodolac (Lodine)

2. The patient is on sumatriptan (Imitrex) for migraines. For which of the following should the nurse instruct the patient to notify his physician immediately?

1. Chest pain
2. GI upset
3. Bleeding
4. Lethargy

3. When a patient is receiving an NSAID, the nurse must assess the patient for:

1. GI upset and bleeding
2. Urinary retention

3. Blurred vision
4. Anorexia, headache

4. The patient is experiencing opioid dependency. Which drug is used to treat this condition?

1. Oxycodone hydrochloride (OxyContin)
2. Propoxyphene hydrochloride (Darvon)
3. Hydromorphone hydrochloride (Dilaudid)
4. Methadone (Dolophine)

5. The nurse understands that pain signals begin at the _____ and proceed through the central nervous system.

1. Spinal cord
2. Viscera
3. Nociceptors
4. Substance P

6. Prior to administering pain medication, what must be assessed?

1. The patient's diagnosis
2. The location, severity, and quality of pain
3. When the patient last had a meal
4. The patient's susceptibility to addiction

7. The patient has been receiving morphine sulfate for pain control. Assessment reveals a decreased level of consciousness and shallow respirations at a rate of 8 per minute. The nurse anticipates what opioid antagonist being ordered?

1. Butorphanol (Stadol)
2. Hydrocodone bitartrate (Hycodan)
3. Naloxone hydrochloride (Narcan)
4. Oxycodone hydrochloride (OxyContin)

8. The patient is allergic to aspirin. Which of the following drugs may be an alternative for relief of mild pain?

1. Acetaminophen
2. Morphine sulfate
3. Etodolac (Lodine)
4. Fentanyl (Sublimaze)

9. Adverse effects of ergotamine (Ergostate) include:

1. Bradycardia, chest pain, and hypertension
2. Nausea, vomiting, chest pain, and tachycardia
3. Urinary retention, hypertension, and peripheral dilation
4. Peripheral constriction, bradycardia, and chest pain

10. Chronic pain is:

1. Intense and lasts less than 3 months
2. Persistent, interferes with daily activities, and lasts longer than 6 months
3. Somatic in nature, which makes it difficult to treat
4. Neuropathic in nature, which makes it difficult to treat

CASE STUDY QUESTIONS

For questions 1– 4 please refer to the following case study, and choose the correct response from choices 1–4.

*M*s. Coidiuf, age 42, sustained a back injury 3 years ago, which responded well to treatment with nonsteroidal anti-inflammatory medication. Over the last 6 months, Ms. Coidiuf has been seeing her physician again with complaints of painful sensations "shooting" down her right hip. Despite careful attention, it appears that Ms. Coidiuf's pain is no longer responding to anti-inflammatory medication. Her physician prescribes a narcotic analgesic (moderate effectiveness) with acetaminophen, hoping this treatment might provide relief. Following three physical therapy sessions, the patient continues to report that she is "still miserable," leading her physician to believe that her condition is worsening. Heat packs, massage, and relaxation therapy have not been successful.

1. The most likely target of pharmacologic intervention for Ms. Coidiuf 3 years ago was:

1. Inhibition of spinal substance P release
2. Release of endorphin neurotransmitters in the central nervous system (CNS)
3. Inhibition of pain transmitted by Aδ fibers
4. Inhibition of cyclooxygenase (COX) enzyme

2. Which of the following narcotic analgesics was probably given to Ms. Coidiuf?

1. Percocet
2. Talwin
3. Dilaudid
4. Demerol

3. Which of the following symptoms has Ms. Coidiuf likely avoided by her physician switching to narcotic therapy?

1. Decreased GI motility
2. GI bleeding
3. Drowsiness
4. Vomiting

4. With continued pharmacologic intervention, which of the following would be less of a concern for Ms. Coidiuf?

1. Tolerance to the medication
2. Withdrawal symptoms
3. Sedation
4. Respiratory depression

FURTHER STUDY

- More information on the following classes of drugs can be found in these chapters: beta-adrenergic blockers (Chapter 8 ⓒⓒ), calcium channel blockers (Chapter 17 ⓒⓒ), antidepressants (Chapter 10 ⓒⓒ), and antiseizure drugs (Chapter 13 ⓒⓒ).

- NSAIDs used for inflammation are presented in Chapter 23 ⓒⓒ.

- The use of acetylcysteine as an antidote for acetaminophen overdose is discussed in Chapter 27 ⓒⓒ.

- Opioids used to treat diarrhea are covered in Chapter 28 ⓒⓒ.

EXPLORE PEARSON mynursingkit™

MyNursingKit is your one stop for online chapter review materials and resources. Prepare for success with additional NCLEX®-style practice questions, interactive assignments and activities, web links, animations and videos, and more!

Register your access code from the front of your book at
www.mynursingkit.com

15 Drugs for Anesthesia

CORE CONCEPTS

15.1 Local anesthesia causes a rapid loss of sensation to a limited part of the body.

15.2 Local anesthetics produce their therapeutic effect by blocking the entry of sodium ions into neurons.

15.3 Local anesthetics are classified by their chemical structures.

15.4 General anesthesia is a loss of sensation occurring throughout the entire body, accompanied by a loss of consciousness.

15.5 General anesthetics are usually administered by the IV or inhalation routes.

15.6 Intravenous anesthetics are important supplements to general anesthesia and include barbiturates, opioids, and benzodiazepines.

15.7 Nonanesthetic drugs are used as adjuncts to anesthesia and include barbiturates, barbiturate-like drugs, opioids, neuromuscular blocking agents, and other miscellaneous drugs.

DRUG SNAPSHOT

The following drugs are discussed in this chapter:

DRUG CLASSES	DRUG PROFILES
Local Anesthesia	
Amides	**Pr** lidocaine (Xylocaine)
Esters	
Miscellaneous agents	
General Anesthesia	
Inhalation agents	

DRUG CLASSES	DRUG PROFILES
Gases	**Pr** nitrous oxide
Volatile liquids	**Pr** halothane (Fluothane)
Intravenous agents	**Pr** thiopental (Pentothal)
Adjuncts to Anesthesia	
Neuromuscular blockers	**Pr** succinylcholine (Anectine)

LEARNING OUTCOMES

After reading this chapter, the student should be able to:

1. Compare and contrast the five major routes for administering local anesthetics.

2. Describe differences between the two major chemical classes of local anesthetics.

3. Explain why epinephrine and sodium hydroxide are sometimes included as part of the local anesthetic medicine.

4. Identify the actions of general anesthetics within the central nervous system (CNS).

5. Compare and contrast the two primary ways that general anesthesia may be induced.

6. Identify the four stages of general anesthesia.

7. For each of the drug classes listed, name representative drugs and explain their mechanisms of action, primary actions, and important adverse effects.

8. Categorize drugs used for anesthesia based on their classifications and actions in the body.

KEY TERMS

amides (AM-ides) *236*

anesthesia (ANN-ess-THEE-zee-uh) *233*

esters (ES-turs) *236*

general anesthesia *233*

local anesthesia *233*

Anesthesia is a medical procedure performed by administering drugs that cause a loss of sensation. **Local anesthesia** occurs when sensation is lost to a limited part of the body without loss of consciousness. **General anesthesia** requires different classes of drugs that cause loss of sensation to the entire body, usually resulting in a loss of consciousness. This chapter examines drugs used for both local and general anesthesia.

an = *without*
thesia = *sensation*

LOCAL ANESTHESIA

Local anesthesia is loss of sensation to a relatively small part of the body without loss of consciousness to the patient. This technique may be necessary when a relatively brief dental or medical procedure is performed.

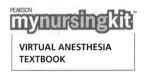

PEARSON
mynursingkit

VIRTUAL ANESTHESIA
TEXTBOOK

Local anesthesia causes a rapid loss of sensation to a limited part of the body.

CORE CONCEPT 15.1

Although local anesthesia often causes a loss of sensation to a small, limited area, it sometimes affects relatively large portions of the body, such as an entire limb. Because of this action, some local anesthetic treatments are more accurately called *surface anesthesia* or *regional anesthesia,* depending on how the drugs are administered and the results they produce.

The five major routes (Figure 15.1 ■) for applying local anesthetics are the following:

1. Topical
2. Infiltration
3. Nerve block
4. Spinal
5. Epidural

Fast Facts Anesthesia and Anesthetics

■ The first medical applications of anesthetics involved ether (in 1842) and nitrous oxide (in 1846).

■ Over 20 million people receive anesthetics each year in the United States.

■ Most of the general public associate use of local anesthetic drugs with the practice of dentistry or topical skin medications.

■ About half of the general anesthetics in medical practice are administered by a nurse anesthetist.

■ Herbal products may interact with anesthetics; for example, St. John's wort may intensify or prolong the effects of some opioids and anesthetics.

FIGURE 15.1

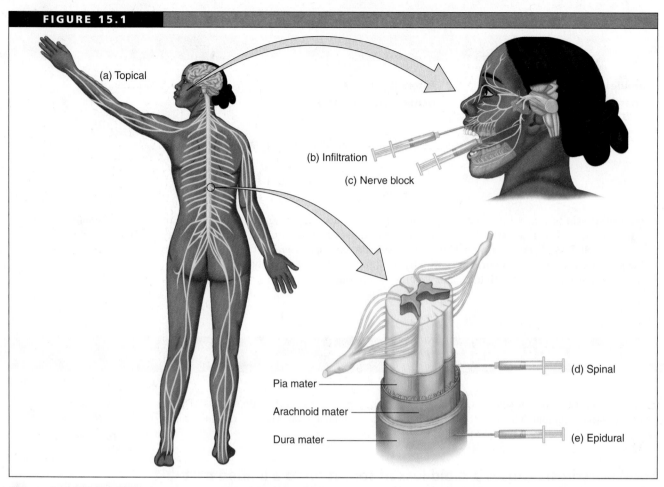

(a) Topical

(b) Infiltration

(c) Nerve block

(d) Spinal

(e) Epidural

Pia mater

Arachnoid mater

Dura mater

Routes for applying local anesthesia include (a) topical, (b) infiltration, (c) nerve block, (d) spinal, and (e) epidural.

The method used depends on the location and amount of anesthesia that is needed. For example, some local anesthetics are applied topically before a needlestick or minor skin surgery. Others are used to block sensations to large areas such as limbs or the lower abdomen. The different methods of local and regional anesthesia are summarized in Table 15.1.

TABLE 15.1 | **Methods of Local and Regional Anesthesia**

ROUTE	FORMULATION/METHOD	DESCRIPTION
Epidural anesthesia	Injection into the epidural space of the spinal cord	Most commonly used in obstetrics during labor and delivery
Infiltration (field block) anesthesia	Direct injection into tissue immediate to the surgical site	Drug diffuses into tissue to block a specific group of nerves in a small area very close to the area to be operated on
Nerve block anesthesia	Direct injection into tissue that may be distant from the operation site	Drug affects the bundle of nerves serving the area to be operated on; used to block sensation in a limb or large area of the face
Spinal anesthesia	Injection into the cerebrospinal spinal fluid (CSF)	Drug affects large, regional area such as the lower abdomen and legs
Topical (surface) anesthesia	Creams, sprays, suppositories, drops, and lozenges	Applied to mucous membranes, including the eyes, lips, gums, nasal membranes, and throat; very safe unless absorbed

■ What is local anesthesia? Name the five general routes for local and regional anesthesia.

Local anesthetics produce their therapeutic effect by blocking the entry of sodium ions into neurons.

CORE CONCEPT **15.2**

The mechanism of action by which neurons conduct electrical impulses is well known. Recall that the concentration of sodium is normally higher outside the neurons compared to the inside. A rapid influx of sodium ions into the cell is necessary for neurons to conduct an action potential and to fire.

Local anesthetics act by blocking sodium channels, as illustrated in Figure 15.2 ■. The blocking of sodium channels is nonselective; therefore, both sensory and motor impulses are affected. Sensation and muscle activity in the treated area will be decreased temporarily. Because of this mechanism of action, local anesthetics are sometimes called *sodium channel blockers*.

During a medical or surgical procedure, it is essential that the anesthetic lasts for at least until the procedure is completed. Small amounts of epinephrine are sometimes added to the anesthetic solution in order to constrict blood vessels in the immediate area (where the local anesthetic is applied). This keeps the drug active at the injected site and lengthens its duration of action. The addition of epinephrine to lidocaine (Xylocaine), for example, increases the anesthetic effect from about 20 minutes to 60 minutes. Prolonging the anesthetic effect is important; otherwise, a second injection would be necessary.

Sometimes an alkaline substance, such as sodium hydroxide or sodium bicarbonate, is added to anesthetic solutions to increase the drug's effectiveness in areas with extensive local infection or abscesses. The reason for this is that bacteria tend to acidify an infected site, and local anesthetics are less effective in an acidic environment. Adding alkaline substances neutralizes the infected region and allows the anesthetic to work better.

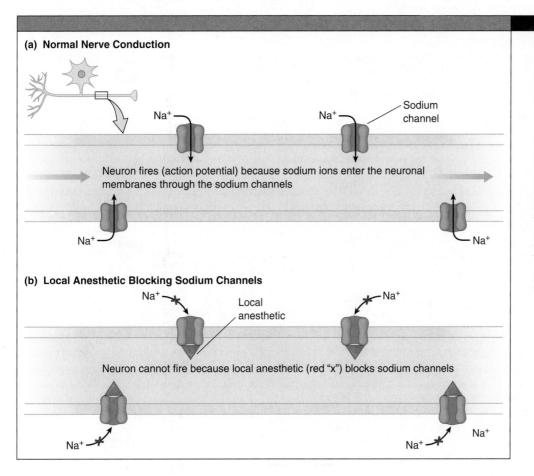

FIGURE 15.2

(a) Normal Nerve Conduction

(b) Local Anesthetic Blocking Sodium Channels

(a) In normal nerve conduction, sodium ions (Na$^+$) enter the sodium channels along a neuron and allow the neuron to fire (set off an action potential) and conduct an impulse. (b) Local anesthetics (represented by the red x) block the sodium channels. Sodium ions are not able to enter the neuronal membrane through the sodium channels. Therefore, no action potential can be conducted along the nerve.

Local anesthetics are classified by their chemical structures.

The two major classes of local anesthetics are **esters** and **amides** (Table 15.2). The terms *ester* and *amide* refer to types of chemical linkages found within the anesthetic molecules, as illustrated in Figure 15.3 ■. A small number of miscellaneous agents are neither esters nor amides.

Cocaine, the first local anesthetic widely used for medical procedures, was used as far back as the 1880s. Cocaine is a natural ester, found in the leaves of the plant *Erythroxylon coca,* native to the Andes Mountains of Peru. As late as the 1980s, cocaine was routinely used for eye surgery, nerve blocks, and spinal anesthesia. Although still available for local anesthesia, cocaine is a Schedule II drug and rarely used therapeutically in the United States. The abuse potential of cocaine is discussed in Chapter 7 ⚭ .

Another ester, procaine (Novocain), was the drug of choice for dental procedures from the mid-1900s to the 1960s. About that time, amide anesthetics were developed, and use of the ester anesthetics declined. One ester, benzocaine (Solarcaine and others), is used as a topical over-the-counter (OTC) agent for treating a large number of painful conditions, including sunburn, insect bites, hemorrhoids, sore throat, and minor wounds.

In most cases, amides have replaced the esters because they produce fewer adverse effects and generally have a longer duration of action. Lidocaine (Xylocaine) is the most widely used amide for short surgical procedures requiring local anesthesia.

TABLE 15.2	**History of Selected Local Anesthetics**	
DRUG	**USE**	**REMARKS**
ESTERS		
benzocaine (Americaine, Anbesol, others) (see page 621 for the Drug Profile box)	Topical anesthesia	For sunburn, sore throat, earache, hemorrhoids, and other minor skins conditions
chloroprocaine (Nesacaine)	Infiltration, nerve block, and epidural anesthesia	Short duration
cocaine	Topical anesthesia	For ear, nose, and throat procedures
procaine (Novocain)	Infiltration, nerve block, epidural, and spinal anesthesia	Short duration
tetracaine (Pontocaine)	Topical and spinal anesthesia	Longer duration
AMIDES		
articaine (Septodont, Septanest)	Infiltration and nerve block anesthesia	Longer duration
bupivicaine (Marcaine)	Infiltration and epidural anesthesia	Longer duration
dibucaine (Nupercaine, Nupercainal)	Topical or spinal anesthesia	Longer duration
etidocaine (Duranest)	Infiltration, nerve block, and epidural anesthesia	Longer duration
Pr lidocaine (Xylocaine)	Topical anesthesia, infiltration, nerve block, epidural, and spinal anesthesia	May be combined as a mixture of lidocaine and prilocaine (EMLA cream) for topical application
mepivacaine (Carbocaine)	Infiltration, nerve block, and epidural anesthesia	Intermediate duration
prilocaine (Citanest)	Infiltration, nerve block, and epidural anesthesia	Intermediate duration
ropivacaine (Naropin)	Infiltration, nerve block, and epidural anesthesia	Longer duration
MISCELLANEOUS AGENTS		
dyclonine (Dyclone)	Topical anesthesia	For ear, nose, and throat procedures
pramoxine (Tronothane)	Topical anesthesia	For minor medical procedures

FIGURE 15.3

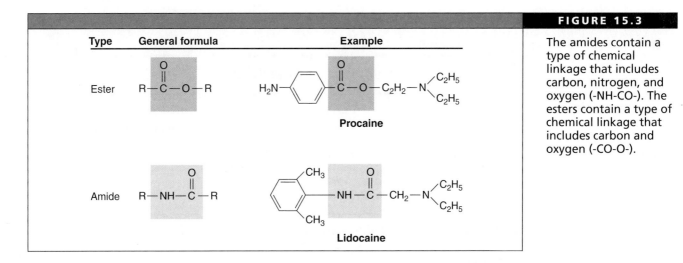

The amides contain a type of chemical linkage that includes carbon, nitrogen, and oxygen (-NH-CO-). The esters contain a type of chemical linkage that includes carbon and oxygen (-CO-O-).

Adverse effects to local anesthesia are uncommon. Allergy is rare. When it does occur, it is often due to sulfites, which are added as preservatives to prolong the shelf life of the anesthetic, or to methylparaben, which may be added to prevent bacterial growth in anesthetic solutions. Early signs of adverse effects of local anesthetics include symptoms of CNS stimulation such as restlessness or anxiety. Later, drowsiness and unresponsiveness may occur due to CNS depression. Cardiovascular effects, including hypotension and dysrhythmias, are possible. Patients with a history of cardiovascular disease are often given forms of local anesthetics that contain no epinephrine to reduce the possible effects of this sympathomimetic on the heart and blood pressure. CNS and cardiovascular adverse effects are rare unless the local anesthetic is absorbed rapidly or is accidentally injected directly into a blood vessel.

Concept Review   15.2

■ How does a local anesthetic work? How does the anesthetic action of lidocaine with epinephrine differ from that of lidocaine without epinephrine?

DRUG PROFILE: ℗ *Lidocaine (Xylocaine)*

Therapeutic Class: Anesthetic (local/regional/topical), antidysrhythmic (class IB)
Pharmacologic Class: Sodium channel blocker; amide

Actions and Uses:

Lidocaine is the most frequently used injectable local anesthetic. It is available in solutions ranging from 0.5% to 2% for infiltration, nerve block, spinal, or epidural anesthesia. A topical form is also available. When given for anesthesia, its onset of action is 5–15 minutes. Several hours may be needed for complete sensation to reappear. Lidocaine is also given IV, IM, or subcutaneously to treat dysrhythmias, as discussed in Chapter 19 ⚭ . Solutions of lidocaine containing preservatives or epinephrine are used for local anesthesia only and must never be given parenterally for dysrhythmias.

Adverse Effects and Interactions:

When used for anesthesia, adverse effects are uncommon. An early symptom of toxicity is excitement, leading to irritability and confusion. Serious adverse effects include convulsions, respiratory depression, and cardiac arrest. Until the effect of the anesthetic diminishes, patients may injure themselves by biting or chewing areas of the mouth that have no sensation following a dental procedure.

Barbiturates may decrease activity of lidocaine. Increased effects of lidocaine occur if taken with cimetidine, quinidine, and beta blockers. If lidocaine is used on a regular basis, its effectiveness may diminish when used with other medications.

Mechanism in Action:

Lidocaine acts as a local anesthetic to block neuronal pain impulses and as an antidysrhythmic to correct ventricular fibrillation and tachycardia. These actions are achieved by blocking sodium channels located within the membranes of neurons and cardiac muscle cells.

Refer to MyNursingKit for a Nursing Process Focus specific to this drug.

NURSING PROCESS FOCUS

Patients Receiving Local Anesthesia

ASSESSMENT
Prior to administration:
- Assess for allergies to amide-type local anesthetics
- Check for the presence of broken skin, infections, burns, and wounds where medication is to be applied
- Assess for character, duration, location, and intensity of pain where medication is to be applied

POTENTIAL NURSING DIAGNOSES
- Risk for Injury related to lack of sensation to a part of the body caused by the drug.
- Pain related to administration of drug.
- Deficient Knowledge related to information about drug therapy.

PLANNING: PATIENT GOALS AND EXPECTED OUTCOMES
The patient will:
- Experience no pain during surgical procedure
- Experience no adverse effects from anesthesia

IMPLEMENTATION

Interventions and (Rationales)	Patient Education/Discharge Planning
Monitor for cardiovascular adverse effects. (These may occur if anesthetic is absorbed.)	Instruct the patient to report any unusual heart palpitations, lightheadedness, drowsiness, or confusion. If using medication on a regular basis, instruct the patient to see the health care provider regularly.
Monitor skin or mucous membranes for infection or inflammation. (Condition could be worsened by the drug.)	Instruct the patient to report irritation or increase in discomfort in areas where medication was used.
Monitor for length of effectiveness. (Local anesthetics are effective for 1–3 hours.)	Instruct the patient to report any discomfort during the procedure.
Obtain information on and monitor the use of other medications.	Instruct the patient to report use of any medications to the health care provider.
Provide for patient safety. (There is a potential for injury related to the fact that the area being treated lacks sensation.)	Inform the patient about having no feeling in the anesthetized area and taking extra caution to avoid injury, including heat-related injury.
Monitor for gag reflex if used in the mouth or throat. (Xylocaine viscous may interfere with the swallowing reflex.)	Instruct the patient to: - Not eat within 1 hour of administration - Not chew gum while any portion of the mouth or throat is anesthetized to prevent biting injuries

EVALUATION OF OUTCOME CRITERIA
Evaluate the effectiveness of drug therapy by confirming that patient goals and expected outcomes have been met (see "Planning").

See Table 15.2 for a list of drugs to which these nursing actions apply.

GENERAL ANESTHESIA

General anesthesia involves loss of sensation to the entire body. General anesthetics are used when it is necessary for patients to remain still and without pain for a period longer than could be achieved with local anesthetics.

Oil of Cloves for Dental Pain

One natural remedy for tooth pain is oil of cloves, a natural substance whose use dates back thousands of years in Chinese medicine. Extracted from the clove plant *Eugenia*, eugenol is the active chemical that produces a numbing effect. It works especially well for dental caries (cavities). The herb is applied by soaking a piece of cotton and packing it around the gums close to the affected tooth. Dentists sometimes recommend it for temporary relief of a toothache. Clove oil has an antiseptic effect that has been reported to kill microorganisms.

Other uses of clove oil that lack reliable scientific evidence include treatment of premature ejaculation, low libido, and fever reduction. Clove oil is very safe, with rash and gastrointestinal (GI) upset being the most common adverse effects. Clove oil may increase the risk for bleeding and should be used cautiously in patients taking anticoagulants.

General anesthesia is a loss of sensation occurring throughout the entire body, accompanied by a loss of consciousness.

CORE CONCEPT 15.4

The goal of general anesthesia is to provide a rapid and complete loss of sensation. Signs of general anesthesia include total analgesia (no feeling of pain) and loss of consciousness, memory, and body movement. Although these signs are similar to those of sleeping, general anesthesia and sleep are not exactly the same. General anesthetics stop most nervous activity in the brain, whereas sleeping stops activity in only very specific areas. If fact, some brain activity actually increases during sleep, as described in Chapter 9 ∞ .

General anesthesia usually requires more than one drug. Multiple medications are used to rapidly cause unconsciousness and muscle relaxation and to maintain deep anesthesia. This approach, called *balanced anesthesia,* allows the dose of inhalation anesthetic to be lower so that the procedure is safer for the patient.

General anesthesia occurs in distinct steps, or stages. The most effective medications can quickly cause all four stages, whereas others are only able to cause stage 1 (light sedation). Most major surgery occurs in stage 3, when skeletal muscles are relaxed and the patient is sedated. Stage 3 anesthesia is called *surgical anesthesia.* When a patient is given surgical anesthesia, the anesthesiologist will try to move quickly through stage 2 because this stage produces symptoms such as hyperactivity and irregular breathing and heart rate. Often an IV agent will be given to calm the patient during this stage. The stages of general anesthesia are shown in Table 15.3.

General anesthetics are usually administered by the IV or inhalation routes.

CORE CONCEPT 15.5

There are two primary methods of causing general anesthesia. Intravenous agents are usually administered first because they act within a few seconds. After the patient loses consciousness, inhaled agents are used to maintain the anesthesia. During short surgical procedures or those requiring lower stages of anesthesia, the IV agents may be used alone.

TABLE 15.3	Stages of General Anesthesia
Stage 1	Loss of pain; the patient loses general sensation but may be awake. This stage proceeds until the patient loses consciousness.
Stage 2	Excitement and hyperactivity; the patient may be delirious and try to resist treatment. Heartbeat and breathing may become irregular, and blood pressure can increase. This is the stage when some IV agents are administered to calm the patient.
Stage 3	Surgical anesthesia; skeletal muscles become relaxed and delirium stabilizes; cardiovascular and breathing respiratory activities stabilize. Eye movements slow down and the patient becomes very still. This is the stage during which surgery occurs.
Stage 4	Paralysis of the medulla region in the brain responsible for controlling respiratory and cardiovascular activity. If breathing or the heart stops, death could result. This stage is usually avoided during general anesthesia.

TABLE 15.4	Inhaled General Anesthetics
DRUG	**USE**
VOLATILE LIQUID	
desflurane (Suprane)	Induction and maintenance of general anesthesia
enflurane (Ethrane)	Induction and maintenance of general anesthesia
Pr halothane (Fluothane)	Induction and maintenance of general anesthesia; use has declined because safer agents are available
isoflurane (Forane)	Induction and maintenance of general anesthesia; most widely used inhalation anesthetic
methoxyflurane (Penthrane)	Used during labor because it does not suppress uterine contractions as much as other agents
sevoflurane (Ultane)	Induction and maintenance of general anesthesia
GAS	
Pr nitrous oxide	Used alone in dentistry, obstetrics, and short medical procedures; used in combination with more potent inhaled anesthetics

Inhaled general anesthetics, shown in Table 15.4, may be gases or volatile liquids. These agents produce their effects by preventing the flow of sodium into neurons in the CNS, thus delaying nerve impulses and producing a dramatic reduction in neural activity. The exact mechanism for how this occurs is not known, although it is likely that gamma-aminobutyric acid (GABA) receptors in the brain are activated. It is not the same mechanism as that of local anesthetics. There is some evidence suggesting that the mechanism may be related to how some antiseizure drugs work; however, this has not been proved. There is not a specific receptor that binds to general anesthetics, and they do not seem to affect neurotransmitter release.

The only gas used routinely for anesthesia is nitrous oxide, commonly called *laughing gas.* Nitrous oxide is used for dental procedures and for brief obstetrical and surgical procedures. It may also be used together with other general anesthetics, making it possible to increase their effectiveness while decreasing their dosages.

DRUG PROFILE: Pr *Nitrous Oxide*

Therapeutic Class: General anesthetic
Pharmacologic Class: Inhalation gaseous agent

Actions and Uses:

The main action of nitrous oxide is analgesia caused by suppression of pain mechanisms in the CNS. This agent has a low potency and does not produce complete loss of consciousness or extreme relaxation of skeletal muscle. Because nitrous oxide does not cause surgical anesthesia (Stage 3), it is commonly combined with other surgical anesthetic agents. Nitrous oxide is ideal for dental procedures because the patient remains conscious and can follow instruction while experiencing full analgesia.

Adverse Effects and Interactions:

When used in low to moderate doses, nitrous oxide produces few adverse effects. At higher doses, patients exhibit some adverse signs of Stage 2 anesthesia, such as anxiety, excitement, and combativeness. Lowering the inhaled dose will quickly reverse these adverse effects. As nitrous oxide is exhaled the patient may temporarily have some difficulty breathing at the end of a procedure. Nausea and vomiting following the procedure are more common with nitrous oxide than with other inhalation anesthetics. Nitrous oxide has the potential to be abused by users (sometimes medical personnel) who enjoy the relaxed, sedated state that the drug produces.

 Refer to MyNursingKit for a Nursing Process Focus specific to this drug.

DRUG PROFILE: 🅟 *Halothane (Fluothane)*

Therapeutic Class: General anesthetic
Pharmacologic Class: Inhalation volatile liquid

Actions and Uses:

Halothane produces a potent level of surgical anesthesia that is rapid in onset. Although potent, halothane does not produce as much muscle relaxation or analgesia as other volatile anesthetics. Therefore, halothane is primarily used with other anesthetic agents, including muscle relaxants and analgesics. Nitrous oxide is sometimes combined with halothane. Patients recover from anesthesia rapidly after halothane is discontinued.

Adverse Effects and Interactions:

Halothane moderately sensitizes the heart muscle to epinephrine; therefore, dysrhythmias are a concern. This agent lowers blood pressure and the respiration rate. It also stops reflex mechanisms that normally keep the contents of the stomach from being aspirated into the lungs. Because of potential liver toxicity, use of halothane has declined.

Malignant hyperthermia is rare, but it can be a fatal adverse effect triggered by all inhalation anesthetics. It causes muscle rigidity and severe temperature elevation (up to 43°C). This risk is greatest when halothane is used with succinylcholine.

Levodopa taken at the same time increases the level of dopamine in the CNS and should be stopped 6 to 8 hours before halothane administration.

Skeletal muscle weakness, respiratory depression, or apnea may occur if halothane is administered with polymyxins, lincomycin, or aminoglycosides.

Refer to MyNursingKit for a Nursing Process Focus specific to this drug.

Nitrous oxide should be used cautiously in patients with myasthenia gravis because it may cause respiratory depression and prolonged hypnotic effects. Patients with cardiovascular disease, especially those with increased intracranial pressure, should be monitored carefully because the hypnotic effects of the drug may be prolonged or more powerful.

The volatile anesthetics are liquid at room temperature but are converted into a vapor and inhaled to produce their anesthetic effects. Commonly administered volatile agents are halothane (Fluothane), enflurane (Ethrane), and isoflurane (Forane). The most potent of these is halothane (Fluothane). Some general anesthetics increase the sensitivity of the heart to drugs such as epinephrine, norepinephrine, dopamine, and serotonin. Most volatile liquids depress cardiovascular and respiratory function. Because isoflurane (Forane) has less effect on the heart and does not damage the liver, it has become the most widely used inhalation anesthetic. The volatile liquids are excreted almost entirely by the lungs through exhalation.

Intravenous anesthetics are important supplements to general anesthesia and include barbiturates, opioids, and benzodiazepines.

Although occasionally used alone, intravenous anesthetics are often administered with inhaled general anesthetics (Table 15.5). Administration of IV and inhaled anesthetics together allows the dose of the inhaled agent to be reduced, thereby lessening the possibility of serious adverse effects. Furthermore, when combined, they provide more analgesia and muscle relaxation than could be provided by the inhaled anesthetic alone. When IV anesthetics are administered without other anesthetics, they are generally used for medical procedures that take less than 15 minutes.

Drugs used as IV anesthetics include barbiturates, opioids, and benzodiazepines. Opioids offer the advantage of superior analgesia. For example, combining the opioid fentanyl (Sublimaze) with the antipsychotic agent droperidol (Inapsine) produces a state known as *neurolept analgesia.* In this state, patients are conscious but insensitive to pain and unaware of their surroundings. The premixed combination of these two agents is marketed as Innovar. A similar conscious, *dissociated* (that is, *unaware*) state is produced with ketamine (Ketalar).

TABLE 15.5	Intravenous Anesthetics
DRUG	**REMARKS**
BARBITURATE AND BARBITURATE-LIKE AGENTS	
etomidate (Amidate)	For induction of anesthesia; for short medical procedures
methohexital sodium (Brevital)	Ultrashort acting; for induction of anesthesia; used as a supplement to other anesthetic agents
propofol (Diprivan)	For induction and maintenance of general anesthesia; for short medical procedures
Pr thiopental (Pentothal)	Ultrashort acting; for induction of anesthesia; used as a supplement to other anesthetic agents
BENZODIAZEPINES	
diazepam (Valium) (see page 199 for the Drug Profile box)	For induction of anesthesia; prototype drug for the benzodiazepines
lorazepam (Ativan) (see page 122 for the Drug Profile box)	For induction of anesthesia and to produce conscious sedation; for short medical procedures or surgery
midazolam hydrochloride (Versed)	For induction of anesthesia and to produce conscious sedation; for short diagnostic procedures
OPIOIDS	
alfentanil hydrochloride (Alfenta)	Rapid onset and short duration of action; for induction of anesthesia; used as a supplement to other anesthetic agents
fentanyl citrate (Sublimaze, others)	Short-acting analgesic used during the operative and perioperative period; used to supplement both general and regional anesthesia
remifentanil hydrochloride (Ultiva)	Approximately seven times more potent than fentanyl; onset and duration of action more rapid than fentanyl; for induction and maintenance of anesthesia
sufentanil citrate (Sufenta)	Approximately 7 times more potent than fentanyl; onset and duration of action more rapid than fentanyl; for induction and maintenance of anesthesia
OTHERS	
ketamine (Ketalar)	For sedation, amnesia, and analgesia; for short diagnostic, therapeutic, or surgical procedures; most often used in children

Concept Review 15.3

■ What is the role of IV anesthetics in surgical anesthesia? Why are these drugs not used alone for general anesthesia?

ADJUNCTS TO ANESTHESIA

A number of drugs are used either to complement the effects of general anesthetics or to treat anticipated adverse effects of the anesthesia. These agents, shown in Table 15.6, are called *adjuncts* to anesthesia. They may be given prior to, during, or after surgery.

CORE CONCEPT 15.7

Nonanesthetic drugs are used as adjuncts to anesthesia and include barbiturates, barbiturate-like drugs, opioids, neuromuscular blocking agents, and other miscellaneous drugs.

pre = *before*
operative = *surgery*

The preoperative drugs given to relieve anxiety and to provide mild sedation include barbiturates or benzodiazepines. Opioids such as morphine may be given to counteract pain that the patient

DRUG PROFILE: Ⓟ Thiopental (Pentothal)

Therapeutic Class: General anesthetic

Pharmacologic Class: Intravenous induction agent; short-acting barbiturate

Actions and Uses:

Thiopental is the oldest IV anesthetic. It is used for brief medical procedures or to rapidly cause unconsciousness prior to administering inhaled anesthetics. It is classified as an ultrashort-acting barbiturate, having an onset time of less than 30 seconds and a duration of only 10 to 30 minutes. Unlike some anesthetic agents, it has very low analgesic properties.

Adverse Effects and Interactions:

Like other barbiturates, thiopental can produce severe respiratory depression when used in high doses. It is used with caution in patients with cardiovascular disease because of its ability to depress the myocardium and cause dysrhythmias. Patients may experience emergence delirium postoperatively. This causes hallucinations, confusion, and excitability.

Thiopental interacts with many other drugs. For example, use of CNS depressants increases respiratory and CNS depression. Phenothiazines increase the risk of hypotension. Use with caution with herbal supplements, such as kava and valerian, which may increase sedation.

Refer to MyNursingKit for a Nursing Process Focus specific to this drug.

TABLE 15.6	Selected Adjuncts to Anesthesia
DRUG	**REMARKS**
BARBITURATE AND BARBITURATE-LIKE AGENTS	
amobarbital (Amytal)	Intermediate duration; for preoperative sedation
butabarbital sodium (Butisol)	Intermediate duration; for preoperative sedation
pentobarbital (Nembutal)	Short duration; for preoperative sedation; potent, causes respiratory depression
secobarbital (Seconal)	Short duration; for preoperative sedation
OPIOIDS	
alfentanil hydrochloride (Alfenta)	Short duration; for induction of anesthesia when endotracheal or mechanical ventilation is needed; provides analgesia
fentanyl citrate (Duragesic, Actiq, others)	For analgesia during or after anesthesia; the combination of fentanyl and droperidol is called Innovar
remifentanil hydrochloride (Ultiva)	For analgesia during or after anesthesia; shorter duration of action than fentanyl
sufentanil citrate (Sufenta)	For primary anesthesia or to provide analgesia during or after anesthesia
DOPAMINE BLOCKERS	
droperidol (Inapsine)	For nausea and vomiting caused by opioids; reduces anxiety and relaxes muscles
promethazine (Phenergan)	For nausea and vomiting associated with obstetric sedation and opioids
NEUROMUSCULAR BLOCKERS	
mivacurium (Mivacron)	short duration; nondepolarizing type
Ⓟ succinylcholine (Anectine)	Short duration; depolarizing type
tubocurarine	Long duration; nondepolarizing type
CHOLINERGIC AGENT	
bethanechol (Duvoid, Urecholine) (see page 99 for the Drug Profile box)	For relief of constipation and urinary retention caused by opioids; stimulates GI motility

DRUG PROFILE: ℗ *Succinylcholine (Anectine)*

Therapeutic Class: Skeletal muscle paralytic agent, neuromuscular blocker
Pharmacologic Class: Depolarizing blocker, acetylcholine receptor blocking agent

Actions and Uses:

Like the natural neurotransmitter acetylcholine, succinylcholine acts on cholinergic receptor sites at neuromuscular junctions. At first, depolarization occurs, and skeletal muscles contract. After repeated contractions, however, the membrane is unable to repolarize as long as the drug stays on the receptor. Effects are first noted as muscle weakness and muscle spasms. Eventually paralysis occurs. Succinylcholine is rapidly broken down by the enzyme pseudocholinesterase; when the IV infusion is stopped, the duration of action is only a few minutes. Use of succinylcholine reduces the amount of general anesthetic needed for procedures.

Adverse Effects and Interactions:

Succinylcholine can cause complete paralysis of the diaphragm and intercostal muscles; thus, mechanical ventilation is necessary during surgery. Bradycardia and respiratory depression are expected adverse effects. If doses are high, tachycardia, hypotension, and urinary retention may occur. Patients with certain genetic defects may experience rapid onset of extremely high fever with muscle rigidity—a serious condition known as malignant hyperthermia.

Additive skeletal muscle blockade will occur if succinylcholine is given concurrently with clindamycin, aminoglycosides, furosemide, lithium, quinidine, or lidocaine.

Increased effect of succinylcholine may occur if given with phenothiazines oxytocin, promazine; tacrine, or thiazide diuretics. Decreased effect of succinylcholine occurs if given with diazepam.

If this drug is given with halothane or nitrous oxide, an increased risk of bradycardia, dysrhythmias, sinus arrest, apnea, and malignant hyperthermia exists. If succinylcholine is given with cardiac glycosides, there is increased risk of cardiac dysrhythmias. If narcotics are given with succinylcholine, there is increased risk of bradycardia and sinus arrest.

Refer to MyNursingKit for a Nursing Process Focus specific to this drug.

PATIENTS NEED TO KNOW

Patients treated with local anesthetic medications need to know the following:

1. When using topical anesthetics for skin conditions, avoid touching the eyes.
2. Never apply topical medications to large patches of skin or to areas where there is an open lesion or cut.
3. Notify the dentist or health care providers of any previous adverse reactions to local anesthesia before being given additional anesthetic medications.
4. After receiving local anesthetic solutions for the mouth, do not consume food and drink until it is clear that the anesthetic has worn off.
5. Do not chew or pick at an area where a dental procedure has been performed while the area is still numb.
6. Be careful not to inhale anesthetic sprays used for topical application.
7. Get immediate assistance if drowsiness, confusion, or blurred vision has occurred after receiving a local anethetic. Other signs/symptoms to look for include lightheadedness, an irregular heartbeat, or feeling faint.
8. Report all medications and conditions to the health care provider before receiving anesthetics.
9. For outpatient dental or medical procedures involving anesthesia, someone should be available to assist with activities such as transportation.
10. Follow postprocedure instructions carefully after anesthesia.
11. Have sufficient pain medication readily available so that postprocedure pain can be managed after the effects of the anesthesia are no longer felt.

will experience after surgery. Anticholinergics such as atropine may be administered to dry secretions and suppress the bradycardia caused by some anesthetics.

During surgery, the primary adjuncts are the *neuromuscular blockers*. These agents cause skeletal muscles to relax totally so that surgical procedures can be carried out safely. Administration of these drugs also allows the amount of anesthetic to be reduced. Neuromuscular blocking agents are classified as *depolarizing blockers* or *nondepolarizing blockers*. The prime depolarizing blocker is succinylcholine (Anectine), which works by binding to acetylcholine receptors at neuromuscular junctions to cause total skeletal muscle relaxation. Succinylcholine is used in surgery for ease of tracheal intubation. Mivacurium (Mivacron) is the shortest acting of the nondepolarizing blockers, whereas tubocurarine is a longer-acting neuromuscular blocking agent. The nondepolarizing blockers cause muscle paralysis by competing with acetylcholine for cholinergic receptors at the neuromuscular junctions. Upon binding to the receptors, nondepolarizing blockers prevent muscle contraction.

Postoperative drugs include analgesics for pain and antiemetics such as promethazine (Phenergan) for the nausea and vomiting that sometimes occur during recovery from the anesthesia. Occasionally, a parasympathomimetic such as bethanechol (Urecholine) is administered to stimulate the smooth muscle of the bowel and urinary tract to begin working again following surgery.

post = *after*
operative = *surgery*

anti = *against*
emetic = *vomiting*

CHAPTER REVIEW

CORE CONCEPTS SUMMARY

15.1 Local anesthesia causes a rapid loss of sensation to a limited part of the body.

Local anesthesia is loss of sensation to a relatively small part of the body without causing loss of consciousness. Sometimes local anesthesia is applied to an entire limb. In these cases, it is more accurately called *surface anesthesia* or *regional anesthesia,* depending on how the drugs are administered and the results they produce.

15.2 Local anesthetics produce their therapeutic effect by blocking the entry of sodium ions into neurons.

Blocking sodium entry into neurons prevents transmission of the electrical impulse along the nerve. Epinephrine is sometimes added to anesthetic solutions to increase the duration of action of the anesthetic. A base such as sodium hydroxide is added to make an infected tissue environment more alkaline.

15.3 Local anesthetics are classified by their chemical structures.

The two major classes of local anesthetics are esters and amides. Benzocaine (Solarcaine, others) is the most commonly used ester; lidocaine (Xylocaine) is the most widely prescribed amide.

15.4 General anesthesia is a loss of sensation occurring throughout the entire body, accompanied by a loss of consciousness.

General anesthesia proceeds in stages from light sedation to total loss of consciousness. The less potent anesthetics cause Stage 1 anesthesia, whereas more potent agents cause surgical anesthesia (Stage 3).

15.5 General anesthetics are usually administered by the IV or inhalation routes.

Two primary methods for producing rapid unconsciousness and total analgesia are IV agents and inhaled general anesthetics. IV agents include barbiturates and barbiturate-like agents, opioids, and benzodiazepines. Inhalation agents include nitrous oxide, the only gaseous agent, and volatile liquids. Many agents may be used alone or in combination with other agents. The mechanism by which general anesthetics produce their effect is not completely known.

15.6 Intravenous anesthetics are important supplements to general anesthesia and include barbiturates, opioids, and benzodiazepines.

Intravenous agents may be used along with inhaled anesthetics to lower the potential for serious adverse effects. Barbiturates, opioids, and benzodiazepines are generally reserved for quick medical procedures and treatments requiring superior analgesia.

15.7 Nonanesthetic drugs are used as adjuncts to anesthesia and include barbiturates, barbiturate-like drugs, opioids, neuromuscular blocking agents, and other miscellaneous drugs.

A number of drugs are given prior to surgery to relieve anxiety, provide mild sedation, counteract pain, and dry secretions. Neuromuscular blockers, given during surgery, relax skeletal muscle and maintain a proper heart rate. Drugs after surgery include agents for pain and vomiting and for activating the bowels and urinary tract.

REVIEW QUESTIONS

The following questions are written in NCLEX-PN® style. Answer these questions to assess your knowledge of the chapter material, and go back and review any material that is not clear to you.

1. This herbal product may prolong or intensify the effects of anesthesia.

1. Kava kava
2. Oil of cloves
3. Anise
4. St. John's wort

2. When toxic, this local anesthetic causes CNS excitement, irritability, and confusion.

1. Isoflurane (Forane)
2. Lidocaine (Xylocaine)
3. Nitrous oxide
4. Epinephrine

3. The patient in labor will most likely receive which type of anesthesia?

1. Nerve block
2. Epidural
3. Spinal
4. Surface

4. During anesthesia, the patient assessment reveals restlessness, blood pressure 196/110, pulse 128, and respirations 38. The patient is most likely in which stage of anesthesia?

1. Stage 1
2. Stage 2
3. Stage 3
4. Stage 4

5. This is the stage of anesthesia when surgery begins.

1. Stage 1
2. Stage 2
3. Stage 3
4. Stage 4

6. The patient being prepared for surgery asks the nurse why he is receiving meperidine (Demerol) and atropine prior to surgery. The nurse's best response would be:

1. "You will need to speak with your physician."
2. "The meperidine (Demerol) will help to control pain before and after surgery, whereas the atropine will help to decrease secretions."
3. "The meperidine (Demerol) and atropine will help your anesthetic work more effectively."
4. "These medications are routinely used before we send a patient to surgery."

7. The patient with a history of cardiovascular disease should receive anesthetics without epinephrine because it can cause:

1. Tachycardia and hypertension
2. Bradycardia and hypotension
3. Tachycardia and hypotension
4. Bradycardia and hypertension

8. The patient receives nitrous oxide in addition to thiopental (Pentothal):

1. To provide the additional anesthesia to put him in a sleep-like state
2. To increase the effectiveness of each drug at lower dosages
3. Because thiopental (Pentothal) is not effective when used alone
4. Because nitrous oxide is not effective when used alone

9. The patient is having a cyst removed under local anesthesia. The physician requests lidocaine (Xylocaine) with epinephrine. The nurse understands the addition of epinephrine is to:

1. Prevent infection
2. Prevent an allergic reaction
3. Increase the duration of the anesthetic
4. Decrease pain after the procedure

10. The patient is experiencing nausea in the recovery room. The nurse anticipates which medication being ordered?

1. Meperidine (Demerol)
2. Bethanechol (Urecholine)
3. Phenergan
4. Succinylcholine

CASE STUDY QUESTIONS

For questions 1–4, please refer to the following case study, and choose the correct answer from choices 1–4.

*M*r. Wand, age 77, has a history of cardiovascular disease. He has collapsed and sustained an injury to his scalp. The wound is substantial, and Mr. Wand is bleeding across his right forehead. The patient is rushed to the emergency department by his nephew. The nephew reports that his uncle is normally very fearful of doctors and nurses. It is unclear why Mr. Wand collapsed. The nurse decides to inject the tissue surrounding the wound with 1% lidocaine with epinephrine for local anesthesia prior to suturing the laceration.

1. The route of drug administration in this case is referred to as:

1. Topical (surface) anesthesia
2. Infiltration (field block) anesthesia
3. Nerve block anesthesia
4. Epidural anesthesia

2. Soon after administering this medication, the nurse should primarily be concerned with which of the following symptoms?

1. Constriction of airways
2. Anxiety
3. Tachycardia
4. Unresponsiveness

3. Would it be advisable to give Mr. Wand a barbiturate to help him calm down due to his fear of doctors and nurses in this case?

1. No, a barbiturate might *increase toxicity symptoms* if Mr. Wand is allergic to lidocaine.
2. Yes, a barbiturate might *increase the effectiveness of lidocaine* in this situation and help the patient calm down.
3. No, a barbiturate might *decrease the effectiveness of lidocaine* in this situation and *make the patient more irritable*.
4. No, a barbiturate might *decrease the effectiveness of lidocaine* in this situation, although the *medication would normally have a calming effect*.

4. Which serious adverse effect of lidocaine coincides with the possible cause of Mr. Wand's collapse and therefore is a reason why the nurse should be very cautious?

1. Convulsions
2. Cardiac arrest
3. Respiratory depression
4. All of the above

FURTHER STUDY

- The abuse potential of cocaine is discussed in Chapter 7 ⦾.

- The use of barbiturates in treating insomnia is included in Chapter 9 ⦾, and for seizures in Chapter 13 ⦾.

- The use of benzodiazepines in treating anxiety is presented in Chapter 9 ⦾, and for seizures in Chapter 13 ⦾.

- The use of opiods in pain management is included in Chapter 14 ⦾, and in treating diarrhea in Chapter 29 ⦾.

- Bethanechol (Urecholine) is a profile cholinergic agent in Chapter 8 ⦾.

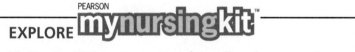

EXPLORE **mynursingkit™** PEARSON

MyNursingKit is your one stop for online chapter review materials and resources. Prepare for success with additional NCLEX®-style practice questions, interactive assignments and activities, web links, animations and videos, and more!

Register your access code from the front of your book at
www.mynursingkit.com

UNIT 3

The Cardiovascular and Urinary Systems

16 Drugs for Lipid Disorders

CORE CONCEPTS

16.1 The three classes of lipids are triglycerides, steroids, and phospholipids.

16.2 Lipoprotein levels are important predictors of cardiovascular disease.

16.3 Lipid levels can often be controlled through lifestyle changes.

16.4 Statins are drugs of choice in reducing blood lipid levels.

16.5 Bile acids can increase cholesterol excretion and reduce LDL levels.

16.6 Nicotinic acid can reduce triglyceride and LDL-cholesterol levels.

16.7 Fibric acid agents lower triglyceride levels but have little effect on LDLs.

16.8 Newer approaches to treating hyperlipidemia include ezetimibe and fixed-dose combination therapy.

DRUG SNAPSHOT

The following drugs are discussed in this chapter:

DRUG CLASSES	DRUG PROFILES
HMG-CoA reductase inhibitors (statins)	**Pr** atorvastatin (Lipitor)
Bile acid resins	**Pr** cholestyramine (Questran)
Nicotinic acid	
Fibric acid agents (fibrates)	**Pr** gemfibrozil (Lopid)

LEARNING OUTCOMES

After reading this chapter, the student should be able to:

1. Summarize the links among high blood cholesterol, low-density lipoprotein (LDL) levels, and cardiovascular disease.

2. Compare and contrast the different types of lipids.

3. Describe how lipids are transported through the body.

4. Compare and contrast the different types of lipoproteins.

5. Give examples of how blood lipid levels can be controlled through nonpharmacologic means.

6. For each of the classes in the Drug Snapshot, identify representative drugs and explain their mechanisms of action, primary actions, and important adverse effects.

7. Categorize antihyperlipidemic drugs based on their classifications and mechanisms of action.

atherosclerosis (ath-ur-oh-skler-OH-sis) *251*

bile acid (BEYE-ul) *257*

high-density lipoprotein (HDL) *253*

HMG-CoA reductase (ree-DUCK-tase) *256*

hypercholesterolemia (HEYE-purr-koh-LESS-tur-ol-EEM-ee-uh) *253*

hyperlipidemia (HEYE-purr-LIP-id-EEM-ee-uh) *253*

lecithin (LESS-ih-thin) *252*

lipoprotein (LIP-oh-PROH-teen) *253*

low-density lipoprotein (LDL) *253*

phospholipid (FOS-foh-LIP-id) *252*

plaque (PLAK) *252*

steroid (STAIR-oyd) *251*

steroid nucleus (STAIR-ol NUK-lee-us) *251*

therapeutic lifestyle changes *254*

triglyceride (tri-GLISS-ur-ide) *251*

very low-density lipoprotein (VLDL) *253*

Research during the 1960s and 1970s brought about a nutritional revolution as new knowledge about lipids and their relationship to obesity and cardiovascular disease allowed people to make more intelligent lifestyle choices. Since then, advances in the diagnosis of lipid disorders have helped to identify those patients at greatest risk for cardiovascular disease, and those most likely to benefit from pharmacologic intervention. Safe, effective drugs for lowering lipid levels are now available that decrease the risk of cardiovascular-related diseases. As a result of this knowledge and from advancements in pharmacology, the incidence of death due to most cardiovascular diseases has been declining. However, these disorders still remain the leading cause of death in the United States.

The three classes of lipids are triglycerides, steroids, and phospholipids.

CORE CONCEPT 16.1

The three classes of lipids are illustrated in Figure 16.1 ■. The most common are the **triglycerides**, or neutral fats. Triglycerides form a large family of different lipids, all having three fatty acids attached to a chemical backbone of glycerol. Triglycerides are the major storage form of fat in the body and the only type of lipid that serves as an important energy source. They account for 90% of the total lipids in the body.

A second class of lipids is the **steroids**, a diverse group of substances having a common chemical structure called the **steroid nucleus** or ring. Cholesterol is the most widely known of the steroids. Its negative role in promoting **atherosclerosis** is well known, but cholesterol also is a natural and vital component of cellular membranes. Cholesterol serves as the building block for a number of essential biochemicals, including vitamin D, bile salts, cortisol, estrogen, and testosterone. Although the body needs only minute amounts of cholesterol and because the body is able to make this lipid from other chemicals, it is not necessary to ingest excess

athero = *fatty*
sclera = *hard*
osis = *condition of*

Fast Facts High Blood Cholesterol

- Thirty million Americans (15% of U.S. adults) are believed to have both hypertension and high blood cholesterol levels.
- The incidence of high blood cholesterol increases until age 65.
- Moderate alcohol intake does not reduce LDL cholesterol, but it does increase high-density lipoprotein (HDL) cholesterol.
- High blood cholesterol occurs more frequently in men than in pre-menopausal women, but after age 50, the disease is more common in women.
- To lower blood cholesterol, dietary intake of both cholesterol and saturated fats must be reduced.
- Familial hypercholesterolemia affects 1 in 500 people and is a genetic disease that predisposes people to high cholesterol levels.

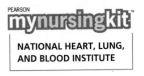

PEARSON
mynursingkit™

NATIONAL HEART, LUNG, AND BLOOD INSTITUTE

FIGURE 16.1

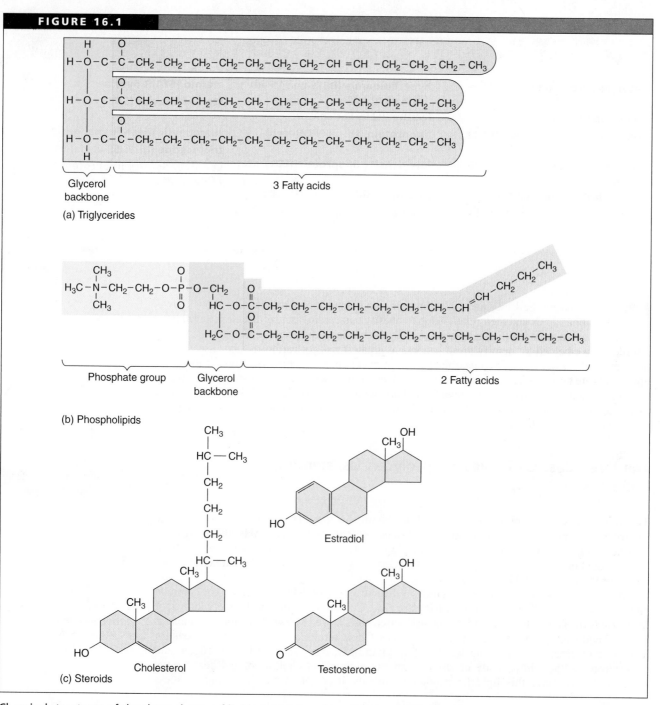

Chemical structures of the three classes of lipids: (a) triglycerides, (b) phospholipids, (c) steroids

amounts of cholesterol in the diet. Dietary cholesterol is obtained solely from animal food products; humans do not absorb the sterols produced by plants. Cholesterol contributes to the fatty **plaque** that narrows arteries, thereby contributing to angina, myocardial infarction (MI), and cerebrovascular accident (CVA), as discussed in Chapter 21 ⬯.

The third class, the **phospholipids**, is formed when a phosphorus group replaces one of the fatty acids in a triglyceride. This class of lipids is essential to building cellular membranes. The best known phospholipids are **lecithins**, which are found in high concentration in egg yolks and soybeans. Once promoted as a natural treatment for high cholesterol levels, controlled studies have not shown lecithin to be of any benefit for this disorder. Likewise, lecithin has been proposed as a remedy for nervous system diseases such as Alzheimer's disease and bipolar disorder, but there is no definite evidence to support these claims.

Several terms are used to describe lipid disorders. **Hyperlipidemia**, the general term referring to high levels of lipids in the blood, is a major risk factor for cardiovascular disease. Elevated
blood cholesterol, or **hypercholesterolemia**, is the type of hyperlipidemia that is most familiar to
the general public. Most patients with these lipid disorders are asymptomatic and do not seek
medical intervention until cardiovascular disease produces symptoms such as chest pain or signs
of hypertension. For most patients, lipid disorders are the result of a *combination* of genetic and
environmental (lifestyle) factors.

hyper = *above*
lipid = *fat*
emia = *blood*

Lipoprotein levels are important predictors of cardiovascular disease.

Knowledge of cholesterol metabolism is important to understanding cardiovascular disease and
the pharmacotherapy of lipid disorders. In simplest terms, the greater the amount of cholesterol
circulating in the blood, the greater the risk of cardiovascular disease. This is because the circulating cholesterol binds to vessel walls, increasing plaque buildup as years pass.

Because it is not soluble in blood, very little cholesterol actually travels through the blood in
its free form. Cholesterol and other lipids are packaged as lipoprotein complexes, which contain
an inner core of lipid surrounded by an outer shell of protein. **Lipoproteins** are water soluble and
can be transported freely throughout the blood. The three most common lipoproteins are named
based on their weight or density, which comes primarily from the amount of protein present in
the complex. Figure 16.2 ■ illustrates the three basic lipoproteins and their composition.

Although cholesterol is packaged in all lipoproteins, **low-density lipoprotein (LDL)** has the
greatest amount: Almost 50% of LDL consists of cholesterol. The liver makes LDL, which is then
transported to tissues and organs, where it is used to build plasma membranes or to synthesize
other steroids. Once in the tissues, cholesterol can also be stored for later use. Storage of cholesterol in the lining of blood vessels, however, contributes to plaque buildup and atherosclerosis.
LDL is often called "bad" cholesterol, because this lipoprotein contributes significantly to plaque
deposits and coronary artery disease.

Under normal circumstances, the body makes all the cholesterol it needs to construct cell
membranes and other vital functions. When cholesterol is ingested, the body simply makes less
to compensate for the increased amounts in the diet. If a person includes too much cholesterol in
the diet, however, this feedback loop fails and LDL-cholesterol builds, eventually resulting in
health problems.

The body has a remarkable method for keeping blood cholesterol levels in check. A second
type of lipoprotein, **high-density lipoprotein (HDL)**, picks up cholesterol in the blood and other
tissues and returns it to the liver. Once in the liver, the cholesterol is used to make bile, which is
essential for digestion of lipids. The cholesterol component of bile is then excreted in the feces,
although some is reabsorbed back into the circulation. Excretion via bile is the only route the body
uses to remove cholesterol. Thus HDL may be thought of as "cholesterol scavengers" that pick
up cholesterol in blood and tissues and transport it for removal from the body. Because HDL transports cholesterol for destruction and removes it from the body, it is considered "good" cholesterol.

Of course, cholesterol is not the only type of lipid that can lead to cardiovascular disease.
Triglycerides must also be monitored and maintained within normal levels. **Very low-density
lipoprotein (VLDL)** is the primary carrier of triglycerides in the blood. VLDL is made in the liver
and converted to LDL as it travels through the bloodstream. Most of the triglycerides in VLDL
are transported to adipose tissue for storage. The health consequences of high blood levels of
VLDL are not as clear as for LDL levels. It has been demonstrated, however, that high levels of
VLDL are associated with an increased risk of pancreatitis.

Lipid levels can often be controlled through lifestyle changes.

When a patient is found to have high LDL-cholesterol levels, a decision must be made regarding
the initiation of drug therapy. Although the drugs used to control lipid levels are generally safe
and effective, other risk factors are considered, such as age, family history of heart disease, hypertension, and cigarette smoking. The stage at which drug therapy is begun depends on the number and extent of these risk factors. The more risk factors present, the more aggressive is the
therapy. Table 16.1 gives the desirable, borderline, and high laboratory values for each of the major lipids and lipoproteins.

Composition of
lipoproteins: (a) HDL;
(b) LDL; (c) VLDL

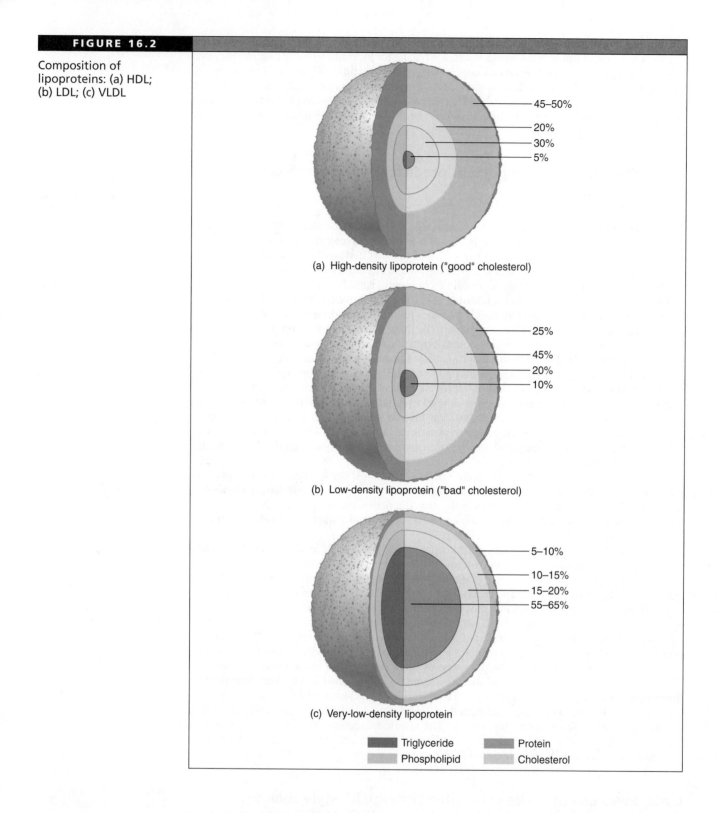

45–50%
20%
30%
5%

(a) High-density lipoprotein ("good" cholesterol)

25%
45%
20%
10%

(b) Low-density lipoprotein ("bad" cholesterol)

5–10%
10–15%
15–20%
55–65%

(c) Very-low-density lipoprotein

Triglyceride   Protein
Phospholipid   Cholesterol

Recommendations for the treatment of high blood cholesterol have been set by the National Cholesterol Education Program (NCEP) of the National Institutes of Health. These recommendations, which are revised periodically, are the gold standard for treating this disorder. In some patients, high blood cholesterol levels can be controlled by initiating **therapeutic lifestyle changes** without drug therapy. Many patients with borderline laboratory values can control their hyperlipidemia entirely through nonpharmacologic means. Even in patients with high risk for whom drug therapy is indicated, using these changes is important for reducing cholesterol levels. Following are the features of therapeutic lifestyle changes:

TABLE 16.1	Standard Laboratory Lipid Profiles	
TYPE OF LIPID	**LABORATORY VALUE (MG/DL)**	**STANDARD**
Total cholesterol	<200	Desirable
	200–239	Borderline high risk
	>239	High risk
LDL cholesterol	<100	Optimal
	100–129	Near optimal/above optimal
	130–159	Borderline high risk
	160–189	High risk
	>190	Very high risk
HDL cholesterol	<40	High risk
	40–59	Borderline high risk
	>60	Desirable
Triglycerides	<150	Normal
	150–199	Borderline high risk
	200–499	High risk
	>500	Very high risk

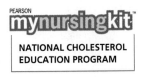

PEARSON
mynursingkit

NATIONAL CHOLESTEROL EDUCATION PROGRAM

- Increase physical activity, which raises HDL levels and lowers triglycerides.
- Maintain optimum weight because obesity is a major risk factor for coronary heart disease.
- Reduce dietary saturated fat intake to 7% of total caloric intake.
- Reduce cholesterol intake to less than 200 mg/day.
- Increase intake of whole grains, vegetables, and fruits so that total dietary fiber is 10 to 25 g/day.
- Reduce or eliminate tobacco use.

In addition to the recommendations of the NCEP, other lifestyle changes may contribute to keeping blood cholesterol levels within normal values and reducing the risk of heart disease. These factors include maintaining blood pressure within normal limits, reducing stress, and limiting the intake of high-sugar foods. The particular type of fat ingested is also thought to play a role in blood cholesterol levels. Omega-3 fatty acids, which are found in high amounts in fatty fish (albacore tuna, salmon, sardines), tofu, and flaxseed oil, have been shown to reduce the risk of cardiovascular disease. Transfatty acids in the diet can raise blood cholesterol levels. Therefore, patients should be advised to avoid foods that are fried or contain vegetable shortening or partially hydrogenated oils.

Concept Review 16.1

- Why is the cholesterol in high-density lipoproteins considered to be "good" cholesterol?

Statins are drugs of choice in reducing blood lipid levels.

CORE CONCEPT 16.4

In the late 1970s, compounds were isolated from various species of fungi that were found to inhibit cholesterol production in human cells in the laboratory. This class of drugs, known as the *statins,* has since revolutionized the treatment of lipid disorders. Statins can produce a dramatic 20% to 40% reduction in LDL-cholesterol levels. In addition to decreasing LDL-cholesterol levels in the blood, statins can also lower triglyceride levels, lower VLDL levels, and raise "good" HDL-cholesterol levels. These effects have been shown to reduce the incidence of serious cardiovascular related events by 25% to 30%. Statins are preferred drugs in the treatment of lipid disorders and are among the most widely prescribed drugs in the United States.

Cholesterol is made in the liver by a series of more than 25 metabolic steps, beginning with acetyl CoA, a two-carbon unit that is produced from the breakdown of fatty acids. Of the many

FIGURE 16.3

Cholesterol biosynthesis
and excretion

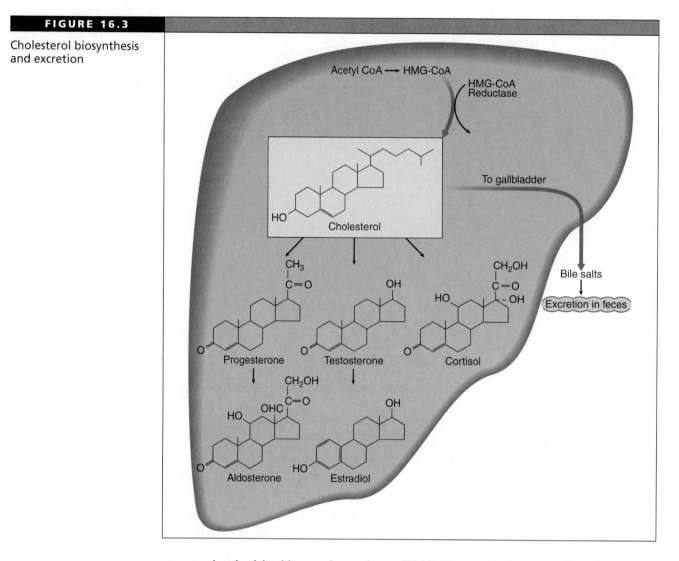

enzymes involved in this complex pathway, **HMG-CoA reductase** (hydroxymethylglutaryl-Coenzyme A reductase) serves as the primary regulator of cholesterol biosynthesis. Under normal conditions, this enzyme is controlled through negative feedback: High levels of LDL cholesterol in the blood will shut down production of HMG-CoA reductase, thus turning off the cholesterol pathway. Figure 16.3 ■ illustrates some of the steps in cholesterol biosynthesis and the importance of HMG-CoA reductase.

The statins act by inhibiting HMG-CoA reductase. As the liver makes less cholesterol, it responds by making more LDL receptors. These receptors remove more LDL from the blood; thus, blood levels of LDL cholesterol are reduced. The drop in lipid levels is not permanent, however, so patients need to remain on these drugs during the remainder of their lives or until their hyperlipidemia can be controlled through lifestyle changes. Statins have been shown to slow the progression of coronary artery disease and to reduce mortality from cardiovascular disease. Doses of the HMG-CoA reductase inhibitors are shown in Table 16.2.

All the statins are given orally. Some statins should be administered in the evening because cholesterol biosynthesis in the body is higher at night. Atorvastatin and rosuvastatin have longer half-lives and are effective regardless of the time of day they are taken.

The statins are generally safe drugs, having few serious adverse effects. Gastrointestinal (GI) disturbances such as indigestion, flatulence, cramping, and constipation are usually mild and disappear with continued use. Statins can cause muscle injury, resulting in symptoms such as weakness, soreness, and pain. Muscle side effects are dose related and tend to occur more often in elderly patients. Patients should be carefully monitored for these symptoms because muscle injury may progress to more serious conditions. In 2001, cerivastatin was removed from the market because of 31 fatalities due to severe rhabdomyolysis associated with the use of the drug. *Rhabdomyolysis* is a medical condition in which muscle tissue becomes extremely inflamed, re-

TABLE 16.2	Drugs for Dyslipidemias	
DRUG	**ROUTE AND ADULT DOSE**	**REMARKS**
HMG-COA REDUCTASE INHIBITORS		
Ⓟ atorvastatin (Lipitor)	PO; 10–80 mg/day	May be taken with or without food any time of the day
fluvastatin (Lescol)	PO; 20 mg/day (max: 80 mg/day)	May be taken with or without food in the evening
lovastatin (Mevacor)	PO; 10–20 mg once daily	Should be taken with meals in the evening
pitavastatin (Livalo)	PO; 1–4 mg once daily (max: 4mg/day)	Newest of the statin drugs
pravastatin (Pravachol)	PO; 10–40 mg/day	May be taken with or without food in the evening
rosuvastatin (Crestor)	PO; 5–40 mg/day	May be taken with or without food at any time of the day
simvastatin (Zocor)	PO; 5–40 mg/day	May be taken with or without food in the evening
BILE ACID-BINDING AGENTS		
Ⓟ cholestyramine (Questran)	PO; 4–8 g bid–qid	Taken with large amounts of fluid; take other drugs 1 hour before or 4 hours after
colesevelam (Welchol)	PO; 1.9 g bid	Taken with meals and with at least 8 oz of fluid
colestipol (Colestid)	PO; 5–20 g/day in divided doses	Taken with large amounts of fluid; take other drugs 1 hour before or 4 hours after
FIBRIC ACID AGENTS		
fenofibrate (Tricor, others)	PO; 54 mg/day (max: 160 mg/day)	Taken with meals. Assess periodically for symptoms of myopathy
fenofibric acid (Triplix)	PO; 45–135 mg once daily	Newest of the fibric acid agents
Ⓟ gemfibrozil (Lopid)	PO; 600 mg bid (max: 1500 mg/day)	Take 30 min before morning and evening meals
OTHER AGENTS		
ezetimibe (Zetia)	PO; 10 mg/day	One of the newest antihyperlipidemics; inhibits cholesterol absorption
niacin (Niac, Nicobid, others)	PO; 1.5–3 g/day (max: 6 g/day)	Also used to treat niacin deficiency (10–20 mg/day). Give with meals

sulting in breakdown of muscle. Patients reporting muscular soreness or weakness may have their statin dosage reduced, or they may be switched to a drug of a different class.

Bile acids resins can increase cholesterol excretion and reduce LDL levels.

CORE CONCEPT **16.5**

Prior to the discovery of the statins, the primary means of lowering blood cholesterol was through use of bile acid resins. **Bile acids** are substances that aid the digestion of fats, which contain a high concentration of cholesterol. Once bound in the intestine, the cholesterol in the bile acids is eliminated in the feces. Although they are no longer considered first-line drugs for hyperlipidemia, they are sometimes combined with statins for patients who are unable to achieve sufficient response from the statins alone. Doses of these drugs are listed in Table 16.2.

Although effective at producing a 20% decrease in LDL-cholesterol levels, the bile acid resins tend to cause more frequent adverse effects than do the statins. Taken orally, bile acid resins are not absorbed into the circulation; therefore, their adverse effects are limited to the GI tract. Many patients, however, experience constipation, bloating, nausea, or indigestion. The newest drug in this class, colesevelam (Welchol), is reported to have fewer adverse effects than the older drugs. Also of concern is that bile acid resins can prevent the absorption of other medications and vitamins that may be taken at the same time. This can be avoided by teaching the patient to take these drugs 1 hour before, or 4 hours after, other medications.

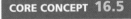

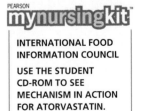

INTERNATIONAL FOOD INFORMATION COUNCIL

USE THE STUDENT CD-ROM TO SEE MECHANISM IN ACTION FOR ATORVASTATIN.

DRUG PROFILE: Pr *Atorvastatin (Lipitor)*

Therapeutic Class: Antilipemic drug
Pharmacologic Class: HMG-CoA reductase inhibitor (statin)

Actions and Uses:

The primary indication for atorvastatin is hypercholesterolemia. Although lovastatin (Mevacor) was the first HMG-CoA reductase inhibitor approved for use in the United States, newer statins have been developed that offer certain advantages. For example, atorvastatin has a longer half-life and may be administered without regard to food or time of day. Maximum effects from atorvastatin are seen in 4–8 weeks, after which time a follow-up measurement of blood lipid levels is taken to determine whether the dosage is optimum. Patients receiving this drug should be placed on a cholesterol-lowering diet, because this will enhance the drug's therapeutic effects. The primary goal in atorvastatin therapy is to reduce the risk of MI and stroke.

Adverse Effects and Interactions:

Adverse effects of atorvastatin are rarely severe enough to cause discontinuation of therapy and include GI complaints such as intestinal cramping, diarrhea, and constipation. A small percentage of patients experience liver damage; thus, liver function is usually monitored periodically during therapy. The most serious adverse effect is rhabdomyolysis. Like other statins, atorvastatin is a pregnancy category X drug. Pregnancy testing should be conducted prior to treatment in women of childbearing years, and the patient should be advised to take precautions to prevent pregnancy during therapy.

Atorvastatin interacts with many other drugs. For example, it may increase digoxin levels by 20%, as well as increase levels of oral contraceptives. Erythromycin may increase atorvastatin levels by 40%.

Grapefruit juice inhibits the metabolism of statins, allowing them to reach toxic levels. Because HMG-CoA reductase inhibitors also decrease the synthesis of coenzyme Q10 (CoQ10), patients may benefit from CoQ10 supplements.

Mechanism in Action:

Atorvastatin slows the biosynthesis of cholesterol by blocking the rate-limiting enzyme, HMG-CoA reductase. This enzyme is necessary for the availability of LDL and VLDL fragments to body cell, including the liver. Atorvastatin also up-regulates LDL receptors in the liver. The net effect is reduced cholesterol and trigylceride blood levels.

 Refer to MyNursingKit for a Nursing Process Focus specific to this drug.

DRUG PROFILE: Pr *Cholestyramine (Questran)*

Therapeutic Class: Antilipemic drug
Pharmacologic Class: Bile acid resin

Actions and Uses:

Cholestyramine is used to treat elevated levels of cholesterol and LDLs. The drug is formulated as a powder that is mixed with fluid before being taken once or twice daily. It is not absorbed or metabolized once it enters the intestine; thus, it does not produce systemic effects. It may take 30 days or longer to produce its maximum effect. Cholestyramine is sometimes combined with other cholesterol-lowering drugs such as the statins or nicotinic acid to produce additive effects.

Adverse Effects and Interactions:

Although cholestyramine rarely produces serious adverse effects, patients may experience constipation, bloating, gas, and nausea that may limit its use. Cholestyramine has the ability to bind to other drugs and interfere with their absorption. Examples include binding to vitamin K, thiazide diuretics, and penicillins. To prevent potential interactions, other medications should be taken 1 hour before or 4 hours after administration of cholestyramine. It should not be taken at the same time as other medications.

Refer to MyNursingKit for a Nursing Process Focus specific to this drug.

NURSING PROCESS FOCUS

Patients Receiving HMG-CoA Reductase Inhibitor (Statin) Therapy

ASSESSMENT

Prior to administration:
- Obtain a complete health history (physical/mental), including allergies, drug history, and possible drug interactions
- Obtain baseline liver function tests, lipid studies, and a pregnancy test in women of childbearing age

POTENTIAL NURSING DIAGNOSES

- Deficient Knowledge related to need for altered lifestyle.
- Noncompliance related to dietary and drug regimen.
- Chronic Pain related to drug-induced myopathy.
- Impaired Health Maintenance related to insufficient knowledge of actions and effects of drug therapy.

PLANNING: PATIENT GOALS AND EXPECTED OUTCOMES

The patient will:
- Immediately report skeletal muscle pain, unexplained muscle soreness, or weakness
- Demonstrate compliance with appropriate lifestyle changes
- Demonstrate an understanding of the drug's action by accurately describing adverse effects and precautions

IMPLEMENTATION

Interventions and (Rationales)	Patient Education/Discharge Planning
Monitor blood cholesterol and triglyceride levels at intervals during therapy (to determine effectiveness of therapy).	Advise the patient of the importance of keeping appointments for laboratory testing.
Monitor patient compliance with dietary regimen. (Maintenance of controlled saturated fat diet is essential to the effectiveness of medications.)	Provide the patient with information needed to maintain a low saturated fat, low cholesterol diet.
Monitor the patient for alcohol abuse. (Excessive alcohol intake may result in liver damage and interfere with drug effectiveness.)	Instruct the patient to avoid or limit alcohol use.
Monitor CPK level. (Elevated CPK may be indicative of impending myopathy.)	Instruct the patient to report symptoms of leg or muscle pain to the health care provider.
Obtain the patient's smoking history. (Smoking increases risk of cardiovascular disease and may decrease HDL levels.)	Encourage smoking cessation if appropriate.

EVALUATION OF OUTCOME CRITERIA

Evaluate the effectiveness of drug therapy by confirming that patient goals and expected outcomes have been met (see "Planning").

See Table 16.2 for a list of drugs to which these nursing actions apply.

Nicotinic acid can reduce triglyceride and LDL-cholesterol levels.

CORE CONCEPT 16.6

Nicotinic acid, or niacin, is a water-soluble B-complex vitamin whose primary action is to decrease VLDL levels. The patient also experiences a reduction in LDL-cholesterol and triglyceride levels. It also has the desirable effects of reducing triglycerides and increasing HDL levels. Thus, niacin is unique in that it can improve all lipoprotein abnormalities. As with other lipid-lowering drugs, maximum therapeutic effects may take a month or longer to achieve.

Its ability to lower lipid levels is unrelated to its role as a vitamin; very high doses are needed to achieve an antilipidemic effect. For lowering cholesterol, the usual dose is 2 to 3 g per day. When taken as a vitamin, the dose is only 25 mg per day.

NATURAL THERAPIES

Coenzyme Q10 for Heart Disease

Coenzyme Q10 (CoQ10) is a vitamin-like substance found in most animal cells. It is an essential component in the cell's mitochondria, which produce energy or ATP. Because the heart requires high levels of ATP, a sufficient level of CoQ10 is essential to that organ. Foods richest in this substance are pork, sardines, beef heart, salmon, broccoli, spinach, and nuts. Elderly people appear to have an increased need for CoQ10.

Reports of the benefits of CoQ10 for treating heart disease began to emerge in the mid-1960s. Subsequent reports have claimed that CoQ10 may be beneficial in angina pectoris, dysrhythmias, periodontal disease, immune disorders, neurologic disease, obesity, diabetes mellitus, and certain cancers. Considerable research has been conducted on this antioxidant.

The statins decrease CoQ10 levels. Indeed, many of the adverse effects of statins may be due to the decrease in CoQ10 levels, including muscle weakness and rhabdomyolysis. Supplementation with CoQ10 may improve myopathy symptoms. Like most dietary supplements, controlled research studies are often lacking and give conflicting results. At this time, evidence to support the use of CoQ10 in treating patients with heart disease, neurologic disorders, or cancer is weak.

Although effective at reducing LDL cholesterol by 20%, nicotinic acid produces more adverse effects than the statins. Flushing and hot flashes occur in almost every patient, although taking one aspirin tablet 30 minutes prior to niacin administration can reduce flushing in many patients. A variety of uncomfortable intestinal effects such as nausea, excess gas, and diarrhea are commonly reported. More serious adverse effects such as liver toxicity and gout are possible. Because of these adverse effects, nicotinic acid is most often used in lower doses in combination with a statin or bile acid resin because the beneficial effects of these drugs are additive. Extended-release niacin, which is taken once daily, causes less flushing and GI adverse effects.

As a vitamin, niacin is available without a prescription. However, patients should be instructed not to attempt self-medication with this drug. One form of niacin, available over the counter as a vitamin supplement called *nicotinamide,* has no lipid-lowering effects. Patients should be informed that if nicotinic acid is used to lower cholesterol, it should be done under medical supervision.

Concept Review 16.2

■ How does the mechanism of the statins differ from that of nicotinic acid?

CORE CONCEPT 16.7

Fibric acid agents lower triglyceride levels but have little effect on LDLs.

Once commonly prescribed to reduce lipid levels, the fibric acid agents, or fibrates, have been largely replaced by the statins. They are sometimes used in combination with the statins. In addition they remain drugs of choice for treating extremely high triglyceride levels. Doses of the fibrates are listed in Table 16.2.

The first fibric acid agent, clofibrate (Atromid-S), was widely prescribed until studies demonstrated it did not reduce mortality from cardiovascular disease. Although clofibrate is no longer available in the United States, the other fibric acid agents, fenofibrate (Tricor), fenofibric acid (Triplix), and gemfibrozil (Lopid), are sometimes prescribed for patients who have excessive triglyceride and VLDL levels. Fibrates are the most effective agents for reducing VLDLs and blood triglyceride levels. Elevation of "good" HDL cholesterol is another effect of fibrate therapy. Unfortunately, these drugs have little effect on LDL-cholesterol levels.

Fibrates cause few serious adverse effects. Rashes and GI complaints are the most common adverse effects. Patients have an increased risk of gallstones. Like the statins, some patients experience muscle pain or weakness; therefore, patients receiving combination therapy with both statins and fibrates should be monitored carefully. The mechanisms of action of the fibrates and other antihyperlipidemic drugs are shown in Figure 16.4 ■. Dosages of these drugs are listed in Table 16.2.

FIGURE 16.4

Mechanisms of action
of lipid-lowering drugs

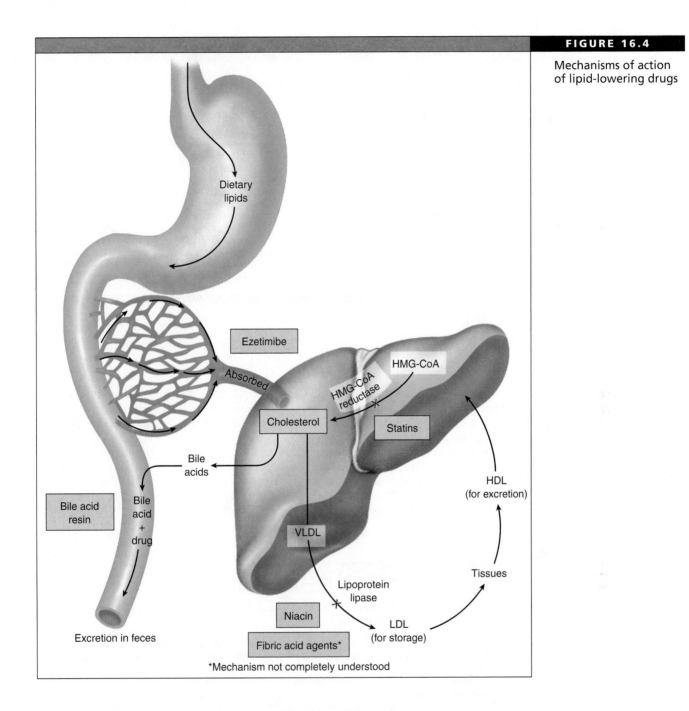

Dietary
lipids

Ezetimibe

HMG-CoA

Absorbed

HMG-CoA
reductase

Cholesterol

Statins

Bile
acids

Bile acid
resin

Bile
acid
+
drug

VLDL

HDL
(for excretion)

Tissues

Lipoprotein
lipase

Niacin

LDL
(for storage)

Fibric acid agents*

Excretion in feces

*Mechanism not completely understood

Newer approaches to treating hyperlipidemia include ezetimibe and fixed-dose combination therapy.

The newer drug for treating high blood cholesterol levels is ezetimibe (Zetia). Ezetimibe acts on the small intestine to block the absorption of dietary cholesterol. LDL-cholesterol and triglyceride levels are reduced, with a slight increase in HDL cholesterol. When used as monotherapy, it can decrease blood cholesterol levels by about 20%. Adding a statin to the therapeutic regimen reduces LDL by an *additional* 15% to 20%. Adverse effects from ezetimibe are uncommon and include abdominal pain, back pain, diarrhea, and arthralgia. The dose for ezetimibe is listed in Table 16.2.

A recent trend in the treatment of hyperlipidemia is to combine drugs from two different classes in a single tablet. Vytorin combines 10 mg of ezetimibe with 10, 20, 40, or 80 mg of simvastatin. Advicor combines 20 mg of lovastatin with 500, 750, or 1000 mg of niacin. These fixed-dose combinations allow for lower doses of each individual agent, potentially resulting in fewer

DRUG PROFILE: ⓟ *Gemfibrozil (Lopid)*

Therapeutic Class: Antihyperlipidemic drug
Pharmacologic Class: Fibric acid agent

Actions and Uses:

Gemfibrozil can cause up to a 50% reduction in VLDL with an increase in HDL. Because it is less effective than the statins, it is not a drug of first choice for reducing LDL-cholesterol levels. However, it is useful for patients with high triglyceride levels who have not responded favorably to diet modification and those at risk for pancreatitis.

Adverse Effects and Interactions:

The most common adverse effects of gemfibrozil are related to the GI system: diarrhea, nausea, and abdominal cramping. The drug produces few serious adverse effects, but it may increase the likelihood of gallstones and occasionally affect liver function.

Using gemfibrozil with oral anticoagulants may increase the risk of bleeding. Concurrent use with statins should be avoided because this increases the risk of myopathy and rhabdomyolysis.

 Refer to MyNursingKit for a Nursing Process Focus specific to this drug.

adverse effects. Taking a single tablet is easier for the patient to remember, which increases increasing compliance. Because the combination agents attack cholesterol levels using two distinct mechanisms of action, it may be possible to get a synergistic, or additive, effect of the drugs on blood cholesterol levels.

A second trend in treating cardiovascular disease is to combine an antihypertensive agent with an antihyperlipidemic drug. For example, Caduet combines the antihypertensive amlodipine with atorvastatin. Several fixed-dose combinations are available with 5 to 10 mg of amlodipine and 10 to 80 mg of atorvastatin. These combination agents are targeted for the estimated 30 million Americans who have both hypertension and elevated blood cholesterol levels.

PATIENTS NEED TO KNOW

Patients treated for lipid disorders need to know the following:

In General

1. Because high cholesterol and triglyceride levels in the blood increase the risk for heart disease and stroke, follow the health care provider's instructions even when feeling well.
2. Continuation of a low-fat, low-cholesterol diet while taking lipid-lowering drugs will provide the best results.

Regarding Statin Medications

3. Atorvastatin and rosuvastatin are effective regardless of the time of day they are taken. Taking other statin drugs in the evening makes them available to work on the higher amount of cholesterol that the body makes at night.
4. The health care provider may prescribe a fibric acid agent to lower triglycerides and another drug to lower cholesterol. One drug should not be stopped when the second drug is ordered, except a practitioner's advice.

Regarding Bile Acid-Binding Agents

5. Self-medication with niacin can cause gout and liver damage from high doses. It will not lower cholesterol at low doses. Supervision by a health care provider supports safe and effective use of this drug.
6. If prescribed bile acid resins, such as psyllium (Metamucil), cholestyramine (Questran), and colestipol (Colestid), take 1 hour after or 4 hours before other drugs to avoid counteracting drug effectiveness. Dissolving the bile acid resin in water and keeping fluid intake high helps to avoid irritation of the mouth and constipation.

CORE CONCEPTS SUMMARY

16.1 The three classes of lipids are triglycerides, steroids, and phospholipids.

The three types of lipids are classified as triglycerides, phospholipids, and steroids. *Hyperlipidemia*, the general term referring to high levels of lipids in the blood, is a major risk factor for cardiovascular disease.

16.2 Lipoprotein levels are important predictors of cardiovascular disease.

Lipids are packaged for travel through the blood in lipoprotein complexes. High VLDL and LDL are associated with an increased incidence of cardiovascular disease, whereas HDL provides a protective effect.

16.3 Lipid levels can often be controlled through lifestyle changes.

Before starting pharmacotherapy for hyperlipidemia, patients are usually advised to control the condition through lifestyle changes such as restriction of dietary saturated fats and cholesterol, increased exercise, and smoking cessation.

16.4 Statins are drugs of choice in reducing blood lipid levels.

Drugs in the statin class inhibit HMG-CoA reductase, a critical enzyme in the biosynthesis of cholesterol. They are safe and effective at lowering LDL cholesterol and are the most widely prescribed class of drugs for hyperlipidemias.

16.5 Bile acids can increase cholesterol excretion and reduce LDL levels.

The bile acid-binding drugs are effective at lowering LDL cholesterol, although they produce more adverse effects than the statins. They should be taken separately from other medications because they can interfere with drug absorption.

16.6 Nicotinic acid can reduce triglyceride and LDL-cholesterol levels.

Nicotinic acid, or niacin, can be effective at lowering LDL cholesterol and triglycerides when given in large amounts. It is not usually a first-choice drug but is sometimes combined in smaller doses with other lipid-lowering agents.

16.7 Fibric acid agents lower triglyceride levels but have little effect on LDLs.

Fibric acids such as gemfibrozil are effective at lowering triglycerides but less effective than the statins at lowering blood lipids. Their use is limited because of frequent adverse effects. However, they are sometimes combined with other agents to produce an additive effect.

16.8 Newer approaches to treating hyperlipidemia include ezetimibe and fixed-dose combination therapy.

Newer approaches to treating hyperlipidemia are emerging. These include ezetimibe, which blocks cholesterol absorption from the intestine, and combination drugs such as Advicor and Vytorin, which attack high blood cholesterol levels using two different mechanisms.

REVIEW QUESTIONS

The following questions are written in NCLEX-PN® style. Answer these questions to assess your knowledge of the chapter material, and go back and review any material that is not clear to you.

1. This lipoprotein is responsible for transporting cholesterol from the blood to the liver.

1. LDL
2. VLDL
3. HDL
4. Triglycerides

2. Which of the HMG-CoA reductase inhibitors should be taken with meals?

1. Atorvastatin (Lipitor)
2. Simvastatin (Zocor)
3. Simvastatin (Mevacor)
4. Digixon (Lanoxin)

3. Statin drugs are most effective when administered:

1. In the morning
2. In the evening
3. With other medications
4. On an empty stomach

4. When asked how an HMG-CoA reductase inhibitor lowers cholesterol, the nurse correctly answers that it is by inhibiting the manufacture of cholesterol or by:

1. Increasing the secretion of bile acids
2. Decreasing triglyceride production
3. Removing cholesterol from the small intestine
4. Promoting the breakdown of cholesterol

5. Which of the following patient concerns would the nurse consider to be an adverse reaction to a bile acid resin?

1. Constipation
2. Headache
3. Anxiety
4. Double vision

6. When administering colestipol (Colestid), the nurse:

1. Administers the drug with meals to prevent GI upset
2. Administers the drug 30 minutes prior to meals
3. Administers the drug at least 1 hour before or 4 hours after meals
4. Administers the drug at bedtime

7. Which of the following antihyperlipidemic medications is most effective in reducing serum triglyceride levels?

1. Gemfibrozil (Lopid)
2. Niacin (Nicotinic acid)
3. Lovastatin (Mevacor)
4. Cholestyramine (Questran)

8. On assessment, the patient is found to have a cholesterol level of 326 mg/dl and an elevated blood pressure. The best treatment for this patient would be a low-fat diet and:

1. An exercise program
2. Cholesterol-lowering medication
3. Niacin
4. An antihypertensive

9. The patient has developed gallstones and elevated liver enzymes. Which of the following cholesterol-lowering medications could cause this?

1. Cholestyramine (Questran)
2. Niacin (Nicotinic acid)
3. Gemfibrozil (Lopid)
4. Lovastatin (Mevacor)

10. The preferred first-choice drugs to treat elevated cholesterol levels are:

1. Statins
2. Bile acids
3. Fibric acids
4. Nicotinic acids

CASE STUDY QUESTIONS

For questions 1–4, please refer to the following case study, and choose the correct answer from choices 1–4.

*M*r. Long is a 50-year-old office worker who has gained 50 pounds over the past 5 years. His blood pressure has consistently been high, but he has declined to take medication for the condition. His LDL-cholesterol level has been above 210 mg/dl on his last three office visits. He claims to have no chronic diseases and is at the office seeking assistance concerning his weight gain.

1. The physician ordered cholestyramine for Mr. Long. This drug acts by:

1. Inhibiting enzymes that make cholesterol
2. Binding bile acids in the intestine, which increases cholesterol excretion
3. Increasing the breakdown of cholesterol in the liver
4. Making more bile acids, which bind cholesterol

2. After 2 months of therapy, the physician switched the prescription to lovastatin (Mevacor). This drug acts by:

1. Inhibiting enzymes that make cholesterol
2. Binding bile acids in the intestine, which increase cholesterol excretion

3. Increasing the breakdown of cholesterol in the liver
4. Making more bile acids, which bind cholesterol

3. After several weeks of lovastatin therapy, Mr. Long returns to the office for follow-up. What question should you ask to determine if he may be suffering from a very serious adverse effect of the statins?

1. Do you have bloody diarrhea more than once a week?
2. Have you felt confused, lethargic, or drowsy since starting the drug?
3. Have you experienced excessive muscle weakness or pain?
4. Have you experienced acid indigestion or nausea?

4. Which of the following is an expected therapeutic effect of lovastatin?

1. Higher LDL level
2. Higher VLDL level
3. Lower HDL level
4. Higher HDL level

FURTHER STUDY

- Chapter 18 discusses fatty plaques that cause angina, myocardial infarction, and cerebrovascular accidents.

- The role of niacin as a vitamin is presented in Chapter 30 .

EXPLORE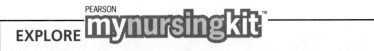

MyNursingKit is your one stop for online chapter review materials and resources. Prepare for success with additional NCLEX®-style practice questions, interactive assignments and activities, web links, animations and videos, and more!

Register your access code from the front of your book at
www.mynursingkit.com

17 Drugs for Hypertension

CORE CONCEPTS

17.1 Hypertension is characterized by the consistent elevation of arterial blood pressure.

17.2 Failure to treat hypertension can lead to stroke, heart failure, or myocardial infarction.

17.3 Blood pressure is caused by the pumping action of the heart.

17.4 The primary factors responsible for blood pressure are cardiac output, the resistance of the small arteries, and blood volume.

17.5 Many nervous and hormonal factors help to keep blood pressure within normal limits.

17.6 Positive lifestyle changes can reduce blood pressure and lessen the need for medications.

17.7 Selection of specific antihypertension drugs depends on the severity of the disease.

17.8 Diuretics are often drugs of first choice for treating mild to moderate hypertension.

17.9 Calcium channel blockers have emerged as important drugs in the treatment of hypertension.

17.10 Blocking the renin-angiotensin-aldosterone system leads to a decrease in blood pressure.

17.11 Alpha- and beta-adrenergic blockers are commonly used to treat hypertension.

17.12 Vasodilators lower blood pressure by relaxing arteriolar smooth muscle.

DRUG SNAPSHOT

The following drugs are discussed in this chapter:

DRUG CLASSES	DRUG PROFILES
Diuretics	**Pr** hydrochlorothiazide (Microzide)
Calcium channel blockers	**Pr** nifedipine (Adalat, Procardia)
Renin-angiotensin system modifiers	**Pr** enalapril (Vasotec)

DRUG CLASSES	DRUG PROFILES
Adrenergic blockers	**Pr** doxazosin (Cardura)
Direct-acting vasodilators	**Pr** hydralazine (Apresoline)

LEARNING OUTCOMES

After reading this chapter, the student should be able to:

1. Define hypertension.
2. Summarize the long-term consequences of untreated hypertension.
3. Describe how the pumping action of the heart creates blood pressure.
4. Explain the effects of cardiac output, peripheral resistance, and blood volume on blood pressure.
5. Discuss how the vasomotor center, baroreceptors, emotions, and hormones influence blood pressure.
6. Discuss the role of therapeutic lifestyle changes in the management of hypertension.
7. Describe general principles guiding the pharmacotherapy of hypertension.
8. For each of the classes listed in the Drug Snapshot, identify representative medications and explain the mechanism of drug action, primary actions, and important adverse effects.

Cardiovascular disease, which includes all conditions affecting the heart and blood vessels, is the most common cause of death in the United States. Hypertension or high blood pressure is the most common of the cardiovascular diseases. Because health care providers encounter numerous patients with this disease, a firm grasp of the underlying principles of antihypertensive therapy is critical.

Hypertension is characterized by the consistent elevation of arterial blood pressure.

CORE CONCEPT 17.1

Hypertension (HTN) is defined as the consistent elevation of arterial blood pressure. The diagnosis of chronic HTN is rarely made on a single blood pressure measurement. Patients are said to have HTN if they present with a sustained systolic blood pressure of greater than 140 mmHg or diastolic pressure of greater than 90 to 99 mmHg after multiple measurements are made over several clinic visits.

Many attempts have been made to further define HTN with the goal of developing guidelines for treatment. In 2003 the National High Blood Pressure Education Program Coordinating Committee of the National Heart, Lung, and Blood Institute of the National Institutes of Health issued guidelines for treating HTN that have become well accepted in the medical community. The Committee classified HTN into three categories—prehypertension, Stage 1, and Stage 2. The recommendations from Committee Report JNC-7 are summarized in Table 17.1.

Blood pressure changes throughout the life span, gradually and continuously rising from childhood through adulthood. What is considered normal blood pressure at one age may be considered abnormal in someone older or younger. Table 17.2 shows the normal variation in blood pressure in people that occurs throughout the life span.

hyper = *high*
tension = *pressure*

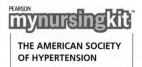

THE AMERICAN SOCIETY OF HYPERTENSION

Failure to treat hypertension can lead to stroke, heart failure, or myocardial infarction.

CORE CONCEPT 17.2

HTN is a complex disease that is caused by a combination of genetic and environmental factors. In 90% of the patients with HTN, no specific cause for the elevated blood pressure can be identified. This type of HTN is called *primary* or *essential*. Although the actual cause of primary HTN is not known, many conditions or risk factors are associated with the disease. Advancing age and weight gain, particularly around the hips and thighs, tends to be associated with HTN. The disease

267

TABLE 17.1	Classification and Management of Hypertension in Adults		
		INITIAL ANTIHYPERTENSIVE THERAPY	
BLOOD PRESSURE CLASSIFICATION	**SYSTOLIC/DIASTOLIC BLOOD PRESSURE (MMHG)**	*WITHOUT* COMPELLING INDICATION*	*WITH* COMPELLING INDICATION*
Normal	119/79 or lower	No antihypertensive indicated	No antihypertensive indicated
Prehypertension	120–139/80–89		
Stage 1 Hypertension	140–159/90–99	Thiazide diuretic (for most patients)	Other antihypertensives, as needed
Stage 2 Hypertension	160 or higher/100 or higher	Two-drug combination anti-hypertensive (for most patients)	

Source: National High Blood Pressure Education Program National Heart, Lung & Blood Institute. (2003). JNC-7 Express: The Seventh Report of the Joint National Committee on Prevention, Detection, Evaluation and Treatment of High Blood Pressure. http://www.nhlbi.nih.gov.

*Compelling indications include: heart failure, postmyocardial infarction, high risk for coronary artery disease, diabetes, chronic kidney disease, and recurrent stroke prevention.

TABLE 17.2	Variation in Blood Pressure Throughout the Life Span	
AGE (YEARS)	**MALES (MMHG)**	**FEMALES (MMHG)**
1	96/66	95/65
5	92/62	92/62
10	103/69	103/70
20–24	123/76	116/72
30–34	126/79	120/75
40–44	129/81	127/80
50–54	135/83	137/84
60–64	142/85	144/85
70–74	145/82	159/85
80+	145/82	157/83

is most prevalent in Blacks and least prevalent in Mexican Americans. Men in all ethnic groups experience more HTN compared to women. The disease also has a hereditary component, with family members of patients with HTN having greater risk of acquiring the disease than nonfamily members. Other factors, such as tobacco use and high-fat diets, clearly contribute to the disease.

In 10% of patients, a specific cause of the HTN *can* be identified. This is called **secondary hypertension**. Certain diseases, such as Cushing's syndrome, hyperthyroidism, and chronic renal disease, cause elevated blood pressure. Certain drugs are also associated with HTN, including corticosteroids, oral contraceptives, and erythropoietin (epoetin alfa). The therapeutic goal for secondary HTN is to treat or remove the underlying condition that is causing the blood pressure elevation. In many cases, correcting this comorbid condition will cure the associated HTN.

Because chronic HTN may produce no identifiable symptoms for as long as 10 to 20 years, many people are not aware of their condition. Convincing patients to control their diets, spend money on medication, and take drugs on a regular basis when they are feeling healthy is a difficult task for the health care practitioner. Failure to control HTN, however, can result in serious consequences. Prolonged high blood pressure can lead to accelerated narrowing of the arteries, resulting in strokes, kidney failure, and even cardiac arrest. One of the most serious consequences of chronic HTN is that the heart must work harder to pump blood to organs and tissues. This excessive workload can cause the heart to fail and the lungs to fill with fluid, a condition known as heart failure (HF). Drug therapy of HF is covered in Chapter 18 ⏎.

The death rate from cardiovascular-related diseases has dropped significantly over the past 20 years because, in large part, of the recognition and treatment of HTN, as well as the acceptance of healthier lifestyle habits. Early treatment is essential; the long-term cardiovascular damage caused by HTN may be irreversible if the disease is allowed to progress unchecked.

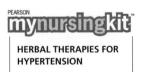

HERBAL THERAPIES FOR HYPERTENSION

Fast Facts Hypertension

- HTN increases with age. It affects approximately:
  30% of those 50 years old and older; 64% of men older than age 65; 75% of women older than age 75
- HTN causes over 54,000 deaths each year.
- High blood pressure affects more than 73 million U.S. adults, or approximately 1 in 3 Americans.
- African American males have the highest rate (51%) of HTN.
- Approximately 65% of Americans diagnosed with HTN do not have their condition under adequate control.
- HTN is the most common complication of pregnancy.

Blood pressure is caused by the pumping action of the heart.

Although pressure can be measured in nearly any vessel in the body, the term *blood pressure* commonly refers to the pressure in the arteries. Because the pumping action of the heart is the source of blood pressure, those arteries closest to the heart, such as the aorta, have the highest pressure. Pressure decreases gradually as the blood travels farther from the heart, until it falls close to zero in the largest veins. This is illustrated in Figure 17.1 ■.

When the ventricles of the heart contract and eject blood, the pressure created in the arteries is called **systolic pressure**. When the ventricles relax and the heart temporarily stops ejecting blood, pressure in the arteries will fall, and this results in **diastolic pressure**. Blood pressure is

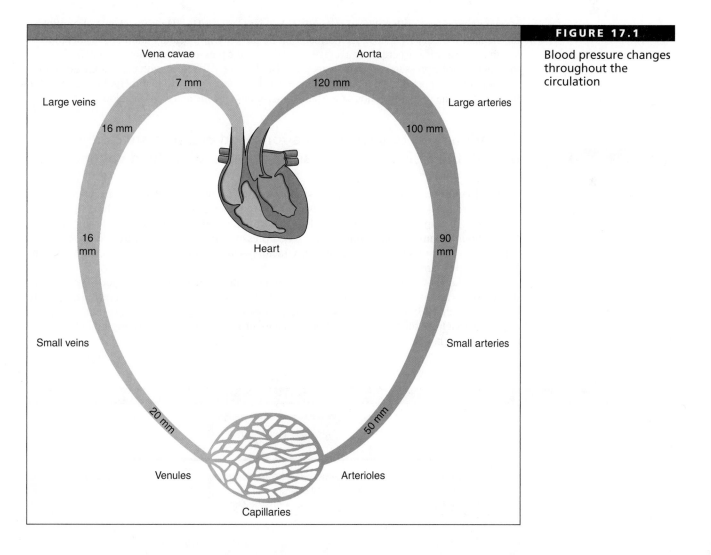

FIGURE 17.1

Blood pressure changes throughout the circulation

FIGURE 17.2

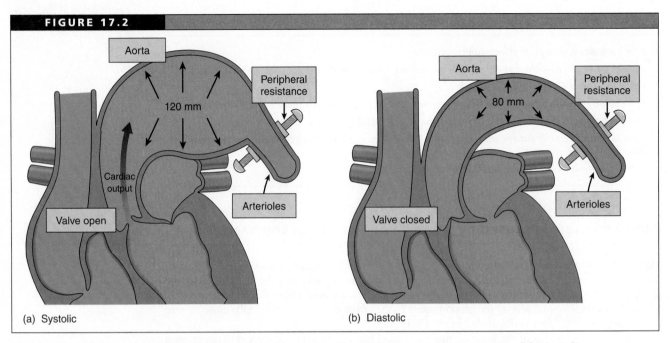

(a) Systolic   (b) Diastolic

(a) Systolic pressure occurs when the heart ejects blood, creating high pressure in the arteries. (b) Diastolic pressure occurs when the heart relaxes, resulting in less pressure in the arteries.

measured in units of millimeters of mercury, abbreviated as mmHg. (Hg is the chemical symbol for the element mercury.) The average normal systolic pressure in a healthy adult is considered to be less than 120 mmHg, whereas the average normal diastolic pressure is less than 80 mmHg. The systolic and diastolic pressures are usually measured and reported together, with the systolic given first. For example, average normal blood pressure is said to be less than 120/80 mmHg. Figure 17.2 ■ illustrates how the pumping action of the heart determines systolic and diastolic blood pressure.

CORE CONCEPT 17.4

The primary factors responsible for blood pressure are cardiac output, the resistance of the small arteries, and blood volume.

In order to understand how drugs affect blood pressure, the student must have an excellent knowledge of cardiovascular physiology. Investing time to understand the details of how this system functions will reap great rewards later when studying the cardiovascular and respiratory drugs.

Although many factors can influence blood pressure, three factors are truly responsible for determining the pressure. The three primary factors—cardiac output, peripheral resistance, and blood volume—are shown in Figure 17.3 ■.

The volume of blood pumped per minute is called the **cardiac output**. Although resting cardiac output is approximately 5 liters per minute (L/min), strenuous exercise can increase this output to as much as 35 L/min. This is important to pharmacology because drugs that change the cardiac output have the potential to influence a patient's blood pressure. It is important to remember that the higher the cardiac output, the higher the blood pressure.

FIGURE 17.3

Primary factors affecting blood pressure

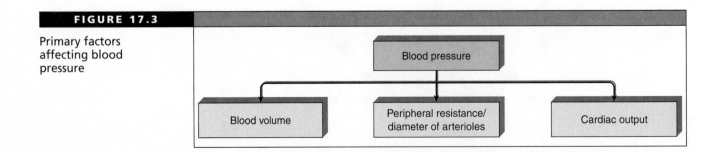

As blood flows at high speeds through the vascular system, it bumps and drags across the walls of the vessels. Although the vessel walls are extremely smooth, this friction reduces the velocity of the blood. This dragging or friction in the arteries is called **peripheral resistance**. Arteries have smooth muscle in their walls that, when constricted, will cause the inside diameter or **lumen** to become smaller, thus creating more resistance and higher pressure. This is how the body controls normal minute-by-minute changes in blood pressure. This is also important to pharmacology because a number of drugs affect vascular smooth muscle, causing vessels to constrict, thus raising blood pressure. Other drugs cause the smooth muscle to relax, thereby opening the lumen and lowering blood pressure. These drugs are among those used to treat HTN. The role of the autonomic nervous system in controlling peripheral resistance is presented in Chapter 8 ∞ .

The third factor responsible for blood pressure is the total amount to blood in the vascular system, or *blood volume*. Although the average person maintains a relatively constant blood volume of approximately 5 L, this can change as a result of certain regulatory factors and with certain disease states. More blood in the vascular system will exert additional pressure on the walls of the arteries and raise blood pressure. For example, high sodium diets cause water to be retained by the body, thus increasing blood volume and raising blood pressure. On the other hand, drugs called **diuretics** can cause fluid loss through urination, thus decreasing blood volume and lowering blood pressure. Diuretics are discussed later in this chapter and in Chapter 23 ∞ .

Many nervous and hormonal factors help to keep blood pressure within normal limits.

It is critical that the body maintains a normal range of blood pressure and that it has the ability to safely and rapidly change pressure as it proceeds through daily activities such as sleep and exercise. Too little blood pressure can cause dizziness and lack of urine formation, whereas too much pressure can cause vessels to rupture. A diagram explaining how the body maintains homeostasis during periods of blood pressure change is shown in Figure 17.4 ■.

Blood pressure is regulated on a minute-to-minute basis by a cluster of neurons in the medulla oblongata called the **vasomotor center**. Nerves travel from the vasomotor center to the arteries, where the smooth muscle is directed to either constrict (raise blood pressure) or relax (lower blood pressure).

Clusters of neurons in the aorta and the carotid artery act as sensors to provide the vasomotor center with vital information on current conditions in the vascular system. Some of these neurons, called **baroreceptors**, have the ability to sense blood pressure within these large vessels.

baro = *pressure*
receptor = *sensor*

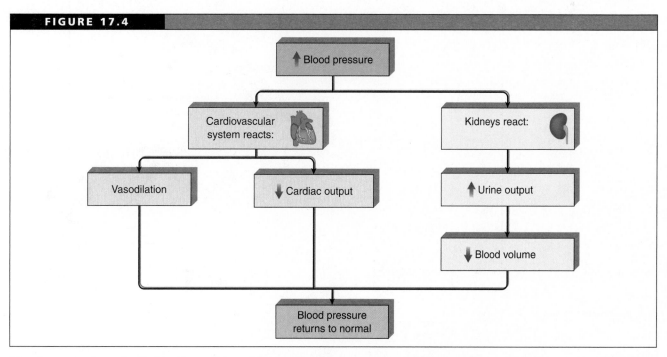

FIGURE 17.4

Blood pressure is controlled by the actions of the cardiovascular system and kidneys.

The baroreceptors are important to the pharmacotherapy of HTN. When a drug is given to lower blood pressure, the baroreceptors respond by trying to return pressure to its original (high) level. The baroreceptor response includes an immediate increase in heart rate, known as **reflex tachycardia**. In time, the body will recognize the lower blood pressure as normal, "reset" the baroreceptors, and reflex tachycardia will diminish. If reflex tachycardia does not decrease, a patient may be administered a beta-adrenergic blocker to prevent heart rate increase.

Emotions can also have a profound effect on blood pressure. Anger and stress can cause blood pressure to rise, whereas mental depression and lethargy may cause it to fall. Strong emotions, if present for a long time, may be important contributors to chronic HTN.

Certain hormones and other agents affect blood pressure on a daily basis. When given as drugs, some of these agents may have a profound effect on blood pressure. For example, an injection of epinephrine or norepinephrine will immediately raise blood pressure. **Antidiuretic hormone (ADH)** is a strong vasoconstrictor that can increase blood pressure by raising blood volume. The **renin-angiotensin-aldosterone system** is particularly important in the drug therapy of HTN and is discussed in Section 17.10. A summary of the various nervous and hormonal factors influencing blood pressure is shown in Figure 17.5 ■.

anti = *against*
diuretic = *urination*

Concept Review   17.1

■ Because hypertension may cause no symptoms, how would you convince a patient to take his or her medication regularly?

FIGURE 17.5

Hormonal and nervous factors influencing blood pressure

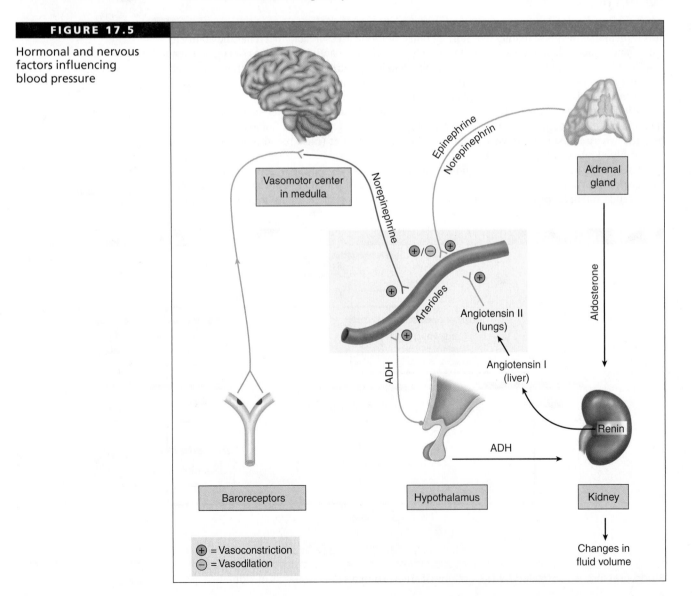

Positive lifestyle changes can reduce blood pressure and lessen the need for medications.

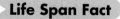

When a patient is first diagnosed with HTN, the health care provider obtains a comprehensive medical history to determine if the disease can be controlled without medications. Therapeutic lifestyle changes should be recommended for all patients with prehypertension or HTN. Of greatest importance is maintaining optimum weight, because obesity is closely associated with blood lipid elevation and HTN. Combining a safe weight loss program with proper nutrition can delay the progression from prehypertension to HTN.

In many cases, implementing positive lifestyle changes may eliminate the need for pharmacotherapy altogether. Even if pharmacotherapy is required, it is important that the patients continue their lifestyle modifications so that dosages can be minimized, thus lowering the potential for drug adverse effects. Important nonpharmacologic methods for controlling HTN are as follows:

- Implement a medically supervised, safe weight-reduction plan, if 20% or more over normal body weight.
- Stop using tobacco.
- Restrict salt (sodium) intake, and eat foods rich in potassium and magnesium.
- Limit alcohol consumption.
- Implement a medically supervised aerobic exercise plan.
- Reduce sources of stress and learn to implement coping strategies.

> **Life Span Fact**

Control of blood pressure is particularly important in aging patients. Age often causes blood vessels to be less elastic, thus impairing their ability to dilate or constrict with activities of daily living. Health care providers should emphasize to their older patients the importance of blood pressure monitoring and control.

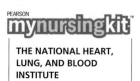

THE NATIONAL HEART, LUNG, AND BLOOD INSTITUTE

Selection of specific antihypertension drugs depends on the severity of the disease.

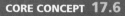

The goal of antihypertensive therapy is to reduce blood pressure to normal levels so that the long-term consequences of HTN may be prevented. Keeping blood pressure within normal limits has been shown to reduce the risk of HTN-related diseases such as stroke and heart failure. Several therapeutic strategies are used to achieve this goal, as summarized in Figure 17.6 ■.

Management of HTN depends on the degree of blood pressure increase, and whether the patient has a compelling indication such as myocardial infarction (MI), heart failure, or stroke (see Table 17.2). Pharmacotherapy usually begins with low doses of a single medication having few adverse effects, usually a diuretic. If this does not control blood pressure in 2 to 4 weeks, the prescriber may increase the dose of the initial drug or substitute another antihypertensive drug from a different drug class. The following drug classes are considered primary antihypertensive agents:

- Diuretics
- Renin-angiotensin-aldosterone inhibitors
- Calcium channel blockers (CCBs)
- Beta-adrenergic blockers

A common strategy used in controlling HTN is known as **stepped care**. This is the use of two drugs from different classes, rather than one. The advantage of this approach is that it allows lower doses of each drug than would be needed if a single one were used. Lower doses usually produce fewer side effects and improve patient adherence to therapy. Adherence decreases when patients need to take more than one drug or when they need to take them more often. For convenience, drug manufacturers often combine two drugs into a single pill or capsule. The diuretic hydrochlorothiazide (Microzide) is the most common drug used in combination antihypertensive products. Examples of antihypertensive combination drugs include Diovan HCT (hydrochlorothiazide and valsartan), Zestoretic (hydrochlorothiazide and lisinopril), and Lotrel (benazepril and amlodipine).

In designing outcomes for patients with HTN, special attention should be placed on African Americans with this disorder. The incidence of HTN is significantly higher in African Americans than in other ethnic groups, and aggressive antihypertensive therapy may be necessary to manage the disorder. Some physicians recommend initiating therapy with two drugs to ensure adequate response. Based on clinical trials in African Americans, the Food and Drug Administration (FDA) recently approved BiDil, a fixed-dose combination of isosorbide dinitrate and hydralazine that appears to be particularly effective at lowering blood pressure in this population.

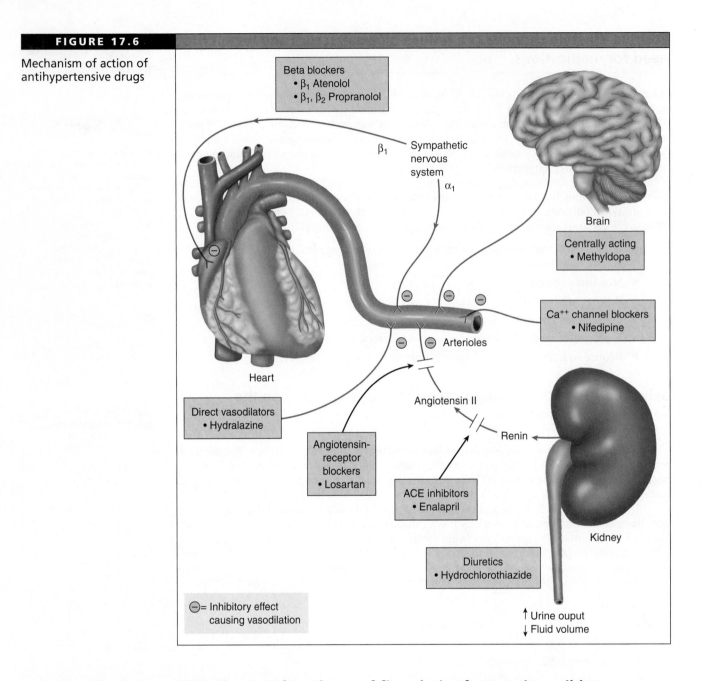

FIGURE 17.6

Mechanism of action of antihypertensive drugs

Diuretics are often drugs of first choice for treating mild to moderate hypertension.

CORE CONCEPT 17.8

Diuretics act by increasing the amount of urine produced by the kidneys. They are widely used in the treatment of HTN and HF. Table 17.3 lists diuretics commonly used to treat HTN.

Diuretics were the first widely prescribed class of drugs used to treat HTN in the 1950s. Despite many advances in drug therapy since then, diuretics are still considered by many physicians to be drugs of first choice because they produce few adverse effects and are very effective at controlling mild to moderate HTN. For more advanced disease, they are prescribed in combination with antihypertensive medications from other classes. Diuretics are also used to treat HF (see Chapter 18 ⊙⊙) and kidney disorders (see Chapter 30 ⊙⊙).

Although many different diuretics are available for HTN, all produce a similar outcome: the reduction of blood volume through the urinary excretion of water and electrolytes. **Electrolytes** are ions such as sodium (Na^+), calcium (Ca^{2+}), chloride (Cl^-), and potassium (K^+). The mechanisms by which diuretics reduce blood volume differ among the various diuretics. Differences among the diuretic classes are presented in Chapter 23 ⊙⊙ .

▶ **Life Span Fact**

Older adults are especially at risk for dyhydration and must be carefully monitored during the initial stages of diuretic therapy.

TABLE 17.3	Diuretics for Hypertension

DRUG	ROUTE AND ADULT DOSE	REMARKS
amiloride (Midamor)	PO; 5–10 mg/day (max: 20 mg/day)	Potassium sparing; acts by directly inhibiting sodium-potassium exchange in the distal tubule
chlorothiazide (Diuril) (see page 374 for the Drug Profile box)	PO/IV; 250 mg–1 g in one to two divided doses (max: 2 g/day)	Thiazide type; acts by inhibiting sodium reabsorption in the distal tubule; decreases blood potassium levels
chlorthalidone (Hygroton)	PO; 12.5–25 mg daily (max: 50 mg/day)	Thiazide type; acts by inhibiting sodium reabsorption in the distal tubule; decreases blood potassium levels
eplerenone (Inspra)	PO; 25–50 mg once daily (max: 100 mg/day)	A newer potassium-sparing diuretic; acts by blocking the aldosterone receptor
furosemide (Lasix) (see page 298 for the Drug Profile box)	PO; 20–80 mg/day (max: 600 mg/day)	Loop diuretic; decreases blood potassium levels; acts by inhibiting sodium and chloride reabsorption in the loop of Henle; IV and IM forms available
Pr hydrochlorothiazide (Microzide)	PO; 25–100 mg in one to two divided doses (max: 50 mg/day)	Thiazide type; acts by inhibiting sodium reabsorption in the distal tubule; decreases blood potassium levels
indapamide (Lozol)	PO; 1.25–5 mg daily (max: 5 mg/day)	Similar to thiazide type; acts by inhibiting sodium reabsorption in the distal tubule; decreases blood potassium levels
spironolactone (Aldactone) (see page 375 for the Drug Profile box)	PO; 25–100 mg 1–2 times/day (max: 400 mg/day)	Potassium-sparing; acts by inhibiting aldosterone in the distal tubule
torsemide (Demadex)	PO/IV; 10–20 mg/day (max: 200 mg/day)	Loop diuretic; acts by inhibiting sodium and chloride reabsorption in the loop of Henle and distal tubule
triamterene (Dyrenium)	PO; 50–100 mg bid (max: 300 mg/day)	Potassium sparing; acts by directly inhibiting sodium-potassium exchange in the distal tubule

One of the most common adverse effects of diuretic therapy is *dehydration*, the excessive loss of water from the body. Early signs of dehydration include thirst, dry mouth, dizziness, lethargy, and a fall in blood pressure.

de = *high*
hydra = *water*
tion = *condition*

Electrolyte imbalances of potassium, sodium, and magnesium ions are additional adverse effects of diuretic therapy. Loss of K^+, or **hypokalemia**, is of particular concern because it can lead to serious abnormalities in cardiac rhythm. When taking thiazide or loop diuretics, patients should be encouraged to include a potassium supplement or to eat foods rich in potassium content, such as bananas, oranges, tomatoes, milk, salmon, and beef.

hyper = *high*
hypo = *low*
ka = *potassium*
emia = *blood*

Certain diuretics such as spironolactone (Aldactone) have fewer tendencies to cause K^+ depletion, and, for this reason, are called *potassium-sparing diuretics*. Taking potassium supplements with potassium-sparing diuretics may lead to dangerously high K^+ levels in the blood, or **hyperkalemia**, which can cause cardiac conduction abnormalities.

Concept Review 17.2

■ State the major reasons why patients should continue lifestyle changes even though their antihypertensive drugs appear to be effective.

Calcium channel blockers have emerged as important drugs in the treatment of hypertension.

CORE CONCEPT **17.9**

Calcium channel blockers (CCBs) comprise a group of about 10 drugs that are used to treat a number of cardiovascular diseases, including angina pectoris, cardiac dysrhythmias, and HTN. When CCBs were first approved for the treatment of angina in the early 1980s, it was quickly noted that a "side effect" of the drugs was the lowering of blood pressure in patients with HTN. CCBs have since become a widely prescribed class of drugs for HTN. Table 17.4 lists CCBs that are commonly used to treat HTN.

DRUG PROFILE: Pr *Hydrochlorothiazide (Microzide)*

Therapeutic Class: Drug for hypertension and edema

Pharmacologic Class: Thiazide diuretic

Actions and Uses:

Hydrochlorothiazide is the most widely prescribed diuretic for HTN, belonging to a class of drugs known as the thiazides. Like many diuretics, it produces few serious adverse effects and is effective at producing a 10–20 mmHg reduction in blood pressure. Patients with severe HTN require the addition of a second drug from a different class to control the disease. Hydrochlorothiazide is approved to treat ascites, edema, HF, and HTN.

Hydrochlorothiazide acts on the kidney tubule to decrease the reabsorption of Na^+. When hydrochlorothiazide blocks this reabsorption, more Na^+ and water are sent into the urine, thus reducing blood volume and decreasing blood pressure. The volume of urine produced is directly proportional to the amount of Na^+ reabsorption blocked by the diuretic.

Adverse Effects and Interactions:

Hydrochlorothiazide has few serious adverse effects. The most common adverse effects involve potential electrolyte imbalances, especially loss of excessive K^+ and Na^+. Because K^+ deficiency may cause cardiac conduction abnormalities, patients are usually asked to increase their intake of dietary potassium as a precaution.

Hydrochlorothiazide increases the action of other antihypertensives and skeletal muscle relaxants. It may reduce the effectiveness of anticoagulants, antigout drugs, and antidiabetic drugs, including insulin.

Central nervous system (CNS) depressants such as alcohol, barbiturates, and opioids may increase the orthostatic hypotension caused by hydrochlorothiazide. Steroids or amphotericin B increase K^+ loss when given in conjunction with hydrochlorothiazide, leading to hypokalemia.

Hydrochlorothiazide increases the risk of serum toxicity of the following drugs: digoxin, lithium, allopurinol, anesthetics, and antineoplastics. It also alters vitamin D metabolism and calcium conservation; use of calcium supplements may cause hypercalcemia. It should be used with caution with herbal supplements, such as ginkgo biloba, which may cause an increase in blood pressure.

Refer to MyNursingKit for a Nursing Process Focus specific to this drug.

TABLE 17.4	Calcium Channel Blockers Used for Hypertension	
DRUG	**ROUTE AND ADULT DOSE**	**REMARKS**
amlodipine (Norvasc)	PO; 5–10 mg once daily (max: 10 mg/day)	Works primarily on peripheral circulation; reduces systolic, diastolic, and mean blood pressure; also for angina
diltiazem (Cardizem, Cartia XT, Dilacor XR, Taztia XT, Tiazac) (see page 346 for the Drug Profile box)	PO; 80–120 mg tid (max: 540 mg/day)	Dilates coronary arteries; affects calcium channels in both heart and blood vessels; sustained-release and IV forms are available; also for angina and specific dysrhythmias
felodipine (Plendil)	PO; 5–10 mg/day (max: 20 mg/day)	Selective for calcium channels in blood vessels; also for angina and heart failure
isradipine (DynaCirc)	PO; 1.25–10 mg bid (max: 20 mg/day)	Affects calcium channels in both heart and blood vessels; also for angina
nicardipine (Cardene)	PO; 20–40 mg tid (max: 120 mg/day)	Selective for calcium channels in blood vessels; also for angina; sustained-release and IV forms are available
Pr nifedipine (Adalat, Procardia)	PO; 10–20 mg tid (max: 180 mg/day)	Selective for calcium channels in blood vessels; decreases peripheral vascular resistance and increases cardiac output; also for angina; sustained-release form is available
nisoldipine (Nisocor)	PO; 10–20 mg bid (max: 60 mg/day)	Structurally similar to nifedipine; affects calcium channels in both the heart and blood vessels; also for angina and heart failure
verapamil (Calan, Isoptin, others) (see page 316 for the Drug Profile box)	PO; 40–80 mg tid (max: 480 mg/day)	Affects calcium channels in both heart and blood vessels; sustained-release form available; IV form available for specific dysrhythmias

DRUG PROFILE: ℗ *Nifedipine (Adalat, Procardia)*

Therapeutic Class: Drug for hypertension and angina
Pharmacologic Class: Calcium channel blocker

Actions and Uses:

Nifedipine is a CCB prescribed for angina as well as for HTN. Nifedipine selectively blocks calcium channels in myocardial and vascular smooth muscle, including that in the coronary arteries. This results in reduced oxygen demands by the heart, an increase in cardiac output, and a fall in blood pressure. Nifedipine is as effective as diuretics and beta-adrenergic blockers at reducing blood pressure.

Adverse Effects and Interactions:

Adverse effects of nifedipine are generally minor and related to vasodilation, such as headache, dizziness, and flushing. Fast-acting forms of nifedipine can cause significant reflex tachycardia. To avoid rebound hypotension, discontinuation of drug therapy should occur gradually.

Nifedipine may increase serum levels of digoxin, cimetidine, and ranitidine, and increase the effects of warfarin, resulting in increased partial thromboplastin time (PTT). It may also increase the effects of fentanyl anesthesia, resulting in severe hypotension and an increased need for fluids. Grapefruit juice may cause greater absorption of nifedipine.

Alcohol increases the vasodilating action of nifedipine and can lead to a severe drop in blood pressure. Nicotine causes vasoconstriction, countering the desired effect of nifedipine. Nifedipine should be used with caution with melatonin because this combination may increase blood pressure and heart rate.

Mechanism in Action:

Blocking calcium influx into smooth muscle cells results in arteriolar vasodilation. When arterioles are dilated, peripheral resistance and cardiac workload are reduced, and the blood pressure returns to normal.

Refer to MyNursingKit for a Nursing Process Focus specific to this drug.

Contraction of a muscle is regulated by the amount of calcium ions inside the muscle cell. Muscular contraction occurs when Ca^{2+} enters the cell through channels in the plasma membrane. CCBs block these channels and prevent Ca^{2+} from entering the cell, thus inhibiting muscular contraction. At low doses, CCBs cause vasodilation in arterioles, thus decreasing blood pressure. Some CCBs, such as nifedipine (Adalat, Procardia), are selective for calcium channels in arterioles, whereas others, such as verapamil (Calan, Isoptin, others), affect channels in both arterioles and cardiac muscle. CCBs vary in their potency and in the frequency and types of

NURSING PROCESS FOCUS

Patients Receiving Calcium Channel Blocker Therapy

ASSESSMENT

Prior to administration:
- Obtain a complete health history (physical/mental), including data on recent cardiac events, allergies, drug history, and possible drug interactions
- Obtain an electrocardiogram (ECG) and vital signs; assess in context of the patient's baseline values
- Assess neurologic status and level of consciousness
- Auscultate chest sounds for rales or rhonchi that indicate pulmonary edema
- Assess lower limbs for edema; note character/level

POTENTIAL NURSING DIAGNOSES

- Ineffective Health Maintenance related to drug therapy regimen.
- Deficient Knowledge related to information about drug therapy.
- Decreased Cardiac Output related to effects of drug therapy.
- Risk for Injury related to possible orthostatic hypotension.

continued . . .

NURSING PROCESS FOCUS (continued)

PLANNING: PATIENT GOALS AND EXPECTED OUTCOMES

The patient will:
- Exhibit a reduction in systolic/diastolic blood pressure
- Demonstrate an understanding of the drug's action by accurately describing adverse effects and precautions

IMPLEMENTATION

Interventions and (Rationales)	Patient Education/Discharge Planning
■ Monitor vital signs and ECG. Obtain blood pressure readings in sitting, standing, and supine positions to monitor fluctuations in blood pressure. (Calcium channel blockers [CCBs] dilate the arteries, reducing blood pressure.)	Instruct the patient to: ■ Monitor vital signs as specified by the nurse, particularly the blood pressure, ensuring proper use of home equipment ■ Withhold medication for severe hypotensive readings as specified by the nurse (e.g., "hold for levels below 88/50 mmHg") ■ Immediately report palpitations or rapid heartbeat
■ Observe for changes in level of consciousness, dizziness, fatigue, postural hypotension (caused by vasodilation). ■ Observe for paradoxical increase in chest pain, angina symptoms, or increase in heart rate (related to severe hypotension).	Instruct the patient to: ■ Report dizziness or lightheadedness ■ Rise slowly from prolonged periods of sitting or lying down ■ Report chest pain or other angina-like symptoms
■ Monitor for signs of HF. (CCBs can decrease myocardial contractility, increasing the risk of HF.)	■ Instruct the patient to immediately report any severe shortness of breath, frothy sputum, profound fatigue, and swelling. These may be signs of HF or fluid accumulation in the lungs.
■ Monitor for fluid accumulation. Measure intake and output, and daily weights. (Edema is an adverse effect of some CCBs.)	Instruct the patient to: ■ Avoid excessive heat, which contributes to excessive sweating and fluid loss ■ Measure and monitor fluid intake and output, and weigh daily ■ Consume enough *plain* water to remain adequately, but not overly, hydrated
■ Observe for hypersensitivity reaction.	■ Instruct the patient to immediately report difficulty breathing, throat tightness, hives or rash, muscle cramps, or tremors.
■ Monitor liver and kidney function. (CCBs are metabolized in the liver and excreted by the kidneys.)	Instruct the patient to: ■ Report signs of liver toxicity: nausea, vomiting, anorexia, bleeding, severe upper abdominal pain, heartburn, jaundice, or a change in the color or character of stools ■ Report signs of renal toxicity: fever, flank pain, changes in urine output, color, or character (cloudy, with sediment, etc.) ■ Adhere to laboratory testing regimens as ordered by the health care provider
■ Observe for constipation. May need to increase dietary fiber or administer laxatives.	Advise the patient to: ■ Maintain adequate fluid and fiber intake to facilitate stool passage ■ Use a bulk laxative or stool softener, as recommended by the health care provider
■ Ensure patient safety. Monitor ambulation until response to the drug is known (because of postural hypotension caused by the drug).	■ Instruct the patient to avoid driving or other activities that require mental alertness or physical coordination until the effects of the drug are known.

EVALUATION OF OUTCOME CRITERIA

Evaluate the effectiveness of drug therapy by confirming that patient goals and expected outcomes have been met (see "Planning").

See Table 17.4 for a list of drugs to which these nursing actions apply.

adverse effects produced. The use of CCBs in the treatment of dysrhythmias and angina is discussed in Chapters 19 and 21 ⚭ , respectively.

The high safety profile of CCBs has contributed to their popularity in treating HTN. Common adverse effects related to their vasodilation action include headache, facial flushing, and dizziness. The CCBs that affect the heart should be used cautiously in patients with preexisting heart disease.

Blocking the renin-angiotensin-aldosterone system leads to a decrease in blood pressure.

CORE CONCEPT 17.10

The renin-angiotensin-aldosterone system (RAAS) is one of the primary homeostatic mechanisms controlling blood pressure and fluid balance in the body. Drugs that modify the RAAS decrease blood pressure and increase urine volume. They are widely used in the treatment of HTN, HF, and MI. Table 17.5 lists the RAAS modifiers commonly used to treat HTN.

Renin is an enzyme secreted by the kidneys when blood pressure falls or when there is a decrease in Na^+ flowing through the kidney tubules. In a series of enzymatic steps, **angiotensin II**, one of the most potent natural vasoconstrictors known, is formed. The enzyme reponsible for the final step of this pathway is called **angiotensin-converting enzyme (ACE)**. The intense vasoconstriction of arterioles caused by angiotensin II raises blood pressure by increasing peripheral resistance.

angio = *vessels*
tensin = *pressure*

TABLE 17.5	ACE Inhibitors and Angiotensin-Receptor Blockers Used for Hypertension	
DRUG	**ROUTE AND ADULT DOSE**	**REMARKS**
ACE INHIBITORS		
benazepril (Lotensin)	PO; 10–40 mg in one to two divided doses (max: 40 mg/day)	May be used in combination with thiazide diuretics
captopril (Capoten)	PO; 6.25–25 mg tid (max: 450 mg/day)	Also for HF and MI
℗ enalapril (Vasotec)	PO; 5–40 mg in 1–2 divided doses (max: 40 mg/day)	Also for HF; IV form available
fosinopril (Monopril)	PO; 5–40 mg daily (max: 80 mg/day)	Also for HF
lisinopril (Prinivil, Zestril) (see page 295 for the Drug Profile box)	PO; 10 mg daily (max: 80 mg/day)	Also for HF and MI
moexipril (Univasc)	PO; 7.5–30 mg daily (max: 30 mg/day)	Approved for HTN only
perindopril (Aceon)	PO; 4 mg once daily (max: 16 mg/day)	Also for heart failure
quinapril (Accupril)	PO; 10–20 mg daily (max: 80 mg/day)	Also for HF
ramipril (Altace)	PO; 2.5–5 mg daily (max: 20 mg/day)	Also for HF
trandolapril (Mavik)	PO; 1–4 mg daily (max: 8 mg/day)	Approved for HTN only; discontinue diuretics 2–3 days before starting therapy
ANGIOTENSIN-RECEPTOR BLOCKERS		
candesartan (Atacand)	PO; start at 16 mg/day (max: 32 mg/day)	Approved for HTN only
eprosartan (Teveten)	PO; 600 mg/day or 400 mg qid–bid (max: 800 mg/day)	Approved for HTN only
irbesartan (Avapro)	PO; 150–300 mg/day (max: 300 mg/day)	Maximum effect may take 6–12 weeks
losartan (Cozaar)	PO; 25–50 mg in one to two divided doses (max: 100 mg/day)	Causes relaxation of smooth vascular muscle
olmesartan (Benicar)	PO; 20–40 mg/day (max: 40 mg/day)	Approved for HTN only
telmisartan (Micardis)	PO; 40–80 mg/day (max: 80 mg/day)	Approved for HTN only
valsartan (Diovan)	PO; 80 mg/day (max: 320 mg/day)	Evidence of effectiveness of therapy in 2–4 weeks

NATURAL THERAPIES

Grape Seed Extract for Hypertension

Grapes and grape seeds have been used for thousands of years. Their primary use has been for cardiovascular conditions such as HTN, high blood cholesterol, atherosclerosis, and to generally improve circulation. Some claim that grape seed extract improves wound healing, prevents cancer, and lowers the risk for the long-term consequences of diabetes.

The grape seeds, usually obtained from winemaking, are crushed and placed into tablet, capsule, or liquid forms. Grape seed extract has antioxidant properties. In general, antioxidants improve wound healing and repair cellular injury. Preliminary evidence suggests that it may have some benefit in repairing blood vessel damage that could lead to atherosclerosis and HTN. Controlled, long-term studies on the effects of grape seed extract on HTN have not been conducted. It has few adverse effects, but caution should be used if taking anticoagulant drugs because increased bleeding may result. Overall, the benefits of grape seed extract are no different than those of a diet balanced with natural antioxidants (and an occasional glass of red wine).

A second, equally important effect of angiotensin II is stimulation of the secretion of **aldosterone**, a hormone from the adrenal gland that increases sodium ion reabsorption in the kidney. This increase in Na^+ reabsorption helps the body retain water, which raises blood volume and increases blood pressure. Drugs that inhibit the RAAS block the effects of angiotensin II, thus decreasing blood pressure through *two* mechanisms: dilating arteries and decreasing blood volume.

NURSING PROCESS FOCUS

Patients Receiving ACE Inhibitor Therapy

ASSESSMENT

Prior to administration:
- Obtain a complete health history (physical/mental), including data on recent cardiac events and any incidence of angioedema, allergies, drug history, and possible drug interactions
- Obtain an ECG and vital signs; assess in context of the patient's baseline values
- Assess neurologic status and level of consciousness
- Obtain blood and urine specimens for laboratory analysis

POTENTIAL NURSING DIAGNOSES

- Risk for Injury related to orthostatic hypotension.
- Deficient Knowledge related to information about drug therapy.
- Ineffective Tissue Perfusion related to decreased blood volume.
- Risk for Imbalanced Nutrition: More than Body Requirements related to hyperkalemia.

PLANNING: PATIENT GOALS AND EXPECTED OUTCOMES

The patient will:
- Exhibit a reduction in systolic/diastolic blood pressure
- Maintain normal serum electrolyte levels during drug therapy
- Demonstrate an understanding of the drug's action by accurately describing adverse effects and precautions

IMPLEMENTATION

Interventions and (Rationales)

- Monitor for first-dose phenomenon of profound hypotension.

Patient Education/Discharge Planning

- Warn the patient about the first-dose phenomenon; reassure that this effect diminishes with continued therapy.

Instruct the patient:
- That changes in consciousness may occur due to rapid reduction in blood pressure and to immediately report feelings of faintness
- That the drug takes effect in approximately 1 hour and peaks in 3–4 hours
- To rest in the supine position beginning 1 hour after administration and for 3 hours after the first dose
- To always rise slowly, avoiding sudden posture changes

continued . . .

NURSING PROCESS FOCUS (continued)

Interventions and (Rationales)	Patient Education/Discharge Planning
■ Observe for hypersensitivity reaction, particularly angioedema. (Angioedema may arise at any time during ACE inhibitor therapy, but it is generally expected shortly after initiation of therapy.)	Instruct the patient: ■ To immediately report difficulty breathing, throat tightness, muscle cramps, hives or rash, or tremors (These symptoms can occur as early as the first dose or much later as a delayed reaction.) ■ That angioedema can be life threatening and to call emergency medical services if severe dyspnea or hoarseness is accompanied by swelling of the face or mouth
■ Monitor for the presence of blood dyscrasia. ■ Observe for signs of infection: fever, sore throat, malaise, joint pain, ecchymoses, profound fatigue, shortness of breath, or pallor. (Bruising is a sign of bleeding that can indicate the presence of a serious blood disorder.)	Instruct the patient to observe for bruising and signs of bleeding from the nose, mouth, gastrointestinal (GI) tract ("coffee ground" vomit or tarry stools) as well as menstrual flooding or bright red rectal bleeding. ■ Instruct the patient to immediately report any flulike symptoms.
■ Monitor for changes in level of consciousness, dizziness, drowsiness, or lightheadedness. (Signs of decreased blood flow to the brain are due to the drug's vasodilating hypotensive action. Sudden syncopal collapse is possible.)	Instruct the patient to: ■ Report dizziness or fainting that persists beyond the first dose as well as unusual sensations (e.g., numbness and tingling) or other changes in the face or limbs ■ Contact the health care provider before the next scheduled dose of the drug if fainting occurs
■ Monitor for persistent dry cough (a possible adverse effect of the drug). Monitor changes in cough pattern. (This may indicate another disease process.)	Instruct the patient to: ■ Expect persistent dry cough ■ Report any change in the character or frequency of cough (Any cough accompanied by shortness of breath, fever, or chest pain should be reported *immediately* because it may indicate MI.) ■ Sleep with the head elevated if cough becomes troublesome when in the supine position ■ Use nonmedicated sugar-free lozenges or hard candies to relieve cough
■ Monitor for dehydration or fluid overload. (Dehydration causes low circulating blood volume and will exacerbate hypotension. Severe dehydration may trigger syncope and collapse. Pitting edema, a sign of fluid retention, can be a sign of HF and may indicate reduced drug effectiveness.)	Instruct the patient to: ■ Observe for signs of dehydration, such as oliguria, dry lips and mucous membranes, or poor skin turgor ■ Report any bodily swelling that leaves sunken marks on the skin when pressed ■ Measure and monitor fluid intake and output, and weigh daily ■ Monitor increased need for fluids caused by vomiting, diarrhea, or excessive sweating ■ Avoid excessive heat that contributes to sweating and fluid loss ■ Consume adequate amounts of *plain* water
■ Monitor for hyperkalemia. (This may occur due to reduced aldosterone levels.)	Instruct the patient to: ■ Immediately report signs of hyperkalemia: nausea, irregular heartbeat, profound fatigue/muscle weakness, and slow or faint pulse ■ Avoid consuming electrolyte-fortified snacks, or sports drinks that may contain potassium ■ Avoid using salt substitute (KCl) to flavor foods ■ Consult the health care provider before taking any nutritional supplements containing potassium

continued . . .

NURSING PROCESS FOCUS *(continued)*

Interventions and (Rationales)

- Monitor for liver and kidney function. (ACE inhibitors are metabolized by the liver and excreted by the kidneys.)

Patient Education/Discharge Planning

Instruct the patient to:
- Report signs of liver toxicity such as nausea; vomiting; anorexia; diarrhea; rash; jaundice; abdominal pain, tenderness, or distension; or change in the color or character of stools
- Discontinue the drug immediately and contact the health care provider if jaundice occurs
- Adhere to laboratory testing regimen as ordered by the health care provider

---

- Ensure patient safety (due to postural hypotension caused by the drug). Monitor ambulation until response to the drug is known.

Instruct the patient to:
- Obtain help prior to getting out of bed or attempting to walk alone
- Avoid driving or other activities that require mental alertness or physical coordination until effects of the drug are known

---

EVALUATION OF OUTCOME CRITERIA

Evaluate the effectiveness of drug therapy by confirming that patient goals and expected outcomes have been met (see "Planning").

See Table 17.5 for a list of drugs to which these nursing actions apply.

DRUG PROFILE: ℗ *Enalapril (Vasotec)*

Therapeutic Class: Drug for hypertension and heart failure
Pharmacologic Class: ACE inhibitor

Actions and Uses:

Enalapril is one of the most common ACE inhibitors prescribed for HTN. Unlike captopril (Capoten), the first ACE inhibitor to be marketed, enalapril has a prolonged half-life, which permits administration once or twice daily. Enalapril acts by reducing angiotensin II and aldosterone levels to produce a significant reduction in blood pressure, with few adverse effects. Enalapril has effectiveness comparable to the thiazide diuretics and the beta-adrenergic blockers. It may be used by itself or in combination with other antihypertensives. Vaseretic is a fixed-dose combination of enalapril and hydrochlorothiazide.

Adverse Effects and Interactions:

Unlike diuretics, ACE inhibitors such as enalapril have little effect on electrolyte balance, and unlike beta-adrenergic blockers, they cause few cardiac adverse effects. Like other antihypertensive drugs, enalapril may cause hypotension, especially when moving quickly from a supine to an upright position. This condition, known as postural or orthostatic hypotension, can cause lightheadedness and even fainting. Care must be taken because a rapid fall in blood pressure may occur following the first dose. Most drugs in this class cause a persistent, dry cough. Other adverse effects include headache, dizziness.

Thiazide diuretics increase the risk of excessive potassium loss when used with enalapril. On the other hand, potassium-sparing diuretics increase the risk of hyperkalemia when used with ACE inhibitors. Renin-releasing antihypertensives increase the action of enalapril and can cause profound hypotension.

Enalapril may induce lithium toxicity by reducing renal clearance of lithium. Nonsteroidal anti-inflammatory drugs (NSAIDs) may reduce the effectiveness of ACE inhibitors.

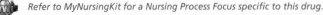

Refer to MyNursingKit for a Nursing Process Focus specific to this drug.

First detected in the venom of pit vipers in the 1960s, drugs that inhibit ACE have been approved for hypertension since the 1980s. Since then, the ACE inhibitors have become important drugs in the treatment of HTN. ACE inhibitors are drugs of choice for patients with both diabetes and HTN because they have been shown to reduce the progression to kidney failure that often occurs in patients with diabetes. Because of cardiovascular changes associated with diabetes, these patients often require therapy with at least two antihypertensive drugs. Adverse effects of ACE inhibitors are relatively minor and include persistent cough and hypotension following the first dose of the drug. Some ACE inhibitors have also been approved for the treatment of HF and MI, and these are discussed in Chapters 18 and 21 ⚭ , respectively.

A second method of modifying the RAAS is blocking the action of angiotensin II *after* it is formed. Several drugs, including irbesartan (Avapro), losartan (Cozaar), and valsartan (Diovan), block the receptors for angiotensin in arteriolar smooth muscle and in the adrenal gland, thus causing blood pressure to fall. Their actions of arteriolar dilation and increased renal Na^+ excretion are quite similar to those of the ACE inhibitors. Angiotensin-receptor blockers (ARBs) have relatively few adverse effects, such as headache, dizziness, and facial flushing, most of which are related to hypotension. Drugs in this class are usually combined with drugs from other classes; for example, the drug Hyzaar combines losartan with the diuretic hydrochlorothiazide.

tachy = *rapid*
cardia = *heart*

Alpha- and beta-adrenergic blockers are commonly used to treat hypertension.

CORE CONCEPT   17.11

Stimulation of the sympathetic division of the autonomic nervous system causes fight-or-flight responses such as faster heart rate, an increase in blood pressure, and bronchodilation. By blocking the sympathetic "fight-or-flight" responses, drugs can cause the heart rate to slow, blood pressure

---

DRUG PROFILE: ℗ *Doxazosin (Cardura)*

Therapeutic Class: Drug for hypertension and BPH
Pharmacologic Class: Alpha₁-adrenergic blocker

Actions and Uses:

Doxazosin is a selective alpha₁-adrenergic blocker available only in oral form. Because it is selective for blocking alpha₁-receptors in vascular smooth muscle, it has few adverse effects on other autonomic organs and is sometimes preferred over nonselective beta blockers such as propranolol (Inderal, InnoPran XL). Doxazosin dilates both arteries and veins and is capable of causing a rapid, profound fall in blood pressure. Although prazosin (Minipress) was the first alpha-adrenergic blocker available for hypertension, other alpha blockers such as doxazosin and terazosin (Hytrin) are more widely used because they have prolonged half-lives that allow them to be taken once daily.

Doxazosin and several other alpha-adrenergic blockers also relax smooth muscle around the prostate gland. Patients who have dificulty urinating due to an enlarged prostate, a condition known as benign prostatic hyperplasia (BPH), sometimes receive these drugs to relieve symptoms of this disease, as discussed in Chapter 32 ⚭ .

Adverse Effects and Interactions:

When starting doxazosin therapy, some patients experience orthostatic hypotension, although tolerance normally develops to this adverse effect after a few doses. Dizziness and headache are also common adverse effects, although they are rarely severe enough to cause discontinuation of therapy. Oral cimetidine may cause a mild increase (10%) in the half-life of doxazosin.

Mechanism in Action:

Doxazosin selectively blocks alpha₁-adrenergic receptors. By dilating vascular smooth muscle, alpha₁-blockers reverse any frictional resistance to lower blood pressure. Alpha₁-blockers relax smooth muscle around the prostate gland.

 Refer to MyNursingKit for a Nursing Process Focus specific to this drug.

to decline, and the bronchi to dilate. Adrenergic antagonists (or blockers) that are important in managing HTN are listed in Table 17.6.

Because of their beneficial effects on the heart and vessels, adrenergic blockers are used for a wide variety of cardiovascular disorders. These drugs can block the effects of the sympathetic division through a number of different mechanisms, although they all have in common the effect of lowering blood pressure. These mechanisms include the following:

- Blockade of alpha$_1$-receptors in the arterioles
- Blockade of beta$_1$-receptors in the heart
- Nonselective blockade of both beta$_1$- and beta$_2$-receptors
- Stimulation of alpha$_2$-adrenergic receptors in the brainstem (centrally acting)

hyper = *high*
plasia = *growth*

Some drugs, such as epinephrine, affect both beta- and alpha-adrenergic receptors and can cause serious adverse effects. Drugs that affect only one receptor subtype produce fewer adverse effects. Prazosin (Minipress), for example, is specific to alpha$_1$-receptors and thus has less effect

TABLE 17.6	Adrenergic Blockers and Central-Acting Agents Used for Hypertension	
DRUG	**ROUTE AND ADULT DOSE**	**REMARKS**
acebutolol (Sectral)	PO; 400–800 mg/day (max: 1200 mg/day)	Selective beta$_1$-blocker; also for premature ventricular beats
atenolol (Tenormin) (see page 345 for the Drug Profile box)	PO; 25–50 mg/day (max: 100 mg/day)	Selective beta$_1$-blocker; IV form available for MI; monitor apical pulse prior to administration
betaxolol (Kerlone)	PO; 10–40 mg/day (max: 40 mg/day)	Selective beta$_1$-blocker; approved for HTN only; discontinue drug gradually to avoid rebound HTN
bisoprolol (Zebeta)	PO; 2.5–5 mg daily (max: 20 mg/day)	Selective beta$_1$-blocker; also for angina; discontinue the drug gradually to avoid rebound HTN
carvedilol (Coreg) (see page 300 for the Drug Profile box)	PO; 6.25 mg bid (max: 50 mg/day)	Blocks both alpha and beta receptors; also for HF
clonidine (Catapres)	PO; 0.1 mg bid–tid (max: 0.8 mg/day)	Central-acting alpha$_2$-adrenergic agent; transdermal patch available; epidural infusion form available for management of cancer pain
(Pr) doxazosin (Cardura)	PO; 1 mg at bedtime; may increase to 16 mg/day in one to two divided doses (max: 16 mg/day)	Selective alpha$_1$-blocker; also for BPH
methyldopa (Aldomet)	PO; 250 mg bid or tid (max: 3 g/day)	Central-acting alpha$_2$-adrenergic agent; IV form available; lowers standing and supine blood pressure
metoprolol (Lopressor, Toprol, others)	PO; 50–100 mg daily or bid (max: 450 mg/day)	Selective beta$_1$-blocker; sustained-release and IV forms available; also for angina and MI
nadolol (Corgard)	PO; 40 mg/day (max: 320 mg/day)	Nonselective beta blocker; also for angina
pindolol (Visken)	PO; 5 mg bid (max: 60 mg/day)	Nonselective beta$_1$- and beta$_2$-blocker; for HTN only
prazosin (Minipress) (see page 107 for the Drug Profile box)	PO; 1 mg at bedtime; increase to 1 mg bid–tid (max: 20 mg/day)	Selective alpha$_1$-blocker used in combination with other antihypertensives; also for BPH, Raynaud's disease, and pheochromocytoma
propranolol (Inderal, InnoPran XL) (see page 314 for the Drug Profile box)	PO; 40 mg bid but may be increased to 160–480 mg/day in divided doses (max: 480 mg/day)	Nonselective beta$_1$- and beta$_2$-blocker; also for angina, MI, dysrhythmias, and migraine prophylaxis; IV form available
terazosin (Hytrin)	PO; 1 mg at bedtime; increase 1–5 mg/day (max: 20 mg/day)	Selective alpha$_1$-blocker; also for BPH
timolol (Timoptic, Timoptic XE) (see page 637 for the Drug Profile box)	PO; 10 mg bid (max: 60 mg/day)	Nonselective beta$_1$- and beta$_2$-blocker; also for MI and migraine prophylaxis and for glaucoma

on the heart, which contains beta$_1$-receptors. On the other hand, atenolol (Tenormin) and metoprolol (Lopressor, Toprol) are selective for beta$_1$-receptors and thus have little effect on the bronchi, which have beta$_2$-receptors. Of the adrenergic antagonists, only the beta-adrenergic blockers are considered first-line drugs for the pharmacotherapy of HTN.

The adverse effects of adrenergic antagonists are quite predictable because they are extensions that would be expected from blocking the fight-or-flight response. The alpha$_1$-blockers tend to cause **orthostatic hypotension** in patients when they move quickly from a supine to an upright position. Dizziness, nausea, **bradycardia**, and dry mouth are also common. Less common, though sometimes a major cause for nonadherence, is their adverse effect on male sexual function (impotence). Because nonselective beta blockers slow the heart rate and cause bronchoconstriction, they should be used with caution in patients with asthma or HF.

Some adrenergic blockers affect the production of neurotransmitters in the *central* nervous system rather than affecting the *peripheral* nervous system. For example, methyldopa (Aldomet) is converted to a **false neurotransmitter** in the brainstem, thus causing a shortage of the "real" neurotransmitter and inhibition of the sympathetic nervous system. Clonidine (Catapres), an alpha$_2$ blocker, affects alpha-adrenergic receptors in the cardiovascular control centers in the brainstem. The central acting agents have a tendency to produce sedation and are infrequently prescribed.

ortho = *straight*
static = *causing to stand*

brady = *slow*
cardia = *heart*

Concept Review   17.3

■ Why is it important for the patient to weigh himself or herself on a regular basis when taking antihypertensive drugs?

Vasodilators lower blood pressure by relaxing arteriolar smooth muscle.

CORE CONCEPT 17.12

Many of the antihypertensive drugs discussed thus far lower blood pressure through indirect means by affecting enzymes (ACE inhibitors), autonomic nerves (alpha and beta blockers), or fluid volume (diuretics). It would seem that a more efficient way to reduce blood pressure would be to cause a direct relaxation of arteriolar smooth muscle. Indeed, drugs that directly affect vascular smooth muscle are highly effective at lowering blood pressure, but they produce too many

---

DRUG PROFILE: ℗ *Hydralazine (Apresoline)*

Therapeutic Class: Drug for hypertension and heart failure
Pharmacologic Class: Direct-acting vasodilator

Actions and Uses:

Hydralazine was one of the first oral antihypertensive drugs marketed in the United States. Therapy is generally begun with low doses, which are gradually increased until the desired therapeutic response is obtained. After several months of therapy, tolerance to the drug develops and a dosage increase may be necessary. Although it produces an effective reduction in blood pressure, drugs in other antihypertensive classes have largely replaced hydralazine because of its many adverse effects. However, this may change due to the recent approval of BiDil, a fixed-dose combination of isosorbide dinitrate and hydralazine that appears to be effective at lowering blood pressure in African Americans.

Adverse Effects and Interactions:

Headache, reflex tachycardia, palpitations, flushing, nausea, and diarrhea are common but may resolve as therapy progresses. Patients taking hydralazine often receive a beta-adrenergic blocker to counteract reflex tachycardia. The drug may produce a lupus-like syndrome with extended use. Sodium and fluid retention is another potentially serious adverse effect. The use of hydralazine is mostly limited to patients whose HTN cannot be controlled with other, safer medications.

Administering hydralazine with other antihypertensives or monoamine oxidase (MAO) inhibitors may cause severe hypotension. This includes all drug classes used as antihypertensives. NSAIDs may decrease the antihypertensive response of hydralazine.

Refer to MyNursingKit for a Nursing Process Focus specific to this drug.

TABLE 17.7	Direct-Acting Vasodilators for Hypertension	
DRUG	**ROUTE AND ADULT DOSE**	**REMARKS**
(Pr) hydralazine (Apresoline)	PO; 10–50 mg qid (max: 300 mg/day)	Diastolic response usually greater than systolic; IV and IM forms available
minoxidil (Loniten)	PO; 5–40 mg/day (max: 100 mg/day)	Reserved for severe hypertension; topical form used to promote hair growth
nitroprusside (Nitropress)	IV; 0.5–10 mcg/kg/min	For hypertensive crisis; produces both arteriolar and venous dilation; infusion not to exceed 10 min

adverse effects to be drugs of first choice. The direct-acting vasodilators used for hypertension are listed in Table 17.7.

Direct vasodilators produce reflex tachycardia, a normal physiologic response to the sudden decrease in blood pressure caused by the drug. Reflex tachycardia forces the heart to work harder, and blood pressure increases, counteracting the effect of the antihypertensive drug. A second potentially serious adverse effect of direct vasodilator therapy is Na^+ and water retention. As the kidney retains more Na^+ and water, blood volume increases, thus raising blood pressure and canceling the antihypertensive action of the vasodilator.

One direct-acting vasodilator, nitroprusside (Nitropress), is a traditional drug of choice for hypertensive emergency, a condition in which diastolic pressure is greater than 120 mmHg and there is evidence of organ damage, usually to the heart, kidney, or brain. This potentially life-threatening condition must be controlled quickly. Nitroprusside has the ability to lower blood pressure almost instantaneously on IV administration. Care must be taken not to decrease blood pressure too quickly because this can result in hypotension and severe restriction of blood flow to the cerebral, coronary, or renal capillaries.

PATIENTS NEED TO KNOW

Patients treated for HTN need to know the following:

1. Take medications as prescribed.
2. Never discontinue the medication without approval from a health care provider.
3. To control HTN, incorporate lifestyle changes such as diet and exercise, even if blood pressure is brought into normal limits by the medication.
4. Check blood pressure on a regular basis and report significant variations to the health care provider.
5. Get out of bed slowly to avoid dizziness.
6. Unless a potassium-sparing diuretic is prescribed, an increased intake of potassium-rich foods such as bananas, dried fruits, and orange juice may be necessary.
7. Take weight measurements regularly and report abnormal weight gains or losses.
8. Do not take any over-the-counter (OTC) medications for colds, flu, or allergies without first checking with a health care provider.

SAFETY ALERT

Drug-to-Food Interactions

Mr. Bruce loves to have grapefruit juice every day because of its "health benefit." Unfortunately, the benefits of eating or drinking certain foods may become risks when taken at the same time of some medications. Examples of this include the combination of grapefruit juice and certain blood pressure-lowering drugs or some cholesterol-lowering drugs, which can cause toxic levels of the drug in the blood. The nurse should ensure that patients are fully informed about how to take their drugs by providing both oral and written instructions. It is also advisable that patients keep their medications in their original, labeled containers so that instructions are readily available.

Retrieved from http://www.fda.gov/ForConsumers/ConsumerUpdates/UCM096386

17.1 Hypertension is characterized by the consistent elevation of arterial blood pressure.

A patient having a sustained blood pressure of 140/90 mmHg after multiple measurements made over several clinic visits is said to have hypertension (HTN). HTN is classified into three categories—prehypertension, Stage 1, and Stage 2.

17.2 Failure to treat hypertension can lead to stroke, heart failure, or myocardial infarction.

HTN is one of the most common diseases. Uncontrolled HTN can cause chronic and debilitating disorders such as stroke, heart attack, and heart failure.

17.3 Blood pressure is caused by the pumping action of the heart.

As the heart pumps, it creates pressure that is greatest in the arteries closest to the heart. The pressure created by the heart's contraction is called systolic pressure, and that present during the heart's relaxation is called diastolic pressure.

17.4 The primary factors responsible for blood pressure are cardiac output, the resistance of the small arteries, and blood volume.

As blood leaves the heart, its pressure depends on how much blood is present in the vessels (blood volume), how much is ejected per minute, and how much resistance it encounters from the small arteries (peripheral resistance). These are considered the primary factors controlling blood pressure.

17.5 Many nervous and hormonal factors help to keep blood pressure within normal limits.

Clusters of neurons in the medulla known as the vasomotor center regulate blood pressure. Feedback is provided to the vasomotor center by baroreceptors in the aorta and carotid arteries. Hormonal agents such as epinephrine or ADH may have profound effects on blood pressure.

17.6 Positive lifestyle changes can reduce blood pressure and lessen the need for medications.

Because antihypertensive drugs may have uncomfortable adverse effects, lifestyle changes such as proper diet and exercise are often implemented prior to and during drug therapy to enable lower drug doses.

17.7 Selection of specific antihypertension drugs depends on the severity of the disease.

Drug therapy of HTN often begins with low doses of a single drug. If ineffective, a second drug from a different class may be added to the regimen. Multi-drug therapy is common.

17.8 Diuretics are often drugs of first choice for treating mild to moderate hypertension.

Diuretics are often drugs of first choice for HTN because they have few adverse effects and can control minor to moderate HTN. Electrolytes should be carefully monitored in patients taking diuretics.

17.9 Calcium channel blockers have emerged as important drugs in the treatment of hypertension.

Calcium channel blockers (CCBs) block calcium ions from entering smooth muscle cells, causing arterioles to relax, thus reducing blood pressure. Some CCBs are also used to treat angina, heart failure, and dysrhythmias.

17.10 Blocking the renin-angiotensin-aldosterone system leads to a decrease in blood pressure.

Blocking angiotensin-converting enzyme (ACE) or the angiotensin II receptor can prevent the intense vasoconstriction caused by angiotensin. These drugs also decrease blood volume, which aids in producing their antihypertensive effect.

17.11 Alpha- and beta-adrenergic blockers are commonly used to treat hypertension.

Autonomic drugs that block alpha$_1$-receptors, block beta$_1$- and/or beta$_2$-receptors, or stimulate alpha$_2$-receptors in the brainstem (centrally acting) to lower blood pressure are available. Although acting by different mechanisms, these drugs all lower blood pressure.

17.12 Vasodilators lower blood pressure by relaxing arteriolar smooth muscle.

A few drugs lower blood pressure by directly relaxing arteriolar smooth muscle. Other than their use in treating hypertensive crisis, drugs in this class are not widely used because of their numerous adverse effects.

REVIEW QUESTIONS

The following questions are written in NCLEX-PN® style. Answer these questions to assess your knowledge of the chapter material, and go back and review any material that is not clear to you.

1. Which of the following is not a nonpharmacologic method of controlling hypertension?

1. Weight loss
2. Smoking cessation
3. Moderate exercise
4. Decreased potassium and magnesium intake

2. An otherwise healthy man has been diagnosed with hypertension. You suspect that the physician will order:

1. Hydrochlorothiazide (Microzide)
2. Captopril (Capoten)
3. Nifedipine (Adalat, Procardia)
4. Enalapril (Vasotec)

3. The patient is on two antihypertensive drugs. The nurse recognizes that the advantage of multidrug treatment is:

1. Blood pressure decreases faster.
2. Adverse effects are fewer and patient adherence is greater.
3. There is less daily medication dosing.
4. Multidrug therapy treats the patient's other medical conditions.

4. The patient is taking furosemide (Lasix) 40 mg bid. The patient should be monitored for:

1. Hyperkalemia
2. Hypokalemia
3. Hypernatremia
4. Hypercalcemia

5. The patient has been taking losartan (Cozaar) for his hypertension. The physician has determined that the current medication regimen is not effective. Which of the following drugs may be added to the treatment plan?

1. Felodipine (Plendil)
2. Methyldopa (Aldomet)

3. Atenolol (Tenormin)
4. Hydrochlorothiazide (Microzide)

6. The patient has been started on antihypertensives. The patient should be monitored for:

1. Nausea and vomiting
2. Diarrhea
3. Dizziness
4. Tetany

7. This antihypertensive medication is a potassium-sparing diuretic.

1. Furosemide (Lasix)
2. Spironolactone (Aldactone)
3. Chlorothiazide (Diuril)
4. Hydrochlorothiazide (Microzide)

8. The type of antihypertensive that affects the renin-angiotensin-aldosterone system to increase urine is the:

1. Calcium channel blocker
2. Adrenergic blocker
3. ACE inhibitor
4. Direct-acting vasodilator

9. The class of antihypertensives that relax smooth muscles in the blood vessels to decrease peripheral resistance are the:

1. Calcium channel blockers
2. Beta-adrenergic blockers
3. ACE inhibitors
4. Direct-acting vasodilators

10. The patient is on an ACE inhibitor. Which of the following may develop as a result of therapy?

1. Hypokalemia
2. Hyperkalemia
3. Hypernatremia
4. Hyperglycemia

CASE STUDY QUESTIONS

For questions 1–4, please refer to the following case study, and choose the correct answer from choices 1–4.

*M*s. Rodriguez was admitted to the emergency department unconscious with a possible stroke. Her blood pressure was measured as 210/120 mmHg, and she was immediately placed on nitroprusside (Nitropress). She stayed in the hospital for 2 days and was discharged with a blood pressure of 135/88 mmHg. She was given a prescription for Aldactazide, a combination drug that contains hydrochlorothiazide and spironolactone.

1. Why was nitroprusside, rather than Aldactazide, used in the emergency department?

1. Nitroprusside is safer.
2. Nitroprusside has a longer duration of action.
3. Nitroprusside has a faster onset of action.
4. Ms. Rodriguez may have been allergic to Aldactazide.

2. What two drug classes are contained in Aldactazide?

1. Thiazide diuretic and beta blocker
2. Thiazide diuretic and potassium-sparing diuretic
3. ACE inhibitor and potassium-sparing diuretic
4. Alpha-adrenergic blocker and ACE inhibitor

3. What instructions should be given to the patient taking Aldactazide?

1. Weigh self regularly and report any abnormal weight gain or loss.
2. Take a daily potassium supplement.
3. Eat plenty of calcium-rich foods such as yogurt.
4. Do not exercise regularly because exercise may interfere with blood pressure regulation.

4. After 8 months on Aldactazide, the physician switched Ms. Rodriguez to nifedipine (Procardia). The patient stopped taking this drug because it made her dizzy, and she felt her heart was racing. This common adverse effect was probably due to:

1. Electrolyte imbalance
2. Overdose of nifedipine
3. Excessive vasodilation of arteries
4. Reflex tachycardia

FURTHER STUDY

- Drugs for heart failure are discussed in Chapter 18.
- The role of the autonomic nervous system in controlling peripheral resistance is covered in Chapter 8.
- Diuretics used in the treatment of kidney disorders are discussed in Chapter 23, and Chapter 18 covers their use in the treatment of heart failure.
- The use of calcium channel blockers (CCBs) in treating dysrhythmias is discussed in Chapter 19; CCBs used to treat angina are covered in Chapter 21.

- ACE inhibitors approved for treating heart failure are covered in Chapter 18; Chapter 21 gives information on their use in myocardial infarction.
- The role of alpha blockers in treating benign prostatic hyperplasia (BPH) is covered in Chapter 32.

EXPLORE PEARSON mynursingkit™

MyNursingKit is your one stop for online chapter review materials and resources. Prepare for success with additional NCLEX®-style practice questions, interactive assignments and activities, web links, animations and videos, and more!

Register your access code from the front of your book at
www.mynursingkit.com

18 Drugs for Heart Failure

CORE CONCEPTS

18.1 Heart failure is closely associated with disorders such as chronic hypertension, coronary artery disease, and diabetes.

18.2 The central cause of heart failure is weakened heart muscle.

18.3 The three primary characteristics of heart function are force of contraction, heart rate, and speed of impulse conduction.

18.4 The specific therapy for heart failure depends on the severity of the disease.

18.5 Angiotensin-converting enzyme (ACE) inhibitors are the preferred drugs for heart failure.

18.6 Diuretics relieve symptoms of heart failure by reducing fluid overload and decreasing blood pressure.

18.7 Cardiac glycosides increase the force of myocardial contraction and were once the traditional drugs of choice for heart failure.

18.8 Beta-adrenergic blockers are used in combination with other drugs to slow the progression of heart failure.

18.9 Vasodilators reduce symptoms of heart failure by decreasing cardiac workload.

18.10 Phosphodiesterase inhibitors and other miscellaneous drugs are used for short-term therapy of advanced heart failure.

DRUG SNAPSHOT

The following drugs are discussed in this chapter:

DRUG CLASSES	DRUG PROFILES
Angiotensin-converting enzyme (ACE) inhibitors	Pr lisinopril (Prinivil, Zestril)
Diuretics	Pr furosemide (Lasix)
Cardiac glycosides	Pr digoxin (Lanoxin)
Beta-adrenergic blockers	Pr carvedilol (Coreg)

DRUG CLASSES	DRUG PROFILES
Vasodilators	
Phosphodiesterase inhibitors and miscellaneous agents	Pr milrinone (Primacor)

LEARNING OUTCOMES

After reading this chapter, the student should be able to:

1. Identify the major risk factors that accelerate the progression to heart failure.

2. Relate how the classic symptoms associated with heart failure may be caused by weakened heart muscle.

3. Identify drug classes that are used for first- and second-choice pharmacotherapy of heart failure.

4. Explain several means by which patients may control their heart failure without drugs.

5. For each of the classes listed in the Drug Snapshot, identify representative medications and explain the mechanism of drug action, primary actions, and important adverse effects.

6. Categorize heart failure drugs based on their classification and mechanism of action.

afterload *292*

contractility (kon-trak-TILL-eh-tee) *292*

heart failure (HF) *291*

inotropic effect (in-oh-TRO-pik) *292*

natriuretic peptide (hBNP) (na-tree-ur-ET-ik) *302*

peripheral edema (purr-IF-ur-ul eh-DEE-mah) *292*

phosphodiesterase (fos-fo-die-ES-tur-ase) *302*

preload *292*

Heart failure (HF) is one of the most common fatal cardiovascular diseases, and its incidence is expected to increase as the population ages. Despite the dramatic decline in death rates for most cardiovascular diseases that has occurred over the past two decades, the death rate for HF has only recently begun to decrease. Although improved treatment of myocardial infarction (MI) and hypertension (HTN) has led to declines in mortality due to HF, approximately one in five patients dies within 1 year of diagnosis of HF, and 50% die within 5 years.

Heart failure is closely associated with disorders such as chronic hypertension, coronary artery disease, and diabetes.

CORE CONCEPT 18.1

Heart failure (HF) is the inability of the ventricles to pump enough blood to meet the body's metabolic demands. It is not usually considered a distinct disease in itself, but is instead caused or worsened by certain underlying disorders. Indeed, although weakening of cardiac muscle is a natural consequence of aging, the process can be accelerated by a number of diseases associated with HF that are shown in Table 18.1. Because there is no cure for HF, the treatment goals are to prevent, treat, or remove the underlying causes, when possible, so that the patient's quality of life

TABLE 18.1	Disorders Commonly Associated with Heart Failure
DISEASE	**DESCRIPTION**
Chronic hypertension	Sustained high systemic blood pressure
Coronary artery disease	Atherosclerosis of the coronary arteries
Diabetes	Lack of insulin or inability to tolerate carbohydrates
Mitral stenosis	Inability of the mitral valve to open fully
Myocardial infarction	Heart muscle death due to coronary artery obstruction

Fast Facts Heart Failure

- HF increases with age. It affects:
  - 2% of those 40–50 years old
  - 5% of those 60–69 years old
  - 10% of those over age 70
- More than 57,000 people die of HF each year.
- Blacks have 1.5 to 2 times the incidence of HF as whites.
- HF occurs slightly more frequently in men than in women.
- HF is twice as frequent in patients with hypertension and five times as frequent in persons who have experienced an MI.

can be improved and life expectancy extended. Effective drug therapy can relieve many of the distressing symptoms of HF and may prolong patients' lives.

CORE CONCEPT 18.2

The central cause of heart failure is weakened heart muscle.

Although a number of diseases can lead to HF, the end result is the same: The heart is unable to pump out the volume of blood required to meet the needs of the other organs. To understand how drugs act on the weakened heart muscle, it is essential to understand the underlying cardiac physiology.

The right side of the heart receives blood from the venous system and sends it to the lungs, where the blood receives oxygen and gives up its carbon dioxide. The blood returns to the left side of the heart, which sends it out to the rest of the body through the aorta. The amount of blood received by the right side should exactly equal that sent out by the left side. If this does not happen, HF may occur. The amount of blood pumped by each ventricle per minute is the cardiac output. The relationship between cardiac output and blood pressure is explained in Chapter 17 ⚭ .

Although many variables affect cardiac output, the two most important factors are preload and afterload. Just before the chambers of the heart contract (systole), they are filled to their maximum capacity with blood. The degree to which the heart fibers are stretched just prior to contraction is **preload**. The more these fibers are stretched, the more forcefully they will contract. This is somewhat analogous to a rubber band: The more it is stretched, the more forcefully it will snap back. This strength of contraction of the heart is called **contractility**.

The second important factor affecting cardiac output is afterload. For the left ventricle to pump blood out of the heart, it must overcome a fairly substantial pressure in the aorta. The **afterload** is the amount of pressure in the aorta that must be overcome for blood to be ejected from the left ventricle.

In HF, the myocardium becomes weakened, and the heart cannot eject all the blood it receives. This weakening may occur on the left side, the right side, or both sides of the heart. If it occurs on the left side, excess blood accumulates in the left ventricle. The wall of the left ventricle may become thicker (hypertrophy) in an attempt to compensate for the extra blood. Because the left ventricle has limits to its ability to compensate, blood "backs up" into the lungs, resulting in the classic symptoms of cough and shortness of breath, particularly when the patient is lying down. Left HF is sometimes called *congestive* HF.

Although left HF is more common, the right side of the heart can also become weak, either simultaneously with the left side or independently from the left side. In right HF, the blood "backs up" into the peripheral veins. This results in swelling of the feet and ankles, a condition known as **peripheral edema**, and engorgement of organs such as the liver. Figure 18.1 ■ illustrates the underlying pathophysiology of HF. Figure 18.2 ■ illustrates the signs and symptoms of the patient in HF.

PEARSON
mynursingkit™

THE BEATING HEART

CORE CONCEPT 18.3

The three primary characteristics of heart function are force of contraction, heart rate, and speed of impulse conduction.

Cardiac physiology is quite complex, particularly when the heart is challenged with a chronic disease such as HF. A simplified method for understanding cardiac function, and one that is quite useful for understanding drug therapy, is to visualize the heart as having three fundamental characteristics:

1. It contracts with a specific force or strength (contractility).
2. It beats at a certain rate (beats per minute).
3. It conducts electrical impulses at a particular speed.

The ability to change the force of contraction, or contractility, is of particular interest to the pharmacotherapy of HF. Because the fundamental cause of HF is a weak myocardium, causing the muscle to beat more forcefully seems to be an ideal solution. The ability to increase the strength of contraction is called a positive **inotropic effect** and is a fundamental characteristic of the class of drugs known as the cardiac glycosides.

The ability of the heart to speed up or slow down is a second characteristic important to pharmacology. A faster heart works harder but not necessarily more efficiently. A slower heart has a longer time to rest between beats, thus decreasing the workload on the heart.

ino = *fiber*
tropic = *to influence*

FIGURE 18.1

Pathophysiology of heart failure

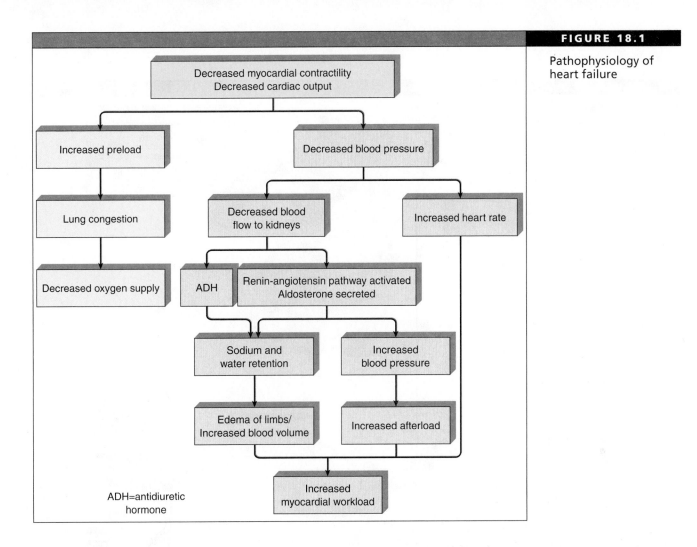

FIGURE 18.2

Signs and symptoms of the patient with heart failure

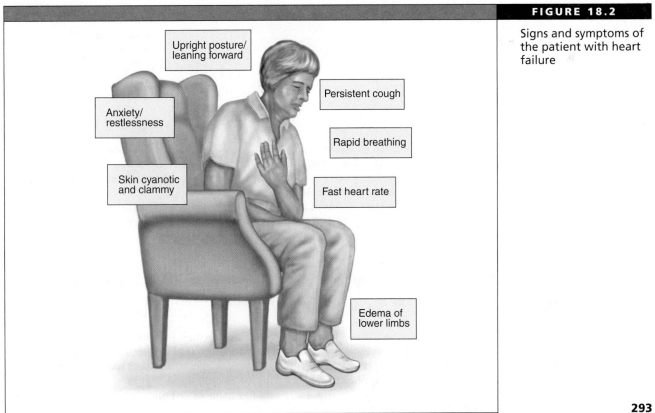

FIGURE 18.3

Mechanisms of action of drugs used to treat heart failure

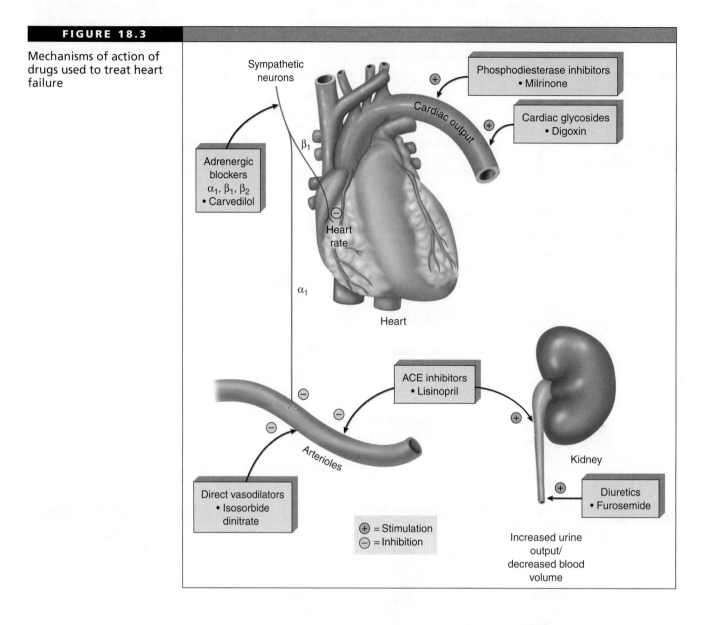

A third fundamental characteristic of cardiac physiology is the electrical conduction through the heart. Some cardiovascular drugs influence the speed of this conduction. Slowing the conduction speed through the heart will cause the heart to beat slower, thus lessening cardiac workload. These drugs are covered in Chapter 19 ⬭.

These primary characteristies of cardiac function can be modified through pharmacotherapy to assist the heart in meeting the body's metabolic demands. The mechanisms by which HF medications accomplish this are shown in Figure 18.3 ■.

The specific therapy for heart failure depends on the severity of the disease.

CORE CONCEPT 18.4

Although HF can be acute and require immediate treatment, it is often considered a progressive, chronic disorder. In its early stages, many of its symptoms can be improved through nonpharmacologic interventions. Through certain lifestyle changes, the patient can experience a higher quality of life either without drug therapy or with lower drug doses that have less risk for adverse effects. Signs and symptoms of HF are shown in Figure 18.2. Following are nonpharmacologic methods for controlling HF:

- Stop using tobacco.
- Limit salt (sodium) intake and be sure to eat foods rich in potassium and magnesium.
- Limit alcohol consumption.
- Implement a medically supervised exercise plan.
- Learn and use effective ways to deal with stress.
- Reduce weight to an optimum level.
- Limit caffeine consumption.

Once heart disease progresses such that it significantly affects activities of daily living, drug therapy is indicated. Drugs for HF may be classified as first- or second-choice drugs. If first-choice drugs are not effective, then second-choice drugs will be tried or added to the regimen. The drugs of first choice are the ACE inhibitors and diuretics. These agents reduce most symptoms of mild to moderate HF and produce the fewest number of adverse effects. Sometimes considered first-choice drugs, the cardiac glycosides are effective but have the potential for serious adverse effects. Drugs of second choice are those used in acute HF, or when the ACE inhibitors and diuretics prove ineffective. Second-choice drugs include the phosphodiesterase inhibitors, vasodilators, and beta-adrenergic blockers. The use of multiple drugs is common in the pharmacotherapy of HF.

Angiotensin-converting enzyme (ACE) inhibitors are the preferred drugs for heart failure.

CORE CONCEPT 18.5

Drugs affecting the renin-angiotensin-aldosterone system lower blood pressure and reduce the workload on the heart. They are drugs of choice in the treatment of HF. Table 18.2 lists the ACE inhibitors approved to treat HF.

The basic pharmacology of the ACE inhibitors and their effects on the renin-angiotensin-aldosterone pathway are discussed in Chapter 17 ⚭ . Approved for the treatment of HTN since the 1980s, ACE inhibitors have since been shown to slow the progression of HF and to reduce deaths from this disease. They have replaced digoxin as the preferred drugs for the treatment of chronic HF.

DRUG PROFILE: ℗ *Lisinopril (Prinivil, Zestril)*

Therapeutic Class: Drug for heart failure and HTN

Pharmacologic Class: ACE inhibitor

Actions and Uses:

Because of its value in the treatment of both HF and HTN, lisinopril has become one of the most frequently prescribed drugs. Like other ACE inhibitors, doses of lisinopril may require 2–3 weeks of adjustment to reach maximum effectiveness, and several months of therapy may be needed for a patient's cardiac function to return to normal. Because of their combined hypotensive action, concurrent therapy with lisinopril and diuretics should be carefully monitored.

Adverse Effects and Interactions:

Lisinopril exhibits few serious adverse effects. The most common adverse effects are cough, headache, dizziness, orthostatic hypotension, and rash. Because high potassium levels may occur during therapy, use of potassium supplements or potassium-sparing diuretics should be avoided during lisinopril therapy. Thus, electrolyte levels are usually monitored periodically. Angioedema is a rare, though potentially serious, adverse effect.

Lisinopril interacts with indomethacin and other nonsteroidal anti-inflammatory drugs (NSAIDs) to cause decreased antihypertensive activity. When taken together with potassium-sparing diuretics, hyperkalemia may result. Lisinopril may increase lithium levels and toxicity.

Mechanism in Action:

ACE causes the conversion of angiotensin I to angiotensin II. Two major physiologic actions result from this conversion: increased water/sodium retention and increased peripheral vascular resistance. Both actions contribute to HTN. Lisinopril lowers blood pressure by blocking ACE.

Refer to MyNursingKit for a Nursing Process Focus specific to this drug.

TABLE 18.2	Drugs for Heart Failure	
DRUG	**ROUTE AND ADULT DOSE**	**REMARKS**
ACE INHIBITORS		
captopril (Capoten)	PO; 6.25–12.5 mg tid (max: 450 mg/day)	Decreases central venous and pulmonary wedge pressure; also for HTN and acute MI
enalapril (Vasotec) (see page 282 for the Drug Profile box)	PO; 2.5 mg qid–bid (max: 40 mg/day)	Increases cardiac output; IV form available; also for HTN
fosinopril (Monopril)	PO; 5–40 mg daily (max: 40 mg/day)	Also for HTN
(Pr) lisinopril (Prinivil, Zestril)	PO; 10 mg daily (max: 80 mg/day)	Therapy should not begin until 2–3 days after diuretics are stopped; also for HTN and acute MI
quinapril (Accupril)	PO; 10–20 mg daily (max: 40 mg/day)	Observe for signs of hyperkalemia; also for HTN
ramipril (Altace)	PO; 2.5–5 mg bid (max: 10 mg/day)	Also for HTN
SELECTED DIURETICS		
bumetanide (Burinex, Bumex)	PO; 0.5–2 mg daily (max: 10 mg/day)	Affects loop of Henle; diuretic activity is 40 times greater and duration of action is shorter than furosemide; IM and IV forms available
eplerenone (Inspra)	PO; 25–50 mg once daily (max: 100 mg/day)	Newer potassium-sparing diuretic; originally approved for HTN
(Pr) furosemide (Lasix)	PO; 20–80 mg in one or more divided doses (max: 600 mg/day)	Monitor for signs and symptoms of hypokalemia; also for HTN; IV and IM forms available; loop diuretic
hydrochlorothiazide (Microzide) (see page 276 for the Drug Profile box)	PO; 25–200 mg in one to three divided doses (max: 200 mg/day)	May bring on diabetes in patients with prediabetes; also for HTN; thiazide diuretic
spironolactone (Aldactone) (see page 375 for the Drug Profile box)	PO; 5–200 mg in divided doses (max: 200 mg/day)	Used for refractory edema with HF; also for HTN; potassium-sparing diuretic
torsemide (Demadex)	PO; 10–20 mg/day (max: 200 mg/day)	Affects loop of Henle; also for HTN; IV form available
CARDIAC GLYCOSIDE		
(Pr) digoxin (Lanoxin)	PO; 0.125–0.5 mg/day (max: 0.5 mg/day)	Increases cardiac output; larger dose is given to initiate therapy; IV form available; also used for dysrhythmias
BETA-ADRENERGIC BLOCKERS		
(Pr) carvedilol (Coreg)	PO; 3.125 mg bid for 2 weeks (max: 25–50 mg bid)	Reduces cardiac workload; dose must be increased very slowly to prevent adverse effects; primary use is for HTN
metoprolol succinate (Toprol-XL)	PO; 25 mg/day for 2 weeks; 12.5 mg/day for severe cases (max: 200 mg/day)	Metoprolol succinate (Toprol XL) and metoprolol tartrate (Lopressor) are also used for HTN angina and MI. Only the succinate salt is approved to treat HF
DIRECT-ACTING VASODILATORS		
hydralazine with isosorbide dinitrate (BiDil)	PO; 1–2 tablets tid (each tablet contains 20 mg isosorbide dinitrate and 37.5 mg hydralazine) (max: 2 tablets/day)	Increases heart rate and cardiac output; decreases myocardial oxygen consumption; hydralazine also for HTN and isosorbide dinitrate for angina
Nesiritide (Natrecor)	IV; 2 mcg/kg bolus followed by continuous infusion at 0.01 mcg/kg/min	Hypotension, increased serum creatine, headache, *dysrhythmias*
PHOSPHODIESTERASE INHIBITORS		
inamrinone (Inocor)	IV; 0.75 mg/kg bolus given slowly over 2–3 min; then 5–10 mcg/kg/min (max: 10 mg/kg/day)	Larger dose is given to initiate therapy; peak effect reached in 10 min
(Pr) milrinone (Primacor)	IV; 50 mcg/kg over 10 min; then 0.375–0.75 mcg/kg/min	Larger dose is given to initiate therapy; peak effect reached in 2 min

NATURAL THERAPIES

Carnitine and Heart Disease

Carnitine is a natural substance structurally similar to amino acids. Its primary function in metabolism is to move fatty acids from the bloodstream into cells, where carnitine assists in the breakdown of lipids and the production of energy. The best food sources of carnitine are organ meat, fish, muscle meats, and milk products. Carnitine is available as a supplement in several forms, including L-carnitine, D-carnitine, and actetyl-carnitine. D-carnitine is associated with potential adverse effects and thus should be avoided.

Carnitine has been claimed to enhance energy and sports performance, heart health, memory, immune function, and male fertility. It is also being marketed as a "fat burner" for weight reduction.

Carnitine has been extensively studied. There is solid evidence to support supplementation in patients who are deficient in carnitine. Certain patients, such as vegetarians or those with heart disease, may need additional amounts. Carnitine supplementation has been shown to improve exercise tolerance in patients with angina. The use of carnitine may prevent the occurrence of dysrhythmias in the early stages of heart disease. Carnitine has also been shown to decrease triglyceride levels while increasing high-density lipoprotein (HDL) serum levels, thus helping to minimize one of the major risk factors associated with heart disease. Research has not shown carnitine supplementation to be of significant benefit in enhancing sports performance or weight loss.

The ACE inhibitors produce their effects by blocking ACE, which prevents the formation of angiotensin, an extremely potent vasoconstrictor. The primary actions of the ACE inhibitors are to lower blood pressure and reduce blood volume by enhancing the excretion of sodium and water. The resultant reduction of arterial blood pressure increases cardiac output. An additional effect of the ACE inhibitors is dilation of the veins returning blood to the heart. This action decreases preload and reduces pulmonary congestion and peripheral edema. The combined actions of ACE inhibitors substantially decrease the workload on the heart and allow it to work more efficiently. Several ACE inhibitors have been shown to reduce mortality following acute MI when therapy is started soon after the onset of symptoms (see Chapter 21 ⨉).

A related group of drugs act by blocking the effects of angiotensin *after* it is formed. Angiotensin-receptor blockers (ARBs) are newer drugs that have similar effectiveness to the ACE inhibitors. Valsartan (Diovan) and candesartan (Atacand) were approved to treat HF in 2005. Because research has not yet demonstrated a clear advantage of ARBs over other medications, their use in the treatment of HF is usually reserved for patients unable to tolerate the adverse effects of ACE inhibitors.

dys = *difficult or bad*
rhythmia = *rhythm*

hypo = *below*
kal = *potassium*
emia = *blood*

Diuretics relieve symptoms of heart failure by reducing fluid overload and decreasing blood pressure.

CORE CONCEPT **18.6**

Diuretics are commonly used for the treatment of HF. They produce few adverse effects and are effective at increasing urine flow, lowering blood volume, and reducing edema and congestion. When diuretics reduce fluid overload and lower blood pressure, the workload on the heart is reduced and cardiac output increases. They are widely used in the treatment of cardiovascular disease in patients with fluid overload (see Table 18.2). When used to treat HF, diuretics are usually prescribed in combination with ACE inhibitors and other HF medications in patients who have edema.

The most common adverse effects from diuretic therapy are electrolyte imbalances. Of greatest concern are the effects of diuretics on potassium levels, because too little or too much potassium can greatly affect a failing heart. This can be especially important in patients taking cardiac glycosides; patients with potassium or magnesium deficiencies are at greater risk for toxicity from digoxin. Potassium or magnesium supplements may be prescribed to prevent this adverse effect. Frequent laboratory testing may be necessary to monitor electrolyte levels in patients with HF.

The mechanism by which diuretics reduce blood volume, specifically where and how the nephron of the kidney is affected, differs among the various drugs. Differences in mechanisms among the classes of diuretics are discussed in Chapter 23 ⨉ . The role of the thiazide diuretics in the treatment of HTN is discussed in Chapter 17 ⨉ .

DRUG PROFILE: ℗ *Furosemide (Lasix)*

Therapeutic Class: Drug for heart failure and HTN
Pharmacologic Class: Diuretic (loop type)

Actions and Uses:

Furosemide is used in the treatment of acute HF because it has the ability to remove large amounts of edema fluid from the patient in a short time. Patients often receive quick relief from their distressing symptoms. Compared to other diuretics, furosemide is particularly beneficial when cardiac output and renal flow are severely diminished.

Adverse Effects and Interactions:

Adverse effects of furosemide, like those of most diuretics, involve potential electrolyte imbalances, the most important of which is hypokalemia. Because hypokalemia may cause dysrhythmias in patients taking cardiac glycosides, combination therapy with furosemide and digoxin must be carefully monitored. When furosemide is given with corticosteroids and amphotericin B, it can increase hypokalemia. When given with lithium, elimination of lithium is decreased, causing higher risk of toxicity. When given with sulfonylureas and insulin, furosemide may diminish their hypoglycemic effects. Because furosemide is such a potent drug, fluid loss must be carefully monitored to prevent possible dehydration and hypotension.

Furosemide should be monitored carefully in patients receiving aminoglycoside antibiotics because additive ototoxicity may result. Patients allergic to sulfur or sulfonamide antibiotics should not receive furosemide because of potential allergic response.

Mechanism in Action:

Furosemide acts by preventing the reabsorption of sodium and chloride in the loop of Henle region of the nephron. By blocking sodium chloride (NaCl) reabsorption, furosemide interferes with water reabsorption. When water reabsorption is blocked, increased urination results.

Refer to MyNursingKit for a Nursing Process Focus specific to this drug.

CORE CONCEPT 18.7

Cardiac glycosides increase the force of myocardial contraction and were once the traditional drugs of choice for heart failure.

The value of the cardiac glycosides in treating heart disorders has been known for over 2000 years. They have been used as arrow poisons by African tribes and as medicines by the ancient Egyptians and Romans.

Extracted from the common plants *Digitalis purpura* (purple foxglove) and *Digitalis lanata* (white foxglove), drugs from this class are sometimes called *digitalis glycosides*. Until the discovery of the ACE inhibitors, the cardiac glycosides were the mainstay of HF treatment. Digoxin (Lanoxin) is the only drug in this class available in the United States. The routes and dose for digoxin are listed in Table 18.2.

The primary action of digoxin is an increase in the force of contraction. This action, a positive inotropic effect, allows the weakened heart to eject more blood per beat, thus increasing cardiac output. The increased cardiac output helps the heart to meet the metabolic demands of the tissues.

A second important action of digoxin is its ability to slow electrical conduction through the heart. This results in fewer beats per minute. The reduced heart rate, combined with more forceful contractions, allows for much greater efficiency of the heart.

Unfortunately, digoxin has the potential to cause serious adverse effects at high doses and in certain patients. The margin of safety between a beneficial dose and a toxic dose is very small; thus, therapy should be closely monitored. Serum digoxin levels above 1.8 ng/ml are considered toxic. Initial adverse effects are gastrointestinal (GI) related and include loss of appetite, vomiting, and diarrhea. Headache, drowsiness, confusion, and blurred vision may occur. Excessive slowing of the heart rate and other cardiac abnormalities can be fatal if not corrected.

DRUG PROFILE: ℗ *Digoxin (Lanoxin)*

Therapeutic Class: Drug for heart failure
Pharmacologic Class: Cardiac glycoside

Actions and Uses:

The primary benefit of digoxin is its ability to increase the strength of cardiac contraction (positive inotropic effect). Digoxin accomplishes this by inhibiting Na^+–K^+ ATPase, an enzyme in myocardial cells.

By increasing myocardial contractility, digoxin directly increases cardiac output, thus alleviating symptoms of HF and improving exercise tolerance. The increased cardiac output also results in increased urine production and a desirable reduction in blood volume, thus relieving the distressing symptoms of lung congestion and peripheral edema.

In addition to its positive inotropic effect, digoxin also affects impulse conduction in the heart. It has the ability to suppress the sinoatrial (SA) node (the pacemaker of the heart) and slow electrical conduction through the atrioventricular (AV) node. Because of these actions, digoxin is sometimes used to treat cardiac rhythm abnormalities known as dysrhythmias, which is discussed in Chapter 19 ⚭ . Pulse rate should be monitored daily, and values less than 60 bpm or greater than 100 bpm should be reported to the health care provider.

Adverse Effects and Interactions:

The most dangerous adverse effect of digoxin is its ability to create dysrhythmias, particularly in patients who have hypokalemia. Because diuretics can cause hypokalemia and are also often used to treat HF, use of digoxin and diuretics together must be carefully monitored. Levels of potassium, magnesium, calcium, blood urea nitrogen (BUN), and creatinine should be monitored frequently (hypokalemia predisposes the patient to digoxin toxicity). Other adverse effects of digoxin therapy include nausea, vomiting, and anorexia and abnormalities of the nervous system such as blurred vision. Periodic serum levels are checked to determine if the digoxin level is within the therapeutic range, and the dosage may be adjusted based on the laboratory results. Digoxin also interacts with many other medications. Concurrent use with beta blockers may result in additive bradycardia. Because small changes in digoxin levels can produce serious adverse effects, the health care provider must constantly be alert for drug–drug interactions.

Mechanism in Action:

The primary action of digoxin is to inhibit the Na^+–K^+ ATPase enzyme. This enzyme is responsible for pumping sodium ions out of the myocardial cell in exchange for potassium ions. As Na^+ accumulates, calcium ions are released from their storage areas in the cell. The release of calcium ions produces a more forceful contraction of the muscle fibers.

Refer to MyNursingKit for a Nursing Process Focus specific to this drug.

The antidote for digoxin toxicity is administration of digoxin immune fab (Ovine). This drug binds digoxin, preventing it from reaching the tissues. Onset of action is rapid—less than 1 minute after the IV infusion is begun.

Concept Review   18.1

■ If cardiac glycosides are so effective at increasing myocardial contraction, why are they no longer drugs of first choice for HF?

Beta-adrenergic blockers are used in combination with other drugs to slow the progression of heart failure.

CORE CONCEPT 18.8

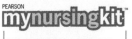

SUPPORT FOR PATIENTS WITH HEART FAILURE AND HEALTH PROFESSIONALS

Drugs that produce a positive inotropic effect, such as the cardiac glycosides and phosphodiesterase inhibitors, play important roles in treating the diminished contractility that is the hallmark of HF. It may seem somewhat unusual then to find medications that exhibit a *negative* inotropic effect prescribed for this disease. Yet such is the case with the beta-adrenergic blockers. Beta blockers have been shown to dramatically reduce the number of hospitalizations and deaths associated with HF.

Beta-adrenergic antagonists block the cardiac actions of the sympathetic nervous system, thus slowing the heart rate and reducing blood pressure. Workload on the heart is decreased. Carvedilol (Coreg) and metoprolol (Toprol XL) are the two beta blockers approved to treat HF. Patients with HF must be carefully monitored when taking beta blockers because these drugs have

DRUG PROFILE: ℗ *Carvedilol (Coreg)*

Therapeutic Class: Drug for heart failure and HTN
Pharmacologic Class: Beta-adrenergic blocker

Actions and Uses:

Carvedilol was the first beta-adrenergic blocker approved for the treatment of HF. It has been found to reduce symptoms, slow the progression of the disease, and increase exercise tolerance when combined with other HF drugs such as ACE inhibitors. Unlike many drugs in this class, carvedilol blocks beta$_1$- and beta$_2$- as well as alpha$_1$-adrenergic receptors. The primary therapeutic effects relevant to HF are a reduction in heart rate and a drop in blood pressure. The lower blood pressure reduces the workload on the heart. The drug is also approved to treat HTN and for reducing cardiac complications following an MI.

Adverse Effects and Interactions:

The most frequent adverse effects of carvedilol include back pain, bradycardia, dizziness, shortness of breath, fatigue, orthostatic hypotension, and weight gain. It should be used with caution in patients with asthma or cardiac dysrhythmias.

Carvedilol's effect in decreasing heart rate and contractility has the potential to worsen HF; therefore, dosage must be carefully monitored. Because of the potential for adverse cardiac effects, beta-adrenergic blockers such as carvedilol are usually given concurrently with other drugs in the treatment of HF.

Carvedilol interacts with many drugs. For example, levels of carvedilol are significantly increased when the drug is taken with rifampin. MAO inhibitors, clonidine, and reserpine can cause hypotension or bradycardia when given with carvedilol. When given with digoxin, carvedilol may increase digoxin levels. It may also enhance the hypoglycemic effects of insulin and oral hypoglycemic agents.

Refer to MyNursingKit for a Nursing Process Focus specific to this drug.

the potential to worsen HF. They are always used in combination with other agents, usually ACE inhibitors. The basic pharmacology of the beta blockers is presented in Chapter 8 ⚭ . Other indications, routes, and dosages of the beta-adrenergic blockers are discussed elsewhere in this text: hypertension in Chapter 17 ⚭ , dysrhythmias in Chapter 19 ⚭ , and angina/myocardial infarction in Chapter 21 ⚭ .

CORE CONCEPT 18.9

Vasodilators reduce symptoms of heart failure by decreasing cardiac workload.

The two direct-acting vasodilators, hydralazine (Apresoline) and isosorbide dinitrate (Isordil), act directly on vascular smooth muscle to relax blood vessels and lower blood pressure. Hydralazine acts on arterioles, whereas isosorbide dinitrate acts on veins. Because the two drugs act synergistically, isosorbide dinitrate is combined with hydralazine in the treatment of HF. BiDil is a fixed-dose combination of 20 mg of isosorbide dinitrate with 37.5 mg of hydralazine. Dosing for the drug is shown in Table 18.2

Because of a high incidence of adverse effects, including reflex tachycardia and orthostatic hypotension, vasodilators play a minor role in the drug therapy of HF. They are generally reserved for patients with more severe disease, or those who cannot tolerate ACE inhibitors. Hydralazine is featured as a profile drug for direct vasodilators in the treatment of HTN in Chapter 17 ⚭ . Isosorbide dinitrate belongs to a class of drugs called organic nitrates that are widely used in the treatment of angina pectoris (see Chapter 21 ⚭).

Concept Review **18.2**

■ Why are the ACE inhibitors preferred over both the nitrates and the diuretics in the treatment of HF?

DRUG PROFILE: Ⓟ *Milrinone (Primacor)*

Therapeutic Class: Drug for heart failure
Pharmacologic Class: Phosphodiesterase inhibitor

Actions and Uses:

Of the two phosphodiesterase inhibitors available, milrinone is generally preferred because it has a shorter half-life and fewer adverse effects. It is given intravenously only and is primarily used for the short-term support of advanced HF. Peak effects occur in 2 minutes. Immediate effects of milrinone include an increased force of contraction and an increase in cardiac output.

Adverse Effects and Interactions:

The most serious adverse effect of milrinone is ventricular dysrhythmia, which can occur in more than 1 of every 10 patients taking the drug. The patient's electrocardiogram (ECG) should be monitored continuously during the infusion of the drug. Less serious adverse effects include headache, nausea, and vomiting.

Use with disopyramide may cause excessive hypotension. Caution should be used when administering milrinone with digoxin, dobutamine, or other inotropic drugs because their positive inotropic effects on the heart may be additive.

 Refer to MyNursingKit for a Nursing Process Focus specific to this drug.

Phosphodiesterase inhibitors and other miscellaneous drugs are used for short-term therapy of advanced heart failure.

CORE CONCEPT 18.10

Phosphodiesterase inhibitors are drugs with a very brief half-life that are occasionally used for the short-term control of acute HF. The doses of phosphodiesterase inhibitors are given in Table 18.2.

PATIENTS NEED TO KNOW

Patients treated for HF need to know the following:

In General

1. Take blood pressure regularly because many drugs for HF affect blood pressure. Report any persistent changes.
2. Take weight measurements regularly and report abnormal weight gains or losses.
3. An increased intake of potassium-rich foods such as bananas, dried fruits, and orange juice, or a potassium supplement, may be necessary if certain diuretics are taken. Taking potassium supplements with food reduces stomach irritation. Salt intake should be limited.

Regarding ACE Inhibitors

4. Avoid sudden position changes because these can cause lightheadedness.

Regarding Cardiac Glycosides

5. Check pulse rate before taking digoxin. If the rate is less than 60 beats per minute or the rate designated by a health care provider, the drug should not be taken.
6. Many drugs interact with digoxin to increase or decrease its effects on the heart. For this reason, it is important to consult with a health care provider before taking any other medication.
7. Report visual disturbances (seeing halos or a yellow-green tinge, blurring), nausea, headaches, or irregular heartbeat without delay because they are signs and symptoms of digoxin toxicity.

Regarding Diuretics

8. Limit salt intake as directed by the health care provider.
9. Drink at least 6 to 8 glasses of water daily.
10. Report any of the following adverse effects: abdominal pain, jaundice, dark urine, flulike symptoms.
11. To prevent dizziness, avoid sudden position changes.

The two drugs in this class block the enzyme **phosphodiesterase** in cardiac and smooth muscle. Blocking phosphodiesterase has the effect of increasing the amount of calcium available for myocardial contraction. The inhibition results in two main actions that benefit patients with HF: an increased force of contraction (positive inotropic response) and vasodilation. Because of their toxicity, however, phosphodiesterase inhibitors are reserved for patients who have not responded to ACE inhibitors or cardiac glycosides, and they are generally used for 2 to 3 days only.

A third vasodilator used for HF is very different from hydralazine or isosorbide dinitrate. Nesiritide (Natrecor) is a small peptide hormone that is structurally identical to a hormone known as beta-type **natriuretic peptide (hBNP)**, which is secreted by the heart. Nesiritide reduces both preload and afterload, improving cardiac efficiency in patients with HF. Nesiritide has limited uses because of its ability to cause severe hypotension. The medication is only given by IV infusion, and patients require continuous monitoring. It is approved for patients with severe HF.

natri = *sodium*
uretic = *urinary excretion*

CHAPTER REVIEW

CORE CONCEPTS SUMMARY

18.1 Heart failure is closely associated with disorders such as chronic hypertension, coronary artery disease, and diabetes.

Heart failure (HF) is not considered a distinct disease in itself. Instead, a number of diseases that affect the heart, such as chronic hypertension (HTN), coronary artery disease, and diabetes, lead to the collection of symptoms known as HF.

18.2 The central cause of heart failure is weakened heart muscle.

HF occurs when the heart cannot pump enough blood to meet the demands of the tissues. This usually occurs when the heart muscle cannot contract with sufficient force. HF may occur on the right side, left side, or both sides of the heart, producing symptoms such as shortness of breath, coughing, and peripheral edema.

18.3 The three primary characteristics of heart function are force of contraction, heart rate, and speed of impulse conduction.

The ability of the heart to effectively pump blood depends on the strength of contraction of the myocardial fibers. Heart rate and the speed of the impulse conduction across the myocardium also directly affect the ability of the heart to pump blood.

18.4 The specific therapy for heart failure depends on the severity of the disease.

Mild HF can be improved through lifestyle changes such as tobacco cessation and maintaining optimum weight. As HF progresses, pharmacotherapy with drugs of first choice, such as ACE inhibitors or diuretics, is indicated. More advanced disease may require therapy with cardiac glycosides, phosphodiesterase inhibitors, beta blockers, or vasodilators.

18.5 Angiotensin-converting enzyme (ACE) inhibitors are the preferred drugs for heart failure.

ACE inhibitors improve HF by reducing peripheral edema and increasing cardiac output. Because of their effectiveness and their relatively low potential for serious adverse effects, they have become first-choice drugs in the treatment of HF.

18.6 Diuretics relieve symptoms of heart failure by reducing fluid overload and decreasing blood pressure.

Diuretics produce few serious adverse effects and are often used in combination with other HF drugs to reduce patients' symptoms. Potent diuretics such as furosemide are particularly valuable in treating acute HF.

18.7 Cardiac glycosides increase the force of myocardial contraction and were once the traditional drugs of choice for heart failure.

Cardiac glycosides, long the mainstay for pharmacotherapy of HF, increase myocardial contractility and are effective. The large number of drug–drug interactions and the potential for serious adverse effects such as dysrhythmias limit their use.

18.8 Beta-adrenergic blockers are used in combination with other drugs to slow the progression of heart failure.

Although beta blockers decrease myocardial contractility, they also lower heart rate and blood pressure, which is beneficial to reducing the symptoms of HF. When administered to treat patients with HF, they are nearly always used in combination with other drugs.

18.9 Vasodilators reduce symptoms of heart failure by decreasing cardiac workload.

Direct vasodilators are effective at relaxing blood vessels, thus reducing myocardial oxygen demand on the heart. BiDil is a combination of two vasodilators: isosorbide dinitrate and hydralazine. Their use is limited by their high incidence of adverse effects.

18.10 Phosphodiesterase inhibitors and other miscellaneous drugs are used for short-term therapy of advanced heart failure.

Phosphodiesterase inhibitors are a relatively new class of drugs used for the short-term treatment of HF. Although effective, they are given IV only and can produce potentially serious adverse effects. Nesiritide (Natrecor) is a small peptide hormone that is approved only for severe HF because of its potentially serious adverse effects.

REVIEW QUESTIONS

The following questions are written in NCLEX-PN® style. Answer these questions to assess your knowledge of the chapter material, and go back and review any material that is not clear to you.

1. The patient has developed a cough and shortness of breath when he lies down. The nurse suspects:

1. Right HF
2. Left HF
3. Liver engorgement
4. Peripheral edema

2. The patient has been started on digoxin (Lanoxin) therapy. Which of the following should be monitored?

1. BUN levels
2. Amylase levels
3. Sodium levels
4. Potassium levels

3. Which of the following should be expected with the use of digoxin (Lanoxin)?

1. Increased weight
2. Decreased edema
3. Increased blood volume
4. Increased heart rate

4. A patient who is taking hydralazine for HF is also experiencing angina. Which of the following drugs would be used in combination with hydralazine to help relieve this patient's symptoms?

1. Isosorbide dinitrate (Isordil)
2. Carvedilol (Coreg)
3. Chlorothiazide (Diuril)
4. Milrinone (Primacor)

5. The patient is admitted with HF. The physician orders IV milrinone (Primacor). The most serious adverse effect of this drug is:

1. Headache
2. Dysrhythmias
3. Confusion
4. Drowsiness

6. Which of the following should not be included in the education provided to a patient on lisinopril (Prinivil)?

1. "It may take several months for your blood pressure to return to normal."
2. "You must have your potassium monitored from time to time."
3. "This medication may change your vision from time to time."
4. "You may notice a change in your sensation of taste."

7. In addition to decreasing cardiac contractility, beta blockers:

1. Lower heart rate and blood pressure
2. Increase heart rate and afterload
3. Produce systemic vasoconstriction
4. Increase the forces of myocardial contraction

8. Which drug would the nurse expect to be ordered for a patient with digoxin toxicity?

1. Digoxin immune fab
2. Milrinone
3. Amrinone
4. Flecainide (Tambocor)

9. A patient is receiving digoxin and furosemide (Lasix). Which of the following electrolyte levels should the nurse most carefully monitor?

1. Potassium
2. Creatinine
3. Sodium
4. Calcium

10. The patient with HF has noted a 5-pound weight gain over the last 3 days. The patient should:

1. Watch his diet
2. Take an additional dose of his medication
3. Notify his physician
4. Increase his exercise regimen

CASE STUDY QUESTIONS

For questions 1–4, please refer to the following case study, and choose the correct answer from choices 1–4.

*M*r. Novi, age 45, has smoked since age 12. He recently has had trouble breathing when mowing the lawn, and he coughs when he lies down to sleep at night. The physician has diagnosed Mr. Novi with early HF.

1. Which of the following drugs would *most* likely be prescribed for Mr. Novi?

1. Isosorbide dinitrate (Isordil)
2. Enalapril (Vasotec)
3. Milrinone (Primacor)
4. Quinapril (Accupril)

2. Which of the following actions would be most desirable for a drug used to treat HF in Mr. Novi?

1. Increase the heart rate
2. Increase the forcefulness of heart contractions
3. Increase arterial blood pressure
4. Increase blood volume by retaining water

3. After a year, Mr. Novi enters the emergency department with acute shortness of breath and severe congestion in both lungs. Which of the following medications would be a likely choice for this patient in the emergency department?

1. Inamrinone (Inocor)
2. Captopril (Capoten)
3. Carvedilol (Coreg)
4. Spironolactone (Aldactone)

4. Mr. Novi has been placed on digoxin and furosemide. Which of the following adverse effects of furosemide could lead to dysrhythmias and other cardiac disease in patients taking digoxin?

1. Hypotension
2. Bradycardia
3. Hypokalemia
4. Hyperkalemia

FURTHER STUDY

- The relationship between cardiac output and blood pressure is explained in Chapter 17 ⬭ .

- Chapter 17 ⬭ describes the pharmacology of ACE inhibitors and how they affect the renin-angiotensin-aldosterone pathway.

- For further discussion of ACE inhibitor therapy in treating acute MI, see Chapter 21 ⬭ .

- More information on the role of hydralazine in the treatment of hypertension is found in Chapter 17 ⬭ .

- The use of isosorbide dinitrate in the treatment of angina pectoris is discussed in Chapter 21 ⬭ .

- Differences in mechanisms of action among diuretics is discussed in Chapter 23 ⬭ .

- Chapter 17 ⬭ discusses how diuretics are used to treat hypertension.

- Chapter 8 ⬭ explains the basic pharmacology of beta blockers.

- Uses, routes, and dosages of beta blockers are discussed in Chapter 17 ⬭ (to treat hypertension), Chapter 19 ⬭ (for dysrhythmias), and Chapter 21 ⬭ (to treat angina and MI).

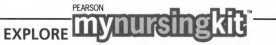

EXPLORE PEARSON **mynursingkit**™

MyNursingKit is your one stop for online chapter review materials and resources. Prepare for success with additional NCLEX®-style practice questions, interactive assignments and activities, web links, animations and videos, and more!

Register your access code from the front of your book at
www.mynursingkit.com

19 Drugs for Dysrhythmias

CORE CONCEPTS

19.1 Some types of dysrhythmias produce no patient symptoms, whereas others may be life threatening.

19.2 Dysrhythmias are classified by their location and type of rhythm abnormality produced.

19.3 The electrical conduction pathway in the myocardium keeps the heart beating in a synchronized manner.

19.4 Most antidysrhythmic drugs act by blocking ion channels in myocardial cells.

19.5 Antidysrhythmic drugs are classified by their mechanisms of action.

19.6 Sodium channel blockers slow the rate of impulse conduction through the heart.

19.7 Beta-adrenergic blockers reduce automaticity and slow conduction velocity in the heart.

19.8 Potassium channel blockers prolong the refractory period of the heart.

19.9 Calcium channel blockers are available to treat supraventricular dysrhythmias.

19.10 Digoxin and adenosine are used for specific dysrhythmias but do not act by blocking ion channels.

DRUG SNAPSHOT

The following drugs are discussed in this chapter:

DRUG CLASSES	DRUG PROFILES	DRUG CLASSES	DRUG PROFILES
Sodium channel blockers	(Pr) procainamide (Procanbid)	Calcium channel blockers	(Pr) verapamil (Calan, Isoptin, others)
Beta-adrenergic blockers	(Pr) propranolol (Inderal, InnoPran XL)	Miscellaneous drugs	
Potassium channel blockers	(Pr) amiodarone (Cordarone)		

LEARNING OUTCOMES

After reading this chapter, the student should be able to:

1. Explain how rhythm abnormalities can affect cardiac function.

2. Illustrate the flow of electrical impulses through the normal heart.

3. Classify dysrhythmias based on their location and type of conduction abnormality.

4. Explain the importance of ion channels to cardiac function and the pharmacotherapy of dysrhythmias.

5. Identify the importance of nonpharmacologic therapies in the treatment of dysrhythmias.

6. Identify basic mechanisms by which antidysrhythmic drugs act.

7. For each of the classes in the Drug Snapshot, identify representative drugs and explain their mechanisms of action, primary actions, and important adverse effects.

8. Categorize antidysrhythmic drugs based on their classifications and mechanisms of action.

KEY TERMS

atrioventricular bundle (ay-tree-oh-ven-TRIK-you-lur BUN-dul) *308*

atrioventricular (AV) node (ay-tree-oh-ven-TRIK-you-lur noad) *308*

automaticity (aw-toh-muh-TISS-uh-tee) *308*

bundle branches (BUN-dul BRAN-chez) *308*

calcium ion channels (KAL-see-um) *309*

cardioversion/defibrillation (kar-dee-oh-VER-shun/dee-fib-ree-LAY-shun) *310*

depolarization (dee-po-lur-eye-ZAY-shun) *309*

dysrhythmias (diss-RITH-mee-uh) *306*

ectopic foci/pacemakers (ek-TOP-ik FO-si) *308*

electrocardiogram (ECG) (e-lek-tro-KAR-dee-oh-gram) *308*

fibrillation (fi-bruh-LAY-shun) *307*

polarized (POLE-uh-rized) *309*

potassium ion channels (po-TASS-ee-um) *309*

Purkinje fibers (purr-KEN-gee FI-burrs) *308*

refractory period (ree-FRAK-tor-ee) *310*

sinoatrial (SA) node (si-no-AYE-tree-ul noad) *308*

sinus rhythm (SI-nuss) *308*

sodium ion channels (SO-dee-um) *309*

supraventricular (sue-prah-ven-TRIK-you-lur) *307*

---

dys = *difficult or bad*
rhythm = *rhythm*
ia = *condition*

Dysrhythmias are abnormalities of electrical conduction or rhythm in the heart. Sometimes called arrhythmias, they encompass a number of different disorders that range from harmless to life threatening. Diagnosis is often difficult because patients usually must be connected to an electrocardiogram (ECG) and be experiencing symptoms to determine the exact type of rhythm disorder. Proper diagnosis and optimum pharmacologic treatment can significantly reduce the frequency of dysrhythmias and their consequences.

CORE CONCEPT 19.1

Some types of dysrhythmias produce no patient symptoms, whereas others may be life threatening.

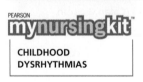

CHILDHOOD
DYSRHYTHMIAS

a = *no or not*
symptomat = *symptoms*
ic = *pertaining to*

Whereas some dysrhythmias produce no symptoms and have negligible effects on heart function, others are life threatening and require immediate treatment. Typical symptoms include dizziness, weakness, decreased exercise tolerance, shortness of breath, and fainting. Many patients report palpitations or a sensation that their heart has skipped a beat. Persistent dysrhythmias are associated with increased risk of stroke and heart failure. Severe dysrhythmias may result in sudden death. Because asymptomatic patients may not seek medical attention, it is difficult to estimate the frequency of the disease, although it is likely that dysrhythmias are quite common in the population.

Fast Facts Dysrhythmias

- Dysrhythmias are responsible for more than 44,000 deaths each year.
- Atrial dysrhythmias occur more commonly in men than in women.
- The incidence of atrial dysrhythmias increases with age. They affect:

    Less than 0.5% of those aged 25–35
    1.5% of those up to age 60
    9% of those over age 75

- About 15% of strokes occur in patients with atrial dysrhythmias.
- A large majority of sudden cardiac deaths are believed to be caused by ventricular dysrhythmias.

Dysrhythmias are classified by their location and type of rhythm abnormality produced.

There are many types of dysrhythmias, and they may be classified by a number of different methods. The simplest method is to name dysrhythmias according to the type of rhythm abnormality produced and their locations. A summary of the different types of dysrhythmias along with a brief description of each abnormality is given in Table 19.1. Dysrhythmias that originate in the atria are sometimes referred to as **supraventricular**. Those that originate in the ventricles are generally more serious because they are more likely to interfere with the normal function of the heart. Although obtaining a correct diagnosis of the type of dysrhythmia is sometimes difficult, it is essential for effective treatment. Atrial **fibrillation**, a complete disorganization of rhythm, is thought to be the most common type of dysrhythmia.

supra = *above*
ventricular = *cardiac ventricle*

Dysrhythmias can occur in both healthy and diseased hearts. Although the actual cause of most dysrhythmias is elusive, dysrhythmias are often associated with certain conditions, primarily heart disease and myocardial infarction. Following are some of the diseases commonly associated with dysrhythmias:

- Hypertension (HTN)
- Cardiac valve disease, such as mitral stenosis
- Coronary artery disease
- Medications such as digoxin
- Low potassium levels in the blood
- Myocardial infarction
- Adverse effect from antidysrhythmic medication
- Stroke
- Diabetes mellitus
- Congestive heart failure

The electrical conduction pathway in the myocardium keeps the heart beating in a synchronized manner.

Although there are many different types of dysrhythmias, all have in common a defect in the formation or conduction of electrical impulses across the myocardium. These electrical impulses carry the signal for cardiac muscle cells to contract and must be coordinated precisely for the chambers to beat in a synchronized manner. For the heart to function properly, the atria must contract simultaneously, sending their blood into the ventricles. Following atrial contraction, the right and left ventricles then must contract simultaneously. Lack of synchronization of the atria and

TABLE 19.1	**Types of Dysrhythmias**
NAME OF DYSRHYTHMIA	**DESCRIPTION**
Atrial or ventricular flutter and/or fibrillation	Very rapid, uncoordinated beats; atrial may require treatment but is not usually fatal; ventricular flutter or fibrillation requires immediate treatment
Atrial or ventricular tachycardia	Rapid heartbeat greater than 100 beats per minute in adults; ventricular tachycardia is more serious than atrial tachycardia
Heart block	Area of nonconduction in the myocardium; may be partial or complete; classified as first, second, or third degree
Premature atrial or premature ventricular contractions (PVCs)	An extra beat often originating from a source other than the sinoatrial (SA) node; not normally serious unless it occurs in high frequency
Sinus bradycardia	Slow heartbeat, less than 60 beats per minute; may require a pacemaker

ventricles or of the right and left sides of the heart may have serious consequences. The normal conduction pathway in the heart is illustrated in Figure 19.1 ∎.

Control of this synchronization begins in a small area of tissue in the wall of the right atrium known as the **sinoatrial (SA) node**. The SA node or pacemaker of the heart has a property called **automaticity**, the ability of certain cells to spontaneously generate an electrical impulse known as an *action potential*, without instructions from the nervous system. The SA node generates a new action potential approximately 75 times every minute under resting conditions. This is referred to as the normal **sinus rhythm**.

On leaving the SA node, the action potential travels quickly across both atria to the **atrioventricular (AV) node**. The AV node also has the property of automaticity, although less so than the SA node. If the SA node malfunctions, the AV node has the ability to spontaneously generate action potentials and continue the heart's contraction.

As the action potential leaves the AV node, it travels rapidly to the **atrioventricular bundle** or bundle of His. The impulse is then conducted down the right and left **bundle branches** to the **Purkinje fibers**, which carry the impulse to all regions of the ventricles almost simultaneously.

The wave of electrical activity across the myocardium can be measured by an **electrocardiogram (ECG)**. The total time for the electrical impulse to travel across the heart is about 0.22 second. A normal ECG and its relationship to impulse conduction in the heart are shown in Figure 19.2 ∎.

Although action potentials normally begin at the SA node and spread across the myocardium in a coordinated manner, other regions of the heart may begin to initiate beats. These areas, known as **ectopic foci** or **ectopic pacemakers**, may send impulses across the myocardium that compete with those from the normal conduction system. Although healthy hearts often experience an extra beat without incident, ectopic foci in diseased hearts have the potential to cause many of the types of dysrhythmias noted in Table 19.1.

It is important to understand that the underlying purpose of this conduction system is to keep the heart beating in a regular, synchronized manner so that cardiac output can be maintained. Some dysrhythmias occur sporadically, produce no symptoms, and cause little or no effect on cardiac output. These types of abnormalities may go unnoticed by the patient and rarely require treatment. Some dysrhythmias, however, seriously affect cardiac output, producing patient symptoms and resulting in potentially serious, if not mortal, consequences. It is these types of dysrhythmias that require pharmacotherapy.

ec = *outside*
top = *place*
ic = *pertaining to*

| **Concept Review** | **19.1** |

∎ Trace the flow of electrical conduction through the heart. What would happen if the impulse never reached the AV node?

FIGURE 19.1

Normal conduction pathway in the heart *Source: Pearson Education/PH College*

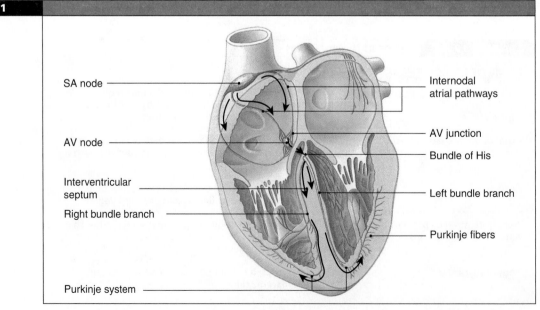

SA node

Internodal atrial pathways

AV node

AV junction

Bundle of His

Interventricular septum

Left bundle branch

Right bundle branch

Purkinje fibers

Purkinje system

FIGURE 19.2

Normal ECG tracing

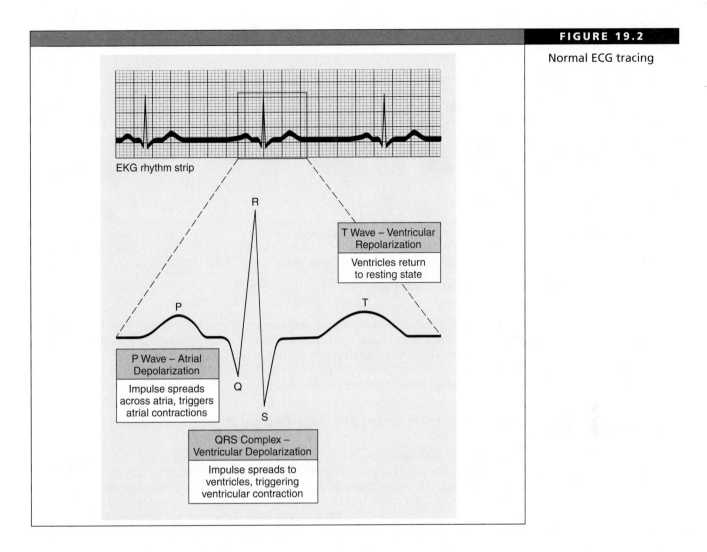

Most antidysrhythmic drugs act by blocking ion channels in myocardial cells.

Because most antidysrhythmic drugs act by interfering with the cardiac action potential, a firm grasp of this phenomenon is necessary for understanding drug mechanisms. Action potentials occur in both neurons and cardiac muscle cells due to differences in the concentration of certain ions found inside and outside the cell. Under resting conditions, sodium ions (Na^+) and calcium ions (Ca^{2+}) are found in higher concentrations *outside* the myocardial cells, whereas potassium ions (K^+) are found in higher concentrations *inside* these cells. These imbalances are, in part, responsible for the inside of a myocardial cell membrane being slightly negatively charged relative to the outside of the membrane. A cell having this negative membrane potential is said to be **polarized**.

An action potential begins when **sodium ion channels** located in the plasma membrane open and Na^+ rushes into the cell, producing a rapid **depolarization**, or loss of membrane potential. During this period, Ca^{2+} also enters the cell through **calcium ion channels**. It is this influx of Ca^{2+} that is responsible for the contraction of cardiac muscle. The cell returns to its polarized state by the removal of Na^+ from the cell via the sodium pump and movement of K^+ back into the cell through **potassium ion channels**. In cells located in the SA and AV nodes, it is the influx of Ca^{2+}, rather than Na^+, that generates the rapid depolarization of the membrane.

Although it may seem complicated to learn the different ions involved in an action potential, this is vital to cardiac pharmacology. Blocking potassium, sodium, or calcium ion channels is the primary pharmacologic strategy used to prevent or terminate dysrhythmias. Figure 19.3 ■ illustrates the flow of ions during the action potential.

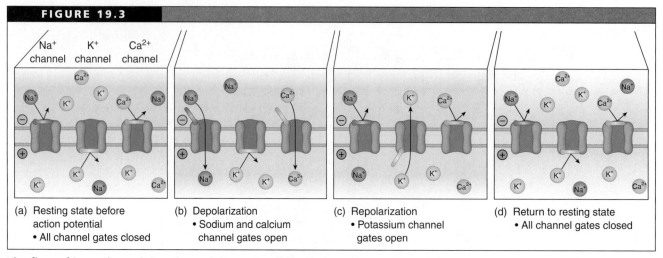

(a) Resting state before action potential
• All channel gates closed

(b) Depolarization
• Sodium and calcium channel gates open

(c) Repolarization
• Potassium channel gates open

(d) Return to resting state
• All channel gates closed

The flow of icons through ion channels in myocardial cells

The pumping action of the heart requires alternating periods of contraction and relaxation. There is a brief period following depolarization when the cell cannot initiate another action potential. This time, known as the **refractory period**, ensures that the myocardial cell finishes contracting before a second action potential begins. Some antidysrhythmic drugs produce their effects by prolonging the refractory period.

CORE CONCEPT 19.5

Antidysrhythmic drugs are classified by their mechanisms of action.

The therapeutic goals of antidysrhythmic pharmacotherapy is to prevent or terminate dysrhythmias in order to decrease the possibility of sudden death, stroke, or other complications resulting from the disease. All antidysrhythmic drugs have the potential to profoundly affect the heart's conduction system. Because they can cause serious adverse effects, antidysrhythmic drugs are normally reserved for patients experiencing symptoms of dysrhythmia or for those whose condition cannot be controlled by other means. Treating asymptomatic dysrhythmias with medications provides little or no benefit to the patient.

Antidysrhythmic drugs are classified by the stage at which they affect the action potential. These drugs fall into four primary classes and a miscellaneous group that does not act by one of the first four mechanisms. Categories of antidysrhythmics include the following:

- Sodium channel blockers (Class I)
- Beta-adrenergic blockers (Class II)
- Potassium channel blockers (Class III)
- Calcium channel blockers (Class IV)
- Miscellaneous antidysrhythmic drugs

The use of antidysrhythmic drugs has significantly declined in the past 20 years. Research studies have found that the use of antidysrhythmic medications for prophylaxis can actually *increase* patient mortality. This is because there is a narrow margin between a therapeutic effect and a toxic effect with drugs that affect cardiac rhythm. They have the ability not only to *correct* dysrhythmias but also to worsen or even *create* new dysrhythmias. The health care provider must carefully monitor patients taking antidysrhythmic drugs. Often, the patient is hospitalized during the initial stages of therapy so that the optimum dose can be accurately determined.

There are several nonpharmacologic strategies that physicians use to eliminate dysrhythmias. Cardiac pacemakers are sometimes inserted to correct the types of dysrhythmias that cause the heart to beat too slowly. The more serious types of dysrhythmias are corrected through electrical shock of the heart, a treatment called **cardioversion** or **defibrillation**. The electrical shock momentarily stops all electrical impulses in the heart, both normal and abnormal. Under ideal conditions, the temporary cessation of electrical activity allows the SA node to automatically return conduction to a normal sinus rhythm. Catheter ablation is a treatment used to identify and destroy the myocardial cells responsible for the abnormal conduction. Implantable cardioverter

NURSING PROCESS FOCUS

Patients Receiving Antidysrhythmic Drugs

ASSESSMENT

Prior to administration:
- Obtain a complete health history (physical/mental), including allergies, drug history, and possible drug interactions
- Assess to determine if cardiac alteration is producing a symptomatic effect on cardiac output, including vital signs, level of consciousness, urinary output, skin temperature, and peripheral pulses
- Obtain baseline ECG to compare throughout therapy

POTENTIAL NURSING DIAGNOSES

- Ineffective Tissue Perfusion related to cardiac conduction abnormality.
- Deficient Knowledge related to information about drug therapy.
- Risk for Injury related to adverse effects of drug therapy.

PLANNING: PATIENT GOALS AND EXPECTED OUTCOMES

The patient will:
- Exhibit improved cardiac output as evidenced by stabilization of heart rate, heart rhythm, sensorium, urinary output, and vital signs
- State expected outcomes of drug therapy
- Demonstrate an understanding of the drug's action by accurately describing drug adverse effects and precautions

IMPLEMENTATION

Interventions and (Rationales)	Patient Education/Discharge Planning
■ Ensure cardiac rate and rhythm are monitored continuously if administering drug IV. (IV route is used when rapid therapeutic effects are needed. Constant monitoring is needed to detect any potential serious dysrhythmias.)	■ Explain the need for continuous ECG monitoring when administering the medication intravenously.
■ Monitor the IV site. Administer all parenteral medication via an infusion pump.	■ Instruct the patient to report any burning or stinging pain, swelling, warmth, redness, or tenderness at the IV insertion site.
■ Investigate possible causes of the dysrhythmia such as electrolyte imbalances, hypoxia, pain, anxiety, caffeine ingestion, and tobacco use.	Instruct the patient to: ■ Maintain a diet low in sodium and fat with sufficient potassium ■ Report illness such as flu, vomiting, diarrhea, and dehydration to the health care provider to avoid adverse effects ■ Restrict use of caffeine and tobacco products
■ Observe for adverse effects specific to the antidysrhythmic used.	Instruct the patient to: ■ Report adverse effects specific to the prescribed antidysrhythmic ■ Report palpitations, chest pain, dyspnea, unusual fatigue, weakness, and visual disturbances
■ Monitor for proper use of medication.	Instruct the patient to: ■ Never discontinue the drug abruptly ■ Take the drug exactly as prescribed, even if feeling well ■ Take the pulse prior to taking the drug (Instruct the patient regarding the normal range and rhythm of pulse; instruct to consult the health care provider regarding "reportable" pulse.)

EVALUATION OF OUTCOME CRITERIA

Evaluate the effectiveness of drug therapy by confirming that patient goals and expected outcomes have been met (see "Planning").

See Tables 19.2 through 19.5 for lists of drugs to which these nursing actions apply.

defibrillators (ICDs) may be placed in a patient to restore normal rhythm by either pacing the heart or giving it an electric shock when dysrhythmias occur.

CORE CONCEPT 19.6

Sodium channel blockers slow the rate of impulse conduction through the heart.

The first medical uses of the sodium channel blockers were recorded in the 18th century. Quinidine, the oldest antidysrhythmic drug, was originally obtained as a natural substance from the bark of the South American *Cinchona* tree. Although a prototype for many decades, quinidine (Quinidex, others) is rarely used today owing to the availability of safer antidysrhythmics. Sodium channel blockers used as antidysrhythmics are listed in Table 19.2.

Sodium channel blockers, the Class I drugs, are the largest group of antidysrhythmics. They are further divided into three subgroups—IA, IB, and IC—based on subtle differences in their mechanisms of action. Because progression of the action potential depends on the opening of sodium ion channels, a blockade of these channels will slow the spread of impulse conduction across the myocardium.

The chemical structures and actions of the sodium channel blockers are similar to those of the local anesthetics. In fact, the antidysrhythmic drug lidocaine is a prototype local anesthetic in Chapter 15 ⊙. This anesthetic-like action slows impulse conduction across the heart. A few, such as quinidine and procainamide, are effective against many different types of dysrhythmias. The remaining Class I drugs are more specific and indicated only for life-threatening ventricular dysrhythmias.

All the sodium channel blockers have the potential to cause new dysrhythmias or worsen existing ones; thus, frequent ECGs should be obtained. The reduced heart rate caused by the drugs can result in hypotension, dizziness, and fainting. Some Class I drugs have significant anticholinergic adverse effects such as dry mouth, constipation, and urinary retention.

Concept Review 19.2

■ Why does slowing the speed of the electrical impulse across the myocardium sometimes correct a dysrhythmia?

TABLE 19.2 Sodium Channel Blockers (Class I)

DRUG	RATE AND ADULT DOSE	REMARKS
disopyramide (Norpace)	PO; 100–200 mg qid (max: 1200–1600 mg/day)	Class 1A; sustained-release form available; usually reserved for serious ventricular dysrhythmias
flecainide (Tambocor)	PO; 100 mg bid (max: 400 mg/day)	Class 1C; usually reserved for serious ventricular dysrhythmias
lidocaine (Xylocaine) (see page 237 for the Drug Profile box)	IV; 1–4 mg/min infusion rate (max: 3 mg/kg per 5–10 min)	Class 1B; usually reserved for rapid control of ventricular dysrhythmias; IM, subcutaneous, and topical forms available; also widely used as a local anesthetic
mexiletine (Mexitil)	PO; 200–300 mg tid (max: 1200 mg/day)	Class 1B; usually reserved for serious ventricular dysrhythmias
phenytoin (Dilantin, Phenytek) (see page 202 for the Drug Profile box)	PO; 100–200 mg tid (max: 625 mg/day) IV; 50–100 mg every 10–15 min until dysrhythmia is terminated (max: 1 g/day)	Class 1B; offlabel use for dysrhythmias induced by cardiac glycosides; oral form is used to treat convulsions
Pr procainamide (Procanbid)	PO; 1-g loading dose followed by 250–500 mg every 3 hours	Class 1A; IM, IV, and sustained-release forms available; for both supraventricular and ventricular dysrhythmias
propafenone (Rythmol)	PO; 150–300 mg tid (max: 900 mg/day)	Class 1C; usually reserved for serious ventricular dysrhythmias
quinidine sulfate	PO; 200–400 mg tid or qid (max: 3–4 g/day)	Class 1A; gluconate salt is also available in IM and IV forms; sustained-release forms available for the sulfate and gluconate salts

DRUG PROFILE: ⓟ *Procainamide (Procanbid)*

Therapeutic Class: Antidysrhythmic (Class 1A)
Pharmacologic Class: Sodium channel blocker

Actions and Uses:

Procainamide is an older drug, approved in 1950, that is chemically related to the local anesthetic procaine. Procainamide blocks sodium ion channels in myocardial cells, thus slowing conduction of the action potential across the myocardium. This slight delay in conduction velocity prolongs the refractory period and can suppress dysrhythmias. Procainamide is referred to as a broad-spectrum drug because it has the ability to correct many different types of dysrhythmias. The most common dosage form is the extended-release tablet; however, procainamide is also available in capsule, IV, and IM formulations.

Adverse Effects and Interactions:

Procainamide has a narrow margin of safety, and dosage must be monitored carefully to avoid serious adverse effects. Nausea, vomiting, abdominal pain, and headache are common during therapy. The drug can cause fever accompanied by anorexia, weakness, and nausea/vomiting. High doses may produce central nervous system (CNS) effects such as confusion or psychosis. Like other antidysrhythmic drugs, procainamide has the ability to produce new dysrhythmias or worsen existing ones. A lupus-like syndrome may occur in 30% to 50% of patients taking the drug over a year.

Additive cardiac depressant effects may occur if procainamide is administered with other antidysrhythmics. Additive anticholinergic adverse effects will occur if procainamide is used concurrently with other medications that have anticholinergic effects.

Refer to MyNursingKit for a Nursing Process Focus specific to this drug.

Beta-adrenergic blockers reduce automaticity and slow conduction velocity in the heart.

CORE CONCEPT 19.7

Beta-adrenergic blockers are used to treat a large number of cardiovascular diseases, including HTN, myocardial infarction (MI), heart failure, and dysrhythmias. Their ability to slow the heart rate and conduction velocity can suppress several types of dysrhythmias. Beta blockers of importance to dysrhythmias are listed in Table 19.3.

The basic pharmacology of beta-adrenergic blockers is explained in Chapter 8 ⊚. Although the effects of beta blockers on the heart are complex, their basic actions are to slow the heart rate and decrease conduction velocity through the AV node. Myocardial automaticity is reduced, and many types of dysrhythmias are stabilized. The main value of beta blockers as antidysrhythmic drugs is to treat atrial dysrhythmias that are associated with heart failure.

Only a few beta blockers are approved for dysrhythmias because of the potential for adverse effects. Blockade of beta receptors in the heart may result in bradycardia, and hypotension may cause dizziness and possible fainting. Beta blockers that affect beta$_2$-receptors will also affect the lungs, thus increasing the risk for bronchospasm. This is of particular concern in patients with asthma and in elderly patients with chronic obstructive pulmonary disease (COPD).

▶ **Life Span Fact**

Special attention should be given to older adults because anticholinergic adverse effects may worsen urinary hesitancy in patients with prostate enlargement.

TABLE 19.3	Beta-Adrenergic Blockers Used for Dysrhythmias (Class II)	
DRUG	**RATE AND ADULT DOSE**	**REMARKS**
acebutolol (Sectral)	PO; 200–600 mg bid (max: 1200 mg/day)	Cardioselective beta$_1$-blocker; usually reserved for ventricular dysrhythmias; also for HTN and angina
esmolol (Brevibloc)	IV; 50 mcg/kg/min maintenance dose (max: 200 mcg/kg/min)	Cardioselective beta$_1$-blocker; usually reserved for immediate control of severe atrial dysrhythmias; very short half-life of 9 min
ⓟ propranolol (Inderal, InnoPran XL)	PO; 10–30 mg tid or qid (max: 480 mg/day) IV; 0.5–3.1 mg every 4 hours	Sustained-release forms available; also for HTN, prevention of MI, angina, and migraines

DRUG PROFILE: Pr *Propranolol (Inderal, InnoPran XL)*

Therapeutic Class: Antidysrhythmic (Class II)
Pharmacologic Class: Beta-adrenergic blocker

Actions and Uses:

Propranolol is a nonselective beta-adrenergic blocker, affecting both beta$_1$-receptors in the heart and beta$_2$-receptors in the lungs. Propranolol reduces heart rate, slows conduction velocity, and lowers blood pressure. Propranolol is most effective in treating tachycardia and is often combined with other drugs such as digoxin (Lanoxin) or quinidine (Quinidex) in the treatment of cardiovascular disease. It is approved to treat a wide variety of disorders, including HTN, angina, and migraine headaches, and to prevent MI.

Adverse Effects and Interactions:

Frequent adverse effects of propranolol include hypotension and bradycardia. Because of its ability to slow the heart rate, patients with serious cardiac disorders such as heart failure must be carefully monitored. Adverse effects such as diminished sex drive and impotence may result in nonadherence.

Propranolol interacts with many other drugs, including phenothiazines, which have additive hypotensive effects. Propranolol should not be given within 2 weeks of a monoamine oxidase (MAO) inhibitor. Beta-adrenergic drugs such as albuterol block the actions of propranolol.

Mechanism in Action:

Propranolol is a nonspecific beta-adrenergic blocker that reduces automaticity and conduction velocity in the heart. These effects are achieved by interfering with the binding of natural adrenergic substances such as dopamine, epinephrine, and norepinephrine, all of which increase cardiac conduction, heart rate, force of contraction, and blood pressure.

Refer to MyNursingKit for a Nursing Process Focus specific to this drug.

Concept Review 19.3

■ Why are selective alpha-adrenergic blockers such as doxazosin (Cardura) of no value in treating dysrhythmias?

CORE CONCEPT 19.8

Potassium channel blockers prolong the refractory period of the heart.

Although a small class of drugs, the potassium channel blockers (Class III) have important applications to the treatment of dysrhythmias. Potassium channel blockers used as antidysrhythmics are listed in Table 19.4.

The drugs in Class III exert their actions by blocking potassium ion channels in myocardial cells. After the action potential has passed and the myocardial cell is in a depolarized state, repolarization depends on removal of potassium from the cell. The Class III drugs prolong the duration of the action potential by lengthening the refractory period (resting stage), which tends to stabilize dysrhythmias. In 2009, a new potassium channel blocker, dronedarone (Multaq), was approved to treat persistent atrial dysrhythmias.

TABLE 19.4 Potassium Channel Blockers (Class III)

DRUG	RATE AND ADULT DOSE	REMARKS
Pr amiodarone (Cordarone)	PO; 400–600 mg/day (max: 1600 mg/day as loading dose)	IV form available; usually reserved for serious ventricular dysrhythmias
dofetilide (Tikosyn)	PO; 125–500 mcg bid based on creatinine clearance	Usually for atrial dysrhythmias
dronedarone (Multaq)	PO; 400 mg bid	Newer drug; given to reduce the risk of cardiovascular hospitalization in patients with atrial dysrythmias
ibutilide (Corvert)	IV; 1 mg (10 ml) infused over 10 min	Usually reserved for atrial flutter or fibrillation
sotalol (Betapace, Betapace AF, Sorine)	PO; 80 mg bid (max: 320 mg/day)	Usually reserved for serious ventricular dysrhythmias; also a nonselective beta-adrenergic blocker

DRUG PROFILE: Pr *Amiodarone (Cardarone)*

Therapeutic Class: Antidysrhythmic (Class III)
Pharmacologic Class: Potassium channel blocker

Actions and Uses:

Amiodarone is approved for the treatment of resistant ventricular tachycardia that may prove life threatening, and it has become a drug of choice for the treatment of atrial dysrhythmias in patients with heart failure. In addition to blocking potassium ion channels, some of amiodarone's actions on the heart relate to its blockade of sodium ion channels. Amiodarone is available as oral tablets and as an IV infusion. IV infusions are limited to short-term therapy, normally only 2 to 4 days. Its onset of action may take several weeks when the drug is given orally. Its effects, however, can last 4–8 weeks after the drug is discontinued because it has an extended half-life that may exceed 100 days.

Adverse Effects and Interactions:

The most serious adverse effect from amiodarone occurs in the lung, with the drug causing a pneumonia-like syndrome. The drug also causes blurred vision, rashes, photosensitivity, nausea, vomiting, anorexia, fatigue, dizziness, and hypotension. Because this medication is concentrated by certain tissues and has a prolonged half-life, adverse effects may be slow to resolve. As with other antidysrhythmics, patients must be closely monitored to avoid serious toxicity.

Amiodarone interacts with many other drugs. For example, it increases digoxin levels in the blood and enhances the actions of anticoagulants. If used together with beta blockers, sinus bradycardia may increase, and sinus arrest and atrioventricular block may occur. Amiodarone increases phenytoin levels two- to threefold.

Use cautiously with herbal supplements such as echinacea, which may cause increased liver toxicity. Aloe may increase the effect of amiodarone.

Mechanism in Action:

Amiodarone is effective in maintaining sinus rhythm in patients with atrial fibrillation, recurrent ventricular tachycardia, and fibrillations that are resistant to other drugs. Amiodarone blocks inactivated sodium and potassium channels and interferes with myocardial cell-to-cell coupling.

Refer to MyNursingKit for a Nursing Process Focus specific to this drug.

Drugs in this class generally have restricted uses because of potentially serious adverse effects. Like other antidysrhythmics, potassium channel blockers slow the heart rate, resulting in bradycardia and possible hypotension. These adverse effects occur in a significant number of patients. These medications can worsen dysrhythmias, especially following the first few doses.

Calcium channel blockers are available to treat supraventricular dysrhythmias.

CORE CONCEPT 19.9

Like the beta blockers, the calcium channel blockers (Class IV) are widely prescribed for various cardiovascular disorders. By slowing conduction velocity, they are able to stabilize certain dysrhythmias. Although about 10 calcium channel blockers (CCBs) are available to treat cardiovascular diseases, only a limited number have been approved for dysrhythmias. Doses for the CCBs used for treating dysrhythmias are listed in Table 19.5. The basic pharmacology of this drug class is presented in Chapter 17 ∞. Diltiazem is featured as a profile drug in Chapter 21 ∞.

Blockade of calcium ion channels has a number of effects on the heart, most of which are similar to those of beta-adrenergic blockers. Effects include reduced automaticity in the SA node and slowed impulse conduction through the AV node. This prolongs the refractory period and stabilizes many types of dysrhythmias. CCBs are only effective against supraventricular dysrhythmias.

CCBs are well tolerated by most patients. As with other antidysrhythmics, patients should be carefully monitored for bradycardia and hypotension. Because their cardiac effects are almost identical to those of beta-adrenergic blockers, patients concurrently taking drugs from both classes are especially at risk for bradycardia and possible heart failure. Because older patients often have multiple cardiovascular disorders, such as HTN, heart failure, and dysrhythmias, it is not unusual to find elderly patients taking drugs from multiple classes.

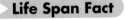 **Life Span Fact**

The health care provider should carefully monitor older adults with preexisting heart failure because these patients are particularly at risk from the cardiac effects of potassium channel blockers.

TABLE 19.5	Calcium Channel Blockers (Class IV) and Miscellaneous Drugs for Dysrhythmias	
DRUG	**RATE AND ADULT DOSE**	**REMARKS**
diltiazem (Cardizem, Cartia XT, Dilacor XR, Taztia XT, Tiazac) (see page 346 for the Drug Profile box)	IV; 5–15 mg/hr continuous infusion for a maximum of 24 hr (max: 15 mg/hr)	Oral and sustained-release forms available for HTN and angina
Pr verapamil (Calan, Isoptin, others)	PO; 240–480 mg/day IV; 5–10 mg direct: may repeat in 15–30 min if needed	Sustained-release and IV forms available; also for HTN, angina, and migraines
MISCELLANEOUS DRUGS		
adenosine (Adenocard, Adenoscan)	IV; 6–12 mg given as a bolus injection every 1–2 min as needed (max: 12 mg/dose)	Usually reserved for atrial dysrhythmias; half-life is only 10 seconds
digoxin (Lanoxin) (see page 299 for the Drug Profile box)	PO; 0.125–0.5 mg qid; dose is individualized for each patient	Usually reserved for atrial dysrhythmias; IV and IM forms available; also for heart failure

DRUG PROFILE: **Pr** *Verapamil (Calan, Isoptin, Others)*

Therapeutic Class: Antidysrhythmic (Class IV)
Pharmacologic Class: Calcium channel blocker

Actions and Uses:

Verapamil was the first CCB approved by the Food and Drug Administration (FDA). The drug acts by inhibiting the flow of Ca^{2+} into myocardial cells and in vascular smooth muscle. In the heart, this action slows conduction velocity and stabilizes dysrhythmias. In the vessels, calcium ion channel inhibition lowers blood pressure. Verapamil also dilates the coronary arteries, an action that is important when the drug is used to treat angina (see Chapter 18 ⬭).

Adverse Effects and Interactions:

Adverse effects are generally minor and may include headache, constipation, and hypotension. Because verapamil can cause bradycardia, patients with heart failure should be carefully monitored. Like many other antidysrhythmics, it has the ability to elevate blood levels of digoxin. Because both digoxin and verapamil have the effect of slowing conduction through the AV node, their concurrent use must be carefully monitored.

Grapefruit juice may increase verapamil levels. The drug should be used cautiously with hawthorn, which may have additive hypotensive effects.

Refer to MyNursingKit for a Nursing Process Focus specific to this drug.

Concept Review 19.4

■ Remembering the effects of digoxin on the heart from Chapter 18 ⬭ , explain why most antidysrhythmic drugs have the potential to cause serious adverse effects in patients taking cardiac glycosides.

CORE CONCEPT 19.10

Digoxin and adenosine are used for specific dysrhythmias but do not act by blocking ion channels.

Two other drugs, adenosine and digoxin, are used to treat specific dysrhythmias, but they do not act by the mechanisms described previously. These drugs are summarized in Table 19.5.

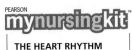

Adenosine (Adenocard, Adenoscan) is given as a 1- to 2-second bolus IV injection to terminate serious atrial tachycardia by slowing conduction through the AV node and decreasing automaticity of the SA node. Its primary indication is a specific dysrhythmia known as paroxysmal supraventricular tachycardia (PSVT), for which it is a drug of choice. Because of its 10-second half-life, adverse effects are generally self-limiting.

Although digoxin (Lanoxin) is primarily used to treat heart failure, it is also prescribed for certain types of atrial dysrhythmias because it decreases automaticity of the SA node and slows conduction through the AV node. Excessive levels of digoxin can produce serious dysrhythmias, and interactions with other medications are common; therefore, patients must be carefully monitored during therapy. The mechanism of action and adverse effects of digoxin are described in Chapter 18 ⚭ .

PATIENTS NEED TO KNOW

Patients treated for dysrhythmias need to know the following recommendations:

In General
1. Monitor heart rate and blood pressure regularly during treatment with adenosine (Adenocard, Adenoscan) or ibutilide (Corvert).
2. Monitor for a decreased heart rate and changes in rhythm while taking antidysrhythmic drugs. Report changes to a health care provider.

Regarding CCBs
3. Notify a health care provider if a very slow heart rate (less than 60 beats per minute), dizziness when standing up quickly, headache, or constipation is experienced.
4. Inform a health care provider if systolic blood pressure is less than 90 mmHg, and do not take the next dose of CCB until instructed to do so.
5. Do not discontinue medication suddenly. It should be stopped gradually under the supervision of a health care provider.

Regarding Beta Blockers
6. Notify dentists, surgeons, and eye doctors if taking propranolol (Inderal, InnoPran XL). This drug lowers intraocular pressure.
7. For those with diabetes, check blood glucose regularly while taking beta blockers. These medications can change how the body uses sugars and starches.

CHAPTER REVIEW

CORE CONCEPTS SUMMARY

19.1 Some types of dysrhythmias produce no patient symptoms, whereas others may be life threatening.

Some dysrhythmias produce no symptoms and are harmless, whereas others are life threatening. The frequency of dysrhythmias is difficult to ascertain, although they are thought to be quite common, particularly in the geriatric population.

19.2 Dysrhythmias are classified by their location and type of rhythm abnormality produced.

Dysrhythmias are classified by their site of origin, either atrial or ventricular, and by the type of rhythm abnormality produced, such as tachycardia, flutter, or fibrillation. Dysrhythmias are associated with diseases such as HTN and heart failure.

19.3 The electrical conduction pathway in the myocardium keeps the heart beating in a synchronized manner.

The normal rhythm of the heart is established by the SA node, which ensures that the chambers beat in a synchronized manner. The central problem with dysrhythmias is their potential to affect the function of the heart, reduce cardiac output, and cause certain consequences such as stroke or heart failure.

19.4 Most antidysrhythmic drugs act by blocking ion channels in myocardial cells.

Antidysrhythmic drugs affect the action potential in myocardial cells. They act by blocking sodium, potassium, or calcium channels in the cell membrane.

19.5 Antidysrhythmic drugs are classified by their mechanisms of action.

All antidysrhythmic drugs have the ability to cause rhythm abnormalities or worsen existing ones. Most antidysrhythmic medications are placed into one of five classes, based on their mechanisms of action. Class I agents are further subdivided into IA, IB, and IC. Nonpharmacologic treatments such as cardioversion or catheter ablation are sometimes preferred over drug therapy.

19.6 Sodium channel blockers slow the rate of impulse conduction through the heart.

Sodium channel blockers stabilize dysrhythmias by slowing the spread of impulse conduction across the myocardium. Quinidine, a Class IA agent, is the oldest antidysrhythmic drug.

19.7 Beta-adrenergic blockers reduce automaticity and slow conduction velocity in the heart.

Beta blockers such as propranolol stabilize dysrhythmias by slowing the heart rate and decreasing the conduction velocity through the AV node.

19.8 Potassium channel blockers prolong the refractory period of the heart.

Potassium channel blockers such as amiodarone stabilize dysrhythmias by prolonging the duration of the action potential and extending the refractory period.

19.9 Calcium channel blockers are available to treat supraventricular dysrhythmias.

Calcium channel blockers such as verapamil have effects similar to those of beta-adrenergic blockers. These include reduced automaticity in the SA node, slowed impulse conduction through the AV node, and a prolonged refractory period.

19.10 Digoxin and adenosine are used for specific dysrhythmias but do not act by blocking ion channels.

Digoxin and adenosine are used for specific dysrhythmias but do not act by the mechanisms of Class I, II, III, or IV drugs. Adenosine is used for short-term, rapid termination of dysrhythmias.

REVIEW QUESTIONS

The following questions are written in NCLEX-PN® style. Answer these questions to assess your knowledge of the chapter material, and go back and review any material that is not clear to you.

1. This electrolyte produces depolarization when it rushes into cardiac cell.
1. Potassium
2. Magnesium
3. Sodium
4. Chloride

2. Sodium channel blockers:
1. Reduce automaticity
2. Slow impulse conduction
3. Prolong the refractory period
4. Increase impulse conduction

3. This antiseizure medication is used off label to treat dysrhythmias.
1. Phenobarbital
2. Topiramate (Topamax)
3. Flecainide (Tambocor)
4. Phenytoin (Dilantin)

4. When the patient is on amiodarone (Cardarone), digoxin must be:
1. Discontinued
2. Increased
3. Decreased
4. Doubled

5. An expected outcome of a patient taking an antidysrhythmic drug would be:
1. Decreased cardiac output
2. Increased cardiac output
3. Increased renal insufficiency
4. Increased hepatic insufficiency

6. The patient taking an antidysrhythmic must be instructed to notify the physician if:
1. Constipation occurs
2. The heart rate is less than 60 beats per minute
3. The heart rate is greater than 90 beats per minute
4. Blood pressure does not decrease

7. Common adverse effects of antidysrhythmic medications include:
1. Dizziness, hypotension, and weakness
2. Headache, hypertension, and fatigue

3. Weakness, fatigue, and hypertension
4. Anorexia, diarrhea, and hypertension

8. Which of the following would be included in the teaching plan for a patient taking an antidysrhythmic medication?

1. "Take the drug only when you are feeling excessively tired."
2. "Take your blood pressure and pulse prior to taking your medication."
3. "Do not drink alcohol unless you have spoken with your physician."
4. "You will need to increase your sodium and potassium intake."

9. This antidysrhythmic also is used to treat angina.

1. Digoxin (Lanoxin)
2. Verapamil (Calan)
3. Adenosine (Adenocard)
4. Quinidine sulfate

10. This antidysrhythmic is also used to treat hypertension and angina.

1. Diltiazem (Cardizem)
2. Digoxin (Lanoxin)
3. Adenosine (Adenocard)
4. Quinidine sulfate

CASE STUDY QUESTIONS

For questions 1–4, please refer to the following case study, and choose the correct answer from choices 1–4.

*M*r. Duncan, who has a history of HTN, has arrived in the emergency department with a life-threatening ventricular dysrhythmia. He has been placed on an IV lidocaine infusion.

1. Lidocaine would be expected to terminate this dysrhythmia primarily by which of the following mechanisms?

1. Speeding up the heart rate
2. Lowering blood pressure
3. Increasing the strength of myocardial contractions
4. Slowing the speed of electrical conduction across the myocardium

2. When Mr. Duncan is discharged from the hospital, he is placed on propranolol. What effect would this drug have on his hypertension?

1. This drug will worsen his hypertension.
2. This drug will lower his hypertension.
3. This drug will have no effect on his hypertension.

3. The physician lowers the dose of propranolol and adds amiodarone (Cordarone) to the drug regimen. Mr. Duncan experiences dizziness, fainting spells, and fatigue. Which of the following would *most likely* explain these symptoms?

1. Mr. Duncan is not eating enough potassium-rich foods.
2. The drug combination is causing bradycardia or hypotension.
3. The drug combination is causing respiratory depression.
4. Mr. Duncan's hypertension is out of control.

4. When taking these medications, Mr. Duncan should be instructed to:

1. Check his pulse rate frequently
2. Keep a log of weight gain or loss
3. Eat plenty of foods containing potassium
4. Avoid taking aspirin, unless instructed to do so by the physician

FURTHER STUDY

- The basic pharmacology of beta-adrenergic blockers is explained in Chapter 8 ⚭ .
- Calcium channel blockers are discussed in Chapters 17 and 21 ⚭ .

- Chapter 21 ⚭ covers the mechanism of action and adverse effects of digoxin.
- A profile feature for lidocaine is presented in Chapter 15 ⚭ .

 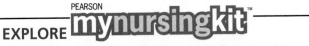

20 Drugs for Coagulation Disorders

CORE CONCEPTS

20.1 Hemostasis is a complex process involving multiple steps and many clotting factors.

20.2 Removing a blood clot is essential to restoring normal circulation.

20.3 Drugs are used to modify the coagulation process.

20.4 Anticoagulants prevent the formation and enlargement of clots.

20.5 Antiplatelet agents prolong bleeding time by interfering with platelet aggregation.

20.6 Thrombolytics are used to dissolve existing clots.

20.7 Hemostatics are used to promote the formation of clots.

DRUG SNAPSHOT

The following drugs are discussed in this chapter:

DRUG CLASSES	DRUG PROFILES
Anticoagulants	℗ heparin
	℗ warfarin (Coumadin)
Antiplatelet drugs	℗ clopidogrel (Plavix)

DRUG CLASSES	DRUG PROFILES
Thrombolytics	℗ alteplase (Activase)
Hemostatics	℗ aminocaproic acid (Amicar)

LEARNING OUTCOMES

After reading this chapter, the student should be able to:

1. Explain the importance of hemostasis.

2. Construct a flow chart diagramming the important steps of hemostasis and fibrinolysis.

3. Describe the types of disorders for which coagulation modifier drugs are prescribed.

4. Identify the primary mechanisms by which coagulation modifier drugs act.

5. For each of the classes in the Drug Snapshot, identify representative drugs and explain their mechanisms of action, primary actions, and important adverse effects.

6. Categorize coagulation modifier drugs based on their classifications and mechanisms of action.

KEY TERMS

activated partial thromboplastin time (aPTT): (throm-bow-PLAS-tin) 325

anticoagulant (ANT-eye-co-AG-you-lent) 323

clotting factors 321

coagulation (co-ag-you-LAY-shun) 321

coagulation cascade (cass-KADE) 321

embolus (EM-boh-luss) 324

fibrin (FEYE-brin) 321

fibrinogen (feye-BRIN-oh-jen) 321

fibrinolysis (feye-brin-OL-oh-sis) 323

glycoprotein IIb/IIIa (GLEYE-koh-proh-teen) 328

hemostasis (hee-moh-STAY-sis) 321

hemostatics (hee-moh-STAT-iks) 324

international normalized ratio (INR) 327

low molecular weight heparins (LMWHs) 325

plasmin (PLAZ-min) 323

plasminogen (plaz-MIN-oh-jen) 323

prothrombin (PRO-throm-bin) 321

prothrombin time (PT) 325

thrombin (THROM-bin) 321

thromboembolic disorder (THROM-bow-EM-bow-lik) 323

thrombolytics (throm-bow-LIT-iks) 324

thrombus (THROM-bus) 324

tissue plasminogen activator (tPA) 323

Everyone is familiar with the bleeding associated with simple cuts and scrapes, and we take for granted that bleeding will stop in a few minutes. **Hemostasis**, or the stopping of blood flow, is an essential mechanism protecting the body from both external and internal injury. Without efficient hemostasis, bleeding from wounds would lead to shock and perhaps death. Too much clotting, however, can be just as deadly as too little. Thus, hemostasis must maintain a delicate balance between blood fluidity and coagulation.

hemo = *blood*
stasis = *stopping*

A number of diseases and conditions can affect hemostasis. Some common disorders that often require pharmacotherapy with coagulation modifiers are described in Table 20.1.

Hemostasis is a complex process involving multiple steps and many clotting factors.

CORE CONCEPT 20.1

Hemostasis is complex and involves a number of substances called **clotting factors**. Hemostasis occurs in a series of sequential steps, sometimes referred to as a *cascade*. Drugs can be used to modify several of these steps.

When an injury occurs, cells lining damaged blood vessels release chemicals that begin the clotting process. The vessel immediately spasms, which limits blood flow to the injured area. Small blood components called platelets become sticky, adhere to the injured area, and aggregate or clump to plug the damaged vessel. Blood flow is further slowed, allowing **coagulation**, the formation of an insoluble clot. The basic steps of hemostasis are shown in Figure 20.1 ■.

The **coagulation cascade** is a complex series of steps that begins when the injured cells release a chemical called *prothrombin activator* or *prothrombinase*. Prothrombin activator converts the clotting factor **prothrombin** to an enzyme called **thrombin**. Thrombin then converts **fibrinogen**, a plasma protein, to long strands of **fibrin**. Thus two of the factors essential to clotting, thrombin and fibrin, are only formed *after* injury to the vessels. The fibrin strands form an insoluble web over the injured area to stop blood loss. Normal blood clotting occurs in about 6 minutes. The primary steps in the coagulation cascade are shown in Figure 20.2 ■.

thrombo = *clot*
plastin = *to form*

pro = *before*
thrombin = *clot*

TABLE 20.1	Disorders Commonly Treated with Coagulation Modifier Drugs
DISORDER/CONDITION	**DESCRIPTION**
angina	pain due to narrowing of the coronary vessels that interferes with blood flow to cardiac muscle
cerebrovascular accident (CVA)/stroke	clot within an artery that blocks blood flow to the brain
deep vein thrombosis (DVT)	clot within a vein in the legs
indwelling devices	mechanical heart valves, stents
myocardial infarction	death of cardiac muscle tissue due to blockage of a coronary artery by a clot
postoperative hemorrhage	bleeding following a surgical procedure
pulmonary embolus	clot within a pulmonary artery that blocks blood flow to the lungs
valvular heart disease	disease of heart valves or replacement of a heart valve

FIGURE 20.1

Basic steps in
hemostasis

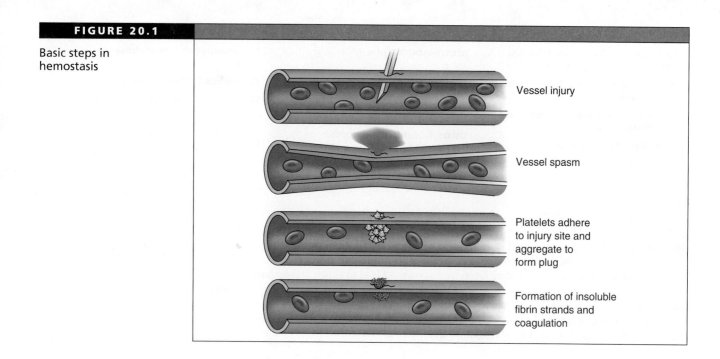

FIGURE 20.2

Major steps in the
coagulation cascade

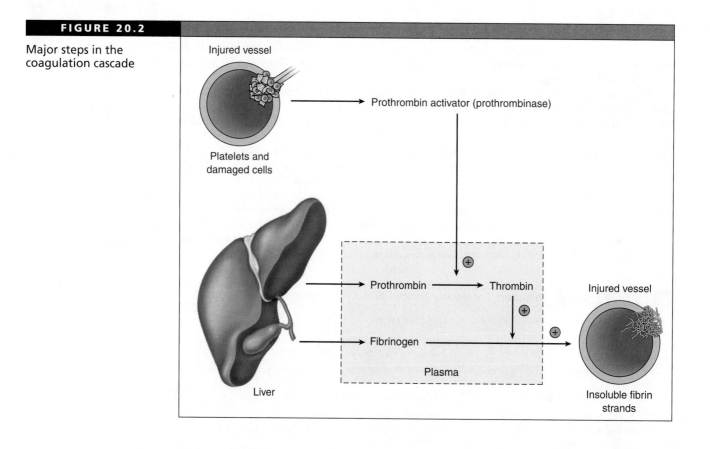

It is important to note that several clotting factors, including thromboplastin and fibrinogen, are proteins made by the liver that are constantly circulating through the blood in an *inactive* form. Vitamin K is required for the liver to make four of the clotting factors. Because the liver supplies many of the clotting factors, liver disease is one of the most common causes of coagulation disorders.

Fast Facts Clotting Disorders

- More than 2 million patients each year develop deep vein thrombosis (DVT).
- More than 60,000 patients die each year of pulmonary emboli.
- Von Willebrand's disease is the most common hereditary platelet disorder and is caused by a deficiency of a clotting protein.
- Hemophilia A, or classic hemophilia, is a hereditary condition in which a person lacks clotting factor VIII; it accounts for 80% of all hemophilia cases.
- More than 15,000 people in the United States have hemophilia.

Removing a blood clot is essential to restoring normal circulation.

CORE CONCEPT 20.2

The goal of hemostasis has been achieved once a blood clot is formed and the body is protected from excessive hemorrhage. The clot, however, may prevent adequate blood flow to the affected area; circulation must eventually be restored so that the tissue can resume normal activities. The process of clot removal is called **fibrinolysis**.

Fibrinolysis also involves several sequential steps. When the fibrin clot is formed, nearby blood vessel cells secrete **tissue plasminogen activator (tPA)**. tPA converts the inactive protein **plasminogen**, which is present in the fibrin clot, to its active form called **plasmin**. Plasmin then digests the fibrin strands to remove the clot. The body normally regulates fibrinolysis such that *unwanted* fibrin clots are removed, whereas fibrin present in wounds is left to maintain hemostasis. The steps of fibrinolysis are shown in Figure 20.3 ■.

fibrin = *fiber*
lysis = *break apart*

Drugs are used to modify the coagulation process.

CORE CONCEPT 20.3

There are many types of disorders in which abnormal coagulation might occur. The term **thromboembolic disorder** is used to describe conditions in which the body forms undesirable clots. Thromboembolic disorders may occur in either veins or arteries and can place patients in extreme danger. Blood clots may become dislodged and move to another part of the body, such as the lungs or the brain.

Drugs can modify hemostasis in a number of ways. The most commonly prescribed coagulation modifiers, the class of drugs known as the **anticoagulants**, are used to prevent the formation of clots. To accomplish clot prevention, drugs can either inhibit specific clotting factors in the coagulation cascade or diminish the clotting action of platelets. Regardless of the mechanism, all anticoagulant drugs will increase the time the body takes to form clots. These drugs are often referred to as *blood thinners*, which is an incorrect term, because they do not change the thickness of the blood.

anti = *against*
coagulation = *clotting*

FIGURE 20.3

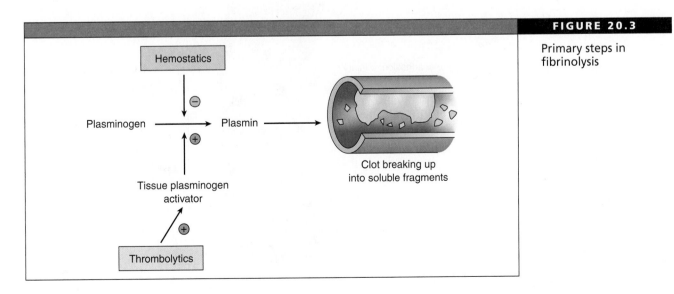

Primary steps in fibrinolysis

thrombo = *clot*
lytic = *remove/destroy*

Once an abnormal clot has formed, it may be critical to quickly remove it in order to restore normal function. This is particularly important for blood vessels serving the heart, lungs, and brain. A specific class of drugs, the **thrombolytics**, is used to dissolve such life-threatening clots.

In some cases, the blood may not clot quickly enough—for example, following surgery. In this case, it is sometimes desirable to administer medications that make the blood clot more quickly in order to prevent excessive bleeding. These drugs, called **hemostatics**, inhibit the normal removal of fibrin, thus keeping the clot in place for a longer period. Hemostatics are used to speed clot formation or to limit bleeding from a surgical site (see Figure 20.3).

Concept Review 20.1

- Which clotting factors are always circulating in the blood? Which are formed only once coagulation is underway?

CORE CONCEPT 20.4

Anticoagulants prevent the formation and enlargement of clots.

Once a stationary clot, or **thrombus**, forms in a vessel, it often grows larger as more fibrin is added. Pieces of the thrombus may break off and travel in the bloodstream to lodge in other vessels. A traveling clot is called an **embolus**. When thrombi or emboli form, drug therapy is indicated.

By inhibiting certain clotting factors, anticoagulants lengthen clotting time and prevent thrombi from forming or growing larger. Because thromboembolic disease can be life threatening, therapy is often begun by administering anticoagulants intravenously or subcutaneously to achieve a very rapid onset of action. As the disease stabilizes, the patient is switched to oral anticoagulants. Anticoagulants act by a number of different mechanisms, which are illustrated in Figure 20.4 ■. Table 20.2 lists the primary anticoagulants.

The most frequent, and potentially serious, adverse effect of anticoagulant and antiplatelet drugs is bleeding. The patient must be observed for signs of hemorrhage, such as bruising, bleeding gums, and blood in the urine or stools. Patients who have recently experienced a traumatic injury or surgery are especially at risk. Any symptoms of bleeding must be immediately reported to the health care provider. Specific blockers may be administered to reverse the anticoagulant effects: Protamine sulfate is used for heparin, and vitamin K is administered for warfarin.

Parenteral anticoagulants: The traditional drug of choice for rapid anticoagulation is heparin. Heparin inactivates thrombin and several other clotting factors within minutes after it is

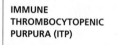

IMMUNE THROMBOCYTOPENIC PURPURA (ITP)

FIGURE 20.4

Mechanism of action of anticoagulants

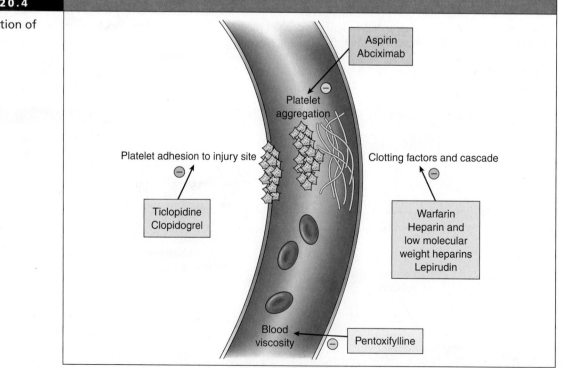

TABLE 20.2	Anticoagulants	
DRUG	**ROUTE AND ADULT DOSE**	**REMARKS**
argatroban (Acova, Novastan)	IV; 2–10 mcg/kg/min	Thrombin inhibitor; for prevention and treatment of thrombosis
bivalirudin (Angiomax)	IV; 0.75 mg/kg initial bolus followed by 1.75 mg/kg/hr for 4 hr	Thrombin inhibitor; used with aspirin to prevent clots during angioplasty
desirudin (Iprivask)	Subcutaneous; 15 mg bid for 9–12 days	Thrombin inhibitor; for DVT prophylaxis in patients undergoing hip replacement surgery
fondaparinux (Arixtra)	Subcutaneous; 2.5 mg/daily	For prevention of DVT and pulmonary embolism
(Pr) heparin	IV infusion; 5000–40,000 units/day subcutaneously; 15,000–20,000 units/bid	For prevention and treatment of venous thrombosis and pulmonary edema; therapy begins with a higher dose, which is gradually reduced
lepirudin (Refludan)	IV; 0.4 mg/kg bolus followed by 0.15 mg/kg/hr for 2–10 days	Thrombin inhibitor; for prevention of clots in patients with heparin-induced thrombocytopenia
(Pr) warfarin (Coumadin)	PO; 2–15 mg/day	Same use as heparin but effect is more prolonged; IV form is available
LOW MOLECULAR WEIGHT (FRACTIONATED) HEPARINS (LMWHS)		
dalteparin (Fragmin)	Subcutaneous; 2500–5000 units/day	For prevention and treatment of DVT following knee or hip replacement or abdominal surgery, unstable angina, or acute coronary syndromes
enoxaparin (Lovenox)	Subcutaneous; 30 mg bid for 7–10 days	
tinzaparin (Innohep)	Subcutaneous; 175 units/kg daily for at least 6 days	

given by the IV route. In recent years the heparin molecule has been shortened and modified to create a newer class of drugs called **low molecular weight heparins (LMWHs)**. LMWHs are parenteral drugs that possess the same anticoagulant activity as heparin but have several advantages. They produce a more predictable anticoagulant response than heparin; therefore, less frequent laboratory monitoring is required. They also exhibit a much longer half-life than heparin that permits once daily dosing, and family members or the patient can be taught to give the necessary subcutaneous injections at home. LMWHs have become the drugs of choice for many clotting disorders, including the prevention of deep vein thrombosis (DVT) following surgery.

Other parenteral anticoagulants include the direct thrombin inhibitors such as lepirudin (Refludan). These drugs bind to the active site of thrombin, preventing the formation of fibrin clots. The thrombin inhibitors have limited therapeutic uses. Bivalirudin (Angiomax) is administered in combination with aspirin to prevent thrombi in patients undergoing angioplasty. Argatroban (Acova, Novastan) and lepirudin are indicated for prevention or treatment of low platelet counts induced by heparin therapy. Desirudin (Iprivask) is a newer antithrombin medication that is given subcutaneously 15 minutes prior to hip replacement surgery for prophylaxis of DVT.

To avoid serious adverse effects, drug therapy with coagulation modifier drugs is individualized to each patient and must be carefully monitored. For heparin the **activated partial thromboplastin time (aPTT)** is used. Baseline values of aPTT range from 25 to 40 seconds. During heparin therapy, the aPTT is maintained at 1.5 to 2 times the baseline level. If the aPTT rises above 80 seconds, the heparin dosage should be reduced. During the first few days of heparin therapy, aPTT is measured every 4 to 6 hours to avoid abnormal bleeding.

Oral anticoagulants: The most frequently prescribed oral anticoagulant is warfarin (Coumadin). Often, patients begin anticoagulation therapy with heparin and are switched to warfarin when their condition stabilizes. When transitioning, the two drugs are administered concurrently for 2 to 3 days because warfarin takes several days of therapy before it achieves optimum anticoagulation effects.

The laboratory test used during therapy with the oral anticoagulants is **prothrombin time (PT)**. Although the normal range for PT is 12 to 15 seconds, this value becomes prolonged with anticoagulant treatment. Daily PT tests may be conducted at the start of pharmacotherapy to ensure optimum dose levels. The frequency of PT tests is decreased to weekly or monthly as

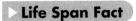

▶ Life Span Fact

Bleeding complications are more likely to occur in older adults. Prescribed doses of anticoagulants are generally lower for older patients, and this group receives more frequent assessments and laboratory testing to avoid serious complications.

NURSING PROCESS FOCUS

Patients Receiving Anticoagulant Therapy

ASSESSMENT

Prior to administration:
- Obtain complete health history (physical/mental), including recent surgeries or trauma, allergies, drug history, and possible drug interactions
- Obtain vital signs; assess in context of patient's baseline values

POTENTIAL NURSING DIAGNOSES

- Risk for Injury (bleeding) related to adverse effects of anticoagulant therapy.
- Ineffective Tissue Perfusion related to altered blood flow.
- Deficient Knowledge related to information about drug therapy.
- Noncompliance related to drug therapy regimen.

PLANNING: PATIENT GOALS AND EXPECTED OUTCOMES

The patient will:
- Experience a decrease in blood coagulability as shown by laboratory values ordered by the health care provider
- Demonstrate an understanding of the drug's action by accurately describing drug adverse effects and precautions

IMPLEMENTATION

Interventions and (Rationales)	Patient Education/Discharge Planning
■ Monitor for adverse clotting reaction(s). (Heparin can cause thrombus formation with thrombocytopenia, or "white clot syndrome." Coumadin may cause cholesterol microemboli, which result in gangrene, localized vasculitis, or "purple toes syndrome." ■ Observe for skin necrosis, blue or purple mottling of the feet that blanches with pressure or fades when the legs are elevated. (Patients on anticoagulant therapy remain at risk for developing emboli resulting in cerebrovascular accident or pulmonary embolism.)	■ Instruct the patient to immediately report sudden dyspnea; chest pain; and temperature or color change in the hands, arms, legs, and feet. (Gangrene may occur between days 3 and 8 of warfarin therapy. Purple toes syndrome usually occurs within weeks 3–10 or later.) Instruct the patient to: ■ Feel pedal pulses daily to check circulation ■ Protect feet from injury by wearing loose-fitting socks; avoid going barefoot
■ Use with caution in patients with GI, renal, and/or liver disease, alcoholism, diabetes, hypertension, hyperlipidemia, and in elderly patients and premenopausal women. (Patients with CAD risk factors are at increased risk of developing cholesterol microemboli.)	■ Advise elderly patients; menstruating women; and those with peptic ulcer disease, alcoholism, or kidney or liver disease that they have an increased risk of bleeding. ■ Advise patients with diabetes and those with high blood pressure or high cholesterol that they are at risk of developing microscopic clots, despite anticoagulant therapy.
■ Monitor for signs of bleeding: flulike symptoms, excessive bruising, pallor, epistaxis, hemoptysis, hematemesis, menorrhagia, hematuria, melena, frank rectal bleeding, or excessive bleeding from wounds or in the mouth. (Bleeding is a sign of anticoagulant overdose.)	Instruct the patient to: ■ Immediately report flulike symptoms (dizziness, chills, weakness, pale skin); blood coming from a cough, the nose, mouth, or rectum; menstrual "flooding"; "coffee grounds" vomit; tarry stools; excessive bruising; bleeding from wounds that cannot be stopped within 10 minutes; and all physical injuries ■ Avoid all contact sports and amusement park rides that cause intense or violent bumping or jostling ■ Use a soft toothbrush and electric shaver ■ Keep a "pad count" during menstrual periods to estimate blood losses
■ Monitor vital signs. (Increase in heart rate accompanied by low blood pressure or subnormal temperature may signal bleeding.)	■ Instruct the patient to immediately report palpitations, fatigue, or feeling faint, which may signal low blood pressure related to bleeding.

continued . . .

NURSING PROCESS FOCUS *(continued)*

Interventions and (Rationales)

- Monitor laboratory values: CBC, especially in premenopausal women, and aPTT, PTT, or INR for therapeutic values. (Heparin may cause significant elevations of SGOT [S-AST] and SGPT [S-ALT] because the drug is metabolized by the liver.)

- Monitor the use of other medications or herbal supplements.

Patient Education/Discharge Planning

Instruct the patient to:
- Always inform laboratory and dental personnel of heparin therapy when providing samples
- Carry a wallet card or wear medical ID jewelry indicating heparin therapy

- Instruct the patient to consult a health care provider before taking any other drugs, including OTC or herbal supplements. Many drugs decrease the action of anticoagulants.

EVALUATION OF OUTCOME CRITERIA

Evaluate the effectiveness of drug therapy by confirming that patient goals and expected outcomes have been met (see "Planning").

See Table 20.2 for a list of drugs to which these nursing actions apply.

therapy progresses and the patient's condition stabilizes. Because the method of performing PT tests varies from laboratory to laboratory, clotting time is sometimes reported as an **international normalized ratio (INR)**, which is the PT multiplied by a correction factor. Recommended post-treatment INR values range from 2 to 4.5.

DRUG PROFILE: 🅟 *Heparin*

Therapeutic Class: Anticoagulant
Pharmacologic Class: Indirect thrombin inhibitor

Actions and Uses:

Heparin is a natural substance found in the lining of blood vessels. Its normal function is to prevent excessive clotting within blood vessels. When given as a drug, heparin provides immediate anticoagulant activity. The binding of heparin to a substance called antithrombin III results in an inactivation of some of the clotting factors and an inhibition of thrombin activity. Because heparin is not absorbed by the gastrointestinal mucosa, it must be given either subcutaneously or through IV infusion. The onset of action for IV heparin is immediate, whereas subcutaneous heparin may take up to an hour for maximum therapeutic effect.

Adverse Effects and Interactions:

Abnormal bleeding is common during heparin therapy. If aPTT becomes prolonged or toxicity is observed, stopping the heparin infusion will result in loss of anticoagulant activity within hours. If serious hemorrhage occurs, a specific blocker, protamine sulfate, may be administered to neutralize the anticoagulant activity of heparin. Protamine sulfate has an onset time of 5 minutes and is also a blocker of the LMWHs.

Heparin-induced thrombocytopenia (HIT) is a serious complication that occurs in up to 30% of patients taking the drug. The patient may experience serious and even life-threatening thrombosis. Although the half-life of heparin is short, it may take a week after the drug is discontinued for platelets to completely recover.

Oral anticoagulants, including warfarin, increase the action of heparin. Ibuprofen, ASA, and other drugs that inhibit platelet aggregation may induce bleeding. Nicotine, digoxin, tetracyclines, or antihistamines may inhibit anticoagulation. Herbal supplements that may affect coagulation, such as ginger, garlic, green tea, feverfew, or ginkgo, should be avoided because they may increase the risk of bleeding.

Refer to MyNursingKit for a Nursing Process Focus specific to this drug.

Antiplatelet drugs prolong bleeding time by interfering with platelet aggregation.

Antiplatelet medications modify coagulation by interfering with various aspects of platelet function. Unlike the anticoagulants, which are used primarily to prevent thrombosis in *veins*, antiplatelet agents are used to prevent clot formation in *arteries*.

Platelets are a key component required for blood clotting. Too few platelets or diminished platelet function can profoundly increase bleeding time. The three primary subclasses of antiplatelet agents are (1) aspirin, (2) adenosine diphosphate (ADP) receptor blockers, and (3) glycoprotein IIb/IIIa receptor blockers. Doses for antiplatelet agents are listed in Table 20.3.

Aspirin deserves special mention as an antiplatelet agent. Because it is available over the counter, patients may not consider aspirin a strong medication. However, its anticoagulant activity is well documented. Aspirin acts by inhibiting thromboxane$_2$, which causes platelet aggregation. The anticoagulant effect of a single dose of aspirin may last for as long as a week. Use of aspirin with other coagulation modifiers should be avoided unless approved by the prescriber. The primary actions and adverse effects of aspirin are described in a Drug Profile in Chapter 14 ⬚.

The ADP receptor blockers are a small group of drugs that interfere with the plasma membrane of platelets, preventing them from aggregating. Both ticlopidine (Ticlid) and clopidogrel (Plavix) are given orally to prevent thrombi formation in patients who have experienced a recent thromboembolic event such as a stroke or MI. Clopidogrel is safer, having adverse effects comparable to those of aspirin. Prasugrel (Effient) is a newer drug in this class, approved in 2009 to reduce thrombotic events in patients undergoing percutaneous coronary intervention (PCI).

Glycoprotein IIb/IIIa inhibitors are relatively new additions to the treatment of thromboembolic disease. **Glycoprotein IIb/IIIa** is an enzyme necessary for platelet aggregation. Inhibition of this enzyme has the effect of preventing thrombus formation in patients experiencing a recent MI, stroke, or PCI. These drugs are very expensive and must be given by the IV route.

TABLE 20.3	Antiplatelet Agents	
DRUG	**ROUTE AND ADULT DOSE**	**REMARKS**
aspirin (Acetylsalicylic Acid, ASA) (see page 222 for the Drug Profile box)	PO; 80 mg/day–650 mg bid	Inhibits platelet aggregation; available without a prescription; higher doses are used to treat inflammation or pain; therapeutic serum level is 10–30 mcg/dl
cilostazol (Pletal)	PO; 100 mg bid	Inhibits platelet aggregation; for intermittent claudication
dipyridamole (Persantine)	PO; 75–100 mg qid	Platelet inhibitor used to prevent embolism in cardiac valve replacement; usually used with warfarin
pentoxifylline (Trental)	PO; 400 mg tid	Reduces blood viscosity and increases the flexibility of red blood cells; for intermittent claudication
ADP RECEPTOR BLOCKERS		
clopidogrel (Plavix)	PO; 75 mg daily	Prolongs bleeding time
prasugrel (Effient)	PO; 60 mg loading dose followed by 10 mg/day	Newer drug used to prevent thrombotic events in patients undergoing PCI
ticlopidine (Ticlid)	PO; 250 mg bid	Platelet aggregation inhibitor; prolongs bleeding time
GLYCOPROTEIN IIB/IIIA BLOCKERS		
abciximab (ReoPro)	IV; 0.25 mg/kg initial bolus over 5 min; then 10 mcg/min for 12 hr	Used to prevent cardiac ischemia during coronary angioplasty; effects continue up to 48 hr after infusion is stopped
eptifibatide (Integrilin)	IV; 180 mcg/kg initial bolus over 1–2 min; then 2 mcg/kg/min for 24–72 hr	Also for unstable angina and other acute coronary syndromes; effects continue up to 8 hr after infusion is stopped
tirofiban (Aggrastat)	IV; 0.4 mcg/kg/min for 30 min; then 0.1 mcg/kg/min for 12–24 hr	Similar to eptifibatide; effects continue up to 8 hr after infusion is stopped

DRUG PROFILE: ℗ *Warfarin (Coumadin)*

Therapeutic Class: Anticoagulant
Pharmacologic Class: Vitamin K antagonist

Actions and Uses:

Warfarin is used to prevent thrombi and emboli formation. Thus it is administered to patients at high risk for CVA, MI, DVT, and pulmonary embolism. This includes patients undergoing hip or knee surgery, those with long-term indwelling central venous catheters or prosthetic heart valves, and those who have experienced a recent MI.

Unlike heparin, the anticoagulant activity of warfarin can take several days to reach its maximum effect. This explains why heparin and warfarin therapy are overlapped. Warfarin inhibits the action of vitamin K that is essential for the synthesis of several clotting factors. Because these clotting factors are normally circulating in the blood, it takes several days for them to clear the plasma and for the anticoagulant effect of warfarin to appear. Another reason for the slow onset is that 99% of warfarin binds to plasma proteins and is unavailable to produce its effect. This high level of protein binding is responsible for a significant number of drug-drug interactions that may occur during warfarin therapy.

Adverse Effects and Interactions:

Like all anticoagulants, the most serious adverse effect of warfarin is abnormal bleeding. On discontinuation of therapy, the activity of warfarin can take up to 10 days to diminish. If life-threatening bleeding occurs during therapy, the anticoagulant effects of warfarin can be reduced in 6 hours through the IM or subcutaneous administration of its blocker, vitamin K. The therapeutic range of serum warfarin levels varies from 1 to 10 mcg/ml to achieve an INR value of 2–3.

Extensive protein binding is responsible for numerous drug interactions, some of which occur with NSAIDs, diuretics, SSRIs and other antidepressants, steroids, antibiotics and vaccines, and vitamins (for example, vitamin K). Use with NSAIDs may increase bleeding risk. During warfarin therapy the patient should not take any other prescription or OTC drugs unless approved by the health care provider. Use of warfarin with herbal supplements such as green tea, ginkgo, feverfew, garlic, cranberry, chamomile, and ginger may increase the risk of bleeding.

Mechanism in Action:

Warfarin inhibits two enzymes involved in the formation of activated vitamin K, which is required for the synthesis of clotting factors II, VII, IX, and X. Warfarin inhibits the synthesis of *new* clotting factors but does not affect clotting factors that are already circulating in the blood. The result is slowed clot formation and increased bleeding time.

Refer to MyNursingKit for a Nursing Process Focus specific to this drug.

NATURAL THERAPIES

Garlic for Cardiovascular Health

Garlic (*Allium sativum*) is one of the best-studied herbs. Several substances have been isolated from garlic and shown to have pharmacologic activity. Dosage forms include eating prepared garlic oil or the fresh bulbs from the plant.

Modern claims for garlic uses have focused on the cardiovascular system: treatment of high blood lipid levels, atherosclerosis, and hypertension. Other modern claims are that garlic reduces blood glucose levels and has antibacterial and antineoplastic activity.

Like many other supplements, garlic likely has some health benefits, but controlled, scientific studies are often lacking and the results are mixed. Garlic has been shown to decrease the aggregation or "stickiness" of platelets, thus producing an anticoagulant effect. There is some research to show that the herb has a small effect on lowering blood cholesterol, although the effects seem to be short term.

Garlic is safe for consumption in moderate amounts. Patients taking anticoagulant medications should limit their intake of garlic to avoid bleeding complications. Patients with diabetes should monitor their blood glucose levels closely if taking high doses of garlic.

Thrombolytics are used to dissolve existing clots.

CORE CONCEPT 20.6

It is often mistakenly believed that the purpose of anticoagulants such as heparin and warfarin is to digest and remove preexisting clots. This is not the case: A totally different type of drug is needed for this purpose. These drugs, called *thrombolytics*, are administered quite differently than

---

DRUG PROFILE: ℗ *Clopidogrel (Plavix)*

Therapeutic Class: Antiplatelet agent
Pharmacologic Class: ADP receptor blocker

Actions and Uses:

Clopidogrel prolongs bleeding time by inhibiting platelet aggregation. It is given orally. Although its only approved use is to reduce the risk of stroke due to thrombi, it may be given off-label to prevent thrombi formation in patients with coronary artery stents and to prevent postoperative deep vein thrombosis. Because it is expensive, it is usually prescribed only for patients unable to tolerate aspirin, which has similar anticoagulant activity. Ticlopidine (Ticlid) acts by the same mechanism as ticlopidine but causes more adverse effects.

Adverse Effects and Interactions:

Clopidogrel has approximately the same tolerability as aspirin. The incidence of GI bleeding is less than that for aspirin. Frequent adverse effects include a flulike syndrome, headache, diarrhea, dizziness, bruising, upper respiratory tract infection, and rash or pruritus. Excessive bleeding is a potential adverse effect, although it only occurs in about 1% of patients. The other drug in this class, ticlopidine, can cause an acute blood disorder known as thrombotic thrombocytopenia purpura, which can be fatal in up to 30% of patients who develop the disorder. Clopidogrel does not exhibit the same degree of toxicity as ticlopidine.

Use with anticoagulants, other antiplatelet agents, thrombolytic agents, or NSAIDS, including aspirin, will increase the risk of bleeding. Barbiturates, rifampin, or carbamazepine may increase the anticoagulant activity of clopidogrel. The azole antifungals, protease inhibitors, erythromycin, verapamil, or zafirlukast may diminish the antiplatelet actions of clopidogrel.

Refer to MyNursingKit for a Nursing Process Focus specific to this drug.

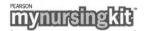

RISK FACTORS AND
PREVENTION OF DEEP
VEIN THROMBOSIS (DVT)

the anticoagulants and produce their effects by different mechanisms. Thrombolytics are prescribed for situations in which a clot has already formed, including the following:

- Acute MI
- Pulmonary embolism
- Cerebrovascular accident (CVA)
- DVT
- Arterial thrombosis
- Coronary thrombosis
- To clear thrombi in arteriovenous cannulas and blocked IV catheters

The goal of thrombolytic therapy is to quickly restore blood flow to the tissue served by the blocked vessel. Delays in reestablishing circulation may result in permanent tissue damage. The therapeutic effect of thrombolytics is greater when they are administered as soon as possible after clot formation occurs, preferably within 4 hours.

Thrombolytics have a narrow margin of safety between dissolving normal and abnormal clots. Vital signs must be monitored continuously, and any signs of bleeding may call for discontinuation of therapy. Because these medications are rapidly destroyed in the bloodstream, discontinuation normally results in the immediate end of thrombolytic activity. After the clot is successfully dissolved by the thrombolytic, coagulation modifier therapy is initiated to prevent the reformation of clots.

Since the discovery of streptokinase, the first thrombolytic, there have been a number of generations of thrombolytics. The newer drugs such as tenecteplase (TNKase) have a more rapid onset and a longer duration and may produce fewer adverse effects than older drugs in this class. Table 20.4 lists the major thrombolytics.

DRUG PROFILE: ℗ *Alteplase (Activase)*

Therapeutic Class: Drug for dissolving clots
Pharmacologic Class: Thrombolytic

Actions and Uses:

Produced through recombinant DNA technology, alteplase is identical to the enzyme human tissue plasminogen activator (tPA). Like other thrombolytics, the primary action of alteplase is to convert plasminogen to plasmin, which then dissolves clots. Alteplase must be given within 6 hours of the onset of symptoms of MI and within 3 hours of thrombotic stroke to be effective. Peak effect occurs in 5–10 minutes. Alteplase is a drug of choice for the treatment of CVA due to thrombus and is used off-label to restore the patency of IV catheters.

Adverse Effects and Interactions:

Thrombolytics such as alteplase are contraindicated in patients with active bleeding or with a history of recent trauma. The patient must be monitored carefully for signs of bleeding every 15 minutes for the first hour of therapy and every 30 minutes thereafter. Signs of bleeding such as bruising, hematomas, or nosebleeds should be reported to the health care provider immediately.

Concurrent use with anticoagulants, antiplatelet agents, or NSAIDs, including aspirin, may increase the risk of bleeding. Use with supplements that affect coagulation, such as feverfew, green tea, ginkgo, fish oil, ginger, or garlic, should be avoided because they may increase the risk of bleeding.

 Refer to MyNursingKit for a Nursing Process Focus specific to this drug.

TABLE 20.4	Thrombolytics	
DRUG	**ROUTE AND ADULT DOSE**	**REMARKS**
℗ alteplase (Activase)	IV; 60 mg initially, then 20 mg/hr infused over next 2 hr	Naturally occurring tissue plasminogen activator; must be given within 6 hours of start of MI or 3 hours of thrombotic stroke
reteplase (Retavase) (see page 348 for the Drug Profile box)	IV; 10 units over 2 min; repeat dose in 30 min	Given during an acute MI to decrease the risk of HF and death
streptokinase (Kabikinase)	IV; 250,000–1.5 million units over 60 min	For acute DVT, pulmonary embolism, and MI
tenecteplase (TNKase)	IV; 30–50 mg infused over 5 sec	Newer thrombolytic with longer half-life and fewer adverse effects

Concept Review 20.2

■ Both warfarin and heparin are effective anticoagulants. Why would a physician choose heparin over warfarin?

Hemostatics are used to promote the formation of clots.

Hemostatics, also called *antifibrinolytics*, have an action opposite to that of anticoagulants: to shorten bleeding time. The name *hemostatics* comes from their ability to slow blood flow. They are used to prevent and treat excessive bleeding following surgical procedures.

All of the hemostatics have very specific indications for use, and none are commonly prescribed. Although their mechanisms differ, all drugs in this class prevent fibrin from dissolving, thus enhancing the stability of the clot. The hemostatics are listed in Table 20.5.

TABLE 20.5	Hemostatics	
DRUG	**ROUTE AND ADULT DOSE**	**REMARKS**
Pr aminocaproic acid (Amicar)	IV; 4–5 g for 1 hr, then 1–1.25 g/hr until bleeding is controlled	For control of excessive bleeding caused by a pathologic condition known as *systemic hyperfibrinolysis;* oral form available
aprotinin (Trasylol)	IV; 2 million KIU (loading dose) followed by 500,000 KIU/hr during procedure	Used to prevent blood loss following cardiopulmonary bypass surgery; considered an investigational new drug
tranexamic acid (Cyklokapron)	PO; 25 mg/kg qid	Used just prior to and following dental surgery; IV form available

NURSING PROCESS FOCUS

Patients Receiving Thrombolytic Therapy

ASSESSMENT

Prior to administration:
- Obtain complete health history (physical/mental), including recent surgeries or trauma, allergies, drug history, and possible drug interactions
- Obtain vital signs; assess in context of patient's baseline values
- Assess lab values: aPTT, PT, Hgb, Hct, platelet count

POTENTIAL NURSING DIAGNOSES

- Risk for Injury (bleeding) related to adverse effects of thrombolytic therapy.
- Ineffective Tissue Perfusion related to increase in size of thrombus, altered blood flow.
- Deficient Knowledge related to information about drug therapy.

PLANNING: PATIENT GOALS AND EXPECTED OUTCOMES

The patient will:
- Undergo a dissolving of preexisting blood clot(s) as evidenced by laboratory values ordered by the health care provider
- Demonstrate an understanding of the drug's action by accurately describing adverse effects and precautions

IMPLEMENTATION

Interventions and (Rationales)	**Patient Education/Discharge Planning**
• If necessary, have IV lines initiated or Foley catheter prior to beginning therapy. (This decreases the risk of bleeding from those sites.)	• Instruct the patient about procedures and why they are necessary prior to beginning thrombolytic therapy.
• Monitor vital signs every 15 minutes during the first hour of infusion, then every 30 minutes during the remainder of infusion. • Patient should be moved as little as possible during the infusion. (This is done to prevent internal injury.)	Advise the patient: • Of the need for frequent monitoring of vital signs • That activity will be limited during infusion and pressure dressing may be needed to prevent any active bleeding
• If given for thrombotic CVA, monitor neurologic status frequently. • Have cardiac rhythm monitored while medication is infusing. (Dysrhythmias may occur with reperfusion of myocardium.)	• Advise the patient about assessments and why they are necessary. • Advise the patient that cardiac rhythm will be monitored during therapy.
• Monitor blood tests (Hct, Hgb, platelet counts) during and after therapy for indications of blood loss due to internal bleeding. (Patient has increased risk of bleeding for 2–4 days postinfusion.)	• Instruct the patient of increased risk for bleeding and of the need for activity restriction and frequent monitoring during this time.

EVALUATION OF OUTCOME CRITERIA

Evaluate the effectiveness of drug therapy by confirming that patient goals and expected outcomes have been met (see "Planning").

See Table 20.4 for a list of drugs to which these nursing actions apply.

DRUG PROFILE: Ⓟ *Aminocaproic Acid (Amicar)*

Therapeutic Class: Clot stabilizer
Pharmacologic Class: Hemostatic/Antifibrinolytic

Actions and Uses:

Aminocaproic acid is prescribed in situations in which there is excessive bleeding as a result of clots being dissolved prematurely. The drug acts by inactivating plasminogen, the precursor of the enzyme plasmin, which dissolves the fibrin clot. During acute hemorrhages, it can be given IV to reduce bleeding in 1–2 hours. It is most commonly prescribed following surgery to reduce postoperative bleeding.

Adverse Effects and Interactions:

Because aminocaproic acid tends to stabilize clots, it should be used cautiously in patients with a history of thromboembolic disease. Adverse effects are generally mild. The therapeutic serum level is 100–400 mcg/ml.

Drug interactions include hypercoagulation when used with estrogens and oral contraceptives.

Refer to MyNursingKit for a Nursing Process Focus specific to this drug.

PATIENTS NEED TO KNOW

Patients treated for coagulation disorders need to know the following:

1. Keep all scheduled appointments for PT, aPTT, and INR laboratory tests. Test results are used in making decisions about drug dose adjustments.
2. Report unusual bruising or bleeding, such as nosebleeds, bleeding gums, black or red stool, heavy menstrual periods, or spitting up blood, to health care providers.
3. Inform dental hygienists and dentists about the use of anticoagulant medication.
4. Use caution when engaged in activities that can cause bleeding, such as shaving, brushing teeth, trimming nails, and using kitchen knives. A soft toothbrush and an electric razor are safe choices. Contact sports, with their high risk for injury, should be avoided.
5. Take medications on time and as directed. Do not skip a dose, double up on doses, or discontinue taking medication without guidance from a health care provider.
6. Do not eat large or inconsistent amounts of foods high in vitamin K when taking warfarin because it interferes with clotting time.
7. Speak with the health care provider before taking any other drugs, including OTC drugs or herbal supplements. Many drugs increase or decrease the action of anticoagulants.

SAFETY ALERT

Medication Label Confusion – Heparin

The morning headlines read, "Fatal Overdose Given to Babies by Nurse." In the fall of 2006, the media reported a story about three premature infants who received fatal overdoses of heparin. Several other babies were affected but survived. Apparently, 1-ml heparin vials with 10,000 units/ml were placed in an automated dispensing unit where 10 units/ml vials were usually kept. The guidelines, known as the "six rights" of drug administration, should always be followed. In this case, checking the drug label for medication amounts would have helped ensure that the correct dosage of heparin was administered to the infants.

CHAPTER REVIEW

CORE CONCEPTS SUMMARY

20.1 **Hemostasis is a complex process involving multiple steps and many clotting factors.**

Hemostasis is an essential mechanism protecting the body from both external and internal injury; it occurs in a sequential series of steps known as the coagulation cascade. The final result of coagulation is formation of a fibrin clot that protects the body from excessive blood loss.

20.2 **Removing a blood clot is essential to restoring normal circulation.**

Blood clots are removed by fibrinolysis. Plasmin digests the fibrin strands, thus restoring circulation to the injured area.

20.3 **Drugs are used to modify the coagulation process.**

Anticoagulants prevent the formation of clots, thrombolytics dissolve existing clots, and hemostatics promote the formation of clots. Coagulation is always carefully monitored through the use of PT or aPTT laboratory tests.

20.4 **Anticoagulants prevent the formation and enlargement of clots.**

Anticoagulants prolong coagulation time by inhibiting platelets or a specific clotting factor in the coagulation cascade. Heparin is given IV or subcutaneously to provide immediate anticoagulation activity, and warfarin is given orally to offer more prolonged action. Protamine sulfate can reverse the anticoagulant activity of heparin, and vitamin K can reverse the effects of warfarin.

20.5 **Antiplatelet agents prolong bleeding time by interfering with platelet aggregation.**

Aspirin, ADP receptor blockers, and glycoprotein IIb/IIIa receptor blockers prolong bleeding time by interfering with platelet function. They are used to prevent thrombus formation in arteries.

20.6 **Thrombolytics are used to dissolve existing clots.**

By dissolving existing clots, thrombolytics restore circulation to an injured area. For maximum effectiveness, they should be given as soon as possible after the thrombus is diagnosed.

20.7 **Hemostatics are used to promote the formation of clots.**

Hemostatics inhibit fibrin in a clot from dissolving and are used primarily to prevent excessive bleeding from surgical sites.

REVIEW QUESTIONS

The following questions are written in NCLEX-PN® style. Answer these questions to assess your knowledge of the chapter material, and go back and review any material that is not clear to you.

1. The patient's INR is 5.5. The nurse will:
1. Recheck the lab value
2. Notify the physician
3. Administer warfarin (Coumadin)
4. Hold the warfarin (Coumadin) and notify the physician

2. The patient has been started on warfarin (Coumadin) for DVT. The patient asks when the medication will break up the clots. The nurse's best response would be:
1. "It will take 7 to 10 days for the clot to break down."
2. "This medication will not break down clots but will make it less likely that the clot will get larger."
3. "It will break down the clot within 8 to 12 hours of administration."
4. "You will need to be on this medication for a long time before it will break down the clot."

3. The patient on IV heparin is started on warfarin (Coumadin) because:
1. Additional medication is needed
2. Warfarin is much more effective than heparin
3. Warfarin is not effective until 12 to 24 hours after the administration of the first dose
4. Heparin has a low molecular weight and is effective for only a short time

4. The patient is receiving enoxaparin (Lovenox) subcutaneously every 12 hours following knee replacement surgery. The nurse should assess for:
1. Gingival hyperplasia
2. Signs and symptoms of bruising and bleeding
3. Clotting at the incision site
4. Increased pain

5. The patient has severe hepatic cirrhosis. The nurse understands the patient's abnormal coagulation times relate to:

1. Inadequate tissue plasminogen activator
2. Inadequate prothrombin activator
3. Inadequate vitamin E
4. Inadequate vitamin K

6. The patient is receiving warfarin (Coumadin). Which of the following laboratory tests should be scheduled?

1. Prothrombin time (PT)
2. International normalized ratio (INR) and PT
3. Partial prothrombin time (PPT)
4. INR

7. The patient on anticoagulant therapy has had a minor surgical procedure. Which of the following would be appropriate for pain control?

1. Ibuprofen (Motrin)
2. Aspirin
3. Acetaminophen (Tylenol)
4. Naproxin sodium (Naprosyn)

8. The patient on intermittent heparin is found to have hematuria and bleeding from old IV sites. The nurse anticipates what being ordered?

1. Protamine sulfate
2. Vitamin K
3. Pentoxifylline (Trental)
4. Ardeparin (Normiflo)

9. Which drug would be appropriate for a patient experiencing an acute MI?

1. Dipyridamole (Persantine)
2. Aminocaproic acid (Amicar)
3. Desmopressin acetate (DDAVP)
4. Alteplase (Activase)

10. A patient is receiving alteplase (Activase), a thrombolytic drug. The nurse must monitor the patient for which of the following possible adverse effects:

1. Temperature of 100.8 F
2. Bruising and epistaxis
3. Skin rash with urticaria
4. Wheezing with labored breathing

CASE STUDY QUESTIONS

For questions 1–4, please refer to the following case study, and choose the correct answer from choices 1–4.

Mr. Hawkins was recently admitted to the hospital with chest pain and suspected pulmonary embolism. He was immediately placed on heparin for 2 days and then switched to warfarin. He is now leaving the hospital with instructions to have laboratory testing every other day for the next 2 weeks.

1. What was the likely goal of placing Mr. Hawkins on heparin?

1. To dissolve pulmonary emboli
2. To prevent excessive bleeding
3. To reduce blood viscosity
4. To prevent additional thrombi from forming

2. Which of the following is the most common and dangerous adverse effect of heparin therapy?

1. Nausea/vomiting
2. MI
3. Bleeding
4. Sedation

3. What was the likely reason why Mr. Hawkins was switched from heparin to warfarin before he was released from the hospital?

1. Warfarin is more effective.
2. Warfarin is given orally.
3. Warfarin causes less risk of hemorrhage.
4. Warfarin is less expensive.

4. What laboratory tests will likely be performed during the 2 weeks after his release?

1. PT/INR
2. Complete blood count (CBC)
3. aPTT
4. White blood cell count

FURTHER STUDY

- The actions and adverse effects of aspirin are described in a Drug Profile in Chapter 12 ⊙.

- The role of thrombolytics in the treatment of MI and cerebrovascular accident is presented in Chapter 18 ⊙.

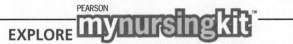

EXPLORE mynursingkit™

MyNursingKit is your one stop for online chapter review materials and resources. Prepare for success with additional NCLEX®-style practice questions, interactive assignments and activities, web links, animations and videos, and more!

Register your access code from the front of your book at
www.mynursingkit.com

21

Drugs for Angina Pectoris, Myocardial Infarction, and Cerebrovascular Accident

CORE CONCEPTS

21.1 Coronary heart disease is caused by a restriction in blood flow to the myocardium.

21.2 Angina pectoris is characterized by severe chest pain caused by lack of sufficient oxygen flow to heart muscle.

21.3 Anginal pain can often be controlled through positive lifestyle changes and surgical procedures.

21.4 The pharmacologic management of angina is achieved by reducing cardiac workload.

21.5 The organic nitrates relieve anginal pain by dilating veins and the coronary arteries.

21.6 Beta-adrenergic blockers are sometimes preferred drugs for reducing the frequency of angina attacks.

21.7 Calcium channel blockers relieve anginal pain by reducing the cardiac workload.

21.8 The early diagnosis and treatment of myocardial infarction (MI) increases chances of survival.

21.9 Thrombolytics dissolve clots blocking the coronary arteries.

21.10 Drugs are used to treat the symptoms and complications of acute MI.

21.11 Aggressive treatment of cerebrovascular accident (CVA) can increase survival.

DRUG SNAPSHOT

The following drugs are discussed in this chapter:

DRUG CLASSES	DRUG PROFILES
Organic nitrates	**Pr** nitroglycerin (Nitrostat, Nitro-Bid, Nitro-Dur, others)
Beta-adrenergic blockers	**Pr** atenolol (Tenormin)
Calcium channel blockers	**Pr** diltiazem (Cardizem, Cartia XT, Dilacor XR, Taztia XT, Tiazac)
Thrombolytics	**Pr** reteplase (Retavase)

LEARNING OUTCOMES

After reading this chapter, the student should be able to:

1. Describe how the myocardium receives its oxygen and nutrient supply.

2. Explain the pathophysiology of angina pectoris.

3. Identify lifestyle changes that may be implemented to manage symptoms of angina.

4. Explain the pathophysiology of MI.

5. Describe the pharmacologic treatment of CVA.

6. For each of drug classes listed in the Drug Snapshot, identify representative drugs and explain the mechanisms of drug action, primary actions, and important adverse effects as they relate to the treatment of angina, MI, or CVA.

7. Categorize drugs used to treat angina, MI, and CVA based on their classification and mechanisms of action.

KEY TERMS

angina pectoris (an-JEYE-nuh PEK-tore-us) *338*

atherosclerosis (ath-ur-oh-skler-OH-sis) *339*

cerebrovascular accident/stroke (sir-ree-bro-VASK-u-lur) *349*

coronary arteries (KOR-un-air-ee AR-tur-ees) *338*

coronary artery bypass graft (CABG) surgery *340*

hemorrhagic stroke (hee-moh-RAJ-ik) *350*

myocardial infarction (MI) (meye-oh-KAR-dee-ul in-FARK-shun) *346*

myocardial ischemia (meye-oh-KAR-dee-ul ik-SKEE-mee-uh) *339*

percutaneous transluminal coronary angioplasty (PTCA) (per-cue-TAIN-ee-us trans-LOO-min-ul KOR-un-air-ee ANN-gee-oh-plas-tee) *340*

plaque (plak) *339*

stable angina *339*

thrombotic stroke (throm-BOT-ik) *349*

unstable angina *339*

vasospastic (Prinzmetal's) angina *339*

All tissues in the body are dependent on a continuous supply of oxygen and other nutrients that are delivered via an extensive arterial system. When these vessels become clogged by fatty deposits or a clot, the tissues served by the affected arteries are starved for oxygen and their function is affected. This chapter covers the pharmacotherapy of three such diseases: angina pectoris, myocardial infarction (MI), and cerebrovascular accident (CVA), also called stroke.

CORE CONCEPT 21.1

Coronary heart disease is caused by a restriction in blood flow to the myocardium.

myo = *muscle*
cardium = *heart*

The heart is the hardest working organ in the body. Whereas the activity of most organs slows considerably during rest and sleep, the heart must continue pumping so that the tissues can receive the nutrients they need and dispose of the wastes they have accumulated. Because it is such a vital organ, the heart muscle or myocardium must receive a continuous supply of oxygen and nutrients. Any disturbance in blood flow to the vital organs or to the myocardium itself—even for brief episodes—can result in life-threatening consequences.

Because the heart chambers fill with blood more than 60 times per minute, one would think that the myocardium would have an ample supply of oxygen and nutrients. The myocardium, however, receives essentially no nutrients from the blood traveling through the heart's chambers. Instead, heart muscle receives its nutrients from the first two arteries branching off the aorta, the right and left **coronary arteries**. As these arteries branch, they circle the heart, bringing cardiac muscle a continuous supply of oxygen and nutrients.

Coronary heart disease (CHD), also called coronary artery disease (CAD), is the term used to describe impaired blood flow in the coronary arteries. Moderate restriction of flow leads to angina pectoris. Severe impairment or complete loss of blood flow causes MI and a high risk of sudden death. CHD can also cause dysrhythmias and lead to heart failure.

ANGINA PECTORIS

Angina pectoris is acute chest pain caused by insufficient oxygen to a portion of the myocardium. Angina is characterized by chest pain on physical exertion or emotional stress. Although it produces many of the same symptoms as a heart attack, its pharmacologic treatment is quite different.

Angina pectoris is characterized by severe chest pain caused by lack of sufficient oxygen flow to heart muscle.

The most common cause of angina is **atherosclerosis**: a buildup of fatty, fibrous material called **plaque** in the walls of arteries. Although plaque may take as long as 40 to 50 years to accumulate to a level that would cause symptoms, plaque deposition actually begins very early in life. If plaque accumulates in a coronary artery, the myocardium downstream from the affected artery begins to receive less oxygen than it needs to perform its metabolic functions. This condition of having a reduced blood supply to cardiac muscle cells is called **myocardial ischemia**. Figure 21.1 ■ illustrates the progressive accumulation of plaque that is characteristic of atherosclerosis.

The classic presentation of angina pectoris is intense pain in the chest, often moving to the left side of the neck and lower jaw and down the left arm. Angina pain is usually preceded by physical exertion or emotional excitement—events associated with *increased myocardial oxygen demand*. The plaque-filled coronary artery is unable to supply the amount of nutrients needed by the stressed myocardium. With rest, anginal pain usually diminishes in less than 15 minutes.

There are several types of angina. Angina pectoris that is predictable in its frequency, intensity, and duration is called **stable angina**. If angina episodes become more frequent or severe and occur during periods of rest, the condition is called **unstable angina**. Unstable angina requires more aggressive medical intervention. It is sometimes considered a medical emergency because it is associated with an increased risk of MI. A third type of angina is known as **vasospastic**, or **Prinzmetal's, angina**. This type is caused by *spasms* of the coronary arteries, which may or may not contain plaque. Vasospastic angina pain occurs most often during periods of rest.

Angina pain may closely mimic that of an MI. It is necessary for the health care provider to quickly distinguish between the two diseases because the pharmacologic treatment of angina is much different than that of MI. Whereas angina is rarely fatal, MI has a high mortality rate if treatment is delayed. Thus, drug therapy must begin immediately.

Chest pain is a common complaint of patients seeking care in physicians' offices and emergency departments. It is also one of the most frightening symptoms for patients, who often equate their pain to having MI with a real risk of sudden death. The pain experienced by the patient, however, is only a symptom of an underlying disorder; a large number of diverse diseases can produce pain in the chest, and some of these are unrelated to the heart. A major goal of the health care provider is to quickly determine the cause of the pain so that the proper treatment can be administered. Table 21.1 lists some of the common diseases that can produce chest pain as a symptom.

athero = *fatty*
sclera = *hard*
osis = *condition of*

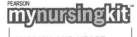

WOMEN AND HEART DISEASE

FIGURE 21.1

Plaque and thrombus formation in the coronary artery
Source: Reprinted by permission of Pearson Education, Inc., Upper Saddle River, NJ

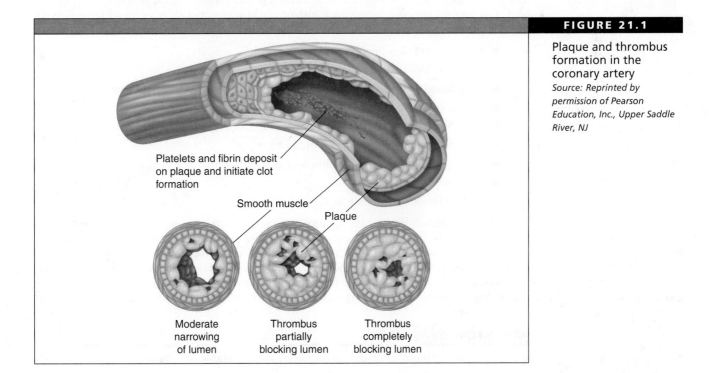

Platelets and fibrin deposit on plaque and initiate clot formation

Smooth muscle

Plaque

Moderate narrowing of lumen

Thrombus partially blocking lumen

Thrombus completely blocking lumen

TABLE 21.1	Examples of Disorders That May Produce Chest Pain
NAME OF DISEASE	**DESCRIPTION**
Mitral stenosis	Inability of the mitral valve to fully open
Myocardial infarction	Cardiac muscle tissue death due to clots in coronary arteries
Hypertension	High systemic blood pressure
Coronary artery disease	Atherosclerosis of the coronary arteries
Diabetes	Lack of insulin or inability to tolerate carbohydrates
Peptic ulcer disease	Erosion of the mucosa of the stomach or small intestine
Gastric reflux	Backflow of stomach contents into the esophagus

Fast Facts Angina Pectoris and Coronary Heart Disease

■ Coronary heart disease causes one out of every five deaths in the United States.

■ Over 9 million Americans have angina pectoris; 500,000 new cases occur each year.

■ Among ethnic groups, the incidence of angina is highest among Blacks, intermediate in Mexican Americans, and lowest in non-Hispanic Whites.

■ Angina occurs more frequently in women than men; Black women have twice the risk of Black men.

CORE CONCEPT 21.3

Anginal pain can often be controlled through positive lifestyle changes and surgical procedures.

A combination of variables influences the development and progression of CHD, including dietary patterns and lifestyle choices. A number of dietary and lifestyle factors are associated with an increased incidence of angina. The health care provider should help the patient control the frequency of anginal episodes by advising him or her to implement some or all of the following lifestyle changes:

- Limit alcohol consumption to small amounts.
- Eliminate foods high in cholesterol or saturated fats.
- Keep blood cholesterol and other lipid indicators within the normal ranges.
- Do not use tobacco.
- Keep blood pressure within the normal range.
- Exercise regularly and maintain optimum weight.
- Keep blood glucose levels within normal range.
- Limit salt (sodium) intake.
- Reduce stress levels as much as possible.

angio = *vessel*
plasty = *shaped or molded by a surgical procedure*

per = *through*
cutaneous = *skin*

When the coronary arteries are significantly obstructed, the two most common interventions are **percutaneous transluminal coronary angioplasty (PTCA)** with stent insertion, and **coronary artery bypass graft (CABG) surgery**. PTCA is a procedure whereby the area of narrowing is dilated using either a balloon catheter or a laser. Because the artery may return to its narrowed state after the procedure, a stent is sometimes used in conjunction with balloon angioplasty. Angioplasty with stenting typically relieves 90% of the original blockage in the artery.

Concept Review 21.1

■ How can a health care provider distinguish between stable angina and unstable angina?

The pharmacologic management of angina is achieved by reducing cardiac workload.

The treatment goals for a patient with angina are twofold: to *reduce the frequency* of anginal episodes and to *terminate* acute anginal pain in progress. Long-term goals include extending the patient's life span by preventing serious consequences of ischemic heart disease, such as dysrhythmias, heart failure, and MI. The primary means by which antianginal drugs act is by reducing the myocardial demand for oxygen. This reduced demand can be accomplished by at least four mechanisms:

- Slowing the heart rate
- Dilating veins so that heart receives less blood (reduced *preload*)
- Causing the heart to contract with less force (reduced *contractility*)
- Lowering blood pressure, thus offering the heart less resistance when ejecting blood from the ventricles (reduced *afterload*)

Three classes of drugs—organic nitrates, beta-adrenergic blockers, and calcium channel blockers—are used to treat angina. Rapid-acting organic nitrates are drugs of choice for *terminating* acute angina pain. Beta-adrenergic blockers are drugs of choice for *preventing* angina pain. Calcium channel blockers are used when beta blockers are not tolerated well by a patient. It is important to understand that the antianginal medications relieve symptoms but do not cure the underlying disorder. A summary of the means used to prevent and treat coronary artery disease is shown in Figure 21.2 ■.

Approved in 2006, ranolazine (Ranexa) is a newer drug for angina. Ranolazine is believed to act by shifting the metabolism of cardiac muscle cells so that they utilize glucose as the primary energy source rather than fatty acids. The drug is approved only for chronic angina that has not responded to other agents.

FIGURE 21.2

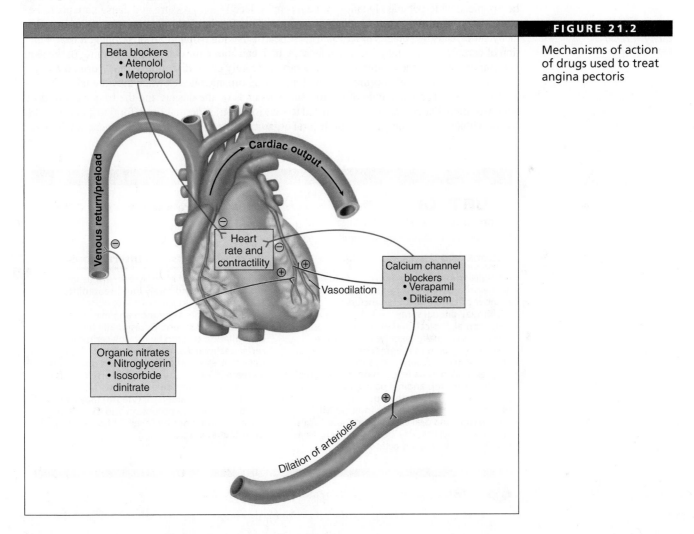

Mechanisms of action of drugs used to treat angina pectoris

The organic nitrates relieve anginal pain by dilating veins and the coronary arteries.

All drugs in this chemical class possess at least one nitrate (NO_2) group. The vasodilation effect of these agents is a result of the conversion of nitrate to its active form, nitric oxide (NO). Another nitrogen-containing drug, nitrous oxide (N_2O), is used in anesthesia (see Chapter 13 ⬭). Organic nitrates used to treat angina are listed in Table 21.2.

Since the discovery of their medicinal properties in 1857, the organic nitrates have been the mainstay for the treatment of angina. The primary therapeutic action of these agents is their ability to relax both arterial and venous smooth muscle. Dilation of veins reduces the amount of blood returning to the heart (preload), so the chambers contain a smaller volume. With less blood for the ventricles to pump, the workload on the heart is decreased, thereby lowering myocardial oxygen demand. The therapeutic outcome is that chest pain is terminated and episodes of angina become less frequent.

Organic nitrates also have the ability to dilate coronary arteries, and this was once thought to be their primary mechanism of action. It seems logical that dilating a partially occluded coronary vessel would allow more oxygen to reach ischemic myocardial tissue. Although this effect does indeed occur, it is not believed to be the primary mechanism of nitrate action in stable angina. This action, however, is important in treating the less common form of angina known as vasospastic angina. The organic nitrates can relax these spasms and stop the pain.

trans = *across or through*
dermis = *skin*

Organic nitrates are of two types: short acting and long acting. The short-acting agents, such as nitroglycerin, are taken sublingually to quickly stop an acute anginal attack in progress. Long-acting nitrates, such as isosorbide dinitrate (Dilatrate SR, Isordil), are taken orally or delivered through a transdermal patch to decrease the frequency and severity of anginal episodes. Long-acting nitrates are also useful in reducing the symptoms of heart failure (see Chapter 18 ⬭).

Although nitrates are safe drugs that have few serious adverse effects, some adverse effects may be troublesome to patients. Dilation of veins can reduce blood pressure and cause patients to become dizzy when moving to a standing position. This fall in blood pressure can result in reflex tachycardia, causing patients to feel as if their heart is having palpitations or skipping a beat. Dilation of cerebral vessels may cause headache, which can sometimes be severe. Flushing of the skin is common. Most of these effects are temporary and rarely cause discontinuation of drug therapy.

tachy = *rapid*
cardia = *heart*

Tolerance commonly occurs with the long-acting organic nitrates when they are taken for extended periods. The magnitude of the tolerance depends on the dosage and the frequency of drug administration. Patients are often instructed to remove the transdermal patch for 6 to 12 hours each day or withhold the nighttime dose of the oral organic nitrate to delay the development of tolerance.

DRUG PROFILE: ℞ *Nitroglycerin (Nitrostat, Nitro-Bid, Nitro-Dur, Others)*
Therapeutic Class: Antianginal drug
Pharmacologic Class: Organic nitrate, vasodilator

Actions and Uses:

Nitroglycerin, the oldest and most widely used of the organic nitrates, can be delivered by a number of different routes, including sublingual, lingual spray, oral, IV, transmucosal, transdermal, topical, and extended-release forms. It is normally taken while an acute anginal episode is in progress or just prior to physical activity. When given sublingually, it reaches peak plasma levels in only 4 minutes and thus can stop anginal pain rapidly. Chest pain that does not respond quickly to sublingual nitroglycerin may indicate MI. The transdermal and oral sustained-release forms are for prophylaxis only, because they have a relatively slow onset of action.

Adverse Effects and Interactions:

Adverse effects of nitroglycerin are usually cardiovascular and rarely life threatening. Because nitroglycerin can dilate vessels in the head, headache is common and may be persistent and severe. Occasionally the venodilation created by nitroglycerin causes *reflex tachycardia*. A beta-adrenergic blocker may be prescribed to diminish this undesirable increase in heart rate. Many adverse effects of nitroglycerin diminish after a few doses.

Using with sildenafil (Viagra) may cause life-threatening hypotension and CV collapse. Nitrates should not be taken 24 hours before or after taking Viagra.

Refer to MyNursingKit for a Nursing Process Focus specific to this drug.

TABLE 21.2	Selected Drugs for Angina and Myocardial Infarction	
DRUG	**ROUTE AND ADULT DOSE**	**REMARKS**
ORGANIC NITRATES		
amyl nitrate	Inhalation; 1 ampule (0.18–0.3 ml) prn	Short acting; onset is 10–30 seconds; may be repeated in 3–5 minutes; also used as treatment for cyanide poisoning
isosorbide dinitrate (Dilatrate SR, Isordil)	PO; 2.5–30 mg qid (max: 480 mg/day)	For both acute attacks and long-term management; sublingual and chewable forms smaller dose is given to initiate therapy; extended-release form available
isosorbide mononitrate (Imdur, Ismo, Monoket)	PO; 20 mg bid (max: 240 mg/day with sustained release)	For the prevention of angina; a smaller dose is given to initiate therapy; extended-release form available
(Pr) nitroglycerin (Nitrostat, Nitro-Bid, Nitro-Dur, others)	Sublingual: 1 tablet (0.3–0.6 mg) or 1 spray (0.4–0.8 mg) every 3–5 min (max: 3 doses in 15 min)	Dilates both arteries and veins; sublingual, oral, translingual, IV, transmucosal, transdermal, and topical forms available; extended-release form available
BETA-ADRENERGIC BLOCKERS		
acebutolol (Sectral)	PO; 400–800 mg daily (max: 1200 mg/day)	Cardioselective $beta_1$-blocker; decreases cardiac output; for hypertension, dysrhythmias, and angina
(Pr) atenolol (Tenormin)	PO; 25–50 mg daily (max: 100 mg/day)	Cardioselective $beta_1$-blocker; reduces rate and force of cardiac contractions; for angina, MI, and hypertension
metoprolol (Lopressor, Toprol XL)	For angina: PO; 100 mg bid (max: 400 mg/day) For MI: IV; 5 mg every 2 min for 3 doses followed by PO doses	Cardioselective $beta_1$-blocker; for angina, MI, and hypertension sustained-release form (Toprol XL) available for heart failure
nadolol (Corgard)	PO; 40 mg daily (max: 240 mg/day)	Nonselective $beta_1$- and $beta_2$-blocker; for long-term prevention of angina and hypertension
propranolol (Inderal, InnoPran XL) (see page 314 for the Drug Profile box)	PO; 10–80 mg bid–tid (max: 320 mg/day)	Nonselective $beta_1$- and $beta_2$-blocker; IV form available; for angina, hypertension, dysrhythmias, MI, and migraine prophylaxis
timolol maleate (Betimol)	PO; 15–45 mg tid (max: 60 mg/day)	Nonselective $beta_1$- and $beta_2$-blocker; for hypertension and angina; topical form available for glaucoma
CALCIUM CHANNEL BLOCKERS		
amlodipine (Norvasc)	PO; 5–10 mg daily (max: 10 mg/day)	Also for hypertension; Lotrel contains amlodipine and the ACE inhibitor benazepril
bepridil (Vascor)	PO; 200 mg daily (max: 400 mg/day)	Also blocks sodium channels; usually reserved for patients unresponsive to safer antianginals
(Pr) diltiazem (Cardizem, Cartia XT, Dilacor XR, Taztia XT, Tiazac)	PO; regular release; 30 mg tid-qid (max: 480 mg/day) Extended release 20–240 mg bid (max: 540 mg/day)	Dilates coronary arteries and decreases coronary artery spasm; also for hypertension; IV form available for dysrhythmias
nicardipine (Cardene)	PO; 20–40 mg tid or 30–60 mg Sustained release: bid (max: 120 mg/day)	Also for hypertension; IV form available
nifedipine (Adalat, Procardia) (see page 277 for the Drug Profile box)	PO; 10–20 mg tid (max: 180 mg/day) Extended release: 30–90 mg once daily	Used in the treatment of vasospastic angina; also for hypertension
verapamil (Calan, Isoptin, others) (see page 316 for the Drug Profile box)	PO; 80 mg tid–qid (max: 480 mg/day) Sustained release: 180 mg once daily	Dilates coronary arteries and inhibits coronary artery spasm; also for hypertension; IV form available for dysrhythmias

NURSING PROCESS FOCUS

Patients Receiving Nitroglycerin

ASSESSMENT

Prior to administration:
- Obtain a complete health history (physical/mental), including allergies, drug history, and possible drug interactions
- Assess vital signs, electrocardiogram (ECG), frequency and severity of angina, and alcohol use
- Obtain history of cardiac disorders and blood testing, including cardiac enzymes, complete blood count (CBC), blood urea nitrogen (BUN), creatinine, and liver function tests
- Assess if the patient has taken erectile dysfunction drugs (e.g., sildenafil [Viagra], vardenafil [Levitra], or tadalafil [Cialis]) within the last 24 hours

POTENTIAL NURSING DIAGNOSES

- Risk for Ineffective Tissue Perfusion related to hypotension from drug.
- Risk for Injury (dizziness or fainting) related to hypotension from drug.
- Acute Pain (headache) related to adverse effects of drug.
- Deficient Knowledge related to information about drug therapy.

PLANNING: PATIENT GOALS AND EXPECTED OUTCOMES

The patient will:
- Experience relief or prevention of chest pain
- Report immediately any chest pain unrelieved by nitroglycerin
- Demonstrate an understanding of the drug's action by accurately describing adverse effects and precautions

IMPLEMENTATION

Interventions and (Rationales)	Patient Education/Discharge Planning
• Ask the patient to describe and rate pain prior to drug administration for description/documentation of anginal episode. • Obtain a 12-lead ECG to differentiate between angina and infarction. (Pharmacotherapy depends on which disorder is presenting.)	Instruct the patient to: • Take 1 tablet every 5 minutes until pain is relieved or for up to 3 doses during an acute anginal attack • Call emergency medical services (EMS) if chest pain is not relieved after 3 doses • Place SL tablet under the tongue or spray under the tongue; do not inhale spray • Explain to the patient the reason and importance for conducting an ECG
• Monitor blood pressure and pulse. Do not administer drug if the patient is hypotensive. (Drug will further reduce blood pressure.) • Monitor alcohol use. (Extremely low blood pressure may result, which could cause death.) • Monitor for headache in response to use of nitrates.	• Instruct the patient to sit or lie down before taking medication and to avoid abrupt changes in position. • Emphasize the importance of avoiding alcohol while taking nitroglycerin. Instruct the patient that: • Headache is a common adverse effect that usually decreases over time • Over-the-counter (OTC) medicines usually relieve the headache
• Monitor for use of erectile dysfunction drugs (e.g., sildenafil) concurrently with nitrates. (Life-threatening hypotension may result with concurrent use of these drugs.)	Instruct the patient to: • Not take erectile dysfunction drugs within 24 hours after taking nitrates • Wait at least 24 hours after taking erectile dysfunction drugs to resume nitrate therapy
• Monitor need for prophylactic nitrates.	• Advise the patient to take medication prior to a stressful event or physical activity to prevent angina

EVALUATION OF OUTCOME CRITERIA

Evaluate the effectiveness of drug therapy by confirming that patient goals and expected outcomes have been met (see "Planning").

See Table 21.2 for a list of drugs to which these nursing actions apply.

Beta-adrenergic blockers are sometimes preferred drugs for reducing the frequency of angina attacks.

Beta-adrenergic blockers reduce the workload on the heart and are used for angina prophylaxis. Drugs for angina include cardioselective beta$_1$-blockers and mixed beta$_1$-beta$_2$-blockers. The beta-adrenergic blockers of importance in treating angina are listed in Table 21.2.

The pharmacology of the beta-adrenergic blockers was presented in Chapter 8 ∞ . Beta blockers are widely used in medicine, including for the treatment of hypertension (see Chapter 17 ∞), heart failure (see Chapter 18 ∞), and dysrhythmias (see Chapter 19 ∞). Because of their ability to reduce the workload on the heart by slowing heart rate and reducing contractility, several beta blockers are used to decrease the frequency and severity of anginal attacks caused by exertion.

Beta-adrenergic antagonists are well tolerated by most patients. In some patients, fatigue, lethargy, and depression occur. Because beta blockers slow the heart rate, they are contraindicated in patients with bradycardia and heart block. Heart rate should be closely monitored so that it does not fall below 50–60 bpm at rest or 100 bpm during exercise. Patients with diabetes should be aware that blood glucose levels should be monitored more frequently and that insulin doses may need to be adjusted accordingly. Patients should be advised against abruptly stopping beta-blocker therapy because this may result in a sudden increase in workload on the heart and acute angina symptoms.

Calcium channel blockers relieve anginal pain by reducing the cardiac workload.

Several calcium channel blockers (CCBs) reduce myocardial oxygen demand by lowering blood pressure and slowing the heart rate. They are widely used in the treatment of cardiovascular diseases. CCBs of importance to angina are listed in Table 21.2.

Blockade of calcium ion channels has a number of effects on the heart, most of which are similar to those of beta-adrenergic blockers. Like beta blockers, the CCBs have been discussed several times in this text for the treatment of hypertension (see Chapter 17 ∞) and dysrhythmias (see Chapter 19 ∞). The first approved use of CCBs was for the treatment of angina.

DRUG PROFILE: ℞ *Atenolol (Tenormin)*

Therapeutic Class: Drug for angina, hypertension or MI
Pharmacologic Class: Beta-adrenergic blocker

Actions and Uses:

Atenolol is one of the most frequently prescribed drugs in the United States due to its relative safety and effectiveness in treating a number of chronic disorders, including heart failure, hypertension, stable angina, and MI. Atenolol selectively blocks beta$_1$-receptors in the heart. Its effectiveness in angina is attributed to its ability to slow heart rate and reduce contractility (negative inotropic effect), both of which lower myocardial oxygen demand. Because of its 7- to 9-hour half-life, it may be taken once a day.

Adverse Effects and Interactions:

As a cardioselective beta$_1$-blocker, atenolol has few adverse effects on the lungs and is useful for patients experiencing bronchospasm. Like other beta blockers, therapy generally begins with low doses, which are gradually increased until the therapeutic effect is achieved. The most frequent adverse effects of atenolol include fatigue, weakness, and hypotension.

Using atenolol together with calcium channel blockers may cause excessive cardiac suppression. Using atenolol together with digoxin may cause slowed atrioventricular conduction leading to heart block. Patients should avoid using this drug with nicotine or caffeine because their vasoconstriction action will diminish the beneficial effects of atenolol.

Refer to MyNursingKit for a Nursing Process Focus specific to this drug.

DRUG PROFILE: ℗ *Diltiazem (Cardizem, Cartia XT, Dilacor XR, Taztia XT, Tiazac)*

Therapeutic Class: Drug for angina and hypertension
Pharmacologic Class: Calcium channel blocker

Actions and Uses:

Diltiazem inhibits the transport of calcium ions into myocardial cells and has the ability to relax both coronary and peripheral blood vessels. It is useful in the treatment of atrial dysrhythmias and hypertension as well as angina. When given as sustained-release capsules, it may be administered once daily.

Adverse Effects and Interactions:

Adverse effects of diltiazem are generally not serious and are related to vasodilation such as headache, dizziness, and edema of the ankles and feet. Although diltiazem produces few adverse effects on the heart or vessels, it should be used with caution in patients taking other cardiovascular medications, particularly digoxin or beta-adrenergic blockers; the combined effects of these drugs may cause heart failure or dysrhythmias.

Diltiazem increases the levels of digoxin or quinidine if taken together. It should be used cautiously with ginger because this combination may interfere with blood clotting.

Refer to MyNursingKit for a Nursing Process Focus specific to this drug.

CCBs cause arteriolar smooth muscle to relax, thus lowering peripheral resistance and reducing blood pressure. This decreases the myocardial oxygen demand, thus reducing the frequency of anginal pain. Some CCBs are selective for arterioles. Others, such as verapamil and diltiazem, have an additional beneficial effect of slowing the heart rate (negative chronotropic effect). An additional effect of the CCBs is their ability to dilate the coronary arteries, bringing more oxygen to the myocardium. This is especially important in patients with vasospastic angina. Because they are able to relieve the acute spasms of vasospastic angina, CCBs are considered drugs of choice for this condition.

Adverse effects of CCBs are generally not serious and are related to vasodilation, such as headache, dizziness, and edema of the ankles and feet. CCBs should be used with caution in patients taking other cardiovascular medications that slow conduction through the atrioventricular (AV) node, particularly digoxin or beta-adrenergic blockers. The combined effects of these drugs may cause partial or complete AV heart block, heart failure, or dysrhythmias.

Concept Review 21.2

■ How does decreasing the workload on the heart result in reduction in anginal pain?

MYOCARDIAL INFARCTION

A myocardial infarction (MI) is the result of a sudden occlusion of a coronary artery. Immediate pharmacologic treatment may reduce patient mortality.

CORE CONCEPT 21.8

The early diagnosis and treatment of myocardial infarction (MI) increases chances of survival.

Myocardial infarctions are responsible for a substantial number of deaths each year. Some patients die before reaching a medical facility for treatment, and many others die within 1 to 2 days after the initial MI. Clearly, MI is a serious and frightening disease and is responsible for a large percentage of sudden deaths.

The primary cause of MI is advanced CAD. Plaque buildup can severely narrow one or more branches of the coronary arteries. Pieces of plaque may break off and lodge in a small vessel that serves a portion of the myocardium. Deprived of its oxygen supply, the affected area of the myocardium becomes ischemic and cardiac muscle cells begin to die unless the blood supply is quickly restored. Figure 21.3 ■ illustrates this blockage and the resulting reperfusion process.

The goals of the pharmacologic treatment of acute MI include the following:

- Restoring blood supply (perfusion) to the damaged myocardium as quickly as possible through the use of thrombolytics
- Reducing myocardial oxygen demand with organic nitrates, beta blockers, or CCBs to prevent another MI

FIGURE 21.3

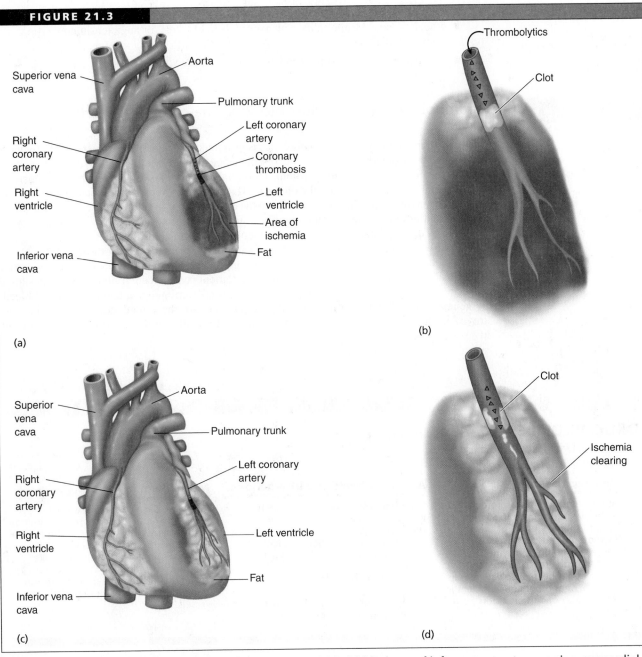

Blockade and reperfusion following myocardial infarction (MI): (a) blockage of left coronary artery causing myocardial ischemia; (b) infusion of thrombolytics; (c) blood supply returning to myocardium; (d) thrombus dissolving and ischemia clearing *Source: (a) and (c) Reprinted by permission of Pearson Education, Inc., Upper Saddle River, NJ*

Fast Facts Myocardial Infarction

- About 1.1 million Americans experience a new or recurrent MI each year.
- About one third of patients experiencing an MI will die.
- About 60% of patients who died suddenly of MI had no previous symptoms of the disease.
- Mortality from MI is slightly higher in men than in women.
- Because women have MIs at older ages, they are more likely to die from them within a few weeks.
- More than 20% of men and 40% of women will die from an MI within 1 year of being diagnosed.

- Controling or preventing MI-associated dysrhythmias with beta blockers or other antidysrhythmics
- Reducing post-MI mortality with aspirin, beta blockers, or angiotensin-converting enzyme (ACE) inhibitors
- Managing severe chest pain and associated anxiety with analgesics

CORE CONCEPT 21.9

Thrombolytics dissolve clots blocking the coronary arteries.

The basic pharmacology of the thrombolytics is presented in Chapter 20 ⊕ . In the treatment of MI, the goal of thrombolytic therapy is to dissolve clots that are obstructing the coronary arteries and restore circulation to the myocardium. Thrombolytics are most effective when administered from 20 minutes to 12 hours after the onset of MI symptoms. Quick restoration of cardiac circulation has been found to reduce mortality from the disease. After the clot is successfully dissolved, anticoagulant or antiplatelet therapy is initiated to prevent the formation of additional thrombi. Dosages and descriptions of the various thrombolytics are given in Chapter 14 ⊕ .

Thrombolytics have a narrow margin of safety. The primary risk of thrombolytics is excessive bleeding from interference in the clotting process. Older adults have an increased risk of serious bleeding and intracranial hemorrhage. Patients with recent trauma or surgery should not receive these drugs. Vital signs must be monitored continuously, and any signs of bleeding generally call for discontinuation of therapy. Because these medications are rapidly destroyed in the blood, stopping the infusion normally results in the rapid termination of any adverse effects.

DRUG PROFILE: ℗ *Reteplase (Retavase)*

Therapeutic Class: Drug for dissolving clots
Pharmacologic Class: Thrombolytic

Actions and Uses:

Like other drugs in this class, reteplase is most effective if given within 30 minutes but not later than 12 hours of the onset of MI symptoms. It usually acts within 20 minutes. A second bolus may be delivered after the first, if necessary. After the clot has been dissolved, therapy with heparin or another anticoagulant is started to prevent additional clots from forming.

Adverse Effects and Interactions:

Reteplase is contraindicated in patients with active bleeding. Health care providers must be vigilant in recognizing and reporting any abnormal bleeding that may occur during thrombolytic therapy.

Drug interactions with anticoagulants and platelet aggregation inhibitors will produce an additive effect and increase the risk of bleeding.

Mechanism in Action:

Reteplase dissolves blood clots by activating plasminogen, a protein found within many body tissues and the general circulation. On activation, plasminogen binds to fibrin, which is the meshlike substance forming the insoluble clot. Thrombolytics remove clots and restore circulation to injured or occluded blood vessels.

 Refer to MyNursingKit for a Nursing Process Focus specific to this drug.

Drugs are used to treat the symptoms and complications of acute MI.

The most immediate needs of the patient with MI are to ensure that the heart continues functioning and that permanent damage from the infarction is minimized. Drugs from several classes are administered soon after the onset of symptoms to prevent reinfarction and, ultimately, to reduce mortality from the episode.

Beta-adrenergic blockers. Beta blockers are used for MI, as they are for angina, to reduce the cardiac workload. Beta blockers have the ability to slow the heart rate, decrease contractility, and reduce blood pressure. These three actions reduce the cardiac oxygen demand, which is beneficial for those who experienced a recent MI. In addition, their ability of beta blockers to slow impulse conduction through the heart tends to suppress dysrhythmias, which can be serious and sometimes fatal complications following MI. Their use has been found to reduce mortality following an MI if given within 8 hours of the MI.

Antiplatelets and anticoagulants. Aspirin has been found to dramatically reduce mortality, as much as 50%, in the weeks following an acute MI. Unless contraindicated, 160 to 324 mg of aspirin is given as soon as possible following a suspected MI. Clopidogrel (Plavix) is another effective antiplatelet agent that has been shown to reduce mortality associated with thrombi formation following an MI. Patients at high risk for thrombi formation may receive anticoagulants such as heparin, low molecular weight heparin, or warfarin (Coumadin) following an MI. Some patients may remain on anticoagulant therapy on a chronic basis after hospital discharge. The various coagulation modifiers are presented in Chapter 20 ⚭ .

Angiotensin-converting enzyme (ACE) inhibitors. The ACE inhibitors captopril (Capoten) and lisinopril (Prinivil, Zestril) have also been found to reduce mortality following MI. These drugs are most effective when therapy is started within 1 or 2 days of the onset of symptoms. Oral therapy with the ACE inhibitors normally begins after thrombolytic therapy has been completed and the patient's condition has stabilized. The pharmacology of the ACE inhibitors is presented in Chapter 17 ⚭ .

Pain management. Pain control is essential following acute MI to ensure the patient's comfort and reduce stress. Opioids such as morphine sulfate are sometimes given to ease the severe pain associated with acute MI and to sedate the anxious patient. Details on the pharmacology of the opioids were presented in Chapter 14 ⚭ .

Concept Review   21.3

- Why is it important to treat an MI within the first 24 hours after symptoms have begun? What classes of drugs are used for this purpose?

CEREBROVASCULAR ACCIDENT

A CVA is caused by a thrombus within or bleeding from a vessel serving the brain. Although drug therapy is limited, immediate treatment may reduce the degree of permanent disability resulting from a CVA.

Aggressive treatment of cerebrovascular accident (CVA) can increase survival.

Cerebrovascular accident (CVA) or **stroke** is a major cause of permanent disability. The majority of strokes are caused by a thrombus in a vessel serving the brain (**thrombotic stroke**). Areas downstream from the clot lose their oxygen supply, and neural tissue will begin to die unless circulation is quickly restored. A smaller percentage of strokes, about 20%, are caused by rupture of a cerebral

cerebro = *head or brain*
vascular = *vessels*

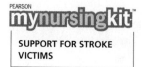

vessel and its associated bleeding into neural tissue (**hemorrhagic stroke**). Symptoms are the same for the two types of strokes. Specific symptoms will vary widely depending on which area of the brain is affected and may include blindness, paralysis, speech problems, coma, and even dementia. Mortality from CVA is very high: As many as 40% of patients will die within the first year of a stroke.

Drug therapy of thrombotic stroke focuses on two main goals: prevention of strokes through the use of anticoagulants and antihypertensive agents, and restoration of blood supply to the affected portion of the brain as quickly as possible after an acute stroke through the use of thrombolytics.

As discussed in Chapter 17 ∞, sustained, chronic hypertension is closely associated with CVA. Antihypertensive therapy with beta-adrenergic blockers, CCBs, diuretics, and ACE inhibitors can help manage blood pressure and reduce the probability of stroke.

In very low doses, aspirin reduces the incidence of CVA by discouraging the formation of thrombi by inhibiting platelet aggregation. Patients are often placed on low-dose aspirin therapy on a continual basis following their first stroke. Clopidogrel (Plavix) is an antiplatelet drug that may be used to provide antiplatelet activity in patients who cannot tolerate aspirin. Other anticoagulants such as warfarin may be given to prevent stroke in high-risk patients such as those with prosthetic heart valves.

The single most important breakthrough in the treatment of stroke was development of the thrombolytic agents. Prior to the discovery of these drugs, the treatment of thrombotic stroke was largely a passive, wait-and-see strategy. Now stroke is aggressively treated with thrombolytics as soon as the patient arrives at the hospital: These agents are most effective if administered within 3 hours of the attack. Use of aggressive thrombolytic therapy can completely restore brain function in a significant number of patients with stroke. Further information on the pharmacology of the thrombolytics can be found in Chapter 20 ∞.

NATURAL THERAPIES

Ginseng and Cardiovascular Disease

Ginseng is one of the oldest known herbal remedies. *Panax ginseng* is distributed throughout China, Korea, and Siberia, whereas *Panax quinquefolius* is native to Canada and the United States. American ginseng is not considered equivalent to Siberian ginseng.

Ginseng has been used for centuries to promote general wellness, boost immune function, and reduce fatigue. There are some claims that the herb lowers blood glucose and can help in the management of hypertension.

Ginseng is thought to have calcium channel blocking actions. The herb appears to improve blood flow to the heart in times of low oxygen supply, such as with myocardial ischemia. Some research has shown that ginseng lowers blood sugar levels in patients with type 2 diabetes. In addition, some studies have found ginseng to boost the immune system. The health care provider should caution patients who take ginseng, because herb–drug interactions are possible with CCBs, oral hypoglycemics, warfarin, and loop diuretics.

Fast Facts Cerebrovascular Accident

- CVA is the third leading cause of death, behind heart disease and cancer.
- The incidence (per 1000 population) of CVA increases with age, although 25% of all CVAs occur in people younger than age 65:

  14% of those 65–74 years old have had a CVA

  25% of those 75–84 years old have had a CVA

  28% of those older than age 85 have had a CVA
- The highest incidence of CVA is in Black men—more than double that of white women.
- CVA occurs more frequently in men than in women, although females account for about 60% of all deaths due to CVAs.
- Over 160,000 Americans die of CVAs each year.

PATIENTS NEED TO KNOW

Patients treated for chest pain need to know the following:

Regarding Antianginals

1. Dissolve one nitroglycerin tablet under the tongue as soon as anginal pain is felt. If pain is not relieved in 5 minutes, use another. Many practitioners recommend a third nitroglycerin tablet for pain not relieved 5 minutes after the second dose. If chest pain/pressure is not relieved by three doses of nitroglycerin, call emergency medical services.
2. Rotate the application site of transdermal patches, and do not apply a new patch until after the old patch has been removed.
3. Change positions slowly. Postural hypotension may cause dizziness and even fainting.
4. Monitor blood pressure regularly, and report any consistent changes to a health care provider.

Regarding Drugs for MI or CVA

5. A variety of drugs are used in the treatment of MI and CVA. It is important to understand and comply with the drug therapy regimen prescribed by the health care provider.

CHAPTER REVIEW

CORE CONCEPTS SUMMARY

21.1 Coronary heart disease is caused by a restriction in blood flow to the myocardium.

The high metabolic rate of the heart requires that a continuous supply of oxygen be maintained in the coronary arteries. Restriction of flow can lead to angina pectoris or MI. Because both of these disorders can cause severe chest pain, the health care provider must quickly determine the cause of the pain, so that the appropriate treatment may be administered.

21.2 Angina pectoris is characterized by severe chest pain caused by lack of sufficient oxygen flow to heart muscle.

The coronary arteries can become partially occluded with plaque, resulting in ischemia. Lack of sufficient oxygen to the myocardium upon emotional or physical exertion causes sharp chest pain, the characteristic symptom of angina.

21.3 Anginal pain can often be controlled through positive lifestyle changes and surgical procedures.

A number of lifestyle changes can reduce the deposition of plaque in the coronary arteries and help prevent coronary heart disease. These include stopping tobacco use, limiting alcohol consumption, and getting adequate exercise. Surgical procedures may be necessary to control severe angina.

21.4 The pharmacologic management of angina is achieved by reducing cardiac workload.

Reducing the workload on the heart can relieve anginal pain. This can be accomplished by slowing the heart rate, dilating the vessels, reducing the force of myocardial contraction, or reducing blood pressure.

21.5 The organic nitrates relieve anginal pain by dilating veins and the coronary arteries.

Fast-acting organic nitrates can quickly terminate anginal pain by causing venodilation, which reduces the workload on the heart. They also dilate the coronary arteries, bringing more oxygen to the myocardium. Long-acting nitrates can prevent acute angina episodes, but the patient may become tolerant to their protective effect.

21.6 Beta-adrenergic blockers are sometimes preferred drugs for reducing the frequency of angina attacks.

Beta blockers lower blood pressure, slow the heart rate, and reduce the force of contraction, thus reducing the workload on the myocardium. They are prescribed to reduce the frequency of acute anginal episodes.

21.7 Calcium channel blockers relieve anginal pain by reducing the cardiac workload.

CCBs are effective at lowering blood pressure, thus reducing the workload on the heart. They are prescribed to reduce the frequency of acute anginal attacks.

21.8 The early diagnosis and treatment of myocardial infarction (MI) increases chances of survival.

Myocardial infarction is caused by a thrombus in a coronary artery and is responsible for a substantial number of sudden deaths. Fast, effective diagnosis and treatment can reduce mortality.

21.9 Thrombolytics dissolve clots blocking the coronary arteries.

When used within hours of the onset of an MI, thrombolytics can dissolve clots and restore circulation to the myocardium.

21.10 Drugs are used to treat the symptoms and complications of acute MI.

Beta blockers can slow the heart rate and reduce blood pressure and have been shown to reduce mortality when given soon after MI symptoms appear. Aspirin and ACE inhibitors have been shown to reduce mortality when given soon after the onset of MI. Narcotic analgesics are sometimes given to reduce the pain and anxiety associated with an MI.

21.11 Aggressive treatment of cerebrovascular accident (CVA) can increase survival.

CVA is now viewed as an emergency condition requiring immediate treatment to improve survival. Thrombolytics, when given quickly after the onset of stroke, can restore some or all brain function. Some degree of stroke prevention can be achieved by using anticoagulants and by controlling blood pressure.

REVIEW QUESTIONS

The following questions are written in NCLEX-PN® style. Answer these questions to assess your knowledge of the chapter material, and go back and review any material that is not clear to you.

1. The patient is being discharged with nitroglycerin (Nitrostat). Patient education would include:
1. "Swallow 3 tablets immediately for pain and call 911."
2. "Put 1 tablet under your tongue for chest pain."
3. "Call your physician when you have chest pain. The physician will tell you how many tablets to take."
4. "Place 3 tablets under your tongue and call 911."

2. The most common adverse effect of nitroglycerin is:
1. Headache
2. Hypertension
3. Diuresis
4. Bradycardia

3. This class of medications decreases heart rate, contractility, and blood pressure, and is used to increase survival rates in post-MI patients.
1. Calcium channel blockers
2. Beta blockers
3. Vasodilators
4. Diuretics

4. The nurse assesses for the most common adverse effect of reteplase (Retavase), which is:
1. Dehydration
2. Bleeding
3. Confusion
4. Increased clotting times

5. The health care provider should be vigilant in observing for which of the following adverse effects during a reteplase infusion?
1. An increase in blood pressure
2. An increase in heart rate
3. Abnormal bleeding
4. Vomiting or diarrhea

6. The patient has a history of CVA. Which of the following drugs would not be recommended for this patient?
1. Aspirin
2. Warfarin (Coumadin)
3. Protamine sulfate
4. Ticlopidine (Ticlid)

7. The patient should remove the transdermal nitroglycerin patch at night to:
1. Prevent overdose
2. Prevent adverse reactions
3. Ensure the dosage is appropriate
4. Delay development of tolerance

8. When treating angina, the nurse knows that the mechanism of action of a beta-adrenergic blocker is:
1. Slowed heart rate and decreased contractility of the heart
2. Relaxation of arterial and venous smooth muscle
3. Increased contractility and heart rate
4. Decreased peripheral resistance

9. The patient taking calcium channel blockers should use extreme caution when taking which of the following medications?

1. Acetaminophen (Tylenol)
2. Ibuprofen (Motrin)
3. Digoxin (Lanoxin)
4. Ranitidine (Zantac)

10. The patient is complaining of a viselike pain in his chest that subsides with rest. The patient is likely experiencing:

1. A stroke
2. A myocardial infarction
3. Angina
4. A cerebral vascular accident

CASE STUDY QUESTIONS

For questions 1–4, please refer to the following case study, and choose the correct answer from choices 1–4.

*M*s. Liu arrives in your office with a complaint of chest pain when she exercises. Subsequent tests show a 10% occlusion of two coronary arteries. Her blood pressure is 125/78 mmHg. The physician prescribes one aspirin per day, sublingual nitroglycerin, and metoprolol.

1. The purpose of the nitroglycerin is to:

1. Prevent acute anginal attacks
2. End an angina attack in progress
3. Prevent MI or stroke
4. Relieve chest pain

2. What instructions should be given for the nitroglycerin?

1. Take before exercising.
2. Take on first indication of chest pain.

3. Take three or four times per day to prevent chest pain.
4. Take before bedtime and when rising.

3. The purpose of the metoprolol is to:

1. Prevent acute anginal attacks
2. End an angina attack in progress
3. Prevent MI or stroke
4. Lower blood pressure

Ms. Liu discontinues her drugs without notifying her physician. Three months later, she arrives in the ED with a possible stroke. Her blood pressure is 186/100 mmHg. The physician orders a reteplase infusion.

4. The function of the reteplase is to:

1. Dissolve existing blood clots
2. Prevent possible formation of blood clots
3. Stabilize blood pressure
4. Reduce workload on the heart

FURTHER STUDY

- The role of long-acting nitrates for treating heart failure is covered in Chapter 18 ⊙ .

- Several chapters include information on beta-adrenergic blockers: Chapter 8 ⊙ discusses their pharmacology; Chapter 17 ⊙ , their use in hypertension; Chapter 18 ⊙ , their use in heart failure; Chapter 19 ⊙ , their use for dysrhythmias.

- Additional information on the use of calcium channel blockers is found in Chapter 17 ⊙ (hypertension) and Chapter 19 ⊙ (dysrhythmias).

- Chapter 20 ⊙ includes information on the basic pharmacology, dosages, and descriptions of thrombolytics, coagulation modifiers, and antiplatelet agents.

- For more information on aspirin, see Chapter 14 ⊙ .

- Chapter 17 ⊙ presents the pharmacology of ACE inhibitors, and Chapter 14 ⊙ provides more information on the opioids.

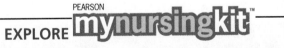

EXPLORE **PEARSON mynursingkit**™

22 Drugs for Shock and Anaphylaxis

CORE CONCEPTS

22.1 Shock is a syndrome characterized by collapse of the circulatory system.

22.2 The initial treatment of shock includes basic life support and identification of the underlying cause.

22.3 Fluid replacement infusions are given to replace fluids lost during shock.

22.4 Vasoconstrictors are administered during shock to maintain blood pressure.

22.5 Inotropic drugs are useful in reversing the decreased cardiac output that occurs during shock.

22.6 Anaphylaxis is a type of shock caused by a hyperresponse of body defense mechanisms.

DRUG SNAPSHOT

The following drugs are discussed in this chapter:

DRUG CLASSES	DRUG PROFILES
Fluid replacement drugs	**Pr** normal serum albumin (Albuminar, Plasbumin, others)
Vasoconstrictors	**Pr** norepinephrine (Levophed)
Inotropic drugs	**Pr** dopamine (Dopastat, Intropin)

LEARNING OUTCOMES

After reading this chapter, the student should be able to:

1. Compare and contrast the different types of shock.
2. Relate the general symptoms of shock to their physiologic causes.
3. Explain the initial treatment of a patient with shock.
4. Compare and contrast the use of blood products, colloids, and crystalloids in the pharmacotherapy of shock.
5. Identify indications for the use of vasoconstrictors and inotropic drugs.
6. For each of the classes in the Drug Snapshot, identify representative drugs and explain their mechanisms of action, primary actions, and important adverse effects.

KEY TERMS

anaphylaxis (ann-ah-fuh-LAK-sis) 355

antigen (ANN-tuh-jen) 362

cardiogenic shock (kar-dee-oh-JEN-ik) 355

colloids (KO-loyds) 359

crystalloids (KRIS-tuh-loyds) 359

hypovolemic shock (high-poh-voh-LEEM-ik) 355

inotropic drug (eye-noh-TROW-pik) 360

neurogenic shock (nyoor-oh-JEN-ik) 355

septic shock (SEP-tik) 355

shock 355

S hock is a condition in which vital organs are not receiving enough blood to function properly. Without adequate oxygen and other nutrients, cells cannot carry on normal metabolism. Shock is a medical emergency; failure to reverse the causes and symptoms of shock may lead to irreversible organ damage and death. This chapter examines how drugs are used to aid in the treatment of different types of shock.

Shock is a syndrome characterized by collapse of the circulatory system.

There are several types of shock, each having different causes. A simple method for classifying shock is by naming the underlying pathologic process or organ system causing the disease. Table 22.1 describes the different types of shock and their primary causes. This chapter focuses on the pharmacologic therapy of three common types of shock: hypovolemic, cardiogenic, and anaphylactic.

Shock is a collection of signs and symptoms, many of which are nonspecific. Although symptoms vary among the different kinds of shock, there are some similarities. The patient may appear pale and claim to feel sick or weak without reporting any specific symptoms. Behavioral changes are often some of the earliest symptoms and may include restlessness, anxiety, confusion, depression, and lack of interest. Thirst is a common complaint. The skin may feel cold or clammy.

Assessing the patient's cardiovascular status may provide important clues for a diagnosis of shock. Blood pressure is usually low, with a diminished cardiac output. Heart rate may be rapid, with a weak pulse. Breathing is rapid and shallow. Figure 22.1 ■ illustrates some of the common symptoms of a patient in shock.

Diagnosis of shock is rarely based on such nonspecific symptoms. A careful medical history, however, will provide the health care provider with valuable clues as to what type of shock may be present. For example, obvious trauma or bleeding combined with the symptoms mentioned previously would suggest **hypovolemic shock.** If trauma to the brain or spinal cord is evident, **neurogenic shock** may be suspected. A history of heart disease would suggest **cardiogenic shock,** whereas a recent infection may indicate **septic shock.** A history of allergy with a sudden onset of symptoms following food or drug intake may suggest **anaphylaxis.**

hypo = *below*
vol = *volume*
emic = *pertaining to the blood*

neuro = *nervous system*
genic = *origin*

The heart and brain are affected early in the progression of shock. Lack of blood to the brain may result in fainting, whereas disruption of blood supply to the myocardium may cause permanent damage to the heart. Immediate treatment is necessary to prevent failure of other organ systems, including respiratory collapse or renal failure.

cardio = *heart*
genic = *origin*

The initial treatment of shock includes basic life support and identification of the underlying cause.

Acute shock is treated as a medical emergency, and the first goal is to provide basic life support. Rapid identification of the underlying cause is essential because the patient's condition

TABLE 22.1	Classification of Shock	
TYPE OF SHOCK	**DEFINITION**	**UNDERLYING PATHOLOGY**
Anaphylactic	Acute allergic reaction	Severe reaction to allergens such as penicillin, nuts, shellfish, or animal proteins
Cardiogenic	Failure of the heart to pump sufficient blood to tissues	Left heart failure, myocardial ischemia, MI, dysrhythmias, pulmonary embolism, and myocardial or pericardial infection
Hypovolemic	Loss of blood volume	Hemorrhage, burns, profuse sweating, excessive urination, vomiting, or diarrhea
Neurogenic	Vasodilation due to overstimulation of the parasympathetic nervous system or understimulation of the sympathetic nervous system	Trauma to the spinal cord or medulla, severe emotional stress or pain, drugs that depress the central nervous system
Septic	Multiple organ dysfunction as a result of pathogenic organisms in the blood	Widespread inflammatory response to bacterial, fungal, or parasitic infection

FIGURE 22.1

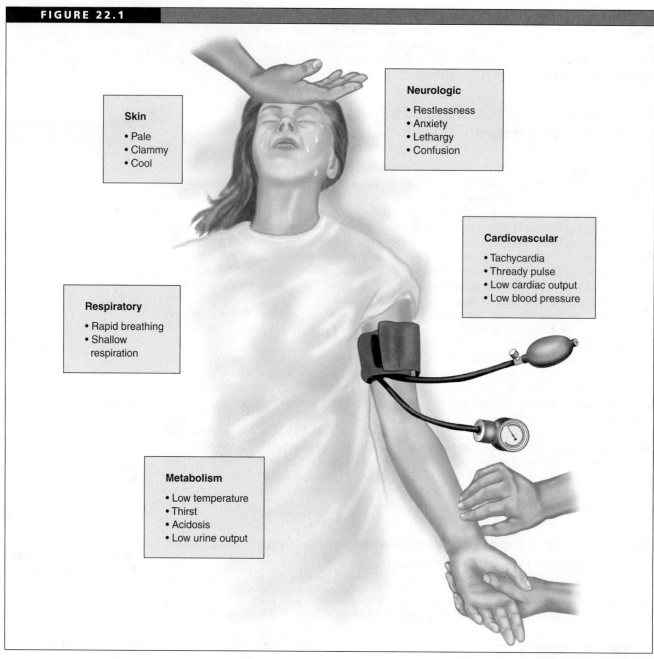

Symptoms of a patient in shock

Fast Facts Shock

- Cardiogenic shock occurs in about 10% of the patients suffering from an acute myocardial infarction (MI).
- Cardiogenic shock is the leading cause of death in patients hospitalized with acute MI, with a mortality rate of 70–80%.
- The mortality rate for patients with sepsis who develop septic shock is 40–70%.
- Incidence of anaphylaxis may be twice as high in women as in men.
- Of the U.S. population, 0.4–0.8% experiences anaphylaxis from insect stings, resulting in approximately 250 deaths per year.

FIGURE 22.2

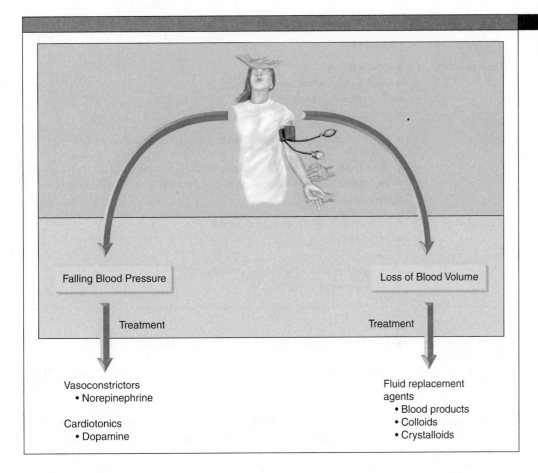

Physiologic changes occurring during shock and their pharmacologic interventions

may deteriorate rapidly without specific, emergency measures. Keeping the patient quiet and warm until specific therapy can be initiated is important. Maintaining the ABCs of life support—airway, breathing, and circulation—is critical. Once basic life support is established, the health care provider can begin more specific treatment of the underlying causes of the shock.

The remaining therapies for shock depend on the specific cause of the condition. The two primary pharmacotherapeutic goals are to restore normal fluid volume and composition and to maintain adequate blood pressure. For anaphylaxis, an additional therapeutic goal is to prevent or stop the hypersensitive inflammatory response. Unless contraindicated, oxygen is administered. Specific pharmacotherapies are illustrated in Figure 22.2 ■.

Concept Review 22.1

■ What signs or symptoms might help a paramedic arriving on the scene of a motorcycle accident determine the cause of the patient's shock?

Fluid replacement infusions are given to replace fluids lost during shock.

CORE CONCEPT 22.3

When a patient loses significant amounts of blood or other body fluids, immediate treatment with fluid replacement drugs is essential. Fluid loss can occur due to hemorrhage, extensive burns, severe dehydration, persistent vomiting or diarrhea, or intensive diuretic therapy. Fluid loss can lead to dehydration and death if the fluid imbalance is not corrected. Fluid replacement drugs are sometimes referred to as *fluid expanders*.

The immediate goal in treating fluid deficiencies is to replace the missing fluid. In mild cases, this may be accomplished by drinking extra water or beverages containing electrolytes. In acute situations, therapy with IV infusions can immediately replace lost fluids. Regardless of how fluids

TABLE 22.2	Fluid Replacement Drugs
AGENT	**EXAMPLES**
Blood products	■ Whole blood ■ Plasma protein fraction ■ Fresh frozen plasma ■ Packed red blood cells
Colloids	■ Plasma protein fraction (Plasmanate, Plasma-Plex, Plasmatein, PPF, Protenate) ■ Normal serum albumin (Albuminar, Plasbumin, others) ■ Dextran 40 (Gentran 40, Hyskon, Rheomacrodex) or dextran 70 (Macrodex) ■ Hetastarch (Hespan)
Crystalloids	■ Normal saline (0.9% sodium chloride) ■ Lactated Ringer's ■ Plasmalyte ■ Hypertonic saline (3% sodium chloride) ■ 5% dextrose in water (D₅W)

are administered, careful attention must be paid to restoring normal levels of electrolytes as well as fluid volume.

Fluid replacement agents may be categorized as blood products, colloids, or crystalloids. Colloid and crystalloid infusions are often used when up to one third of an adult's blood volume is lost. Examples of fluid replacement drugs are listed in Table 22.2.

Blood products. Whole blood may be used for the treatment of acute, massive blood loss when there is the need to replace plasma volume and supply red blood cells. The supply of blood products, however, depends on human donors and requires careful cross-matching to ensure compatibility between the donor and patient. Furthermore, the use of whole blood has the potential to transmit serious infections such as hepatitis or HIV. The administration of whole blood has been largely replaced with the use of specific blood components, colloids, and crystalloids.

DRUG PROFILE: Ⓟ *Normal Serum Albumin (Albuminar, Plasbumin, Others)*

Therapeutic Class: Fluid replacement agent
Pharmacologic Class: Blood product, colloid

Actions and Uses:

Normal serum albumin is a protein extracted from whole blood or plasma. Albumin naturally comprises about 60% of all blood proteins. Its normal functions are to maintain plasma osmotic pressure and to shuttle certain substances through the blood, including a substantial number of drug molecules. After extraction from blood or plasma, albumin is sterilized to remove possible contamination by the hepatitis viruses or HIV.

Administered IV, albumin is used to restore plasma volume during hypovolemic shock or to restore blood proteins in patients with hypoproteinemia. It has an immediate onset of action and is available in concentrations of 5% and 25%.

Adverse Effects and Interactions:

Because albumin is a natural blood product, the patient may have antibodies to the donor's albumin, and allergic reactions are possible. Signs of allergy include fever, chills, rash, dyspnea, and possibly hypotension. Protein overload may occur if excessive albumin is infused.

No clinically significant drug interactions have been identified.

See the Nursing Process Focus in Chapter 28 ⊕ for "Patients Receiving Fluid Replacement Agents."
Refer to MyNursingKit for a Nursing Process Focus specific to this drug.

A single unit of whole blood can be separated into its specific constituents (red and white blood cells, platelets, plasma proteins, fresh frozen plasma, and globulins). This allows a single blood donation to be used to treat more than one patient.

Colloids. **Colloids** are proteins or other large molecules that stay suspended in the blood for a long period and draw water molecules from the body's cells and tissues into the blood vessels. Colloids include normal human serum albumin, dextran, and hetastarch (Hespan).

Crystalloids. **Crystalloids** are IV solutions that contain electrolytes in amounts resembling those of natural plasma. Unlike colloids, crystalloid solutions leave the blood and enter cells. They are used to replace fluids that have been lost and to increase urine output. Common crystalloids include normal saline, lactated Ringer's, hypertonic saline, and 5% dextrose in water (D_5W).

NURSING PROCESS FOCUS

Patients Receiving Fluid Replacement Therapy

ASSESSMENT

Prior to administration:
- Obtain a complete health history (physical/mental), including allergies, drug history, and possible drug interactions
- Assess lung sounds and vital signs
- Assess level of consciousness
- Assess renal function (blood urea nitrogen [BUN] and creatinine)

POTENTIAL NURSING DIAGNOSES

- Risk for Injury related to allergic reaction to drug.
- Ineffective Tissue Perfusion related to adverse effects of drug.
- Excess Fluid Volume related to increased intravascular volume.
- Deficient Knowledge related to information about drug therapy.

PLANNING: PATIENT GOALS AND EXPECTED OUTCOMES

The patient will:
- Maintain urinary output of at least 50 ml/hr and maintain a systolic blood pressure greater than 90 mmHg
- Demonstrate an understanding of the drug's action by accurately describing adverse effects and precautions
- Immediately report any signs of allergic reactions such as difficulty breathing, itching, and flushing

IMPLEMENTATION

Interventions and (Rationales)	Patient Education/Discharge Planning
■ Monitor respiratory status. (Effects of drugs and rapid infusion may result in fluid overload.)	Instruct the patient to: ■ Report any signs of respiratory distress ■ Report changes in sensorium such as lightheadedness, drowsiness, or dizziness
■ Monitor fluid intake and output for changes in renal function. (Renal function changes with an increase or decrease in fluid volume. A decrease is seen with shock.)	■ Instruct the patient concerning the rationale for monitoring fluid intake and output and possible Foley catheter insertion.
■ Monitor electrolytes. (Crystalloid drugs may cause hypernatremia and the resulting fluid retention.)	■ Instruct the patient to report any evidence of edema or weight gain.
■ Observe the patient for signs of allergic reactions. (Administration of blood and blood products could cause allergic reactions.)	Instruct the patient: ■ To report itching, rash, chills, and difficulty breathing ■ That frequent blood draws are necessary to monitor possible complications of drug administration
■ Observe urine for changes in color. (Adverse reaction to blood could cause hematuria.)	■ Instruct the patient to notify the health care provider if changes in urine color occur.

EVALUATION OF OUTCOME CRITERIA

Evaluate the effectiveness of drug therapy by confirming that patient goals and expected outcomes have been met (see "Planning").

CORE CONCEPT 22.4

Vasoconstrictors are administered during shock to maintain blood pressure.

In the early stages of shock, the body compensates for the initial fall in blood pressure by activating the sympathetic nervous system. This sympathetic activity causes vasoconstriction, which raises blood pressure and increases the heart rate and force of myocardial contractions. These compensatory measures help to maintain blood flow to vital organs such as the heart and brain and to decrease flow to "less essential" organs such as the kidneys and liver.

The body's ability to compensate is limited, however, and profound hypotension may develop as shock progresses. In severe cases vasoconstrictors, also called vasopressors, may be needed to help stabilize blood pressure. Because of the potential for serious adverse effects and potential organ damage due to the rapid and intense vasoconstriction, vasopressors are used only after fluid infusions have failed to raise blood pressure. Patients receiving these agents must be monitored continuously during the infusion to avoid hypertension.

Vasoconstrictors used to treat shock include dopamine (Dopastat, Intropin), norepinephrine (Levophed), phenylephrine (Neo-Synephrine), and epinephrine. Because dopamine also affects the strength of myocardial contraction, it is considered both a vasopressor and an inotropic agent (see Section 22.5). Epinephrine is usually associated with the treatment of anaphylaxis (Section 22.6). The basic pharmacology of the sympathomimetic drugs is presented in Chapter 8 ⬭. Table 22.3 gives the dosages for these agents.

CORE CONCEPT 22.5

Inotropic drugs are useful in reversing the decreased cardiac output that occurs during shock.

As shock progresses, the heart begins to fail and cardiac output declines. This lowers the amount of blood reaching vital tissues and deepens the degree of shock. **Inotropic drugs,** also called cardiotonic drugs, have the potential to reverse the cardiac symptoms of shock by increasing the force of myocardial contraction. The role of the cardiotonic drug digoxin (Lanoxin) in treating patients with heart failure was presented in Chapter 18 ⬭. Digoxin increases myocardial contractility and cardiac output, thus rapidly bringing tissues their needed oxygen. Chapter 18 ⬭ should be reviewed because drugs prescribed for heart failure are sometimes used for the treatment of shock.

Dopamine is often a drug of choice for increasing cardiac output in acute situations because it has both inotropic and vasoconstriction actions. Dobutamine (Dobutrex) is a beta$_1$-adrenergic agent that has value in the short-term treatment of certain types of shock because of its ability to

TABLE 22.3	Vasoconstrictors and Inotropic Drugs for Shock	
DRUG	**RATE AND ADULT DOSE**	**REMARKS**
digoxin (Lanoxin, Lanoxicaps) (see page 299 for the Drug Profile box)	IV; digitalizing dose 2.5–5 mcg every 6 hours for 24 hr; maintenance dose 0.125–0.5 mg/day	Doses are highly individualized for each patient; oral forms available; also for dysrhythmias and heart failure
dobutamine (Dobutrex)	IV infused at a rate of 2.5–40 mcg/kg/min for a max of 72 hr	Selective to beta$_1$-adrenergic receptors; for cardiac decompensation
Pr dopamine (Dopastat, Intropin)	IV; 2–5 mcg/kg/min initial dose; may be increased to 20–50 mcg/kg/min	May activate dopaminergic, beta$_1$- or alpha$_1$-adrenergic receptors, depending on dose
Pr epinephrine (Adrenalin)	Subcutaneous 0.1–0.5 ml of 1:100 every 10–15 min; IV 0.1–0.25 ml of 1:1000 every 10–15 min	Nonselective adrenergic drug; available by other routes for cardiac arrest and asthma and as an adjunct to local anesthesia
Pr norepinephrine (Levophed)	IV; Initial 0.5–1 mcg/min, titrate to response; usual range 8–30 mcg/min	Activates alpha- and beta$_1$-adrenergic receptors; also for cardiac arrest
phenylephrine (Neo-Synephrines) (see page 104 for the Drug Profile box)	IV 0.1–0.18 mg/min until pressure stabilizes, then 0.04–0.06 mg/min for maintenance	Selective to alpha$_1$-receptors; used to maintain blood pressure during general anesthesia; also for certain dysrhythmias, nasal congestion, and glaucoma, and to dilate the pupil during eye exams; subcutaneous, IM, ophthalmic, and intranasal forms available

DRUG PROFILE: ℗ *Norepinephrine (Levophed)*

Therapeutic Class: Drug for shock
Pharmacologic Class: Sympathomimetic, vasoconstrictor

Actions and Uses:

Norepinephrine acts directly on alpha-adrenergic receptors in the smooth muscle of blood vessels to immediately raise blood pressure. Its stimulation of beta$_1$-receptors in the heart increases the force of contraction and increases cardiac output. It is given by the IV route and has a duration of only 1 to 2 minutes after the infusion is terminated.

Adverse Effects and Interactions:

Norepinephrine is a powerful vasoconstrictor; thus, continuous monitoring of blood pressure is required to prevent the development of hypertension. When first administered, reflex bradycardia is sometimes experienced. It also has the ability to produce various types of dysrhythmias. Because of its potent effects on the cardiovascular system, it should be used with great caution in patients with heart disease. If extravasation occurs, the drug may cause serious skin and soft tissue injury.

Norepinephrine interacts with many drugs, including alpha and beta blockers, which may decrease the drug's effects on blood pressure. Conversely, ergot alkaloids and tricyclic antidepressants may increase vasopressor effects. Halothane and cyclopropane may increase the risk of dysrhythmias.

Refer to MyNursingKit for a Nursing Process Focus specific to this drug.

DRUG PROFILE: ℗ *Dopamine (Dopastat, Intropin)*

Therapeutic Class: Drug for shock
Pharmacologic Class: Nonselective adrenergic agonist, inotropic agent

Actions and Uses:

Dopamine is the immediate metabolic precursor to norepinephrine. Although classified as a sympathomimetic, the mechanism of dopamine's action is dependent on the dose. At low doses, dopamine selectively increases blood flow through the kidneys. This makes dopamine of particular value in treating hypovolemic and cardiogenic shock. At higher doses, dopamine stimulates beta$_1$-adrenergic receptors, causing the heart to beat with more force and increasing cardiac output. Another beneficial effect of dopamine when given in higher doses is its ability to stimulate alpha-adrenergic receptors, thus causing vasoconstriction and raising blood pressure.

Adverse Effects and Interactions:

Because of its intense effects on the cardiovascular system, patients receiving dopamine are continuously monitored for signs of dysrhythmias and hypotension. Adverse effects are normally self-limiting because of the short half-life of the drug.

Dopamine interacts with many other drugs. For example, administering it with monoamine oxidase (MAO) inhibitors and ergot alkaloids increases alpha-adrenergic effects. Phenytoin may decrease dopamine action. Beta blockers may block the cardiac effects of dopamine. Alpha blockers decrease peripheral vasoconstriction. Halothane increases the risk of hypertension and ventricular dysrhythmias.

Mechanism in Action:

Dopamine is a naturally occurring neurotransmitter that relieves symptoms of heart failure or shock by increasing the force of cardiac contraction. This is accomplished through activation of beta$_1$-adrenergic receptors and an influx of calcium into myocardial cells.

Refer to MyNursingKit for a Nursing Process Focus specific to this drug.

cause the heart to beat more forcefully without significantly increasing heart rate. The resulting increase in cardiac output assists in maintaining blood flow to vital organs. Although very effective, dobutamine has a half-life of only 2 minutes, and therapy is limited to 72 hours.

Anaphylaxis is a type of shock caused by a hyperresponse of body defense mechanisms.

an = *without or against*
phylaxis = *protection*

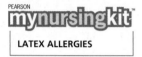

LATEX ALLERGIES

Anaphylaxis is a condition in which the natural body defenses produce a hyperresponse to an antigen. An **antigen** may be defined as anything that is recognized as foreign by the body. Certain foods, industrial chemicals, drugs, pollen, animal proteins, and even latex gloves can be antigens. A more detailed discussion of the immune system and the pharmacotherapy of immune disorders is included in Chapter 24 ⬭.

Following exposure to an antigen, the body responds with actions such as inflammation, antibody production, and activation of lymphocytes that rid the body of the foreign agent. During anaphylaxis, however, the body responds quickly—usually within minutes after exposure to the antigen—by releasing massive amounts of histamine and other inflammatory mediators. The patient may experience itching, hives, and a tightness in the throat or chest. Swelling occurs around the larynx, causing a hoarse voice and a nonproductive cough. As anaphylaxis progresses, the patient experiences a rapid fall in blood pressure and difficulty breathing due to bronchoconstriction. The fall in blood pressure causes *reflex tachycardia*, a rebound speeding up of the heart. Untreated anaphylactic shock may result in death. Figure 22.3 ■ illustrates the signs and symptoms of anaphylaxis.

It is always easier to *prevent* anaphylaxis than it is to *treat* it. Patients should be strongly advised to avoid substances that might trigger acute allergic reactions. This includes carefully reading all food and cosmetic labels to avoid exposure to known allergens. Individuals with known allergies to insect stings or food should carry a portable form of epinephrine, such as an EpiPen. The health care provider should always obtain a comprehensive drug allergy history before administering medications. Common allergens include the penicillin antibiotics and iodine-based contrast media used for radiologic exams. The patient should be observed in the outpatient setting for 20 to 60 minutes after a drug injection because delayed anaphylactic reactions are possible.

DRUG PROFILE: ℗ *Epinephrine (Adrenalin)*
Therapeutic Class: Drug for anaphylaxis and shock
Pharmacologic Class: Sympathomimetic, vasoconstrictor

Actions and Uses:

Subcutaneous or IV epinephrine is a drug of choice for acute anaphylactic shock because it can reverse many of the distressing symptoms within minutes. Epinephrine is nonselective and activates both alpha- and beta-adrenergic receptors. Almost immediately after injection, blood pressure rises due to stimulation of alpha$_1$-receptors. Activation of beta$_2$-receptors in the bronchi opens the airways to relieve shortness of breath. Cardiac output increases due to stimulation of beta$_1$-receptors in the heart. Epinephrine can also be administered topically, by inhalation, or by the intracardiac route.

Adverse Effects and Interactions:

The most common adverse effects of epinephrine are nervousness, tremors, palpitations, dizziness, headache, and stinging/burning at the site of application. When administered parenterally, hypertension and dysrhythmias may occur rapidly; therefore, the patient is monitored continuously following IV or subcutaneous injections.

Epinephrine interacts with many drugs. For example, it may increase hypotension with phenothiazines and oxytocin. There may be additive toxicities with other sympathomimetics. MAO inhibitors, tricyclic antidepressants, and alpha- and beta-adrenergic agents inhibit the actions of epinephrine.

 Refer to MyNursingKit for a Nursing Process Focus specific to this drug.

FIGURE 22.3

Symptoms of
anaphylaxis

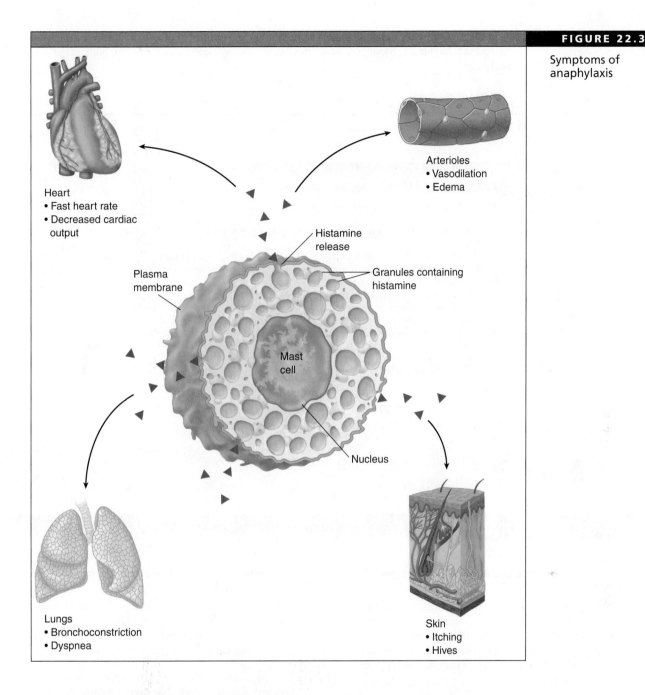

Heart
• Fast heart rate
• Decreased cardiac
  output

Arterioles
• Vasodilation
• Edema

Histamine
release

Plasma
membrane

Granules containing
histamine

Mast
cell

Nucleus

Lungs
• Bronchoconstriction
• Dyspnea

Skin
• Itching
• Hives

The pharmacotherapy of anaphylaxis is symptomatic and involves supporting the cardiovascular system and preventing further hyperresponse by body defenses. Various medications are used to treat the symptoms of anaphylaxis, depending on the severity of the symptoms.

At the first suspicion of anaphylaxis, epinephrine is administered and fluid infusions are begun. Epinephrine is an initial drug of choice because it causes vasoconstriction and can rapidly relieve symptoms of bronchoconstriction. It may be necessary to use other vasoconstrictors (see Table 22.3) to overcome severe hypotension. Infusion of large amounts of fluids may be needed to overcome circulatory shock. These may include blood products, colloids, or crystalloids. Fluid infusions continue until systolic blood pressure reaches at least 90 mmHg and is stable.

A number of other drugs are useful in treating symptoms of anaphylaxis. Oxygen is usually administered immediately. Antihistamines such as diphenhydramine (Benadryl) may be administered IM or IV to prevent additional release of histamine. A bronchodilator such as albuterol (Ventolin, Proventil) is sometimes administered by inhalation to relieve the acute shortness of breath caused by histamine release. Corticosteroids such as hydrocortisone may be administered to dampen the inflammatory response. Corticosteroids may be administered for 24 hours or longer to prevent the possibility of delayed anaphylactic reactions. Additional effects of antihistamines are discussed in Chapter 24, bronchodilators in Chapter 28, and corticosteroids in Chapter 31 ⚭, respectively.

| **Concept Review** | **22.2** |

■ How can cardiotonic drugs reduce the symptoms of shock without causing vasoconstriction?

PATIENTS NEED TO KNOW

Patients treated for shock need to know the following:

1. Seek emergency medical assistance immediately if signs or symptoms of shock are being experienced.
2. While waiting for medical assistance, keep warm by using blankets.
3. Have a caregiver, if present, monitor temperature, pulse, and blood pressure until emergency medical assistance arrives.
4. Do not move around. Lie down and elevate the feet.
5. Report any changes in mental status, such as depression, confusion, or anxiety, to the health care provider immediately.
6. If allergies to bee or wasp stings are known, carry medications such as an EpiPen for all outside activities. Inform others of any allergies, where medications are kept, and how to administer them.
7. Take medications for shock (such as epinephrine) exactly as prescribed.

CHAPTER REVIEW

CORE CONCEPTS SUMMARY

22.1 Shock is a syndrome characterized by collapse of the circulatory system.

Basic types of shock include cardiogenic, hypovolemic, neurogenic, septic, and anaphylactic shock. Nonspecific symptoms of shock include hypotension, cold or clammy skin, reduced cardiac output, and behavioral changes such as confusion, apathy, or disorientation.

22.2 The initial treatment of shock includes basic life support and identification of the underlying cause.

Shock may be life threatening if allowed to proceed without medical intervention. Immediate therapy is targeted at restoring or maintaining vital processes such as respiratory function, blood pressure, and cardiac output. Immediate drug therapy includes vasoconstrictors, cardiotonic agents, and fluid replacement agents.

22.3 Fluid replacement infusions are given to replace fluids lost during shock.

Fluid replacement agents include blood products, colloids, and crystalloids. These agents help to maintain circulation and raise blood pressure.

22.4 Vasoconstrictors are administered during shock to maintain blood pressure.

An immediate concern for the patient in shock is falling blood pressure. A variety of adrenergic agents, both selective and nonselective, are used to maintain blood pressure and cardiac function.

22.5 Inotropic drugs are useful in reversing the decreased cardiac output that occurs during shock.

Circulatory failure can occur during shock if the cardiac output falls below a critical level. A number of cardiotonic drugs are used to strengthen myocardial function and improve cardiac output.

22.6 Anaphylaxis is a type of shock caused by a hyperresponse of body defense mechanisms.

When the body mounts a hyperresponse to an antigen, anaphylactic shock may result. Epinephrine is a drug of choice for immediately reversing the cardiovascular symptoms. Fluid replacement agents, antihistamines, and corticosteroids also serve roles in treating this form of shock.

REVIEW QUESTIONS

The following questions are written in NCLEX-PN® style. Answer these questions to assess your knowledge of the chapter material, and go back and review any material that is not clear to you.

1. The patient with severe burns must be monitored for:

1. Cardiogenic shock
2. Hypovolemic shock
3. Septic shock
4. Anaphylactic shock

2. The most important intervention for a patient experiencing shock is assessing:

1. Temperature
2. Heart rate
3. Respirations rate
4. Blood pressure

3. Which IV solution would be most appropriate for a patient experiencing hypovolemic shock?

1. D$_5$ 0.45% NS
2. Normal serum albumin
3. 0.33% NS
4. Dextran

4. Which of the following is not correct regarding dopamine?

1. At low doses, dopamine causes increased blood flow to the kidneys.
2. At high doses, dopamine increases cardiac output.
3. Dopamine causes vasoconstriction and increases blood pressure.
4. At high doses, dopamine is used to treat anaphylaxis.

5. The patient is experiencing anaphylaxis. Which drug is used to increase blood pressure and treat bronchospasm related to anaphylaxis?

1. Epinephrine
2. Dobutamine (Dobutrex)
3. Digoxin (Lanoxin)
4. Dopamine

6. Which of the following medications is not used to treat anaphylaxis?

1. Antihistamines
2. Corticosteroids
3. Bronchodilators
4. Vasodilators

7. Use of cardiotonic agents in the treatment of shock:

1. Decreases cardiac output
2. Increases cardiac output
3. Slows the heart rate
4. Increases afterload

8. When using norepinephrine (Levophed):

1. Tachycardia may occur
2. Hypotension may occur
3. Hypertension may occur
4. Liver failure may occur

9. Dobutamine (Dobutrex) is used to treat shock because:

1. It increases myocardial contractility and heart rate
2. It increases myocardial contractility without increasing the heart rate
3. It decreases cardiac output
4. It is a powerful vasoconstrictor

10. When treating a patient with shock, it is important to:

1. Keep the patient cool
2. Keep the patient warm
3. Elevate the patient's head
4. Monitor renal failure

CASE STUDY QUESTIONS

For questions 1–4, please refer to the following case study, and choose the correct answer from choices 1–4.

Mr. Hanks arrives in the emergency department having lost a considerable amount of blood in an automobile accident. His blood pressure is 60/30 mmHg. His skin is clammy, and he is going in and out of consciousness. He is gasping for breath. The physician orders an infusion of D$_5$W, IV dobutamine, IM hydrocortisone, and subcutaneous epinephrine.

1. The health care provider notices that Mr. Hanks' breathing becomes less labored and he appears less anxious. Which drug most likely reduced Mr. Hanks' bronchospasm?

1. D$_5$W
2. Dobutamine
3. Hydrocortisone
4. Epinephrine

2. Which drug was given to replace the fluids lost during Mr. Hanks' accident?

1. D₅W
2. Dobutamine
3. Hydrocortisone
4. Epinephrine

3. Within 2 minutes, Mr. Hanks' blood pressure increases to 100/60 mmHg. Which drug most likely caused this effect?

1. D₅W
2. Dobutamine
3. Hydrocortisone
4. Epinephrine

4. After 4 hours, Mr. Hanks has stabilized, but he still has some difficulty breathing. Which of the following would most likely be prescribed for this symptom?

1. Diphenhydramine (Benadryl)
2. Hydrocortisone
3. Phenylephrine (Neo-Synephrine)
4. Albuterol (Ventolin)

FURTHER STUDY

- Chapter 8 ⊙⊙ discusses the basic pharmacology of the adrenergic agents, or sympathomimetics.

- Chapter 18 ⊙⊙ discusses the role of the cardiotonic drug digoxin (Lanoxin) in treating patients with heart failure.

- Fluid replacement agents are presented in greater detail in Chapter 23 ⊙⊙ .

- Chapter 24 ⊙⊙ provides a detailed discussion of the immune system and the pharmacology of immune disorders.

- See Chapter 28 ⊙⊙ for more information on antihistamines and bronchodilators; and Chapter 31 ⊙⊙ for corticosteroids.

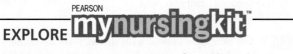

EXPLORE **PEARSON mynursingkit**™

MyNursingKit is your one stop for online chapter review materials and resources. Prepare for success with additional NCLEX®-style practice questions, interactive assignments and activities, web links, animations and videos, and more!

Register your access code from the front of your book at **www.mynursingkit.com**

23 Diuretics and Drugs for Electrolyte and Acid-Base Disorders

CORE CONCEPTS

23.1 The kidneys regulate fluid volume, electrolytes, acids, and bases.

23.2 The composition of filtrate changes dramatically as a result of the processes of reabsorption and secretion.

23.3 Renal failure significantly impacts pharmacotherapy.

23.4 Diuretics are used to treat hypertension, heart failure, and fluid retention disorders.

23.5 The most effective diuretics are those that affect the loop of Henle.

23.6 The thiazides are the most widely prescribed class of diuretics.

23.7 Although less effective than the loop diuretics, potassium-sparing diuretics may help prevent hypokalemia.

23.8 Several less commonly prescribed diuretics have specific indications.

23.9 Electrolytes are charged substances that play important roles in body chemistry.

23.10 Acidic and basic drugs can be administered to maintain normal body pH.

DRUG SNAPSHOT

The following drugs are discussed in this chapter:

DRUG CLASSES	DRUG PROFILES
Loop (high-ceiling) diuretics	
Thiazide diuretics	**Pr** chlorothiazide (Diuril)
Potassium-sparing diuretics	**Pr** spironolactone (Aldactone)
Miscellaneous diuretics	
Electrolytes	**Pr** potassium chloride (KCl)
Acid-base agents	**Pr** sodium bicarbonate (NaHCO$_3$

LEARNING OUTCOMES

After reading this chapter, the student should be able to:

1. Explain the role of the kidneys in maintaining fluid, electrolyte, and acid-base balance.

2. Compare and contrast the loop, thiazide, and potassium-sparing diuretics.

3. Explain the pharmacotherapy of sodium and potassium imbalances.

4. Identify common causes of alkalosis and acidosis and the drugs used to treat these conditions.

5. For each of the classes in the Drug Snapshot, identify representative drugs and explain their mechanisms of action, primary actions, and important adverse effects.

6. Categorize drugs used in the treatment of urinary system electrolyte and acid-base disorders based on their classifications and mechanisms of action.

KEY TERMS

acidosis (ah-sid-OH-sis) *379*

aldosterone (al-DOH-stair-own) *375*

alkalosis (al-kah-LOH-sis) *379*

carbonic anhydrase (kar-BON-ik an-HY-drase) *375*

diuretic (dye-your-ET-ik) *371*

electrolytes (ee-LEK-troh-lites) *377*

erythropoietin (ee-rith-ro-po-EE-tin) *371*

filtrate (FIL-trate) *368*

hyperkalemia (Heye-purr-kah-LEE-mee-ah) *374*

hypernatremia *378*

hypokalemia (heye-poh-kah-LEE-mee-uh) *372*

hyponatremia (hy-po-nay-TREE-mee-uh) *378*

hypernatremia *378*

nephron (NEF-ron) *368*

pH *379*

reabsorption *369*

renal failure *370*

secretion *369*

The volume and composition of fluids in the body must be maintained within narrow limits. Excess fluid volume can lead to hypertension or heart failure, whereas depletion may result in dehydration or shock. Body fluids must also contain specific amounts of essential ions or electrolytes and be maintained at specific pH values. The kidneys serve a remarkable role in keeping the volume and composition of body fluids within normal limits. This chapter examines diuretics and drugs used to reverse electrolyte and acid-base imbalances.

CORE CONCEPT 23.1   The kidneys regulate fluid volume, electrolytes, acids, and bases.

When most people think of the kidneys, they think of excretion. Although this is certainly one of their roles, the kidneys have many other essential functions. The kidneys are the primary organs for regulating fluid balance, electrolyte composition, and the acid-base balance of body fluids. They also secrete the enzyme renin, which helps to control blood pressure (see Chapter 17 ⬀), and erythropoietin, a hormone that stimulates red blood cell production. In addition, the kidneys are responsible for the production of calcitriol, the active form of vitamin D, which helps maintain bone homeostasis (see Chapter 33 ⬀). It is not surprising that the overall health of a patient is strongly dependent on proper functioning of the kidneys.

The urinary system consists of two kidneys, two ureters, a urinary bladder, and a urethra. These structures are shown in Figure 23.1 ■. Each kidney contains more than 2 million **nephrons**, the functional units of the kidney. As blood enters a nephron, it is filtered through a semipermeable membrane known as *Bowman's capsule*. Water and other small molecules readily pass through Bowman's capsule and enter the first section of the nephron, called the *proximal tubule*. Once in the nephron, the fluid is called **filtrate**. After leaving the proximal tubule, the filtrate travels through the *loop of Henle* and, subsequently, the *distal tubule*. Nephrons empty their filtrate into tubes called *common collecting ducts*, and then into larger and larger collecting structures inside the kidney. Fluid leaving the collecting ducts and entering subsequent portions of the kidney is called *urine*. The parts of the nephron are illustrated in Figure 23.2 ■.

Fast Facts Renal Disorders

- Although more than 17,000 kidney transplants are performed annually, more than 70,000 people are on a waiting list for kidney transplants.
- One out of every 750 people is born with a single kidney. A single kidney is larger and more vulnerable to injury from heavy contact sports.
- About 260,000 Americans suffer from chronic kidney failure, and 50,000 die annually from causes related to the disease.
- Type 2 diabetes is the leading cause of chronic kidney failure, accounting for 30–40% of all new cases each year.

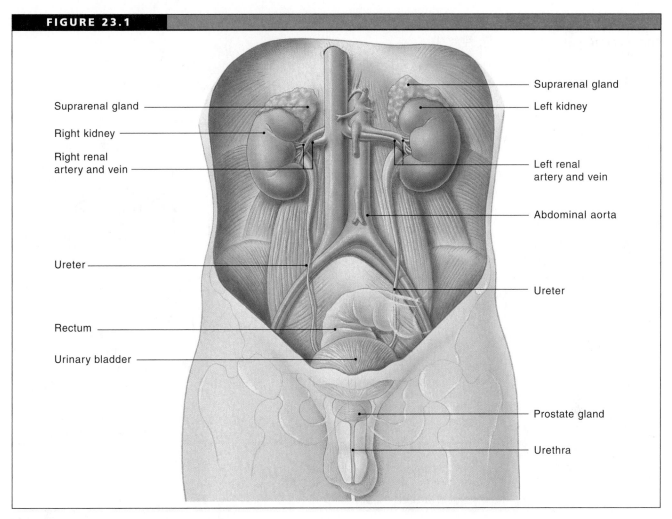

FIGURE 23.1

Suprarenal gland

Right kidney

Right renal
artery and vein

Ureter

Rectum

Urinary bladder

Suprarenal gland

Left kidney

Left renal
artery and vein

Abdominal aorta

Ureter

Prostate gland

Urethra

The urinary system   *Source: Pearson Education/PH College*

The composition of filtrate changes dramatically as a result of the processes of reabsorption and secretion.

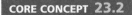

CORE CONCEPT 23.2

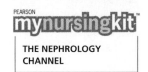

THE NEPHROLOGY CHANNEL

When filtrate enters Bowman's capsule, its composition is very similar to that of plasma. Plasma proteins such as albumin, however, are too large to pass through the filter and will not be present in the filtrate or in the urine of healthy patients. As filtrate travels through the nephron, its composition changes dramatically. Some substances in the filtrate cross the walls of the nephron to reenter the blood, a process known as **reabsorption**. Water is the most important molecule reabsorbed in the tubule. For every 180 liters (47 gallons) of water entering the filtrate each day, 178.5 liters (45.5 gallons) are reabsorbed, leaving only 1.5 liters to be excreted in the urine. Glucose, amino acids, and electrolytes such as sodium, chloride, calcium, and bicarbonate are also reabsorbed.

Certain ions and molecules too large to pass through Bowman's capsule can still enter the urine by crossing from the blood to the filtrate through a process known as tubular **secretion**. Potassium, phosphate, hydrogen, and ammonium ions enter the filtrate through secretion. Examples of drugs secreted in the proximal tubule include penicillin G, ampicillin, nonsteroidal anti-inflammatory drugs (NSAIDs), furosemide, epinephrine, and trimethoprim.

Reabsorption and secretion are critical to the pharmacokinetics of many drugs. Some drugs are reabsorbed, whereas others are secreted into the filtrate. For example, approximately 90% of a dose of penicillin G enters the urine through secretion. When the kidney is damaged, reabsorption and secretion mechanisms are impaired and serum drug levels may be dramatically affected. The processes of reabsorption and secretion are depicted in Figure 23.2.

FIGURE 23.2

The nephron

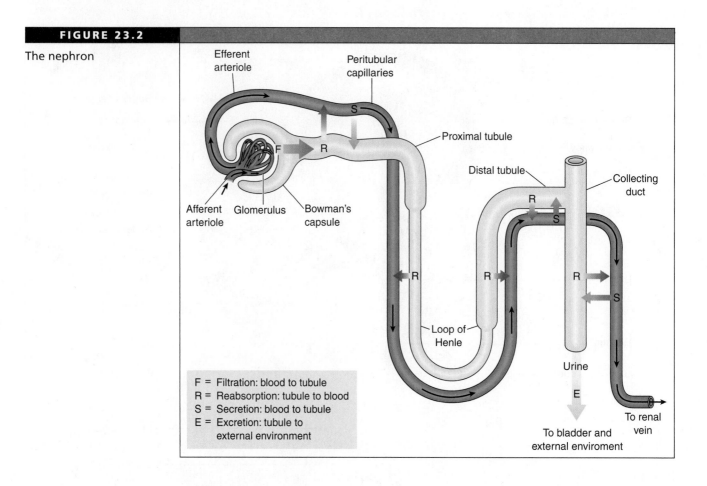

F = Filtration: blood to tubule
R = Reabsorption: tubule to blood
S = Secretion: blood to tubule
E = Excretion: tubule to external environment

Concept Review   23.1

■ How does the composition of filtrate differ from that of blood?

CORE CONCEPT 23.3

Renal failure significantly impacts pharmacotherapy.

Renal failure is a decrease in the kidneys' ability to maintain electrolyte and fluid balance and to excrete waste products. If renal excretion is impaired, drugs will accumulate to high concentrations in the blood and tissues, resulting in toxicity. Because the kidneys excrete most drugs, the majority of medications will require a significant dosage reduction in patients with moderate to severe renal failure. *The importance of this cannot be overemphasized: Administering the "average" dose to a patient in severe renal failure can kill a patient.*

The health care provider has a critical role in preventing serious adverse drug effects in patients with renal impairment. Monitoring kidney function tests such as urinalysis and serum creatinine helps to identify impending renal failure. Notifying the prescriber at the first indication of renal failure allows drug dosages to be lowered, thereby preventing toxicity. Because health care providers frequently encounter patients with renal failure, special note should be taken of nephrotoxic drugs when learning pharmacology. Once a diagnosis of renal impairment is established, all nephrotoxic medications should be either discontinued or used with extreme caution.

Renal failure can be acute or chronic, depending on its onset. Acute renal failure requires immediate treatment because accumulation of waste products such as urea and creatinine can result in death if untreated. The cause of acute renal failure must be quickly identified and corrected. The most common cause of acute renal failure is lack of sufficient blood flow through the kidneys due to underlying conditions such as heart failure, dysrhythmias, hemorrhage, or dehydration.

Chronic renal failure occurs over a period of months or years. More than half of patients with chronic renal failure have a medical history of long-standing hypertension (HTN) or diabetes

NATURAL THERAPIES

Cranberry for Urinary System Health

Nearly everyone is familiar with the bright red cranberries that are eaten during holiday times. Native Americans used the colorful, ripe berries to treat wounds and to cure anorexia and for other digestive complaints. In the 1900s, it was noted that the acidity of the urine increases after eating cranberries; thus began the belief that cranberry juice is a natural cure for urinary tract infections.

Cranberry juice or berries contain a significant amount of vitamin C and other antioxidants that can promote health. They contain a substance that can prevent bacteria from sticking on the walls of the bladder. Research suggests that cranberries can prevent symptomatic urinary tract infections in some patients, especially in women who have recurrent infections.

Cranberry is a safe supplement, although large amounts may cause GI upset and diarrhea. The juice should be 100% cranberry and not "cocktail" juice because that contains sugar, which enhances bacteria growth and may be contraindicated in patients with diabetes. Some individuals may prefer to take cranberry capsules, which are available at most drug stores.

mellitus. Because of its long development and nonspecific symptoms, chronic renal failure may go undiagnosed for many years until the impairment becomes irreversible.

Pharmacotherapy of renal impairment includes administering diuretics, which can increase urine output. Cardiovascular agents are commonly administered to treat underlying HTN or heart failure.

Many patients with chronic renal failure will also have a deficiency of **erythropoietin**, a hormone secreted by the kidney. Erythropoietin serves as a primary signal to increase red blood cell production in the bone marrow. A synthetic form of erythropoietin, epoetin alfa (Epogen, Procrit) is effective in treating several disorders caused by a deficiency in red blood cells. Epoetin is sometimes given to patients undergoing cancer chemotherapy to counteract the anemia caused by antineoplastic agents (see Chapter 27 ⊕). It is occasionally prescribed for patients prior to blood transfusions or surgery and to treat anemia in HIV-infected patients. Epoetin alfa is usually administered three times per week until an increase in the number of red blood cells is achieved.

Diuretics are used to treat hypertension, heart failure, and fluid retention disorders.

CORE CONCEPT 23.4

A **diuretic** is a drug that increases urine output. The goal of most diuretic therapy is to reverse abnormal fluid retention by the body. Excretion of excess fluid in the body is particularly desirable in the following conditions:

dia = *thoroughly*
uretic = *to urinate*

- Hypertension (see Chapter 17 ⊕)
- Heart failure (see Chapter 18 ⊕)
- Kidney failure
- Pulmonary edema
- Liver failure or cirrhosis

The most common way in which diuretics act is by blocking sodium ion (Na^+) reabsorption in the nephron, thus sending more Na^+ to the urine. Chloride ion (Cl^-) follows Na^+. Because water molecules also tend to stay with sodium, blocking the reabsorption of Na^+ will increase the volume of urination, or diuresis. Some drugs, such as furosemide (Lasix), act by preventing the reabsorption of Na^+ in the loop of Henle, and thus they are called loop diuretics. Because of the abundance of Na^+ in the loop of Henle, furosemide is capable of producing large increases in urine output. Other drugs, such as the thiazides, act on the distal tubule. Because most Na^+ has already been reabsorbed from the filtrate by the time it reaches this point in the nephron, the thiazides produce less diuresis than does furosemide. The sites at which the various diuretics act are shown in Figure 23.3 ■.

FIGURE 23.3

Sites of action of
diuretics

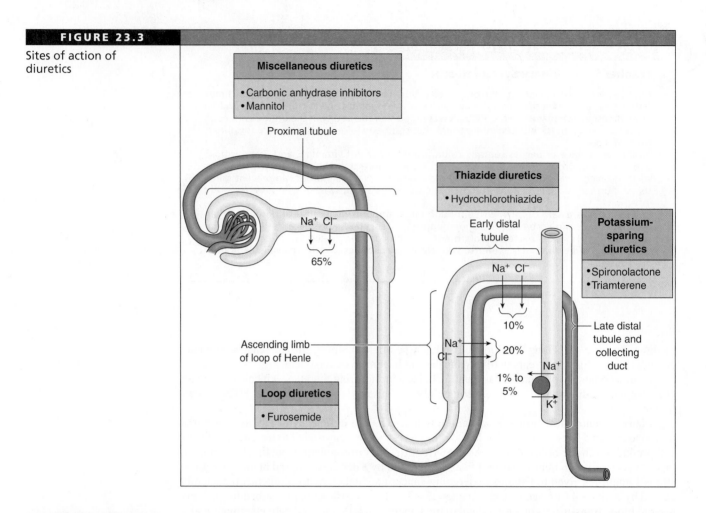

FIGURE 23.3

Sites of action of
diuretics

CORE CONCEPT 23.5

The most effective diuretics are those that affect the loop of Henle.

The most effective diuretics are the *loop* or *high-ceiling diuretics*. Drugs in this class act by blocking the reabsorption of sodium and chloride ions in the loop of Henle. When given IV, they have the ability to cause large amounts of fluid to be excreted by the kidney in a very short time. Loop diuretics are used to reduce the fluid accumulation associated with heart failure, hepatic cirrhosis, or chronic renal failure. Furosemide (Lasix) and torsemide (Demadex) are also approved for HTN.

Furosemide is the most frequently prescribed loop diuretic. A drug profile for furosemide is included in Chapter 17 ⚭ . Unlike the thiazide diuretics, furosemide is able to increase urine output even when blood flow to the kidneys is diminished. Torsemide (Demadex) has a longer half-life than furosemide, which offers the advantage of once-a-day dosing. Bumetanide (Bumex) is 40 times more potent than furosemide but has a shorter duration of action.

The rapid excretion of large amounts of water caused by loop diuretics may produce adverse effects such as dehydration and electrolyte imbalances. Signs of dehydration include thirst, dry mouth, weight loss, and headache. Hypotension, dizziness, and even fainting can result from the rapid fluid loss. Potassium loss, or **hypokalemia**, may cause dysrhythmias, and thus potassium supplements may be indicated during loop diuretic therapy. Potassium loss is of particular concern to patients who are also taking digoxin (Lanoxin). Although rare, ototoxicity is possible. Because of the potential for serious adverse effects, the loop diuretics are normally reserved for patients with moderate to severe fluid retention, or when other diuretics have failed to achieve therapeutic goals. Information on the loop diuretics is given in Table 23.1.

de = *not/without*
hydration = *water*

hypo = *low or below normal*
kal = *potassium*
emia = *blood condition*

Concept Review **23.2**

■ Why are drugs that block Na⁺ reabsorption at the loop of Henle more effective than those that act on the distal tubule?

TABLE 23.1	Loop Diuretics	
DRUG	**ROUTE AND ADULT DOSE**	**REMARKS**
bumetanide (Bumex)	PO; 0.5–2 mg daily (max: 10 mg/day)	IV form available; this drug is 40 times more potent than furosemide
ethacrynic acid (Edecrin)	PO; 50–100 mg once or twice per day (max: 400 mg/day)	IV form available; exhibits the most ototoxicity of the drugs in this class
furosemide (Lasix) (see page 298 for the Drug Profile box)	PO; 20–80 mg daily (max: 600 mg/day)	IV and IM forms available
torsemide (Demadex)	PO; 4–20 mg daily (max: 200 mg/day)	IV form available; exhibits the lowest risk of ototoxicity of the drugs in this class

The thiazides are the most widely prescribed class of diuretics.

CORE CONCEPT 23.6

The thiazides comprise the largest, most frequently prescribed class of diuretics. These drugs act on the distal tubule to block sodium reabsorption and increase water excretion. Their primary use is for the treatment of mild to moderate HTN. They are less effective at producing diuresis than the loop diuretics and they are ineffective in patients with severe renal disease. All the thiazide diuretics are available by the oral route and have equivalent efficacy and safety profiles. Three drugs—chlorthalidone (Hygroton), indapamide (Lozol), and metolazone (Zaroxolyn)—are not true thiazides, although they are included with this drug class because they have similar mechanisms of action and adverse effects. The thiazide and thiazide-like diuretics are listed in Table 23.2.

The frequency of adverse effects with the thiazides is much lower than that of the loop diuretics. As happens with other diuretics, dehydration is possible because of fluid loss, and patients may experience dizziness due to hypotension when moving from a supine to an upright position. Electrolyte levels are monitored periodically to prevent hypokalemia. To avoid adverse effects from the drug, patients taking thiazides should be advised to drink plenty of water and beverages containing electrolytes and to eat a balanced diet.

Although less effective than the loop diuretics, potassium-sparing diuretics may help prevent hypokalemia.

CORE CONCEPT 23.7

Potassium loss is a potentially serious adverse effect of the thiazide and loop diuretics. The therapeutic advantage of the potassium-sparing diuretics is that they are able to increase diuresis without adversely affecting blood potassium levels. These diuretics are shown in Table 23.3.

Normally, sodium and potassium ions are exchanged in the distal tubule; Na^+ is reabsorbed into the bloodstream and K^+ is secreted into the tubule. Potassium-sparing diuretics block this exchange, causing sodium to stay in the tubule and ultimately leave through the urine. When Na^+ is

TABLE 23.2	Thiazide and Thiazide-like Diuretics	
DRUG	**ROUTE AND ADULT DOSE**	**REMARKS**
bendroflumethiazide and nadolol (Corzide)	PO; 1 tablet/day (40–80 mg nadolol/5 mg bendroflumethiazide)	Intermediate acting
ⓟ chlorothiazide (Diuril)	PO; 250–500 mg one or two times/day	IV form available; short acting
chlorthalidone (Hygroton)	PO; 50–100 mg/day	Thiazide-like; long acting
hydrochlorothiazide (Microzide) (see page 276 for the Drug Profile box)	PO; 25–100 mg/day	Short acting
indapamide (Lozol)	PO; 1.25–2.5 mg once daily	Thiazide-like; long acting
methyclothiazide (Aquatensen, Enduron)	PO; 2.5–10 mg/day	Long acting
metolazone (Zaroxolyn)	PO; 2.5–10 mg once daily	Thiazide-like; intermediate acting

DRUG PROFILE: (Pr) *Chlorothiazide (Diuril)*

Therapeutic Class: Antihypertensive, agent for reducing edema
Pharmacologic Class: Thiazide diuretic

Actions and Uses:

Chlorothiazide is prescribed for mild to moderate HTN and may be combined with other antihypertensives in the treatment of severe HTN. It is also used to treat edema due to heart failure, liver disease, and corticosteroid or estrogen therapy. When given orally, it may take as long as 4 weeks to obtain the optimum therapeutic effect. When given IV, results are seen in 15 to 30 minutes.

Adverse Effects and Interactions:

Excess loss of water and electrolytes can occur. Symptoms may include thirst, weakness, lethargy, muscle cramping, hypotension, or tachycardia. Due to the potentially serious consequences of hypokalemia, patients taking digoxin should be carefully monitored. The intake of potassium-rich foods should be increased, and potassium supplements may be indicated.

Chlorothiazide interacts with several drugs. For example, when administered with amphotericin B or corticosteroids, the risk for hypokalemia increases. Antidiabetic medications such as sulfonylureas and insulin may be less effective when taken with chlorothiazide. Cholestyramine and colestipol decrease the absorption of chlorothiazide. Alcohol increases the hypotensive action of some thiazide diuretics, and caffeine may increase diuresis. When chlorothiazide is given concurrently with other antihypertensives, additive effects on blood pressure will occur.

Some herbal supplements may interact with thiazide diuretics. Licorice and oral aloe, in large amounts, may worsen hypokalemia. When used with chlorothiazide, ginkgo biloba may increase blood pressure. Use with hawthorn may result in additive hypotensive effects.

Refer to MyNursingKit for a Nursing Process Focus specific to this drug.

TABLE 23.3	Potassium-Sparing Diuretics	
DRUG	**ROUTE AND ADULT DOSE**	**REMARKS**
amiloride (Midamor)	PO; 5 mg/day (max: 20 mg/day)	Moduretic is a fixed-dose combination of amiloride and hydrochlorothiazide.
eplerenone (Inspra)	PO; 25–50 mg once daily	Newest drug in class; actions very similar to spironolactone
(Pr) spironolactone (Aldactone)	PO; 25–100 mg one or two times/day	Used in combination with other antihypertensives to increase diuresis; monitor serum potassium level carefully
triamterene (Dyrenium)	PO; 50–100 mg bid	Dyazide is a fixed-dose combination of triamterene and hydrochlorothiazide.

blocked, the body retains more K^+. Because most of the Na^+ has already been removed by the time the filtrate reaches the distal tubule, potassium-sparing diuretics produce only a mild diuresis. Their primary use is in combination with thiazide or loop diuretics to minimize potassium loss.

Unlike the loop and thiazide diuretics, patients taking potassium-sparing diuretics should not take potassium supplements and should not add potassium-rich foods to their diet. Intake of excess potassium when taking these medications may lead to **hyperkalemia**.

hyper = *high or above normal*
kal = *potassium*
emia = *blood condition*

Several less commonly prescribed diuretics have specific indications.

A few miscellaneous diuretics have very limited and specific indications. Two of these drugs inhibit **carbonic anhydrase**, an enzyme that affects acid-base balance by its ability to form carbonic acid from water and carbon dioxide. Acetazolamide (Diamox) is a carbonic anhydrase inhibitor used to decrease intraocular pressure in patients with glaucoma (see Chapter 35 ⬭). Unrelated to its diuretic effect, acetazolamide also has applications as an anticonvulsant, in treating motion sickness, and for treating acute mountain sickness in patients at very high altitudes. The carbonic anhydrase inhibitors are not commonly used as diuretics, because they produce a very weak diuresis and have a higher incidence of adverse effects than other diuretics.

The osmotic diuretics also have very specific applications. Mannitol is used to maintain urine flow in patients with acute renal failure or during prolonged surgery. Mannitol can also be used to lower intraocular pressure in certain types of glaucoma. It is a very potent diuretic that is only given by the IV route. Osmotic diuretics are rarely drugs of first choice due to their potential toxicity. Table 23.4 lists some of the miscellaneous diuretics.

intra = *within*
ocular = *eye*

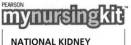

NATIONAL KIDNEY
FOUNDATION

TABLE 23.4	Miscellaneous Diuretics	
DRUG	**ROUTE AND ADULT DOSE**	**REMARKS**
acetazolamide (Diamox)	PO; 250–375 mg/day in a.m.	Carbonic anhydrase inhibitor; IV form available
glycerin (Colace, Osmoglyn)	PO; 1–1.8 g/kg, 1–2 hr before ocular surgery	Osmotic type; also used to treat constipation and acute glaucoma
mannitol	IV; 100 g infused over 2–6 hr	Osmotic type
methazolamide (Neptazane)	PO; 50–100 mg bid or tid	Carbonic anhydrase inhibitor
urea (Ureaphil)	IV; 1–1.5 g/kg over 1–2.5 hr	Osmotic type

DRUG PROFILE: ℗ *Spironolactone (Aldactone)*

Therapeutic Class: Antihypertensive, drug for reducing edema
Pharmacologic Class: Potassium-sparing diuretic, aldosterone antagonist

Actions and Uses:

Spironolactone, the most frequently prescribed potassium-sparing diuretic, is primarily used to treat mild HTN, often in combination with other antihypertensives. It may also be used to reduce edema associated with kidney or liver disease, and it is effective in slowing the progression of heart failure.

Spironolactone blocks sodium reabsorption in the distal tubule by inhibiting aldosterone. **Aldosterone** is a hormone secreted by the adrenal cortex that is responsible for increasing the renal reabsorption of Na^+ in exchange for K^+, thus causing water retention. When blocked by spironolactone, sodium and water excretion is increased, and the body retains more potassium.

Adverse Effects and Interactions:

Spironolactone does such an efficient job of retaining potassium that hyperkalemia may develop. The risk of hyperkalemia is increased if the patient takes potassium supplements or is also taking angiotensin-converting enzyme (ACE) inhibitors, as described in Chapter 17 ⬭ . Signs and symptoms of hyperkalemia include muscle weakness, fatigue, and bradycardia. When potassium levels are monitored carefully and maintained within normal values, adverse effects from spironolactone are uncommon. Spironolactone is contraindicated during pregnancy and lactation.

When spironolactone is combined with ammonium chloride, acidosis may occur. Aspirin and other salicylates may decrease the diuretic effect of the medication. Use of spironolactone with digoxin may decrease the effects of digoxin. When taken with potassium supplements, ACE inhibitors, and angiotensin-receptor blockers, hyperkalemia may result.

Refer to MyNursingKit for a Nursing Process Focus specific to this drug.

NURSING PROCESS FOCUS

Patients Receiving Diuretic Therapy

ASSESSMENT

Prior to administration:
- Obtain a complete health history (physical/mental), including data on recent surgeries or trauma
- Obtain vital signs; assess in context of the patient's baseline values
- Obtain the patient's medication history, including nicotine and alcohol consumption and use of herbal supplements or alternative therapies, to determine possible drug allergies and/or interactions
- Obtain blood and urine specimens for laboratory analysis

POTENTIAL NURSING DIAGNOSES

- Fluid Volume, Excess, related to effects of medical condition.
- Fluid Volume, Deficient, Risk for, related to effects of drug therapy.
- Urinary Elimination, Impaired, related to diuretic use.

PLANNING: PATIENT GOALS AND EXPECTED OUTCOMES

The patient will:
- Exhibit normal fluid balance and maintain electrolyte levels within normal limits during drug therapy
- Demonstrate an understanding of the drug's actions by accurately describing drug side effects and precautions
- Immediately report symptoms of hyperkalemia or hypokalemia and hypersensitivity reactions

IMPLEMENTATION

Interventions and (Rationales)	Patient Education/Discharge Planning
■ Monitor for fluid overload by measuring intake, output, and daily weights. (Intake, output, and daily body weight are indications of the effectiveness of diuretic therapy.)	Instruct the patient to: ■ Immediately report any severe shortness of breath, frothy sputum, profound fatigue, edema in extremities, potential signs of heart failure, or pulmonary edema ■ Accurately measure fluid intake, fluid output, and body weight, and report weight gain of 2 lb or more within 2 days or decrease in output ■ Avoid excessive heat, which contributes to fluid loss through perspiration ■ Consume adequate amounts of *plain water*
■ Monitor laboratory values, especially potassium and sodium. (Diuretics can cause electrolyte imbalances.)	■ Instruct the patient to inform laboratory personnel of diuretic therapy when providing blood or urine samples.
■ Monitor vital signs, especially blood pressure. (Diuretics reduce blood volume, resulting in lowered blood pressure.)	Instruct the patient to: ■ Monitor blood pressure as specified by the health care provider and ensure proper use of home equipment ■ Stop medication if severe hypotension exists, as specified by the health care provider (e.g., "hold for levels below 88/50 mmHg")
■ Observe for changes in level of consciousness, dizziness, fatigue, and postural hypotension. (Reduction in blood volume due to diuretic therapy may produce changes in level of consciousness or syncope.)	Instruct the patient to: ■ Immediately report any change in consciousness, especially feeling faint ■ Change positions slowly ■ Obtain blood pressure readings in sitting, standing, and lying positions

continued...

NURSING PROCESS FOCUS *(continued)*

Interventions and (Rationales)	Patient Education/Discharge Planning
■ Monitor potassium intake. (Potassium is vital to maintaining proper electrolyte balance and can become depleted with thiazide or loop diuretics.)	Instruct patients: ■ Receiving *loop* or *thiazide diuretics* to eat foods high in potassium ■ Receiving *potassium-sparing diuretics* to avoid foods high in potassium ■ To consult with health care provider before using vitamin/mineral supplements or electrolyte-fortified sports drinks
■ Observe for signs of hypersensitivity reaction. (Allergic responses may be life threatening.)	Instruct the patient or caregiver to report: ■ Difficulty breathing, throat tightness, hives or rash, or bleeding ■ Flulike symptoms such as shortness of breath, fever, sore throat, malaise, joint pain, profound fatigue
■ Monitor hearing and vision. (Loop diuretics are ototoxic. Thiazide diuretics increase serum digoxin levels; elevated levels produce visual changes.)	Instruct the patient to report any changes in hearing or vision such as ringing or buzzing in the ears, becoming "hard of hearing," or experiencing dimness of sight, seeing halos, or having "yellow vision."
■ Monitor reactivity to light exposure. (Some diuretics cause photosensitivity.)	Instruct the patient to: ■ Limit exposure to the sun ■ Wear dark glasses and light-colored loose-fitting clothes when outdoors

EVALUATION OF OUTCOME CRITERIA

Evaluate the effectiveness of drug therapy by confirming that patient goals and expected outcomes have been met (see "Planning").

See Tables 23.1 through 23.4 for lists of drugs to which these nursing actions apply.

Electrolytes are charged substances that play important roles in body chemistry.

CORE CONCEPT 23.9

Minerals are inorganic substances needed in very small amounts by the body (see Chapter 30 ⊂⊃). When placed in water, some of these minerals become ions and possess a positive or negative charge. Small, inorganic molecules possessing a positive or negative charge are called **electrolytes**. Electrolytes are essential to many body functions, including nerve conduction, muscle contraction, and bone growth and remodeling. Too little or too much of an electrolyte may result in serious disease and must be quickly corrected.

electro = *conducts electricity*
lyte = *solution*

Levels of electrolytes in body fluids are maintained within very narrow ranges, primarily by the kidney and gastrointestinal (GI) tract. As electrolytes are lost due to normal excretory functions, they must be replaced by adequate intake; otherwise, electrolyte imbalances can result. Although imbalances can occur in any ion, sodium, potassium, and calcium are of greatest importance. Calcium homeostasis is presented in Chapter 33 ⊂⊃ because it is often associated with the pharmacotherapy of bone disorders. Sodium and potassium are discussed in the following paragraphs. The major electrolyte imbalances and their treatments are described in Table 23.5.

An electrolyte imbalance is a sign of an underlying medical condition that needs attention. The most common cause is renal impairment. In some cases, drug therapy itself can cause the electrolyte imbalance. For example, aggressive therapy with loop diuretics such as furosemide (Lasix) can rapidly deplete the body of Na^+ and K^+. Treatment includes correcting the electrolyte imbalance as well as treating the underlying medical condition. Treatments for electrolyte imbalances range from simple changes in dietary intake for mild imbalances to rapid electrolyte infusions in severe cases.

TABLE 23.5	Electrolyte Imbalances		
ION	**CONDITION**	**ABNORMAL SERUM VALUE (mEq/L)**	**SUPPORTIVE TREATMENT***
Calcium	Hypercalcemia	Greater than 11	Hypotonic fluid or calcitonin
	Hypocalcemia	Less than 4	Calcium supplements or vitamin D
Chloride	Hyperchloremia	Greater than 112	Hypotonic fluid
	Hypochloremia	Less than 95	Hypertonic salt solution
Magnesium	Hypermagnesemia	Greater than 4	Hypotonic fluid
	Hypomagnesemia	Less than 0.8	Magnesium supplements
Phosphate	Hyperphosphatemia	Greater than 6	Dietary phosphate restriction
	Hypophosphatemia	Less than 1	Phosphate supplements
Potassium	Hyperkalemia	Greater than 5	Hypotonic fluid, buffers, or dietary potassium restriction
	Hypokalemia	Less than 3.5	Potassium supplements
Sodium	Hypernatremia	Greater than 145	Hypotonic fluid or dietary sodium restriction
	Hyponatremia	Less than 135	Hypertonic salt solution or sodium supplement

*For all electrolyte imbalances, the primary therapeutic goal is to identify and correct the cause of the imbalance.

hyper = *high or above normal*
natri = *sodium*
emia = *blood condition*

Sodium imbalances. Because Na^+ is the major electrolyte in extracellular fluid, imbalances of this ion can have serious consequences. Sodium excess, or **hypernatremia**, is most commonly caused by kidney disease; Na^+ accumulates in the blood due to decreased excretion. Another cause of hypernatremia is high net water losses, such as occur from inadequate water intake, watery diarrhea, fever, or burns. A high serum Na^+ level can cause cellular dehydration with symptoms such as thirst, fatigue, weakness, muscle twitching, convulsions, and a decreased level of consciousness. For minor hypernatremia, a salt-restricted diet may be effective in returning serum Na^+ to normal levels. In patients with acute hypernatremia, however, IV fluids such as 5% D_5W or diuretics may be administered to quickly remove sodium from the body.

Sodium deficiency, or **hyponatremia**, may occur when Na^+ is lost because of disorders of the skin (serious burns), GI tract (vomiting or diarrhea), or kidneys, and with conditions associated with excessive sweating or prolonged fever. Symptoms of hyponatremia include nausea, vomiting, anorexia, abdominal cramping, confusion, lethargy, convulsions, coma, and muscle twitching or tremors. Hyponatremia is usually treated with solutions of sodium chloride or with IV fluids containing salt, such as normal saline or lactated Ringer's. Various concentrations of sodium chloride may be infused, depending on the severity of the deficiency. In most cases, concentrations of 0.45% or 0.9% are used to reverse hyponatremia.

Potassium imbalances. Potassium levels must be carefully balanced between adequate dietary intake and renal excretion. Levels of K^+ in the blood must be maintained within narrow limits because too little or too much of this electrolyte is associated with fatal cardiac dysrhythmias and serious neuromuscular disorders.

Hyperkalemia may be caused by high consumption of potassium-rich foods or dietary supplements, particularly when patients are taking potassium-sparing diuretics such as spironolactone. Excess potassium may also accumulate when renal excretion is diminished due to kidney pathology. The most serious consequences of hyperkalemia are cardiac dysrhythmias.

In mild cases of hyperkalemia, K^+ levels may be returned to normal by restricting major dietary sources of potassium such as bananas, dried fruits, peanut butter, broccoli, and green leafy vegetables. If the patient is taking a potassium-sparing diuretic, the dose is lowered or an alternate drug is considered. In severe cases, serum potassium levels may be lowered by administering sodium polystyrene sulfate (Kayexalate), a resin that removes K^+ by exchanging them for Na^+ in the large intestine. This agent is given concurrently with a laxative to promote rapid evacuation of the potassium. Sodium polystyrene sulfate is available in oral and enema formulations. An alternative method of treating hyperkalemia is to administer glucose and insulin, which causes potassium to leave the extracellular fluid and enter cells.

DRUG PROFILE: ℗ *Potassium Chloride (KCl)*

Therapeutic Class: Potassium supplement
Pharmacologic Class: Electrolyte

Actions and Uses:

Potassium is one of the most important electrolytes in body fluids, and levels must be maintained within a narrow range of values between 3.5 and 5.5 mEq/L. Too much or too little K^+ may lead to serious consequences and must be immediately corrected. Neurons and muscle fibers are most sensitive to potassium loss. Muscle weakness, dysrhythmias, and cardiac arrest are possible consequences. KCl is also used to treat mild forms of alkalosis.

KCl is the drug of choice for treating or preventing hypokalemia. Therapy with loop or thiazide diuretics is the most common cause of excessive potassium loss. Patients taking thiazide or loop diuretics are usually instructed to take oral potassium supplements to prevent hypokalemia. Oral forms include tablets, powders, and liquids, usually heavily flavored because of the unpleasant taste of the drug. Intravenous forms may be given in critical care situations.

Adverse Effects and Interactions:

KCl irritates the GI mucosa; therefore, nausea and vomiting are common. The drug may be taken with meals or antacids to lessen the gastric distress. Taking too much KCl can cause hyperkalemia, especially when it is combined with a diet that contains potassium-rich foods.

Potassium supplements interact with potassium-sparing diuretics and ACE inhibitors to increase the risk of hyperkalemia. If patients are taking these drugs, the health care provider should warn them not to take over-the-counter (OTC) potassium supplements.

Refer to MyNursingKit for a Nursing Process Focus specific to this drug.

Hypokalemia is a relatively common adverse effect resulting from high doses of loop diuretics such as furosemide. Strenuous muscular activity and severe vomiting or diarrhea can also result in significant potassium loss. Mild hypokalemia is treated by increasing the dietary intake of potassium-rich foods. More severe deficiencies require oral or parenteral potassium supplements. Potassium chloride (KCl) is available in IV and a wide variety of oral formulations to increase blood potassium levels.

Acidic and basic drugs can be administered to maintain normal body pH.

CORE CONCEPT 23.10

One of the most important homeostatic functions of the blood is to neutralize strong acids and bases. Much of the food we eat is either more acidic or more alkaline than body fluids. Furthermore, during the breakdown of food, the body generates significant amounts of acid. If body fluids become too acidic or too alkaline, enzymes will not function efficiently and cells may be injured.

The degree of acidity or alkalinity of a solution is measured by its pH. A **pH** of 7.0 is defined as neutral, above 7.0 as basic or alkaline, and below 7.0 as acidic. To maintain homeostasis, the pH of plasma and most body fluids must be kept within the very narrow range of 7.35 to 7.45. At pH values above 7.45, **alkalosis** develops, and symptoms of central nervous system (CNS) stimulation occur that include nervousness and convulsions. **Acidosis** occurs below a pH of 7.35, and symptoms of CNS depression may result in coma. In either alkalosis or acidosis, death may result if large changes in pH are not corrected immediately.

alkal = *basic*
osis = *condition*

Acidosis and alkalosis are not diseases; they are symptoms of an underlying disorder. Primary treatment of acid-base disorders is always targeted to correcting the underlying cause. Drugs are administered to support the patient's vital functions while the disease is being treated. Common causes of alkalosis and acidosis are listed in Table 23.6.

Treatment of alkalosis is directed toward addressing the underlying condition that is causing the excess bases to be retained. In mild cases, alkalosis may be corrected by administering sodium

TABLE 23.6	Causes of Alkalosis and Acidosis

ACIDOSIS	ALKALOSIS
RESPIRATORY ORIGINS OF ACIDOSIS	***RESPIRATORY ORIGIN OF ALKALOSIS***
▪ Hypoventilation or shallow breathing	▪ Hyperventilation due to asthma, anxiety, or high altitude
▪ Airway constriction	
▪ Damage to respiratory center in medulla	
METABOLIC ORIGINS OF ACIDOSIS	***METABOLIC ORIGINS OF ALKALOSIS***
▪ Severe diarrhea	▪ Constipation for prolonged periods
▪ Kidney failure	▪ Ingestion of excess sodium bicarbonate
▪ Diabetes mellitus	▪ Diuretics that cause potassium depletion
▪ Excess alcohol ingestion	▪ Severe vomiting
▪ Starvation	

chloride concurrently with KCl. This combination increases the renal excretion of bicarbonate ion (a base), which indirectly increases the acidity of the blood. For acute patients, acidifying agents may be used. Hydrochloric acid and ammonium chloride are two drugs that can quickly lower the pH in patients with severe alkalosis.

In patients with acidosis, the goal is to quickly reverse the level of acids in the blood. The treatment of choice for acute acidosis is to administer infusions of sodium bicarbonate. Bicarbonate ion acts as a base to quickly neutralize acids in the blood and other body fluids. The patient must be carefully monitored during infusions because this drug can "over-correct" the acidosis, causing blood pH to turn alkaline. The correction of acid-base imbalances is illustrated in Figure 23.4 ▪.

DRUG PROFILE: ⓅⓇ *Sodium Bicarbonate (NaHCO₃)*

Therapeutic Class: Agent to treat acidosis or bicarbonate deficiency
Pharmacologic Class: Electrolyte

Actions and Uses:

Acidosis is a more common event than alkalosis, occurring during shock, cardiac arrest, or diabetes mellitus. Sodium bicarbonate is the drug of choice for correcting acidosis: The bicarbonate ion (HCO_3^-) directly raises the pH of body fluids. Sodium bicarbonate may be given orally, if acidosis is mild, or IV, in cases of acute disease. Although sodium bicarbonate neutralizes gastric acid, it is rarely used to treat peptic ulcers because of its tendency to cause gas and gastric distention.

Sodium bicarbonate may also be used to make the urine more basic. An alkaline urine will speed the excretion of acidic drugs such as the barbiturates and aspirin.

Adverse Effects and Interactions:

Most of the adverse effects of sodium bicarbonate therapy are the result of alkalosis caused by *too much* bicarbonate ion. Symptoms may include confusion, irritability, slow respiration rate, and vomiting. Simply discontinuing the sodium bicarbonate infusion often reverses these symptoms; however, potassium chloride or ammonium chloride may be administered to reverse the alkalosis.

Sodium bicarbonate may decrease the absorption of ketoconazole and may decrease elimination of dextroamphetamine, ephedrine, pseudoephedrine, and quinidine. Sodium bicarbonate may increase the elimination of lithium, salicylates, and tetracyclines. Chronic use of sodium bicarbonate with milk or calcium supplements may cause milk–alkali syndrome, a condition characterized by very high serum calcium levels and possible kidney failure.

 Refer to MyNursingKit for a Nursing Process Focus specific to this drug.

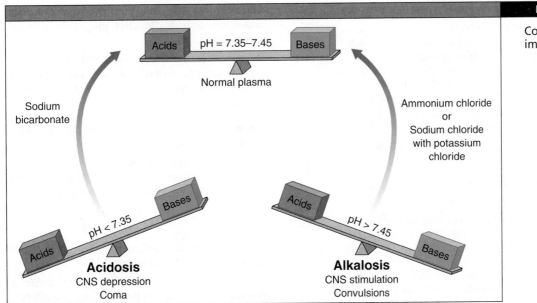

FIGURE 23.4

Correction of acid-base imbalances

PATIENTS NEED TO KNOW

Patients treated for urinary, acid-base, and fluid disorders need to know the following:

Regarding Diuretics

1. When taking diuretics, drink plenty of water if dry mouth or thirst develops, unless otherwise directed by a health care provider.
2. Take diuretics at least 2 hours before bedtime to avoid nighttime diuresis.
3. If diabetes is present, monitor blood sugar levels very closely when taking loop diuretics because these drugs may elevate blood glucose levels.
4. Do not take thiazide diuretics during pregnancy or when breast-feeding.
5. When taking loop or thiazide diuretics, increase intake of potassium-rich foods such as dark leafy vegetables, nuts, citrus fruits, bananas, and potatoes. If taking a potassium-sparing diuretic, avoid these foods unless otherwise instructed by a health care provider.
6. Avoid caffeinated beverages when taking diuretics. The diuretic effect of the caffeine combined with the effects of these medications may cause dehydration.

Regarding Potassium Supplements

7. Because KCl tablets are irritating to the GI mucosa, they should be taken with food. Do not crush or suck the tablets. If nausea or heartburn occurs, take antacids along with the KCl.

CHAPTER REVIEW

CORE CONCEPTS SUMMARY

23.1 **The kidneys regulate fluid volume, electrolytes, acids, and bases.**

The kidneys are essential to the overall health of the patient, and to controlling fluid volume, electrolyte composition, and acid-base balance. The functional unit of the kidney is the nephron.

23.2 **The composition of filtrate changes dramatically as a result of the processes of reabsorption and secretion.**

Filtrate entering the proximal tubule resembles plasma without proteins. Through the processes of reabsorption and secretion, the filtrate composition changes, producing urine.

23.3 Renal failure significantly impacts pharmacotherapy.

Because the kidneys excrete most drugs, a large number of medications require a significant dosage reduction in patients with moderate to severe renal failure. Renal failure is classified as acute or chronic. Pharmacotherapy of renal failure attempts to cure the cause of the dysfunction. Diuretics may be used to maintain urine output. Epoetin alfa is a form of erythropoietin used to treat anemias in which there is a deficiency in red blood cell production.

23.4 Diuretics are used to treat hypertension, heart failure, and fluid retention disorders.

Diuretics are drugs that increase urine output, usually by blocking sodium reabsorption. Indications for diuretics include hypertension, heart failure, kidney failure, and liver disease.

23.5 The most effective diuretics are those that affect the loop of Henle.

The high-ceiling or loop diuretics such as furosemide act by blocking sodium reabsorption in the loop of Henle. They are the most effective diuretics but are more likely to cause dehydration and electrolyte loss.

23.6 The thiazides are the most widely prescribed class of diuretics.

The thiazide diuretics block sodium reabsorption in the distal tubule. Although less effective than the loop diuretics, the thiazides are more frequently prescribed because of their lower incidence of serious adverse effects.

23.7 Although less effective than the loop diuretics, potassium-sparing diuretics may help prevent hypokalemia.

Potassium-sparing diuretics act on the distal tubule and are more effective than the loop diuretics. Their primary advantage is that they do not cause potassium loss.

23.8 Several less commonly prescribed diuretics have specific indications.

Carbonic anhydrase inhibitors and osmotic diuretics are not commonly prescribed. They have specific applications, such as decreasing intraocular pressure and maintaining urine flow during renal failure.

23.9 Electrolytes are charged substances that play important roles in body chemistry.

Electrolyte imbalances can cause serious problems. Hypokalemia is a serious potential adverse effect of drug therapy with certain diuretics. Oral or IV potassium chloride can reverse symptoms of hypokalemia. Although less common, hyperkalemia may be just as serious and may be reversed by administration of glucose or insulin.

23.10 Acidic and basic drugs can be administered to maintain normal body pH.

Sodium chloride with potassium chloride may be administered to reverse mild to moderate alkalosis. Hydrochloric acid or ammonium chloride may be administered for acute alkalosis. Sodium bicarbonate is used to reverse acidosis.

REVIEW QUESTIONS

The following questions are written in NCLEX-PN® style. Answer these questions to assess your knowledge of the chapter material, and go back and review any material that is not clear to you.

1. Which of the following is not a function of the kidneys?
1. Acid-base balance
2. Secretion of renin
3. Production of white blood cells
4. Production of calcitriol

2. When assessing for dehydration, the nurse will look for:
1. Headache and increased urinary output
2. Weight gain and edema
3. Hypertension and decreased urinary output
4. Hypotension, headache, and dry mucous membranes

3. A patient newly diagnosed with hypertension will most likely be started on which of the following medications?
1. Ethacrynic acid (Edecrin)
2. Chlorothiazide (Diuril)
3. Spironolactone (Aldactone)
4. Mannitol

4. The patient recently started on diuretic therapy should be taught to:
1. Take medication at night
2. Rise slowly from a sitting position
3. Increase sodium intake
4. Decrease fluid intake

5. When too much ammonium chloride is administered, the blood becomes:
1. Alkalotic
2. Acidotic
3. Neutralized
4. Normalized

6. The patient is exhibiting signs and symptoms of metabolic acidosis. Which of the following is not a cause of metabolic acidosis?

1. Severe diarrhea
2. Hyperventilation
3. Starvation
4. Diabetes mellitus

7. Which of the following is appropriate treatment if the patient is experiencing hypernatremia?

1. Diuretics
2. Potassium
3. IV fluids
4. Increasing fluid intake

8. The patient is receiving IV normal saline because of hyponatremia. The hyponatremia may have been caused by:

1. Constipation
2. Severe nausea and vomiting
3. Dehydration
4. Hemorrhage

9. If taking diuretics, the patient should be instructed to decrease her intake of:

1. Dark green, leafy vegetables
2. Nuts
3. Fruits
4. Caffeine

10. The patient taking torsemide (Demadex) must closely monitor his _____ levels.

1. Glucose
2. Magnesium
3. Calcium
4. Selenium

CASE STUDY QUESTIONS

For questions 1–4, please refer to the following case study, and choose the correct answer from choices 1–4.

*M*r. Grant has been placed on hydrochlorothiazide (Microzide) for high blood pressure, and potassium chloride as a dietary supplement. His wife tells him to eat lots of bananas because she read that this was necessary when taking diuretics. After a few weeks, Mr. Grant becomes weak and feels as if his heart is skipping beats. His blood pressure remains high, despite the diuretic.

1. Which of the following should have been explained to Mr. Grant regarding his medication?

1. Never eat bananas when taking Microzide.
2. Eat lots of bananas when taking Microzide.
3. Limit potassium-rich foods when taking potassium supplements.
4. Never eat bananas and take Microzide at the same meal.

2. Given the previous information, it is quite possible that Mr. Grant's cardiac symptoms and weakness were caused by:

1. Hyperkalemia
2. Hypokalemia
3. Hypernatremia
4. Hyponatremia

3. The physician examines Mr. Grant and decides to administer a dose of sodium polystyrene sulfonate (Kayexalate). The rationale for administering this drug is to:

1. Increase fluid volume
2. Decrease fluid volume
3. Increase serum potassium levels
4. Decrease serum potassium levels

4. After Mr. Grant's condition stabilized, the physician decided to select a more effective diuretic to treat the hypertension. Which class is more effective than the thiazides and would most likely be selected for Mr. Grant?

1. Potassium-sparing
2. Loop/high-ceiling
3. Osmotic
4. Carbonic anhydrase inhibitors

FURTHER STUDY

- Chapter 33 ⚭ contains information on calcium homeostasis and on calcitriol, the active form of vitamin D.

- ACE inhibitors for treating hypertension are discussed in Chapter 17 ⚭.

- The use of spironolactone in the pharmacotherapy of heart failure is presented in Chapter 18 ⚭.

- The use of diuretics in the pharmacotherapy of hypertension is discussed in Chapter 17 ⚭. A drug profile for furosemide is contained in Chapter 17 ⚭.

- The use of acetazolamide in treating open-angle glaucoma is discussed in Chapter 35 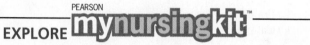 .

- Chapter 30 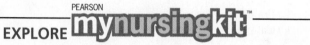 includes additional information on the pharmacology of minerals, some of which are electrolytes.

EXPLORE PEARSON **mynursingkit™**

MyNursingKit is your one stop for online chapter review materials and resources. Prepare for success with additional NCLEX®-style practice questions, interactive assignments and activities, web links, animations and videos, and more!

Register your access code from the front of your book at **www.mynursingkit.com**

UNIT 4

The Immune System

UNIT CONTENTS

24 Drugs for Inflammation and Immune Modulation

CORE CONCEPTS

24.1 Inflammation is a body defense that limits the spread of invading microorganisms and injury.

24.2 The body reacts to injury by releasing chemical mediators that cause inflammation.

24.3 Inflammation may be treated with nonpharmacologic and pharmacologic therapies.

24.4 NSAIDs are the primary drugs for the treatment of mild inflammation.

24.5 Glucocorticoids are effective in treating severe inflammation.

24.6 The immune response results from activation of the humoral and cell-mediated immune systems.

24.7 Vaccines are biologic agents used to prevent illness.

24.8 Biologic response modifiers are used to boost the immune response.

24.9 Immunosuppressants are primarily used to avoid tissue rejection following organ transplant.

DRUG SNAPSHOT

The following drugs are discussed in this chapter:

DRUG CLASSES	DRUG PROFILES
Nonsteroidal anti-inflammatory drugs (NSAIDs)	(Pr) naproxen (Naprosyn) and naproxen sodium (Aleve, Anaprox)
Glucocorticoids	(Pr) prednisone
Vaccines	(Pr) hepatitis B vaccine (Energix-B, Recombivax HB)
Immunosuppressants	(Pr) cyclosporine (Neoral, Sandimmune)

LEARNING OUTCOMES

After reading this chapter, the student should be able to:

1. Identify common signs and symptoms of inflammation.

2. Outline the basic steps in the acute inflammatory response.

3. Describe the central role of histamine in inflammation.

4. Outline general strategies for treating inflammation.

5. Compare and contrast the humoral and cell-mediated immune responses.

6. For each of the drug classes in the Drug Snapshot, identify representative drugs and explain the mechanisms of drug action, primary actions related to inflammation and/or the immune system, and important adverse effects.

7. Categorize drugs used in the treatment of inflammation, allergies, and immune disorders based on their classifications and mechanisms of action.

8. For each of the major vaccines, give the recommended dosage schedule.

KEY TERMS

active immunity 396

alternate-day therapy 394

anaphylaxis (ANN-ah-fah-LAX-iss) 388

antibodies (ANN-tee-BOD-ee) 395

antigens (ANN-tih-jen) 394

B cell 394

biologic response modifiers 399

boosters 396

Cushing's syndrome (KUSH-ings) 394

cyclooxygenase (COX) (SYE-klo-OK-sah-jen-ays) 390

cytokines (SYE-toh-kines) 395

cytotoxic T cells 395

helper T cells 395

histamine (HISS-tuh-meen) 388

humoral immunity (HYOU-mor-ul eh-MEWN-uh-tee) 394

immunoglobulins (Ig) (ih-MEW-noh-GLOB-you-lin) 395

immunosuppressants (ih-MEW-noh-suh-PRESS-ent) 400

inflammation (IN-flah-MAY-shun) 388

lymphocyte (LIM-foh-site) 394

mast cells 388

passive immunity 396

plasma cells 395

salicylism (sal-IH-sill-izm) 391

T cells 395

titer (TIE-ter) 396

toxoids (TOX-oid) 396

transplant rejection 400

vaccines (vaks-EEN) 396

vaccination/immunization (VAK-sin-AYE-shun/IH-mewn-ize-AYE-shun) 396

The pain and redness of inflammation following minor abrasions and cuts is something everyone has experienced. Although there may be discomfort from such scrapes, inflammation is a normal and expected part of our body's defense against injury. For some diseases, however, inflammation can rage out of control, producing severe pain, fever, and other distressing symptoms. It is these sorts of conditions for which drug therapy may be needed.

Similarly, our bodies come under continuous attack from a host of foreign invaders that include viruses, bacteria, fungi, and even multicellular organisms. In defending the body, our immune system is capable of mounting a rapid and effective response against many of these pathogens. In some cases, vaccines or other drugs are given to stimulate body defenses so that disease can be prevented or controlled. On other occasions it is desirable to decrease the immune response to allow a transplanted organ to survive. The purpose of this chapter is to examine the pharmacotherapy of diseases and conditions affecting our body defenses.

Fast Facts Inflammatory and Allergic Disorders

- Arthritis, the most common inflammatory disorder, is the leading cause of disability in the United States.
- Inflammatory bowel disease affects 300,000–500,000 Americans each year.
- In the United States, approximately 70 million NSAID prescriptions are written, and 30 billion over-the-counter NSAID tablets are sold, each year.
- More than 1% of the U.S. population uses NSAIDs on a daily basis.
- Worldwide, more than 30 million people consume NSAIDs daily, and, of these, 40% are older than 60 years.
- It is estimated that NSAIDS cause 16,500 deaths in the United States annually, largely as a result of GI complications. This is more mortality than is caused from gastric cancer.

INFLAMMATION

Inflammation is a body defense that limits the spread of invading microorganisms and injury.

The human body has developed complex ways to defend itself against physical injury and invasion by microorganisms. Inflammation is one of these defense mechanisms. **Inflammation** occurs in response to many different stimuli, including physical injury; exposure to toxic chemicals, extreme heat, or invading microorganisms; or death of cells. The central purpose of inflammation is to contain the injury or destroy the microorganism. By removing cellular debris and dead cells, repair of the injured area can move at a faster pace. Inflammation proceeds in the same manner, regardless of the cause that triggered it. Signs of inflammation include swelling, pain, warmth, and redness of the affected area.

Inflammation may be classified as *acute* or *chronic*. Acute inflammation has an immediate onset and lasts 1 to 2 weeks. During acute inflammation, 8 to 10 days are normally needed for the symptoms to resolve and for repair to begin. If the body cannot contain or neutralize the damaging agent, inflammation may continue for long periods and become chronic. In chronic diseases such as lupus and rheumatoid arthritis, inflammation may persist for years, with symptoms becoming progressively worse over time. Other disorders such as seasonal allergy arise at predictable times each year, and inflammation may produce only minor, annoying symptoms.

The body reacts to injury by releasing chemical mediators that cause inflammation.

Whether the injury is due to pathogens, chemicals, or physical trauma, the damaged tissue releases a number of chemical mediators that act as "alarms" that notify the surrounding area of the injury. Chemical mediators of inflammation include histamine, leukotrienes, bradykinin, complement, and prostaglandins. Table 24.1 describes the sources and actions of these mediators.

Histamine is a key chemical mediator of inflammation. It is primarily stored within **mast cells** located in tissue spaces under epithelial membranes such as the skin, in the bronchial tree and digestive tract, and along blood vessels. Mast cells detect foreign agents or injury and respond by releasing histamine, which initiates the inflammatory response within seconds. In addition, histamine directly stimulates pain receptors.

When released at an injury site, histamine and other mediators dilate nearby blood vessels, causing the capillaries to become more permeable or leaky. Plasma and components such as complement proteins and phagocytes can then enter the area to neutralize foreign agents. The affected area may become congested with blood because of the permeable capillaries, which can lead to significant swelling and pain. Figure 24.1 ■ shows the basic steps in acute inflammation.

Rapid release of histamine on a larger scale throughout the body is responsible for **anaphylaxis**, a life-threatening allergic response that may result in shock and death. A number of chemicals, insect stings, foods, and some therapeutic drugs can cause this widespread release of histamine from mast cells. Drug therapy of anaphylactic shock is discussed in Chapter 19 ⌒ .

TABLE 24.1	Chemical Mediators of Inflammation
Bradykinin	Present in an inactive form in plasma and mast cells; vasodilator that causes pain; effects are similar to those of histamine
Complement	Series of at least 20 proteins that combine in a cascade fashion to neutralize or destroy an antigen
Histamine	Stored and released by mast cells; causes dilation of blood vessels, smooth muscle constriction, tissue swelling, and itching
Leukotrienes	Stored and released by mast cells; effects are similar to those of histamine
Prostaglandins	Present in most tissues; stored and released by mast cells; increase capillary permeability, attract white blood cells to site of inflammation, and cause pain

FIGURE 24.1

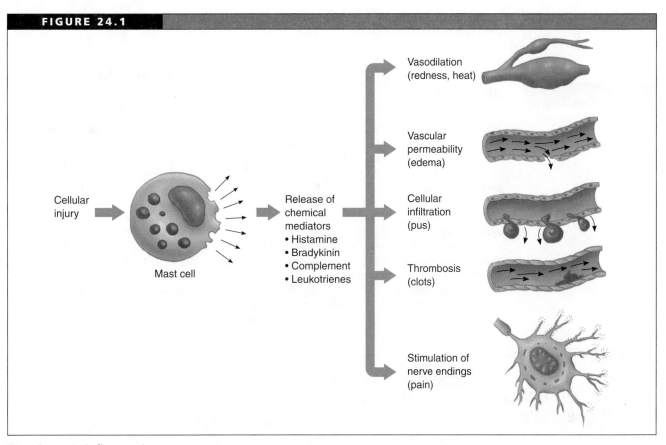

Steps in acute inflammation   *Source: Pearson Education/PH College*

Inflammation may be treated with nonpharmacologic and pharmacologic therapies.

CORE CONCEPT **24.3**

PEARSON
mynursingkit

POLLEN AND ALLERGIC RHINITIS

Because inflammation is a nonspecific process and may be caused by such a variety of etiologies, it may occur in nearly any tissue or organ system. When treating inflammation, the following general principles apply:

- Inflammation is not a disease but a symptom of an underlying disorder. Whenever possible, the *cause* of the inflammation is identified and treated.

- Inflammation is a natural process for ridding the body of foreign agents, and it is usually self-limiting. For mild symptoms, nonpharmacologic therapies such as ice packs and rest should be used whenever applicable.

- Topical drugs should be used when applicable because they cause fewer adverse effects. Inflammation of the skin and mucous membranes of the mouth, nose, rectum, and vagina are best treated with topical drugs. Many of these are available over-the-counter (OTC).

The goal of pharmacotherapy with anti-inflammatory drugs is to prevent or decrease the intensity of the inflammatory response and reduce fever, if present. Most anti-inflammatory agents are nonspecific; the drug will exhibit the same inhibitory actions regardless of the cause of the inflammation. Common diseases that benefit from anti-inflammatory agents include allergic rhinitis, anaphylaxis, ankylosing spondylitis, contact dermatitis, Crohn's disease, glomerulonephritis, Hashimoto's thyroiditis, peptic ulcer disease, rheumatoid arthritis, systemic lupus erythematosus, and ulcerative colitis.

The two primary drug classes used for inflammation are the nonsteroidal anti-inflammatory drugs (NSAIDs) and the glucocorticoids (also called corticosteroids). For mild to moderate pain, inflammation, and fever, NSAIDs are the preferred drugs. Should inflammation become severe, glucocorticoids therapy is begun. Due to their serious long-term adverse effects, glucocorticoids

rhin = *nose*
itis = *inflammation*

are usually used for only 1–3 weeks to bring inflammation under control, and then the patient is switched to NSAIDs.

NSAIDs are the primary drugs for the treatment of mild inflammation.

NSAIDs such as aspirin and ibuprofen have analgesic, antipyretic, and anti-inflammatory effects. They are drugs of choice in the treatment of mild to moderate inflammation. Some NSAIDs used for inflammation are listed in Table 24.2.

The analgesic action of NSAIDs is discussed in Chapter 14 ∞. This class includes some of the most widely used drugs, such as aspirin and ibuprofen. Although acetaminophen can reduce pain and fever, it has no anti-inflammatory action and is thus not considered an NSAID.

Aspirin is useful in treating inflammation because it inhibits **cyclooxygenase (COX)**, a key enzyme in the pathway of prostaglandin synthesis that is found in every tissue. Aspirin causes irreversible inhibition of both forms of cyclooxygenase, COX-1 and COX-2. Because it is readily available, inexpensive, and effective, aspirin is sometimes a drug of first choice for treating mild inflammation. The basic pharmacology and a drug profile of aspirin are presented in Chapter 14 ∞.

Unfortunately, large doses of aspirin are necessary to suppress severe inflammation, and these doses result in a greater incidence of serious adverse effects. The most common adverse effects observed during high-dose therapy relate to the digestive system. By increasing gastric acid

TABLE 24.2	Selected Nonsteroidal Anti-inflammatory Drugs (NSAIDs)	
DRUG	**ROUTE AND ADULT DOSE**	**REMARKS**
aspirin (Acetylsalicylic Acid, ASA) (see page 222 for the Drug Profile box)	PO; 350–650 mg every 4 hours (max: 4 g/day)	Inhibits the formation of prostaglandins; also for fever, pain, and prevention of stroke and myocardial infarction (MI)
celecoxib (Celebrex)	PO; 100–200 mg bid (max: 400 mg/day)	Selective COX-2 inhibitor
diclofenac (Cataflam, Solaraze, Voltaren)	PO; 50 mg bid–qid (max: 200 mg/day)	Extended-release form available
diflunisal	PO; 250–500 mg bid (max: 1500 mg/day)	Similar to ibuprofen
etodolac	PO; 200–400 mg tid–qid (max: 1200 mg/day)	Extended-release form available
fenoprofen (Nalfon)	PO; 300–600 mg tid–qid (max: 3200 mg/day)	Similar to ibuprofen
flurbiprofen (Ansaid)	PO; 50–100 tid–qid (max: 300 mg/day)	Similar to ibuprofen
ibuprofen (Advil, Motrin, others)	PO; 400–800 mg tid–qid (max: 3200 mg/day)	Blocks prostaglandin synthesis as well as modulates T-cell function; also for dysmenorrhea
ketoprofen	PO; 75 mg tid or 50 mg qid (max: 300 mg/day)	Extended-release form available; similar to ibuprofen; also for dysmenorrhea
nabumetone	PO; 1000 mg daily (max: 2000 mg/day)	Inhibits COX-2 more than COX-1
Pr naproxen (Naprosyn) and naproxen sodium (Aleve, Anaprox)	PO; 250–500 mg bid (max: 1000 mg/day)	Also for dysmenorrhea
oxaprozin (Daypro)	PO; 600–1200 mg daily (max: 1800 mg/day)	Similar to naproxen; once-a-day dosage
piroxicam (Feldene)	PO; 10–20 mg once or twice a day (max: 20 mg/day)	Has prolonged half-life
tolmetin (Tolectin)	PO; 400 mg tid (max: 2 g/day)	Exact mode of anti-inflammatory action unknown

DRUG PROFILE: Ⓟ *Naproxen (Naprosyn) and Naproxen Sodium (Aleve, Anaprox)*

Therapeutic Class: Analgesic, anti-inflammatory drug, antipyretic

Pharmacologic Class: Nonsteroidal anti-inflammatory drug (NSAID)

Actions and Uses:

Naproxen is an older NSAID that is prescribed for the treatment of mild to moderate pain, fever, and inflammation. Its efficacy at relieving pain and inflammation is similar to that of aspirin. Common indications include treating the pain associated with rheumatoid arthritis and osteoarthritis, gout, and bursitis. In treating rheumatoid arthritis, the therapeutic effects may take 3 to 4 weeks to appear.

Adverse Effects and Interactions:

Adverse effects of naproxen are generally not serious and include GI upset, dizziness, and drowsiness. Administration with food will decrease the incidence of stomach upset, which is the most common adverse effect. Because naproxen may prolong bleeding time, the drug should be administered with caution to those with bleeding disorders. Patients taking naproxen should notify their dental hygienist before dental procedures are performed.

Using naproxen concurrently with oral anticoagulants can prolong bleeding time. Lithium levels may be increased. Bleeding potential increases when used with herbal agents such as feverfew, garlic, ginger, and ginkgo biloba.

Mechanism in Action:

Naproxen is an NSAID that inhibits prostaglandin synthesis through the nonselective inhibition of cyclooxygenase type-1 (COX-1) and cyclooxygenase type-2 (COX-2) enzymes. It also inhibits platelet aggregation and prolongs bleeding time without affecting whole blood clotting, prothrombin time, or platelet count.

Refer to MyNursingKit for a Nursing Process Focus specific to this drug.

secretion and irritating the stomach lining, aspirin may cause pain, heartburn, and even bleeding due to ulceration. In some patients, even small doses may cause gastrointestinal (GI) bleeding. Some aspirin formulations are buffered or given an enteric coating to minimize GI adverse effects. Because aspirin also has an antiplatelet effect (see Chapter 20 ⚭), the potential for bleeding must be carefully monitored by the health care provider. High doses may produce **salicylism**, a syndrome that includes symptoms such as ringing in the ears, dizziness, headache, and sweating. Patients with preexisting kidney disease should be monitored carefully because aspirin and other NSAIDs may affect kidney function.

Ibuprofen and ibuprofen-like drugs are available as alternatives to aspirin. Like aspirin, they exhibit their effects through inhibition of COX-1 and COX-2. Because of their similar mechanisms, they all have similar pharmacologic properties and a relatively low incidence of adverse effects. The most common adverse effects of these drugs are nausea and vomiting, although the incidence of gastric ulceration and bleeding is less than that of aspirin. Most have no significant effect on blood coagulation and are safe to use for patients who may be at risk for bleeding.

Selective inhibition of COX-2 produces the analgesic, anti-inflammatory, and antipyretic effects seen with the NSAIDs without causing some of the serious adverse effects of the older NSAIDs. Because they have no GI adverse effects and do not affect blood coagulation, these drugs quickly became the treatment of choice for moderate to severe inflammation.

However, in 2004, research data revealed that one NSAID, rofecoxib (Vioxx), doubled the risk of heart attack and stroke in patients taking rofecoxib for extended periods. Based on these reports, the drug manufacturer voluntarily removed the drug from the market. Shortly afterward, a second COX-2 inhibitor, valdecoxib (Bextra), was also voluntarily withdrawn, leaving celecoxib (Celebrex) the sole drug in this class.

Glucocorticoids are effective in treating severe inflammation.

CORE CONCEPT 24.5

Glucocorticoids, or corticosteroids, are natural hormones released by the cortex of the adrenal gland that have powerful effects on nearly every cell in the body. One of their most useful actions is their ability to suppress severe inflammation. When used to treat inflammatory disorders, the drug doses are many times higher than those naturally present in the blood. Glucocorticoids have

NURSING PROCESS FOCUS

Patients Receiving NSAID Therapy

ASSESSMENT

Prior to administration:
- Obtain a complete health history (physical/mental), including allergies, drug history, and possible drug interactions
- Determine pain and analgesic usage patterns
- Identify infectious agents or other factors responsible for inflammation or pain

POTENTIAL NURSING DIAGNOSES

- Acute Pain related to injury or surgical procedure.
- Chronic Pain related to injury.
- Deficient Knowledge related to information about drug therapy.
- Ineffective Health Maintenance related to chronic pain.

PLANNING: PATIENT GOALS AND EXPECTED OUTCOMES

The patient will:
- Report pain relief or a reduction in pain intensity
- Demonstrate an understanding of the drug's action by accurately describing drug adverse effects and precautions
- Report ability to manage activities of daily living
- Immediately report effects such as unresolved, untoward, or rebound pain; persistent fever; blurred vision; tinnitus; bleeding; changes in color of stool or urine

IMPLEMENTATION

Interventions and (Rationales)	Patient Education/Discharge Planning
■ NSAIDs may be administered PO or PR. When using suppositories, monitor integrity of rectum; observe for rectal bleeding.	Inform the patient: ■ Not to cut or crush enteric-coated tablets. Regular tablets may be broken or pulverized and mixed with food. ■ To take liquid ASA immediately after mixing because it breaks down rapidly ■ Not to take different drugs and formulations, such as ibuprofen and naproxen, concurrently. Consult the health care provider regarding appropriate OTC analgesics for specific types of pain. ■ To consult the nurse regarding ASA therapy following surgery. (ASA is an anticoagulant. The body needs time to manufacture new platelets to make clots that promote wound healing.) ■ To advise laboratory personnel of aspirin therapy when providing urine samples
■ Monitor vital signs, especially temperature. (Increased pulse and blood pressure may indicate discomfort; if accompanied by pallor and/or dizziness, may indicate bleeding.)	Instruct the patient to: ■ Report rapid heartbeat, palpitations, dizziness, or pallor ■ Monitor blood pressure and temperature, ensuring proper use of home equipment
■ Monitor for signs of GI bleeding, GI elimination, or hepatic toxicity. (NSAIDs can be a local irritant to the GI tract with anticoagulant action that is metabolized in the liver.) Conduct guaiac stool testing for occult blood and monitor complete blood count (CBC) for anemia-related blood loss.	Instruct the patient to: ■ Report any bleeding, abdominal pain, anorexia, heartburn, nausea, vomiting, jaundice, or change in the color or character of stools ■ Know the proper method of obtaining stool samples and home testing for occult blood ■ Adhere to a regimen of laboratory testing as ordered by the health care provider ■ Take NSAIDs with food to reduce stomach upset
■ Assess for character, duration, location, and intensity of pain and the presence of inflammation.	Instruct the patient to: ■ Report pain and/or inflammation that remains unresolved ■ Take only the prescribed amount of NSAIDs to decrease the potential for adverse effects

continued . . .

NURSING PROCESS FOCUS *(continued)*

Interventions and (Rationales)

- Monitor for hypersensitivity reaction.
- Monitor urinary output and edema in feet/ankles. (Medication is excreted through the kidneys. Long-term use may lead to renal dysfunction.)
- Monitor for sensory changes indicative of drug toxicity: tinnitus, blurred vision.
- Evaluate blood salicylate levels.

Patient Education/Discharge Planning

- Advise the patient to immediately report shortness of breath, wheezing, throat tightness, itching, or hives. If these occur, stop taking ASA immediately and inform the health care provider.
- Instruct the patient to report changes in urination, flank pain, or pitting edema.
- Immediately report sensory changes in sight or hearing, especially blurred vision or ringing in the ears.
- Return to the health care provider for prescribed follow-up appointments.

EVALUATION OF OUTCOME CRITERIA

Evaluate the effectiveness of drug therapy by confirming that patient goals and expected outcomes have been met (see "Planning").

See Table 24.2 for a list of drugs to which these nursing actions apply.

numerous therapeutic applications. The uses of glucocorticoids in treating hormonal imbalances are presented in detail in Chapter 31. Doses for the glucocorticoids used to treat severe inflammatory disease are listed in Table 24.3.

Glucocorticoids affect inflammation in multiple ways. They suppress the actions of chemical mediators of inflammation such as histamine and prostaglandins. In addition, they inhibit the immune system by suppressing certain functions of phagocytes and lymphocytes. These multiple effects have the ability to markedly reduce inflammation, making glucocorticoids the most effective medications for the treatment of severe inflammatory disorders.

Unfortunately, the glucocorticoids have a number of serious adverse effects that limit their therapeutic use. These include suppression of the normal functions of the adrenal gland (adrenal insufficiency), elevated blood glucose, mood changes, cataracts, peptic ulcers, electrolyte imbalances, and osteoporosis. Because of their effectiveness at reducing the signs and symptoms of inflammation, glucocorticoids can mask infections that may be present in the patient. This combination of masking inflammation and suppressing the immune system creates a potential for existing infections to grow rapidly and undetected. An active infection is usually a contraindication for glucocorticoid therapy.

Because the appearance of these adverse effects is a function of the dose and duration of therapy, treatment is often limited to the short-term control of acute disease. When longer therapy is

TABLE 24.3	Selected Glucocorticoids for Severe Inflammation	
DRUG	**ROUTE AND ADULT DOSE**	**REMARKS**
betamethasone (Celestone)	PO; 0.6–7.2 mg/day	Topical, IM, and IV forms available
cortisone	PO; 20–300 mg/day in divided doses	IM form available; also for adrenal insufficiency
dexamethasone	PO; 0.25–4 mg bid–qid	IM and IV forms available; also for adrenal insufficiency and immunosuppression
hydrocortisone (Cortef, Hydro-cortone, Solu-Cortef, others) (see page 562 for the Drug Profile box)	Topical 0.5% cream applied 1–4 times daily; PO 10–320 mg tid–qid	Used widely for skin inflammation; IM, PO, rectal, and IV forms available; may be injected intra-articular
methylprednisolone (Depo-Medrol, Medrol)	PO; 4–48 mg/day in divided doses	Available in IM, IV, and rectal forms; also for neoplasia and adrenal insufficiency
prednisolone (Orapred, Prelone)	PO; 5–60 mg 1–4 times daily	Available in IM and IV forms; also for neoplasia and adrenal insufficiency
Pr prednisone	PO; 5–60 mg 1–4 times daily	Available in oral form only; also for neoplasia
triamcinolone (Aristospan, Kenalog)	PO; 4–48 mg 1–4 times daily	Available in IM, subcutaneous, intradermal, intra-articular, and aerosol forms

DRUG PROFILE: 🅿️ *Prednisone*

Therapeutic Class: Anti-inflammatory agent
Pharmacologic Class: Glucocorticoid

Actions and Uses:

Prednisone is a synthetic glucocorticoid. Its actions are the result of being metabolized to an active form, which is also available as a drug called prednisolone (Orapred, Prelone). When used for inflammation, a 4- to 10-day duration for therapy is common. Alternate-day dosing is used for longer-term therapy. Prednisone is occasionally used to terminate acute bronchospasm in patients with asthma (see Chapter 28 ⬭) and for patients with certain cancers such as Hodgkin's disease, acute leukemia, and lymphomas (see Chapter 27 ⬭).

Adverse Effects and Interactions:

When used for short-term therapy, prednisone has few adverse effects. Long-term therapy may result in Cushing's syndrome, a condition that includes elevated blood glucose, fat redistribution to the shoulders and face, muscle weakness, bruising, and bones that easily fracture. Glucocorticoids can raise blood glucose levels. Patients with diabetes may require an adjustment in insulin dose. Gastric ulcers may occur with long-term therapy, and an antiulcer medication may be prescribed prophylactically. Patients must report any potential infections immediately. This drug should be discontinued gradually.

Barbiturates, phenytoin, and rifampin increase the metabolism of prednisone: Increased doses of prednisone may be needed. Amphotericin B and diuretics together with prednisone can increase potassium loss. Prednisone may inhibit antibody response to vaccines and toxoids. In patients with myasthenia gravis, use of prednisone with ambenonium, neostigmine, or pyridostigmine can cause severe muscle weakness.

🌐 *Refer to MyNursingKit for a Nursing Process Focus specific to this drug.*

indicated, doses are kept as low as possible and **alternate-day therapy** is sometimes used; the medication is taken every other day to encourage the patient's adrenal glands to function on the days when no drug is taken. During long-term therapy, the health care provider must be alert for signs of overtreatment, a condition called **Cushing's syndrome.** Signs include bruising and a characteristic pattern of fat deposits in the cheeks (moon face), shoulders (buffalo hump), and abdomen. The body becomes accustomed to the high doses of glucocorticoids, and patients must discontinue the drug gradually because abrupt withdrawal can result in lack of adrenal function.

IMMUNE DISORDERS

Although inflammation is *nonspecific,* the body has also developed elaborate mechanisms of protection that target *specific* foreign agents. Drugs may be used to either *boost* the immune system (vaccines, biologic response modifiers) or *dampen* the immune system (immunosuppressants).

The immune response results from activation of the humoral and cell-mediated immune systems.

CORE CONCEPT 24.6

anti = *against*
gen = *formation*

Foreign substances that cause a specific immune response are called **antigens.** Proteins such as those present on the surfaces of pollen grains, bacteria, and viruses are the strongest antigens. The primary cell of the immune system that interacts with antigens is the **lymphocyte.** Two basic types of lymphocytes are responsible for activating two very different branches of the immune system.

Humoral immunity is initiated when an antigen encounters a type of lymphocyte known as a **B cell.** The antigen activates the B cell, which then divides rapidly to form many copies, or clones, of itself. Most cells in this clone are called *plasma cells*. The primary function of the **plasma cells** is to secrete **antibodies**, also called **immunoglobulins (Ig)**, which are specific to the antigen that initiated the immune response. As they circulate through the body, antibodies physically interact with the antigens to neutralize or target them for destruction by other cells of the immune response. Peak production of antibodies occurs about 10 days after an immune response. Figure 24.2 ■ shows the basic steps in the humoral immune response.

After the antigen challenge, *memory B cells* are formed that will remember the specific antigen-antibody interaction. Should the body be exposed to the same antigen in the future, the body will be able to manufacture even higher levels of antibodies in a shorter period, approximately 2 to 3 days. For some antigens, such as those for measles, mumps, or chickenpox, memory can be retained for an entire lifetime. Vaccines, discussed later in this chapter, are sometimes administered to produce these memory cells in advance of exposure to the antigen, so that when the body is exposed to the real organism it can mount a fast, effective response.

The second branch of the immune response involves lymphocytes called **T cells**. Two major types of T cells are **helper T cells** and **cytotoxic T cells**. These cells are often named after a protein receptor on their plasma membrane; the helper T cells have a CD4 receptor, and the cytotoxic T cells have a CD8 receptor. Helper T cells are particularly important because they are responsible for activating most other immune cells, including B cells. Cytotoxic T cells travel throughout the body, directly killing certain bacteria, parasites, virus-infected cells, and cancer cells.

T cells rapidly form clones when they encounter their specific antigen. Unlike B cells, however, T cells do not produce antibodies. Instead, T cells produce huge amounts of **cytokines**, which are hormone-like proteins. Some cytokines kill foreign organisms directly, whereas others act as messengers to the immune system, stimulating T cells, B cells, and other white blood cells

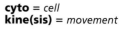

cyto = *cell*
kine(sis) = *movement*

FIGURE 24.2

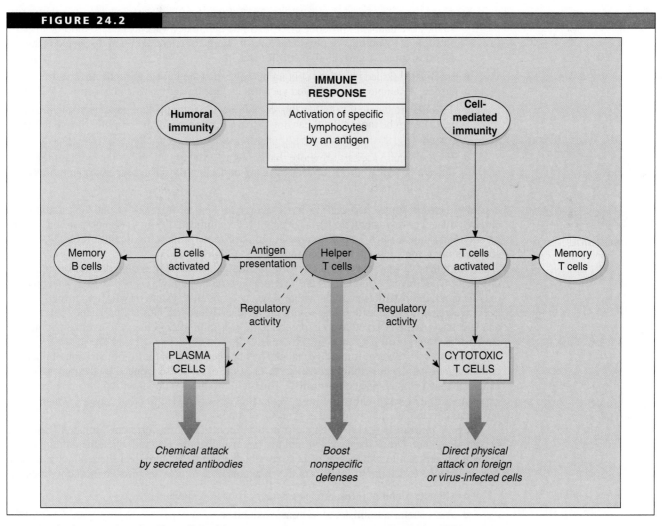

Steps in the humoral and cell-mediated immune responses   *Source: Pearson Education/PH College*

to rid the body of the foreign agent. Specific cytokines released by activated T cells include several interleukins, gamma interferon, and tumor necrosis factor (TNF). Some of these cytokines have been used to treat certain immune disorders and cancers. This class of medications, called *biologic response modifiers,* is discussed in Section 24.8 and in Chapter 25 ⚭ .

Like B cells, some of the activated T cells become memory cells. If the person encounters the same antigen in the future, the memory T cells will assist in mounting a more rapid immune response.

CORE CONCEPT 24.7

Vaccines are biological agents used to prevent illness.

Vaccination, or **immunization**, is the process of introducing a foreign substance into the body to trigger immune activation *before* the patient is exposed to the real pathogen. These biologic immune stimulators are called **vaccines**. As a result of the vaccination, memory B cells are formed. When the patient is later exposed to the actual infectious organism, these cells will react quickly by producing large quantities of antibodies that will help to neutralize or destroy the pathogen. Some immunizations require follow-up doses, called **boosters**, to provide sustained protection. The effectiveness of most vaccines can be assessed by measuring the amount of antibody produced after the vaccine has been administered, a quantity called a **titer**. If the titer falls below a specified protective level over time, a booster is indicated.

The goal of vaccine administration is to induce long-lasting immunity to a pathogen *without* producing an illness in an otherwise healthy person. Therefore, the microorganisms and other substances used as vaccines must be able to strongly activate the immune system but be modified to pose no significant risk of disease development. The four methods of producing safe and effective vaccines include the following:

- Attenuated (live) vaccines contain microbes that are alive but weakened (attenuated) so they are unable to produce disease. Some attenuated vaccines cause mild or subclinical symptoms of the disease. An example of a live attenuated vaccine is the measles, mumps, and rubella (MMR) vaccine.
- Inactivated (killed) vaccines contain microbes that are unable to replicate or cause disease. Examples of inactivated vaccines include the influenza and hepatitis A vaccines.
- **Toxoids** are types of vaccines that contain bacterial toxins that have been chemically modified to be incapable of causing disease. Examples include diphtheria and tetanus toxoids.
- Recombinant vaccines are those that contain partial organisms or bacterial proteins that are generated in the laboratory using biotechnology. The best example of this type is the hepatitis B vaccine.

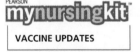

VACCINE UPDATES

The widespread use of vaccines has prevented illness in millions of patients, particularly children. One disease—smallpox—has been virtually eliminated from the planet through immunization, and others, such as polio, have diminished to extremely low levels. Table 24.4 gives some common vaccines and their recommended schedules.

Common adverse effects of vaccine administration include redness and discomfort at the site of injection and fever. Although severe reactions are rare, anaphylaxis is possible. Vaccinations may be contraindicated for patients with a weakened immune system or who are currently experiencing symptoms such as diarrhea, vomiting, or fever. Most vaccines are pregnancy category C, and vaccinations are often delayed in pregnant patients until after delivery to avoid any potential harm to the fetus.

There are two types of immunity that can be obtained through the administration of pharmacologic agents, as illustrated in Figure 24.3 ■. The type of response induced by the real pathogen, or its vaccine, is called **active immunity**: The body produces its own antibodies in response to exposure. The active immunity induced by vaccines closely resembles that caused by natural exposure to the antigen, including the generation of memory cells.

Passive immunity occurs when preformed antibodies are transferred or "donated" from one person to another. Drugs for passive immunity are usually administered when the patient has already been exposed to a pathogen or is at very high risk to exposure, and there is not sufficient time to develop active immunity. Examples of agents used to provide passive immunity include:

- Gamma globulin infused to counteract exposure to hepatitis
- Antivenoms administered to treat snake bites
- Sera used to treat botulism, tetanus, and rabies

TABLE 24.4	Selected Vaccines and Their Schedules
VACCINE	**SCHEDULE**
Diphtheria, tetanus, and pertussis (Daptacel, DTaP, Infanrix, Tripedia)	Ages 2 months, 4 months, 6 months, and 18 months
Haemophilus influenza type B conjugate (ActHIB, HibTITER, PedvaxHIB) Comvax is a combination of *Haemophilus* and hepatitis B vaccines	Ages 2 months, 4 months, 6 months, and 15 months
Hepatitis A (Havrix, VAQTA)	Children: Age 12 months, followed by a booster 6–12 months later Adults: First dose followed by a booster 6–12 months later
Hepatitis B (Engerix-B, Recombivax HB) Twinrix is a combination of hepatitis A and hepatitis B vaccines	Children: At birth; then at 1–4 mo and 6–18 mo Adults: Three doses, with the second dose 30 days after the first, and the final dose 6 months after the first
Human papillomavirus (Gardasil)	Children (females): first dose at age 11 or 12 years. Second dose 2 months after the first dose and the third dose 6 months after the first dose
Influenza vaccine (Afluria, Fluarix, FluLaval, Fluvirin, Fluzone)	Children: Two doses 1 month apart; then annual dose Adults: single annual dose
Measles, mumps, and rubella (MMR II) Proquad is a combination of MMR and varicella vaccines	Children: first dose at age 12–15 months with booster at age 4–6 years
Pneumococcal, polyvalent (Pneumovax 23), or 7-valent (Prevnar)	Children (Prenvar): Ages 2 months, 4 months, 6 months, and 12–15 months Adults: single dose
Poliovirus, inactivated (IPOL)	Children: Ages 4–8 weeks, 2–4 months, and 6–12 months
Rotavirus (Rotarix, RotaTeq)	Children: three 2-ml doses at 2 months, 4 months, and 6 months (Rotarix does not require a dose at 6 months)
Varicella (Varivax)	Younger than 12 months: single dose Patients 12 months and older: two doses given 4–8 weeks apart

Because these medications do not stimulate the patient's immune system, their protective effects last only until the antibodies disappear from the body, usually 2 to 3 weeks.

One vaccine that has received considerable attention in recent years is that for anthrax. Anthrax is caused by the bacterium *Bacillus anthracis,* which normally affects domestic and wild animals. In the fall of 2001, however, five people in the United States died as a result of exposure to anthrax due to purposeful, bioterrorist actions. Anthrax spores can remain viable in soil for hundreds, and perhaps thousands, of years. Anthrax spores are resistant to drying, heat, and some harsh chemicals and can easily be applied to envelopes or other personal items to transmit disease.

NATURAL THERAPIES

Echinacea for Boosting the Immune System

Echinacea purpurea, or purple coneflower, is one of the most popular medicinal botanicals. This plant is native to the midwestern United States and central Canada; its flowers, leaves, and stems are harvested and dried. Preparations include dried powder, tinctures, fluid extracts, and teas. No single ingredient seems to be responsible for the herb's activity; many active chemicals have been identified from the extracts.

Echinacea was used by Native Americans to treat various wounds and injuries. Echinacea is claimed to boost the immune system by increasing phagocytosis and inhibiting bacterial enzymes. Some substances in echinacea appear to have antiviral activity; the herb is sometimes taken to prevent and treat the common cold and influenza, an indication for which it has received official approval in Germany. In general, it is used as a supportive treatment for any disease involving inflammation and to enhance the immune system.

FIGURE 24.3

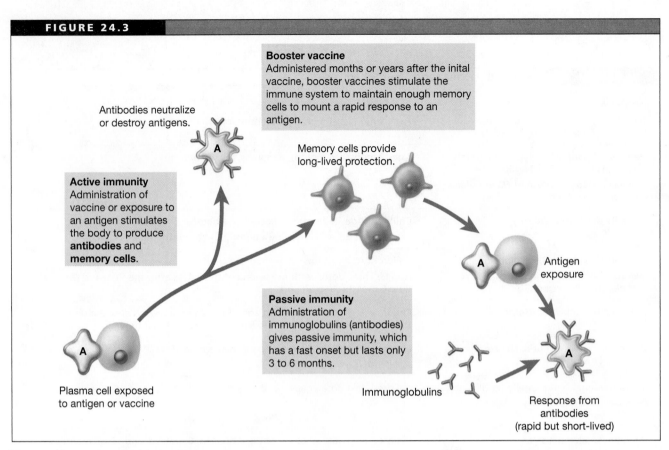

Booster vaccine
Administered months or years after the inital vaccine, booster vaccines stimulate the immune system to maintain enough memory cells to mount a rapid response to an antigen.

Antibodies neutralize or destroy antigens.

Memory cells provide long-lived protection.

Active immunity
Administration of vaccine or exposure to an antigen stimulates the body to produce **antibodies** and **memory cells**.

Antigen exposure

Passive immunity
Administration of immunoglobulins (antibodies) gives passive immunity, which has a fast onset but lasts only 3 to 6 months.

Plasma cell exposed to antigen or vaccine

Immunoglobulins

Response from antibodies (rapid but short-lived)

Mechanisms of active and passive immunity

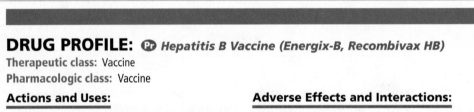

DRUG PROFILE: ⓟ *Hepatitis B Vaccine (Energix-B, Recombivax HB)*

Therapeutic class: Vaccine
Pharmacologic class: Vaccine

Actions and Uses:

Hepatitis B vaccine is administered IM to provide prophylaxis against exposure to the hepatitis B virus, which is of special interest because it is transmitted through infected blood and body fluids. Following injection, the body produces antibodies against the virus. The Centers for Disease Control and Prevention (CDC) strongly recommends that all health care providers (including students) who have the potential for exposure to the virus receive the vaccine. The regimen involves three doses of the vaccine, usually followed by a titer to confirm that active immunity has been achieved.

Hepatitis B vaccine is sometimes given to patients *after* they have been exposed to the virus. In this case, it is often combined with hepatitis B immune globulin (HBIG), which will provide passive immunity while the body is building its own antibodies to the virus. Once a hepatitis B infection is acquired, it is difficult to eliminate; therefore, prevention is the best treatment.

Adverse Effects and Interactions:

The adverse effects of hepatitis B vaccine are similar to those of other vaccines. Pain and inflammation may appear at the injection site. A fever may develop, and the patient may feel tired and lethargic. Although anaphylaxis is rare, epinephrine should be kept available. No clinically significant interactions have been found.

Refer to MyNursingKit for a Nursing Process Focus specific to this drug.

Fast Facts Vaccines and Organ Transplants

■ Vaccines have eliminated smallpox from the world and the poliovirus from the Western Hemisphere.

■ Vaccines lowered the number of measles cases in the United States from more than 503,000 in 1962 to about 100 annually.

■ The most common transplanted organs are the kidney, liver, and heart.

■ More than 79,000 patients are waiting for organ transplants, with about 3,000 added to the list every month.

■ Because of the lack of available transplants, many patients die every year. This includes about:
  ■ 2,000 kidney patients
  ■ 1,300 liver patients
  ■ 450 heart patients
  ■ 360 lung patients

Anthrax immunization (vaccination) has been approved by the Food and Drug Administration (FDA) for more than 30 years, but it has not been widely used because of the extremely low incidence of this disease in the United States. In addition, there is an ongoing controversy regarding the safety of the anthrax vaccine and whether it is effective at preventing the disease. At this time, the Centers for Disease Control and Prevention (CDC) is recommending vaccination for only a few select populations:

■ Laboratory personnel who work with anthrax

■ Military personnel deployed to high-risk areas

■ Individuals who deal with animal products imported from areas with a high incidence of the disease

Biologic response modifiers are used to boost the immune response.

CORE CONCEPT 24.8

When challenged by antigens, certain cells in the immune system secrete chemicals called cytokines that help fight the invading organism. Several of these natural chemicals are now available as medications to treat certain disorders. Drugs in this class, the **biologic response modifiers**, are administered to boost certain functions of the immune system. Only a few such medications have been approved.

Interferons (IFNs) are cytokines secreted by lymphocytes and macrophages that have been infected with a virus. IFNs slow the spread of viral infections and enhance the activity of existing leukocytes. In addition to antiviral properties, these drugs exhibit anticancer and anti-inflammatory actions. Alpha IFNs have the widest therapeutic application (when used as medications, the spelling is changed to *alfa*). Indications for IFN alpha therapy include cancers, such as hairy cell leukemia and AIDS-related Kaposi's sarcoma, and chronic hepatitis virus B or C infections. Interferon alfa-2b (Intron A) is featured as a profile antineoplastic drug in Chapter 27 ⬭ . Interferon beta is primarily used for treatment of severe multiple sclerosis (see Chapter 12 ⬭).

Interleukins are another class of cytokines secreted by lymphocytes, monocytes, and macrophages. Although 30 different interleukins have been identified, only a few are available as medications. The interleukins have widespread effects on immune function, and all of them boost the activity of natural defense mechanisms. Interleukin-2 is available as aldesleukin (Proleukin), which is approved for the treatment of metastatic renal carcinoma. Interleukin-11, which is derived from bone marrow cells, is a growth factor with multiple hematopoietic effects. It is marketed as oprelvekin (Neumega) for its ability to stimulate platelet production in patients with weakened immune systems.

In addition to IFNs and interleukins, a few additional biologic response modifiers are available to enhance the immune system. Levamisole (Ergamisole) is used to stimulate B cells, T cells, and macrophages in patients with colon cancer. Bacille Calmette-Guérin (BCG) vaccine (TICE, TheraCys) is an attenuated strain of *Mycobacterium tuberculosis* used for the pharmacotherapy of certain types of bladder cancer.

Immunosuppressants are primarily used to avoid tissue rejection following organ transplant.

The immune system is normally viewed as a life saver, protecting us from destructive pathogens in the environment. For those receiving organ or tissue transplants, however, the immune system is the enemy. Transplanted organs always contain some antigens that trigger the recipient's immune response. This response, called **transplant rejection**, is sometimes acute, with antibodies rushing to destroy the transplanted tissue within a few days. The cell-mediated immune system reacts more slowly to the transplant, attacking it about 2 weeks following surgery. Even if the organ survives these attacks, chronic rejection of the transplant may occur months or even years after surgery.

Immunosuppressants are medications given to lessen the immune response. One or more of these agents are administered at the time of transplantation and continued for several months following surgery. In some cases, they are continued indefinitely at low doses. Transplantation would be impossible without the use of effective immunosuppressant drugs. In addition, these drugs may be prescribed for severe cases of rheumatoid arthritis or other serious inflammatory disorders. Unlike transplant recipients who may receive immunosuppressants indefinitely, patients with acute inflammatory disorders usually are given these drugs only for brief periods to control relapses.

The mechanism of action of each of the immunosuppressant drugs differs, although nearly all are toxic to bone marrow. Because the immune system is suppressed, infections are common and the patient must be protected from situations in which exposure to pathogens is likely. Long-term survivors of transplants are also at increased risk of developing cancers, especially lymphoma, skin cancer, cervical cancer, and Kaposi's sarcoma. Doses for these drugs are listed in Table 24.5.

TABLE 24.5	**Selected Immunosuppressants**	
DRUG	**ROUTE AND ADULT DOSE**	**REMARKS**
anakinra (Kineret)	Subcutaneous; 100 mg once daily	For rheumatoid arthritis that has not responded to safer drugs
azathioprine (Imuran)	PO/IV; 3–5 mg/kg daily	Inhibits DNA, RNA, and protein synthesis; also for severe rheumatoid arthritis
basiliximab (Simulect)	IV; 20 mg times two doses (first dose 2 hr before surgery; second dose 4 days after transplant)	Antibody against the CD25 receptor on T cells; approved for use in patients with kidney transplant
(Pr) cyclosporine (Neoral, Sandimmune)	PO; initial dose 14–18 mg/kg just prior to surgery; after 2 weeks, then 5–10 mg/kg/day	IV form available; inhibits T cells; also for rheumatoid arthritis, severe psoriasis, and other severe inflammatory disorders
lymphocyte immune globulin or antithymocyte globulin (Atgam)	IV; 10–30 mg/kg daily for 1–2 weeks	Polyclonal antibodies that alter the formation of T cells and reduce their numbers
methotrexate (Rheumatrex, Trexall) (see page 466 for the Drug Profile box)	PO; 15–30 mg/day for 5 days; repeat every 12 weeks for three courses	IV, IM, and intrathecal forms available; blocks metabolism of folic acid; also for neoplasia, severe psoriasis, and severe rheumatoid arthritis
muromonab-CD3 (Orthoclone OKT 3)	IV; 5 mg/day administered for 10–14 days	Antibodies against the CD3 receptor on T cells; often a treatment of choice to prevent renal transplant rejection
mycophenolate (CellCept, Myfortic)	PO/IV; 720 mg bid in combination with corticosteroids and cyclosporine, within 24 hr of transplant	IV form available; inhibits B cells, T cells, and antibody formation
sirolimus (Rapamune)	PO; 6 mg loading dose, then 2 mg/day	Suppresses antibody production and acute transplant rejection
tacrolimus (Prograf)	PO; 0.15–0.3 mg/kg/day in two divided doses every 12 hours	IV form available; inhibits T cells; also for severe psoriasis
Temsirolimus (Torisel)	IV; 25 mg once weekly over 30–60 min	Newer drug that is metabolized to sirolimus; very toxic to the hematologic system

DRUG PROFILE: Pr Cyclosporine (Neoral, Sandimmune)

Therapeutic Class: Immunosuppressant
Pharmacologic Class: Calcineurin inhibitor

Actions and Uses:

Cyclosporine is a complex chemical obtained from a soil fungus, that inhibits helper T cells. It is approved for the prophylaxis of kidney, heart, and liver transplant rejection and psoriasis, although it may be prescribed for other severe inflammatory conditions. Compared to some of the other immunosuppressants, it is less toxic to bone marrow cells. When prescribed for transplant recipients, it is often used in combination with high doses of glucocorticoids such as prednisone. Cyclosporine is normally administered by the oral route.

Adverse Effects and Interactions:

The primary adverse effect of cyclosporine occurs in the kidney, with up to 75% of patients experiencing reduction in urine output. Frequent laboratory tests of kidney function are necessary. Other common adverse effects are tremor, hypertension, and elevated hepatic enzyme values. Although opportunistic infections are common during cyclosporine therapy, they are fewer than with other immunosuppressants. Periodic blood counts are necessary to be certain that white blood cells (WBCs) do not fall below 4,000 or platelets below 75,000.

Because cyclosporine is extensively metabolized in the liver, many drug interactions are possible. The following drugs increase the metabolism of cyclosporine, making the drug *less effective:* phenytoin, carbamazepine, TMP-SMZ, and phenobarbital. The following drugs decrease the metabolism of cyclosporine, causing the drug to build high concentrations and become *potentially toxic:* macrolide antibiotics, azole antifungals, and amphotericin B. Because cyclosporine can damage the kidneys, other nephrotoxic drugs such as amphotericin B, NSAIDs, or aminoglycosides should be administered with great caution.

Refer to MyNursingKit for a Nursing Process Focus specific to this drug.

Concept Review   24.1

■ Why are oral glucocorticoids usually used concurrently with immunosuppressant drugs following a transplant operation?

SAFETY ALERT

Know How to Use the Equipment

The EpiPen is an autoinjector containing epinephrine that is used to prevent and treat anaphylaxis and severe allergic reactions to insect stings, foods, or drugs. The device is easy to operate, although the word "auto" sometimes gives people a false sense of security. An Australian study in 2007 reported that of 100 hospital-based pediatricians, only two were able to demonstrate the correct way to administer the drug using the EpiPen. Even after reading instructions, only 40% got most of the steps right. In 37% of cases, epinephrine would not have reached the patient's circulation. The nurse has a key responsibility in teaching parents and older children the correct use of the EpiPen.

Mehr, S., Robinson, M., & Tang, M. (2007).

PATIENTS NEED TO KNOW

Patients treated for inflammatory or immune disorders need to know the following:

Regarding Anti-inflammatory Medications

1. Take NSAIDs with food to decrease stomach irritation.
2. Avoid drinking alcohol when taking high doses of NSAIDs or aspirin because it increases stomach irritation.
3. If ringing in the ears, dizziness, headache, or signs of bleeding or bruising occur, discontinue aspirin use immediately and report the incident to the health care provider.
4. Take glucocorticoids exactly as prescribed because improper use may lead to serious adverse effects.

Regarding Vaccines

5. Maintain an accurate, written record of vaccinations, including the date of the vaccination, route and site of vaccination, type of vaccine (including manufacturer and lot number), and the address of the physician's office where the vaccination occurred.
6. Keep immunizations up to date to prevent illness. Because recommendations can change, seek current information from a health care provider periodically.
7. Vaccines may contain a number of additives, including antibiotics, formaldehyde, thimersol, and monosodium glutamate. If an allergy is known or suspected to any of these additives, notify a health care provider before getting a vaccination.
8. Never take cyclosporine with grapefruit juice; blood levels of the drug are increased by this combination.

Regarding Immunosuppressants

9. Reduce risk of illness by avoiding crowds, avoiding those with colds/infections, and washing hands frequently.
10. Keep scheduled laboratory and doctor appointments. Regular laboratory testing is extremely important, especially monitoring complete blood count (CBC), electrolytes, hormone levels, and urine studies.
11. Immediately report an elevation in temperature, unusual bleeding, sore throat, mouth ulcers, and fatigue to the health care provider.

CHAPTER REVIEW

CORE CONCEPTS SUMMARY

24.1 Inflammation is a body defense that limits the spread of invading microorganisms and injury.

Inflammation is a nonspecific response designed to rid the body of invading pathogens or to contain the spread of injury. Acute inflammation occurs over a period of several days, whereas chronic inflammation may continue for months or years.

24.2 The body reacts to injury by releasing chemical mediators that cause inflammation.

Inflammation is initiated by chemical mediators, the most important of which is histamine. Release of these meditators causes vasodilation, allowing capillaries to become leaky, thus causing tissue swelling. Extremely rapid release of histamine throughout the body can trigger anaphylaxis.

24.3 Inflammation may be treated with nonpharmacologic and pharmacologic therapies.

When possible, topical drugs are used because they produce fewer adverse effects than oral or parenteral drugs. The two primary drug classes used for inflammation are the NSAIDs and glucocorticoids.

24.4 NSAIDs are the primary drugs for the treatment of mild inflammation.

NSAIDs are drugs that inhibit the enzyme cyclooxygenase. Nonselective cyclooxygenase inhibitors, including aspirin, are effective at reducing inflammation and pain but cause significant GI adverse effects in some patients.

24.5   Glucocorticoids are effective in treating severe inflammation.

Glucocorticoids are hormones that are extremely effective at reducing inflammation. Because overtreatment with these drugs can cause Cushing's syndrome, glucocorticoid therapy for inflammation is generally short term.

24.6   The immune response results from activation of the humoral and cell-mediated immune systems.

B cells become plasma cells and secrete large quantities of antibodies. The antibodies are specific to the antigen and neutralize the foreign agent or destroy it. Some B cells remember the antigen for many years. T cells also recognize specific antigens, but instead of producing antibodies, they produce cytokines, some of which rid the body of the foreign agent. Memory B and T cells remember the antigen for many years and mount a faster immune response on subsequent exposures.

24.7   Vaccines are biological agents used to prevent illness.

Vaccines are usually given to prevent a serious infectious disease. Vaccines may be live, attenuated, or toxoids. They are effective when taken according to schedule and rarely produce serious adverse effects.

24.8   Biologic response modifiers are used to boost the immune response.

Several drugs are available to boost a patient's immune function. Interleukins, interferons, and other agents enhance the body's natural defenses, primarily in the pharmacotherapy of cancer.

24.9   Immunosuppressants are primarily used to avoid tissue rejection following organ transplant.

For an organ or tissue transplant to be successful, the patient's immune system must be suppressed following surgery. Immunosuppressants are effective at lessening the immune response but must be monitored carefully because loss of immune function can lead to infections and cancer.

REVIEW QUESTIONS

The following questions are written in NCLEX-PN® style. Answer these questions to assess your knowledge of the chapter material, and go back and review any material that is not clear to you.

1. A patient is getting ready to go home from the hospital and the health care provider and patient are discussing the types of over-the-counter NSAID medications that are available. The health care provider states that an OTC medication that is not classified as an NSAID is:

1. Aspirin
2. Ibuprofen
3. Acetaminophen
4. Motrin

2. The patient has been taking aspirin for several days for headache. While assessing the patient, the health care provider discovers that the patient is experiencing ringing in the ears and dizziness. The most appropriate action by the nurse is:

1. To question the patient about history of sinus infection
2. To determine if the patient has mixed the aspirin with other medications
3. To tell the patient not to take any more aspirin
4. To tell the patient to take the aspirin with food or milk

3. The most common adverse effect of NSAIDs is:

1. Edema
2. Rash
3. GI upset
4. Bleeding

4. The patient taking glucocorticoids is at risk for:

1. Bleeding
2. Respiratory distress
3. Dehydration
4. Infection

5. The patient with diabetes taking prednisone states that his blood sugar is higher than normal. The health care provider's most appropriate response would be:

1. "You must not be following your diet for diabetes."
2. "Prednisone can cause blood sugar levels to increase."
3. "You must be developing an illness."
4. "Your diabetes must be getting worse."

6. Which type of immunity occurs when the patient's immune system is stimulated to produce antibodies after exposure to a vaccine?

1. Passive
2. Attenuated
3. Live
4. Active

7. The patient on immunosuppressants must be assessed for:

1. Hyperglycemia
2. Infection
3. Hypoglycemia
4. Bleeding

8. Cytokines:

1. Produce antibodies
2. Are memory cells
3. Can rid the body of foreign agents
4. Reduce inflammation

9. Which of the following statements by a patient taking cyclosporine (Neoral, Sandimmune) would indicate the need for more teaching?

1. "I will report any reduction in urine output to my health care provider."
2. "I will wash my hands frequently."
3. "I will take my blood pressure at home every day."
4. "I will take my cyclosporine at breakfast with a glass of grapefruit juice."

10. The health care provider should monitor a transplant patient for the major adverse effect of cyclosporine (Neoral, Sandimmune) therapy by assessing which of the following laboratory tests?

1. CBC
2. Serum creatinine
3. Liver enzymes
4. Electrolytes

CASE STUDY QUESTIONS

For questions 1–4, please refer to the following case study, and choose the correct answer from choices 1–4.

*M*rs. Greene, 50 years old, has been experiencing a gradual increase in pain and swelling of her hands. Her knuckles have also become red and warm to the touch. She enjoys gardening and playing tennis, but over the last 6 months she has not been able to participate in these activities because it is "too painful." Mrs. Greene has been treating herself with NSAIDs, specifically ibuprofen and Naprosyn.

1. Regarding Mrs. Greene's use of NSAIDs, what question should you ask to determine potential adverse effects?

1. "Have you experienced excessive drowsiness?"
2. "Have you experienced GI upset?"
3. "Have you experienced excessive dryness or stinging sensations in your nose?"
4. "Have you experienced any rashes or dryness of the skin?"

2. To help Mrs. Greene alleviate the adverse effects of NSAIDs, the nurse would advise her to:

1. Take NSAIDs with food
2. Take NSAIDs on an empty stomach

3. Take both types of NSAIDs at the same time. It is okay.
4. There are no adverse effects of most NSAIDs

3. Mrs. Greene is diagnosed with rheumatoid arthritis. She experiences a "flare-up" (acute exacerbation) of her disease. Because Mrs. Greene has experienced a "flare-up" of her condition, which of the following drug classes would likely be prescribed over a 10-day period?

1. Biologic response modifiers
2. Intranasal glucocorticoids
3. Systemic glucocorticoids
4. Sympathomimetics

4. Her health care provider prescribes prednisone. Mrs. Greene asks why she was given this medication. The health care provider tells her that:

1. He just wanted to try something different
2. Prednisone markedly reduces inflammation and is beneficial for short-term use
3. Prednisone is used only for pain control
4. Prednisone has very few adverse effects, even when used for long periods

FURTHER STUDY

- Drug therapy for anaphylaxis is discussed in Chapter 22 ∞.

- The analgesic action of NSAIDs and the basic pharmacology of aspirin are presented in Chapter 14 ∞.

- Chapter 31 ∞ presents details of glucocorticoids in treating hormonal imbalances.

- Chapter 28 ∞ discusses the use of prednisone to stop acute bronchospasm in asthma; Chapter 27 ∞ details its use in the treatment of certain cancers.

PEARSON
EXPLORE mynursingkit™

MyNursingKit is your one stop for online chapter review materials and resources. Prepare for success with additional NCLEX®-style practice questions, interactive assignments and activities, web links, animations and videos, and more!

Register your access code from the front of your book at
www.mynursingkit.com

25 Drugs for Bacterial Infections

CORE CONCEPTS

25.1 Pathogens are organisms that cause disease by invading tissues or secreting toxins.

25.2 Anti-infective drugs are classified by their chemical structures or by their mechanisms of action.

25.3 Anti-infective drugs act by selectively targeting a pathogen's metabolism or life cycle.

25.4 Acquired resistance is a major clinical problem that is worsened by improper use of anti-infectives.

25.5 Careful selection of the correct antibiotic is essential for effective pharmacotherapy and to limit adverse effects.

25.6 The penicillins are one of the oldest and safest groups of anti-infectives.

25.7 The cephalosporins are similar in structure and function to the penicillins and are one of the most widely prescribed anti-infective classes.

25.8 The tetracyclines have broad spectrums but are drugs of choice for few diseases.

25.9 The macrolides are safe alternatives to penicillin for many infections.

25.10 The aminoglycosides are narrow-spectrum drugs that have the potential to cause serious toxicity.

25.11 Fluoroquinolones have wide clinical applications because of their broad spectrum of activity and relative safety.

25.12 Sulfonamides are traditional drugs of choice for urinary tract infections.

25.13 A number of additional anti-infectives have distinct mechanisms of action and specific indications.

25.14 The pharmacotherapy of tuberculosis requires special dosing regimens and schedules.

DRUG SNAPSHOT

The following drugs are discussed in this chapter:

DRUG CLASSES	DRUG PROFILES
Penicillins	**Pr** penicillin G Sodium/ Potassium
Cephalosporins	**Pr** cefotaxime (Claforan)
Tetracyclines	**Pr** tetracycline (Sumycin, others)
Macrolides	**Pr** erythromycin (E-Mycin, Erythrocin)
Aminoglycosides	**Pr** gentamicin

DRUG CLASSES	DRUG PROFILES
Fluoroquinolones	**Pr** ciprofloxacin (Cipro)
Sulfonamides	**Pr** trimethoprim-sulfamethoxazole (Bactrim, Septra)
Miscellaneous antibacterials	**Pr** vancomycin (Vancocin)
Antitubercular agents	**Pr** isoniazid (INH, Nydrazid)

LEARNING OUTCOMES

After reading this chapter, the student should be able to:

1. Distinguish between the terms pathogenicity and virulence.

2. Explain how bacteria are described and classified.

3. Compare and contrast the terms bacteriostatic and bacteriocidal.

4. Using a specific example, explain how resistance can develop to an anti-infective drug.

5. Explain the importance of culture and sensitivity testing to anti-infective chemotherapy.

6. Identify the mechanism of development and symptoms of superinfections caused by anti-infective therapy.

7. For each of the classes in the Drug Snapshot, identify representative drugs and explain the mechanisms of drug action, primary actions, and important adverse effects.

8. Explain how the pharmacotherapy of tuberculosis differs from that of other infections.

KEY TERMS

acquired resistance *410*

antagonism *412*

antibiotic (ann-tie-bye-OT-ik) *409*

anti-infective (ann-tie-in-FEK-tive) *409*

bacteriocidal (bak-teer-ee-oh-SY-dall) *409*

bacteriostatic (bak-teer-ee-oh-STAT-ik) *409*

beta-lactamase/penicillinase (bay-tuh-LAK-tam-ace/pen-uh-SILL-in-ace) *412*

beta-lactam ring (bay-tuh LAK-tam) *412*

broad-spectrum antibiotic *412*

chemoprophylaxis (kee-moh-pro-fill-AX-is) *411*

culture and sensitivity (C&S) testing *412*

host flora (host FLOR-uh) *412*

mutations (myou-TAY-shuns) *409*

narrow-spectrum antibiotic *412*

nephrotoxicity (NEF-row-toks-ISS-ih-tee) *420*

nosocomial infections (noh-soh-KOH-mee-ul) *410*

ototoxicity (OH-toh-toks-ISS-ih-tee) *420*

pathogen (PATH-oh-jen) *407*

pathogenicity (path-oh-jen-ISS-ih-tee) *407*

photosensitivity *417*

plasmids (PLAZ-mid) *410*

red-man syndrome *424*

superinfections *412*

toxins (TOX-in) *408*

tubercles (TOO-burr-kyouls) *426*

virulence (VEER-you-lens) *407*

The human body has adapted quite well to living in a world teeming with microorganisms (microbes). Present in the air, water, food, and soil, microbes are an essential component to life on the planet. In some cases, microorganisms such as those in the colon play a beneficial role in human health. When in an unnatural environment or when present in unusually high numbers, however, microorganisms can cause a variety of ailments ranging from mildly annoying to fatal. The development of the first anti-infective drugs in the mid-1900s was a milestone in the field of medicine. In the last 60 years, pharmacologists have attempted to keep pace with microbes that rapidly become resistant to therapeutic agents. This chapter examines two groups of anti-infectives: the antibacterial agents and the specialized drugs used to treat tuberculosis.

Fast Facts Bacterial Infections

■ Infectious diseases are the third most common cause of death in the United States and the most common cause of death worldwide.

■ Foodborne illness is responsible for 76 million illnesses, 300,000 hospitalizations, and 5,000 deaths each year. About 500 people die of food poisoning each year in the United States.

■ Urinary tract infections (UTIs) are the most common infection acquired in hospitals. Nearly all are associated with the insertion of a urinary catheter. Hospital-acquired urinary infections add an average of 3.8 days to a hospital stay and can cost over $3,800 per infection.

■ More than 2 million nosocomial infections are acquired each year. These infections add 1 day for UTI, 7 to 8 days for surgical site infections, and 6 to 30 days for pneumonia.

■ Up to 30% of all *Streptococcus pneumoniae* found in some areas of the United States are resistant to penicillin.

■ Nearly all strains of *Staphylococcus aureus* in the United States are resistant to penicillin.

■ About 73,000 cases of *Escherichia coli* poisoning are reported annually in the United States, with the most common source being ground beef.

Pathogens are organisms that cause disease by invading tissues or secreting toxins.

An organism that can cause disease in humans is called a **pathogen**. Human pathogens include viruses, bacteria, fungi, unicellular organisms (protozoans), and multicellular animals. Examples of these pathogens are illustrated in Figure 25.1 ■. To infect humans, pathogens must bypass a number of elaborate body defenses, such as those described in Chapter 24 ⌾. Pathogens may enter through broken skin, or by ingestion, inhalation, or contact with a mucous membrane such as the nasal, urinary, or vaginal mucosas.

path = *disease*
gen = *producing*

Some pathogens are extremely infectious and life threatening to humans, whereaas others simply cause annoying symptoms or none at all. The ability of an organism to cause infection is called its **pathogenicity**. Pathogenicity depends on an organism's ability to bypass or overcome the body's immune system. Fortunately for us, only a few dozen pathogens commonly cause disease in humans. Some of these are listed in Table 25.1. Another common word used to describe a pathogen is **virulence**. A highly virulent organism is one that can produce disease when present in very small numbers.

After gaining entry, pathogens generally cause disease by one of two basic mechanisms. Invasiveness is the ability of a pathogen to grow extremely rapidly and damage surrounding tissues

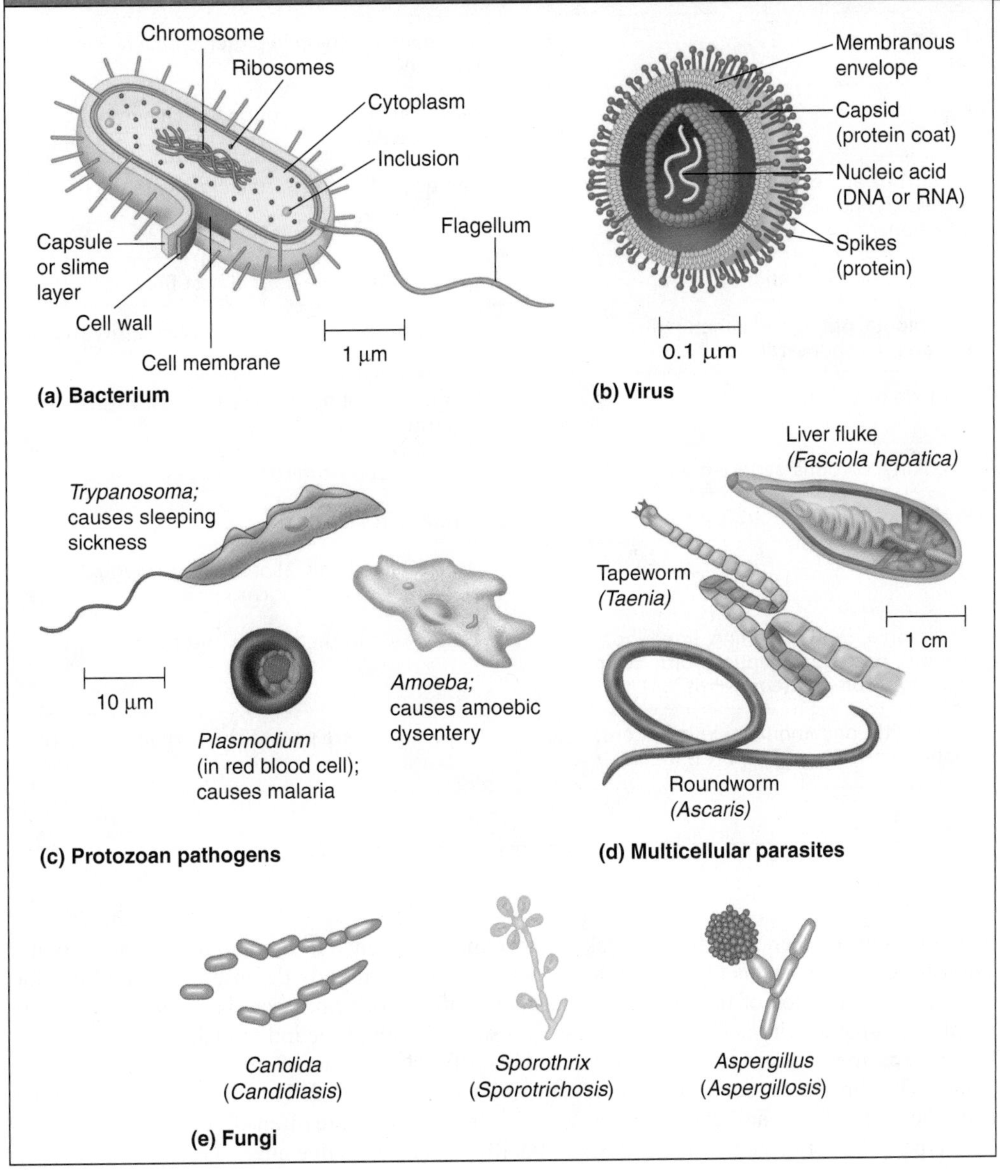

FIGURE 25.1

Types of pathogenic organisms: (a) bacterium; (b) virus; (c) protozoan pathogens; (d) multicellular parasites; (e) fungi   *Source: Reprinted by permission of Pearson Education, Inc., Upper Saddle River, NJ*

TABLE 25.1	Common Bacterial Pathogens	
NAME OF ORGANISM	**DISEASE(S)**	**REMARKS**
Bacillus anthracis	Anthrax	Aerobe; appears in cutaneous and respiratory forms
Borrelia burgdorferi	Lyme disease	Acquired from tick bites
Chlamydia trachomatis	Venereal disease, eye infection	Most common cause of sexually transmitted disease in the United States
Enterococcus	Wounds, UTI, endocarditis, bacteremia	Common opportunistic microbe, part of normal flora of the urogenital and intestinal tracts
Escherichia coli	Traveler's diarrhea, UTI, bacteremia, meningitis in children	Part of normal flora of the intestinal tract
Haemophilus	Pneumonia, meningitis in children, bacteremia, otitis media, sinusitis	Some species are part of the normal host flora of the upper respiratory tract
Klebsiella pneumoniae	Pneumonia, UTI	Common opportunistic microbe
Mycobacterium leprae	Leprosy	Most cases in the United States occur in immigrants from Africa or Asia
Mycobacterium tuberculosis	Tuberculosis	Incidence very high in patients infected with HIV
Mycoplasma pneumoniae	Pneumonia	Most common cause of pneumonia in patients ages 5 to 35
Neisseria gonorrhoeae	Gonorrhea and other sexually transmitted diseases, endometriosis, neonatal eye infection	Can be part of the normal host flora
Neisseria meningitidis	Meningitis in children	Can be part of the normal host flora
Pneumococcus	Pneumonia, otitis media, meningitis, bacteremia, endocarditis	Part of normal flora in upper respiratory tract
Proteus mirabilis	UTI, skin infections	Part of normal flora in the gastrointestinal (GI) tract
Pseudomonas aeruginosa	UTI, skin infections, septicemia	Common opportunistic microbe
Rickettsia rickettsii	Rocky Mountain spotted fever	Acquired from tick bites
Salmonella enteritidis	Food poisoning	From infected animal products, raw eggs, or undercooked meat or chicken
Staphylococcus aureus	Pneumonia, food poisoning, impetigo, wounds, bacteremia, endocarditis, toxic shock syndrome, osteomyelitis, UTI	Can be part of the normal host flora
Streptococcus	Pharyngitis, pneumonia, skin infections, septicemia, endocarditis, otitis media	Some species are part of the normal host flora

UTI = urinary tract infection

by their sheer numbers. Because a week or more may be needed to mount an immune response against the organism, this rapid growth can easily overwhelm body defenses. A second mechanism is the production of **toxins**. Even very small amounts of some bacterial toxins may disrupt normal cellular activity and, in extreme cases, result in death of the individual.

Several methods are used to describe and classify the millions of species of bacteria on the planet. The three most common methods are shown in Table 25.2. Health care providers must learn these organizational schemes because anti-infective drugs are often effective only for a specific type of bacteria, such as gram-positive bacilli or gram-negative anaerobes.

TABLE 25.2	Methods of Describing and Classifying Bacteria
METHOD	**DESCRIPTION**
Staining	Gram positive or gram negative
Shape	Bacilli (rods), cocci (spheres), and spirilla (spirals)
Ability to use O_2	Aerobic (uses O_2) or anaerobic grows (without O_2)

Anti-infective drugs are classified by their chemical structures or by their mechanisms of action.

CORE CONCEPT 25.2

Anti-infective is a general term that applies to any drug that is effective against pathogens. In its broadest sense, an anti-infective drug may be used to treat bacterial, fungal, viral, or parasitic infections. The most frequent term used to describe an anti-infective drug is *antibiotic*. Technically, **antibiotic** refers to a natural substance produced by bacteria that can kill other bacteria. In clinical practice, however, the terms *antibacterial, anti-infective, antimicrobial,* and *antibiotic* are often used interchangeably.

anti = *against*
bio = *life*
ic = *pertaining to*

With more than 300 anti-infective drugs available, it is helpful to group these drugs into classes that have similar properties. Two means of grouping are widely used: chemical classes and pharmacologic classes.

Chemical class names such as aminoglycosides, fluoroquinolones, and sulfonamides refer to the fundamental chemical structure of the anti-infectives. Anti-infectives belonging to the same chemical class usually share similar antibacterial properties and adverse effects. Although chemical names are often long and difficult to pronounce, placing drugs into chemical classes will assist the student in mentally organizing these drugs into distinct therapeutic groups.

Pharmacologic classes are used to group anti-infectives by their *mechanism of action*. Examples include cell wall inhibitors, protein synthesis inhibitors, folic acid inhibitors, and reverse trancriptase inhibitors. These classifications are used in this text, where appropriate.

Anti-infective drugs act by selectively targeting a pathogen's metabolism or life cycle.

CORE CONCEPT 25.3

The primary goal of antimicrobial therapy is to assist the body's defenses in eliminating a pathogen. Drugs that accomplish this goal by *killing* bacteria are called **bacteriocidal**. Some medications do not kill the bacteria but instead *slow their growth,* allowing the body's natural defenses to eliminate the microorganisms. These growth-slowing drugs are called **bacteriostatic**.

bacteria = *bacteria*
cidal = *killing*
static = *staying the same*

Bacterial cells are quite different from human cells. Bacteria have cell walls and contain certain enzymes that human cells lack. Antibiotics exert selective toxicity on bacterial cells by targeting these unique differences. Through this selective action, pathogens can be killed or their growth severely hampered without major effects on human cells. Of course there are limits to this selective toxicity, depending on the specific antibiotic and the dose used, and adverse effects can be expected from all the anti-infectives. The basic mechanisms of action of antimicrobial drugs are shown in Figure 25.2 ■.

Acquired resistance is a major clinical problem that is worsened by improper use of anti-infectives.

CORE CONCEPT 25.4

Microorganisms have the ability to replicate extremely rapidly. For example, under ideal conditions *E. coli* can produce a million cells every 20 minutes. During this rapid replication, bacteria make frequent errors, or **mutations**, while duplicating their genetic code. These mutations occur spontaneously and randomly in the bacterial cell. Although most mutations are harmful to the organism, mutations occasionally result in a bacterial cell that has reproductive advantages over its neighbors. The mutated bacterium may be able to survive in harsher conditions or perhaps grow faster than surrounding cells. One such mutation of particular importance to medicine is that which confers drug resistance on a microorganism.

Antibiotics help promote the appearance of drug-resistant bacterial strains by killing the masses of bacteria that are sensitive to the drug. Consequently, the only bacteria remaining are

FIGURE 25.2

Mechanisms of action
of antimicrobial drugs

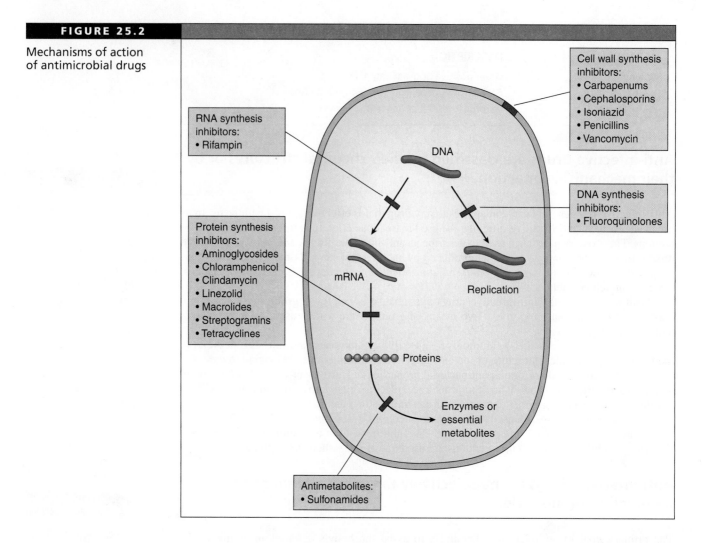

RNA synthesis
inhibitors:
• Rifampin

Cell wall synthesis
inhibitors:
• Carbapenums
• Cephalosporins
• Isoniazid
• Penicillins
• Vancomycin

DNA

Protein synthesis
inhibitors:
• Aminoglycosides
• Chloramphenicol
• Clindamycin
• Linezolid
• Macrolides
• Streptogramins
• Tetracyclines

DNA synthesis
inhibitors:
• Fluoroquinolones

mRNA

Replication

Proteins

Enzymes or
essential
metabolites

Antimetabolites:
• Sulfonamides

those microbes that possess mutations that make them *insensitive* to the effects of the antibiotic. These drug-resistant bacteria are then free to grow unrestrained by their neighbors that were killed by the antibiotic. Soon the patient develops an infection that is resistant to conventional drug therapy. This phenomenon, called **acquired resistance**, is illustrated in Figure 25.3 ■. Bacteria may pass the resistance gene to other bacteria by transferring small pieces of circular DNA called **plasmids**.

The widespread and sometimes unwarranted use of antibiotics has led to many resistant strains. For example, 60% of all *Staphylococcus* bacteria are now resistant to penicillin. The longer an antibiotic is used in the population and the more often it is prescribed, the larger will be the percentage of resistant strains. Infections acquired in a hospital or other health care setting, called **nosocomial infections**, are often resistant to common antibiotics. Two particularly serious resistant infections are those caused by methicillin-resistant *Staphylococcus aureus* (MRSA) and vancomycin-resistant enterococci (VRE).

Health care providers play important roles in delaying the emergence of resistance. The following are four principles recommended by the Centers for Disease Control and Prevention (CDC):

■ Prevent infections whenever possible. It is always easier to prevent an infection than to treat one. This includes teaching the patient the importance of getting immunizations.

■ Restrict the use of antibiotics to those conditions deemed medically necessary. Antibiotics should be prescribed only when there is a clear rationale for their use.

■ Advise the patient to take anti-infectives for the full length of therapy, even if symptoms disappear before the regimen is finished. Prematurely stopping antibiotic therapy allows some pathogens to survive, thus promoting the development of resistant strains.

FIGURE 25.3
Acquired resistance

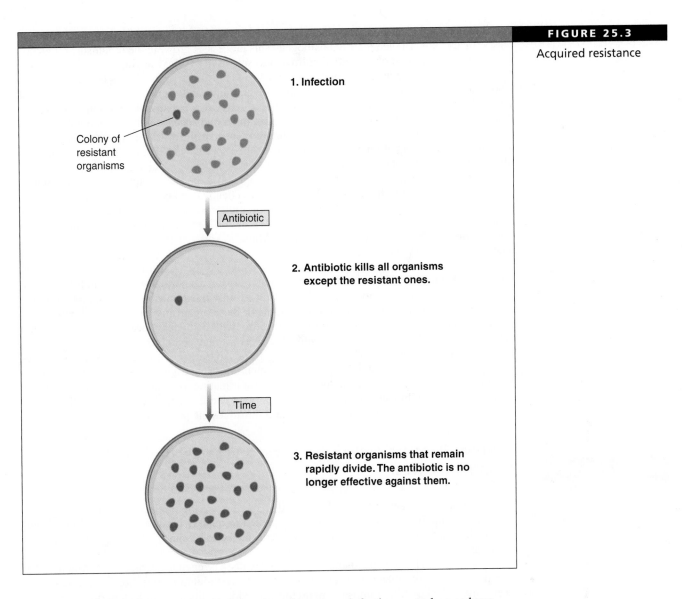

1. Infection

Colony of resistant organisms

Antibiotic

2. Antibiotic kills all organisms except the resistant ones.

Time

3. Resistant organisms that remain rapidly divide. The antibiotic is no longer effective against them.

■ Prevent transmission of the pathogen by using proper infection control procedures. This includes the use of standard precautions and teaching patients methods of proper hygiene for preventing transmission in the home and community settings.

In most cases, antibiotics are given when there is clear evidence of bacterial infection. Some patients, however, receive antibiotics to *prevent* an infection, a practice called *prophylactic use,* or **chemoprophylaxis**. Examples of patients who might receive prophylactic antibiotics include those who have suppressed immune systems, have experienced deep puncture wounds such as dog bites, and have prosthetic heart valves and are about to undergo medical or dental surgery.

Careful selection of the correct antibiotic is essential for effective pharmacotherapy and to limit adverse effects.

CORE CONCEPT 25.5

Selection of an antibiotic that will be effective against a specific pathogen is an important task of the health care provider. Selecting an incorrect drug will delay proper treatment, giving the microorganisms more time to invade. Prescribing ineffective antibiotics also promotes the development of resistance and may cause unnecessary adverse effects in the patient.

Ideally, laboratory tests should be conducted to identify the organism prior to beginning antiinfective therapy. Laboratory tests may include examination of body specimens such as urine, sputum, blood, or pus for microorganisms. Organisms isolated from the specimens are grown in the laboratory and identified. The laboratory then tests several antibiotics to determine which is most effective against the identified pathogen. This process of growing the organism and identifying the effective antibiotic is called **culture and sensitivity (C&S) testing**.

Ideally, the pathogen should be identified *before* anti-infective therapy is begun. However, laboratory testing and identification may take several days and, in the case of viruses, several weeks. If the infection is severe, therapy is often begun with a **broad-spectrum antibiotic**, one that is effective against a wide variety of different microbial species. After laboratory testing is completed, the drug may be changed to a **narrow-spectrum antibiotic**, one that is effective against a smaller group of microbes or only the isolated species. In general, narrow-spectrum antibiotics have less effect on normal host flora, thus causing fewer adverse effects.

In most cases, anti-infective therapy uses a single drug, because combining two antibiotics may actually decrease each drug's effectiveness. This phenomenon is known as **antagonism**. Use of multiple antibiotics also has the potential to promote resistance. Multidrug therapy is warranted, however, if the patient's infection is caused by different organisms or if therapy must be started before C&S testing has been completed. Multidrug therapy is common in the treatment of tuberculosis and HIV infection.

One common adverse effect of anti-infective therapy is the appearance of secondary infections, called **superinfections**, that occur when microorganisms normally present in the body are killed by the drug. These normal microorganisms, or **host flora**, inhabit the skin and the upper respiratory, urogenital, and intestinal tracts. Some of these organisms serve a useful purpose by producing antibacterial substances and by competing with pathogenic organisms for space and nutrients. Removal of host flora by an antibiotic gives pathogenic microorganisms space to grow or allows for overgrowth of nonaffected normal flora. Appearance of a new infection while receiving anti-infective therapy is suspicious of a superinfection. Signs and symptoms of a superinfection may include diarrhea, bladder pain, painful urination, or abnormal vaginal discharges. Broad-spectrum antibiotics are more likely to cause superinfections because they kill so many different species of microorganisms. Figure 25.3 illustrates the production of a superinfection.

The penicillins are one of the oldest and safest groups of anti-infectives.

CORE CONCEPT 25.6

Although not the first anti-infective discovered, penicillin was the first *mass-produced* antibiotic. Isolated from the fungus *Penicillium* in 1941, penicillin quickly became a miracle drug by preventing thousands of deaths from what are now considered to be minor infections. The penicillins are listed in Table 25.3.

Penicillins kill bacteria by disrupting their cell walls. The chemical structure of penicillin that is responsible for its antibacterial activity is called the **beta-lactam ring**. Some bacteria secrete an enzyme, called **beta-lactamase** or **penicillinase**, which splits the beta-lactam ring. This structural change allows these bacteria to become resistant to the effects of most penicillins. The action of penicillinase is illustrated in Figure 25.4 ■. Since their discovery, large numbers of resistant bacterial strains that limit the therapeutic usefulness of the penicillins have emerged.

Chemical modifications to the natural penicillin molecule produced drugs offering several advantages.

- *Penicillinase-resistant penicillins*   Oxacillin and cloxacillin (Cloxapen) are examples of drugs that are effective against penicillinase-producing bacteria. These are sometimes called antistaphylococcal penicillins.

- *Broad-spectrum penicillins*   Ampicillin (Principen) and amoxicillin (Amoxil, Trimox) are effective against a wide range of microorganisms and are called *broad-spectrum* penicillins. These are sometimes referred to as aminopenicillins.

- *Extended-spectrum penicillins*   Carbenicillin (Geocillin) and piperacillin are effective against even more microbial species than the aminopenicillins, including *Pseudomonas*, *Enterobacter*, *Klebsiella*, and *Bacteroides fragilis*.

Several drugs are available that inhibit the bacterial beta-lactamase enzyme. When combined with a penicillin, these agents protect the penicillin molecule from destruction, extending its spectrum of activity. The three beta-lactamase inhibitors—clavulanate, sulbactam, and tazobactam—are only available in fixed-dose combinations with specific penicillins. These include Augmentin (amoxicillin plus clavulanate), Timentin (ticarcillin plus clavulanate), Unasyn (ampicillin plus sulbactam), and Zosyn (piperacillin plus tazobactam).

TABLE 25.3 — Penicillins

DRUG	ROUTE AND ADULT DOSE	REMARKS
amoxicillin (Amoxil, Trimox)	PO; 250–500 mg tid	Broad spectrum; IV form available; amoxicillin plus clavulanate is called Augmentin
ampicillin (Principen)	PO; 250–500 mg qid	Broad spectrum; IM and IV forms available
bacampicillin (Spectrobid)	PO; 400–800 mg bid	Broad spectrum
carbenicillin (Geocillin)	PO; 382–764 mg qid	Extended spectrum; IM and IV forms available
cloxacillin (Cloxapen)	PO; 250–500 mg qid	Penicillinase resistant
dicloxacillin	PO; 125–500 mg qid	Penicillinase resistant
nafcillin	PO; 250 mg–1 g qid (max: 12 g/day)	Penicillinase resistant; IM and IV forms available
oxacillin	PO; 250 mg–1 g qid (max: 12 g/day)	Penicillinase resistant; IV and IM forms available
penicillin G benzathine (Bicillin)	IM; 1.2 million units as a single dose	Prolonged duration of action
penicillin G procaine (Wycillin)	IM; 600,000–1.2 million units daily	Prolonged duration of action
Pr penicillin G sodium/potassium	PO; 2–24 million units divided every 4–6 hours	IM and IV forms available; ineffective against most forms of S. aureus
penicillin V (Pen-Vee K, Veetids, Vee-Cillin-K)	PO; 125–250 mg qid	Acid stable
piperacillin	IM; 2–4 g tid–qid (max: 24 g/day)	Extended spectrum
piperacillin/tazobactam (Zosyn)	IV; 3.375 g qid over 30 min	Extended spectrum
ticarcillin (Ticar)	IM; 1–2 g qid (max: 24 g/day)	Extended spectrum

FIGURE 25.4 — Action of penicillinase

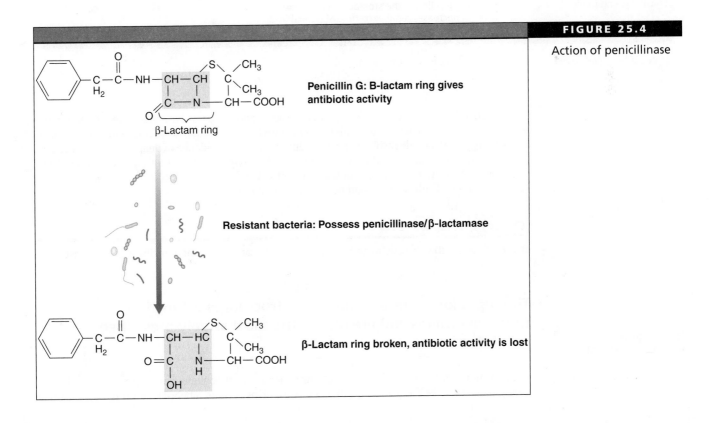

Penicillin G: B-lactam ring gives antibiotic activity

β-Lactam ring

Resistant bacteria: Possess penicillinase/β-lactamase

β-Lactam ring broken, antibiotic activity is lost

NATURAL THERAPIES

The Antibacterial Properties of Goldenseal

Goldenseal (*Hydrastis canadensis*) was once a common plant found in woods in the eastern and midwestern United States. As word spread of its medicinal properties, the plant was harvested to near extinction. In particular, goldenseal was reported to mask the appearance of drugs in the urine of patients wanting to hide their drug abuse. This claim has been proven false.

The roots and leaves of goldenseal are dried and available as capsules, tablets, salves, and tinctures. One of the primary ingredients in goldenseal is hydrastine, which is reported to have antibacterial and antifungal properties. When used topically or locally, it is claimed to be of value in treating bacterial and fungal skin infections and oral conditions such as gingivitis and thrush. Other possible indications include hypertension, duodenal ulcers, and conjunctivitis.

DRUG PROFILE: ℗ *Penicillin G Sodium/Potassium*

Therapeutic Class: Antibacterial
Pharmacologic Class: Cell wall inhibitor, natural penicillin

Actions and Uses:

Similar to penicillin V, penicillin G is sometimes a drug of first choice against *streptococcal, pneumococci,* and *staphylococcal* organisms that do not produce penicillinase and are shown to be susceptible by C&S testing. It is also a preferred drug for gonorrhea and syphilis caused by susceptible strains. Penicillin V is more acid stable; over 70% is absorbed after an oral dose compared to the 15% to 30% from penicillin G. Because of its low oral absorption, penicillin G is often given by the IV or IM routes. Penicillinase-producing organisms inactivate both penicillin G and penicillin V.

Adverse Effects and Interactions:

Penicillin G has few adverse effects. Although not serious, diarrhea, nausea, and vomiting are the most common adverse effects. Anaphylaxis is the most serious adverse effect, although its incidence is very low. Pain at the injection site may occur, and superinfections are possible.

Penicillin G may decrease the effectiveness of oral contraceptives. Colestipol decreases absorption of penicillin G. Potassium-sparing diuretics may cause hyperkalemia with penicillin G. Food increases the breakdown of penicillin in the stomach. Probenecid decreases renal excretion of penicillin G.

Mechanism in Action:

Penicillin G is a narrow-spectrum antibiotic that attaches to the penicillin-binding protein (PBP) at the active site of selected bacterial cell walls. Following attachment, penicillin G prevents the synthesis of new peptide bridges, causing fragmentation of the peptidoglycan cell wall matrix. Death of the bacterium soon follows.

 Refer to MyNursingKit for a Nursing Process Focus specific to this drug.

In general, the adverse effects of penicillins are minor, and this has contributed to their widespread use for more than 60 years. Allergy is the most common adverse effect. Symptoms of penicillin allergy may include rash, fever, and anaphylaxis. The incidence of anaphylaxis is quite low, ranging from 0.04% to 2%. Allergy to one penicillin increases the risk of allergy to other drugs in the same class. Other less common adverse effects of the penicillins include skin rashes and lowered red blood cell, white blood cell, or platelet counts.

Concept Review 25.1

■ Why does antibiotic resistance become more of a problem when antibiotics are prescribed too often?

CORE CONCEPT 25.7

The cephalosporins are similar in structure and function to the penicillins and are one of the most widely prescribed anti-infective classes.

Isolated shortly after the penicillins, the four generations of cephalosporins comprise the largest antibiotic class. Like the penicillins, the cephalosporins contain a beta-lactam ring that is primarily responsible for their antimicrobial activity. The cephalosporins are bacteriocidal and inhibit bacterial cell wall synthesis. Table 25.4 lists the cephalosporins and their dosages.

More than 20 cephalosporins are available, all having similar sounding names that can challenge even the best memory. They are classified by their "generation." The first-generation drugs contain a beta-lactam ring, and bacteria producing beta-lactamase will normally be resistant to these agents. The second-generation cephalosporins are more potent and more resistant to beta-lactamase and exhibit a broader spectrum than the first-generation drugs. The third-generation cephalosporins generally have a longer duration of action, an even broader spectrum, and are resistant to beta-lactamases. Third-generation cephalosporins are preferred drugs against infections by *Pseudomonas, Klebsiella, Neisseria, Salmonella, Proteus,* and *Haemophilus influenzae.* Newer, fourth-generation drugs are more effective against organisms that have developed resistance to earlier cephalosporins. There are not always clear distinctions among the generations.

The primary therapeutic use of the cephalosporins is for gram-negative infections and for patients who cannot tolerate the less expensive penicillins. Like the penicillins, allergic reactions are the most common adverse effect. Skin rashes are a common sign of allergy and may appear several days following the initiation of therapy. GI complaints are common. Earlier generation cephalosporins exhibited kidney toxicity, but this is diminished with the newer drugs. The nurse must be aware that some patients (5% to 10%) who are allergic to penicillin will also be allergic to cephalosporins. Despite this small incidence of cross allergy, cephalosporins offer a reasonable alternative for *most* patients who are unable to take penicillins. However, cephalosporins are contraindicated if the patient has previously experienced a *severe* allergic reaction to a penicillin.

TABLE 25.4	Selected Cephalosporins	
DRUG	**ROUTE AND ADULT DOSE**	**REMARKS**
FIRST GENERATION		
cefadroxil (Duricef)	PO; 500 mg–1 g once or twice daily (max: 2 g/day)	Binds to bacterial cell walls; bacteriocidal
cefazolin (Ancef, Kefzol)	IM; 250 mg–2 g tid (max: 12 g/day)	IV form available
cephalexin (Keflex)	PO; 250–500 mg qid	Binds to bacterial cell walls; bacteriocidal; broad spectrum
SECOND GENERATION		
cefaclor (Ceclor)	PO; 250–500 mg tid	Binds to bacterial cell walls; extended-release form available; bacteriocidal
cefotetan (Cefotan)	IM; 1–2 g every 12 hours	IV form available
cefprozil (Cefzil)	PO; 250–500 mg once or twice daily	Binds to bacterial cell walls; bacteriocidal
cefuroxime (Ceftin, Zinacef)	PO; 250–500 mg bid	Binds to bacterial cell walls; IM and IV forms available; bacteriocidal
THIRD AND FOURTH GENERATIONS		
cefdinir (Omnicef)	PO; 300 mg bid	Third generation; broad spectrum
cefditoren (Spectracef)	PO; 400 mg bid for 10 days	Third generation
cefepime (Maxipime)	IM; 0.5–1 g bid (max: 3 g/day)	Fourth generation; IV form available
cefixime (Suprax)	PO; 400 mg daily or 200 mg bid	Third generation; binds to bacterial cell walls; bacteriocidal
(Pr) cefotaxime (Claforan)	IM; 1–2 g bid–tid (max: 12 g/day)	Third generation; binds to bacterial cell walls; bacteriocidal; IV form available
ceftriaxone (Rocephin)	IM; 1–2 g once or twice daily (max: 4 g/day)	Third generation; binds to bacterial cell walls; IV form also available; bacteriocidal

---

DRUG PROFILE: ℞ *Cefotaxime (Claforan)*

Therapeutic Class: Antibacterial
Pharmacologic Class: Cell wall inhibitor; third-generation cephalosporin

Actions and Uses:

Cefotaxime is a third-generation cephalosporin with a broad spectrum of activity against gram-negative organisms. It is effective against many organisms that have developed resistance to earlier-generation cephalosporins and to other classes of anti-infectives. Cefotaxime exhibits bacteriocidal activity by inhibiting cell wall synthesis. It is prescribed for serious infections of the lower respiratory tract, central nervous system (CNS), urogenital system, bones, and joints. It may also be used for blood infections such as bacteremia or septicemia. Like many of the cephalosporins, cefotaxime is not absorbed from the GI tract and must be given by the IM or IV routes.

Adverse Effects and Interactions:

For most patients, cefotaxime and the other cephalosporins are safe medications. Hypersensitivity is the most common adverse effect, although symptoms may include only a minor rash and itching. Anaphylaxis is possible; thus, the health care provider should be alert for this reaction. GI-related adverse effects such as diarrhea, vomiting, and nausea may occur. Some patients experience considerable pain at the injection site.

Probenecid decreases elimination by the kidneys. Alcohol interacts with cefotaxime to produce a disulfiram–like reaction. Cefotaxime interacts with nonsteroidal anti-inflammatory drugs (NSAIDs) to cause an increase in platelet inhibition.

Refer to MyNursingKit for a Nursing Process Focus specific to this drug.

CORE CONCEPT 25.8

The tetracyclines have broad spectrums but are drugs of choice for few diseases.

The first tetracyclines were extracted from *Streptomyces* soil microorganisms in 1948. Their widespread use in the 1950s and 1960s has resulted in a large number of resistant bacterial strains that now limits their therapeutic usefulness. Table 25.5 lists the tetracyclines and their dosages.

Tetracyclines exert a bacteriostatic effect by inhibiting bacterial protein synthesis. They are effective against a wide range of gram-negative and gram-positive organisms and have one of the broadest spectrums of any class of antibiotics. They are drugs of first choice for relatively few diseases, including Rocky Mountain spotted fever, typhus, cholera, Lyme disease, ulcers caused by *Helicobacter pylori,* and *Chlamydia* infections. Drugs in this class are occasionally used for the treatment of acne vulgaris, for which they are given topically or PO at low doses. The newest tetracycline, tigecycline (Tygacil), was approved in 2005 to treat drug-resistant intra-abdominal infections and complicated skin infections, especially those caused by MRSA.

TABLE 25.5	Tetracyclines	
DRUG	**ROUTE AND ADULT DOSE**	**REMARKS**
demeclocycline (Declomycin)	PO; 150–300 mg bid–qid (max: 2.4 g/day)	Intermediate duration of action; broad spectrum
doxycycline (Vibramycin, others)	PO; 100 mg bid on day 1, then 100 mg daily (max: 200 mg/day)	Long duration of action; IV form available; subgingival form available for periodontitis
minocycline (Minocin, others)	PO; 200 mg as one dose followed by 100 mg bid	Long duration of action; IV form available; available as microsphere powder for periodontitis and as extended-release tablet for acne
℞ tetracycline (Sumycin)	PO; 250–500 mg bid–qid (max: 2 g/day)	Short acting; inhibits protein synthesis; bacteriostatic; IM and topical forms available
tigecycline (Tygacil)	IV; 100 mg, followed by 50 mg every 12 hours	Newest tetracycline; very limited indications

DRUG PROFILE: ℗ *Tetracycline (Sumycin, Others)*

Therapeutic Class: Antibacterial

Pharmacologic Class: Tetracycline, protein synthesis inhibitor

Actions and Uses:

Tetracycline is effective against many different microorganisms, including some protozoans. Its use has increased over the past decade due to its effectiveness against *H. pylori* in the treatment of peptic ulcer disease. It is given orally and has a short half-life. A topical preparation is available for treating acne. It should be administered 1–2 hours before or after meals to avoid drug interactions.

Adverse Effects and Interactions:

As a broad-spectrum antibiotic, tetracycline has a tendency to affect vaginal, oral, and intestinal flora and cause superinfections. Diarrhea may be severe enough to cause discontinuation of therapy. Other common adverse effects include nausea, vomiting, and photosensitivity.

Tetracycline can decrease the effectiveness of oral contraceptives, and thus alternative precautions should be taken during therapy to prevent pregnancy. Pregnant patients and those who are breastfeeding should not take tetracyclines because they are pregnancy category D medications.

Refer to MyNursingKit for a Nursing Process Focus specific to this drug.

The tetracyclines cause few serious adverse effects. Gastric distress is relatively common with tetracyclines, however, and patients tend to take tetracyclines *with* food. Patients should be urged *not* to drink milk with these medications because tetracyclines bind ions such as calcium and iron, thereby decreasing the drug's absorption by as much as 50%. Patients should be advised to avoid direct exposure to sunlight because tetracyclines can cause **photosensitivity**, which makes the skin particularly susceptible to sunburn. Unless suffering from a life-threatening infection, patients younger than 9 years are not given tetracyclines because these drugs may cause permanent yellow-brown teeth discoloration in young children. These drugs are pregnancy category D agents; tetracyclines should not be used during pregnancy. Because of their broad spectrum, the risk for superinfection is relatively high, and nurses should always be observant for signs of a secondary infection. Outdated tetracycline may deteriorate and become nephrotoxic; therefore, unused prescriptions should be discarded promptly.

The macrolides are safe alternatives to penicillin for many infections.

CORE CONCEPT 25.9

Erythromycin (E-Mycin, Erythrocin), the first macrolide antibiotic, was isolated from *Streptomcyes* in a soil sample in 1952. Macrolides are prescribed for infections that are resistant to penicillins. Commonly prescribed macrolides are listed in Table 25.6.

TABLE 25.6	Macrolides	
DRUG	**ROUTE AND ADULT DOSE**	**REMARKS**
azithromycin (Zithromax)	PO; 500 mg for one dose, then 250 mg daily for 4 days	Inhibits protein synthesis; bacteriostatic; IV form available
clarithromycin (Biaxin)	PO; 250–500 mg bid	Inhibits protein synthesis; bacteriostatic
dirithromycin (Dynabac)	PO; 500 mg daily	Should be taken with food to enhance its activity
℗ erythromycin (E-Mycin, Erythrocin)	PO; 250–500 mg qid or 333 mg tid	Bacteriostatic or bactericidal (E-Mycin, Erythrocin), depending on nature of organism and drug concentration; IV form available

DRUG PROFILE: ℗ *Erythromycin (E-Mycin, Erythrocin)*

Therapeutic Class: Antibacterial

Pharmacologic Class: Macrolide protein synthesis inhibitor

Actions and Uses:

Erythromycin is inactivated by stomach acid and is thus administered as coated tablets or capsules that dissolve in the small intestine. The drug's main application is for patients who are allergic to penicillins or who may have a penicillin-resistant infection. It is a preferred drug for infections by *Bordetella pertussis* (whooping cough), *Legionella pneumophila* (Legionnaire's disease), *M. pneumoniae,* and *Corynebacterium diphtheriae.*

Adverse Effects and Interactions:

The most common adverse effects from erythromycin are nausea, abdominal cramping, and vomiting, although these are rarely serious enough to cause discontinuation of therapy. Concurrent administration with food reduces these symptoms. Its spectrum of activity is similar to that of the penicillins.

Anesthetic agents and anticonvulsant drugs may interact to cause serum drug levels to rise and result in toxicity. This drug interacts with cyclosporine, increasing the risk for kidney toxicity. It may increase the effects of warfarin. The concurrent use of erythromycin with lovastatin or simvastatin is not recommended because it may increase the risk of muscle toxicity.

Refer to MyNursingKit for a Nursing Process Focus specific to this drug.

The macrolide antibiotics inhibit bacterial protein synthesis and may be either bacteriocidal or bacteriostatic, depending on the dose and the target organism. Macrolides are considered safe alternatives to penicillin, although they are drugs of first choice for relatively few infections. Common uses of macrolides include the treatment of whooping cough, Legionnaire's disease, and infections by *Streptococcus, H. influenzae, M. pneumoniae,* and *Chlamydia.* Clarithromycin is one of several antibiotics used to treat peptic ulcer disease.

The macrolides exhibit no serious adverse effects. Mild GI upset, diarrhea, and abdominal pain are the most common adverse effects. Because macrolides are broad-spectrum agents, patients should be observed for signs of superinfection. Like most of the older antibiotics, macrolide-resistant strains are becoming more common. Other than prior allergic reactions to macrolides, there are no contraindications to therapy.

The newer macrolides have a longer half-life and cause less GI irritation than erythromycin. For example, azithromycin (Zithromax) has such an extended half-life that it can be administered for only 5 days, rather the 10 days required for most antibiotics. The shorter duration of therapy is thought to increase patient adherence.

Concept Review 25.2

■ If penicillins are inexpensive, why might a physician prescribe a more expensive cephalosporin or macrolide antibiotic?

CORE CONCEPT 25.10

The aminoglycosides are narrow-spectrum drugs that have the potential to cause serious toxicity.

The aminoglycosides, first isolated from soil organisms in 1942, share a common chemical structure of an amino group (NH_2) and a sugar group. Although more toxic than most other antibiotic classes, they have important therapeutic applications for the treatment of a number of aerobic gram-negative bacteria, mycobacteria, and some protozoans. Table 25.7 lists the aminoglycosides and their dosages.

Aminoglycosides are bacteriocidal and act by inhibiting bacterial protein synthesis. They are normally reserved for serious aerobic gram-negative infections, including those caused by *E. coli, Serratia, Proteus, Klebsiella,* and *Pseudomonas.* When used for systemic bacterial infections, they

TABLE 25.7	Aminoglycosides	
DRUG	**ROUTE AND ADULT DOSE**	**REMARKS**
amikacin (Amikin)	IM; 5–7.5 mg/kg as a loading dose, then 7.5 mg/kg bid	Broader spectrum than others in this class; usually bacteriocidal; IV form available
Pr gentamicin	IM; 1.5–2 mg/kg as a loading dose, then 1–2 mg/kg bid–tid	IV, topical, and ophthalmic forms available
kanamycin (Kantrex)	IM; 5–7.5 mg/kg bid–tid	Also used to sterilize the bowel prior to colon surgery; oral, inhalation, and IV forms available
neomycin	PO; 4–12 g/day in divided doses	Oral, topical, and IV forms available
paromomycin (Humatin)	PO; 7.5–12.5 mg/kg tid	For parasitic infections of the intestine; also used to treat hepatic coma
streptomycin	IM; 15 mg/kg up to 1 g as a single dose	For tuberculosis, tularemia, and plague
tobramycin (Nebcin)	IM; 1 mg/kg tid (max: 5 mg/kg/day)	Most effective against *P. aeruginosa;* IV form available

are given parenterally because they are poorly absorbed from the GI tract. They are occasionally given orally to sterilize the bowel before intestinal surgery. Neomycin is available for topical infections of the skin, eyes, and ears. Paromomycin (Humatin) is given orally for the treatment of parasitic infections. The first aminoglycoside, streptomycin, was once widely prescribed, but its use is now limited to the treatment of tuberculosis due of the development of a large number of resistant strains. The student should note the differences in spelling of some of these drugs, from -*mycin* to -*micin*, which reflects the different organisms from which the drugs were originally isolated.

The clinical applications of the aminoglycosides are limited by their potential to cause serious adverse effects. The degree and types of potential toxicity are similar for all drugs in this class.

DRUG PROFILE: **Pr** *Gentamicin*

Therapeutic Class: Antibacterial
Pharmacologic Class: Aminoglycoside, protein synthesis inhibitor

Actions and Uses:

Gentamicin is a broad-spectrum, bacteriocidal antibiotic usually prescribed for serious urinary, respiratory, nervous, or GI infections. Activity includes *Enterobacter, E. coli, Klebsiella, Citrobacter, Pseudomonas,* and *Serratia*. It is often used in combination with other antibiotics or when other antibiotics have proven ineffective. A topical formulation (Genoptic) is available for infections of the external eye.

Adverse Effects and Interactions:

As with other aminoglycosides, adverse effects from gentamicin may be severe. Ototoxicity is possible and may become permanent with continued use. Ringing in the ears, dizziness, and persistent headaches are early signs of ototoxicity. Frequent hearing tests should be conducted so that gentamicin may be discontinued if early signs of ototoxicity are detected. The health care provider must also be alert for signs of nephrotoxicity because this may limit drug therapy with gentamicin. Signs of reduced kidney function include low urine output, proteinuria, and elevated BUN and creatinine levels.

Using this drug together with amphotericin B, capreomycin, cisplatin, polymyxin B, or vancomycin increases the risk of nephrotoxicity. The risk of ototoxicity increases if the patient is currently taking amphotericin B, furosemide, aspirin, bumetanide, ethacrynic acid, cisplatin, or paromomycin.

Refer to MyNursingKit for a Nursing Process Focus specific to this drug.

oto = *ear*
toxicity = *poison*
nephron = *kidney*

Of greatest concern are their effects on the inner ear and the kidney. Damage to the inner ear, or **ototoxicity**, causes hearing impairment, dizziness, loss of balance, persistent headache, and ringing in the ears. Because permanent deafness may occur, aminoglycosides are usually discontinued when symptoms of hearing impairment first appear. Kidney damage, or **nephrotoxicity**, is recognized by abnormal urinary function tests, such as elevated serum creatinine or blood urea nitrogen (BUN). Nephrotoxicity caused by aminoglycosides is usually reversible.

CORE CONCEPT 25.11

Fluoroquinolones have wide clinical applications because of their broad spectrum of activity and relative safety.

The class of drugs called fluoroquinolones was once reserved only for UTIs because of their toxicity. However, the development of safer drugs in this class began in the late 1980s and has continued to the present day. Newer fluoroquinolones have a broader spectrum of activity and are used for a variety of infections. The fluoroquinolones are listed in Table 25.8.

The first drug in this class, nalidixic acid (NegGram), was approved in 1962, but its use is restricted to UTIs. Four generations of fluoroquinolones have since become available. All fluoroquinolones have activity against gram-negative pathogens; the newer ones are significantly more effective against gram-positive microbes.

The fluoroquinolones are bacteriocidal and act by inhibiting bacterial DNA synthesis. These antibiotics are extensively used as alternatives to other antibiotics. Clinical applications include infections of the respiratory, GI, and gynecologic tracts, and some skin and soft-tissue infections.

The most widely used drug in this class, ciprofloxacin (Cipro), is a drug of choice for exposure to anthrax (*B. anthracis*), a potential bioterrorist threat. If exposure to anthrax is *suspected*, 500 mg of ciprofloxacin is administered by the oral route every 12 hours for 60 days. If exposure has been *confirmed*, ciprofloxacin is immediately administered IV, 400 mg every 12 hours. Other antibiotics are also effective against anthrax, including penicillin, vancomycin, ampicillin, erythromycin, tetracycline, and doxycycline.

A major advantage of the fluoroquinolones is that most are well absorbed orally and may be administered either once or twice a day. They should not be taken together with multivitamins or mineral supplements because these interact to reduce the absorption of some fluoroquinolones by as much as 90%.

Fluoroquinolones are safe for most patients, with nausea, vomiting, and diarrhea being the most frequent adverse effects. The most serious adverse effects are dysrhythmias (for gatifloxacin and moxifloxacin) and potential hepatotoxicity. Because fluoroquinolones may affect cartilage development, these drugs are not approved for children under age 18.

TABLE 25.8	**Fluoroquinolones**	
DRUG	**ROUTE AND ADULT DOSE**	**REMARKS**
cinoxacin (Cinobac)	PO; 250–500 mg bid–qid	For UTI
Pr ciprofloxacin (Cipro)	PO; 250–750 mg bid	For lung, skin, bone, and joint infections, and for anthrax; broad spectrum
gatifloxacin (Zymar)	PO; 400 mg tid	For respiratory infections, UTI, and gonorrhea; IV form available
gemifloxacin (Factive)	PO; 320 mg daily	For respiratory infections
levofloxacin (Levaquin)	PO; 250–500 mg daily	For respiratory tract and skin infections; IV form available
moxifloxacin (Avelox)	PO; 400 mg daily	For sinus and respiratory tract infections
nalidixic acid (NegGram)	PO; acute therapy: 1 g qid; PO; chronic therapy: 500 mg qid	For UTI
norfloxacin (Noroxin)	PO; 400 mg bid	For UTI; ophthalmic form available
ofloxacin (Floxin)	PO; 200–400 mg bid	For UTI, respiratory tract infections, and gonorrhea

DRUG PROFILE: ℗ *Ciprofloxacin (Cipro)*

Therapeutic Class: Antibacterial

Pharmacologic Class: Fluoroquinolone, bacterial DNA synthesis inhibitor

Actions and Uses:

Ciprofloxacin (Cipro), a second-generation fluoroquinolone, is the most widely used drug in this class. Ciprofloxacin inhibits bacterial replication and DNA repair and is more effective against gram-negative than gram-positive organisms. It is prescribed for respiratory infections, bone and joint infections, GI infections, ophthalmic infections, sinusitis, and prostatitis. It is rapidly absorbed after oral administration, and an IV form is available for severe infections. An extended-release form of the drug, Proquin XR, is administered for only 3 days and is approved for bladder infections.

Adverse Effects and Interactions:

Ciprofloxacin is well tolerated by most patients, and serious adverse effects are uncommon. Nausea, vomiting, and diarrhea may occur in as many as 20% of patients. Ciprofloxacin may be administered with food to lessen adverse GI effects; however, it should not be taken with antacids or mineral supplements because drug absorption will be diminished. Some patients report headache and dizziness.

Using this drug with warfarin may increase warfarin's anticoagulant effects and result in bleeding. Antacids, ferrous sulfate, and sucralfate decrease the absorption of ciprofloxacin. Caffeine should be restricted to avoid excessive nervousness, anxiety, or tachycardia.

Refer to MyNursingKit for a Nursing Process Focus specific to this drug.

Sulfonamides are traditional drugs of choice for urinary tract infections.

The discovery of the sulfonamides in the 1930s heralded a new era in the treatment of infectious disease. With their wide spectrum of activity, the sulfonamides significantly reduced deaths due to infections and earned their discoverer a Nobel Prize in medicine. The sulfonamides are listed in Table 25.9. Sulfonamides suppress bacterial growth by inhibiting folic acid, an essential substance in cellular metabolism.

Although initially very effective, several factors led to a significant decline in the use of sulfonamides. Their widespread availability over many decades produced a substantial number of resistant bacterial strains. The development of the penicillins, cephalosporins, and macrolides gave physicians greater choices of safer agents. Approval of the combination antibiotic trimethoprim-sulfamethoxazole (Bactrim, Septra) marked a resurgence in the use of sulfonamides in treating

TABLE 25.9	Sulfonamides	
DRUG	**ROUTE AND ADULT DOSE**	**REMARKS**
sulfacetamide (Cetamide, others)	Ophthalmic; one to three drops of 10%, 15%, or 30% solution	10% ointment also available
sulfadiazine (Microsulfon)	PO; 2–4 g daily in four to six divided doses	For malaria, toxoplasmosis, and prophylaxis of rheumatic fever
sulfadoxine–pyrimethamine (Fansidar)	PO; 1 tablet weekly (500 mg sulfadoxine, 25 mg pyrimethamine)	For prevention and treatment of malaria
sulfasalazine (Azulfidine)	PO; 1–2 g/day in four divided doses (max: 8 g/day)	For ulcerative colitis and rheumatoid arthritis
sulfisoxazole (Gantrisin)	PO; 2–4 g initially, followed by 1–2 g qid	For UTI; short acting; vaginal form available
℗ trimethoprim-sulfamethoxazole (Bactrim, Septra)	PO; 160 mg TMP/800 mg SMZ bid	Combination drug; for UTI, *Pneumocystis*, and ear infections; IV form available

---

DRUG PROFILE: Ⓟ *Trimethoprim-sulfamethoxazole (Bactrim, Septra)*

Therapeutic Class: Antibacterial
Pharmacologic Class: Sulfonamide, folic acid inhibitor

Actions and Uses:

The combination of sulfamethoxazole (SMZ), a sulfonamide, with the anti-infective trimethoprim (TMP) is most frequently used in the pharmacotherapy of UTIs. It is also approved for the treatment of *Pneumocystis carinii* pneumonia, *Shigella* infections of the small bowel, and acute episodes of bronchitis.

Both SMZ and TMP are inhibitors of the bacterial metabolism of folic acid. Combining the two drugs produces a greater bacterial kill than would be achieved with either drug used separately. Another advantage of the combination is that development of resistance is lower than is observed when either of the agents is used alone.

Adverse Effects and Interactions:

Nausea and vomiting are the most frequent adverse effects of TMP-SMZ therapy. Hypersensitivity is relatively common and usually manifests as skin rash, itching, and fever. This medication should be used cautiously in patients with preexisting kidney disease, because sulfonamides can adversely affect renal function. Periodic laboratory evaluations are usually performed to identify early signs of adverse blood effects.

TMP and SMZ may increase the effects of oral anticoagulants. These drugs may also increase methotrexate toxicity. Potassium supplements should not be taken during therapy, unless directed by the health care provider.

Refer to MyNursingKit for a Nursing Process Focus specific to this drug.

UTIs. In communities with high resistance rates, trimethoprim-sulfamethoxazole is no longer a preferred drug, unless C&S testing determines it to be the most effective drug for the specific pathogen.

Sulfonamides are classified by their route of administration: systemic or topical. Systemic agents, such as sulfisoxazole (Gantrisin) and trimethoprim-sulfamethoxazole, are rapidly absorbed when given orally and excreted rapidly by the kidney. Other sulfonamides such as sulfadiazine (Microsulfon) are used only for topical infections. The topical sulfonamides are not preferred drugs because many patients are allergic to substances containing sulfur. One drug in this class, sulfadoxine-pyrimethamine (Fansidar), has an exceptionally long half-life and is occasionally prescribed for malarial prophylaxis.

In general, the sulfonamides are safe medications; however, some adverse effects may be serious. Adverse effects include the formation of crystals in the urine, allergic reactions, nausea, and vomiting. Although not common, potentially fatal blood abnormalities, such as aplastic anemia, acute hemolytic anemia, and agranulocytosis, can occur.

A number of additional anti-infectives have distinct mechanisms of action and specific indications.

CORE CONCEPT 25.13

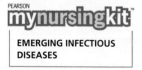

EMERGING INFECTIOUS DISEASES

Some anti-infectives cannot be grouped into classes, or the class is too small to warrant separate discussion. That is not to diminish their importance in medicine; some of these miscellaneous anti-infectives are critical drugs for specific infections. For example, clindamycin (Cleocin) is sometimes the drug of choice for oral infections caused by *Bacteroides* species. It is considered to be appropriate treatment when less toxic alternatives are not effective. Vancomycin (Vancocin) is an antibiotic usually reserved for severe infections from gram-positive organisms such as *S. aureus* and *S. pneumoniae*. It is often used after bacteria have become resistant to other, safer antibiotics. Vancomycin is the most effective drug for treating MRSA infections.

Several miscellaneous agents represent newer classes of antibiotics. Linezolid (Zyvox) is the first drug in a class called the oxazolidinones. This drug is effective against MRSA infections. Quinupristin/dalfopristin (Synercid) is a combination drug that is the first in an antibiotic class called streptogramins. This drug is primarily indicated for treatment of vancomycin-resistant *Enterococcus faecalis* infections. Daptomycin (Cubicin) is the first in a newer class of antibiotics called the cyclic lipopeptides. It is approved for the treatment of serious skin and skin-structure

TABLE 25.10	Miscellaneous Anti-infectives	
DRUG	**ROUTE AND ADULT DOSE**	**REMARKS**
aztreonam (Azactam)	IM; 0.5–2 g bid–qid (max: 8 g/day)	Monobactam class; for gram-negative aerobic bacteria; IV form available
chloramphenicol	PO; 50 mg/kg qid	Broad spectrum; for typhoid fever and meningitis; IV form available
clindamycin (Cleocin)	PO; 150–450 mg qid	Bacteriostatic; effective against anaerobic organisms; topical, IM, and IV forms available
daptomycin (Cubicin)	IV; 4 mg/kg once every 24 hours for 7–14 days	Bacteriocidal; for serious skin infections
ertapenem (Invanz)	IV/IM: 1 g/day	Carbapenem class; very broad spectrum
fosfomycin (Monurol)	PO; 3 g sachet dissolved in 3–4 oz of water as a single dose	Bacteriocidal; for UTI
imipenem-cilastatin (Primaxin)	IV; 250–500 mg tid–qid (max: 4 g/day)	Carbapenum class; combination drug; IM form available; one of the broadest spectrums of any anti-infective
lincomycin (Lincocin)	PO; 500 mg tid–qid (max: 8 g/day)	Bacteriostatic; effective against anaerobic organisms; IM form available
linezolid (Zyvox)	PO; 600 mg bid (max: 1,200 mg/day)	For vancomycin-resistant *Enterococcus;* IV form available
meropenem (Merrem IV)	IV; 1–2 g tid	Carbapenum class; for intra-abdominal infections, bacterial meningitis
methenamine (Mandelamine, Hiprex, Urex)	PO; hippurate 1 g bid; mandelate 1 g qid	For chronic UTI; broad spectrum
metronidazole (Flagyl) (see page 450 for the Drug Profile box)	PO; 7.5 mg/kg qid	For serious infections with anaerobic bacteria; also for protozoan infections; IV form available
nitrofurantoin (Furadantin, Macrobid, Macrodantin)	PO; 50–100 mg qid	For UTI; extended-release form available; interferes with bacterial enzymes
quinupristin-dalfopristin (Synercid)	IV; 7.5 mg/kg infused over 50 min every 8 hours	Streptogamins class; for serious infections resistant to vancomycin
spectinomycin (Trobicin)	IM; 2 g as single dose	Bacteriostatic; for gonorrhea
teicoplanin (Targocid)	IV; 6 mg/kg/day after two loading doses 12 hours apart	Glycopeptide class; for serious infections of the blood and heart
telithromycin (Ketek)	PO; 800 mg daily	Ketolide class; for community-acquired respiratory tract infections
(Pr) vancomycin (Vancocin)	IV; 500 mg qid–1 g bid	For *Staph*-resistant infections

infections such as major abscesses, postsurgical skin-wound infections, and infected ulcers. Table 25.10 lists some of these miscellaneous antibiotics and their dosages.

Imipenem (Primaxin), ertapenem (Invanz), and meropenem (Merrem IV) belong to a newer class of antibiotics called *carbapenems*. These drugs are bacteriocidal and have some of the broadest antimicrobial spectrums of any class of antibiotics. Imipenem, the most widely prescribed drug in this small class, is administered in a fixed-dose combination with cilastatin, which increases the serum levels of the antibiotic. Meropenem is approved only for peritonitis and bacterial meningitis. Ertapenem is approved for the treatment of serious abdominopelvic and skin infections, community-acquired pneumonia, and complicated UTI. Diarrhea, nausea, rashes, and thrombophlebitis at injection sites are the most frequent adverse effects of the carbapenems.

DRUG PROFILE: Ⓟ *Vancomycin (Vancocin)*

Therapeutic Class: Antibiotic
Pharmacologic Class: Bacterial cell wall synthesis inhibitor

Actions and Uses:

Vancomycin is usually reserved for severe infections from gram-positive organisms such as *S. aureus* and *Streptococcus pneumoniae.* It is often used after bacteria have become resistant to other, safer antibiotics. It is bacteriocidal, inhibiting bacterial cell-wall synthesis. Because vancomycin was not used frequently during the first 30 years following its discovery, the incidence of vancomycin-resistant organisms is smaller than with other antibiotics. Vancomycin is the most effective drug for treating MRSA infections, which have become a major problem in the United States. Vancomycin-resistant strains of *S. aureus,* however, have begun to appear in recent years. Vancomycin is normally given IV because it is not absorbed from the GI tract.

Adverse Effects and Interactions:

Frequent, minor side effects include flushing, hypotension, and rash on the upper body, sometimes called **red-man syndrome**. More serious adverse effects are possible with higher doses, including nephrotoxicity and ototoxicity. Some patients experience an acute allergic reaction and even anaphylaxis.

Vancomycin adds to toxicity of aminoglycosides, amphotericin B, cisplatin, cyclosporine, polymyxin B, and other ototoxic and nephrotoxic medications. Cholestyramine and colestipol can decrease the absorption of vancomycin.

Refer to MyNursingKit for a Nursing Process Focus specific to this drug.

NURSING PROCESS FOCUS

Patients Receiving Antibacterial Therapy

ASSESSMENT

Prior to administration:
- Obtain a complete health history (physical/mental), including allergies, drug history, and possible drug interactions
- Obtain specimens for C&S before initiating therapy
- Perform infection-focused physical examination, including vital signs, white blood cell count, and sedimentation rate

POTENTIAL NURSING DIAGNOSES

- Infection related to inadequate primary defenses.
- Risk for Injury related to tissue destruction and adverse effects of drug therapy.
- Deficient Knowledge related to information about disease process, transmission, and drug therapy.
- Noncompliance related to therapeutic regimen.

PLANNING: PATIENT GOALS AND EXPECTED OUTCOMES

The patient will:
- Report reduction in symptoms related to the diagnosed infection and have negative results for laboratory and diagnostic tests for the presenting infection
- Demonstrate an understanding of the drug's action by accurately describing drug adverse effects and precautions
- Immediately report significant adverse effects such as shortness of breath, swelling, fever, stomatitis, loose stools, vaginal discharge, or cough
- Complete full course of antibiotic therapy and comply with follow-up care

IMPLEMENTATION

Interventions and (Rationales)

- Monitor vital signs and symptoms of infection to determine antibacterial effectiveness. (Another drug or different dosage may be required.)

Patient Education/Discharge Planning

- Instruct the patient to notify the health care provider if symptoms persist or worsen.

continued . . .

NURSING PROCESS FOCUS *(continued)*

Interventions and (Rationales)	Patient Education/Discharge Planning
■ Monitor for hypersensitivity reaction. (Immediate hypersensitivity reaction may occur within 2–30 minutes; accelerated reaction occurs in 1–72 hours; and delayed reaction after 72 hours.)	■ Instruct the patient to discontinue the medication and inform the health care provider if symptoms of hypersensitivity reaction develop such as wheezing; shortness of breath; swelling of face, tongue, or hands; or itching or rash.
■ Monitor for severe diarrhea. (The condition may occur due to superinfection or the possible adverse effect of antibiotic-associated pseudomembranous colitis, or AAPMC.)	Instruct the patient to: ■ Consult the health care provider before taking antidiarrheal drugs, which could cause retention of harmful bacteria ■ Consume cultured dairy products with live active cultures, such as kefir, yogurt, or buttermilk, to help maintain normal intestinal flora
■ Administer drug around the clock (to maintain effective blood levels).	Instruct the patient to: ■ Take the medication on schedule ■ Complete the entire prescription even if feeling better to prevent development of resistant bacteria
■ Monitor for superinfection, especially in elderly, debilitated, or immunosuppressed patients. (Increased risk for superinfections is due to elimination of normal flora.)	■ Instruct the patient to report signs and symptoms of superinfection, such as fever; black hairy tongue; stomatitis; loose, foul-smelling stools; vaginal discharge; or
■ Monitor intake of over-the-counter (OTC) products such as antacids, calcium supplements, iron products, and laxatives containing magnesium. (These products interfere with absorption of many antibiotics.)	■ Advise the patient to consult with the health care provider before using OTC medications or herbal products.
■ Monitor for photosensitivity. (Tetracyclines, fluoroquinolones, and sulfonamides can increase the patient's sensitivity to ultraviolet light and increase risk of sunburn.)	Encourage the patient to: ■ Avoid exposure to direct sunlight during and after therapy ■ Wear protective clothing, sunglasses, and sunscreen when outdoors
■ Determine the interactions of the prescribed antibiotics with various foods and beverages.	Instruct the patient regarding foods and beverages that should be avoided with specific antibiotic therapies: ■ No acidic fruit juices with penicillins ■ No alcohol intake with cephalosporins ■ No dairy product/calcium products with tetracyclines
■ Monitor the IV site for signs and symptoms of tissue irritation, severe pain, and extravasation.	■ Instruct the patient to immediately report pain or other symptoms of discomfort during intravenous infusion.
■ Monitor for adverse effects specific to various antibiotic therapies. (See "Nursing Considerations" for each antibiotic classification in this chapter.)	■ Instruct the patient to report adverse effects specific to the antibiotic therapy prescribed.
■ Monitor renal function such as intake and output ratios and urine color and consistency. Monitor laboratory work, including serum creatinine and BUN. (Some antibiotics such as the aminoglycosides are nephrotoxic.)	Inform the patient: ■ About the purpose of required laboratory tests and scheduled follow-ups with the health care provider ■ To increase fluid intake to 2000–3000 ml/day
■ Monitor for symptoms of ototoxicity. (Some antibiotics, such as the aminoglycosides and vancomycin, may cause vestibular or auditory nerve damage.)	Instruct the patient to notify the health care provider of: ■ Changes in hearing, ringing in the ears, or full feeling in the ears ■ Nausea and vomiting with motion, ataxia, nystagmus, or dizziness
■ Monitor the patient for compliance with antibiotic therapy.	Instruct the patient in the importance of: ■ Completing the prescription as ordered ■ Follow-up care after antibiotic therapy is completed

EVALUATION OF OUTCOME CRITERIA

Evaluate the effectiveness of drug therapy by confirming that patient goals and expected outcomes have been met (see "Planning").

See Tables 25.3 through 25.10 for lists of drugs to which these nursing actions apply.

TUBERCULOSIS

Tuberculosis (TB) is a highly contagious infection caused by the organism *Mycobacterium tuberculosis*. Although the microorganisms typically invade the lungs, they may also enter other body systems, particularly bone. The slow-growing mycobacteria activate cells of the immune response, which attempt to isolate the pathogens by creating a wall around them. The mycobacteria usually become dormant, lying inside cavities called **tubercles**. They may remain dormant during an entire lifetime, or they may become reactivated if the immune system becomes suppressed. When active, TB can be quite infectious, being spread by contaminated sputum. With the immune suppression characteristic of AIDS, the incidence of TB has greatly increased: As many as 20% of all patients with AIDS develop active TB.

Two other types of mycobacteria infect humans. *Mycobacterium leprae* is responsible for leprosy, a disease rarely seen in the United States and Canada. *M. leprae* is treated with multiple drugs, usually beginning with rifampin. *Mycobacterium avium* complex (MAC) causes an infection of the lungs, most commonly observed in patients with AIDS. The most effective drugs against MAC are the macrolides azithromycin (Zithromax) and clarithromycin (Biaxin).

CORE CONCEPT 25.14

The pharmacotherapy of tuberculosis requires special dosing regimens and schedules.

Drug therapy of tuberculosis differs from that of most other infections. Mycobacteria have a cell wall that is resistant to penetration by anti-infective drugs. For medications to reach the microorganisms isolated in the tubercles, therapy must continue for 6 to 12 months. Although the patient may not be infectious this entire time and may have no symptoms, it is critical that therapy continue the entire period. Some patients develop multidrug-resistant infections and require therapy for as long as 24 months.

A second feature of the pharmacotherapy of TB is that at least two—and sometimes four or more—antibiotics must be administered concurrently. During the 6- to 24-month treatment period, different combinations of drugs may be used. Multidrug therapy is necessary because the mycobacteria grow slowly, and resistance is common. Using multiple drugs and switching the

DRUG PROFILE: ℗ *Isoniazid (INH, Nydrazid)*
Therapeutic Class: Antituberculosis agent
Pharmacologic Class: Mycolic acid inhibitor

Actions and Uses:
Isoniazid is a drug of choice for the treatment of *M. tuberculosis* because decades of experience have shown it to have a superior safety profile and to be the most effective single drug for the disease. Isoniazid acts by inhibiting the synthesis of mycolic acid, an essential cell-wall component of mycobacteria. It is bacteriocidal for actively growing organisms but bacteriostatic for dormant mycobacteria. It is selective for *M. tuberculosis*. Isoniazid is used alone for chemoprophylaxis, or in combination with other antitubercular drugs for treating active disease.

Adverse Effects and Interactions:
The most common adverse effects of isoniazid are numbness of the hands and feet, rash, and fever. Although rare, liver toxicity is a serious adverse effect; thus, the health care provider should be alert for signs of jaundice, fatigue, elevated hepatic enzymes, or loss of appetite. Liver enzyme tests are usually performed monthly during therapy to identify early hepatotoxicity.

Aluminum-containing antacids should not be administered concurrently because they can decrease the absorption of isoniazid. When disulfiram is taken with INH, lack of coordination or psychotic reactions may result. Drinking alcohol with INH increases the risk of liver toxicity.

 Refer to MyNursingKit for a Nursing Process Focus specific to this drug.

TABLE 25.11	First-Line Antitubercular Drugs	
DRUG	**ROUTE AND ADULT DOSE**	**REMARKS**
ethambutol (Myambutol)	PO; 15–25 mg/kg daily	Used in combination with other antituberculars
Pr isoniazid (INH, Nydrazid)	PO; 15 mg/kg daily	Used in combination with other antituberculars; IM form available
pyrazinamide (PZA)	PO; 5–15 mg/kg tid–qid	Rifater is a fixed-dose combination of pyrazinamide with isoniazid and rifampin
rifabutin (Mycobutin)	PO; 300 mg once daily (for prophylaxis) or 5 mg/kg/day (for active TB) (max: 300 mg/day)	Very similar to rifampin and rifapentine
rifampin (Rifadin, Rimactane)	PO; 600 mg daily as a single dose or 900 mg twice weekly for 4 months	Used in combination with other antituberculars; IV form available; also for leprosy, *H. influenzae,* and meningococcus infections
rifapentine (Priftin)	PO; 600 mg twice a week for 2 months, then once a week for 4 months	Used in combination with other antituberculars

combinations during the long treatment period lowers the potential for resistance and increases therapeutic success. Although many different drug combinations are used, a typical regimen for patients with no complicating factors includes the following:

- *Initial phase*   2 months of daily therapy with isoniazid, rifampin (Rifadin, Rimactane), pyrazinamide (PZA), and ethambutol (Myambutol). If laboratory test results show that the strain is sensitive to the first three drugs, ethambutol is dropped from the regimen.
- *Continuation phase*   4 months of therapy with isoniazid and rifampin, two to three times per week.

There are two broad categories of antitubercular agents. One category consists of primary, first-line drugs, which are safer and generally the most effective. Secondary (second-line) drugs, more toxic and less effective than the first-line agents, are used when resistance develops. Table 25.11 lists drugs used as first-choice therapy of TB.

NURSING PROCESS FOCUS

Patients Receiving Antitubercular Drugs

ASSESSMENT

Prior to administration:
- Obtain a complete health history (physical/mental), including allergies, drug history, and possible drug interactions
- Perform complete physical examination, including vital signs
- Assess for presence/history of the following:
  - Positive tuberculin skin test
  - Positive sputum culture or smear
  - Close contact with person recently infected with TB
  - HIV infection or AIDS
  - Immunosuppressant drug therapy
  - Alcohol abuse
  - Liver or kidney disease
  - Cognitive ability to comply with long-term therapy

POTENTIAL NURSING DIAGNOSES

- Risk for Infection related to inadequate primary defenses, environmental exposure.
- Risk for Injury related to tissue destruction and adverse effects of drug therapy.
- Deficient Knowledge related to information about drug therapy.
- Noncompliance related to therapeutic regimen.

continued . . .

PLANNING: PATIENT GOALS AND EXPECTED OUTCOMES

The patient will:
- Report reduction in tuberculosis symptoms and have negative results for laboratory and diagnostic tests indicating TB infection
- Demonstrate an understanding of the drug's action by accurately describing adverse effects and precautions
- Immediately report effects such as visual changes, difficulty voiding, changes in hearing, and symptoms of liver or kidney impairment
- Complete full course of antitubercular therapy and comply with follow-up care

IMPLEMENTATION

Interventions and (Rationales)	Patient Education/Discharge Planning
■ Monitor for hepatic adverse effects. (Antituberculosis agents, such as isoniazid and rifampin, cause hepatic impairment.)	■ Instruct the patient to report yellow eyes and skin, loss of appetite, dark urine, and unusual tiredness.
■ Monitor for neurologic adverse effects such as numbness and tingling of the extremities. (Antituberculosis agents, such as isoniazid, cause peripheral neuropathy and depletion of vitamin B_6.)	Instruct the patient to: ■ Report numbness and tingling of extremities ■ Take supplemental vitamin B_6 as ordered to reduce risk of adverse effects
■ Collect sputum specimens as directed by the health care provider. (This will determine the effectiveness of the antituberculosis agent.)	■ Instruct the patient in technique needed to collect a quality sputum specimen.
■ Monitor for dietary compliance when patient is taking isoniazid. (Foods high in tyramine can interact with the drug and cause palpitations, flushing, and hypertension.)	■ Advise patients taking isoniazid to avoid foods containing tyramine, such as aged cheese, smoked and pickled fish, beer and red wine, bananas, and chocolate.
■ Monitor for adverse effects specific to various antituberculosis drugs.	Instruct the patient to report adverse effects specific to the antituberculosis therapy prescribed, such as: ■ Blurred vision or changes in color or vision field (ethambutol) ■ Difficulty in voiding (pyrazinamide) ■ Fever, yellowing of skin, weakness, dark urine (isoniazid, rifampin) ■ GI system disturbances (rifampin) ■ Changes in hearing (streptomycin) ■ Numbness and tingling of extremities (isoniazid) ■ Red discoloration of body fluids (rifampin) ■ Dark concentrated urine, weight gain, edema (streptomycin)
■ Establish therapeutic environment to ensure adequate rest, nutrition, hydration, and relaxation. (Symptoms of TB are manifested when the immune system is suppressed.)	Instruct the patient: ■ Concerning infectious control measures, such as frequent handwashing, covering the mouth when coughing or sneezing, and proper disposal of soiled tissues ■ To incorporate health-enhancing activities, such as adequate rest and sleep, intake of essential vitamins and nutrients, and intake of six to eight glasses of water/day
■ Monitor the patient's ability and motivation to comply with therapeutic regimen. (Treatment must continue for the full length of therapy to eliminate all *M. tuberculosis* organisms.)	Explain the importance of complying with the entire therapeutic plan, including: ■ Taking all medications as directed by health care provider ■ Not discontinuing medication until so instructed ■ Wearing a medical alert bracelet ■ Keeping all appointments for follow-up care

EVALUATION OF OUTCOME CRITERIA

Evaluate the effectiveness of drug therapy by confirming that patient goals and expected outcomes have been met (see "Planning").

See Table 25.11 for a list of drugs to which these nursing actions apply.

A third feature of anti-TB therapy is that drugs are used extensively for *preventing* the disease in addition to treating it. Chemoprophylaxis is common for close contacts or family members of patients recently infected with TB. Therapy usually begins immediately after a patient receives a positive tuberculin test. Patients with immunosuppression, such as those with AIDS or those receiving immunosuppressant drugs, may receive preventive treatment with anti-TB drugs. A short-term therapy of 2 months, consisting of a combination treatment with isoniazid (INH, Nydrazid) and pyrazinamide, is approved for TB prophylaxis in patients positive for HIV.

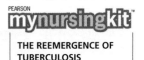

PEARSON
mynursingkit™

THE REEMERGENCE OF
TUBERCULOSIS

Concept Review 25.3

■ How does drug therapy of tuberculosis differ from that of conventional anti-infective chemotherapy? What are the rationales for these differences?

PATIENTS NEED TO KNOW

Patients treated for bacterial infections need to know the following:

In General

1. Take the entire prescription of anti-infective medication exactly as directed because partial doses, skipped doses, and shortened length of treatment encourage the development of resistant organisms.
2. Some antibiotics may cause GI upset. If this occurs, take the drug with food or milk as directed. Check prescription label for specific directions.
3. Eating active-culture yogurt or buttermilk may decrease the risks for diarrhea and vaginitis associated with antibiotic destruction of normal flora.
4. Antibiotics are most effective if taken around the clock, rather than just during normal waking hours.

Regarding Penicillins

5. It may be necessary to stay in the office for at least 30 minutes after receiving an injection of penicillin so the health care providers can monitor you for possible allergic reactions.
6. Avoid intake of caffeinated beverages, citrus fruits, and fruit juices for at least 1 hour before and 2 hours after taking oral penicillin to maximize the drug's absorption.

Regarding Sulfonamides and Tetracyclines

7. Take oral cephalosporins and oral lincomycin with food, and oral sulfonamides with food or milk, to decrease GI upset. Drink a glass of water with each dose of sulfonamide, tetracycline, lincomycin, or fluoroquinolone, and drink a total of 2–3 L of fluid a day.
8. Avoid sun/tanning exposure while taking sulfonamides and tetracyclines because these drugs cause photosensitivity.
9. Antacids, dairy products, iron, baking soda, and kaolin-pectin bind and inactivate tetracycline. Separate intake by 2–3 hours for full antibiotic effectiveness.
10. Sulfonamides, tetracycline, and other antibiotics may interfere with the effectiveness of oral contraceptives. Ask a health care provider about the advisability of using an additional form of contraception.

SAFETY ALERT

Allergic Reactions and Antibiotics

Last night, Mrs. Jones received the first dose of levofloxacin (Levaquin). While receiving the medication, she reported itching and a slight swelling of the tongue and lips (angioedema). However, later that day she had no discomfort or presence of the previous symptoms. Prior to the initial administration of the drug, the nurse checked the patient's chart for the presence of allergies, but it is imperative that the nurse *reassess* the patient for drug allergies. Even though patients may initially report their drug allergies to their health care providers, they sometimes forget to mention these during stressful times. Secondly, before the patient receives another dose of this antibiotic, the health care provider should be notified of the reaction, preferably when it occurred but certainly before the second dosage. Hypersensitivity reactions can worsen with each exposure to an antigen (the antibiotic). The next dose could cause a life-threatening anaphylactic response.

CHAPTER REVIEW

CORE CONCEPTS SUMMARY

25.1 Pathogens are organisms that cause disease by invading tissues or secreting toxins.

Pathogens can overwhelm natural immune defenses by growing extremely rapidly and invading normal tissues or by producing potent toxins. Bacteria are classified on the basis of their staining ability and structural and functional characteristics.

25.2 Anti-infective drugs are classified by their chemical structures or by their mechanisms of action.

Because of the large number of anti-infectives available, it is advantageous for the student to understand how to classify these drugs because medications in the same class exhibit similar pharmacologic activity. Anti-infective drugs are classified based on similarities in their chemical structures or by their mechanisms of action.

25.3 Anti-infective drugs act by selectively targeting a pathogen's metabolism or life cycle.

Bacteria multiply rapidly, and drugs have been designed to take advantage of this characteristic. Anti-infectives may be bacteriocidal or bacteriostatic, or both, depending on the organism and dose.

25.4 Acquired resistance is a major clinical problem that is worsened by improper use of anti-infectives.

Errors during replication result in random mutations of the bacterial DNA. Although rare, an occasional mutation may confer antibiotic resistance to a bacterium. Therapy with antibiotics kills the affected bacteria, leaving the resistant ones to multiply and spread within the patient. To limit this problem, antibiotics should be prescribed only when medically necessary.

25.5 Careful selection of the correct antibiotic is essential for effective pharmacotherapy and to limit adverse effects.

Culture and sensitivity tests are used to identify the type of bacteria present and determine which antibiotics are most effective. Until test results are obtained, the patient may be started on a broad-spectrum antibiotic. Because broad-spectrum drugs are more likely to affect the patient's normal flora, a narrow-spectrum drug may be prescribed after the organism is identified.

25.6 The penicillins are one of the oldest and safest groups of anti-infectives.

Penicillins have been widely used because of their high margin of safety and effectiveness. Some patients are allergic to this class of drugs, and many bacterial species have become resistant to penicillins, thus limiting their use.

25.7 The cephalosporins are similar in structure and function to the penicillins and are one of the most widely prescribed anti-infective classes.

The cephalosporins consist of a large class of antibiotics, classified by generation, that are considered alternatives to penicillin. In general, they are used for serious gram-negative infections and for patients who are resistant to or cannot tolerate the penicillins.

25.8 The tetracyclines have broad spectrums but are drugs of choice for few diseases.

The tetracyclines have a broader spectrum of action and produce more adverse effects than the penicillins. Their use is limited to a small number of diseases such as Rocky Mountain spotted fever, typhus, cholera, Lyme disease, and chlamydial infections.

25.9 The macrolides are safe alternatives to penicillin for many infections.

The macrolides are generally prescribed when a patient is allergic to penicillin or has a penicillin-resistant infection. They produce few adverse effects.

25.10 The aminoglycosides are narrow-spectrum drugs that have the potential to cause serious toxicity.

The aminoglycosides are usually reserved for severe gram-negative infections of the urinary tract because they have the potential to cause serious adverse effects. Most of them are poorly absorbed from the GI tract and must be given parenterally.

25.11 Fluoroquinolones have wide clinical applications because of their broad spectrum of activity and relative safety.

Although fluoroquinolones are an older class of antibacterials, newer drugs in this class have been developed to greatly expand their use. They are effective oral alternatives to other antibiotics for both gram-negative and gram-positive organisms. Ciprofloxacin (Cipro) is one of the few agents approved for the treatment of anthrax.

25.12 Sulfonamides are traditional drugs of choice for urinary tract infections.

In the 1930s, the sulfonamides revolutionized the treatment of infectious disease. Present-day use of these agents is limited by bacterial resistance. The fixed combination of trimethoprim-sulfamethoxazole (Bactrim, Septra) is an important drug in the pharmacotherapy of UTIs.

25.13 A number of additional anti-infectives have distinct mechanisms of action and specific indications.

A number of important antibiotics do not belong to any of the previous classes. The streptogramins and oxazolidinones are small groups of drugs having specific applications. Vancomycin is known as the "last chance" antibiotic for use when resistance has developed to most other anti-infectives.

25.14 The pharmacotherapy of tuberculosis requires special dosing regimens and schedules.

Drug therapy of tuberculosis involves taking multiple drugs for prolonged periods. Patients exhibiting a new, positive TB test are often given these drugs prophylactically, even if no signs of the disease are apparent.

REVIEW QUESTIONS

The following questions are written in NCLEX-PN® style. Answer these questions to assess your knowledge of the chapter material, and go back and review any material that is not clear to you.

1. The patient is taking amoxicillin (Amoxil). Which of the following statements by the patient demonstrates that he or she needs additional instruction?

1. "I will take this medication until it is gone."
2. "I will call my doctor if I develop a fever or a rash."
3. "Before I take my medication, I will avoid orange juice."
4. "I will take the medication until I feel better."

2. Children younger than 9 years should not be given tetracyclines because:

1. Photosensitivity may occur
2. Children's teeth may become discolored
3. Superinfections may occur
4. Children become dehydrated easily

3. The patient on tetracyclines should be instructed:

1. To take it with food or milk
2. That it is safe for pregnancy
3. To take it 1–2 hours before or after meals
4. That it has no adverse effects

4. The patient on aminoglycosides should be monitored for:

1. Nephrotoxicity
2. Hepatic failure
3. Superinfection
4. Hypertension and rash

5. If ciprofloxin (Cipro) is administered with antacids, absorption is:

1. Increased
2. Decreased
3. Not affected
4. Delayed

6. The patient has a urinary tract infection. The nurse anticipates which of the following medications being ordered?

1. Sulfacetamide (Cetamide)
2. Sulfadiazine (Microsulfon)
3. Trimethoprim-sulfamethoxazole (Septra)
4. Vancomycin (Vancocin)

7. The patient with tuberculosis is now on isoniazid (INH). Which laboratory test should be monitored at least monthly?

1. PT and PTT
2. CBC
3. BUN
4. Liver enzymes

8. The patient asks why he must take two medications for his tuberculosis. The nurse's best response would be:

1. "You have TB throughout your body. It will take additional medications to cure you."
2. "You will need to speak with your physician."
3. "Taking multiple drugs increases the chances that therapy will be successful."
4. "With multiple drugs, we can decrease the time you need to take the medications."

9. Prophylactic treatment of TB in the patient with HIV would include which of these drugs?

1. Streptomycin and isoniazid (INH)
2. Pyrazinamide and rifampin
3. Rifampin and streptomycin
4. Isoniazid (INH) and pyrazinamide

10. Patients on antibiotics should be instructed to:

1. Take the medication with food
2. Increase fluid intake to 2–3 L per day
3. Take all medication on an empty stomach
4. Take medication until symptoms subside

CASE STUDY QUESTIONS

For questions 1–4, please refer to the following case study, and choose the correct answer from choices 1–4.

Mr. Wu is a new patient at your clinic. Six months ago, he had a kidney transplant and is taking immunosuppressant drugs. Recently, he has been experiencing repeated bacterial infections due to resistant strains and has been switched to different antibiotics throughout the last 6 months. The physician suspects a kidney infection.

1. Mr. Wu is admitted to the hospital and is administered gentamicin 300 mg daily by IV infusion. Which of the following tests should you monitor?

1. Input and output ratio
2. Serum transaminase levels
3. Visual acuity tests
4. Fasting blood glucose levels

2. Mr. Wu is showing signs of hearing loss due to gentamicin therapy and he is switched to ciprofloxacin (Cipro) 200 mg every 12 hours. For which common adverse effect of ciprofloxacin therapy should you monitor?

1. Hearing loss
2. Diminished liver function

3. Nausea and vomiting
4. Nephrotoxicity

3. Mr. Wu is discharged from the hospital with a prescription for 4 g daily PO sulfisoxazole (Gantrism). The primary use of this sulfonamide is for the pharmacotherapy of:

1. UTI
2. Resistant staph infections (MRSA)
3. Respiratory infections
4. Gonorrhea and other sexually transmitted bacterial infections

4. A year later, Mr. Wu returns for a follow-up and you note in the chart that he has been taking rifampin (Rifidin) and ethambutol (Myambutol) for the last 3 months. You can conclude that Mr. Wu:

1. Is being treated for tuberculosis
2. Has a severe respiratory infection
3. Is being treated for a resistant staph infection (MRSA)
4. Needs to have his medications reevaluated by the physician

FURTHER STUDY

- Body defenses that pathogens must bypass to infect humans are discussed in detail in Chapter 24 ⊂⊃ .

- Chapter 34 ⊂⊃ discusses some of the anti-infective agents for skin disorders.

- Chapter 26 ⊂⊃ discusses anti-infective drugs used to treat viral, fungal, and parasitic infections.

26 Drugs for Fungal, Viral, and Parasitic Diseases

CORE CONCEPTS

26.1 Fungal infections are classified as superficial or systemic.

26.2 Systemic antifungal drugs are used for serious infections of internal organs.

26.3 Superficial infections of the skin, nails, and mucous membranes are effectively treated with topical and oral antifungal drugs.

26.4 Viruses are infectious agents that require a host to replicate.

26.5 Antiretroviral drugs do not cure HIV-AIDS, but they do help many patients live longer.

26.6 Antiviral drugs are available to treat herpes simplex, influenza, and hepatitis infections.

26.7 Infections caused by helminths and protozoans cause significant disease worldwide.

DRUG SNAPSHOT

The following drugs are discussed in this chapter:

DRUG CLASSES	DRUG PROFILES
Antifungal drugs for systemic infections	**Pr** amphotericin B (AmBisome, Fungizone, others)
Antifungal drugs for superficial infections	**Pr** nystatin (Mycostatin, Nystop, others)
Antiretroviral drugs for HIV-AIDS	**Pr** zidovudine (AZT, Retrovir)
Antiviral drugs for herpes simplex and influenza	**Pr** acyclovir (Zovirax)
Antiprotozoans and antihelmintics	**Pr** metronidazole (Flagyl)

LEARNING OUTCOMES

After reading this chapter, the student should be able to:

1. Compare and contrast the pharmacotherapy of superficial and systemic fungal infections.

2. Identify the types of patients most likely to acquire serious fungal infections.

3. Describe the basic structure of a virus.

4. Identify specific viral infections that benefit from pharmacotherapy.

5. Explain the purpose and expected outcomes of HIV pharmacotherapy.

6. Define HAART, and explain why it is commonly used in the pharmacotherapy of HIV infection.

7. Identify protozoan and helminth infections that may benefit from pharmacotherapy.

8. For each of the drug classes listed in the Drug Snapshot, identify representative drugs and explain the mechanisms of drug action, primary actions, and important adverse effects.

9. Categorize drugs used in the treatment of fungal, viral, protozoan, and helminth infections based on their classifications and mechanisms of action.

433

antiretroviral (an-tie-RET-roh-veye-ral) *442*

capsid (CAP-sid) *438*

dermatophytic (der-MAT-oh-FIT-ik) *435*

dysentery (DISS-en-tare-ee) *448*

fungi (FUN-jeye) *434*

helminth (HELL-minth) *448*

highly active antiretroviral therapy (HAART) *442*

host *441*

influenza (in-flew-EN-zah) *447*

intracellular parasite *441*

malaria (mah-LARE-ee-ah) *448*

mycoses (my-KOH-sees) *434*

protozoan (PRO-toh-ZOH-en) *448*

reverse transcriptase (ree-VERS trans-CRIP-tace) *442*

superficial mycoses *435*

systemic mycoses *435*

virus *438*

yeast (YEEST) *434*

Fungi, protozoans, and multicellular parasites are exceedingly more complex than bacteria. Most antibacterial drugs are ineffective against these organisms because their structure and biochemistry are so different from that of bacteria. Although there are fewer medications to treat these diseases, the available medications are usually effective.

Viruses, on the other hand, are nonliving particles that infect by entering a host cell and using the host's internal machinery to replicate itself. Antiviral drugs are the least effective of all the anti-infective classes. Although the number of antiviral medications has increased dramatically in recent years, they are relatively ineffective at preventing or treating viral infections.

CORE CONCEPT 26.1

Fungal infections are classified as superficial or systemic.

Fungi are single-celled or multicellular organisms that are much more complex than bacteria. Several species of fungi grow on skin and mucosal surfaces and are part of the normal host flora. The human body is remarkably resistant to infection by these organisms; patients with healthy immune systems rarely experience serious fungal diseases. Those with a suppressed immune system, however, such as patients infected with HIV, may acquire frequent fungal infections, some of which may require intensive drug therapy.

Fungal infections are called **mycoses**. Most exposure to pathogenic fungi occurs through inhalation of fungal spores or by handling contaminated soil. Thus, many fungal infections involve the respiratory tract, skin, hair, and nails. An additional common source of fungal infections, especially of the mouth or vagina, is overgrowth of normal flora. **Yeasts**, which include the common pathogen *Candida albicans,* are single-celled fungi. Table 26.1 lists the most common fungal pathogens.

myc = *fungus*
oses = *conditions*

Fast Facts Fungal, Viral, and Parasitic Diseases

- Ninety percent of human fungal infections are caused by just a few dozen species.
- Of all human fungal infections, 86% are caused by *Candida albicans.* The second most common (1.3%) is caused by species of *Aspergillus.*
- About 45 million Americans are infected with genital herpes—1 of every 5 of the total adolescent and adult population.
- More than 400,000 Americans are currently living with HIV infections; about 40,000 new infections occur each year.
- Approximately 70% of new HIV infections occur in men, with the largest risk category being men who have sex with other men.
- Of the new HIV infections in women, 75% are acquired through heterosexual contact.
- Since the beginning of the AIDS epidemic, more than 520,000 Americans have died of AIDS.
- Between 300 million and 500 million cases of malaria occur worldwide each year, with an estimated 2.7 million deaths resulting from the disease.

TABLE 26.1	Fungal Pathogens
NAME OF FUNGUS	**DISEASE AND PRIMARY ORGAN SYSTEM**
SYSTEMIC	
Aspergillus fumigatus and others	Aspergillosis: opportunistic; most commonly affects the lungs but can spread to other organs
Blastomyces dermatitidis	Blastomycosis: begins in the lungs and spreads to other organs
Candida albicans and others	Candidiasis: most common opportunistic fungal infection; may occur in mucous membranes and nearly any organ
Coccidioides immitis	Coccidioidomycosis: begins in the lungs and spreads to the skin and other organs
Cryptococcus neoformans	Cryptococcosis: opportunistic; begins in the lungs but is the most common cause of meningitis in patients with AIDS
Histoplasma capsulatum	Histoplasmosis: begins in the lungs and spreads to other organs
Pneumocystis carinii	Pneumocystis pneumonia: opportunistic; primarily causes pneumonia but can spread to other organs
SUPERFICIAL	
Candida albicans and others	Candidiasis: affects the skin, nails, oral cavity (thrush), vagina
Epidermophyton floccosum	Athlete's foot (tinea pedis), jock itch (tinea cruris), and other skin disorders
Microsporum species	Ringworm of the scalp (tinea capitus)
Sporothrix schenckii	Sporotrichosis: affects primarily the skin and superficial lymph nodes
Trichophyton species	Affects the scalp, skin, and nails

A simple and useful method of classifying fungal infections is to consider them as either superficial or systemic. **Superficial mycoses** typically affect the scalp, skin, nails, and mucous membranes such as the oral cavity and vagina. Mycoses of this type are often treated with topical drugs because the incidence of adverse effects is much lower by using this route of administration. Superficial fungal infections are sometimes called **dermatophytic**.

Systemic mycoses are those affecting internal organs, typically the lungs, brain, and digestive organs. Although much less common than superficial mycoses, systemic fungal infections affect multiple body systems and are sometimes fatal to patients with suppressed immune systems. Mycoses of this type often require aggressive oral or parenteral medications that produce more adverse effects than the topical agents.

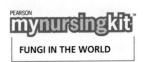

PEARSON
mynursingkit™

FUNGI IN THE WORLD

derma = *skin*
phyto = *something that grows*

Systemic antifungal drugs are used for serious infections of internal organs.

CORE CONCEPT 26.2

Systemic or invasive fungal infections require intensive pharmacotherapy for extended periods. Amphotericin B and fluconazole are the most frequently prescribed drugs for these types of infections. Table 26.2 lists the primary antifungal drugs.

Opportunistic fungal disease in patients with AIDS prompted the development of several new drugs for systemic fungal infections in the past 20 years. Others who may experience systemic infections include patients receiving prolonged therapy with corticosteroids (see Chapters 24 and 31 ⊕), those with extensive burns, those receiving antineoplastic drugs (see Chapter 27 ⊕), and those who have recently received organ transplants (see Chapter 24 ⊕). Systemic antifungal medications have little or no antibacterial activity, and pharmacotherapy often continues for several months.

Amphotericin B (AmBisome, Fungizone, others) has been the preferred drug for treating systemic fungal infections since the 1960s. However, the newer *azole* drugs such as fluconazole (Diflucan) and itraconazole (Sporanox) are safer and have become drugs of choice for the treatment of less severe systemic infections. Ketoconazole has become a drug of choice for less severe systemic mycoses or for the prophylaxis of fungal infections. The *azole* drugs have a spectrum of activity similar to that of amphotericin B, are considerably less toxic, and have the major advantage that they can be administered orally. Several are available for both superficial and systemic mycoses.

TABLE 26.2   Selected Antifungal Drugs

DRUG	ROUTE AND ADULT DOSE	REMARKS
Pr amphotericin B (AmBisome, Fungizone, others)	IV; 0.3–1.5 mg/kg/day, infused over 2–4 hr (max: 1.5 mg/kg/day)	Cream, lotion, and PO suspension forms available for topical mycoses; must infuse a test dose first; has potential for severe adverse effects
butenafine (Mentax)	Topical; apply daily for 4 weeks	For athlete's foot
butoconazole (Femstat)	Topical; one applicator intravaginally at bedtime for 3 days	For vaginal mycoses
anidulafungin (Eraxis)	IV; Loading dose 100 mg on day 1 followed by 50 mg/day	Newer drug for advanced *Candida* infections
caspofungin acetate (Cancidas)	IV; 70 mg infused over 1 hr on day 1, followed by 50 mg infused over 1 hr qid for 30 days	Newer drug for invasive *Candida* and *Aspergillus* infections
ciclopirox cream, gel, shampoo (Loprox) or nail lacquer (Penlac)	Topical; apply bid for 4 weeks	For skin and nail mycoses
clotrimazole (Gyne-Lotrimin, Mycelex, Femizole)	Topical; for skin mycoses apply bid for 4 weeks; for vaginal mycoses, insert one applicatorful intravaginally at bedtime for 7 days	For vaginal and skin mycoses, athlete's foot, and candidiasis; vaginal tablet form also available
econazole (Spectazole)	Topical; apply bid for 4 weeks	For skin mycoses
fluconazole (Diflucan)	PO; 200–400 mg on day 1, then 100–200 mg daily for 2–4 weeks	For both systemic and superficial mycoses; 1% cream available for topical infections; IV form available
flucytosine (Ancobon)	PO; 50–150 mg/kg in divided doses	For severe systemic infections such as candidiasis or cryptococcosis; IV form available
griseofulvin (Fulvicin)	PO; 500 mg microsize or 330–375 mg ultramicrosize daily	For ringworm and other skin and nail infections
itraconazole (Sporanox)	PO; 200 mg daily; may increase to 200 mg bid (max: 400 mg/day)	For severe systemic lung mycoses and superficial nail mycoses
ketoconazole (Nizoral)	PO; 200–400 mg daily	For severe systemic mycoses; topical form available for superficial mycoses
micafungin (Mycamine)	IV; 50–150 mg/kg/day	Newer drug for advanced *Candida* infections
miconazole (Micatin, Monistat)	Topical; apply bid for 2–4 weeks	For vaginal and skin mycoses; also available as vaginal suppositories and tampons
naftifine (Naftin)	Topical; apply cream daily or gel bid for 4 weeks	For skin mycoses
Pr nystatin (Mycostatin, Nystop, others)	PO; 500,000–1,000,000 units tid	For candidiasis; vaginal tablet form available
oxiconazole (Oxistat)	Topical; apply daily in the evening for 2 months	For skin mycoses
sertaconazole (Ertaczo)	Topical; 2% cream bid for 4 weeks	For tinea pedis
terbinafine (Lamisil)	Topical; apply daily or bid for 7 weeks; PO; 250 mg daily for 6–13 weeks	For skin and nail mycoses
terconazole (Terazol)	Topical; insert one applicator intravaginally at bedtime for 3–7 days	For vulvovaginal candidiasis; vaginal suppository form available
tioconazole (Vagistat)	Topical; insert one applicator intravaginally at bedtime for 1 day	For vulvovaginal candidiasis
tolnaftate (Aftate, Tinactin)	Topical; apply bid for 4–6 weeks	For skin mycoses, ringworm, athlete's foot
undecylenic acid (Fungi-Nail, Gordochom)	Topical; apply once or twice daily	For athlete's foot, diaper rash
voriconazole (Vfend)	IV; 6 mg/kg every 12 hours on day 1, then 3–4 mg/kg every 12 hours	For systemic aspergillosis; oral form available

---

DRUG PROFILE: ℗ *Amphotericin B (AmBisome, Fungizone, Others)*

Therapeutic Class: Antifungal (systemic type)
Pharmacologic Class: Polyene

Actions and Uses:

Amphotericin B has a wide spectrum of activity and is effective against most of the fungi pathogenic to humans; thus, it is a preferred drug for many severe systemic mycoses. It acts by binding to fungal cell membranes and causing them to become permeable or leaky. Because amphotericin B is not absorbed from the gastrointestinal (GI) tract, it is normally given by IV infusion. Topical preparations are available for superficial mycoses. Several months of pharmacotherapy may be required for a complete cure. Unlike antibiotics, resistance to amphotericin B is not common.

To reduce the toxicity of amphotericin B, the original drug molecule has been formulated with several lipid molecules. These include liposomal amphotericin B (AmBisome), amphotericin B lipid complex (Abelcet), and amphotericin B cholesteryl sulfate complex (Amphotec). These newer forms are very expensive and usually reserved for serious fungal infections.

Adverse Effects and Interactions:

Amphotericin B can cause a number of serious adverse effects. Many patients develop fever and chills at the beginning of therapy, which subside as treatment continues. Phlebitis, or inflammation of the veins, is common during IV therapy. Some degree of nephrotoxicity is observed in most patients, and laboratory tests of kidney function are normally performed throughout the treatment period.

Amphotericin B interacts with many drugs. For example, therapy with aminoglycosides, vancomycin, carboplatin, and furosemide, which reduce renal function, is not recommended. Use with corticosteroids, skeletal muscle relaxants, and thiazole may cause hypokalemia. Use with digoxin increases the risk of digoxin toxicity in patients with preexisting hypokalemia.

Refer to MyNursingKit for a Nursing Process Focus specific to this drug.

A newer class of antifungals called *echinocandins* has been added to the treatment options for systemic mycoses. The first drug in this class, caspofungin, has become an important alternative to amphotericin B in the treatment of aspergillosis. Approved in 2006, anidulafungin (Eraxis) is approved for invasive candidiasis. The echinocandins are less toxic than amphotericin B.

Concept Review 26.1

■ Why has the number of antifungal and antiviral drugs increased significantly over the past 20 years?

Superficial infections of the skin, nails, and mucous membranes are effectively treated with topical and oral antifungal drugs.

CORE CONCEPT 26.3

Superficial fungal infections of the hair, scalp, nails, and the mucous membranes of the mouth and vagina are rarely medical emergencies. Infections of the nails and skin, for example, may be ongoing for months or even years before a patient seeks treatment. Unlike systemic fungal infections, superficial infections may occur in any patient, not just those who have suppressed immune systems.

Antifungal medications applied topically are much safer than their systemic counterparts because only small amounts are absorbed into the circulation. Many are available as over-the-counter (OTC) creams, gels, solutions, and ointments. Although a fungal infection may be diagnosed as superficial, oral antifungal drugs are occasionally prescribed along with the topical agents to be certain that the infection is completely eliminated from the deeper skin layers. The length of pharmacotherapy varies widely among the different types of superficial mycoses. Vaginal infections are sometimes treated successfully with a single vaginal tablet of clotrimazole, whereas nail mycoses may require several months of therapy with itraconazole or terbinafine.

DRUG PROFILE: ℗ *Nystatin (Mycostatin, Nystop, Others)*

Therapeutic Class: Topical antifungal
Pharmacologic Class: Polyene

Actions and Uses:

Although it belongs to the same chemical class as amphotericin B, nystatin is available in a wider variety of formulations, including cream, ointment, powder, tablets, and lozenges. It is used as a topical agent against *Candida* infections of the vagina, skin, and mouth. It may also be used orally to treat candidiasis of the intestine because it travels through the GI tract without being absorbed.

Adverse Effects and Interactions:

When given topically, nystatin produces few adverse effects other than minor skin irritation. When given orally, it may cause diarrhea, nausea, and vomiting.

 Refer to MyNursingKit for a Nursing Process Focus specific to this drug.

Adverse effects from topical antifungal therapy are generally minor. If applied to the skin, irritation, redness, and itching may be experienced. Vaginal administration may result in burning, itching, or irritation. Antifungal drugs should not be applied to open sores or severely abraded skin because this may result in undesirable absorption of the drug and additional adverse effects.

CORE CONCEPT 26.4

Viruses are infectious agents that require a host to replicate.

Viruses are nonliving agents that infect bacteria, plants, and animals. Viruses contain none of the vital organelles that are present in the cells of living organisms. In fact, the structure of viruses is primitive compared to even the simplest cell. Surrounded by a protective protein coat or **capsid**, a virus contains only a few dozen genes—either in the form of ribonucleic acid (RNA) or deoxyribonucleic acid (DNA)—that contain the information needed for viral replication. Figure 26.1 ■ shows the basic structure of one important virus: HIV.

FIGURE 26.1

Structure of the human immunodeficiency virus (HIV)

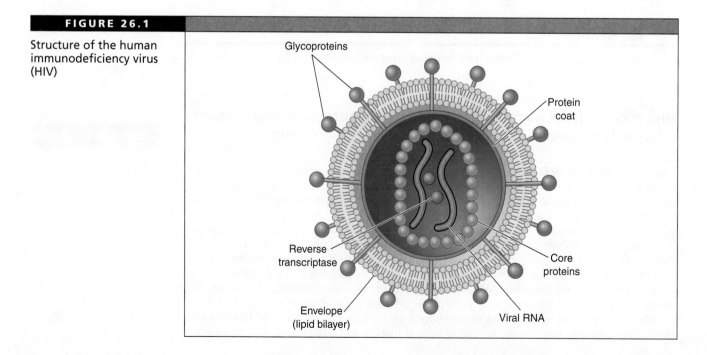

NURSING PROCESS FOCUS

Patients Receiving Superficial Antifungal Therapy

ASSESSMENT

Prior to administration:
- Obtain a complete health history (physical/mental), including allergies, drug history, and possible drug interactions
- Obtain a culture and sensitivity of the suspected area of infection to determine need for therapy
- Obtain baseline liver function tests

POTENTIAL NURSING DIAGNOSES

- Risk for Injury (rash) related to adverse effect of drug therapy.
- Deficient Knowledge related to information about drug therapy.
- Risk for Impaired Skin Integrity.

PLANNING: PATIENT GOALS AND EXPECTED OUTCOMES

The patient will:
- Report healing of fungal infection
- Demonstrate an understanding of the drug's action by accurately describing drug adverse effects and precautions
- Immediately report effects such as hepatoxicity, GI distress, rash, or decreased urine output

IMPLEMENTATION

Interventions and (Rationales)	Patient Education/Discharge Planning
■ Monitor for possible adverse effects or hypersensitivity.	Instruct the patient to report: ■ Burning, stinging, dryness, itching, erythema, urticaria, angioedema, and local irritation (for superficial drugs) ■ Symptoms of hepatic toxicity—jaundice, dark urine, light-colored stools, and pruritus ■ Nausea, vomiting, and diarrhea ■ Signs and symptoms of hypo- or hyperglycemia
■ Encourage compliance with instructions when taking oral antifungals (to increase medication effectiveness).	Instruct the patient to: ■ Swish the oral suspension to coat all mucous membranes, and then swallow the medication ■ Spit out the medication instead of swallowing if GI irritation occurs ■ Allow troche to dissolve completely, rather than chewing or swallowing; it may take 30 min for it to completely dissolve ■ Avoid food or drink for 30 min following administration ■ Remove dentures prior to using the oral suspension ■ Take ketoconazole with water, fruit juice, coffee, or tea to enhance dissolution and absorption
■ Administer and monitor topical application.	Instruct the patient to: ■ Avoid wearing tight-fitting undergarments if using ointment in the vaginal or groin area ■ Avoid occlusive dressings. (Dressings increase moisture in the infected areas and encourage development of additional yeast infections.)
■ Monitor for contact dermatitis with topical formulations. (This is related to the preservatives found in many of the formulations.)	■ Instruct the patient to report any redness or skin rash.
■ Encourage infection control practices. Ensure that the patient, family members, and other visitors also practice infection control techniques such as handwashing and avoiding the affected area (to prevent the spread of infection).	Instruct the patient to: ■ Clean the affected area daily ■ Apply medication while wearing a glove ■ Wash hands properly before and after application ■ Change socks daily if rash is on the feet ■ Avoid sharing personal care items with family members/guests

EVALUATION OF OUTCOME CRITERIA

Evaluate the effectiveness of drug therapy by confirming that patient goals and expected outcomes have been met (see "Planning").

See Table 26.2 for a list of drugs to which these nursing actions apply.

TABLE 26.3   Antiretroviral Drugs for HIV-AIDS

DRUG	ROUTE AND ADULT DOSE	REMARKS
NONNUCLEOSIDE REVERSE TRANSCRIPTASE INHIBITORS (NNRTI)		
delavirdine (Rescriptor)	PO; 400 mg tid	Used in combination with other antivirals
efavirenz (Sustiva)	PO; 600 mg daily	Used in combination with other antivirals; a once-daily form is available
etravirine (Intelence)	PO; 200 mg bid	Newer drug in this class; less central nervous system (CNS) toxicity and hepatotoxicity than others
nevirapine (Viramune)	PO; 200 mg daily for 14 days, then increase to bid	Used in combination with other antivirals
NUCLEOSIDE AND NUCLEOTIDE REVERSE TRANSCRIPTASE INHIBITORS		
abacavir (Ziagen)	PO; 300 mg bid	A preferred drug for HIV therapy in combination with other drugs
didanosine (Videx EC)	PO; 125–300 mg bid	For use in patients who are intolerant to AZT
emtricitabine (Emtriva)	PO; 200 mg daily	A preferred drug for HIV therapy in combination with other drugs
lamivudine (Epivir)	PO; 150 mg bid	Widely used because it exhibits fewer adverse effects than other drugs; also used to treat hepatitis B.
stavudine (d4T, Zerit)	PO; 40 mg bid	Usually reserved for advanced HIV infections
tenofovir (Viread)	PO; 300 mg/day	A nucleotide reverse transcriptase inhibitor; a preferred drug for HIV therapy in combination with other drugs
Pr zidovudine (AZT, Retrovir)	PO; 200 mg every 4 hours for 1 month, then 100 mg every 4 hours	For symptomatic or asymptomatic HIV; off-label use: postexposure chemoprophylaxis; IV form available
PROTEASE INHIBITORS		
atazanavir (Reyataz)	PO; 400 mg/day	A preferred drug for HIV therapy in combination with other drugs
darunavir (Prezista)	PO; 600 mg taken with ritonavir 100 mg bid	Usually reserved for advanced HIV infections
fosamprenavir (Lexiva)	PO; 700–1400 mg bid in combination with 100–200 mg ritonavir bid	A preferred drug for HIV therapy in combination with other drugs
idinavir (Crixivan)	PO; 800 mg tid	Has short half-life; administer with a high-fat meal to increase absorption
lopinavir/ritonavir (Kaletra)	PO; 400/100 mg (three capsules or 5 ml of suspension) bid	A preferred drug for HIV therapy in combination with other drugs
nelfinavir (Viracept)	PO; 750 mg tid	Infrequently used due to adverse effects and three doses per day
ritonavir (Norvir)	PO; 600 mg bid	Always used in small doses to boost the effectiveness of other PIs
saquinavir (Invirase)	PO; 1000 mg bid	Usually a second choice drug
tipranavir (Aptivus)	PO; 500 mg taken with 200 mg of ritonavir bid	Usually a second choice drug; administer with a high-fat meal to increase absorption
MISCELLANEOUS DRUGS		
enfuvirtide (Fuzeon)	Subcutaneous; 90 mg bid	Fusion inhibitor; usually reserved for advanced HIV infections
maraviroc (Selzentry)	PO; 150–600 mg bid	CCR5 receptor inhibitor; newer drug usually reserved for advanced HIV infections
raltegravir (Isentress)	PO; 400 mg bid	Integrase inhibitor; newer drug usually reserved for advanced HIV infections

TABLE 26.4	Antiviral Drugs for Herpes and Influenza Infections	
DRUG	**ROUTE AND ADULT DOSE**	**REMARKS**
HERPES VIRUS DRUGS		
(Pr) acyclovir (Zovirax)	PO; 400 mg tid	For HSV-1, HSV-2, and varicella-zoster; topical and IV forms available
cidofovir (Vistide)	IV; 5 mg/kg once weekly for 2 consecutive weeks	For cytomegalovirus retinitis in patients with AIDS; must give probenecid before and after infusion
docosanol (Abreva)	Topical; 10% cream applied to lesion up to five times/day	For herpes simplex lesions on the face and lips
famciclovir (Famvir)	PO; 500 mg tid for 7 days	For HSV-2 varicella-and zoster
foscarnet (Foscavir)	IV; 40–60 mg/kg infused over 1–2 hours tid	For cytomegalovirus retinitis; for the treatment of acyclovir-resistant herpesvirus
ganciclovir (Cytovene)	PO; 1 g tid IV; 5 mg/kg infused over 1 hr bid	Preferred drug for cytomegalovirus; oral form available
penciclovir (Denavir)	Topical; 0.5 inch of ointment to each eye every 3 hours	For herpes simplex lesions on the face and lips
trifluridine (Viroptic)	Topical; one drop in each eye every 2 hours during waking hours (max: nine drops/day)	For herpes eye infections
valacyclovir (Valtrex)	PO; 1 g tid	For HSV-1, HSV-2, and varicella-zoster
INFLUENZA DRUGS		
amantadine (Symmetrel)	PO; 100 mg bid	For treatment and prevention of influenza A; also for Parkinson's disease
oseltamivir (Tamiflu)	PO; 75 mg bid × 5 days	For treatment of influenza
rimantadine (Flumadine)	PO; 100 mg bid	For treatment and prevention of influenza
zanamivir (Relenza)	Inhalation; two inhalations/day × 5 days	For treatment of influenza

Although nonliving and structurally simple, viruses are capable of remarkable feats. They infect an organism, called the **host**, by entering a target cell and using the enzymes inside that cell to replicate. Thus viruses are called **intracellular parasites**, meaning that they must be inside a host cell to cause infection. The host organism and cell are often very specific: It may be a single species of plant, bacteria, or animal, or even a single type of cell within that species. Most often, viruses that affect one species do not affect others, although cases have been documented in which viruses can mutate and cross species, as is likely the case for HIV.

intra = *within*
cellular = *cell*

Many viral infections, such as the rhinoviruses that cause the common cold, are self-limiting and require no medical treatment. Although symptoms may be annoying, the virus disappears in 7 to 10 days and causes no permanent damage if the patient is otherwise healthy. Other viruses, such as HIV, can cause serious and ultimately fatal disease and require aggressive drug therapy. Antiviral therapy is extremely challenging because of the rapid mutation rate of viruses, which can quickly render drugs ineffective. Also complicating therapy is the intracellular nature of the virus, which makes it difficult for medications to find their targets without giving excessively high doses that injure normal cells. The antiviral medications are listed in Tables 26.3 and 26.4. Each of the antiviral drugs is specific to one particular virus. The three basic strategies used for antiviral pharmacotherapy are as follows:

- Prevent viral infections through the administration of vaccines (see Chapter 32 ⊂⊃).
- Treat active infections with drugs such as acyclovir (Zovirax) that interrupt an aspect of the virus's replication cycle.
- For long-term infections, use drugs that boost the patient's immune response (immunostimulants) so that the virus remains in latency and the patient symptom free.

CORE CONCEPT 26.5

Antiretroviral drugs do not cure HIV-AIDS, but they do help many patients live longer.

Drugs for viral infections are classified into those used to treat HIV-AIDS and those used for other viral disorders such as herpes and influenza. Antiviral medications for HIV-AIDS have been developed that slow the growth of HIV by different mechanisms.

The widespread appearance of HIV infection in 1981 created enormous challenges for public health and for the development of new antiviral drugs. HIV-AIDS is unlike any other infectious disease because it is uniformly fatal and demands a continuous supply of new drugs for patients' survival. The challenges of HIV-AIDS have been met by the development of more than 20 new antiviral drugs. Unfortunately, the initial hope of curing HIV-AIDS through antiviral therapy or vaccines has not been realized; none of these medications produces a cure for this disease. Stopping antiretroviral therapy almost always results in a rapid rebound in HIV replication. HIV mutates extremely rapidly, and resistant strains develop so quickly that the creation of novel approaches to antiretroviral drug therapy must remain an ongoing process.

After initial exposure, HIV may remain dormant for several months to many years. During this *latent phase*, patients are asymptomatic and may not even realize they are infected. Once diagnosis is established, however, a decision must be made as to when to begin pharmacotherapy. The advantage of beginning during the latent stage is that early treatment may delay the onset of acute symptoms and the development of AIDS.

Unfortunately, the decision to begin treatment during the latent phase has some negative consequences. Medications for HIV-AIDS are expensive; treatment with some of the newer drugs may cost more than $20,000 per year. These drugs produce uncomfortable and potentially serious adverse effects. Therapy over many years promotes viral resistance; when the acute stage eventually develops, the medications may no longer be effective.

The decision to begin therapy during the acute phase is much easier because the severe symptoms of AIDS can rapidly lead to death. Thus, therapy is nearly always initiated during this phase, when the CD4 T-cell count falls below 200 cells/mcL or when AIDS-defining symptoms become apparent.

The therapeutic goals for the pharmacotherapy of HIV-AIDS include the following:

- Reduce HIV-related morbidity and prolong survival
- Improve the quality of life
- Restore and preserve natural functions of the immune system
- Suppress the viral load to the extent possible
- Prevent the transmission from mother to child in pregnant patients infected with HIV

Although drug therapy for HIV-AIDS has not produced a cure, it has resulted in a number of therapeutic successes. For example, many patients with HIV are able to live symptom free with their disease for a much longer time because of antiviral therapy. Furthermore, the transmission of the virus from a mother infected with HIV to her offspring has been reduced dramatically because of drug therapy of the mother prior to delivery and of the baby immediately following birth. These two factors have resulted in a significant decline in the death rate due to HIV-AIDS in the United States.

Antiviral medications used for HIV-AIDS are called **antiretrovirals** because they block the replication cycle of HIV, which is classified as a retrovirus. The standard treatment for HIV-AIDS includes aggressive treatment with three to four drugs at a time, a regimen called **highly active antiretroviral therapy (HAART)**. The goal of HAART is to reduce the amount of HIV in the plasma to its lowest possible level. It must be understood, however, that HIV is harbored in locations other than the blood, such as in lymph nodes; therefore, elimination of the virus from the blood is not a cure.

The replication of HIV is illustrated in Figure 26.2 ■. Antiretroviral drugs are classified into groups based on how they inhibit HIV replication.

- *Nucleoside and nucleotide reverse transcriptase inhibitors (NRTIs and NtRTIs)* The oldest antiretroviral drug, zidovudine, belongs to the NRTI class. Drugs in this group are structurally similar to nucleosides, the building blocks of DNA. NRTIs inhibit the action of **reverse transcriptase**, the viral enzyme that converts viral RNA into viral DNA.

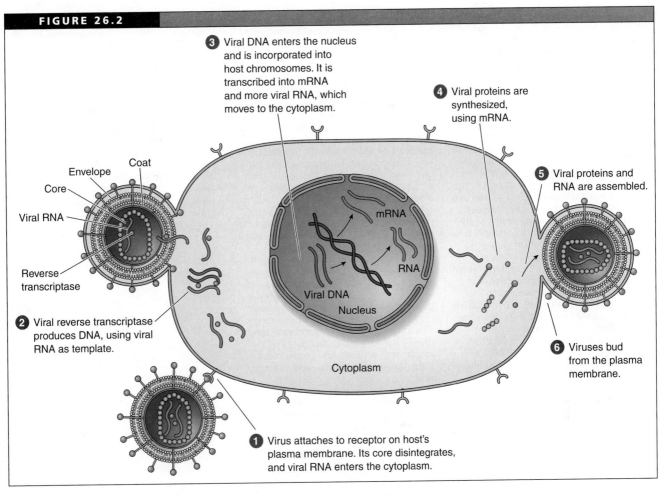

FIGURE 26.2

③ Viral DNA enters the nucleus and is incorporated into host chromosomes. It is transcribed into mRNA and more viral RNA, which moves to the cytoplasm.

④ Viral proteins are synthesized, using mRNA.

⑤ Viral proteins and RNA are assembled.

Coat
Envelope
Core
Viral RNA
Reverse transcriptase

mRNA
RNA
Viral DNA
Nucleus

② Viral reverse transcriptase produces DNA, using viral RNA as template.

Cytoplasm

⑥ Viruses bud from the plasma membrane.

① Virus attaches to receptor on host's plasma membrane. Its core disintegrates, and viral RNA enters the cytoplasm.

Replication of HIV

- *Nonnucleoside reverse transcriptase inhibitors (NNRTIs)* This class also inhibits the viral enzyme reverse transcriptase, but these drugs are not structurally similar to the building blocks of DNA. Instead, these agents bind directly to the reverse transcriptase molecule and inhibit its ability to build viral DNA.
- *Protease inhibitors* These drugs block the final assembly of the HIV particle. They are effective at reducing plasma HIV to very low levels, although resistance develops quickly.
- *Miscellaneous agents* Newer drugs are being developed as scientists discover more about the HIV replication cycle. Enfuvirtide (Fuzeon) blocks the fusion of HIV to the CD4 receptor on the lymphocyte. Raltegravir (Isentress) prevents HIV from inserting its genes into uninfected DNA.

Research into HIV-AIDS is constantly evolving as clinicians strive to determine the most effective combinations of antiretroviral agents. Current clinical guidelines recommend that the initial treatment of patients infected with HIV include one of the following therapies:

- A protease inhibitor (boosted with small amounts of ritonavir) plus two NRTIs
- A nonnucleoside reverse transcriptase inhibitor plus two NRTIs

Concept Review **26.2**

- Why are viral infections difficult to treat with current drugs?

DRUG PROFILE: ℗ *Zidovudine (AZT, Retrovir)*

Therapeutic Class: Antiretroviral

Pharmacologic Class: Nucleoside reverse transcriptase inhibitor (NRTI)

Actions and Uses:

Zidovudine was first discovered in the 1960s, and its antiviral activity was demonstrated prior to the AIDS epidemic. As the HIV reverse transcriptase enzyme begins to synthesize viral DNA, it mistakenly uses zidovudine as one of the building blocks, thus creating a defective DNA strand. Because of its widespread use over the past 25 years, strains of HIV resistant to zidovudine are common. It is usually used in combination with other antiretrovirals because this slows the development of resistance and allows HIV to be attacked by several mechanisms. Combination products containing zidovudine include Combivir (zidovudine and lamivudine) and Trizivir (zidovudine, lamivudine, and abacavir).

Zidovudine is one of the few HIV-AIDS drugs that can prevent HIV infection. By administering zidovudine to a mother infected with HIV starting at 14 weeks of gestation and to the newborn for 6 weeks following delivery, the risk of transmission of the virus to the child can be significantly reduced. Zidovudine is also administered as prophylaxis to health care providers following an accidental needlestick or other exposure to HIV.

Adverse Effects and Interactions:

Zidovudine can result in severe toxicity to blood cells at high doses. Reduced numbers of red blood cells (anemia) and white blood cells (leukopenia) are common and may limit therapy. Lactic acidosis and severe hepatomegaly with steatosis have been reported, including a few fatal cases. Many patients report GI symptoms such as anorexia, nausea, and diarrhea. Patients may experience fatigue and report generalized weakness. Headache will occur in the majority of patients taking zidovudine, and more serious CNS effects have been reported.

Zidovudine interacts with many drugs. Acetaminophen and ganciclovir may worsen bone marrow suppression. The following drugs may increase the risk of AZT toxicity: atovaquone, amphotericin B, aspirin, doxorubicin, fluconazole, methadone, and valproic acid.

Use with caution with herbal supplements such as St. John's wort, which may cause a decrease in antiretroviral activity.

Mechanism in Action:

Zidovudine resembles the chemical structure of thymidine, one of the building blocks of DNA. With the help of reverse transcriptase, the drug becomes incorporated into the infective strand of viral DNA. Once incorporated, zidovudine slows synthesis of HIV, thereby reducing symptoms associated with this infection.

Refer to MyNursingKit for a Nursing Process Focus specific to this drug.

CORE CONCEPT 26.6

Antiviral drugs are available to treat herpes simplex, influenza, and hepatitis infections.

Other than the drugs used to treat HIV, only a few antivirals are available to treat serious viral infections. These include drugs to treat infections with the herpesviruses, the influenza virus, and the hepatitis virus.

Treatment of herpesvirus infection. Herpes simplex viruses (HSV) are a family of viruses that cause repeated, blisterlike lesions on the skin, genitals, and other mucosal surfaces. Herpesviruses are acquired through sexual intercourse or other direct physical contact with an infected person. The herpesvirus family includes the following:

- HSV-type 1—primarily causes infections of the eye, mouth, and lips, although the incidence of genital infections is increasing
- HSV-type 2—genital infections
- Cytomegalovirus (CMV)—affects multiple body systems, usually in patients with immunosuppression

NURSING PROCESS FOCUS

Patients Receiving Antiretroviral Agents

ASSESSMENT

Prior to administration:
- Obtain a complete health history (physical/mental), including allergies, drug history, and possible drug interactions
- Obtain a complete physical examination
- Assess for the presence/history of HIV infection
- Obtain the following laboratory studies:
  - HIV RNA assay/CD4 count
  - Complete blood count (CBC)
  - Liver function
  - Renal function
  - Blood glucose

POTENTIAL NURSING DIAGNOSES

- Risk for Infection related to compromised immune system.
- Decisional Conflict related to therapeutic regimen.
- Fear related to HIV diagnosis.
- Risk for Injury related to adverse effects of drug therapy.
- Deficient Knowledge related to information about disease process, transmission, and drug therapy.

PLANNING: PATIENT GOALS AND EXPECTED OUTCOMES

The patient will:
- Exhibit a decrease in viral load and an increase in CD4 counts
- Demonstrate knowledge of disease process, transmission, and treatment
- Identify adverse effects and report to the health care provider
- Complete full course of therapy and comply with follow-up care

IMPLEMENTATION

Interventions and (Rationales)	Patient Education/Discharge Planning
■ Monitor for symptoms of hypersensitivity reactions. (Zalcitabine may cause anaphylactic reaction.)	■ Instruct the patient to discontinue the medication and inform the health care provider if symptoms of hypersensitivity reaction develop, such as wheezing; shortness of breath; swelling of face, tongue, or hands; or itching or rash.
■ Monitor vital signs, especially temperature, and for symptoms of infection. Monitor white blood cell count. (Antiretroviral drugs such as delavirdine may cause neutropenia.)	Instruct the patient: ■ To report symptoms of infections such as fever, chills, sore throat, and cough ■ On methods to minimize exposure to infection such as frequent handwashing; avoiding crowds and people with colds, flu, and other infections; limiting exposure to children and animals; increasing fluid intake; emptying the bladder frequently; and coughing and deep breathing several times per day
■ Monitor the patient for signs of stomatitis. (Immunosuppression may result in the proliferation of oral bacteria.) ■ Monitor blood pressure. (Antiviral agents such as abacavir may cause significant decrease in blood pressure.)	Instruct the patient to: ■ Be alert for mouth ulcers and to report their appearance ■ Rise slowly from lying or sitting position to minimize effects of postural hypotension ■ Report changes in blood pressure
■ Monitor HIV RNA assay, CD4 counts, liver function, kidney function, CBC, blood glucose, and serum amylase and triglyceride levels. (These will determine effectiveness and toxicity of drug.)	Instruct the patient: ■ On the purpose of required laboratory tests and scheduled follow-ups with the health care provider ■ To monitor weight and presence of swelling ■ To keep all appointments for laboratory tests

continued . . .

NURSING PROCESS FOCUS *(continued)*

Interventions and (Rationales)	Patient Education/Discharge Planning
■ Determine potential drug–drug and drug–food interactions. (Antiretroviral medications have multiple drug–drug interactions and must be taken as prescribed.)	Instruct the patient: ■ When to take the specific medication in relationship to food intake ■ About foods or beverages to avoid when taking medication; some antiretrovirals should not be taken with acidic fruit juice ■ To take medication exactly as directed; do not skip any doses ■ To consult with the health care provider before taking any OTC medications or herbal supplements
■ Monitor for symptoms of pancreatitis, including severe abdominal pain, nausea, vomiting, and abdominal distention. (Antiretroviral agents such as didanosine may cause pancreatitis.)	■ Instruct the patient to report the following immediately: fever, severe abdominal pain, nausea/vomiting, and abdominal distention.
■ Monitor the skin for rash; withhold medication and notify the physician at the first sign of rash. (Several antiretroviral drugs may cause Stevens-Johnson syndrome, which may be fatal.)	■ Advise the patient to check the skin frequently and to notify the health care provider at the first sign of any rash.
■ Establish therapeutic environment to ensure adequate rest, nutrition, hydration, and relaxation. (Support of the immune system is essential in patients with HIV to minimize opportunistic infections.)	Teach the patient to incorporate the following health-enhancing activities: ■ Adequate rest and sleep ■ Proper nutrition that provides essential vitamins and nutrients ■ Intake of six to eight glasses of water per day
■ Monitor blood glucose levels. (Antiretroviral drugs may cause hyperglycemia, especially in patients with type 1 diabetes.)	■ Instruct the patient to report excessive thirst, hunger, and urination to the health care provider. ■ Instruct patients with diabetes to monitor blood glucose levels regularly.
■ Monitor for neurologic adverse effects such as numbness and tingling of the extremities. (Many NRTI agents cause peripheral neuropathy.)	Instruct the patient to: ■ Report numbness and tingling of extremities ■ Use caution when in contact with heat and cold due to possible peripheral neuropathy
■ Determine the effect of the prescribed antiretroviral agents on oral contraceptives. (Many agents reduce the effectiveness of oral contraceptives.)	■ Instruct the patient to use an alternate form of birth control while taking antiretroviral medications.
■ Provide resources for medical and emotional support.	■ Advise the patient on community resources and support groups.
■ Assess the patient's knowledge level regarding use and effect of the medication.	Advise the patient: ■ That the medication may decrease the level of HIV infection in the blood but will not prevent transmitting the virus ■ To use barrier protection during sexual activity ■ To avoid sharing needles ■ To not donate blood

EVALUATION OF OUTCOME CRITERIA

Evaluate the effectiveness of drug therapy by confirming that patient goals and expected outcomes have been met (see "Planning").

See Tables 26.3 and 26.4 for lists of drugs to which these nursing actions apply.

- Varicella-zoster virus—shingles (zoster) and chickenpox (varicella)
- Epstein-Barr virus—mononucleosis and Burkitt's lymphoma, a form of cancer

Following its initial entrance into the human host, HSV may remain in a latent, nonreplicating state in nerve cells for many years. Immunosuppression, physical challenge, or emotional stress can activate the virus and cause the characteristic lesions to reappear. Although herpes lesions are often mild and require no drug therapy, patients who experience frequent recurrences may benefit from low doses of prophylactic antiviral therapy. Topical drugs are available for application on active lesions, but they are not as effective as oral medications. It should be noted that the antiviral drugs used to treat herpesviruses do not cure the patient; the virus remains in the patient for life. Drugs for treating herpesviruses are listed in Table 26.4.

Treatment of influenza virus infection. **Influenza** is a viral infection characterized by acute symptoms that include sore throat, sneezing, coughing, fever, and chills. The virus is easily spread via airborne droplets. In patients who are immunosuppressed, an influenza infection may be fatal.

The best approach to influenza infection is prevention through annual vaccination. Those who benefit greatly from vaccinations include residents of long-term care facilities, those with chronic cardiopulmonary disease, women who will be in their second or third trimester during the peak flu season, and healthy adults older than age 50. Adequate immunity is achieved about 2 weeks after vaccination and lasts for several months up to a year. Additional details on vaccines are presented in Chapter 24 ⬭ .

Antivirals may be used to prevent influenza or decrease the severity of influenza symptoms. The drug amantadine (Symmetrel) has been available to prevent and treat influenza for many years. Amantadine or rimantadine is indicated for unvaccinated high-risk patients after a confirmed outbreak of influenza type A. Therapy with these antivirals is sometimes started at the same time as vaccination; the antiviral offers protection during the period before antibody titers are achieved from the vaccine. Antivirals for influenza are shown in Table 26.4.

The *neuroamidase inhibitors* are used to treat active infections. If given within 48 hours of the onset of symptoms, oseltamivir (Tamiflu) and zanamivir (Relenza) are reported to shorten the normal 7-day duration of influenza symptoms to 5 days. Because these influenza antivirals produce only modest benefits for patients with an active infection, prevention through vaccination remains the best alternative.

Treatment of hepatitis B virus infection. Hepatitis B virus (HBV) is transmitted primarily through exposure to contaminated blood and body fluids. Major risk factors for HBV

DRUG PROFILE: ℗ *Acyclovir (Zovirax)*

Therapeutic Class: Antiviral for herpesviruses
Pharmacologic Class: Nucleoside analog

Actions and Uses:

The antiviral activity of acyclovir is limited to the herpesviruses, for which it is the drug of choice. It is most effective against HSV-1 and HSV-2 and effective only at high doses against CMV and varicella-zoster. By inhibiting viral DNA synthesis, acyclovir decreases the duration and severity of herpes episodes. Resistance has developed to the drug, particularly in patients with HIV-AIDS. When given for prophylaxis, it may decrease the frequency of active herpes episodes, but it does not cure the patient. It is available in topical form for placing directly on active lesions, in oral form for prophylaxis, and as an IV for particularly severe disease.

Adverse Effects and Interactions:

There are few adverse effects to acyclovir when administered topically or orally. When given IV, the drug may cause painful inflammation of vessels at the site of infusion. Because nephrotoxicity is possible, especially when the drug is given by the IV route, kidney function should be carefully monitored.

Acyclovir interacts with several drugs. For example, probenecid decreases acyclovir elimination, and zidovudine may cause increased drowsiness and lethargy.

 Refer to MyNursingKit for a Nursing Process Focus specific to this drug.

include injected drug abuse, sex with a partner infected with HBV, and sex between men. Health care workers are at risk because of accidental exposure to HBV-contaminated needles or body fluids.

Treatment of *acute* HBV infection is symptomatic because 90% of these infections resolve with complete recovery and do not progress to chronic disease. Symptoms of *chronic* HBV, however, may develop as long as 10 years following exposure. The final stage of the infection is hepatic cirrhosis. In addition, chronic HBV infections are associated with an increased risk of hepatocellular carcinoma.

The best treatment for HBV infection is *prevention* through vaccination: HBV vaccine (Recombivax HB, Engerix-B) provides up to 90% of patients with protection against HBV following exposure to the virus. Once chronic hepatitis becomes active, three different therapies are approved for pharmacotherapy:

■ Interferon alfa or peginterferon: these drugs are natural proteins that suppress viral replication and enhance body defenses

■ Lamivudine (Epivir): resembles a building block for DNA; inhibits viral DNA synthesis

■ Adefovir (Hepsera): blocks viral DNA synthesis; primarily used for patients with viruses resistant to lamivudine.

Infections caused by helminths and protozoans cause significant disease worldwide.

CORE CONCEPT 26.7

proto = *first*
zoans = *animals*

Other pathogens that may infect humans include single-celled organisms, or **protozoans**, and multicellular animals such as mites, ticks, and worms. Some of these parasites thrive in conditions in which sanitation and personal hygiene are poor and population density is high. Although many of these diseases are rare in the United States and Canada, travelers to Africa, Asia, and South America may acquire infections overseas and return home with them. Table 26.5 lists selected antiparasitics. Scabicides and pediculicides are covered in Chapter 31 ⚭ .

With a few exceptions, antibiotics, antifungal, and antiviral drugs are ineffective against these complex organisms. Drugs prescribed for parasitic diseases may be classified as antimalarials, antiprotozoans (other than antimalarial agents), antihelmintics, and scabicides/pediculicides.

Malaria is a disease caused by four species of the protozoan *Plasmodium.* Although rare in the United States and Canada, malaria is the second most common fatal infectious disease in the world, with 300–500 million cases occurring annually. The Centers for Disease Control and Prevention (CDC) recommends that travelers to infected areas receive prophylactic antimalarial drugs prior to and during their visit and for 1 week after leaving. Chloroquine (Aralen) is the drug of choice, unless travel is to a region known to have a high incidence of chloroquine-resistant strains.

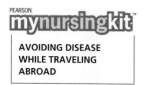

AVOIDING DISEASE
WHILE TRAVELING
ABROAD

Malaria begins with a bite from an infected female *Anopheles* mosquito, which is a carrier for *Plasmodium.* Once a person is infected, *Plasmodium* grows in the liver and eventually travels to red blood cells. Rupture of infected red blood cells causes severe fever and chills. Drug therapy is successful early in the course of the disease but becomes increasingly difficult because *Plasmodium* enters different stages of its life cycle in the body. Dormant parasites may remain in the liver for years and become resistant to medications. Chloroquine (Aralen) is the preferred drug for acute malaria; however, many other agents are also available because resistance to chloroquine is common. Primaquine is one of the few drugs available that can eliminate latent forms of *Plasmodium* residing in the liver. In 2009, the FDA approved the fixed-dose combination drug artemether/lumefantrine (Coartem) to treat acute, uncomplicated malaria infections. Coartem is significant because it offers an additional option for treating patients with chloroquine-resistant infections.

Other species of protozoans that cause significant disease worldwide include *Entamoeba, Giardia, Leishmania, Pneumocystis, Toxoplasma,* and *Trypanosoma.* Amebiasis is a disease caused by *Entamoeba histolytica,* commonly found in Africa, Latin America, and Asia, where it frequently causes serious disease. Although primarily an intestinal disease, *E. histolytica* can invade the liver, where it causes abscesses. The primary sign of amebiasis is a severe form of diarrhea known as amebic **dysentery**. Drugs used to treat amebiasis include those that act directly on amebas in the intestine and those that are administered for their systemic effects on the liver and other organs.

dys = *difficult or painful*
enter = *intestine*

Helminths consist of various species of parasitic worms, including hookworms, pinworms, roundworms, tapeworms, and flukes. Many of these worms attach to the mucosa of the human

TABLE 26.5	Drugs for Helminth and Protozoan Infections	
DRUG	**ROUTE AND ADULT DOSE**	**REMARKS**
ANTIHELMINTICS		
albendazole (Albenza)	PO; 400 mg bid (max: 800 mg/day)	Only antihelmintic drug active against all stages of the helminth life cycle
ivermectin (Stromectol)	PO; 150–200 mcg/kg for one dose	Preferred drug for many helminth infections
mebendazole (Vermox)	PO; 100 mg for one dose or 100 mg bid for 3 days	For the treatment of whipworm, roundworm, hookworm, and pinworm
praziquantel (Biltricide)	PO; 5 mg/kg for one dose or 25 mg/kg tid	For all stages of schistosomiasis; bitter tablet
pyrantel (Antiminth, Ascarel, Pin-X, Pinworm Caplets)	PO; 11 mg/kg for one dose (max: 1 g)	For the treatment of hookworm and roundworm
ANTIMALARIALS		
Artemether and lumefantrine (Coartem)	Oral; 3–6 doses for 3 days (20 mg of artemether and 120 mg of lumefantrine per dose)	Newer drug for patients with chloroquine-resistant malaria.
atovaquone and proguanil (Malarone)	PO; for prophylaxis; one tablet/day starting 1–2 days before travel, and continuing until 7 days after return	Also for *Pneumocystis*
chloroquine (Aralen)	PO; 600 mg initial dose, then 300 mg weekly	Preferred drug for malaria; also for amebiasis and rheumatoid arthritis; IM form available; if administered IV, oral medication is ineffective
hydroxychloroquine (Plaquenil) (see page 607 for the Drug Profile box)	PO; 620 mg initial dose, then 310 mg weekly	Also for rheumatoid arthritis and lupus erythematosus
mefloquine (Lariam)	PO; prevention: begin with 250 mg once a week for 4 weeks, then 250 mg every other week; treatment: 1250 mg as a single dose	For prevention and treatment of malaria
primaquine	PO; 15 mg daily for 2 weeks	Removes *Plasmodium vivax* from the liver; used for malaria suppression
pyrimethamine (Daraprim)	PO; 25 mg once per week for 10 weeks	Also antiprotozoan; drug of choice for toxoplasmosis
quinine (Quinamm)	PO; 260–650 mg tid for 3 days	Largely replaced by other antimalarials; also for nocturnal leg cramps
ANTIPROTOZOANS (NONMALARIAL)		
doxycycline (Vibramycin)	PO; 100 mg/day	For traveler's diarrhea; used also for malaria prophylaxis; a tetracycline antibiotic
ⓟ metronidazole (Flagyl)	PO; 250–750 mg tid	For many parasitic infections; IV form available
nifurtimox (Lampit)	PO; 2–2.5 mg/kg every 6 hours	Preferred drug for American trypanosomiasis
paromomycin (Humatin)	PO; 25–35 mg/kg divided in three doses for 5–10 days	For acute and chronic amebiasis; an aminoglycoside antibiotic
pentamidine (Pentam, NebuPent)	IV; 4 mg/kg daily for 14–21 days; infuse over 60 min	For *Pneumocystis carinii* active infections and prophylaxis; IM and inhalation forms available
suramin (Germanin)	IV; 1 g on days 1, 3, 7, 14, and 21	Preferred drug for early stages of African trypanosomiasis
tinidazole (Tindamax)	PO; 2 grams per day for 3 days	Newer drug for amebiasis giardiasis, or trichomoniasis

---

DRUG PROFILE: ℗ *Metronidazole (Flagyl)*

Therapeutic Class: Anti-infective, antiprotozoan
Pharmacologic Class: Agent that disrupts nucleic acid synthesis

Actions and Uses:

Metronidazole is a preferred drug for amebiasis because it is effective against amebas in the intestine and in other organs. Metronidazole is also a drug of choice for two other protozoan infections: giardiasis from *Giardia lamblia* and trichonomiasis due to *Trichomonas vaginalis*.

Metronidazole is somewhat unique in that it also has antibiotic activity against anaerobic bacteria and thus is used to treat a number of respiratory, bone, skin, and CNS infections. Topical forms are used to treat rosacea, a disease characterized by reddening of the sebaceous glands in the skin around the nose and face. It is used in combination with bismuth and tetracycline to eradicate *H. pylori* infection, which is associated with peptic ulcer disease.

Adverse Effects and Interactions:

Although adverse effects are relatively common, most are not serious enough to cause discontinuation of therapy. The most common adverse effects of metronidazole are anorexia, nausea, diarrhea, dizziness, and headache. Dryness of the mouth and an unpleasant metallic taste may be experienced.

Metronidazole interacts with several drugs. For example, oral anticoagulants increase hypoprothombinemia. In combination with alcohol and medications that contain alcohol, metronidazole may cause a disulfiram reaction. It may also elevate lithium levels.

Refer to MyNursingKit for a Nursing Process Focus specific to this drug.

PATIENTS NEED TO KNOW

Patients treated for fungal, viral, or parasitic infections need to know the following:

Regarding Antifungals

1. Avoid alcohol and other drugs toxic to the liver while taking azole-type antifungals.
2. Griseofulvin, used to treat superficial mycoses, can decrease the effectiveness of oral contraceptives. An alternative method of contraception is advised.
3. Older children and adult patients should swish oral antifungal drugs around in their mouths and swallow them. Caregivers should swab the mouths of infants and toddlers. Wait at least 10 minutes after antifungal treatment to put anything else in the mouth.
4. Rinse the mouth after use of glucocorticoid inhalers to avoid a decrease in local immune defenses against oral candidiasis.
5. While taking antifungal drugs for a vaginal infection, refrain from sexual intercourse until the infection is resolved.

Regarding Antivirals

6. When taking antivirals, it is important to report symptoms of hypersensitivity reactions.
7. When taking antivirals, do not take any other medications or dietary supplements without consulting a health care provider because of the risk for interactions.

Regarding Helminths and Protozoans

8. Course of treatment depends on the nature of the infection/infestation, and treatment plan is to be followed completely as prescribed.
9. Take showers instead of baths. Change underwear, linens, and towels daily.
10. Handwashing is very important in the prevention of pinworms/roundworms.

intestinal tract. Helminth diseases are quite common in areas of the world lacking high standards of sanitation. Helminth infections in the United States and Canada are generally neither common nor fatal, although drug therapy may be indicated. The most common helminth disease worldwide is caused by the roundworm *Ascaris;* however, infection by the pinworm *Enterobius* is more common in the United States. For ascariasis, oral mebendazole (Vermox) for 3 days is the standard treatment. Pharmacotherapy of enterobiasis includes a single dose of mebendazole, albendazole (Albenza), or pyrantel (Antiminth).

Concept Review 26.3

■ How do most patients in the United States and Canada acquire protozoan infections?

CHAPTER REVIEW

CORE CONCEPTS SUMMARY

26.1 **Fungal infections are classified as superficial or systemic.**

Fungi are multicellular organisms. Because most are unaffected by antibiotics, they require different classes of medications. Fungal infections are usually a serious problem only in patients with compromised immune systems. Mycoses are classified as superficial or systemic.

26.2 **Systemic antifungal drugs are used for serious infections of internal organs.**

Systemic mycoses affect the internal organs and may require prolonged and aggressive drug therapy. Systemic antifungal agents may cause serious adverse effects.

26.3 **Superficial infections of the skin, nails, and mucous membranes are effectively treated with topical and oral antifungal drugs.**

Superficial mycoses of the hair, skin, nails, and mucous membranes are very common, though rarely serious. Antifungals given topically as powders, troches, and ointments produce few adverse effects.

26.4 **Viruses are infectious agents that require a host to replicate.**

Viruses take over the cellular machinery of host cells and use it to replicate themselves. Although most viral infections require no pharmacotherapy,

patients with infections by HIV, herpesviruses, and the influenza virus may benefit from drug treatment.

26.5 **Antiretroviral drugs do not cure HIV-AIDS, but they do help many patients live longer.**

Drugs used to treat HIV infections include the nucleoside and nonnucleoside reverse transcriptase inhibitors, protease inhibitors, and fusion inhibitors. These drugs may produce significant toxicity. Although none are able to cure the disease, they may extend the symptom-free period.

26.6 **Antiviral drugs are available to treat herpes simplex, influenza, and hepatitis infections.**

Drug therapy is used to extend the latent period of genital herpes and to speed the recovery from active lesions. A few antivirals are available to prevent influenza, and these are most useful when combined with vaccines. New drugs have been developed to shorten the discomfort period for influenza symptoms, although these drugs have limited effectiveness.

26.7 **Infections caused by helminths and protozoans cause significant disease worldwide.**

Malaria is one of the most common infections in the world, and a significant number of drugs are available to disrupt the *Plasmodium* life cycle. Similarly, amebiasis is a common protozoan disease requiring intensive drug treatment. Diseases caused by helminths are common in areas of the world lacking adequate sanitation.

REVIEW QUESTIONS

The following questions are written in NCLEX-PN® style. Answer these questions to assess your knowledge of the chapter material, and go back and review any material that is not clear to you.

1. The patient on amphotericin B must be monitored for:

1. Ototoxicity
2. Hepatic toxicity
3. Nephrotoxicity
4. Anoxia

2. The patient has oral candidiasis. Which of the following medications does the nurse expect to be ordered?

1. Terbinafine (Lamisil)
2. Clotrimazole (Mycelex)
3. Ketoconazole (Nizoral)
4. Nystatin (Mycostatin)

3. The patient with a fungal infection of her toenails asks how long treatment must occur. The best response would be:

1. "Treatment is very quick, requiring only one tablet of clotrimazole."
2. "Treatment will occur daily for 3 days."
3. "Treatment will last for several months."
4. "You will need to speak to your physician."

4. Patient teaching for a patient on zidovudine (AZT) would include the:

1. Importance of taking the medication every 4 hours
2. Fact that medication is taken daily for 1 month only
3. Information that, if taken correctly, this medication will cure the disease
4. Fact that the medication is used to treat influenza

5. Which of the following drugs would be used to treat genital herpes?

1. Trifluridine (Viroptic)
2. Doxycycline (Vibramycin)
3. Acyclovir (Zovirax)
4. Foscarnet (Foscavir)

6. The patient complains of flulike symptoms that started 24 hours ago. Which of the following class of medications would the nurse anticipate being ordered?

1. Protease inhibitors
2. Nonnucleoside reverse transcriptase inhibitors
3. Nucleoside reverse transcriptase inhibitors
4. Neuroamidase inhibitors

7. The preferred drug to treat *Trichomonas vaginalis* is:

1. Nifurtimox (Lampit)
2. Zidovudine (Retrovir)
3. Nystatin (Mycostatin)
4. Metronidazole (Flagyl)

8. When applying topical antivirals, which of the following statements is true?

1. No other antivirals should be administered.
2. Gloves should be worn to prevent transmission.
3. Antivirals should not be applied to open areas.
4. Vital signs should be assessed prior to administration.

9. A patient on an antiretroviral for HIV has developed anemia. This could indicate which of the following?

1. The patient is most likely being abused.
2. The patient is experiencing minor adverse reactions.
3. The patient is not taking the medications as ordered.
4. The patient may be experiencing severe toxicity due to high doses of the drug.

10. The nurse is providing education to a mother of a young patient about pinworms and roundworms. Which of the following should be included in this teaching?

1. Handwashing is very important in preventing the spread of pinworms and roundworms.
2. Play habits do not contribute to the transmission of pinworms and roundworms.
3. It is not important that children wear shoes when playing outside.
4. Once the child has had worms, reinfection cannot occur.

CASE STUDY QUESTIONS

For questions 1–4, please refer to the following case study, and choose the correct answer from choices 1–4.

*M*s. Davis is a 78-year-old retired auto worker who is frail and in ill health and comes to the health care provider's office for advice.

1. What is her best option to avoid a potential life-threatening bout with the flu?

1. Begin taking oseltamivir (Tamiflu) 1 month before the flu season begins
2. Take zanamavir (Relenza) within 48 hours of the onset of flu symptoms
3. Receive a flu vaccination 30–60 days prior to the start of the flu season
4. Take acyclovir (Zovirax) during the flu season

2. During the flu season, Ms. Davis reports vaginal itching and abnormal discharges, and the physician diagnoses vaginal candidiasis. Which of the following would be the most likely drug therapy?

1. Amphotericin B (Fungizone)
2. Clotrimazole (Gyne-Lotrimin)
3. Acyclovir (Zovirax)
4. Tinidazole (Tindamax)

Mr. Walker attends the local health department clinic for treatment of a chronic disorder.

3. While examining Mr. Walker's medical records, you note that he is taking saquinavir (Invirase), abacavir (Ziagen), and efavirenz (Sustiva). Mr. Walker is most likely suffering from what type of infection?

1. HIV
2. Systemic fungal
3. Malaria
4. Herpes simplex

4. The type of drugs taken by Mr. Walker is called an:

1. Antiviral
2. Antiretroviral
3. Antifungal
4. Antiprotozoan

FURTHER STUDY

- Drugs that suppress the immune system and which may place the patient at higher risk for viral and protozoan infections are discussed in Chapter 24 ∞ .

- Antineoplastic drugs that may place the patient at higher risk for viral and protozoan infections are discussed in Chapter 27 ∞ .

- Information on vaccines is included in Chapter 24 ∞ .

- Chapter 34 ∞ discusses scabicides and pediculicides.

27 Drugs for Neoplasia

CORE CONCEPTS

27.1 Cancer is characterized by rapid, uncontrolled growth of cells.

27.2 The causes of cancer may be chemical, physical, or biological.

27.3 Personal risk of cancer may be lowered by a number of lifestyle factors.

27.4 The three primary goals of chemotherapy are cure, control, and palliation.

27.5 To achieve a total cure, every malignant cell must be removed or killed.

27.6 Use of multiple drugs and special dosing schedules improves the success of chemotherapy.

27.7 Serious toxicity limits therapy with most of the antineoplastic agents.

27.8 Alkylating agents act by changing the structure of DNA in cancer cells.

27.9 Antimetabolites disrupt critical cellular pathways in cancer cells.

27.10 A few cytotoxic antibiotics are used to treat cancer rather than infections.

27.11 Some plant extracts kill cancer cells by preventing cell division.

27.12 Some hormones and hormone antagonists are effective against prostate and breast cancer.

27.13 Biologic response modifiers and some additional antineoplastic drugs are effective against specific tumors.

DRUG SNAPSHOT

The following drugs are discussed in this chapter:

DRUG CLASSES	DRUG PROFILES
Alkylating agents	(Pr) cyclophosphamide (Cytoxan)
Antimetabolites	(Pr) methotrexate (Rheumatrex, Trexall)
Antitumor antibiotics	(Pr) doxorubicin (Adriamycin)
Plant alkaloids/ natural products	(Pr) vincristine (Oncovin)

DRUG CLASSES	DRUG PROFILES
Hormones and hormone antagonists	(Pr) tamoxifen
Biologic response modifiers	(Pr) interferon alfa-2b (Intron A)
Miscellaneous drugs for cancer patients	(Pr) epoetin alfa (Epogen, Procrit)

LEARNING OUTCOMES

After reading this chapter, the student should be able to:

1. Explain differences between normal cells and cancer cells.

2. Identify factors associated with an increased incidence of cancer.

3. Describe lifestyle factors associated with a reduced risk of acquiring cancer.

4. Differentiate among the terms neoplasm, benign, malignant, and carcinoma.

5. Identify the three primary treatments for cancer.

6. Explain why cancer is difficult to cure.

7. Explain how combination therapy and special dosing schedules increase the effectiveness of chemotherapy.

8. Describe the general adverse effects of antineoplastic drugs.

9. For each of the drug classes listed in the Drug Snapshot, explain the mechanisms of drug action, primary actions, and important adverse effects.

10. Categorize anticancer drugs based on their classifications and mechanisms of action.

ancer is one of the most feared diseases for a number of valid reasons. It may be silent, producing no symptoms until it is too large to cure. It sometimes requires painful and disfiguring surgery. It may occur at an early age—even during childhood—depriving people of a normal lifespan. Perhaps worst of all, the medical treatment of cancer often cannot offer a cure, and progression to death is sometimes slow, painful, and psychologically difficult for the patient and his or her loved ones.

Many advances have been made in the diagnosis, understanding, and treatment of cancer. Some types of cancer are now curable, and therapies may provide the patient a longer, symptom-free life. This chapter examines the role of drugs in the treatment of cancer. Medications used to treat this disease are called anticancer drugs, antineoplastics, or cancer chemotherapeutic agents.

Cancer is characterized by rapid, uncontrolled growth of cells.

CORE CONCEPT 27.1

Cancer is a disease characterized by abnormal, uncontrolled cell division. Cell division is a normal process occurring extensively in most body tissues from conception to late childhood. At some point, however, most cells stop dividing at such a rapid rate. Indeed, some adult cells such as muscle cells and brain cells have a total lack of ability to divide. In other cells, the genes controlling growth can be turned back on whenever it is necessary to replace worn-out cells, as is the case for blood cells and cell lining the digestive tract.

Fast Facts Cancer

- It is estimated that more than 1,400,000 new cancer cases occur each year, in the United States with 563,700 deaths (over 1,500 people every day).
- Cancer is the leading cause of death by disease in children younger than 15 years.
- Leukemia is the most common childhood cancer and is responsible for one quarter of all cancers occurring before age 20.
- Lung cancer has the highest mortality rate: It is responsible for 28% of all cancer deaths.
- Prostate cancer is the second leading cause of cancer death in men.
- The highest 5-year survival rates are for cancers of the prostate, testes, and thyroid. The lowest survival rates are for pancreatic and liver cancers.
- Among ethnic groups, African Americans have the highest incidence rates in many types of cancers, including lung, breast, and prostate cancer. Since 1990, this gap has been narrowing.
- Although breast cancer is predominant in women (second in cancer deaths), almost 2,000 men are diagnosed with the disease each year.

FIGURE 27.1

Invasion and metastasis
by cancer cells

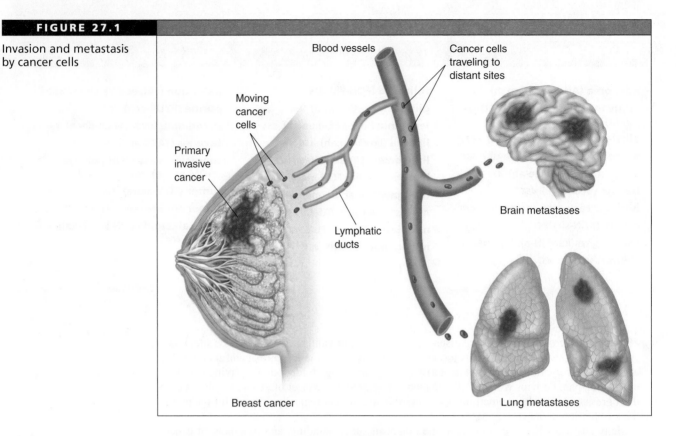

Cancer is thought to result from damage to genes controlling cell growth. Once damaged, the cell is no longer responsive to normal chemical signals checking its growth. The cancer cells lose their normal functions, divide rapidly, and invade surrounding cells. The abnormal cells often travel to distant sites, where they populate new tumors, a process called **metastasis**. Figure 27.1 ■ illustrates some characteristics of cancer cells.

neo = *new*
plasm = *thing formed*

The word **tumor** means swelling, abnormal enlargement, or mass. **Neoplasm** is often used interchangeably with tumor. The suffix –*oma* signifies tumor. Tumors may be either benign or malignant.

Benign tumors grow slowly, do not metastasize, and rarely require drug treatment. Although they do not kill patients, their growth may cause pressure on nerves, blood vessels, or other tissues. When this occurs, they may be surgically removed; they do not normally grow back. Examples include **adenomas**, which are benign tumors of glandular tissue, and **lipomas**, which are tumors of adipose tissue.

adeno = *gland*
oma = *tumor*
lip = *fat*

Malignant tumors are called cancer. The word **malignant** refers to a disease that grows rapidly worse, becomes resistant to treatment, and normally results in death. The two major divisions of malignant neoplasms are carcinomas and sarcomas. Other types include cancer of the blood-forming cells in bone marrow (**leukemia**), cancers of lymphatic tissue (**lymphomas**), and cancers of the central nervous system (**gliomas**).

leuk = *white*
emia = *blood condition*

CORE CONCEPT 27.2

The causes of cancer may be chemical, physical, or biological.

A large number of factors have been found to cause cancer or to be associated with a higher risk for acquiring the disease. Substances that cause cancer are known as **carcinogens**.

Many chemical carcinogens have been identified. For example, chemicals in tobacco smoke are responsible for about one third of all cancers in the United States. Some chemicals, such as asbestos and benzene, have been associated with a higher incidence of cancer in the workplace. The actual site of the cancer may be distant from the site of exposure, as is the case of bladder cancer caused by the inhalation of certain industrial chemicals.

A number of physical factors are also associated with cancer. For example, exposure to large amounts of X-rays is associated with a higher risk of leukemia. Ultraviolet (UV) light from the sun is a known cause of skin cancer.

Viruses are associated with about 15% of all human cancers. Examples include herpes simplex viruses types I and II, Epstein-Barr virus, human papillomavirus (HPV), cytomegalovirus, and human T-lymphotrophic viruses. Factors that suppress the immune system, such as HIV or drugs given after transplant surgery, may encourage the growth of cancer cells.

Some cancers have a strong genetic component. The fact that close relatives may acquire the same type of cancer suggests that the patient may have certain genes that predispose him or her to the condition. These abnormal genes interact with chemical, physical, and biological agents to promote cancer formation in the patient. Other genes, called **tumor suppressor genes**, may inhibit the formation of tumors. If these suppressor genes are damaged, cancer may result. Damage to the suppressor gene known as p53 is associated with cancers of the breast, lung, brain, colon, and bone.

Concept Review 27.1

■ What is the fundamental feature that makes a cancer cell different from a normal cell?

Personal risk of cancer may be lowered by a number of lifestyle factors.

CORE CONCEPT 27.3

Fortunately, adopting healthy lifestyle habits such as those shown in the following list may reduce the risk of acquiring cancer. Eliminating tobacco use is the most important means of reducing cancer risk. Limiting exposure to exhaled, or secondhand, smoke is also thought to be important. Intake of alcoholic beverages and saturated fats should be limited, and body weight kept within medically recommended ranges. The following list indicates some actions that health care providers can recommend to their patients to reduce their risk of cancer:

- Eliminate tobacco use and exposure to secondhand tobacco smoke.
- Limit or eliminate alcoholic beverage use.
- Maintain a healthy diet low in fat and high in fresh vegetables and fruit.
- Choose most of the foods from plant sources; increase fiber in the diet.
- Exercise regularly and keep body weight within optimum guidelines.
- Self-examine your body monthly for abnormal lumps and skin lesions.
- When exposed to direct sun, use skin lotions with the highest sun protection factor (SPF) value.
- For women, have periodic mammograms, as directed by the health care provider.
- For men, have annual prostate exams after age 50.
- Receive screening colonoscopy, according to the schedule recommended by the health care provider.
- For women who are sexually active or have reached age 18, have an annual Pap test and pelvic examination.

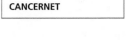

PEARSON
mynursingkit

CANCERNET

The three primary goals of chemotherapy are cure, control, and palliation.

CORE CONCEPT 27.4

Pharmacotherapy of cancer is sometimes simply referred to as **chemotherapy**. Because drugs are transported through the blood, chemotherapy has the potential to reach cancer cells in virtually any location. Chemotherapy has three general goals: cure, control, or palliation.

When diagnosed with cancer, the primary goal desired by most patients is to achieve a complete cure: permanent removal of all cancer cells from the body. The possibility for cure is much greater if a cancer is identified and treated in its early stages, when the tumor is small and localized to a well-defined region. Examples in which chemotherapy has been used successfully as curative treatments include Hodgkin's lymphoma, certain leukemias, and choriocarcinoma.

When cancer has progressed and cure is not possible, a second goal of chemotherapy is to control or manage the disease. Although the cancer is not eliminated, preventing the growth and spread of the tumor may extend the patient's life. Essentially, the cancer is managed as a chronic disease, as is hypertension or diabetes.

In its advanced stages, cure or control of the cancer may not be achievable. For these patients, chemotherapy is used as **palliation**. Chemotherapy drugs are administered to reduce the size of the tumor, easing the severity of pain and other tumor symptoms, thus improving the quality of life.

Chemotherapy may be used alone or in combination with surgery or radiation therapy. Surgery is especially useful for removing solid tumors that are localized. Surgery lowers the number of cancer cells in the body so that radiation therapy and pharmacotherapy can be more successful. Surgery is not an option for tumors of blood cells or when it would not be expected to extend a patient's life span or to improve the quality of life.

Approximately 50% of patients with cancer receive radiation therapy as part of their treatment. Radiation therapy is most successful for cancers that are localized. Radiation treatments are frequently prescribed postoperatively to kill cancer cells that may remain following an operation. Radiation is sometimes given as palliation for inoperable cancers to shrink the size of a tumor that may be pressing on vital organs and to relieve pain, difficulty breathing, or difficulty swallowing.

Adjuvant chemotherapy is the administration of antineoplastic drugs *after* surgery or radiation therapy. The purpose of adjuvant chemotherapy is to rid the body of any cancerous cells that were not removed during the surgery or to treat any microscopic metastases that may be developing. In a few cases, drugs are given as *chemoprophylaxis* with the goal of preventing cancer from occurring. For example, some patients who have had a primary breast cancer removed may receive tamoxifen, even if there is no evidence of metastases, because there is a high likelihood that the disease will recur. Chemoprophylaxis of cancer is uncommon, because most of these drugs have potentially serious adverse effects.

CORE CONCEPT 27.5

To achieve a total cure, every malignant cell must be removed or killed.

To cure a patient, it is believed that every single cancer cell must be eliminated from the body. Even one malignant cell could potentially produce enough offspring to kill the patient. Eliminating every cancer cell, however, is a very difficult task.

Consider that a 1-cm breast tumor may contain 1 billion cancer cells before it is detected. A drug that kills 99% of these cells would be considered a very effective drug. Yet even with this fantastic achievement, 10 million cancer cells would still remain, any one of which could cause the tumor to return and kill the patient. The relationship between cell kill and chemotherapy is shown in Figure 27.2 ■.

It is likely that no antineoplastic drug (or combination of drugs) will kill 100% of the tumor cells. The large burden of cancer cells, however, may be lowered sufficiently to permit the patient's immune system to control or eliminate the remaining cancer cells. Because the immune system is able to eliminate only a relatively small number of cancer cells, it is important that as many cancerous cells as possible be eliminated during treatment. This example reinforces the need to diagnose and treat tumors at an *early* stage, when the number of cancer cells is smaller.

NATURAL THERAPIES

Selenium's Role in Cancer Prevention

Selenium is an essential trace element that is necessary to maintain healthy immune function. It is a vital antioxidant, especially when combined with vitamin E. It protects the immune system by preventing the formation of free radicals, which can damage cells.

Selenium can be found in meat and grains, Brazil nuts, brewer's yeast, broccoli, brown rice, dairy products, garlic, molasses, and onions. The amount of selenium in food, however, has a direct correlation to the selenium content of the soil. The soil of much American farmland is low in selenium, resulting in selenium-deficient produce. Low dietary intake of selenium is associated with increased incidence of several cancers, including lung, colorectal, skin, and prostate cancers. Selenium supplementation has resulted in increased natural killer cell activity, and studies have shown its promise as protection against prostate and colorectal cancers, especially among smokers.

FIGURE 27.2

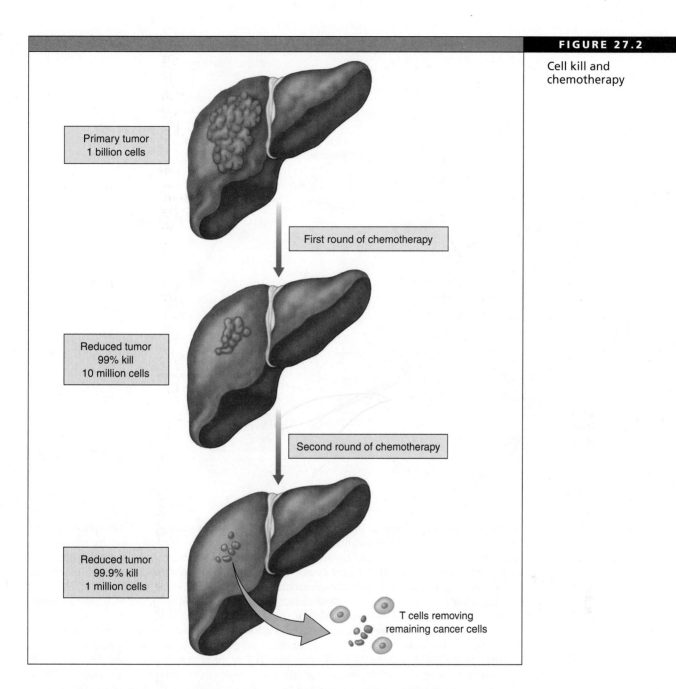

Cell kill and
chemotherapy

Primary tumor
1 billion cells

First round of chemotherapy

Reduced tumor
99% kill
10 million cells

Second round of chemotherapy

Reduced tumor
99.9% kill
1 million cells

T cells removing
remaining cancer cells

Use of multiple drugs and special dosing schedules improves the success of chemotherapy.

CORE CONCEPT **27.6**

Because of their rapid cell division, tumor cells express a high mutation rate. This causes the tumor to change its genetic make-up as it grows, resulting in hundreds of different clones with different growth rates and physiologic properties. An antineoplastic drug may kill only a small portion of the tumor, leaving some clones unaffected. Complicating the chances for a cure is that cancer cells often develop resistance to antineoplastic drugs. Thus a therapy that was very successful in reducing the tumor mass at the start of chemotherapy may become less effective over time.

A number of treatment strategies have been found to increase the effectiveness of anticancer drugs. In most cases, multiple medications from different antineoplastic classes are given concurrently during a course of chemotherapy. Multiple classes will affect different stages of the cancer cell's life cycle, as illustrated in Figure 27.3 ■. This allows the tumor to be attacked through

FIGURE 27.3

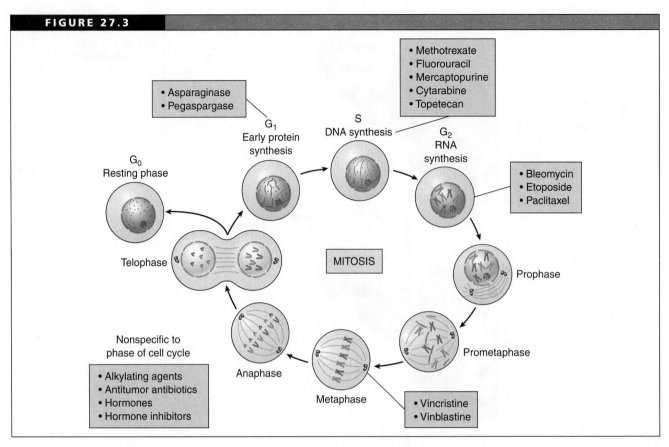

Antineoplastic agents and the cell cycle

several mechanisms of action, thus increasing the cell kill percentage. Using multiple drugs also allows the dosages of each individual agent to be lowered, thereby reducing toxicity and slowing the development of resistance. Examples of common therapies include cyclophosphamide-methotrexate-fluorouracil (CMF) for breast cancer, cyclophosphamide-doxorubicin-vincristine (CAV) for lung cancer, and cyclophosphamide-doxorubicin-vincristine-prednisone (CHOP) for non-Hodgkin's lymphoma. Each type of cancer has its own individual protocol, which is continually being revised based on recent research.

Specific dosing schedules or cycles have been found to increase the effectiveness of antineoplastic agents. For example, some anticancer drugs are given as single doses or perhaps a couple of doses over a few days. Several weeks may pass before the next series of doses. This gives normal cells time to recover from the adverse effects of the drugs, especially bone marrow suppression. It also allows tumor cells that may not have been replicating at the time of the first dose to begin dividing and become more sensitive to the next round of chemotherapy.

Concept Review 27.2

■ Why is it important to kill or remove 100% of the cancer cells to effect a cure?

CORE CONCEPT 27.7

Serious toxicity limits therapy with most of the antineoplastic drugs.

All anticancer drugs have the potential to cause serious toxicity. These drugs are often pushed to their maximum possible dosages so that the greatest cell kill can be obtained. Such high dosages always result in adverse effects in the patient. A list of typical adverse effects of anticancer drugs is given in Table 27.1.

TABLE 27.1	Adverse Effects of Anticancer Drugs	
BLOOD TOXICITY	**GI TOXICITY**	**OTHER EFFECTS**
Anemia (low red blood cell count)	Anorexia (loss of appetite)	Alopecia (loss of hair)
Leukopenia (low white blood cell count)	Bleeding	Fatigue
Thrombocytopenia (low platelet count)	Diarrhea	Fetal birth defects
	Nausea and vomiting	Opportunistic infections
		Ulceration and bleeding of the lips and gums

Normal tissues that are rapidly dividing in the adult are most susceptible to adverse effects. Hair follicles are damaged, resulting in hair loss or **alopecia**. The lining of the digestive tract is affected, sometimes resulting in bleeding, difficulty eating, or severe diarrhea. The vomiting center in the medulla is triggered by many antineoplastics, resulting in severe nausea and vomiting. Vomiting is often so severe that patients may be treated with antiemetic drugs such as prochlorperazine (Compazine) or odansetron (Zofran) before beginning antineoplastic therapy. Blood cells in the bone marrow may be destroyed, causing a reduction in the number of red blood cells, white blood cells, and platelets. Severe effects on blood cells often cause discontinuation of chemotherapy. Efforts to minimize this toxicity may include therapy with growth factors such as filgrastim (Neupogen) or sargramostim (Leukine). These drugs stimulate the production of white blood cells within the bone marrow.

Antineoplastic drugs act by many mechanisms, most of which involve cell killing, or cytotoxicity. Classification is quite variable because some drugs kill cancer cells by several mechanisms and have characteristics from more than one class. Furthermore, the mechanisms by which some of these medications act are not completely understood. A simple method of classifying this complex group of drugs includes six groups:

- Alkylating agents
- Antimetabolites
- Antitumor antibiotics
- Plant alkaloids/natural products
- Hormones and hormone blockers
- Biologic response modifiers

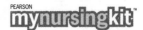

CURRENT INDICATIONS FOR ANTINEOPLASTICS

Alkylating agents act by changing the structure of DNA in cancer cells.

CORE CONCEPT 27.8

Alkylating agents act by chemically binding to nucleic acids and inhibiting cell division. They are some of the most widely used antineoplastic drugs. Table 27.2 lists the alkylating agents and their dosages.

The first alkylating agents, the **nitrogen mustards**, were developed in secrecy as chemical warfare agents during World War I. Although the drugs in this class have quite different chemical structures, all have the common characteristic of being able to form bonds or linkages with DNA. These agents physically attach to DNA, a process called **alkylation**. Alkylation changes the shape of DNA and prevents it from functioning normally. Although each alkylating agent attaches to DNA in a different manner, collectively they have the effect of killing—or at least slowing—the replication of tumor cells. The alkylation may occur in any cancer cell; however, the killing action does not occur until the affected cell attempts to divide. Figure 27.4 ■ illustrates the process of alkylation.

Blood cells are particularly sensitive to alkylating agents, and bone marrow suppression is the primary dose-limiting adverse effect of drugs in this class. Within days of administration, the numbers of red blood cells, white blood cells, and platelets begin to decline. Cells lining the gastrointestinal (GI) tract are also damaged, resulting in nausea, vomiting, and diarrhea. Alopecia is expected from most of the alkylating agents.

TABLE 27.2	Alkylating Agents	
DRUG	**ROUTE AND ADULT DOSE**	**REMARKS**
NITROGEN MUSTARDS		
bendamustine (Treanda)	IV; 90–120 mg/m² (variable schedule)	Newer antineoplastic drug; for chronic lymphocytic leukemia and non-Hodgkin's lymphoma
busulfan (Busulflex, Myleran)	PO; 4–8 mg daily	For chronic myelogenous leukemia; also available IV, prior to stem transplant
chlorambucil (Leukeran)	PO; initial dose 0.1–0.2 mg/kg daily; maintenance dose 4–10 mg daily	For chronic lymphocytic leukemia; non-Hodgkin's lymphoma, and cancer of the breast and ovary
ⓟ cyclophosphamide (Cytoxan)	PO; initial dose 1–5 mg/kg daily; maintenance dose 1–5 mg/kg every 7–10 days	For Hodgkin's disease, non-Hodgkin's lymphoma, leukemias, multiple myeloma, and cancer of the breast, ovary, and lung; IV form available
estramustine (Emcyt)	PO; 14 mg/kg/day in three to four divided doses	For palliative treatment of advanced prostate cancer
ifosfamide (Ifex)	IV; 1.2 g/m² daily for five consecutive days	For testicular cancer
mechlorethamine (Mustargen)	IV; 6 mg/m² on days 1 and 8 of a 28-day cycle	For Hodgkin's disease, non-Hodgkin's lymphoma, and lung cancer
melphalan (Alkeran)	PO; 6 mg daily for 2–3 weeks	For multiple myeloma
NITROSOUREAS		
carmustine (BiCNU, Gliadel)	IV; 200 mg/m² every 6 weeks	For Hodgkin's disease, malignant melanoma, multiple myeloma, and brain cancer
lomustine (CeeNU)	PO; 130 mg/m² as a single dose	For Hodgkin's disease and brain cancer
streptozocin (Zanosar)	IV; 500 mg/m² for five consecutive days	For pancreatic cancer
MISCELLANEOUS ALKYLATING AGENTS		
carboplatin (Paraplatin)	IV; 360 mg/m² every 4 weeks	For cancer of the ovary
cisplatin (Platinol)	IV; 20 mg/m² daily for 5 days	For testicular, bladder, ovarian, uterine, head, and neck carcinomas
dacarbazine (DTIC-Dome)	IV; 2–4.5 mg/kg daily for 10 days	For Hodgkin's disease and malignant melanoma
oxaliplatin (Eloxatin)	IV; 85 mg/m² infused over 120 min once every 2 weeks	For metastatic colorectal cancer
temozolomide (Temodar)	PO; 150 mg/m² daily for five consecutive days	For brain cancer
thiotepa (Thioplex)	IV; 0.3–0.4 mg/kg every 1–4 weeks	For Hodgkin's disease and breast and ovarian cancer

CORE CONCEPT 27.9

Antimetabolites disrupt critical cellular pathways in cancer cells.

Rapidly growing cancer cells require large amounts of nutrients to build proteins and nucleic acids. Antimetabolites are drugs that chemically resemble essential building blocks of the cell. When cancer cells attempt to construct proteins or DNA, they use the antimetabolite drugs instead of the normal building blocks. By disrupting metabolic pathways in this manner, antimetabolites can kill cancer cells or slow their growth. The antimetabolite drugs are listed in Table 27.3.

Several of these antimetabolites resemble **purines** and **pyrimidines**, chemicals that are the building blocks of DNA and RNA. These antimetabolites are called *purine* or *pyrimidine analogs*.

FIGURE 27.4

Mechanism of action of
alkylating agents

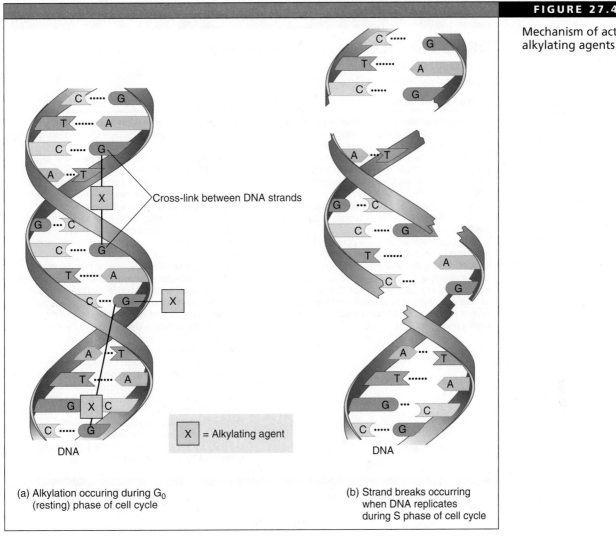

Cross-link between DNA strands

X = Alkylating agent

DNA

DNA

(a) Alkylation occuring during G_0
(resting) phase of cell cycle

(b) Strand breaks occurring
when DNA replicates
during S phase of cell cycle

For example, floxuridine (FUDR) and fluorouracil (Adrucil) are able to block the formation of thymidylate, an essential chemical needed to make DNA. After becoming activated and incorporated into DNA, cytarabine (Cytosar) blocks DNA synthesis. Figure 27.5 ■ illustrates the similarities of some of these analogs to their natural counterparts.

A few cytotoxic antibiotics are used to treat cancer rather than infections.

Antitumor antibiotics are drugs obtained from bacteria that have the ability to kill cancer cells. Although they are not widely prescribed, they are very effective against certain tumors. Table 27.4 lists the primary antitumor antibiotics.

Several substances isolated from bacteria have been found to possess antitumor properties. These chemicals are more toxic than the traditional antibiotics; thus, their use is restricted to treating specific cancers. All the antitumor antibiotics interact with DNA in a manner similar to the alkylating agents. Because of this, their general actions and adverse effects are similar to those of the alkylating agents. Unlike the alkylating agents, however, all the antitumor antibiotics must be administered intravenously or through direct instillation into a body cavity using a catheter. A major dose-limiting adverse effect of drugs in this class is bone marrow suppression.

DRUG PROFILE: Ⓟ *Cyclophosphamide (Cytoxan)*

Therapeutic Class: Antineoplastic
Pharmacologic Class: Alkylating agent

Actions and Uses:

Cyclophosphamide is a commonly prescribed nitrogen mustard. It is used alone or in combination with other drugs against a wide variety of cancers, including Hodgkin's disease, lymphoma, multiple myeloma, breast cancer, and ovarian cancer. Cyclophosphamide acts by attaching to DNA and disrupting cell replication, particularly in rapidly dividing cells. It is one of only a few anticancer drugs that are well absorbed when given orally.

Cyclophosphamide is a powerful immunosuppressant. Although this is considered an adverse effect during cancer chemotherapy, the drug is used to *intentionally* cause immunosuppression for the prophylaxis of organ transplant rejection and to treat severe rheumatoid arthritis and systemic lupus erythematosus (SLE).

Adverse Effects and Interactions:

Bone marrow suppression is a potentially life-threatening adverse reaction that occurs during days 9–14 of therapy; the patient is at dangerous risk for severe infection and sepsis during this period. Thrombocytopenia is common; thus bleeding and bruising may be observed. Nausea, vomiting, and diarrhea are frequently experienced. Fifty percent of patients will develop total baldness, although this effect is usually reversible. Unlike other nitrogen mustards, cyclophosphamide causes little neurotoxicity.

Cyclophosphamide interacts with many drugs. For example, immunosuppressant agents may increase the risk of infections and promote the development of neoplasms. There is an increased chance of bone marrow toxicity if cyclophosphamide is used together with allopurinol. There is an increased risk of bleeding if given with anticoagulants.

If used with digoxin, decreased serum levels of digoxin occur. Using it with insulin may lead to increased hypoglycemia. Phenobarbital, phenytoin, or glucocorticoids may lead to an increased rate of cyclophosphamide metabolism by the liver. Thiazide diuretic use with cyclophosphamide may lead to leukopenia.

St. John's wort may increase the toxic effects of cyclophosphamide.

Refer to MyNursingKit for a Nursing Process Focus specific to this drug.

CORE CONCEPT 27.11

Some plant extracts kill cancer cells by preventing cell division.

Plants have been a valuable source for antineoplastic agents. The primary plant extracts or alkaloids, used as antineoplastics, are listed in Table 27.5.

Chemicals with antineoplastic activity have been isolated from a number of plants, including the common periwinkle (*Vinca rosea*), the Pacific yew, the mandrake plant (May apple), and the shrub *Campothecus acuminata*. Although structurally very different, drugs in this class have the common ability to arrest cell division; thus they are sometimes called *mitotic inhibitors.*

The **vinca alkaloids**, vincristine (Oncovin) and vinblastine (Velban), are older medications derived from the periwinkle plant. Their biological properties were described in folklore for many years in various parts of the world prior to their use as anticancer drugs.

Native Americans described uses of the May apple long before teniposide (Vumon) and etoposide (VePesid) were isolated from this plant and used for chemotherapy. These agents are called **topoisomerase** inhibitors because they block the enzyme topoisomerase, which helps repair DNA damage. Bone marrow suppression is a serious adverse effect of most natural product drugs. More recently isolated topoisomerase inhibitors include topotecan (Hycamtin), which is used to treat metastatic ovarian cancer and lung cancer, and irinotecan (Camptosar), which is indicated for metastatic cancer of the colon.

The **taxanes**, which include paclitaxel (Taxol) and docetaxel (Taxotere), were isolated from the Pacific yew, an evergreen found throughout the Western United States. Paclitaxel is approved for metastatic ovarian and breast cancer and for Kaposi's sarcoma; however, off-label uses include many other cancers. Bone marrow toxicity is usually the dose-limiting factor for the taxanes.

TABLE 27.3 | Antimetabolites

DRUG	ROUTE AND ADULT DOSE	REMARKS
FOLIC ACID ANTAGONISTS		
(Pr) methotrexate (Rheumatrex, Trexall)	PO; 10–30 mg/day for 5 days	For acute lymphoblastic leukemia, choriocarcinoma, lymphoma, head and neck cancer, testicular cancer, bone cancer; IV and IM forms available
pemetrexed (Alimta)	IV; 500 mg/m^2 on day 1 of each 21-day cycle	For malignant mesothelioma and non-small cell lung cancer
pralatrexate (Folotyn)	IV; 30 mg/m^2 administered over 3–5 minutes	For refractory T-cell lymphoma
PYRIMIDINE AND PURINE ANALOGS		
capecitabine (Xeloda)	PO; 2500 mg/m^2 daily for 2 weeks	For metastatic breast cancer and colon cancer
cladribine (Leustatin)	IV; 0.09 mg/m^2	For hairy cell leukemia
clofarabine (Clolar)	IV; 52 mg/m^2 over 2 hours for five consecutive days	For childhood acute lymphoblastic leukemia
cytarabine (Cytosar, Cytosine arabinoside, Depot-Cyt)	IV; 200 mg/m^2 as a continuous infusion over 24 hours	For various leukemias and lymphomas; subcutaneous and intrathecal forms available
fludarabine (Fludara)	IV; 25 mg/m^2 daily	For chronic lymphocytic leukemia
floxuridine (FUDR)	Intra-arterial; 0.1–0.6 mg/kg daily as a continuous infusion	For metastasis from the GI tract to the liver
fluorouracil (5-FU, Adrucil, Efudex, Fluorodex)	IV; 12 mg/kg daily for four consecutive days	For cancer of the breast, colon, rectum, stomach, and pancreas; topical form available for basal cell carcinoma
gemcitabine (Gemzar)	IV; 1000 mg/m^2 every week	For advanced cancers of the pancreas, breast, ovaries, and lung
mercaptopurine (6-MP, Purinethol)	PO; 2.5 mg/kg daily	For childhood acute leukemia
nelarabine (Arranon)	IV; 1500 mg/m^2 on days 1, 3, and 5; repeat every 21 days	Newer drug for leukemias and lymphomas
pentostatin (Nipent)	IV; 4 mg/m^2 every other week	For hairy cell leukemia
thioguanine (6-TG, Tabloid)	PO; 2 mg/kg daily	For remission induction in adult acute leukemia

FIGURE 27.5

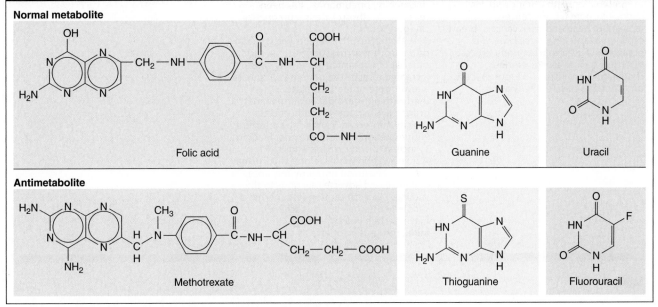

Normal metabolite — Folic acid, Guanine, Uracil

Antimetabolite — Methotrexate, Thioguanine, Fluorouracil

Structural similarities between antimetabolites and their natural counterparts

TABLE 27.4	Antitumor Antibiotics	
DRUG	**ROUTE AND ADULT DOSE**	**REMARKS**
bleomycin (Blenoxane)	IV; 0.25–0.5 units/kg every 4–7 days	For squamous cell carcinoma, Hodgkin's disease, lymphomas, and testicular cancer
dactinomycin (Cosmegen)	IV; 500 mcg/day for a maximum of 5 days	For Wilms' tumor and rhabdomyosarcoma
daunorubicin (Cerubidine)	IV; 30–60 mg/m^2 daily for 3–5 days	For leukemias and lymphomas
daunorubicin liposomal (DaunoXome)	IV; 40 mg/m^2 every 2 weeks	For Kaposi's sarcoma
Pr doxorubicin (Adriamycin)	IV; 60–75 mg/m^2 as a single dose	For lymphomas, sarcomas, acute leukemia, and cancer of the breast, lung, testes, thyroid, and ovary
doxorubicin liposomal (Doxil, Evacet)	IV; 20 mg/m^2 every 3 weeks	For Kaposi's sarcoma
epirubicin (Ellence)	IV; 100–120 mg/m^2 as a single dose	For breast cancer
idarubicin (Idamycin)	IV; 8–12 mg/m^2 daily for 3 days	For acute myelogenous leukemia
mitomycin (Mutamycin)	IV; 2 mg/m^2 as a single dose	For cancer of the colon, stomach, lung, head and neck, rectum, bladder, pancreas, and breast; also for malignant melanoma
mitoxantrone (Novantrone)	IV; 12 mg/m^2 daily for 3 days	For acute nonlymphocytic leukemia

DRUG PROFILE: **Pr** *Methotrexate (Rheumatrex, Trexall)*

Therapeutic Class: Antineoplastic

Pharmacologic Class: Antimetabolite, folic acid analog

Actions and Uses:

Methotrexate blocks folic acid metabolism in rapidly growing tumor cells. **Folic acid** is a water-soluble vitamin found in eggs, veal, liver, whole grains, and dark green vegetables. Folic acid is part of a coenzyme essential to the synthesis of nucleic acids.

Methotrexate is prescribed alone or in combination with other drugs for choriocarcinoma, bone cancers, leukemias, head and neck cancers, breast carcinoma, and lung carcinoma. It is occasionally used to treat non-neoplastic disorders such as severe psoriasis, rheumatoid arthritis, and lupus that are unresponsive to safer medications.

Adverse Effects and Interactions:

Methotrexate has many adverse effects, some of which can be life threatening. The drug can cause fatal bone marrow toxicity at high doses. Hemorrhage and bruising due to low platelet counts are often observed. Nausea, vomiting, and anorexia are common. Although rare, pulmonary toxicity, including life-threatening pneumonitis, has been reported. Methotrexate is a pregnancy category X drug.

Methotrexate interacts with several drugs. Bone marrow suppressants such as other antineoplastic agents may cause increased effects; the patient will require a lower dose of methotrexate. When used with nonsteroidal anti-inflammatory drugs (NSAIDs), severe methotrexate toxicity may occur. Aspirin may interfere with excretion of methotrexate, leading to increased serum levels and toxicity. Administration with live oral vaccine may result in decreased antibody response and increased adverse reactions to the vaccine. Use with caution with herbal supplements, such as echinacea, which may interfere with the drug's immunosuppressant effects.

Mechanism in Action:

Methotrexate interferes with the synthesis of folate. Folate is necessary for the synthesis of DNA, RNA, and protein in rapidly dividing cancer cells. By blocking the synthesis of folic acid, methotrexate is able to inhibit replication, particularly in rapidly dividing cells.

Refer to MyNursingKit for a Nursing Process Focus specific to this drug.

DRUG PROFILE: ℗r *Doxorubicin (Adriamycin)*

Therapeutic Class: Antineoplastic
Pharmacologic Class: Antitumor antibiotic

Actions and Uses:

Doxorubicin attaches to DNA, causing the double strands to be distorted, thus preventing cancer cell division. It is prescribed for solid tumors of the lung, breast, ovary, and bladder, and for certain types of leukemias and lymphomas. It is structurally similar to daunorubicin (Cerubidine). Doxorubicin is one of the most effective single agents against solid tumors.

A novel delivery method has been developed for both doxorubicin and daunorubicin. The drug is enclosed in small sacs, or vesicles, of lipids called **liposomes**. The liposomal vesicle opens and releases the antitumor antibiotic when it reaches a cancer cell. The goal is to deliver a higher concentration of drug directly to the cancer cells, thus sparing normal cells. Doxorubicin liposomal is approved for use in patients with Kaposi's sarcoma, refractory ovarian tumors, and relapsed multiple myeloma.

Adverse Effects and Interactions:

The most serious dose-limiting adverse effect of doxorubicin is delayed cardiac toxicity that may result in irreversible heart failure. Like many of the anticancer medications, doxorubicin may seriously lower blood cell counts. Leaking from an injection site can cause severe pain and serious tissue damage. Nausea, vomiting, diarrhea, and hair loss are common.

Doxorubicin interacts with many drugs. If digoxin is taken at the same time, the patient will have decreased serum digoxin levels. Phenobarbital leads to increased plasma clearance of doxorubicin and decreased effectiveness. Using doxorubicin with phenytoin may lead to decreased phenytoin levels and possible seizure activity. Liver toxicity may occur if mercaptopurine is taken at the same time. Using with verapamil may increase serum doxorubicin levels, leading to doxorubicin toxicity.

Refer to MyNursingKit for a Nursing Process Focus specific to this drug.

TABLE 27.5	Plant Extracts/Natural Products	
DRUG	**ROUTE AND ADULT DOSE**	**REMARKS**
VINCA ALKALOIDS		
vinblastine (Velban)	IV; 3.7–18.5 mg/m² every week	For cancer of the breast and testes; Hodgkin's disease
℗r vincristine (Oncovin)	IV; 1.4 mg/m² every week (max: 2 mg/m²)	For lymphomas, Hodgkin's disease, Wilms' tumor, and childhood acute leukemia
vinorelbine (Navelbine)	IV; 30 mg/m² every week	For lung cancer
TAXANES		
docetaxel (Taxotere)	IV; 60–100 mg/m² every 3 weeks	For ovarian cancer, metastic breast and prostate cancer, advanced stomach cancer and lung cancer
paclitaxel (Taxol)	IV; 135–175 mg/m² every 3 weeks	For Kaposi's sarcoma, ovarian cancer, metastatic breast cancer and certain other solid tumors
TOPOISOMERASE INHIBITORS		
etoposide (VePesid)	IV; 50–100 mg/m² daily for 5 days	For testicular and lung cancer; choriocarcinomas; PO form available
irinotecan (Camptosar)	IV; 125 mg/m² every week for 4 weeks	For colorectal cancer
teniposide (Vumon)	IV; 165 mg/m² every 3–4 days for 4 weeks	For acute lymphocytic leukemia
topotecan (Hycamtin)	IV; 1.5 mg/m² daily for 5 days	For ovarian cancer

DRUG PROFILE: ℗ *Vincristine (Oncovin)*

Therapeutic Class: Antineoplastic
Pharmacologic Class: Vinca alkaloid, plant extract

Actions and Uses:

Vincristine affects rapidly growing cells by inhibiting their ability to complete mitosis. Although it must be given IV, a major advantage of vincristine is that it causes minimal immunosuppression. It is usually prescribed in combination with other antineoplastics for the treatment of lymphoma, leukemias, Kaposi's sarcoma, Wilms' tumor, bladder carcinoma, and breast carcinoma.

Adverse Effects and Interactions:

The major dose-limiting adverse effect of vincristine is neurotoxicity. Symptoms include numbness and tingling in the limbs, muscular weakness, loss of neural reflexes, and pain. Central nervous system (CNS) effects may include seizures, depression, hallucinations, and coma. Severe constipation is common. Immunosuppression may occur, though it is less serious than with vinblastine. Reversible alopecia occurs in most patients. Leaking from the injection site can cause serious tissue damage.

Vincristine interacts with many drugs. Asparaginase used together with or before vincristine may cause increased neurotoxicity secondary to decreased liver clearance of vincristine. Doxorubicin or prednisone may increase bone marrow suppression. Calcium channel blockers may increase vincristine accumulation in cells. When used with digoxin, the patient may need an increased digoxin dose. When vincristine is given with methotrexate, the patient may need lower doses of methotrexate. Vincristine may decrease serum phenytoin levels, leading to increased seizure activity.

Refer to MyNursingKit for a Nursing Process Focus specific to this drug.

CORE CONCEPT 27.12

Some hormones and hormone antagonists are effective against prostate and breast cancer.

PEARSON
mynursingkit™

CLINICAL TRIALS

Use of natural or synthetic hormones or their antagonists as antineoplastic agents is a strategy used to slow the growth of hormone-dependent tumors. Hormone therapy is limited to treating hormone-sensitive tumors of the breast or prostate. The major hormones and hormone antagonists prescribed for cancer are given in Table 27.6.

The growth of certain tumors of reproductive tissues is greatly stimulated by natural hormones. Administering high doses of specific hormones or hormone antagonists can block these receptors and slow tumor growth. For example, administering the male hormone testosterone or the antiestrogen drug tamoxifen can slow specific types of breast cancer that depend on estrogen for growth. Tamoxifen is one of the most widely used drugs for this type of cancer. Administration of the female sex hormone estrogen slows the growth of prostate cancer. The other major class of hormones used for chemotherapy is the corticosteroids. When used for chemotherapy, the doses of these hormones are much higher than the levels normally found in the body. Additional indications for hormone pharmacotherapy are discussed in Chapters 31 and 32 ∞.

As a group, hormones and hormone antagonists are the least toxic of the antineoplastic classes, and they produce few of the toxic adverse effects seen with other antineoplastics. They can, however, cause serious adverse effects when given at high doses for prolonged periods. Because they rarely produce cancer cures when used singly, these agents are normally given for palliation.

TABLE 27.6 — Hormones and Hormone Antagonists

DRUG	ROUTE AND ADULT DOSE	REMARKS
HORMONES		
dexamethasone (Decadron, others)	PO; 0.25 mg bid–qid	For palliative treatment of leukemias and lymphomas
diethylstilbestrol (DES, Stilbestrol)	PO; for treatment of prostate cancer, 500 mg tid; for palliation, 1–15 mg daily	For cancer of the prostate and breast
ethinyl estradiol (Estinyl, others)	PO; for treatment of breast cancer, 1 mg tid for 2–3 months; for palliation of prostate cancer, 0.15–3 mg/day	For cancer of the prostate and breast
fluoxymesterone (Halotestin)	PO; 10 mg tid	For breast cancer
medroxyprogesterone (Provera) (see page 581 for the Drug Profile box)	IM; 400–1000 mg every week	For uterine and renal cancer
megestrol (Megace)	PO; 40–160 mg bid–qid	For advanced cancer of the prostate and breast
prednisone (see page 394 for the Drug Profile box)	PO; 20–100 mg/m² daily	For acute leukemia, Hodgkin's disease, lymphomas
testolactone (Teslac)	PO; 250 mg qid	For breast cancer
testosterone (Andro 100, Histerone, Testred, Delatest)	IM; 200–400 mg every 2–4 weeks	For breast cancer
HORMONE ANTAGONISTS		
anastrozole (Arimidex)	PO; 1 mg daily	For advanced breast cancer
bicalutamide (Casodex)	PO; 50 mg daily	For metastatic prostate cancer
degarelix (Firmagon)	Subcutaneous; 240 mg loading dose followed by 80 mg every 28 days	Newer drug; for advanced prostate cancer
exemestane (Aromasin)	PO; 25 mg daily after a meal	For advanced breast cancer
flutamide (Eulexin)	PO; 250 mg tid	For prostate cancer
goserelin (Zoladex)	Subcutaneous; 3.6 mg every 28 days	For palliation of advanced prostate and breast cancer
histrelin (Vantas)	Implant; one implant every 12 months (50 mg)	For palliation of advanced prostate cancer
letrozole (Femara)	PO; 2.5 mg daily	For advanced breast cancer
leuprolide (Lupron)	Subcutaneous; 1 mg daily	For palliation of advanced prostate cancer
nilutamide (Nilandron)	PO; 300 mg/daily for 30 days, then 150 mg daily	For metastatic prostate cancer
raloxifene (Evista) (see page 603 for the Drug Profile box	PO; 60 mg once daily	For prophylaxis of breast cancer in postmenopausal women who are at high risk for developing the disease
(Pr) tamoxifen	PO; 10–20 mg bid	For breast cancer
toremifene (Fareston)	PO; 60 mg daily	For metastatic breast cancer
Triptorelin (Trelstar)	IM; 3.75 mg once monthly	For palliation of advanced prostate cancer

DRUG PROFILE: ℗ *Tamoxifen*

Therapeutic Class: Antineoplastic

Pharmacologic Class: Hormonal agent, estrogen receptor blocker

Actions and Uses:

Because it blocks estrogen receptors in cancer cells, tamoxifen is sometimes classified as an antiestrogenic. Tamoxifen is effective against breast tumors that require estrogen for their growth. These susceptible cancer cells are known as estrogen receptor (ER)-positive cells. Tamoxifen is given orally and is a preferred drug for treating breast cancer.

A unique feature of tamoxifen is that it is the only antineoplastic that is approved for prophylaxis of breast cancer—for high-risk patients who are at risk of developing the disease. In addition, it is approved as adjunctive therapy in women following mastectomy to decrease the potential for cancer in the other breast.

Adverse Effects and Interactions:

Other than nausea and vomiting, tamoxifen produces little of the serious toxicity observed with other antineoplastics. Of concern, however, is the association of tamoxifen therapy with an increased risk of uterine cancer. Hot flashes, fluid retention, venous blood clots, and abnormal vaginal bleeding are relatively common.

Tamoxifen interacts with several other drugs. For example, anticoagulants may increase the risk of bleeding. Using this drug with cytotoxic agents may increase the risk of blood clots.

Refer to MyNursingKit for a Nursing Process Focus specific to this drug.

CORE CONCEPT 27.13

Biologic response modifiers and some additional antineoplastic drugs are effective against specific tumors.

A number of anticancer drugs act through mechanisms other than those previously described. For example, asparaginase deprives cancer cells of an essential amino acid. Mitotane (Lysodren) is similar to the insecticide DDT; it poisons cancer cells by forming links to proteins. Lenalidomide (Revlimid) is an angiogenesis inhibitor that prevents the formation of new blood vessels that are vital to the growth of new tumors. The uses of these miscellaneous antineoplastics are given in Table 27.7.

Biologic response modifiers are a relatively new class of drugs that do not kill tumor cells directly but instead stimulate the body's immune system to fight the cancer. These treatments are sometimes called immunotherapy. The immunostimulants are less toxic than most other classes of antineoplastics. The three classes of biologic response modifiers include the following:

- *Interferons*   These are natural proteins produced by the immune system in response to viral infection. Peginterferon alfa-2a (Pegasys) and interferon alfa-2b (Intron A) are approved to treat hairy cell leukemia, chronic myelogenous leukemia, Kaposi's sarcoma, and chronic hepatitis B or C.

- *Interleukin-2*   A natural protein that activates the immune response. Aldesleukin (Proleukin) is an interleukin indicated for metastatic renal cell carcinoma.

- *Monoclonal antibodies (MABs)*   These drugs are engineered to attack only one *specific* type of tumor cell. Examples include trastuzumab (Herceptin) for breast cancer cells and alemtuzumab (Campath) for chronic lymphocytic leukemia. The key point about MABs is that the tumor cells must possess the specific protein receptor; otherwise, the MAB will be ineffective.

Patients with neoplastic disorders have a high frequency of blood abnormalities. Some miscellaneous drugs are given to patients undergoing chemotherapy to limit or counteract this toxicity. Oprelvekin (Neumega) stimulates platelet production and helps to prevent severe thrombocytopenia. Epoetin alfa (Epogen, Procrit) stimulates red blood cell production and is used

TABLE 27.7   Selected Biologic Response Modifiers and Miscellaneous Anticancer Drugs

DRUG	ROUTE AND ADULT DOSE	REMARKS
alemtuzumab (Campath)	IV; 3–30 mg/day	For chronic lymphocytic leukemia
altretamine (Hexalen)	PO; 65 mg/m^2/day	For ovarian cancer
arsenic trioxide (Trisenox)	IV; 0.15 mg/kg/day	For acute promyelocytic leukemia
asparaginase (Elspar)	IV; 200 units/kg daily	For acute lymphocytic leukemia
bevacizumab (Avastin)	IV; 5 mg/kg every 14 days	For metastatic colorectal cancer
cetuximab (Erbitux)	IV; 400 mg/m^2 over 2 hr, then 250 mg/m^2 over 1 hr weekly	For metastatic colorectal cancer
erlotinib (Tarceva)	PO; 150 mg once daily	For metastatic non-small cell lung cancer
gefitinib (Iressa)	PO; 250–500 mg/day	Advanced or metastatic lung cancer
hydroxyurea (Hydrea)	PO; 20–30 mg/kg daily	For palliative treatment of malignant melanoma and chronic granulocytic leukemia
imatinib (Gleevec)	PO; 400–600 mg daily	For chronic myeloid leukemia after failure with interferon alfa therapy
Pr interferon alfa-2 (Intron A)	Subcutaneous or IM; 2–3 million units daily for leukemia; 36 million units daily for Kaposi's sarcoma	For hairy cell leukemia, Kaposi's sarcoma non-Hodgkin's lymphoma and malignant melanoma; also for chronic hepatitis B and C viral infections
levamisole (Ergamisol)	PO; 50 mg tid for 3 days	For colon cancer
mitotane (Lysodren)	PO; 3–4 mg tid–qid	For adrenal cortex cancer
ofatumumab (Arzerra)	IV; 300 mg initial dose followed by 2,000 mg weekly for 7 doses	Newer antineoplastic drug; for chronic lymphocytic leukemia
pazopanib (Votrient)	PO; 800 mg once daily	Newer antineoplastic drug; for advanced renal carcinoma
pegaspargase (Oncaspar, PEG-L-asparaginase)	IV; 2500 international units/m^2 every 14 days	For acute lymphocytic leukemia; IM form available
procarbazine (Matulane)	PO; 2–4 mg/kg daily	For Hodgkin's disease
rituximab (Rituxan)	IV; 375 mg/m^2 daily as a continuous infusion	For non-Hodgkin's lymphomas
scinitinib (Sutent)	PO; 50 mg once daily for 4 weeks followed by 2 weeks off	For gastrointestinal and advanced renal carcinoma
trastuzumab (Herceptin)	IV; 4 mg/kg as a single dose, then 2 mg/kg every week	For metastatic breast cancer
zoledronic acid (Zometa)	IV; 4 mg over at least 15 min	For multiple myeloma, severe hypercalcemia caused by malignancy, and Paget's disease

to limit **anemia**, the loss of red blood cells, caused by certain antineoplastics. Administration of filgrastim (Neupogen) increases neutrophil production in patients with cancer whose bone marrow has been suppressed by antineoplastic agents. Low white blood cell counts (neutropenia) often result in severe bacterial and fungal infections in patients during chemotherapy or following organ transplants.

Concept Review   27.3

■ Why are the biologic response modifiers less toxic to normal body cells than other antineoplastics?

DRUG PROFILE: ⓟ *Interferon alfa-2b (Intron A)*

Therapeutic Class: Immunostimulant

Pharmacologic Class: Interferon, biologic response modifier

Actions and Uses:

Interferon alfa-2b is a biologic response modifier that is prepared by recombinant DNA technology and is approved to treat cancers (hairy cell leukemia, malignant melanoma, non-Hodgkin's lymphoma, AIDS-related Kaposi's sarcoma), as well as viral infections (HPV, chronic hepatitis virus B and C). It is available for IV, IM, and subcutaneous administration.

Rebetron is a combination drug containing interferon alfa-2b and ribavirin, an antiviral agent. Rebetron is indicated for pharmacotherapy of hepatitis C infection. Peginterferon alfa-2b (PegIntron) has a molecule of polyethylene glycol (PEG) attached to the interferon molecule, which gives the drug an extended half-life. Peginterferon alfa-2b is approved to treat chronic hepatitis C virus infections.

Adverse Effects and Interactions:

A flulike syndrome of fever, chills, dizziness, and fatigue occurs in 50% of patients, although this usually diminishes as therapy progresses. Headache, nausea, vomiting, diarrhea, and anorexia are relatively common. Depression and suicidal ideation have been reported and may be severe enough to require discontinuation of the drug. With prolonged therapy, immunosuppression, and serious toxicity such as hepatotoxicity and neurotoxicity may be observed.

Use with ethanol may cause excessive drowsiness and dehydration. Zidovudine may increase hematologic toxicity.

 Refer to MyNursingKit for a Nursing Process Focus specific to this drug.

DRUG PROFILE: ⓟ *Epoetin Alfa (Epogen, Procrit)*

Therapeutic Class: Drug for anemia

Pharmacologic Class: Hematopoietic growth factor, erythropoietin

Actions and Uses:

Epoetin alfa is made through recombinant DNA technology and functions like human erythropoietin. Because of its ability to stimulate red blood cell formation, epoetin alfa is effective in treating specific disorders caused by a deficiency in the number of red blood cells. Patients with chronic renal failure often cannot secrete enough erythropoietin and thus will benefit from epoetin administration. Epoetin is sometimes given to patients undergoing cancer chemotherapy to counteract the anemia caused by antineoplastic agents. It is occasionally prescribed for patients prior to blood transfusions or surgery and to treat anemia in patients infected with HIV. Epoetin alfa is usually administered three times per week until a therapeutic response is achieved.

Adverse Effects and Interactions:

The most common adverse effect of epoetin alfa is hypertension, which may occur in as many as 30% of patients receiving the drug. Blood pressure should be monitored during therapy, and an antihypertensive drug may be indicated. The risk of thromboembolic events is increased.

Patients who are on dialysis may require increased doses of heparin. Transient ischemic attacks (TIAs), heart attacks, and strokes have occurred in patients with chronic renal failure who are on dialysis and who are also being treated with epoetin alfa.

The effectiveness of epoetin alfa will be greatly reduced in patients with iron deficiency or other vitamin-depleted states because erythropoiesis cannot be enhanced without these vital nutrients.

There are no clinically significant drug interactions with epoetin alfa.

 Refer to MyNursingKit for a Nursing Process Focus specific to this drug.

NURSING PROCESS FOCUS

Patients Receiving Antineoplastic Therapy

ASSESSMENT

Prior to administration:
- Obtain a complete health history (physical/mental), including laboratory values such as platelets, hematocrit (Hct), leukocyte count, liver and kidney function tests, and serum electrolytes
- Obtain drug history to determine possible drug interactions and allergies
- Assess neurologic status, including mood and/or sensory impairment
- Assess for history or presence of herpes zoster or chickenpox (Immunosuppressive effects of cyclophosphamide and vincristine can cause life-threatening exacerbations.)

POTENTIAL NURSING DIAGNOSES

- Risk for Infection related to compromised immune system.
- Imbalanced Nutrition, Less than Body Requirements, related to nausea, vomiting, diarrhea, and anorexia as a result of drug adverse effects.
- Impaired Skin Integrity related to extravasation.
- Risk for Disturbed Body Image related to physical changes as a result of drug adverse effects.
- Fatigue related to adverse effects of drug therapy.

PLANNING: PATIENT GOALS AND EXPECTED OUTCOMES

The patient will:
- Undergo a reduction in tumor mass and/or progression of abnormal cell growth
- Demonstrate an understanding of the drug's action by accurately describing drug adverse effects, precautions, and therapeutic goals

IMPLEMENTATION

Interventions and (Rationales)

- Monitor hematologic/immune status. Observe for signs and symptoms of bone marrow suppression. (This could indicate overdose.)
- Monitor complete blood count and temperature. Collect stool samples for guaiac testing of occult blood. (Antineoplastics may cause anemia.)

Patient Education/Discharge Planning

Instruct the patient to:
- Immediately report profound fatigue, fever, sore throat, epigastric pain, coffee-grounds vomit, bruising, tarry stools, or frank bleeding
- Avoid persons with active infections
- Monitor vital signs (especially temperature) daily, ensuring proper use of home equipment
- Avoid consuming aspirin
- Anticipate fatigue and balance daily activities to prevent exhaustion
- Avoid activities requiring mental alertness and physical strength until effects of the drug are known

- Monitor cardiorespiratory status, including vital signs and chest/heart sounds. (Cyclophosphamide may cause myopericarditis and lung fibrosis. Doxorubicin may cause sinus tachycardia, cardiac depression, and delayed onset heart failure [HF].) Ensure that ECGs are monitored for T-wave flattening, ST depression, or voltage reduction. Monitor for shortness of breath and pitting edema.

Instruct the patient:
- To immediately report dyspnea; chest, arm, neck, or back pain; tachycardia; cough; frothy sputum; swelling; or activity intolerance
- To maintain a regular schedule of ECGs as advised by the health care provider
- That heart changes may be a sign of drug toxicity; heart failure may not appear for up to 6 months after completion of doxorubicin therapy

- Monitor renal status, urinary output, intake and output, and daily weights. (Cyclophosphamide may cause renal toxicity and/or hemorrhagic cystitis. Vincristine and methotrexate increase uric acid levels, contributing to renal calculi and gout. Vincristine may also cause water retention and highly concentrated urine.)

Instruct the patient:
- To immediately report the following: changes in thirst; changes in color, quantity, and character of urine (e.g., "cloudy," with odor or sediment); joint, abdominal, flank, or lower back pain; difficult urination; and weight gain
- That doxorubicin will turn urine red-brown for 1 to 2 days after administration; blood in the urine may occur several months after cyclophosphamide has been discontinued
- To consume 3 L of fluid on the day before treatment and daily for 72 hr after treatment (when patient has no prescribed fluid restriction)

continued . . .

NURSING PROCESS FOCUS *(continued)*

Interventions and (Rationales)	Patient Education/Discharge Planning
■ Monitor GI status and nutrition. Administer antiemetics 30 to 45 minutes prior to antineoplastic administration or at the first sign of nausea. (Profound nausea, dry heaves, and/or vomiting are common with antineoplastic therapy. Dry mouth can also occur.)	Instruct the patient to: ■ Report loss of appetite, nausea/vomiting, diarrhea, mouth redness, soreness, or ulcers ■ Consume frequent small meals and drink plenty of cold liquids; avoid strong odors and spicy foods to control nausea ■ Examine mouth daily for changes ■ Use a soft toothbrush; avoid toothpicks
■ Monitor for constipation. (Ileus or constipation and fecal impaction may occur with vincristine use, especially among older adults.)	Instruct the patient to: ■ Report changes in bowel habits ■ Increase activity, fiber, and fluids to reduce constipation
■ Monitor neurologic/sensory status. (Antineoplastics may cause peripheral neuropathy and mental depression. Vincristine may cause ataxia and hand/foot drop. Tamoxifen may cause photophobia and decreased vision. Such neurologic changes may be irreversible.)	Instruct the patient to: ■ Report changes in skin color, vision, hearing; report numbness or tingling, staggering gait, or depressed mood; obtain no self-harm contract ■ Limit sun exposure; wear sunscreen, sunglasses, and long sleeves when outdoors
■ Monitor genitourinary status. (Antineoplastic agents—including hormones, and especially tamoxifen—may alter menstrual cycles in women and may produce impotence in men. Tamoxifen increases the risk of endometrial cancer.)	Instruct the patient to: ■ Report changes in menstruation, sexual functioning, and/or vaginal discharge ■ Recognize the risk of endometrial cancer before taking tamoxifen
■ Monitor for hypersensitivity or other adverse reactions.	■ Instruct the patient to immediately report chest or throat tightness, difficulty swallowing, swelling (especially facial), abdominal pain, headache, or dizziness.
■ Monitor hair and skin status. (Alopecia is associated with most chemotherapy and may be a sign of overdosage. Methotrexate can cause a variety of skin eruptions.)	Instruct the patient to: ■ Immediately report desquamation of skin on hands and feet, rash, pruritus, acne, or boils ■ Wear a cold gel cap during chemotherapy to minimize hair loss
■ Monitor for conjunctivitis. (Doxorubicin may cause conjunctivitis.)	■ Instruct the patient or caregiver to immediately report eye redness, stickiness, or pain or weeping.
■ Monitor liver function tests. (Antineoplastics are metabolized by the liver, increasing the risk of hepatotoxicity.)	Instruct the patient to: ■ Report jaundice, abdominal pain, tenderness or bloating, or change in stool color ■ Adhere to laboratory testing regimen for serum blood level tests of liver enzymes, as directed
■ Administer with caution to patients with diabetes mellitus. (Hypoglycemia may occur secondary to combination of cyclophosphamide and insulin.)	Instruct the patient to: ■ Report signs and symptoms of hypoglycemia (e.g., sudden weakness, tremors) ■ Monitor blood glucose daily; consult the health care provider regarding reportable results (e.g., less than 70 mg/dl)

EVALUATION OF OUTCOME CRITERIA

Evaluate the effectiveness of drug therapy by confirming that patient goals and expected outcomes have been met (see "Planning").

See Tables 27.2–27.7 for lists of drugs to which these nursing actions apply.

PATIENTS NEED TO KNOW

Patients treated for cancer need to know the following:

1. If hair loss is expected, cut long hair and be fitted for a wig or hairpiece before starting treatment. Select hats, scarves, or turbans. Use mild shampoo and conditioner.
2. Limit sun exposure; wear sunscreen, sunglasses, and long sleeves when outdoors. When hair is lost, protect the scalp from sunburn with sunscreen or a hat.
3. Eat foods that appeal in small amounts at frequent intervals if appetite is decreased. A health care provider may provide an appetite stimulant such as megestrol acetate (Megace).
4. Discuss drugs to control nausea with a health care provider if nausea is a problem. Drink liquids between meals rather than with food.
5. Because the mouth may become irritated or ulcerated, avoid alcohol-based mouthwash, and use plain water or mild salt solution instead. Use a soft toothbrush. Avoid spicy foods and very hot or very cold food and drink. Ask about a mouth rinse to coat, soothe, and numb, such as BMX (Benadryl, Maalox, and Xylocaine).
6. Because chemotherapy may decrease sperm production or increase the risk of genetic damage to sperm, consider sperm banking prior to receiving chemotherapy.
7. Increase fluid intake to decrease the risk of kidney damage and uric acid crystal formation.
8. Avoid exposure to crowds and individuals with infections or recent vaccinations because the immune system may be less able to protect you. Report temperatures of 101°F (38°C) or higher.
9. Follow a neutropenic diet if white blood cell count is significantly reduced. Avoid raw fruits and vegetables, peppercorns, and raw fish and meat.
10. Report easy bruising, blood in the stool or urine, vomiting, severe fatigue, epigastric pain, and difficulty clotting. Many chemotherapeutic agents reduce production platelets needed for clot formation.

CHAPTER REVIEW

CORE CONCEPTS SUMMARY

27.1 Cancer is characterized by rapid, uncontrolled growth of cells.

Cancer cells grow rapidly, seemingly unaffected by their host surroundings. Cancer cells continue dividing until they invade normal tissues and eventually metastasize. Benign neoplasms grow slowly and rarely result in death. Malignant neoplasms, also known as cancer, are fast-growing and often fatal.

27.2 The causes of cancer may be chemical, physical, or biological.

Many factors have been found to cause or promote cancer. These include industrial chemicals, X-rays, UV light, and viruses. The genetic make-up of the patient plays an important role in whether or not cancer will develop after exposure to carcinogens.

27.3 Personal risk of cancer may be lowered by a number of lifestyle factors.

Eliminating tobacco use and limiting the intake of saturated fats and alcohol are important factors in reducing the risk of developing cancer. Periodic self-examinations and physician check-ups are important in catching cancer at an early, more treatable stage.

27.4 The three primary goals of chemotherapy are cure, control, and palliation.

Surgery, radiation, and chemotherapy are the therapies used for treating cancer. The three primary goals of chemotherapy are cure, control, and palliation. Antineoplastic drugs may also be administered as adjuvant or neoadjuvant chemotherapy, prophylaxis, or myeloablation.

27.5 To achieve a total cure, every malignant cell must be removed or killed.

A single cancer cell may be able to divide rapidly enough to kill its host. Therefore, to achieve a complete cure, every single cancer cell must be eliminated by surgery, radiation, drugs, or the patient's immune system.

27.6 Use of multiple drugs and special dosing schedules improves the success of chemotherapy.

Combinations of antineoplastic drugs are often used to attack cancer cells through several mechanisms and to allow lower doses than if a single agent were used. The schedule of drug administration is critical to the success of the chemotherapy.

27.7 Serious toxicity limits therapy with most of the antineoplastic agents.

Antineoplastic drugs are among the most toxic medications available. Adverse effects are expected and may be severe. Whereas each agent has somewhat different toxicities, common adverse effects include thrombocytopenia, anemia, leukopenia, alopecia, severe nausea, vomiting, and diarrhea.

27.8 Alkylating agents act by changing the structure of DNA in cancer cells.

Alkylating agents are some of the oldest and most reliable of the antineoplastic drugs. By attaching to DNA, they prevent cancer cells from replicating.

27.9 Antimetabolites disrupt critical cellular pathways in cancer cells.

Antimetabolites block a specific step in cancer cell metabolism. By blocking the synthesis of critical cellular molecules, the drugs can slow the growth of cancer cells.

27.10 A few cytotoxic antibiotics are used to treat cancer rather than infections.

Antitumor antibiotics attach to the DNA of cancer cells, thereby inhibiting their growth. Their properties and adverse effects resemble those of the alkylating agents.

27.11 Some plant extracts kill cancer cells by preventing cell division.

Natural products of the periwinkle plant and the Pacific yew have provided several important antineoplastic agents. Drugs in this class also include the topoisomerase inhibitors.

27.12 Some hormones and hormone antagonists are effective against prostate and breast cancer.

A number of estrogens, androgens, corticosteroids, and hormone inhibitors have antitumor activity. They have very specific uses, usually for tumors of reproductive-related organs such as the breast, prostate, or uterus.

27.13 Biologic response modifiers and some additional antineoplastic drugs are effective against specific tumors.

Biologic response modifiers are a small group of drugs used to stimulate the immune system. Although much research has focused on this approach to chemotherapy, these drugs have only limited success.

REVIEW QUESTIONS

The following questions are written in NCLEX-PN® style. Answer these questions to assess your knowledge of the chapter material, and go back and review any material that is not clear to you.

1. When should the nurse administer antiemetic drugs to a patient receiving chemotherapy?
1. When vomiting occurs
2. Once the treatment is completed
3. Prior to treatment
4. Only if the patient requests to be medicated

2. The patient with testicular cancer is receiving cisplatin (Platinol) IV. The health care provider understands that she must assess for:
1. Irreversible heart failure
2. Bone marrow suppression
3. Cardiac toxicity
4. Peripheral neuropathy

3. Which classification of antineoplastic drugs functions to disrupt metabolic pathways to kill or slow cancer growth?
1. Biologic response modifiers
2. Plant alkaloids
3. Antitumor antibiotics
4. Antimetabolites

4. The patient with breast cancer has been receiving IV doxorubicin (Adriamycin). The patient is now complaining of severe pain at the injection site. The nurse understands that the following most likely occurred:
1. An allergic reaction
2. Leaking at the injection site
3. Loss of neural reflexes
4. Development of a blood clot

5. The patient with prostate cancer is receiving leuprolide (Lupron). This is what type of antineoplastic drug?

1. Hormone/hormone antagonist
2. Antitumor antibiotic
3. Alkylating agent
4. Antimetabolite

6. The patient on cyclosphosphamide (Cytoxan) should be taught:

1. That alopecia is irreversible
2. About signs and symptoms of neurotoxicity
3. About signs and symptoms of renal toxicity
4. That nausea, vomiting, and diarrhea may occur 1 or 2 days after treatment

7. Rheumatoid arthritis may be treated with which of the following antineoplastic agents?

1. Fluorouracil (5-FU)
2. Methotrexate
3. Tamoxifen
4. Leuprolide (Lupron)

8. This antineoplastic drug is given to prevent breast cancer in high-risk patients.

1. Rituximab (Rituxan)
2. Paclitaxel (Taxol)
3. Tamoxifen
4. Vincristine (Oncovin)

9. The patient with a decreased white blood cell count should be instructed to:

1. Use alcohol-based mouthwash for mouth sores
2. Increase liquid intake with meals
3. Avoid raw foods
4. Ask his physician about ordering megestrol acetate (Megace)

10. The patient on tamoxifen must be assessed for:

1. Flulike symptoms
2. Uterine cancer
3. Alopecia
4. Thrombocytopenia

CASE STUDY QUESTIONS

For questions 1–4, please refer to the following case study, and choose the correct answer from choices 1–4.

*M*s. *Novak is being treated for invasive cancer and is receiving the following drugs:*

vincristine (Oncovin)
interferon alfa-2b (Intron A)
tamoxifen (Soltamox)
epoetin alfa (Epogen)

1. Which drug acts by boosting the patient's immune system?

1. Vincristine (Oncovin)
2. Epoetin alfa (Epogen)
3. Interferon alfa-2b (Intron A)
4. Tamoxifen

2. Epoetin alfa (Epogen) is likely being administered to:

1. Boost the patient's immune system
2. Boost the number of red blood cells
3. Reduce possible neurotoxicity
4. Kill cancer cells

3. During vincristine (Oncovin) therapy, the nurse must regularly assess:

1. Blood glucose levels
2. For signs of peripheral neuropathy
3. For ototoxicity
4. For confusion and hallucinations

4. With interferon alfa-2b (Intron A), the nurse should monitor for which common adverse effect?

1. Flulike syndrome
2. Decreases in platelets and white blood cells
3. Anemia
4. Weakness or loss of sensation in the extremities

FURTHER STUDY

- Additional indications for hormone pharmacotherapy are discussed in Chapters 31 and 32 ⚬ .

- Drugs for nausea and vomiting (antiemetics) are presented in Chapter 29 ⚬ .

- The use of glucocorticoids in the pharmacotherapy of pulmonary disorders is covered in Chapter 28 ⚬ .

EXPLORE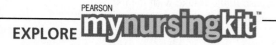

MyNursingKit is your one stop for online chapter review materials and resources. Prepare for success with additional NCLEX®-style practice questions, interactive assignments and activities, web links, animations and videos, and more!

Register your access code from the front of your book at www.mynursingkit.com

5 The Respiratory and Digestive Systems

UNIT CONTENTS

28 Drugs for Respiratory Disorders

CORE CONCEPTS

28.1 The respiratory system supplies oxygen for the body and provides protection against inhaled organisms.

28.2 The inhalation route of drug administration quickly delivers medications directly to their sites of action.

28.3 Allergic rhinitis is characterized by sneezing, watery eyes, and nasal congestion.

28.4 Antihistamines are widely used to treat allergic rhinitis and other minor allergies.

28.5 Intranasal corticosteroids are drugs of choice in treating allergic rhinitis.

28.6 Decongestants are used to reduce nasal congestion caused by allergic rhinitis and the common cold.

28.7 Antitussives and expectorants are used to treat symptoms of the common cold.

28.8 Asthma is a chronic inflammatory disease characterized by bronchospasm.

28.9 Beta-adrenergic agents are the most effective drugs for relieving acute bronchospasm.

28.10 Corticosteroids are the most effective drugs for the long-term prophylaxis of asthma.

28.11 Mast cell stabilizers and leukotriene modifiers are alternative anti-inflammatory drugs for the prophylaxis of asthma.

28.12 Chronic obstructive pulmonary disease is a progressive disorder treated with multiple drugs.

DRUG SNAPSHOT

The following drugs are discussed in this chapter:

DRUG CLASSES	DRUG PROFILES
Antihistamines (H_1-receptor blockers)	Pr diphenhydramine (Benadryl, others)
Intranasal corticosteroids	Pr fluticasone (Flonase, Veramyst)
Decongestants (sympathomimetics)	Pr oxymetazoline (Afrin, others)
Antitussives, expectorants, and mucolytics	

DRUG CLASSES	DRUG PROFILES
Beta-adrenergic agents	Pr salmeterol (Serevent)
Anticholinergics	
Inhaled corticosteroids	
Xanthines	
Mast cell stabilizers	
Leukotriene modifiers	

LEARNING OUTCOMES

After reading this chapter, the student should be able to:

1. Identify major anatomic structures associated with the respiratory system.

2. Explain why inhalation is an effective route of drug administration for respiratory medicines.

3. Describe the types of devices used to deliver medications via the inhalation route.

4. Describe some common causes and symptoms of allergic rhinitis, asthma, and chronic obstructive pulmonary disease.

5. Explain the pharmacologic management of allergic rhinitis, asthma, and chronic obstructive pulmonary disease.

6. Identify drugs that are used to bring symptomatic relief from the common cold.

7. For each of the classes in the Drug Snapshot, identify representative drugs and explain the mechanisms of drug action, primary actions on the respiratory system, and important adverse effects.

8. Categorize drugs used in the treatment of respiratory disorders based on their classifications and mechanisms of action.

KEY TERMS

aerosol (AIR-oh-sol) *483*

allergic rhinitis (rye-NYE-tis) *484*

alveoli (al-VEE-oh-lie) *481*

antitussive (anti-TUSS-ive) *492*

asthma (AZ-muh) *493*

bronchi (BRON-ky) *481*

bronchioles (BRON-key-oles) *481*

bronchoconstriction (BRON-koh-kun-STRIK-shun) *493*

bronchodilation (BRON-koh-dye-LAY-shun) *495*

bronchospasm (bron-koh-SPAZ-um) *493*

chronic bronchitis (KRON-ik bron-KEYE-tis) *500*

dry powder inhaler (DPI) *483*

dyspnea (DISP-nee-uh) *493*

emphysema (em-fuss-EE-muh) *501*

expectorant (eks-PEK-tor-ent) *493*

H₁-receptor blocker *486*

metered-dose inhaler (MDIs) *483*

mucolytic *483*

nebulizer (NEB-you-lyes-ur) *483*

perfusion (purr-FEW-shun) *482*

rebound congestion *491*

respiration (res-purr-AY-shun) *481*

status asthmaticus (STAT-us az-MAT-ik-us) *493*

ventilation (ven-tah-LAY-shun) *482*

The respiratory system is one of the most important organ systems; a mere 5 to 6 minutes without breathing may result in death. When functioning properly, the respiratory system filters incoming air and provides the body with the oxygen critical for all cells to function. Measuring respiration rate and depth and listening to chest sounds with a stethoscope give the health care provider valuable clues as to what may be happening internally. The respiratory system also provides a means by which the body can rid itself of excess acids and bases, a topic that is covered in Chapter 23 ∞ .

The respiratory system supplies oxygen for the body and provides protection against inhaled organsims.

CORE CONCEPT 28.1

The primary function of the respiratory system is to bring oxygen into the body and to remove carbon dioxide. The process by which gases are exchanged is called **respiration**. The basic structures of the respiratory system are shown in Figure 28.1 ■. This system is sometimes divided into two anatomic divisions: the upper and lower respiratory tracts.

Upper respiratory tract (URT). The URT consists of the nose, nasal cavity, pharynx, and paranasal sinuses. These passageways warm, humidify, and clean the air before it enters the lungs. The URT traps and removes particulate matter and many pathogens before they reach the lower portions of the lungs, where they would be able to access the capillaries of the systemic circulation.

The nasal mucosa is a dynamic structure, richly supplied with vascular tissue, under the control of the autonomic nervous system. For example, certain drugs can reduce the thickness of the mucosal layer, thus relieving nasal congestion (see Section 28.5). The nasal mucosa is also the first line of immune defense. Up to a quart of nasal mucus is produced daily, and this fluid is rich with substances that are able to neutralize airborne pathogens. Unfortunately, these cells can over-react to some substances and cause symptoms typical of seasonal allergies, such as nasal congestion, watery eyes, and sneezing.

Lower respiratory tract (LRT). The LRT consists of the lungs and associated structures. Air leaving the URT travels into trachea and **bronchi**, which divide into smaller and smaller passages called **bronchioles**. The bronchial tree ends in dilated sacs called **alveoli**. Although they

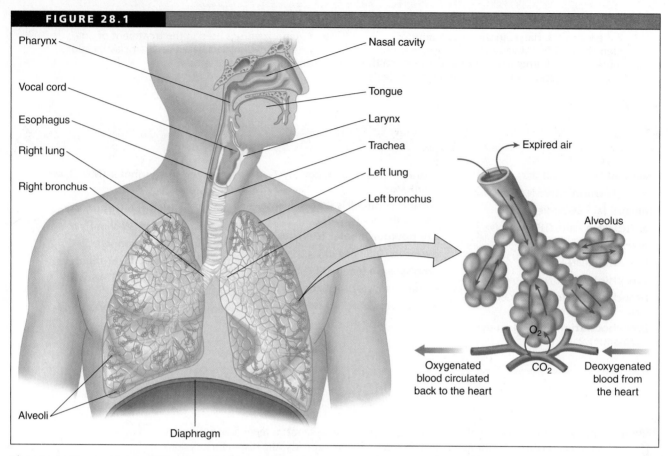

FIGURE 28.1

Pharynx

Nasal cavity

Vocal cord

Tongue

Esophagus

Larynx

Right lung

Trachea

Left lung

Right bronchus

Left bronchus

Expired air

Alveolus

O_2

CO_2

Oxygenated
blood circulated
back to the heart

Deoxygenated
blood from
the heart

Alveoli

Diaphragm

The respiratory system and the process of gas exchange

have no smooth muscle, the alveoli are abundantly rich in capillaries. An extremely thin membrane in the alveoli allows gases to readily move between the internal environment of the blood and the inspired air. As oxygen crosses this membrane, it is exchanged for carbon dioxide, a cellular waste product that travels from the blood to the air. The lung is richly supplied with blood. Blood flow through the lung is called **perfusion**. The process of gas exchange is depicted in Figure 28.1 ■.

Ventilation is the process of moving air into and out of the lungs. As the muscular diaphragm contracts and lowers in position, it creates a negative pressure that draws air into the lungs. This process, known as inspiration, requires energy to produce the contraction. During expiration, the diaphragm relaxes and air leaves the lung passively, with no energy expenditure required. Ventilation is a purely mechanical process that occurs approximately 12–18 times per minute in adults, a rate determined by neurons in the brainstem. This rate may be modified by a number of factors, including emotions, fever, stress, and the pH of the blood.

Concept Review **28.1**

■ What is the difference between ventilation and perfusion?

The inhalation route of drug administration quickly delivers medications directly to their sites of action.

CORE CONCEPT 28.2

The respiratory system offers a rapid and efficient mechanism for delivering drugs. The enormous surface area of the bronchioles and alveoli, and the rich blood supply to these areas, results in an almost instantaneous onset of action for inhaled substances.

Medications are delivered to the respiratory system by aerosol therapy. An **aerosol** is a suspension of very small liquid droplets or fine solid particles within a gas. Aerosol therapy can give immediate relief for bronchospasm. Drugs may also be given to loosen thick mucus in the bronchial tree. The major advantage of aerosal therapy is that it delivers the medications to their immediate site of action, thus reducing systemic adverse effects. To produce the same therapeutic action, an oral medication would have to be given at higher doses and would be distributed to all body tissues.

It should be clearly understood that agents delivered by inhalation can produce systemic effects due to absorption. For example, anesthetics such as nitrous oxide and halothane (Fluothane) are delivered via the inhalation route and are rapidly distributed to cause central nervous system (CNS) depression, as presented in Chapter 15 ⬭. Solvents such as paint thinners and glues are sometimes intentionally inhaled and can cause serious adverse effects on the nervous system, and even death.

Several devices are used to deliver medications via the inhalation route. **Nebulizers** are small machines that vaporize a liquid drug into a fine mist that can be inhaled, often using a facemask. If the drug is a solid, it may be administered using a **dry powder inhaler (DPI)**. A DPI is a small device that is activated by the process of inhalation to deliver a fine powder directly to the bronchial tree. Turbohalers and rotahalers are types of DPIs. **Metered-dose inhalers (MDIs)** are a third type of device commonly used to deliver respiratory medicines. MDIs use a propellant to deliver a measured dose of drugs to the lungs during each breath. The patient times the inhalation to the puffs of drug emitted from the MDI. Patients must be carefully instructed on the correct use of these devices because drug dose depends on their correct use. In addition, swallowing medication that has been deposited in the oral cavity may cause the drug to be absorbed in the gastrointestinal (GI) tract, causing potential adverse effects. Devices used to deliver respiratory agents are shown in Figure 28.2 ■.

The primary goal of drug therapy for many respiratory disorders is to keep the airways open. Drugs include bronchodilators, which directly open the airways, and anti-inflammatory drugs, which prevent their closure. Drugs may be used to act on excessive mucus blocking the airways, either by causing it to become thinner or by breaking up thick mucous plugs. These and other types of drugs used to treat respiratory disorders are illustrated in Figure 28.3 ■.

Concept Review   28.2

■ Name the three types of devices used to deliver drugs by the inhalation route. What are the differences among them?

FIGURE 28.2

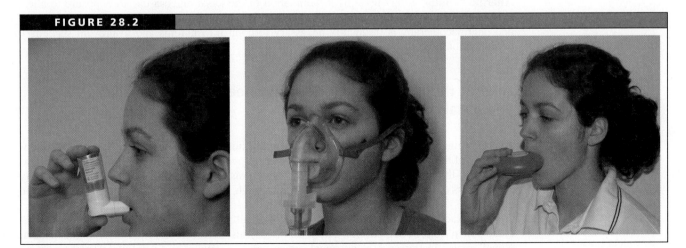

Devices used to deliver respiratory drugs

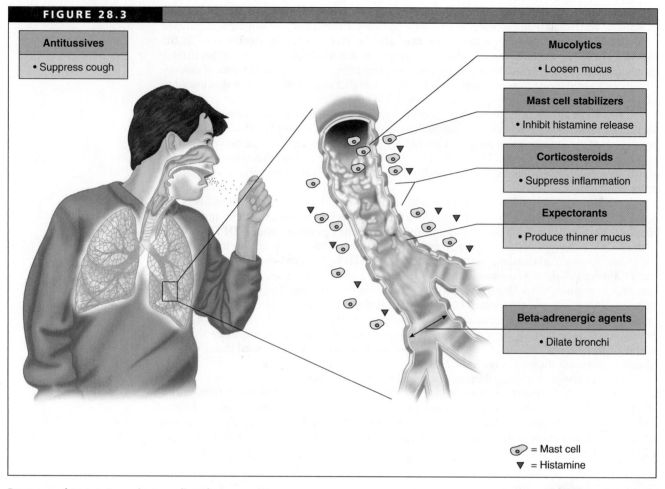

FIGURE 28.3

Drugs used to treat respiratory disorders

ALLERGIC RHINITIS

Allergic rhinitis, or hay fever, is inflammation of the nasal mucosa due to exposure to allergens. Although not life threatening, allergic rhinitis is a condition affecting millions of patients, and pharmacotherapy is frequently necessary to control symptoms and to prevent secondary complications.

Allergic rhinitis is characterized by sneezing, watery eyes, and nasal congestion.

CORE CONCEPT 28.3

Allergic rhinitis is a common disorder affecting millions of people annually. Symptoms resemble those of the common cold: tearing eyes, sneezing, nasal congestion, postnasal drip, and itching of the throat. In addition to the acute symptoms, complications of allergic rhinitis may include loss of taste or smell, sinusitis, chronic cough, hoarseness, and middle ear infections in children.

The exact cause of allergic rhinitis is often difficult to pinpoint; however, common causes include pollen from weeds, grasses, and trees; molds; dust mites; certain foods; and animal dander. Nonallergenic factors such as chemical fumes, tobacco smoke, or air pollutants such as ozone may contribute to the symptoms. Although some patients experience symptoms at specific times of the year, when pollen and mold are at high levels in the environment, others are bothered throughout the year.

The fundamental problem of allergic rhinitis is inflammation of the mucous membranes in the nose, throat, and airways. Chemical mediators such as histamine are released and initiate the distressing symptoms. The pathophysiology of allergic rhinitis is illustrated in Figure 28.4 ■.

The therapeutic goals of treating allergic rhinitis are to prevent its occurrence and to relieve symptoms. Drugs used to treat allergic rhinitis may thus be grouped into two basic categories: preventers and relievers. Preventers are used for prophylaxis and include antihistamines, intranasal corticosteroids, and mast cell stabilizers. Relievers are used to provide immediate, though temporary, relief for allergy symptoms once they have occurred. Relievers include the oral and intranasal sympathomimetics that are used as nasal decongestants.

FIGURE 28.4

Pathophysiology of allergic rhinitis

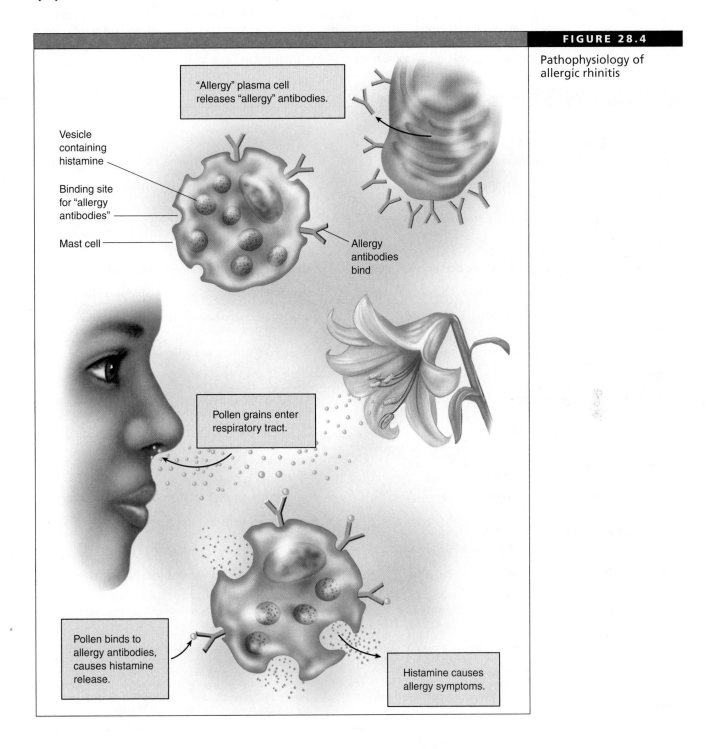

Fast Facts Allergies

- About 175 people die from food allergies each year in the United States.
- Of food allergies, 85% are related to milk, eggs, and nuts.
- About 3 million Americans (1.1%) are allergic to nuts.

CORE CONCEPT 28.4

Antihistamines are widely used to treat allergic rhinitis and other minor allergies.

Antihistamines, also called **H$_1$-receptor blockers**, are drugs that selectively block the actions of histamine at the H$_1$-receptor, thus alleviating allergic symptoms. They are widely used over the counter (OTC) for relief of allergy symptoms, motion sickness, and insomnia. Common H$_1$-receptor blockers used to treat allergies and other disorders are listed in Table 28.1.

TABLE 28.1	H$_1$-Receptor Blockers (Antihistamines)	
DRUG	**ROUTE AND ADULT DOSE**	**REMARKS**
FIRST-GENERATION AGENTS		
azelastine (Astelin)	Intranasal; two sprays per nostril bid	First-generation antihistamine; for nonallergic rhinitis
brompheniramine (Dimetapp, others)	PO; 4–8 mg tid–qid (max: 40 mg/day)	Less sedative effect than diphenhydramine; combined with other drugs for OTC use
chlorpheniramine (Chlor-Trimeton, others)	PO; 2–4 mg tid–qid (max: 24 mg/day)	Usually combined with a decongestant to treat cold, flu, and allergy symptoms; available for OTC use
clemastine (Tavist)	PO; 1.34–2.68 mg bid (max: 8.04 mg/day)	Central sedative effects are generally mild
cyproheptadine	PO; 4–20 mg tid or qid (max: 0.5 mg/kg/day)	Significant antipruritic and CNS depression effects
dexbrompheniramine (Drixoral)	PO; 6 mg bid (max: 12 mg/day)	Usually used in combination with pseudoephedrine and dextromethorphan as an OTC drug for cold and allergy
dexchlorpheniramine (Dexchlor, Poladex, others)	PO; 2 mg every 4–6 hours (max: 12 mg/day)	For seasonal rhinitis and other allergy disorders
(Pr) diphenhydramine (Benadryl, others)	PO; 25–50 mg tid–qid (max: 300 mg/day)	Topical, IV, IM, and subcutaneous forms available; also for motion sickness, Parkinson's disease, vertigo, and as an OTC sleep aid
promethazine (Phenergan)	PO; 12.5–25 mg/day (max: 100 mg/day)	IV, IM, and rectal suppository forms available; also for preoperative sedation, motion sickness, nausea, and vertigo
triprolidine (Aprodine, Zymine, others)	PO; 2.5 mg bid or tid (max: 10 mg/day)	Long acting; combined with other drugs for allergies
SECOND-GENERATION AGENTS		
cetirizine (Zyrtec)	PO; 5–10 mg/day (max: 10 mg/day)	Nonsedating; became available OTC in 2007
desloratadine (Clarinex)	PO; 5 mg/day (max: 5 mg/day)	Nonsedating; the active metabolite of loratadine
fexofenadine (Allegra)	PO; 60 mg twice daily or 180 mg once daily	Once-a-day dosing; nonsedating
levocetirizine (Xyzal)	PO; 5 mg (1 tablet or 2 teaspoons) once daily	Newer drug, approved in 2007; very similar to cetirizine
loratadine (Claritin)	PO; 10 mg daily	Nonsedating; became available OTC in 2001
olopatadine (Patanase)	Intranasal; two sprays per nostril twice daily	Newer drug, approved in 2007; the first second-generation nasal spray for allergic rhinitis

TABLE 28.2	Selected OTC Antihistamine Combinations		
BRAND NAME	**ANTIHISTAMINE**	**DECONGESTANT**	**ANALGESIC**
Actifed Cold and Allergy tablets	chlorpheniramine	phenylephrine	—
Actifed Cold and Allergy	chlorpheniramine	phenylephrine	—
Benadryl Allergy/Cold caplets	diphenhydramine	phenylephrine	acetaminophen
Chlor-Trimeton Allergy/Decongestant tablets	chlorpheniramine	pseudoephedrine	—
Dimetapp Children's Cold and Allergy	brompheniramine	phenylephrine	—
Sudafed PE Sinus and Allergy tablets	chlorpheniramine	phenylephrine	—
Sudafed PE Nighttime Cold	diphenhydramine	phenylephrine	acetaminophen
Tavist Allergy tablets	clemastine	—	—
Triaminic Cold/Allergy	chlorpheniramine	phenylephrine	—
Tylenol Allergy Sinus caplets	chlorpheniramine	phenylephrine	acetaminophen
Tylenol PM Gelcaps	diphenhydramine	—	acetaminophen

Because the term *antihistamine* is nonspecific and does not specify which of the two histamine receptors are affected, *H_1-receptor blocker* is the more accurate term. Although a large number of H_1-receptor blockers are available for use, their effectiveness, therapeutic uses, and adverse effects are similar. A simple classification of these drugs is based on their ability to cause sedation. Older, first-generation H_1-receptor blockers have the potential to cause significant drowsiness, whereas the newer, second-generation agents lack this effect in most patients. Care must be taken to avoid alcohol and other CNS depressants when taking antihistamines because their sedating effects may be additive.

The most common therapeutic use of H_1-receptor blockers is for the treatment of allergies. These drugs provide relief from the characteristic sneezing, runny nose, and itching of the eyes, nose, and throat of allergic rhinitis. Many H_1-receptor blockers are used in OTC cold and sinus medicines, often in combination with decongestants and antitussives. Some common OTC antihistamine combinations used to treat allergies are listed in Table 28.2.

DRUG PROFILE: Ⓟ *Diphenhydramine (Benadryl, Others)*

Therapeutic Class: Drug to treat allergies

Pharmacologic Class: H_1-receptor blocker, antihistamine

Actions and Uses:

Diphenhydramine is a first-generation H_1-receptor blocker whose primary use is to treat symptoms of allergy and the common cold such as sneezing, runny nose, and tearing of the eyes. Diphenhydramine is often combined with an analgesic, a decongestant, or an expectorant in OTC cold and flu products. Diphenhydramine is also used as a topical agent to treat rashes, and IM/IV forms are available for severe allergic reactions. Other indications for diphenhydramine include Parkinson's disease, motion sickness, and insomnia.

Adverse Effects and Interactions:

First-generation H_1-receptor blockers such as diphenhydramine cause significant drowsiness, although this usually diminishes with long-term use. Occasionally, a patient will exhibit CNS stimulation and excitability rather than drowsiness. Excitation is more frequent in children than in adults. Anticholinergic effects such as dry mouth, tachycardia, and mild hypotension are seen in some patients.

Use of diphenhydramine with alcohol, CNS depressants, or monoamine oxidase (MAO) inhibitors may cause additive CNS depression. Use with other OTC cold preparations may increase anticholinergic adverse effects.

Mechanism in Action:

Diphenhydramine acts by competing with histamine for binding to histamine (H_1) receptor sites. It does not prevent the release of histamine. It reduces inflammation by blocking H_1-receptors found within smooth muscle cells of the respiratory tract and the cells lining blood vessels located in the skin.

Refer to MyNursingKit for a Nursing Process Focus specific to this drug.

Antihistamines are most effective when taken prophylactically to prevent allergic symptoms. Their effectiveness may diminish with long-term use. It should be noted that during severe allergic reactions such as anaphylaxis, histamine is just one of several chemical mediators released; thus, H_1-receptor blockers are not very effective in treating this disorder.

Although most antihistamines are given orally, two are available by the intranasal route. Azelastine (Astelin) is approved for nonallergic rhinitis. Although a first-generation agent, azelastine causes less drowsiness than others in its class because it is applied locally to the nasal mucosa, and limited systemic absorption occurs. Olopatadine (Patanase) is a newer second-generation antihistamine approved in 2008 for allergic rhinitis.

H_1-receptor blockers are effective in treating a number of other disorders. Motion sickness responds well to these medications. It is also one of the few classes of drugs available to treat *vertigo*, a form of dizziness that causes significant nausea. Some of the older antihistamines are marketed as OTC sleep aids, taking advantage of their ability to cause drowsiness. A few are used to treat tremors associated with Parkinson's disease.

Concept Review 28.3

- Why are the antihistamines most effective if given *before* inflammation occurs?

NURSING PROCESS FOCUS

Patients Receiving Antihistamine Therapy

ASSESSMENT

Prior to administration:
- Obtain a complete health history (physical/mental), including data on anaphylaxis, asthma, or cardiac disease, plus allergies, drug history, and possible drug interactions
- Obtain ECG and vital signs; assess in context of patient's baseline values
- Assess respiratory status: breathing pattern
- Assess neurologic status and level of consciousness (LOC)

POTENTIAL NURSING DIAGNOSES

- Ineffective Airway Clearance related to difficulty swallowing and coughing.
- Ineffective Breathing Pattern related to retained secretions and discomfort.
- Disturbed Sleep Pattern related to somnolence or agitation.

PLANNING: PATIENT GOALS AND EXPECTED OUTCOMES

The patient will:
- Report relief from allergic symptoms such as congestion, itching, or postnasal drip
- Demonstrate an understanding of the drug's action by accurately describing drug adverse effects and precautions

IMPLEMENTATION

Interventions and (Rationales)

- Auscultate breath sounds before administering drug therapy. Use with extreme caution in patients with asthma or chronic obstructive pulmonary disease (COPD). Keep resuscitative equipment accessible. (Anticholinergic effects of antihistamines may trigger bronchospasm.)

- Monitor vital signs (including ECG) before administering drug therapy. Use with extreme caution in patients with a history of cardiovascular disease. (Anticholinergic effects can increase heart rate and lower blood pressure. Fatal dysrhythmias and cardiovascular collapse have been reported in some patients receiving antihistamines.)

Patient Education/Discharge Planning

- Instruct the patient to immediately report wheezing or difficulty breathing.
- Advise patients with asthma to consult the nurse regarding the use of injectable epinephrine in emergency situations.

Instruct the patient to:
- Immediately report dizziness, palpitations, headache, or chest, arm, or back pain accompanied by nausea/vomiting and/or sweating
- Monitor vital signs daily, ensuring proper use of home equipment

continued . . .

NURSING PROCESS FOCUS *(continued)*

Interventions and (Rationales)	Patient Education/Discharge Planning
■ Monitor thyroid function. Use with caution in patients with a history of hyperthyroidism. (Antihistamines exacerbate CNS-stimulating effects of hyperthyroidism and may trigger thyroid storm.)	■ Instruct the patient to immediately report nervousness or restlessness, insomnia, fever, profuse sweating, thirst, and mood changes.
■ Monitor for vision changes. Use with caution in patients with narrow-angle glaucoma. (Antihistamines can increase intraocular pressure and cause photosensitivity.)	Instruct the patient to: ■ Immediately report head or eye pain and visual changes ■ Wear dark glasses, use sunscreen, and avoid excessive sun exposure
■ Monitor neurologic status, especially LOC. Use with caution in patients with a history of seizure disorder. (Antihistamines lower the seizure threshold. Older adults are at increased risk of serious sedation and other anticholinergic effects.)	Instruct the patient to: ■ Immediately report seizure activity, including any changes in character and pattern of seizures ■ Avoid driving or performing hazardous activities until effects of the drug are known
■ Observe for signs of renal toxicity. Measure intake and output. Use with caution in patients with a history of kidney or urinary tract disease. (Antihistamines promote urinary retention.)	■ Instruct the patient to immediately report flank pain, difficulty urinating, reduced urine output, and changes in the appearance of urine (cloudy, with sediment, odor, etc.).
■ Use with caution in patients with diabetes mellitus. Monitor serum glucose levels with increased dosing frequency. (Antihistamines decrease serum glucose levels.)	Instruct the patient to: ■ Immediately report symptoms of hypoglycemia ■ Consult the health care provider regarding timing of glucose monitoring and reportable results (e.g., "less than 70 mg/dl")
■ Monitor for GI adverse effects. Use with caution in patients with a history of GI disorders, especially peptic ulcers or liver disease. (Antihistamines block H_1-receptors, altering the mucosal lining of the stomach. These drugs are metabolized in the liver, increasing the risk of hepatotoxicity.)	Instruct the patient to: ■ Immediately report nausea, vomiting, anorexia, bleeding, chest or abdominal pain, heartburn, jaundice, or a change in the color or character of stools ■ Avoid substances that irritate the stomach, such as spicy foods, alcoholic beverages, and nicotine; take drug with food to avoid stomach upset
■ Monitor for adverse effects such as dry mouth; observe for signs of anticholinergic crisis.	Instruct the patient to: ■ Immediately report fever or flushing accompanied by difficulty swallowing ("cotton mouth"), blurred vision, and confusion ■ Avoid mixing OTC antihistamines; always consult the health care provider before taking any OTC drugs or herbal supplements ■ Suck on hard candy to relieve dry mouth and maintain adequate fluid intake

EVALUATION OF OUTCOME CRITERIA

Evaluate the effectiveness of drug therapy by confirming that patient goals and expected outcomes have been met (see "Planning").

See Tables 24.4 and 24.5 for lists of drugs to which these nursing actions apply.

Intranasal corticosteroids are drugs of choice in treating allergic rhinitis.

Corticosteroids, also known as glucocorticoids, may be applied directly to the nasal mucosa to prevent symptoms of allergic rhinitis. When applied consistently, they decrease the secretion of inflammatory mediators, reduce tissue edema, and cause mild vasoconstriction. They have begun to replace antihistamines in the treatment of chronic allergic rhinitis. The intranasal corticosteroids and their doses are listed in Table 28.3. All have equal effectiveness and can require 2–3 weeks of therapy before optimum benefits are attained. When delivered by oral inhalation (not intranasal) some of these medications are also used to treat asthma.

Intranasal corticosteroids are administered with a metered-spray device that delivers a consistent dose of drug per spray. Intranasal corticosteroids produce none of the potentially serious adverse effects that are observed when these hormones are given orally. The most frequently reported adverse effects are an intense burning sensation in the nose immediately after spraying and drying of the nasal mucosa.

TABLE 28.3	Intranasal Corticosteroids	
DRUG	**ROUTE AND ADULT DOSE**	**REMARKS**
beclomethasone (Beconase AQ, QVAR)	Intranasal; one spray bid–qid	Oral inhaler available (Beclovent) for asthma
budesonide (Rhinocort Aqua)	Intranasal; two sprays bid	Oral inhaler available (Pulmicort) for asthma
ciclesonide (Omnaris)	Intranasal; two sprays once daily (max: 200 mcg/day)	Newer drug approved in 2006; less likely to cause steroid adverse effects than others in this class
flunisolide (Nasalide, Nasarel)	Intranasal; two sprays bid, may increase to tid if needed	Oral inhaler available (AeroBid) for asthma
Pr fluticasone (Flonase, Veramyst)	Intranasal; one spray in each nostril once (Veramyst) or twice (Flonase) daily	Oral inhaler available (Flovent) for asthma; topical form available (Cutivate) for dermatologic use
mometasone (Nasonex)	Intranasal; two sprays daily	Topical form available (Elocon) for dermatologic use
triamcinolone (Nasacort AQ)	Intranasal; two to four sprays qid	Oral inhaler available (Nasacort) for asthma; also available in IM, subcutaneous, intradermal, and intra-articular forms

DRUG PROFILE: **Pr** *Fluticasone (Flonase, Veramyst)*

Therapeutic Class: Drug for allergic rhinitis
Pharmacologic Class: Intranasal corticosteroid

Actions and Uses:

Fluticasone is typical of the intranasal corticosteroids used to treat allergic rhinitis. Therapy usually begins with two sprays in each nostril twice daily, and decreases to one dose per day. Fluticasone acts to decrease local inflammation in the nasal passages, thus reducing nasal stuffiness.

Adverse Effects and Interactions:

Adverse effects of fluticasone are rare. Small amounts of the intranasal corticosteroids are sometimes swallowed, which increases their potential for causing systemic adverse effects. Nasal irritation and bleeding occur in a few patients.

 Refer to MyNursingKit for a Nursing Process Focus specific to this drug.

Decongestants are used to reduce nasal congestion caused by allergic rhinitis and the common cold.

Decongestants are drugs that relieve nasal congestion. They are administered by either the oral or intranasal routes and are often combined with antihistamines in the pharmacotherapy of allergies or the common cold. Most decongestants are sympathomimetics—agents that activate the sympathetic nervous system. Doses for the decongestants are given in Table 28.4.

Sympathomimetics are effective at relieving the nasal congestion associated with allergic rhinitis and the common cold. Both oral and intranasal preparations are available. The intranasal drugs such as oxymetazoline (Afrin, others) are available OTC as sprays or drops and produce an effective response within minutes. Because of their local action, intranasal sympathomimetics produce few systemic effects. The most serious, limiting adverse effect of the intranasal preparations is **rebound congestion**; prolonged use causes hypersecretion of mucus and worsened nasal congestion once the drug effects wear off. This rebound effect sometimes leads to a cycle of increased drug use as the condition worsens. Because of rebound congestion, intranasal sympathomimetics should be used for no longer than 3 to 5 days. Patients with allergic rhinitis who develop tolerance to the effects of decongestants should be gradually switched to intranasal corticosteroids because they do not cause rebound congestion.

When administered orally, sympathomimetics do not produce rebound congestion. Their onset of action by this route, however, is much slower than the intranasal preparations, and they are less effective at relieving severe congestion. The possibility of systemic adverse effects is also greater with the oral drugs. Potential adverse effects include hypertension and CNS stimulation that may lead to insomnia or anxiety.

Prior to 2000, pseudoephedrine was the most common decongestant found in oral OTC cold and allergy medicines. Pseudoephedrine, however, is the starting chemical for the synthesis of illegal methamphetamine by drug traffickers. Although still OTC, pharmacists are required to monitor distribution of the drug by keeping a log of patients' names and addresses and checking the photo identification of the buyer. Most manufacturers have reformulated their OTC cold medicines to contain phenylephrine rather than pseudoephedrine. A drug prototype feature for phenylephrine is included in Chapter 8 ⊙.

Because sympathomimetics relieve nasal congestion only, they are often combined with antihistamines to control the sneezing and tearing of allergic rhinitis. It is interesting to note that some OTC drugs having the same basic name (Neo-Synephrine, Afrin, Visine) may contain different sympathomimetics. For example, Neo-Synephrine preparations with a 12-hour duration contain the drug oxymetazoline; preparations with the same name that last 4 to 6 hours contain phenylephrine.

TABLE 28.4	Decongestants	
DRUG	**ROUTE AND ADULT DOSE**	**REMARKS**
ephedrine (Pretz-D)	Intranasal (0.25%); two to three sprays/nostril, not more frequently than every 4 hours	Oral, IV, IM, and subcutaneous forms available. Also for acute asthma, hypotension, myasthenia gravis, and urinary incontinence
ipratropium (Atrovent)	Nasal spray; two sprays in each nostril 3–4 times/day up to 4 days	Anticholinergic agent; also available by the inhalation route for asthma
naphazoline (Privine)	Intranasal; two drops every 3–6 hours	Also available as spray
Pr oxymetazoline (Afrin, others)	Intranasal (0.05%); two to three sprays bid for up to 3–5 days	Also available as drops
phenylephrine (Neo-Synephrine) (see page 104 for the Drug Profile box)	Intranasal (0.25–0.5%); one or two sprays every 3–4 hours	Also available as drops, chewable tablets, and hemorrhoidal cream; also available by the subcutaneous, IM and IV routes for severe hypotension and shock
pseudoephedrine (Actifed, Sudafed, others)	PO; 60 mg every 4–6 hours (max: 120 mg/day)	Produces little congestive rebound or irritation; also available as drops and in extended-release form
tetrahydrozoline (Tyzine)	Intranasal (0.1%); two to four drops every 3 hours	Ophthalmic solution is available for allergic reactions of the eye
xylometazoline (Otrivin)	Intranasal (0.1%); one or two sprays bid (max: 3 doses/day)	Also available as drops

---

DRUG PROFILE: ℗ *Oxymetazoline (Afrin, Others)*

Therapeutic Class: Decongestant
Pharmacologic Class: Sympathomimetic

Actions and Uses:

Oxymetazoline activates alpha-adrenergic receptors of the sympathetic nervous system. This stimulation causes arterioles in the nasal passages to constrict, producing a drying of the mucous membranes. Relief from the symptoms of nasal congestion occurs within minutes and lasts for 10–12 hours. The drug is administered with a metered-spray device or by nose drops.

Oxymetazoline (Visine LR) is also available as eyedrops. It causes vasoconstriction of vessels in the eye and is used to relieve redness and provide relief from dryness and minor eye irritations.

Adverse Effects and Interactions:

Rebound congestion is common when oxymetazoline is used for longer than 3–5 days. Minor stinging and dryness in the nasal mucosa may be experienced. Systemic adverse effects are unlikely, unless a considerable amount of the medicine is swallowed. Patients with thyroid disorders, hypertension, diabetes, or heart disease should use sympathomimetics only on the direction of their health care provider.

No clinically significant interactions have been found.

 Refer to MyNursingKit for a Nursing Process Focus specific to this drug.

Ipratropium (Atrovent) is an anticholinergic drug sometimes used as a decongestant. Given by the intranasal route, ipratropium has no serious adverse effects. Its actions are limited to runny nose; it does not stop the sneezing, postnasal drip, or itchy throat or eyes characteristic of allergic rhinitis or the common cold. A more common indication for ipratropium is for the pharmacotherapy of asthma.

Concept Review   28.4

■ The sympathomimetics are the most effective drugs for relieving nasal congestion, but physicians often prefer to prescribe antihistamines or intranasal corticosteroids. Why?

Antitussives and expectorants are used to treat symptoms of the common cold.

CORE CONCEPT 28.7

In addition to congestion, cough is a symptom that causes patients to take OTC remedies or to seek medical attention. Cough is a reflex mechanism controlled by neurons in the cough center, which is located in the medulla oblongata of the brain. In some diseases such as emphysema and bronchitis, or when liquids have been aspirated into the bronchi, it is not desirable to suppress the normal cough reflex. Because cough is merely a symptom, the ultimate therapeutic goal is to identify and treat the underlying disorder whenever possible.

There are many possible causes of cough, ranging from the acute cough of an upper respiratory infection to the chronic cough of tobacco smoking. Some drugs, such as the angiotensin-converting enzyme (ACE) inhibitors and beta-adrenergic blockers, can trigger persistent cough. In many cases, keeping the throat moist with sugar-free candy, "cough drops," or frequent sips of water is sufficient to suppress cough. However, a dry, hacking, nonproductive cough can be quite irritating to the membranes of the throat and can deprive a patient of much-needed rest. It is these types of conditions in which therapy with drugs that control cough, or **antitussives**, may be warranted.

anti = *against*
tussive = *pertaining to a cough*

Opioids, the most effective class of antitussives, act by raising the cough threshold in the cough center, thereby decreasing both the frequency and intensity of cough. Hydrocodone and codeine are the most frequently used opioid antitussives. Doses needed to suppress the cough reflex are low; thus there is minimal potential for dependence. Most codeine cough mixtures are classified as Schedule III, IV, or V drugs and are reserved for more serious cough conditions. The amount of codeine in cough mixtures is low and rarely causes serious adverse effects. However, care must be taken not to give these mixtures to patients allergic to codeine or other opioids. In addition, the drug must be kept secure from children because accidental overdose of opioids in infants can cause severe respiratory depression and even death. Opioids may be combined with other agents such as antihistamines, decongestants, and nonopioid antitussives in the therapy of severe cold or flu symptoms.

The most frequently used OTC antitussive is dextromethorphan, which is included in most severe cold and flu preparations. Dextromethorphan is chemically similar to the opioids and also acts on the CNS to raise the cough threshold. Although it does not have the abuse potential of opioids, in large amounts dextromethorphan can cause slurred speech, dizziness, drowsiness, euphoria, and lack of motor coordination.

Benzonatate (Tessalon) is a nonopioid antitussive that does not act on the cough center. Instead, benzonatate has a local anesthetic-like effect on stretch receptors in the lung, which essentially interrupts the cough message. The patient must be instructed not to chew the soft capsules because they will cause numbness of the throat and tongue.

Expectorants are drugs that reduce the thickness or viscosity of bronchial secretions. They stimulate mucus flow, which thins bronchial secretions, allowing them to be removed with less forceful coughing. The most effective OTC expectorant is guaifenesin. Like dextromethorphan, guaifenesin produces few adverse effects and is a common ingredient in many OTC cold and flu preparations. Higher doses of guaifenesin are available by prescription. Nonprescription cough and cold products (including those containing guaifenesin) should not be used in children under 2 years of age.

Acetylcysteine (Mucomyst) is one of the few drugs available to directly loosen thick, viscous bronchial secretions by breaking down the chemical structure of mucus molecules. Drugs of this type are called **mucolytics**. Acetylcysteine is delivered by the inhalation route and is not available OTC. It is used in patients who have cystic fibrosis or other diseases that produce large amounts of thick bronchial secretions. Acetylcysteine (Acetadote) is also given as a 5% oral solution for acetaminophen overdose. When given within 24 hours of the overdose, acetylcysteine prevents acute liver damage by blocking the formation of toxic metabolites of acetaminophen.

muco = *mucus*
lytic = *destruction or disintegration*

ASTHMA

Asthma is a chronic pulmonary disease with both inflammatory and bronchospasm components. Drugs are given to either decrease the frequency of asthmatic attacks or terminate attacks in progress. Asthma is one of the most common chronic conditions in the United States, affecting 20 million Americans.

Asthma is a chronic inflammatory disease characterized by bronchospasm.

CORE CONCEPT 28.8

Asthma is characterized by chronic inflammation that occurs when potent mediators of the immune and inflammatory responses are released by mast cells lining the bronchial passageways. The result of this inflammation is increased mucus secretion, which narrows the airways and makes breathing more difficult.

The second characteristic of asthma is acute **bronchoconstriction** or **bronchospasm** during which bronchiolar smooth muscle contracts and the airway diameter narrows. This condition is illustrated in Figure 28.5 ■. The inflammatory conditions in the airway make the smooth muscle hyperresponsive to a variety of stimuli. Stimuli such as breathing smoke, pollutants, or cold air may trigger acute bronchospasm. Specific triggers are listed in Table 28.5. Some patients experience bronchospasm on exertion, a condition called *exercise-induced asthma.*

The patient with asthma will exhibit symptoms such as evening cough, **dyspnea** (shortness of breath), chest tightness, and wheezing. Intervals between symptoms may vary from days to weeks to months. **Status asthmaticus** is a severe, prolonged form of asthma that is unresponsive to drug treatment and may lead to respiratory failure.

Because asthma has both a bronchoconstriction component and an inflammatory component, drug therapy of the disease focuses on one or both of these mechanisms. The goals of drug

dys = *painful or difficult*
pnea = *breathing*

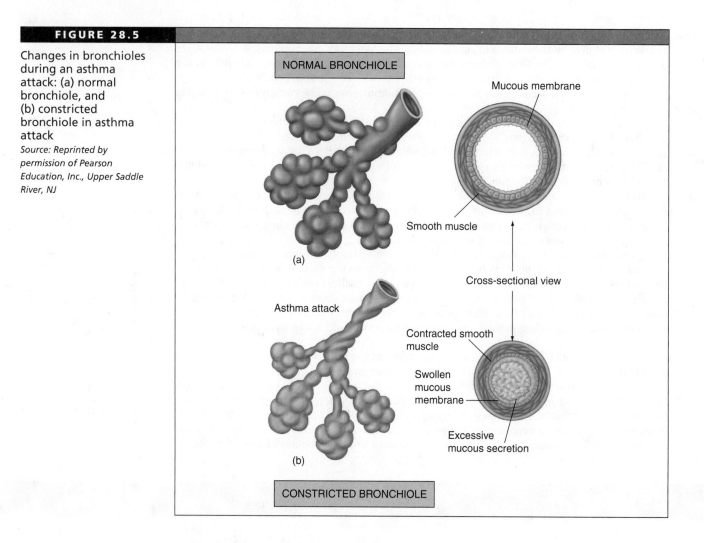

FIGURE 28.5

Changes in bronchioles
during an asthma
attack: (a) normal
bronchiole, and
(b) constricted
bronchiole in asthma
attack
*Source: Reprinted by
permission of Pearson
Education, Inc., Upper Saddle
River, NJ*

NORMAL BRONCHIOLE

Mucous membrane

Smooth muscle

(a)

Cross-sectional view

Asthma attack

Contracted smooth
muscle

Swollen
mucous
membrane

Excessive
mucous secretion

(b)

CONSTRICTED BRONCHIOLE

TABLE 28.5	Common Triggers of Asthma
air pollutants	Tobacco smoke
	Ozone
	Nitrous and sulfur oxides
	Fumes from cleaning fluids or solvents
	Burning leaves
allergens	Pollen from trees, grasses, and weeds
	Animal dander
	Household dust
	Mold
chemicals and food	Drugs such as aspirin, ibuprofen, and beta blockers
	Sulfite preservatives
	Food such as nuts, monosodium glutamate (MSG), shellfish, and dairy products
respiratory infections	Bacterial, fungal, and viral
stress	Emotional stress or anxiety
	Exercise in dry, cold climates

FIGURE 28.6

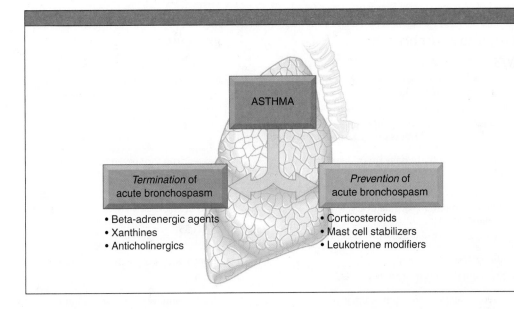

Drug classes used in the pharmacotherapy of asthma

therapy are twofold: to terminate acute bronchospasms in progress and to reduce the frequency of acute asthma attacks. Different drugs are usually needed to achieve each of these goals. The various classes of drugs used for asthma are shown in Figure 28.6 ∎.

Beta-adrenergic agents are the most effective drugs for relieving acute bronchospasm.

CORE CONCEPT 28.9

Recall from Chapter 8 ⚭ that the smooth muscle lining the bronchioles is under the control of the autonomic nervous system. Changes in the airway diameter are made possible by the contraction or relaxation of the bronchiolar smooth muscle. During the fight-or-flight response, beta$_2$-adrenergic receptors of the sympathetic nervous system are stimulated, the bronchiolar smooth muscle relaxes, and **bronchodilation** results. This allows more air to enter the alveoli, thus increasing the oxygen supply to the body during periods of stress or exercise. In practical terms, drugs that enhance bronchodilation will cause the patient to breathe easier; these are some of the most common medications for treating pulmonary disorders.

Bronchodilators are medications from several drug classes that are used to rapidly relieve the acute bronchospasm characteristic of an asthmatic attack. Although the beta-adrenergic agents are the most commonly prescribed types of bronchodilators, theophylline and ipratropium may also be used. Bronchodilators used for asthma are listed in Table 28.6.

Beta-adrenergic agents, or sympathomimetics, are the most effective drugs for the treatment of acute bronchospasm. In most cases, the agents used for pulmonary disease are selective for beta$_2$-receptors in the lung; thus, they produce fewer cardiac adverse effects than the nonselective beta agents. There are two basic classes of beta-adrenergic agents, and each has different indications.

Fast Facts Asthma

- Asthma is responsible for more than 1.5 million emergency department visits and more than 500,000 hospitalizations each year.
- More than 5,500 patients die of asthma each year.
- The incidence of asthma has been dramatically increasing each year since 1980 in all age, gender, and ethnic groups. The highest rate of increase has been among African Americans.
- The highest incidence of asthma is in those younger than age 18. From 7% to 10% of children have the disease.
- In adults, asthma is 35% more common in women than in men. In children, however, the disease affects twice as many boys as girls.

TABLE 28.6	Bronchodilators	
DRUG	**ROUTE AND ADULT DOSE**	**REMARKS**
BETA-ADRENERGIC AGENTS		
albuterol (Proventil, Ventolin, VoSpire)	MDI; two inhalations every 4–6 hours as needed (max: 12 inhalations/day) Nebulizer; 1.25–5 mg every 4–8 hours as needed PO; 2–4 mg tid-qid (max: 32 mg/day); Extended-release tablets: 8 mg every 12 hours (max: 32 mg/day divided)	Relaxes smooth muscle of the bronchial tree; nebulizer form available
arformoterol (Brovana)	Nebulizer; 15 mcg twice daily (max: 30 mcg/day)	Newer drug (approved in 2007) for COPD; long acting; very similar to formeterol
formoterol (Foradil, Perforomist)	DPI; 12 mcg inhalation capsule every 12 hours (max: 24 mcg/day) Nebulizer; 20 mcg bid (max: 40 mcg/day)	Long acting
levalbuterol (Xopenex)	Nebulizer; 0.63 mg tid–qid MDI; two inhalations every 4–6 hours	Short acting; very similar to albuterol
pirbuterol (Maxair)	MDI; two inhalations four times a day (max: 12 inhalations/day)	Short acting; very similar to albuterol
Pr salmeterol (Serevent)	DPI; two aerosol inhalations bid or one powder diskus bid	Long acting
terbutaline (Brethine)	PO; 2.5–5 mg tid (max: 15 mg/day) Subcutaneous; 250 mcg (may be repeated in 15 min) Inhalation; two inhalations (200 mcg/spray) every 4–6 hours	Also used to delay premature labor
XANTHINES		
aminophylline (Truphylline)	PO; 380 mg/day in divided doses every 6–8 hours (max: 928 mg/day)	IV form available
theophylline (Theo-dur)	PO; 300–600 mg/day in divided doses (max: 900 mg/day)	IV and extended-release form available
ANTICHOLINERGICS		
ipratropium (Atrovent, Combivent)	MDI; two inhalations qid (max: 12 inhalations/day) Nebulizer; 500 mcg every 6–8 hours as needed	Combivent is a combination of ipratropium and albuterol
tiotropium (Spiriva)	DPI; one capsule inhaled/day	Handihaler device is used to puncture capsule

- *Short-acting beta agents* Short-acting beta agonists are the most frequently prescribed drugs for aborting or terminating an acute asthma attack because they begin to act within minutes. Their effects, however, last only 2–6 hours.
- *Long-acting beta agents* Because long-acting beta agents take 20–60 minutes to act, they are not used to terminate bronchospasm. They are used in combination with inhaled corticosteroids for the prophylaxis of severe, persistent asthma.

Inhaled beta-adrenergic agents produce little toxicity because only small amounts of the drugs are absorbed. When given orally, a longer duration of action is achieved, but systemic adverse effects such as tachycardia and tremor are more frequently experienced. Tolerance may develop to the therapeutic effects of the beta-adrenergic agents; therefore, the patient must be instructed to seek medical attention if the drugs prove to be less effective with continued use.

As discussed in Chapter 8 ⬡, blocking the parasympathetic nervous system produces similar effects to stimulation of the sympathetic nervous system. It is predictable, then, that anticholinergic drugs would cause bronchodilation and have potential use in the pharmacotherapy of asthma and other pulmonary diseases. The most widely used drug in this class, ipratropium (Atrovent, Combivent), is taken via inhalation to rapidly relieve bronchospasm. Because it is not read-

DRUG PROFILE: *Salmeterol (Serevent)*

Therapeutic Class: Bronchodilator
Pharmacologic Class: Beta-adrenergic agent

Actions and Uses:

Salmeterol is approved for prevention of bronchospasm in patients with asthma and for the prevention of exercise-induced bronchospasm. Its 12-hour duration of action is longer than that of many other bronchodilators, thus making it best suited for the prophylaxis of chronic asthma. Because salmeterol takes 15–25 minutes to act, it should never be used for the termination of acute bronchospasm.

Adverse Effects and Interactions:

Serious adverse effects from salmeterol are uncommon. Some patients may experience headaches, nervousness, and restlessness. Because of its potential to cause tachycardia, patients with heart disease or dysrhythmias should be monitored regularly.

Concurrent use with beta blockers will inhibit the bronchodilation effect of salmeterol.

Mechanism in Action:

Salmeterol relieves bronchospasm by binding selectively with beta$_2$-receptors located on the cellular membranes of bronchiolar smooth muscle. Because salmeterol is a selective beta$_2$-stimulator, there is less potential for activating beta$_1$-cardiac receptors, especially if it is administered as an aerosol. It is primarily used to treat asthma.

Refer to MyNursingKit for a Nursing Process Focus specific to this drug.

ily absorbed from the lungs, it produces few adverse effects, although it is considered less effective than beta-adrenergic agents. Inhaled anticholinergics are more effective when used with other bronchodilators; Combivent is a combination of ipratropium and albuterol in a single MDI canister. In 2005, a new anticholinergic, tiotropium (Spiriva), was approved. Tiotropium has a long duration of action that allows for once-daily dosing.

The third class of bronchodilators is the xanthines (sometimes called methylxanthines). Chemically related to caffeine, theophylline (Theo-dur, others) and aminophylline (Truphylline) were drugs of choice for bronchoconstriction 20 years ago. Theophylline, however, has a narrow margin of safety and interacts with a large number of other drugs. Adverse effects such as nausea, vomiting, and CNS stimulation are relatively common, and dysrhythmias may occur at high doses. Having been largely replaced by safer and more effective drugs, theophylline is now primarily used for the long-term oral prophylaxis of persistent asthma.

NURSING PROCESS FOCUS

Patients Receiving Bronchodilators

ASSESSMENT

Prior to administration:
- Obtain a complete health history (physical/mental), including allergies, drug history, and possible drug reactions
- Assess for symptoms related to respiratory deficiency, such as dyspnea, orthopnea, cyanosis, nasal flaring, wheezing, and weakness
- Obtain vital signs
- Auscultate bilateral breath sounds for air movement and adventitious sounds (crackles, rhonchi, wheezes)
- Assess pulmonary function with pulse oximeter, peak expiratory flowmeter, and/or arterial blood gases to establish baseline

POTENTIAL NURSING DIAGNOSES

- Impaired Gas Exchange related to bronchial constriction.
- Activity Intolerance related to ineffective drug therapy.
- Deficient Knowledge related to information about drug therapy.
- Anxiety related to difficulty in breathing.
- Disturbed Sleep Pattern related to adverse effects of drugs.
- Ineffective Tissue Perfusion related to adverse effects of drugs.

continued . . .

NURSING PROCESS FOCUS *(continued)*

PLANNING: PATIENT GOALS AND EXPECTED OUTCOMES

The patient will:
- Exhibit adequate oxygenation as evidenced by improved lung sounds and pulmonary function values
- Report a reduction in subjective symptoms of respiratory deficiency
- Demonstrate an understanding of the drug's action by accurately describing drug adverse effects and precautions
- Report at least 6 hours of uninterrupted sleep

IMPLEMENTATION

Interventions and (Rationales)	Patient Education/Discharge Planning
■ Monitor vital signs, including pulse, blood pressure, and respiratory rate.	Instruct the patient to: ■ Use medication as directed even if asymptomatic ■ Report difficulty with breathing
■ Ensure pulmonary function is monitored using pulse oximeter, peak expiratory flowmeter, and/or arterial blood gases. (Monitoring is necessary to assess drug effectiveness.)	■ Instruct the patient to report symptoms of deteriorating respiratory status such as increased dyspnea, breathlessness with speech, and/or orthopnea.
■ Monitor the patient's ability to use the inhaler. (Proper use ensures correct dosage.)	Instruct the patient: ■ In proper use of MDI ■ To use the medication strictly as prescribed; do not "double up" on doses ■ To rinse the mouth thoroughly following use
■ Observe for adverse effects specific to the medication used.	■ Instruct the patient regarding adverse effects and to report specific drug adverse effects.
■ Maintain the environment free of respiratory contaminants such as dust, dry air, flowers, and smoke. (These substances may exacerbate bronchial constriction.)	Instruct the patient to: ■ Avoid respiratory irritants ■ Maintain a "clean air environment" ■ Stop smoking and avoid secondhand smoke, if applicable
■ Maintain dietary intake adequate in essential nutrients and vitamins. (Dyspnea interferes with proper nutrition.)	Instruct the patient to: ■ Maintain nutrition with foods high in essential nutrients ■ Consume small frequent meals to prevent fatigue
■ Ensure that the patient maintains adequate hydration of 3 to 4 L/day (to liquefy pulmonary secretions).	Instruct the patient to: ■ Consume 3 to 4 L of fluid/day if not contraindicated ■ Avoid caffeine (increases CNS irritability)
■ Provide emotional and psychosocial support during periods of shortness of breath.	■ Instruct the patient in relaxation techniques and controlled breathing techniques.
■ Monitor patient compliance. (Maintaining therapeutic drug levels is essential to effective therapy.)	■ Inform the patient of the importance of ongoing medication compliance and follow-up.

EVALUATION OF OUTCOME CRITERIA

Evaluate the effectiveness of drug therapy by confirming that patient goals and expected outcomes have been met (see "Planning").

See Table 28.2 for a list of drugs to which these nursing actions apply.

Corticosteroids are the most effective drugs for the long-term prophylaxis of asthma.

The role of intranasal corticosteroids as first-line agents in the treatment of allergic rhinitis is discussed in Section 28.5. When given by the inhalation route, corticosteroids are also prime drugs for the management of asthma.

Because asthma has a major inflammatory component, several classes of anti-inflammatory drugs are used for asthma prophylaxis. The inhaled corticosteroids are most commonly used for this purpose, although mast cell stabilizers and leukotriene inhibitors are also effective. Doses of the anti-inflammatory drugs used for asthma are given in Table 28.7.

Corticosteroids are the most effective drugs available for the *prevention* of acute asthmatic episodes. When inhaled on a daily schedule, corticosteroids suppress inflammation without producing major adverse effects. Mucus production and edema is diminished, thus reducing airway obstruction. Patients should be informed that inhaled corticosteroids must be taken daily to produce their therapeutic effect and that these medications are not effective at terminating episodes in progress. Although symptoms will improve in the first 1 to 2 weeks of therapy, 4 to 8 weeks may be required for maximum benefit. For some patients, a beta-adrenergic agent may be prescribed along with an inhaled corticosteroid because this permits the dose of the corticosteroid to be reduced by as much as 50%.

For severe, persistent asthma that is unresponsive to other treatments, oral corticosteroids may be prescribed. Treatment time is limited to the shortest length possible, usually 5 to 7 days. If taken for longer than 10 days, oral corticosteroids may produce significant adverse effects such as adrenal gland suppression, peptic ulcers, and hyperglycemia. Other uses and adverse effects of corticosteroids are presented in Chapters 24 and 31 ⬭ .

TABLE 28.7	Anti-Inflammatory Drugs for Asthma	
DRUG	**ROUTE AND ADULT DOSE**	**REMARKS**
INHALED CORTICOSTEROIDS		
beclomethasone (Beconase AQ, Qvar)	MDI; one or two inhalations tid or qid (max: 20 inhalations/day)	Intranasal form available for allergic rhinitis
budesonide (Pulmicort Turbuhaler)	DPI; one or two inhalations (200 mcg/inhalation) daily (max: 800 mcg/day)	Intranasal form available for allergic rhinitis
ciclesonide (Alvesco)	MDI; one or two inhalations/day (max: 320–640 mcg/day)	Newer drug; for asthma prophylaxis, not for acute bronchospasm
flunisolide (AeroBid)	MDI; two or three inhalations bid or tid (max: 12 inhalations/day)	Intranasal form available for allergic rhinitis
fluticasone (Flovent)	MDI (44 mcg); two inhalations bid (max: 10 inhalations/day)	Intranasal form available for allergic rhinitis; also available in 110 and 120 mcg inhalers
mometasone (Asmanex)	DPI; one inhalation daily (max: two inhalations daily)	Intranasal form available for allergic rhinitis and topical form for skin inflammation
triamcinolone (Azmacort)	MDI; two inhalations tid or qid (max: 16 inhalations/day)	Also available in IM, subcutaneous, intradermal, topical, and oral forms
MAST CELL STABILIZERS		
cromolyn (Intal)	MDI; one inhalation qid	Intranasal form available OTC for ophthalmic use
nedocromil sodium (Tilade)	MDI; two inhalations qid	Topical form available for ophthalmic use
LEUKOTRIENE MODIFIERS		
montelukast (Singulair)	PO; 10 mg/day in evening	Not for acute bronchospasm; also for allergic rhinitis
zafirlukast (Accolate)	PO; 20 mg bid 1 hour before or 2 hours after meals	Not for acute bronchospasm; also for allergic rhinitis
Zileuton (Zyflo)	PO; 1200 mg bid	Not for acute bronchospasm

CORE CONCEPT 28.11

Mast cell stabilizers and leukotriene modifiers are alternative anti-inflammatory drugs for the prophylaxis of asthma.

Two mast cell inhibitors play a limited though important role in the prophylaxis of asthma. These drugs act by inhibiting the release of histamine from mast cells.

Cromolyn (Intal) is an anti-inflammatory drug that is useful in preventing asthma attacks. When administered via an MDI or a nebulizer, cromolyn is a safe alternative to the corticosteroids. Maximum therapeutic benefit may take several weeks. Patients must be informed that cromolyn should be taken on a daily basis and should not be used to terminate acute attacks. An intranasal form of cromolyn (Nasalcrom) is used in the treatment of seasonal allergies.

Nedocromil (Tilade) is an anti-inflammatory drug that has actions and uses similar to cromolyn. The drug has few adverse effects when administered with an MDI, although some patients experience an unpleasant taste.

The leukotriene modifiers are relatively new drugs used to reduce inflammation and ease bronchoconstriction. They modify the action of leukotrienes, which are mediators of the inflammatory response in patients with asthma. Leukotriene modifiers are alternative drugs used for the management of persistent asthma that cannot be controlled with inhaled corticosteroids or short-acting beta agents.

The leukotriene modifiers are approved for the prophylaxis of chronic asthma; they are ineffective in relieving acute bronchospasm. They are all given orally. Zileuton has a more rapid onset of action (2 hours), whereas the other two leukotriene modifiers take as long as a week to provide therapeutic benefit. Few serious adverse effects are associated with the leukotriene modifiers. Headache, cough, nasal congestion, or GI upset may occur.

Concept Review 28.5

■ Distinguish the classes of drugs that *prevent* asthma attacks from those that can *terminate* an attack in progress. Name at least one drug in each class.

NATURAL THERAPIES

Horehound for Respiratory Disorders

Horehound has been used as an herbal remedy since the days of ancient Egyptians and was popular with Native Americans. In folklore, it was reported to aid in a number of respiratory disorders, including asthma, bronchitis, whooping cough, and infections such as tuberculosis. Nonrespiratory uses include bowel disorders, jaundice, and wound healing.

Active ingredients of horehound are found throughout the flowering plant. The chief constituent is a bitter substance called *marrubium* that stimulates secretions. Formulations include tea, dried or fresh leaves, and liquid extracts. Horehound has an expectorant action when treating colds and is also available as cough drops. It is claimed to restore normal secretions to the lungs and other organs.

CHRONIC OBSTRUCTIVE PULMONARY DISEASE (COPD)

COPD includes progressive lung disorders primarily caused by tobacco smoking. COPD is a major cause of death and disability. Drugs may bring symptomatic relief but do not cure the disorders.

CORE CONCEPT 28.12

Chronic obstructive pulmonary disease is a progressive disorder treated with multiple drugs.

The two primary disorders classified as COPD are chronic bronchitis and emphysema. Both are strongly associated with smoking tobacco products and, secondarily, air pollutants. In **chronic**

bronchitis, excess mucus is produced in the respiratory tree due to inflammation and irritation from smoke or pollutants. The airway becomes partially obstructed with mucus, resulting in the classic signs of dyspnea and coughing. Because microbes enjoy the mucus-rich environment, pulmonary infections are common. Gas exchange may be impaired.

bronch = *bronchus*
itis = *inflammation*

COPD is a progressive disease, with the terminal stage being **emphysema**. After years of chronic inflammation, the bronchioles lose their elasticity, and the alveoli dilate to maximum size to get more air into the lungs. The patient suffers from extreme dyspnea from even the slightest physical activity.

Patients with COPD may receive a number of pulmonary drugs for symptomatic relief of their disorder. The goals of pharmacotherapy are to treat infections and to control cough and bronchospasm. Most patients receive bronchodilators such as ipratropium, beta$_2$-agents, or inhaled corticosteroids. Mucolytics and expectorants are sometimes indicated to reduce the thickness of the bronchial mucus and to aid in its removal. Oxygen therapy may also be used in patients with emphysema. Patients should be taught to avoid taking any drugs that have beta-blocking activity or that otherwise cause bronchoconstriction. Respiratory depressants should be avoided. It is important to note that none of the pharmacotherapies offer a cure for COPD; they only treat the symptoms of a progressively worsening disease.

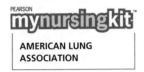

PEARSON
mynursingkit
AMERICAN LUNG ASSOCIATION

PATIENTS NEED TO KNOW

Patients treated for pulmonary disorders need to know the following:

In General

1. Because tolerance to some medications may occur, if medication is no longer effective, report this tolerance to a health care provider. Do not take extra medication without notifying a health care provider.

Regarding Inhaled Medications

2. When using MDIs or DPIs, allow an interval of at least 1 minute to pass between puffs.
3. When taking more than one respiratory medicine, take the bronchodilator first. This opens the airways and increases the effectiveness of the second medication.
4. Rinse the mouth thoroughly following inhaler use to reduce the oral absorption of inhaled medicines.
5. Take inhaled corticosteroids on a regular basis—not as needed. These medications are not used to stop acute asthma attacks.
6. Do not use decongestant nasal sprays for more than 2 or 3 days unless instructed to do so by a health care provider.

Regarding Bronchodilators

7. Avoid caffeine-containing foods and beverages if taking theophylline.
8. Immediately report any abnormalities in pulse rate, changes in blood pressure, or sensations of palpitations when taking beta-adrenergic stimulators.

Regarding Antihistamines and Decongestants

9. If taking antihistamines for the first time, avoid operating machinery or performing other tasks requiring alertness because drowsiness may occur.
10. Use hard candies, chewing gum, or ice chips to reduce the dry mouth caused by some decongestants and antihistamines.
11. Stop taking antihistamines and notify a health care provider if excessive sedation, wheezing, chest tightness, or bleeding/bruising occur.
12. Do not take OTC cold or allergy medicines containing antihistamines at the same time as prescription antihistamines.

CHAPTER REVIEW

CORE CONCEPTS SUMMARY

28.1 The respiratory system supplies oxygen for the body and provides protection against inhaled organisms.

The URT warms the incoming air and reacts to particles or pathogens that attempt to enter the body. The LRT brings needed oxygen into the body and removes carbon dioxide through expiration. The process of moving air into and out of the lungs, or ventilation, is distinct from the process of gas exchange across the alveoli, a process known as respiration.

28.2 The inhalation route of drug administration quickly delivers medications directly to their sites of action.

Inhalation is frequently used as a route of drug administration for those medications targeted for the respiratory system. Nebulizers, DPIs, and MDIs are used to deliver drugs via the inhalation route.

28.3 Allergic rhinitis is characterized by sneezing, watery eyes, and nasal congestion.

Allergic rhinitis, also known as hay fever, is a chronic allergy triggered by a wide variety of antigens. The release of chemicals mediating the immune response can result in seasonal symptoms for some patients, and chronic, continuous symptoms for others.

28.4 Antihistamines are widely used to treat allergic rhinitis and other minor allergies.

The H_1-receptor blockers, or antihistamines, are used to treat allergies, motion sickness, and insomnia. Newer drugs in this class are nonsedating and offer the advantage of once-a-day dosing.

28.5 Intranasal corticosteroids are drugs of choice in treating allergic rhinitis.

Intranasal corticosteroids are the treatment of choice for allergic rhinitis because of their high effectiveness and wide margin of safety. When used by this route, they do not produce the serious adverse effects observed when they are given orally or parenterally.

28.6 Decongestants are used to reduce nasal congestion caused by allergic rhinitis and the common cold.

Oral and intranasal sympathomimetics are effective at relieving nasal congestion. The intranasal agents act more rapidly and are more effective. Use of the intranasal preparations, however, is usually limited to 3 to 5 days because of the potential for rebound congestion.

28.7 Antitussives and expectorants are used to treat symptoms of the common cold.

Antitussives are effective at inhibiting the cough reflex. Although opioids are the most effective, there is some risk of physical dependence. Guaifenesin is an OTC drug used to increase bronchial secretions so that cough may be more productive. Mucolytics loosen mucus so that it may be more easily removed from the bronchial tree.

28.8 Asthma is a chronic inflammatory disease characterized by bronchospasm.

Asthma is a common disease characterized by bronchospasm and chronic airway inflammation. Exposure to a number of factors, including allergens, can cause an acute episode.

28.9 Beta-adrenergic agents are the most effective drugs for relieving acute bronchospasm.

Inhaled $beta_2$-adrenergic agents are drugs of choice for relieving bronchospasm. Anticholinergics are sometimes used for bronchodilation, but fewer are available because of their incidence of adverse effects. Xanthines, once widely used in pulmonary medicine, are now second-choice drugs for relieving bronchospasm because of their higher potential for adverse effects.

28.10 Corticosteroids are the most effective drugs for the long-term prophylaxis of asthma.

Inhaled corticosteroids are the drugs of choice for asthma prophylaxis. The inhaled corticosteroids, even when used on a long-term basis, produce few adverse effects compared to oral corticosteroids.

28.11 Mast cell stabilizers and leukotriene modifiers are alternative anti-inflammatory drugs for the prophylaxis of asthma.

Mast cell stabilizers such as cromolyn are sometimes used for asthma prophylaxis, although they are not as effective as the corticosteroids. The leukotriene modifiers offer another option for the prophylaxis of chronic asthma.

28.12 Chronic obstructive pulmonary disease is a progressive disorder treated with multiple drugs.

Chronic bronchitis and emphysema are two disorders of COPD that often require multiple drug therapy. Bronchodilators, expectorants, mucolytics, antibiotics, and oxygen may offer symptomatic relief.

REVIEW QUESTIONS

The following questions are written in NCLEX-PN® style. Answer these questions to assess your knowledge of the chapter material, and go back and review any material that is not clear to you.

1. The patient is having an acute asthma attack. Which of the following drugs would be most appropriate?
1. Pirbuterol (Maxair)
2. Budesonide (Pulmicort)
3. Fluticasone (Flovent)
4. Zafirlukast (Accolate)

2. Theophylline (Theo-Dur) has been added to your patient's treatment regimen. Which of the following would be highest-priority teaching for patients?
1. Nausea and vomiting may be adverse effects.
2. It is important to monitor for tachycardia.
3. The drug causes nervousness.
4. Avoid caffeine-containing foods and beverages.

3. When teaching a patient on multiple inhalers how to properly use this medication, which of the following would be correct?
1. Take inhaled corticosteroids only for acute attacks.
2. Do not use for more than 3 days unless instructed by the physician.
3. Space inhalers throughout the day to prevent adverse effects.
4. Use bronchodilators first.

4. The physician has ordered montelukast (Singulair). The patient wants to know how soon the medication will begin working. The best response would be:
1. "The medication has a rapid onset—within 2 hours."
2. "It will take about a week to become effective."
3. "This medication is used to treat acute bronchospasms only."
4. "Therapeutic benefits may take several weeks."

5. The patient asks what the difference is between antitussives and mucolytics. The nurse's best reply would be:
1. "Antitussives loosen bronchial secretions, and mucolytics stimulate removal of bronchial secretions."
2. "Antitussives suppress cough, whereas mucolytics loosen bronchial secretions."
3. "The terms are interchangeable."
4. "Both types of drugs work to loosen and remove secretions."

6. The most commonly used antitussive is:
1. Guaifenesin
2. Benzonatate (Tessalon)
3. Acetylcysteine (Mucomyst)
4. Dextromethorphan

7. The patient complains of numbness of the throat and tongue after taking benzonatate (Tessalon). The health care provider should instruct the patient:
1. To swallow, not chew, the medication
2. To decrease the dosage of medication
3. To stop taking the medication immediately
4. That this is a common adverse effect and that will subside over time.

8. Which of the following causes histamine release?
1. Prostaglandins
2. Leukotrienes
3. Bradykinin
4. Mast cells

9. Patients taking intranasal corticosteroids may develop which of the following adverse effects?
1. Rebound congestion
2. Nose bleeds
3. Drowsiness
4. Nervousness

10. Education for a patient using Afrin would include:
1. Not to use it for longer than 3–5 days to prevent rebound congestion from occurring
2. The importance of monitoring for hypertension
3. To notify the physician if nervousness occurs
4. Not to mix with any other medications

CASE STUDY QUESTIONS

For questions 1–4, please refer to the following case study, and choose the correct answer from choices 1–4.

*M*r. Thomas arrives at your office with what appears to be an acute upper respiratory tract infection. He is complaining of nonproductive cough, low-grade fever, and shortness of breath when walking. He is 60 years old and smokes a pack of cigarettes daily. The physician prescribes Hycotuss, a combination drug containing hydrocodone and guaifenesin, acetaminophen, and an ipratropium (Atrovent) inhaler.

1. Which of the prescribed drugs will directly benefit Mr. Thomas's shortness of breath?
1. Hydrocodone
2. Acetaminophen
3. Guaifenesin
4. Ipratropium

2. Which of the prescribed drugs would increase bronchial secretions?

1. Hydrocodone
2. Acetaminophen
3. Guaifenesin
4. Ipratropium

3. Mr. Thomas calls the office the next day, complaining that he is unable to drive his car because of excessive drowsiness. Which drug most likely is causing this drowsiness?

1. Hydrocodone
2. Acetaminophen
3. Guaifenesin
4. Ipratropium

4. Mr. Thomas also has asthma, which has become worse over the past few months. He stated that when an acute asthma attack occurs, budesonide (Pulmicort Turbuhaler) does not stop the episode. The nurse should advise Mr. Thomas:

1. To use four inhalations of budesonide instead of two
2. That budesonide must be taken on a regular schedule, not just during acute episodes
3. To request a tablet form of corticosteroid, rather than an inhaler
4. To always gently clear his nose just prior to using budesonide

FURTHER STUDY

- Drugs for maintaining acid and base balance are covered in Chapter 23 ⊂⊃ .

- Anti-infectives, used in the treatment of lung infections, are discussed in Chapters 25 and 26 ⊂⊃ .

- Chapter 15 ⊂⊃ presents information on anesthetics such as nitrous oxide and halothane (Fluothane), which are delivered via the inhalation route.

- Chapter 8 ⊂⊃ discusses in further detail the autonomic nervous system and its effects on the respiratory system.

- Uses and adverse effects of the corticosteroids are detailed in Chapters 24 and 31 ⊂⊃ .

29 Drugs for Gastrointestinal Disorders

CORE CONCEPTS

29.1 The digestive system breaks down food, absorbs nutrients, and eliminates wastes.

29.2 Peptic ulcer disease is caused by an erosion of the mucosal layer of the stomach or duodenum.

29.3 Peptic ulcer disease is treated by a combination of lifestyle changes and pharmacotherapy.

29.4 Proton-pump inhibitors are effective at reducing gastric acid secretion.

29.5 H_2-receptor blockers reduce the secretion of gastric acid.

29.6 Antacids rapidly neutralize stomach acid and reduce the symptoms of peptic ulcer disease and GERD.

29.7 Antibiotics are administered to eliminate *Helicobacter pylori,* the cause of many peptic ulcers.

29.8 Several miscellaneous drugs are also beneficial in treating peptic ulcer disease.

29.9 Laxatives are used to promote defecation.

29.10 Opioids are the most effective drugs for controlling severe diarrhea.

29.11 Antiemetics are prescribed to treat nausea, vomiting, and motion sickness.

29.12 Anorexiants and lipase inhibitors are used for the short-term management of obesity.

29.13 Pancreatic enzymes are administered as replacement therapy for patients with pancreatitis or malabsorption syndromes.

DRUG SNAPSHOT

The following drugs are discussed in this chapter:

DRUG CLASSES	DRUG PROFILES
Proton-pump inhibitors	(Pr) omeprazole (Prilosec)
H_2-receptor blockers	(Pr) ranitidine (Zantac)
Antacids	
Antibiotics for *H. pylori*	
Laxatives	(Pr) psyllium mucilloid (Metamucil, others)

DRUG CLASSES	DRUG PROFILES
Antidiarrheals	(Pr) diphenoxylate with atropine (Lomotil)
Antiemetics	(Pr) prochlorperazine (Compazine)
Antiobesity drugs	(Pr) sibutramine (Meridia)
Pancreatic enzyme replacement	

LEARNING OUTCOMES

After reading this chapter, the student should be able to:

1. Describe the major anatomic structures of the digestive system.

2. Identify common causes, signs, and symptoms of peptic ulcer disease and gastroesophageal reflux disease (GERD).

3. Identify the major classes of drugs used to treat peptic ulcer disease and GERD.

4. Explain why two or more antibiotics are used concurrently in the treatment of *H. pylori.*

5. Explain the conditions in which the drug treatment of constipation is warranted.

6. Identify the major classes of laxatives.

7. Explain the conditions in which the drug treatment of diarrhea is warranted.

8. Identify the major classes of antiemetics.

9. Describe the types of drugs used in the short-term management of obesity and their effectiveness.

10. Describe the pharmacotherapy of pancreatic insufficiency.

11. For each of the following classes listed in the Drug Snapshot, identify representative drugs and explain the mechanisms of drug action, primary actions related to the digestive system, and important adverse effects.

12. Categorize drugs used in the treatment of digestive system disorders based on their classifications and mechanisms of action.

KEY TERMS

alimentary canal (AL-uh-MEN-tare-ee) *507*

anorexia (AN-oh-REX-ee-uh) *509*

anorexiant (AN-oh-REX-ee-ant) *522*

antacid (an-TASS-id) *515*

antiemetic (AN-tie-ee-MET-ik) *520*

antiflatulent (an-tie-FLAT-u-lent) *515*

cathartic (kah-THAR-tik) *516*

constipation (kon-stah-PAY-shun) *516*

Crohn's disease (KROHNS) *510*

defecation (def-ah-KAY-shun) *516*

diarrhea *518*

dietary fiber *516*

digestion (dye-JES-chun) *507*

emesis (EM-eh-sis) *520*

emetic (ee-MET-ik) *520*

gastroesophageal reflux disease (GERD) (GAS-troh-ee-SOF-ah-JEEL REE-flux) *510*

H$^+$, K$^+$-ATPase *510*

H$_2$-receptor blocker *511*

***Helicobacter pylori* (hee-lick-oh-BAK-tur py-LOR-eye)** *509*

pancreatic insufficiency *523*

peptic ulcer *508*

peristalsis (pair-ih-STAL-sis) *507*

proton-pump inhibitor (PPI) *510*

ulcerative colitis (UL-sir-ah-tiv koh-LIE-tuss) *510*

Zollinger-Ellison syndrome (ZOLL-in-jer ELL-ih-sun) *513*

Very little of the food we eat is directly available to body cells. Food must be broken down, absorbed, and chemically modified before it is in a form useful to cells. The digestive system performs these functions and more. Some disorders of the digestive system are mechanical in nature, slowing or speeding up the transit of substances through the gastrointestinal tract. Other disorders are metabolic, affecting the secretion of digestive enzymes and fluids or the absorption of essential nutrients. Many signs and symptoms are nonspecific and may be caused by any number of different disorders. This chapter examines the drug therapy of common conditions affecting the digestive system.

Fast Facts Gastrointestinal Tract Disorders

- Sixty to seventy million Americans are affected by a digestive disease.
- Thirteen percent of all hospitalizations are for digestive disorders.
- Ulcers are responsible for about 40,000 surgeries annually.
- More than 400,000 new cases of peptic ulcer disease are diagnosed each year.
- Colorectal cancer is the second leading cause of cancer deaths, killing more than 55,000 Americans annually.
- Irritable bowel syndrome affects 10 to 20% of adults.
- Americans spend more than $33 billion annually on weight-reduction products and services.

The digestive system breaks down food, absorbs nutrients, and eliminates wastes.

The digestive system consists of two basic anatomic divisions: the alimentary canal and the accessory organs. The **alimentary canal**, or gastrointestinal (GI) tract, is a long, continuous, hollow tube that extends from the mouth to the anus. The accessory organs of digestion include the liver, gallbladder, and pancreas. The structure of the digestive system is shown in Figure 29.1 ■.

Digestion is the process by which the body breaks down ingested food into small molecules that can be absorbed. The primary functions of the GI tract are to physically transport ingested food and to provide the necessary enzymes and surface area for chemical digestion and absorption. The inner surface is lined with a mucosa layer that secretes acids, bases, mucus, and enzymes important to digestion. The mucosa of the small intestine is lined with tiny projections called *villi* and *microvilli* that provide a huge surface area for the absorption of food and medications.

Substances are propelled along the GI tract by the contractions of several layers of smooth muscle, a process known as **peristalsis**. The speed of transit is critical to the absorption of nutrients and water and for the removal of wastes. If peristalsis is too fast, substances will not have sufficient contact with the mucosa to be absorbed. In addition, the large intestine will not have enough time to absorb water, and diarrhea may result. Abnormally slow transit times may result in constipation or even obstructions in the small or large intestine.

peri = *around*
stalsis = *contraction*

To chemically break down ingested food, a large number of enzymes and other substances are required. Digestive enzymes are secreted by the salivary glands, stomach, small intestine, and pancreas. The liver makes bile, which is stored in the gallbladder until needed for lipid digestion. Because these digestive substances are not common targets for drug therapy, their discussion in this chapter is limited, and the student should refer to anatomy and physiology texts for additional information.

FIGURE 29.1

The digestive system

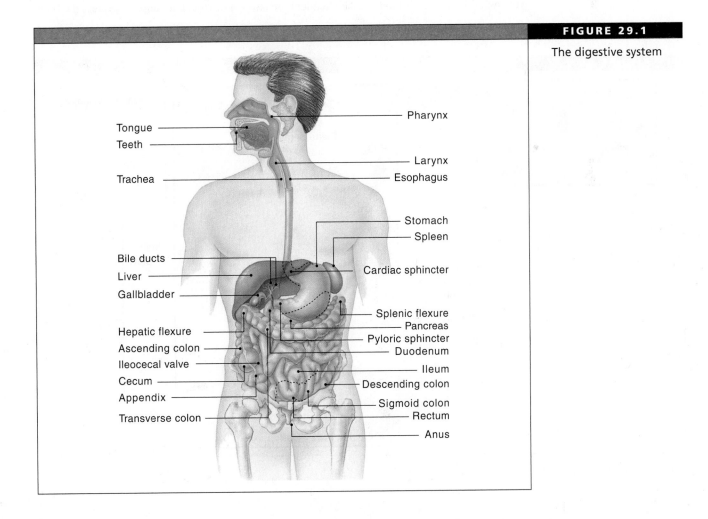

PEPTIC ULCER DISEASE

An ulcer is a sore or erosion of the mucosal layer of the GI tract. Although ulcers may occur in any portion of the GI tract, the duodenum is the most common site.

Peptic ulcer disease is caused by an erosion of the mucosal layer of the stomach or duodenum.

CORE CONCEPT 29.2

pept = *to digest*
ic = *pertaining to*

The term **peptic ulcer** refers to a lesion located in either the stomach (gastric) or small intestine (duodenal). Peptic ulcer disease (PUD) is associated with the following risk factors:

- Close family history of PUD
- Blood group O
- Smoking tobacco
- Alcoholic beverages
- Beverages and food containing caffeine
- Drugs, including corticosteroids, aspirin, and nonsteroidal anti-inflammatory drugs (NSAIDs)
- Excessive psychological stress
- Infection with the bacterium *H. pylori*

One to three liters of hydrochloric acid are secreted each day by cells in the stomach mucosa. Although this strong acid aids in the chemical breakdown of food and helps to protect the body

FIGURE 29.2

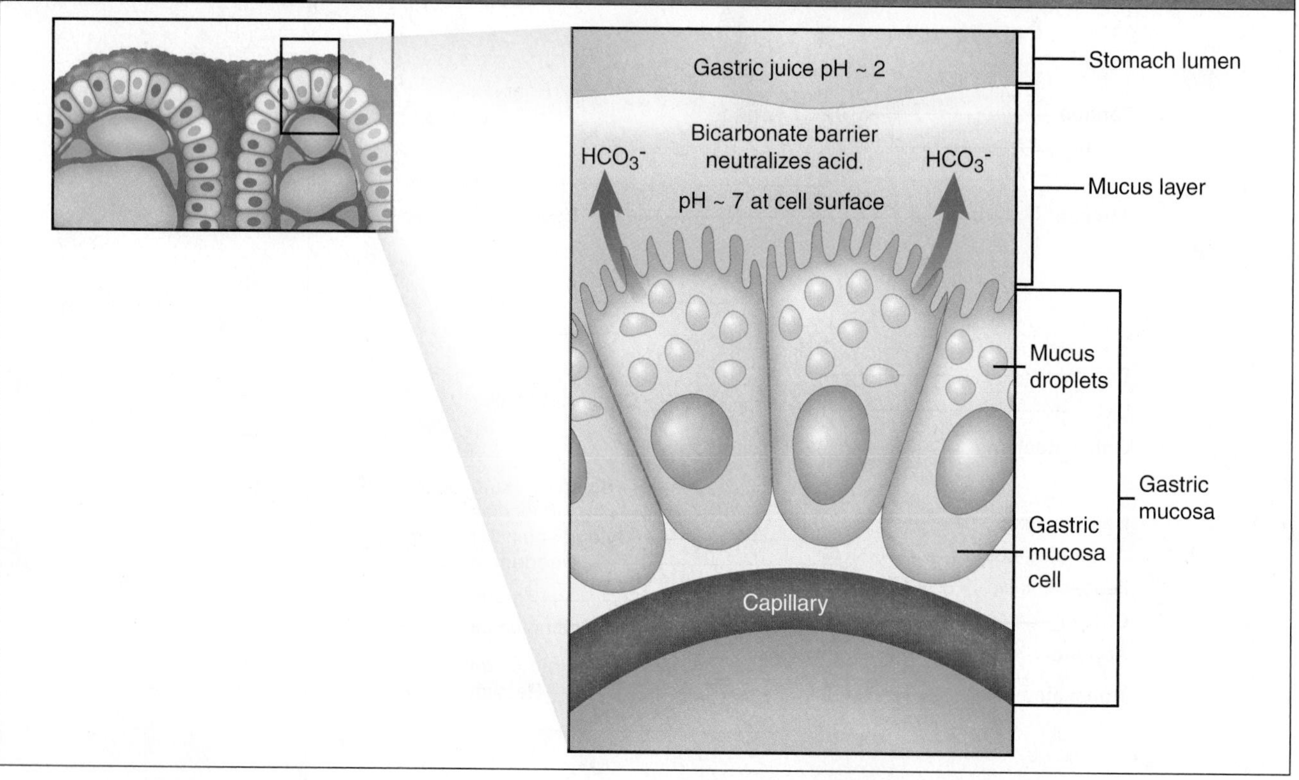

Natural defenses against stomach acid

from ingested microbes, it may be quite damaging to stomach cells. A number of natural defenses protect the stomach lining against this extremely acidic fluid. Certain cells lining the surface of the stomach secrete a thick mucous layer and bicarbonate, a basic ion that neutralizes acid. These provide a protective layer such that the pH at the mucosal surface is nearly neutral. Once reaching the duodenum, the stomach contents are further neutralized by bicarbonate from pancreatic and biliary secretions. These natural defenses are depicted in Figure 29.2 ■.

The primary cause of peptic ulcers is infection by the bacterium ***Helicobacter pylori***. In non-infected patients, duodenal ulcers are commonly caused by therapy with NSAIDs. Secondary factors that contribute to ulcer and the subsequent inflammation include secretion of excess stomach acid and hyposecretion of adequate mucous protection. Figure 29.3 ■ illustrates the mechanism of peptic ulcer formation.

The characteristic symptom of duodenal ulcer is a gnawing or burning upper abdominal pain that occurs 1 to 3 hours after a meal. The pain is worse when the stomach is empty and often disappears following ingestion of food. Nighttime pain, nausea, and vomiting are uncommon. If the erosion progresses deeper into the mucosa, bleeding will occur, and this may be evident as bright red blood in vomit or black, tarry stools. Many duodenal ulcers heal spontaneously, although they often reoccur after months of remission.

Gastric ulcers are less common than the duodenal type and have different symptoms. Although relieved by food, pain may continue even after a meal. Loss of appetite (known as **anorexia**), weight loss, and vomiting are more common. Remissions may be infrequent or absent. Medical follow-up of gastric ulcers sometimes proceeds for many years because a small

an = *not or without*
orexia = *appetite*

FIGURE 29.3

Mechanism of peptic ulcer formation
Reprinted by permission of Pearson Education, Inc., Upper Saddle River, NJ

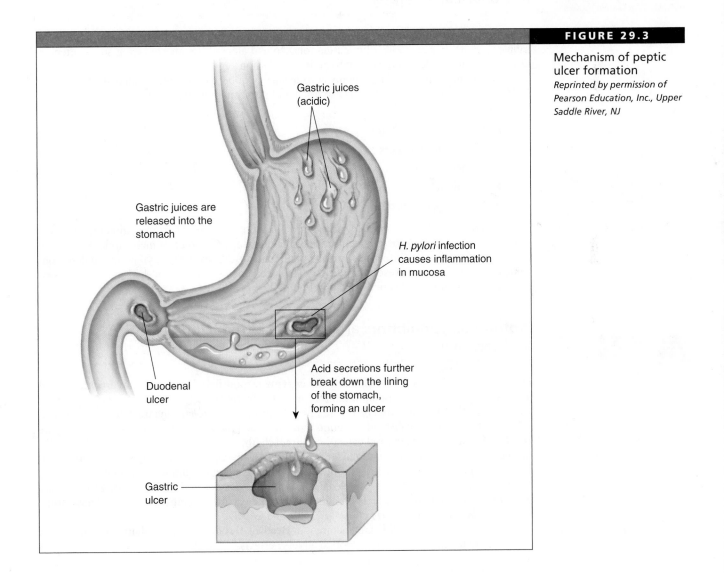

Gastric juices (acidic)

Gastric juices are released into the stomach

H. pylori infection causes inflammation in mucosa

Duodenal ulcer

Acid secretions further break down the lining of the stomach, forming an ulcer

Gastric ulcer

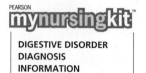

DIGESTIVE DISORDER
DIAGNOSIS
INFORMATION

percentage of the erosions become cancerous. The most severe ulcers may penetrate through the wall of the stomach and cause death. Whereas duodenal ulcers occur most frequently in the 30- to 50-year-old age group, gastric ulcers are more common in those older than age 60.

Ulceration in the lower small intestine is known as **Crohn's disease**, and erosions in the large intestine are called **ulcerative colitis**. These diseases are categorized as inflammatory bowel disease and are treated with the anti-inflammatory medications discussed in Chapter 21 ⌾ . Particularly severe cases may require immunosuppressant drugs such as cyclosporine (Neoral, Sandimmune) or methotrexate (Folex, Mexate, others).

Gastroesophageal reflux disease (GERD) is a common condition in which the acidic contents of the stomach move upward into the esophagus. This causes an intense burning known as *heartburn* and may lead to ulcers in the esophagus. The cause of GERD is usually a loosening of the sphincter located between the esophagus and the stomach. GERD is strongly associated with obesity, and losing weight may eliminate the symptoms. Many of the drugs prescribed for peptic ulcers are also used to treat GERD.

Concept Review 29.1

■ What are the similarities and differences between duodenal ulcers and gastric ulcers?

CORE CONCEPT 29.3

Peptic ulcer disease is treated by a combination of lifestyle changes and pharmacotherapy.

Before starting drug therapy, patients are usually advised to change lifestyle factors that contribute to PUD. For example, eliminating tobacco and alcohol use and reducing stress often allow healing of the ulcer and cause it to go into remission.

For patients requiring drug therapy, a wide variety of both prescription and over-the-counter (OTC) medications are available. These drugs fall into four primary classes, plus one miscellaneous group:

- Proton-pump inhibitors
- H₂-receptor blockers
- Antacids
- Antibiotics
- Miscellaneous agents

The goals of pharmacotherapy are to provide immediate relief from symptoms, promote healing of the ulcer, and prevent recurrence of the disease. The choice of medication depends on the source of the disease (infectious versus inflammatory), the severity of symptoms, and the convenience of OTC versus prescription drugs. The mechanisms of action of the four major classes of drugs used to treat PUD are depicted in Figure 29.4 ■.

CORE CONCEPT 29.4

Proton-pump inhibitors are effective at reducing gastric acid secretion.

Proton-pump inhibitors act by blocking the enzyme responsible for secreting hydrochloric acid in the stomach. The proton-pump inhibitors are listed in Table 29.1.

Proton-pump inhibitors (PPIs) are often the drugs of choice for the treatment of PUD and GERD. These drugs reduce acid secretion in the stomach by binding irreversibly to the enzyme H^+, K^+**-ATPase**. In the mucosal cells of the stomach, this enzyme acts as a pump to release acid (also called H^+, or protons) onto the surface of the GI mucosa. PPIs reduce acid secretion to a greater extent than do the H₂-receptor blockers and have a longer duration of action.

PPIs heal more than 90% of duodenal ulcers within 4 weeks, and about 90% of gastric ulcers in 6 to 8 weeks. Beneficial effects of PPIs last 3 to 5 days after therapy is stopped. These drugs are used only for the *short-term* control of PUD and GERD.

Adverse effects from PPIs are uncommon. Headache, abdominal pain, diarrhea, nausea, and vomiting are the most frequently reported adverse effects.

FIGURE 29.4

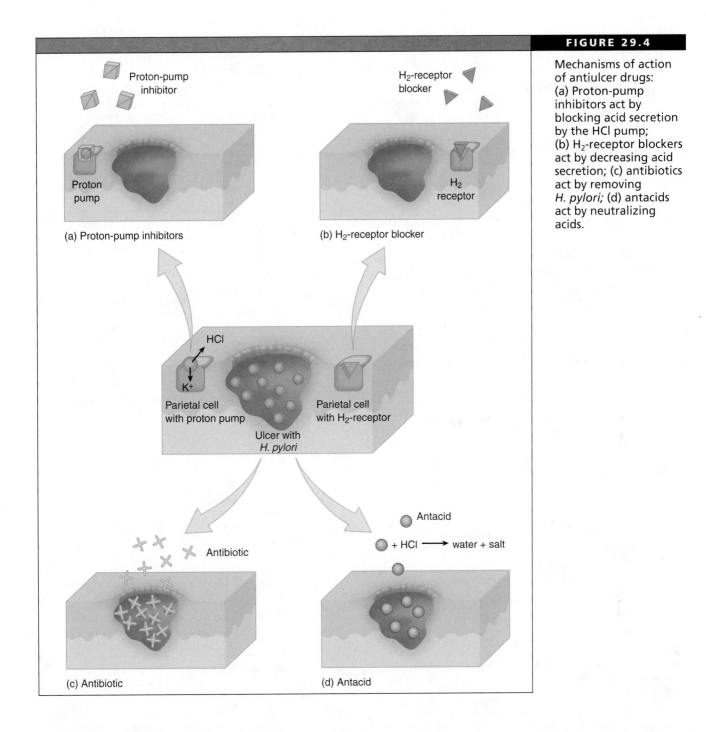

Mechanisms of action of antiulcer drugs: (a) Proton-pump inhibitors act by blocking acid secretion by the HCl pump; (b) H$_2$-receptor blockers act by decreasing acid secretion; (c) antibiotics act by removing *H. pylori;* (d) antacids act by neutralizing acids.

H$_2$-receptor blockers reduce the secretion of gastric acid.

CORE CONCEPT 29.5

The discovery of the H$_2$-receptor blockers in the 1970s marked a major breakthrough in the treatment of peptic ulcer disease. Since then they have become available OTC and are widely used in the treatment of PUD. Doses of the H$_2$-receptor blockers are given in Table 29.1.

Histamine has two types of receptors: H$_1$ and H$_2$. Activation of H$_1$-receptors produces the classic symptoms of allergy, whereas the H$_2$-receptors are responsible for increasing acid secretion in the stomach. Cimetidine (Tagamet), the first **H$_2$-receptor blocker**, and other drugs in this class are quite effective at suppressing the volume and acidity of stomach acid. These drugs are also used to treat the symptoms of GERD.

TABLE 29.1	Drugs for Peptic Ulcer Disease	
DRUG	**ROUTE AND ADULT DOSE**	**REMARKS**
H₂-RECEPTOR BLOCKERS		
cimetidine (Tagamet)	PO; 300 mg every 6 hours or 800 mg at bedtime or 400 mg bid with food	For short-term treatment; decreases the metabolism of many medications; IM and IV forms available
famotidine (Pepcid, Mylanta AP)	PO; 20 mg bid or 40 mg at bedtime	No identified drug interactions; IV form available
nizatidine (Axid)	PO; 150–300 mg at bedtime	Newest drug in this class; rapid onset with few adverse effects
Pr ranitidine (Zantac)	PO; 100–150 mg bid or 300 mg at bedtime	IM and IV forms available; ranitidine with bismuth citrate is given together with clarithromycin for *Helicobacter* infections
PROTON-PUMP INHIBITORS		
esomeprazole (Nexium)	PO; 20–40 mg/day	Also for GERD
lansoprazole (Prevacid)	PO; 15–60 mg/day	Often used in combination with antibiotics for *Helicobacter* infections; Prevac combines lansoprazole, amoxicillin, and clarithromycin
Pr omeprazole (Prilosec)	PO; 20–60 mg once or twice daily	Often used in combination with antibiotics for *Helicobacter* infections; also for GERD
pantoprazole (Protonix)	PO; 40 mg/day	Primarily for GERD; IV form available
rabeprazole sodium (AcipHex)	PO; 20 mg/day	Also for GERD
ANTACIDS		
aluminum hydroxide (AlternaGEL, others)	PO; 600 mg tid–qid	Not absorbed; may cause constipation
calcium carbonate (Titralac, Tums)	PO; 1–2 g bid–tid	Also for calcium replacement therapy; may cause constipation
calcium carbonate with magnesium hydroxide (Mylanta Gel-caps, Rolaids)	PO; two to four capsules or tablets prn (max: 12 tablets/day)	Common OTC therapy
magaldrate (Riopan)	PO; 540–1080 mg (5–10 ml suspension or one or two tablets) daily (max: 20 tablets or 100 ml/day)	Lower incidence of bowel adverse effects than magnesium or aluminum antacids
magnesium hydroxide (Milk of Magnesia)	PO; 5–15 ml or two to four tablets as needed up to four times daily	Also used as a laxative; may cause diarrhea
magnesium hydroxide and aluminum hydroxide with simethicone (Mylanta, Maalox Plus)	PO; 10–20 ml prn (max: 120 ml/day) or two to four tablets prn (max: 24 tablets/day)	Common OTC therapy
sodium bicarbonate (NAHCO₃) (see page 380 for the Drug Profile box)	PO; 325 mg–2 g one to four times/day	IV form available to treat metabolic acidosis and cardiac arrest

Adverse effects of the H₂-receptor blockers are minor and rarely cause discontinuation of therapy. Patients taking high doses, or those with renal or hepatic disease, may experience confusion, restlessness, hallucinations, or depression. Patients should be advised not to take antacids at the same time as H₂-receptor blockers because the absorption of these drugs will be lessened.

Concept Review **29.2**

■ Explain the following statement: All H₂-receptor blockers are antihistamines, but not all antihistamines are H₂-receptor blockers.

DRUG PROFILE: Pr *Omeprazole (Prilosec)*

Therapeutic Class: Antiulcer drug
Pharmacologic Class: Proton-pump inhibitor

Actions and Uses:

Omeprazole was the first proton-pump inhibitor approved for PUD; both prescription and OTC forms are available. Although this agent may take 2 hours to reach therapeutic levels, its effects last up to 72 hours. It is used for the short-term, 4- to 8-week therapy of peptic ulcers and GERD. Most patients are symptom-free after 2 weeks of therapy. It is used for longer periods in patients who have chronic hypersecretion of gastric acid, a condition known as **Zollinger-Ellison syndrome**. It is the most effective drug for this syndrome. Omeprazole is available in oral form only. Zegerid is a combination drug containing omeprazole and the antacid sodium bicarbonate.

Adverse Effects and Interactions:

Adverse effects are generally minor and include headache, nausea, diarrhea, and abdominal pain. The main concern with PPIs is that long-term use has been associated with an increased risk of gastric cancer in laboratory animals. Because of this potential effect, therapy is generally limited to 2 months.

Omeprazole interacts with several drugs. For example, using it together with diazepam, phenytoin, and central nervous system (CNS) depressants will cause increased blood levels of these drugs. Concurrent use with warfarin may increase the risk of bleeding.

 Refer to MyNursingKit for a Nursing Process Focus specific to this drug.

DRUG PROFILE: Pr *Ranitidine (Zantac)*

Therapeutic Class: Antiulcer drug
Pharmacologic Class: H_2-receptor blocker

Actions and Uses:

Ranitidine has become one of the most frequently used drugs in the treatment of mild to moderate PUD and GERD. It has a higher potency than cimetidine, which allows it to be administered once daily, usually at bedtime. Adequate healing of the ulcer takes 4 to 8 weeks. Patients with persistent disease may continue on drug maintenance for long periods to prevent recurrence. Gastric ulcers heal more slowly than duodenal ulcers and require longer drug therapy. IV and IM forms are available for the treatment of acute stress-induced bleeding ulcers. Ranitidine is available in a dissolving tablet form (EFFERdose) for treating GERD in children and infants older than 1 month of age.

Adverse Effects and Interactions:

Adverse effects are uncommon and mild. Ranitidine does not cross the blood-brain barrier to any appreciable extent, so the confusion and CNS depression observed with cimetidine does not occur with ranitidine. Ranitidine has fewer drug–drug interactions than cimetidine. Although rare, severe reductions in the number of red and white blood cells and platelets are possible; thus, periodic laboratory blood counts may be performed. High doses may result in impotence or a loss of libido in men.

Although ranitidine has fewer drug–drug interactions than cimetidine, it interacts with several drugs. For example, ranitidine may reduce the absorption of cefpodoxime, ketoconazole, and itraconazole. Antacids should not be given within 1 hour of H_2-receptor antagonists because effectiveness may be decreased due to reduced absorption.

Mechanism in Action:

Ranitidine blocks the H_2-receptor and provides relief of pain due to gastric acid secretion in patients with peptic ulcer disease or GERD.

Refer to MyNursingKit for a Nursing Process Focus specific to this drug.

NURSING PROCESS FOCUS

Patients Receiving Drug Therapy for Peptic Ulcer Disease

ASSESSMENT

Prior to administration:
- Obtain a complete health history (physical/mental), including allergies, drug history, and possible drug interactions
- Assess patient for signs of GI bleeding
- Obtain vital signs
- Assess level of consciousness
- Obtain results of complete blood count (CBC) and liver, and renal function tests

POTENTIAL NURSING DIAGNOSES

- Risk for Falls related to adverse effect of drug therapy.
- Deficient Knowledge related to information about drug therapy.
- Acute Pain related to gastric irritation from ineffective drug therapy.
- Imbalanced Nutrition: Less than Body Requirements related to adverse effects of drug.

PLANNING: PATIENT GOALS AND EXPECTED OUTCOMES

The patient will:
- Report episodes of drowsiness, dizziness
- Demonstrate an understanding of drug therapy
- Report reoccurrence of abdominal pain or discomfort during drug therapy
- Maintain body weight throughout the course of treatment

IMPLEMENTATION

Interventions and (Rationales)	Patient Education/Discharge Planning
- Monitor use of OTC drugs to avoid drug interactions, especially with cimetidine therapy.	- Instruct the patient to consult with the health care provider before taking other medications or herbal products.
- Monitor level of abdominal pain or discomfort to assess effectiveness of drug therapy.	- Advise the patient that pain relief may not occur for several days after beginning therapy.
- Monitor patient use of alcohol. (Alcohol can increase gastric irritation.)	- Instruct the patient to avoid alcohol use.
- Discuss possible drug interactions. (Antacids can decrease the effectiveness of other drugs taken concurrently.)	- Instruct the patient to take H_2-receptor antagonists and other medications at least 1 hour before antacids. Patients taking antacids should avoid taking other medications for at least 2 hours.
- Administer PPIs before meals.	- Teach the patient to take PPIs before meals, preferably before breakfast.
- Institute effective safety measures regarding falls. (Drugs may cause drowsiness or dizziness.)	- Instruct the patient to avoid driving or performing hazardous activities until drug effects are known.
- Explain need for lifestyle changes. (Smoking and certain foods increase gastric acid secretion.)	Encourage the patient to: - Stop smoking; provide information on smoking cessation programs - Avoid foods that cause stomach discomfort
- Observe the patient for signs of GI bleeding. - Monitor liver function and serum gastrin during long-term use of PPIs. Monitor serum phosphorus and calcium levels during use of antacids. - Do not use antacids with sodium for patients who have heart failure/high blood pressure or those with magnesium for patients who have kidney disease. - Monitor for pregnancy or breastfeeding (Women who are breastfeeding should not take these medications.)	- Instruct the patient to immediately report episodes of blood in the stool or vomitus, increase in abdominal discomfort, or diarrhea. - Encourage the patient to keep all scheduled doctor and laboratory visits. - Explain guidelines for the use of antacids to patients. - Instruct the patient to report possible pregnancy and plans for breastfeeding.

EVALUATION OF OUTCOME CRITERIA

Evaluate the effectiveness of drug therapy by confirming that patient goals and expected outcomes have been met (see "Planning").
See Table 29.1 for a list of drugs to which these nursing actions apply.

Antacids rapidly neutralize stomach acid and reduce the symptoms of peptic ulcer disease and GERD.

CORE CONCEPT 29.6

Antacids are alkaline substances that have been used to neutralize stomach acid for hundreds of years. Doses of the antacids are listed in Table 29.1.

Prior to the development of H₂-receptor blockers and PPIs, **antacids** were the mainstay of peptic ulcer and GERD pharmacotherapy. Indeed, many patients still use these inexpensive and readily available OTC medications. Antacids, however, are no longer recommended as the sole medication for peptic ulcer disease because they do not promote healing of the ulcer.

Antacids are alkaline, inorganic compounds of aluminum, magnesium, or calcium. Combinations of aluminum hydroxide and magnesium hydroxide are the most common type. Both aluminum hydroxide and magnesium hydroxide are bases that are capable of rapidly neutralizing stomach acid. A few products combine antacids and H₂-receptor blockers into a single tablet; for example, Pepcid Complete contains calcium carbonate, magnesium hydroxide, and famotidine.

Simethicone is sometimes added to antacid preparations because it reduces gas bubbles that cause bloating and discomfort. For example, Mylanta contains simethicone, aluminum hydroxide, and magnesium hydroxide. Simethicone is classified as an **antiflatulent** because it reduces gas. It also is available by itself in OTC products such as Gas-X and Mylanta Gas.

anti = *against*
flatus = *gas in the GI tract*

Self-medication with antacids is safe when taken in doses directed on the labels. Although they act within 10 to 15 minutes, their duration of action is only 2 hours. Therefore, they must be taken often during the day. Products containing sodium, calcium, or magnesium can result in absorption of these minerals to the general circulation. When given in high doses, aluminum compounds may interfere with phosphate metabolism and cause constipation. Magnesium compounds may cause diarrhea. Patients should follow the label instructions very carefully and not take more than the recommended dosages.

Antibiotics are administered to eliminate *Helicobacter pylori*, the cause of many peptic ulcers.

CORE CONCEPT 29.7

The bacterium *H. pylori* is associated with 80% of all duodenal ulcers and 70% of all gastric ulcers. This organism has adapted well as a human pathogen by devising ways to neutralize the high acidity surrounding it and by making chemicals called *adhesins* that allow it to stick tightly to the GI mucosa. *H. pylori* infections can remain active for life if not treated appropriately. Elimination of this organism causes ulcers to heal more rapidly and to remain in remission longer. The following antibiotics are commonly used for this purpose:

- Amoxicillin (Sumycin, others)
- Clarithromycin (Biaxin)
- Metronidazole (Flagyl)
- Tetracycline (Achromycin, others)

Two or more antibiotics are given concurrently to increase the effectiveness of therapy and to lower the potential for bacterial resistance. Antibiotic therapy generally continues for 7 to 14 days. Bismuth compounds (Pepto-Bismol, Tritec) are sometimes added to the antibiotic regimen. Although not antibiotics, bismuth compounds do inhibit bacterial growth and prevent *H. pylori* from adhering to the surface of the gastric mucosa. Dosages and additional information for these anti-infectives can be found in Chapters 25 and 26 ∞.

Several miscellaneous drugs are also beneficial in treating peptic ulcer disease.

CORE CONCEPT 29.8

Three additional drugs are beneficial in treating PUD. Sucralfate (Carafate) consists of sucrose (a sugar) plus aluminum hydroxide (an antacid). The drug produces a thick, gel-like substance that coats the ulcer, protecting it against further erosion and promoting healing. Very little of the drug is absorbed from the GI tract. Other than constipation, adverse effects are minimal. A major disadvantage of sucralfate is that it must be taken four times a day.

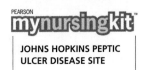

Misoprostol (Cytotec) is a prostaglandin-like substance that inhibits gastric acid secretion and stimulates the production of protective mucus. Its primary use is for the prevention of peptic ulcers in patients taking high doses of NSAIDs or glucocorticoids. Diarrhea and abdominal cramping are relatively common. Classified as a pregnancy category X drug, misoprostol is contraindicated during pregnancy. In fact, misoprostol is sometimes used to terminate pregnancies, as discussed in Chapter 32 ⚭.

Metoclopramide (Reglan) is occasionally used for the short-term therapy of PUD in patients who fail to respond to first-line agents. It is more commonly prescribed to treat nausea/vomiting associated with surgery or cancer chemotherapy. Metoclopramide is available for the oral, IM, or IV routes. CNS adverse effects such as drowsiness, fatigue, confusion, and insomnia may occur in a significant number of patients.

Concept Review 29.3

■ Is peptic ulcer disease considered an infection, an inflammation, or both?

CONSTIPATION

▶ **Life Span Fact**

Constipation occurs more frequently in older adults because fecal transit time through the colon slows with aging; this population also exercises less and has more chronic disorders that cause constipation.

A major function of the large intestine is to reabsorb water from stools. If the waste material remains in the colon for an extended period, however, too much water will be reabsorbed, leading to small, hard stools. The normal frequency of bowel movements varies widely among individuals, from two to three per day to as few as one per week. Difficult or infrequent bowel movements, known as **constipation**, is a common problem with a large number of different causes that include lack of exercise, insufficient food or fluid intake, and lack of sufficient insoluble **dietary fiber**. Certain medications such as opioids, antihistamines, certain antacids, and iron supplements promote constipation. Dietary adjustments and increased physical activity should be considered before drugs are used to treat constipation.

CORE CONCEPT 29.9

Laxatives are used to promote defecation.

Occasional constipation is common and does not require drug therapy. However, chronic, infrequent, and painful bowel movements, accompanied by severe straining, may justify pharmacotherapy. Also, pharmacotherapy may be indicated following surgical procedures to prevent the patient from straining or bearing down when attempting a bowel movement. Drugs are given to cleanse the bowel prior to surgery or for diagnostic procedures of the colon, such as a colonoscopy or barium enema.

laxat = to loosen
ive = nature of, quality of

Laxatives are drugs that promote emptying of the bowel, or **defecation**. **Cathartic** is a related term that implies a stronger and more complete bowel emptying. When taken in prescribed amounts, laxatives have few adverse effects. Selected medications used to treat constipation are listed in Table 29.2. These drugs are often classified into four primary groups and a miscellaneous category.

- *Bulk-forming*   absorb water, thus adding size to the fecal mass. These are agents of choice for the prevention and treatment of chronic constipation. They have a slow onset of action and are not used when a rapid and complete bowel evacuation is necessary.

- *Stimulants*   promote peristalsis by irritating the bowel. Although drugs in this class are effective and act rapidly, they are more likely to cause diarrhea and cramping than the other types of laxatives. They should only be used occasionally because they may cause laxative dependence and depletion of fluid and electrolytes.

- *Saline/osmotic*   cause water to be retained in the fecal mass, causing a more liquid stool. These drugs produce a bowel movement in 1–6 hours, and they should not be used on a regular basis because of the possibility of fluid and electrolyte depletion.

- *Stool softeners/surfactants*   cause more water and fat to be absorbed into the stools. They are most often used to *prevent* constipation, especially in patients who have undergone recent surgery.

- *Miscellaneous*   act by mechanisms other than those just described.

TABLE 29.2	Laxatives	
DRUG	**ROUTE AND ADULT DOSE**	**REMARKS**
bisacodyl (Correctol, Dulcolax, others)	PO; 10–15 mg daily prn	Stimulant type; also available as a rectal suppository
calcium polycarbophil (FiberCon, Equalactin, others)	PO; 1 g/day	Bulk-forming type
castor oil (Emulsoil, Neoloid, Purge)	PO; 15–60 ml daily	Stimulant type; the only laxative to act on the small intestine
docusate (Colace)	PO; 50–500 mg daily	Stool softener/surfactant type
lubiprostone (Amitiza)	PO; 24 mcg bid	Stool softener type
magnesium hydroxide (Milk of Magnesia)	PO; 20–60 ml daily	Saline type
methylcellulose (Citrucel)	PO; 5–20 ml tid in 8–10 oz water	Bulk-forming type
mineral oil	PO; 45 ml bid	Miscellaneous type; lubricates the stools
℗ psyllium muciloid (Metamucil, Naturacil, others)	PO; 1–2 tsp in 8 oz water daily	Bulk-forming type; also used for diarrhea and as an aid in lowering blood cholesterol
senna (Ex Lax, Senokot, others)	8.6-17.2 mg/day	Stimulant type; considered an herbal product

Although laxatives are safe drugs, there are several conditions and potential adverse effects that must be monitored carefully. Laxatives are contraindicated in any patient with a suspected bowel obstruction because their use could cause the bowel to perforate. If acute abdominal cramping or diarrhea occurs, laxatives should be discontinued. Patients should be advised not to overuse laxatives because the smooth muscle in the colon can lose its tone. Chronic constipation is the result.

▶ **Life Span Fact**

Because of their reduced food intake and diminished physical activity, elderly patients are most prone to laxative misuse. Health care providers should advise these patients to increase their fluid intake, fiber consumption, and level of exercise.

Concept Review   29.4

■ Bismuth compounds are used to treat several digestive disorders. Describe these agents and their uses.

DRUG PROFILE: ℗ *Psyllium Mucilloid (Metamucil, Others)*
Therapeutic Class: Agent for constipation
Pharmacologic Class: Bulk-type laxative

Actions and Uses:

Like other bulk-forming laxatives, psyllium is an insoluble fiber that is indigestible and not absorbed from the GI tract. When taken with plenty of water, psyllium swells and increases the size of the fecal mass by drawing water into the intestine. The larger the size of the fecal mass, the more the defecation reflex will be stimulated to promote bowel movements. Several doses of psyllium may be needed to produce a therapeutic effect. More frequent doses of psyllium (7 g/day) may cause a small reduction in blood cholesterol level.

Adverse Effects and Interactions:

Psyllium is a safe laxative and rarely produces adverse effects. It causes less cramping than the stimulant-type laxatives and produces a more natural bowel movement. If taken with insufficient water, it may cause obstructions in the esophagus or intestine.

Psyllium may decrease absorption and the clinical effects of antibiotics, warfarin, digoxin, nitrofurantoin, and salicylates.

Refer to MyNursingKit for a Nursing Process Focus specific to this drug.

NURSING PROCESS FOCUS

Patients Receiving Laxative Therapy

ASSESSMENT

Prior to administration:

- Obtain a complete health history (physical/mental), including allergies, drug history, and possible drug interactions
- Assess bowel elimination pattern
- Assess bowel sounds

POTENTIAL NURSING DIAGNOSES

- Risk for Injury (intestinal obstruction) related to adverse effects from drug therapy.
- Constipation related to diet, medications, or inactivity.

PLANNING: PATIENT GOALS AND EXPECTED OUTCOMES

The patient will:

- Report relief from constipation
- Demonstrate an understanding of the drug's action by accurately describing drug adverse effects and precautions
- Immediately report effects such as nausea, vomiting, diarrhea, abdominal pain, and lack of bowel movement

IMPLEMENTATION

Interventions and (Rationales)	Patient Education/Discharge Planning
■ Monitor frequency, volume, and consistency of bowel movements. (Changes in bowel habits can indicate a serious condition.)	Advise the patient to: ■ Discontinue laxative use if diarrhea occurs ■ Notify the health care provider if constipation continues ■ Take medication as prescribed ■ Increase fluids and dietary fiber, such as whole grains, fibrous fruits, and vegetables ■ Expect results from medication within 2 to 3 days of initial dose
■ Monitor the patient's ability to swallow. (Bulk laxatives can swell and cause obstruction in the esophagus.)	■ Instruct the patient to discontinue the medication and notify the health care provider if having difficulty swallowing.
■ Monitor the patient's fluid intake. (Esophageal or intestinal obstruction may result if the patient does not take in adequate amounts of fluid with the medication.)	Instruct the patient to: ■ Drink six 8-oz glasses of fluid per day ■ Mix medication in a full 8 oz of liquid ■ Drink at least 8 oz of additional fluid

EVALUATION OF OUTCOME CRITERIA

Evaluate the effectiveness of drug therapy by confirming that patient goals and expected outcomes have been met (see "Planning").

See Table 29.2 for a list of drugs to which these nursing actions apply.

DIARRHEA

dia = *through/between*
rrhea = *flow/discharge*

Occasionally, the colon does not reabsorb enough water from the fecal mass, and stools become watery. **Diarrhea** is an increase in the frequency and fluidity of bowel movements. Like constipation, occasional diarrhea is a common, self-limiting disorder that does not require drug therapy. When prolonged or severe, especially in children, diarrhea can result in significant loss of body fluids, and medications may be indicated. Prolonged diarrhea may lead to acid-base or electrolyte disorders, as discussed in Chapter 23 ∞.

Diarrhea is not a disease; it is a symptom of an underlying disorder. Diarrhea may be caused by certain medications, infections of the bowel, inflammatory bowel disorders such as Crohn's disease or ulcerative colitis, and substances such as lactate. Superinfections occurring during anti-infective therapy are common causes of diarrhea because they disrupt the normal microbial flora in the colon.

Opioids are the most effective drugs for controlling severe diarrhea.

Drug therapy of diarrhea depends on the severity of the condition and whether or not a specific cause can be identified. If the cause is an infectious disease, then an antibiotic or antiparasitic drug such as metronidazole (Flagyl) is indicated. If the cause is inflammatory in nature, anti-inflammatory drugs are needed. If the cause appears to be drug induced, the medication should be discontinued and another substituted.

Antidiarrheals act by relaxing the colon's smooth muscle, thus relieving cramping. Slower transit through the large intestine allows for better-formed stools. The selection of a particular agent depends on the severity of the diarrhea. Some antidiarrheals are listed in Table 29.3.

TABLE 29.3 Antidiarrheals

DRUG	ROUTE AND ADULT DOSE	REMARKS
bismuth salts (Pepto-Bismol)	PO; two tablets or 30 ml prn	OTC adsorbent
camphorated opium tincture (Paregoric)	PO; 5–10 mL one to four times daily	Contains morphine: Schedule III drug; Also used to prevent severe opiod withdrawal symptoms in neonates
difenoxin with atropine (Motofen)	PO; one to two mg after each diarrhea episode (max: 8 mg/day)	Opioid; Schedule IV drug
Pr diphenoxylate with atropine (Lomotil)	PO; one or two tablets or 5–10 ml tid–qid	Opioid; Schedule V drug
loperamide (Imodium)	PO; 4 mg as a single dose, then 2 mg after each diarrhea episode (max: 16 mg/day)	Opioid with no physical dependence; abuse is so low, it is not classified as a controlled substance
octreotide (Sandostatin)	Subcutaneous/IV; 100–600 mcg/day in two to four divided doses	For severe diarrhea associated with cancer

DRUG PROFILE: Pr Diphenoxylate with Atropine (Lomotil)

Therapeutic Class: Antidiarrheal
Pharmacologic Class: Opioid

Actions and Uses:

The primary antidiarrheal ingredient in Lomotil is diphenoxylate. Like other opioids, diphenoxylate slows peristalsis, resulting in additional water being reabsorbed from the colon and formation of more solid stools. It is effective for moderate to severe diarrhea. The atropine in Lomotil is not added for its anticholinergic effect; it is added to discourage patients from taking too much of the drug. Diphenoxylate is discontinued as soon as the diarrhea symptoms resolve.

Adverse Effects and Interactions:

Unlike most opioids, diphenoxylate has no analgesic properties and has an extremely low potential for abuse. The drug is well tolerated at normal doses. Some patients experience dizziness or drowsiness, and care should be taken not to operate machinery until the effects of the drug are known. At higher doses, the anticholinergic effects of atropine may be observed, which include drowsiness, dry mouth, and tachycardia.

Other CNS depressants, including alcohol, will cause additive CNS depressant/sedative effects. Monoamine oxidase (MAO) inhibitors may cause hypertensive crisis. Alcohol and other CNS depressants may enhance CNS effects.

Refer to MyNursingKit for a Nursing Process Focus specific to this drug.

Acute or long-lasting diarrhea can lead to serious and even life-threatening conditions. The opioids are drugs of choice for this type of diarrhea because of their rapid onset and effectiveness. At doses used for diarrhea, opioids do not produce dependence or serious adverse effects. The most common opioid antidiarrheal is diphenoxylate (Lomotil), which is a Schedule V controlled substance. Loperamide (Imodium) is an opioid that carries no risk for dependence and is available OTC.

Nonopioid antidiarrheals include bismuth subsalicylate (Pepto-Bismol), which acts by binding and absorbing toxins. The psyllium and pectin preparations slow diarrhea by absorbing large amounts of fluid to form bulkier stools. Intestinal flora modifiers are supplements that help to correct the altered GI flora; a good source of healthy bacteria is yogurt with active cultures.

Refer to MyNursingKit for a Nursing Process Focus specific to this drug.

NAUSEA AND VOMITING

Nausea is an uncomfortable, subjective sensation that is sometimes accompanied by dizziness and an urge to vomit. Vomiting, or **emesis**, is a reflex primarily controlled by the vomiting center, which is located in the medulla oblongata of the brain. Nausea and vomiting are commonly associated with a wide variety of conditions such as food poisoning, early pregnancy, extreme pain, migraines, trauma to the head or abdominal organs, inner ear disorders, and emotional disturbances. In treating nausea or vomiting, an important therapeutic goal is to remove the cause whenever feasible.

CORE CONCEPT 29.11

Antiemetics are prescribed to treat nausea, vomiting, and motion sickness.

Drugs from several pharmacologic classes are prescribed to prevent nausea and vomiting. Patients receiving antineoplastic medications may receive three or more antiemetics to reduce the nausea and vomiting due to the anticancer drugs. The individual antiemetic drugs are listed in Table 29.4.

Many drugs *cause* nausea or vomiting as an adverse effect. The most extreme example of this is the antineoplastic agents, almost all of which cause some degree of nausea or vomiting. In fact, therapy with antineoplastic drugs is one of the most common reasons why **antiemetic** medications are prescribed. When cancer chemotherapy is initiated, it is common for a patient to receive three or more antiemetics. Antiemetic drugs belong to a number of different classes, including the following:

anti = *against*
emetic = *vomit*

- Antipsychotics
- Antihistamines
- Serotonin-receptor blockers
- Glucocorticoids (corticosteroids)
- Benzodiazepines

To avoid losing antiemetic medication because of vomiting, many of these agents are available through the IM, IV, and/or suppository routes. The most effective antiemetics are serotonin-receptor blockers.

Motion sickness is a disorder that affects a portion of the inner ear known as the vestibular apparatus that is associated with significant nausea. The most common drug used for motion sickness is scopolamine, which is administered as a transdermal patch placed behind the ear. Antihistamines such as dimenhydrinate (Dramamine) and meclizine (Antivert) are also effective but may cause significant drowsiness in some patients. Drugs used to treat motion sickness are most effective when taken 20 to 60 minutes before travel is expected.

On some occasions, it is desirable to *stimulate* the vomiting reflex with drugs called **emetics**. Indications for emetics include ingestion of poisons and overdoses of oral drugs. Ipecac syrup, given orally, or apomorphine, given subcutaneously, will induce vomiting in about 15 minutes. Drugs used to stimulate emesis should be used only in emergency situations under the direction of a health care provider.

TABLE 29.4	Selected Antiemetics	
DRUG	**ROUTE AND ADULT DOSE**	**REMARKS**
cyclizine (Marezine)	PO; 50 mg every 4 hours–qid	Antihistamine; for prevention of motion sickness and postoperative nausea and vomiting; IM form available
dexamethasone (Decadron)	IV; 10–20 mg before chemotherapy	Glucocorticoid; IM, inhalation, and IV forms available; also for inflammatory disorders, severe allergies, acute asthma, and neoplasia
dimenhydrinate (Dramamine, others)	PO; 50–100 mg every 4 hours–qid (max: 400 mg/day)	Antihistamine; also used for allergies and cold/flu symptoms; IM and IV forms available
diphenhydramine (Benadryl, others) (see page 487 for the Drug Profile box)	PO; 25–50 mg tid–qid (max: 300 mg/day)	Antihistamine; IM, IV, and topical forms available; also for allergies, Parkinson's disease, and anaphylaxis
dolasetron (Anzemet)	PO; 100 mg 1 hour before chemotherapy	Serotonin-receptor blocker; IV form available
granisetron (Kytril)	IV; 10 mcg/kg 30 minutes before chemotherapy	Serotonin-receptor blocker; oral form available
hydroxyzine (Atarax, Vistaril)	PO; 25–100 mg tid or qid	Antihistamine; IM form available; also for anxiety and as a preoperative medication
lorazepam (Ativan) (see page 122 for the Drug Profile box)	IV; 1.0–1.5 mg before chemotherapy	Benzodiazepine; IM and IV forms available; also for anxiety, insomnia, and as a preoperative medication
meclizine (Antivert, Bonine)	PO; 25–50 mg/day, 1 hour before travel	Antihistamine; for motion sickness and nausea associated with vertigo
methylprednisolone (Medrol, Solu-medrol)	IV; two doses of 125–500 mg 6 hours apart before chemotherapy	Glucocorticoid; IM and IV forms available; also for inflammatory disorders, severe allergies, acute asthma, and neoplasia
metoclopramide (Reglan)	PO; 2 mg/kg 1 hour before chemotherapy	Phenothiazine-like; IV and IM forms available; also for GERD, facilitation of small-bowel intubation, and gastric stasis
ondansetron (Zofran)	IV; 4 mg tid prn	Serotonin-receptor blocker; IM and PO forms available
perphenazine (Phenazine, Trilafon)	PO; 8–16 mg bid–qid	Phenothiazine; IM and IV forms available; also for psychoses
Pr prochlorperazine (Compazine)	PO; 5–10 mg tid or qid	Phenothiazine; IM, IV, and suppository forms available; also for treatment of psychoses
promethazine (Phenergan)	PO; 12.5–25 mg every 4 hours–qid	Both a phenothiazine and an antihistamine; IM, IV, and suppository forms available; also for allergic disorders and as an adjunct to anesthesia and surgery
scopolamine (Hyoscine, Transderm Scop)	Transdermal patch; 0.5 mg every 72 hours	Anticholinergic; oral, IV, IM, and subcutaneous forms available

WEIGHT LOSS

Hunger occurs when the hypothalamus in the brain responds to the levels of certain chemicals (glucose) or hormones (insulin) in the blood. Hunger is a normal physiologic response that drives people to seek nourishment. Appetite is somewhat different than hunger. Appetite is a psychological response that drives food intake based on associations and memory. For example, people often eat not because they are experiencing hunger, but because it is a particular time of day or they find the act of eating pleasurable or social.

DRUG PROFILE: ℗ *Prochlorperazine (Compazine)*

Therapeutic Class: Antiemetic, antipsychotic
Pharmacologic Class: Phenothiazine

Actions and Uses:

Prochlorperazine is a phenothiazine, a class of drugs usually prescribed for psychotic disorders, as discussed in Chapter 11 ◯◯ . The phenothiazines are the largest class of medications prescribed for severe nausea and vomiting, and prochlorperazine is the most frequently prescribed antiemetic drug in its class. Prochlorperazine depresses the vomiting center in the medulla oblongata. As an antiemetic, it is frequently given by the rectal route, where absorption is rapid. It is also available in tablet, extended-release capsule, and IM formulations.

Adverse Effects and Interactions:

Prochlorperazine produces dose-related anticholinergic adverse effects such as dry mouth, constipation, and tachycardia. When used for prolonged periods at higher doses, extrapyramidal symptoms resembling those of Parkinson's disease are a serious concern (see Chapters 11 and 12 ◯◯).

Prochlorperazine interacts with alcohol and other CNS depressants to cause additive sedation. Antacids and antidiarrheals inhibit absorption of prochlorperazine. When taken with phenobarbital, metabolism of prochlorperazine is increased.

Refer to MyNursingKit for a Nursing Process Focus specific to this drug.

NATURAL THERAPIES

Ginger for Nausea

Ginger is obtained from the roots of the herb *Zingiber officinale*, which grows in a wide variety of places across the world. Active ingredients include aromatic oils that give the herb its characteristic scent and antiemetic activity. Because of its widespread use as a spice in Asian cooking, ginger is widely available in a number of forms, including tincture, tea, dried and fresh root, and capsules. Commercial products that use ginger as a flavoring include ginger cookies, gingerbread, and ginger ale. Consumers should check the product ingredients to be certain that the item truly contains ginger extract, rather than artificial ginger flavoring.

Ginger has been used in Chinese medicine for thousands of years. Indications relating to the digestive system include nausea, vomiting, morning sickness, and motion sickness. Studies have shown its effectiveness to be comparable to OTC medications.

Ginger is purported to have other significant benefits. The herb is said to have anti-inflammatory properties that are of benefit to patients with arthritis. It is sometimes given to patients with flu symptoms to help coughs and lower fever. Because of a possible effect on blood clotting, patients taking anticoagulants should avoid ginger unless otherwise directed by their health care provider.

CORE CONCEPT 29.12

Anorexiants and lipase inhibitors are used for the short-term management of obesity.

Despite the public's desire for effective agents to promote weight loss, there are few such drugs available. The approved drugs are used for the treatment of obesity, although they produce only modest weight loss.

Obesity may be defined as being more than 20% above ideal body weight. Because of the prevalence of obesity in society and the difficulty that most patients experience when following weight-reduction plans for extended periods, drug manufacturers have long sought to develop safe drugs that cause weight loss. In the 1970s, amphetamine and dextroamphetamine (Dexedrine) were widely prescribed as **anorexiants** to reduce appetite. These drugs, however, are addictive, and amphetamines are rarely prescribed for this purpose today. In the 1990s, the combination of fenfluramine and phenteramine, known as fen-phen, was widely prescribed until fenfluramine was removed from the market for causing heart valve defects.

The two antiobesity drugs currently available are sibutramine (Meridia) and orlistat (Xenical). Sibutramine is the most widely prescribed anorexiant for the short-term control of obesity. It suppresses appetite, probably by affecting the hunger center in the brain. Orlistat acts by a totally different mechanism—blocking the enzyme lipase in the GI tract, which blocks the absorp-

DRUG PROFILE: ℞ *Sibutramine (Meridia)*

Therapeutic Class: Antiobesity agent, appetite suppressant
Pharmacologic Class: Anorexiant, SSRI

Actions and Uses:

Sibutramine, a selective serotonin reuptake inhibitor (SSRI), is the most widely prescribed appetite suppressant for the short-term control of obesity. When combined with a reduced calorie diet, sibutramine may produce a gradual weight loss of at least 10% of initial body weight over a period of a year. Sibutramine therapy is not recommended for longer than 1 year. It is not approved for patients under age 16.

Adverse Effects and Interactions:

Headache is the most common complaint reported during sibutramine therapy, although insomnia and dry mouth are also possible. The drug should be used with great care in patients with cardiac disorders because it may cause tachycardia and raise blood pressure. It is a Schedule IV drug with low potential for dependence.

Sibutramine interacts with several other drugs. For example, decongestants and cough and allergy medications may cause elevated blood pressure. Ketoconazole and erythromycin may inhibit the metabolism of sibutramine. Using it together with an MAO inhibitor or SSRI may cause serotonin syndrome.

Refer to MyNursingKit for a Nursing Process Focus specific to this drug.

tion of fats. Unfortunately, orlistat may also decrease absorption of other substances, including fat-soluble vitamins and coumadin. The effectiveness of sibutramine and orlistat is very limited, producing only a small increase in weight reduction compared to placebos.

PANCREATIC ENZYMES

The pancreas is responsible for the secretion of essential digestive enzymes. Lack of secretion, or **pancreatic insufficiency**, will result in malabsorption disorders. Replacement therapy with pancreatic enzymes is sometimes necessary.

Pancreatic enzymes are administered as replacement therapy for patients with pancreatitis or malabsorption syndromes.

CORE CONCEPT 29.13

The pancreas secretes more than 1 L of pancreatic juice daily, which contains enzymes that split proteins, fats, and carbohydrates. Because these nutrients must be broken down into simpler molecules before they can be absorbed, lack of sufficient pancreatic juice can cause malabsorption syndromes. Lipase, the enzyme that digests fats, is most affected. The most common cause of pancreatic insufficiency is chronic pancreatitis. This disorder also occurs in most patients with cystic fibrosis.

Symptoms of pancreatic insufficiency include upper abdominal pain, loss of appetite, nausea, vomiting, and weight loss. *Steatorrhea*, the passing of bulky, foul-smelling fatty stools, occurs because dietary fats are passing through the GI tract without being broken down.

Pancreatic enzyme supplements include pancrelipase (Cotazym, Pancrease, others) and pancreatin (Entozyme, Viokase, others). These drugs are obtained from either pig or bovine pancreas and contain the necessary enzymes to digest fats, carbohydrates, and proteins. Pancrelipase is generally preferred because it has significantly more enzyme activity. To avoid destruction by stomach acid, capsules are made with an enteric coating. Dosing is individualized to the degree of pancreatic insufficiency in each patient. Administration of the drug is timed to coincide with meals so that the enzymes are available when food reaches the duodenum. Overtreatment can cause nausea, vomiting, and diarrhea.

PATIENTS NEED TO KNOW

Patients treated for digestive disorders need to know the following:

Regarding Antiulcer Medications

1. Do not smoke tobacco when taking H_2-receptor blockers because this interferes with the drug action.
2. Because drowsiness may occur when starting therapy with H_2-receptor blockers or proton-pump inhibitors, monitor operating equipment and the use of alcohol or other CNS drugs carefully.
3. When taking medications for peptic ulcer, avoid drugs that may cause stomach irritation such as aspirin or NSAIDs.
4. Shake liquid antacids well before pouring. Chewable tablets should be thoroughly chewed before swallowing.

Regarding Laxatives

5. Because bulk-forming laxatives and stool softeners may take several days for results, be patient and do not take more than prescribed.
6. Take bulk-forming laxatives with at least two full glasses of water because this aids in forming larger stools.
7. If constipation is a frequent problem, try drinking more fluids and adding fiber to the diet rather than taking laxatives on a continual basis. Foods rich in fiber include all fruits and vegetables, bran cereals, and whole grain breads.

Regarding Antiemetics

8. Before taking antiemetic medications, try other methods of relieving nausea, such as drinking flat carbonated beverages or weak tea or eating small amounts of crackers or dry toast.
9. When taking phenothiazines or antihistamines as antiemetics, use sugarless candy, gum, or ice chips to minimize dry mouth.
10. Recall that medications taken to suppress hunger produce only modest weight loss and are not effective without a reduced-calorie diet. True, sustained weight loss can only be achieved by modification of dietary habits.

CHAPTER REVIEW

CORE CONCEPTS SUMMARY

29.1 The digestive system breaks down food, absorbs nutrients, and eliminates wastes.

The alimentary canal provides a large surface area for the absorption of nutrients and drugs. Substances are propelled through the GI tract by peristalsis. Abnormally fast or slow peristalsis can affect nutrient, drug, and water absorption.

29.2 Peptic ulcer disease is caused by an erosion of the mucosal layer of the stomach or duodenum.

Infection with *H. pylori* and therapy with NSAIDs are the most common causes of peptic ulcers. A gnawing pain in the upper abdomen that is relieved by eating is the most common symptom of duodenal ulcer. Though less common, gastric ulcers may be more serious and require longer treatment and follow-up. GERD has symptoms similar to those of peptic ulcers and is treated with some of the same medications.

29.3 Peptic ulcer disease is treated by a combination of lifestyle changes and pharmacotherapy.

Before beginning drug therapy, the patient should eliminate tobacco and alcohol use and reduce stress levels because these changes will favor remission of peptic ulcer disease. Goals of drug therapy include relief of symptoms, promotion of ulcer healing, and prevention of recurrences.

29.4 Proton-pump inhibitors are effective at reducing gastric acid secretion.

Proton-pump inhibitors diminish gastric acid secretion by interfering with the enzyme H^+, K^+-ATPase, which is present in the mucosal cells in the stomach. Although very effective, use is usually limited to 2 months because of the possibility of long-term adverse effects.

29.5 H₂-receptor blockers reduce the secretion of gastric acid.

H_2-receptor blockers reduce the volume and acidity of stomach acid. Healing of duodenal ulcers occurs in 4 to 8 weeks, and adverse effects are uncommon.

29.6 Antacids rapidly neutralize stomach acid and reduce the symptoms of peptic ulcer disease and GERD.

Once drugs of choice for treating peptic ulcer disease, antacids are now primarily used to give immediate relief for the heartburn associated with GERD or peptic ulcers.

29.7 Antibiotics are administered to eliminate *Helicobacter pylori*, the cause of many peptic ulcers.

Elimination of *H. pylori* using combination therapy with different antibiotics has been found to promote more rapid ulcer healing and longer remissions.

29.8 Several miscellaneous drugs are also beneficial in treating peptic ulcer disease.

Sucralfate produces a gel-like substance that provides a protective coating for ulcers. Misoprostol inhibits gastric acid secretion and promotes the secretion of protective mucus. Pirenzepine inhibits acid secretion by blocking cholinergic receptors.

29.9 Laxatives are used to promote defecation.

Laxatives are given to promote emptying of the colon. Laxatives act by stimulating peristalsis or by adding more bulk or water to the fecal mass.

29.10 Opioids are the most effective drugs for controlling severe diarrhea.

Diarrhea is treated by addressing its cause, which may include anti-inflammatory drugs or anti-

infectives. Opioids are the most effective drugs for relieving severe diarrhea, but they have some abuse potential. OTC bismuth compounds can help with simple diarrhea.

29.11 Antiemetics are prescribed to treat nausea, vomiting, and motion sickness.

Symptomatic treatment of nausea and vomiting involves drugs from many different classes, including phenothiazines, antihistamines, corticosteroids, benzodiazepines, and serotonin-receptor blockers. Motion sickness can be controlled through medications such as transdermal scopolamine or dimenhydrinate (Dramamine).

29.12 Anorexiants and lipase inhibitors are used for the short-term management of obesity.

Only a few drugs are available for the short-term management of obesity, and these drugs produce only modest weight loss. The anorexiant sibutramine and the lipase inhibitor orlistat are used to help obese patients lose weight.

29.13 Pancreatic enzymes are administered as replacement therapy for patients with pancreatitis or malabsorption syndromes.

Pancreatic insufficiency leads to lack of breakdown and absorption of sufficient quantities of fats, carbohydrates, and proteins. This can lead to malabsorption syndromes. Pancrelipase and pancreatin are used to restore the deficient enzymes.

REVIEW QUESTIONS

The following questions are written in NCLEX-PN® style. Answer these questions to assess your knowledge of the chapter material, and go back and review any material that is not clear to you.

1. The primary cause of peptic ulcers is:

1. Stress
2. Smoking
3. *H. pylori* bacteria
4. Family history

2. The patient with a gastric ulcer has been started on ranitidine (Zantac). Instructions should include:

1. Drug therapy will extend over several weeks or months.
2. Information about the signs and symptoms of CNS depression.
3. Drug therapy will extend over a few days.

4. Information about the signs and symptoms of hepatic disease.

3. Your patient is taking nizatidine (Axid) and magaldrate (Riopan). The patient should:

1. Not take the medications at the same time
2. Take the medications at the same time
3. Switch to another antacid that is safer with this drug
4. Not be taking magaldrate because it is not effective

4. Important teaching to be included for a patient on omeprazole (Prilosec) should include which of the following?

1. This drug is safe for long-term use.
2. This drug should not be taken for more than 2 months.
3. Therapeutic effects may take weeks.
4. This drug must be used with antacids to be effective.

5. When the patient is receiving magnesium hydroxide (Mylanta), the nurse must assess for:

1. Diarrhea
2. Peripheral disease
3. Neuropathy
4. Respiratory disorders

6. The nurse instructs patients using laxatives to:

1. Use daily for best results
2. Not overuse them because they can cause chronic constipation
3. Decrease fluid intake
4. Decrease food intake

7. After administering an antiemetic, the patient should be placed in what position?

1. Face up
2. Side lying
3. Upright
4. Face down

8. Which of the following substances should be avoided when the patient has a peptic ulcer?

1. Aspirin
2. Raw foods
3. Anorexiants
4. Antiemetics

9. The patient on sibutramine (Meridia) must be assessed for:

1. Hepatic toxicity
2. Renal disease
3. Hypertension and tachycardia
4. Severe diarrhea

10. The patient demonstrates an understanding of pancrelipase (Cotazym) when she states:

1. "I will take this medication with meals."
2. "I will take this medication on an empty stomach."
3. "I will only take this medication when I am eating carbohydrates."
4. "If I develop nausea, vomiting, or diarrhea, I will increase my dosage."

CASE STUDY QUESTIONS

For questions 1–4 please refer to the following case study, and choose the correct answer from choices 1–4.

Ms. Han is a 32-year-old stock broker with a very stressful job. She has just been diagnosed with a duodenal ulcer. Initially, the physician prescribed ranitidine (Zantac), clarithromycin, and amoxicillin, with OTC antacids as needed.

1. Which drug was prescribed primarily to reduce the inflammation caused by the ulcer?

1. Ranitidine
2. Antacid
3. Clarithromycin
4. Amoxicillin

2. Which drug was prescribed to eradicate *H. pylori?*

1. Ranitidine
2. Clarithromycin
3. Amoxicillin
4. Both 2 and 3

3. In the treatment of *H. pylori*, the nurse understands that the use of two or more antibiotics is essential for what reason?

1. To lower the potential for bacterial resistance
2. To decrease the chances of development of duodenal ulcers
3. To increase the likelihood of eliminating redevelopment of gastric ulcers
4. To decrease the cost of future drug therapy

4. Ms. Han has been taking aluminum-based antacids for her ulcer and is experiencing constipation. Which of the following would you recommend that she obtain OTC to promote bowel movements?

1. Methylcellulose (Citrucel)
2. Famotidine (Pepcid)
3. Omeprazole (Prilosec)
4. Bismuth salts (Pepto-Bismol)

FURTHER STUDY

- Chapter 24 ⬤ discusses anti-inflammatory medications that can be used in treating inflammatory bowel disease.
- Histamine is discussed in Chapter 24 ⬤.
- Chapter 25 ⬤ contains dosages and additional information for anti-infectives.
- Acid-base and electrolyte disorders are discussed in Chapter 23 ⬤.

- Antipsychotic drugs are discussed in Chapter 11 ⬤. Extrapyramidal symptoms resembling those of Parkinson's disease are discussed in Chapters 11 and 12 ⬤.
- Antineoplastic drugs that cause significant nausea and vomiting are presented in Chapter 27 ⬤.
- Additional applications for opioids are presented in Chapter 14 ⬤.

EXPLORE **PEARSON mynursingkit™**

MyNursingKit is your one stop for online chapter review materials and resources. Prepare for success with additional NCLEX®-style practice questions, interactive assignments and activities, web links, animations and videos, and more!

Register your access code from the front of your book at
www.mynursingkit.com

30 Vitamins, Minerals, and Nutritional Supplements

CORE CONCEPTS

30.1 Vitamins are needed to promote growth and maintain health.

30.2 Vitamins are classified as fat soluble or water soluble.

30.3 Recommended dietary allowances (RDAs) for vitamins have been established for the average healthy adult.

30.4 Vitamin therapy is indicated for specific conditions.

30.5 Minerals are inorganic substances needed in very small amounts to maintain normal body metabolism.

30.6 Enteral and total parenteral nutrition are therapies that deliver essential nutrients to patients with deficiencies.

DRUG SNAPSHOT

The following drugs are discussed in this chapter:

DRUG CLASSES	DRUG PROFILES
Vitamins	**Pr** cyanocobalamin (Crystamine, others)
Minerals	**Pr** ferrous sulfate (Feosol, Feostat, others)
Nutritional Supplements	
Enteral nutrition	
Total parenteral nutrition	

LEARNING OUTCOMES

After reading this chapter, the student should be able to:

1. Identify characteristics that differentiate vitamins from other nutrients.

2. Describe the functions of vitamins and minerals.

3. Explain the rationale behind recommended dietary allowances (RDAs).

4. Describe the role of vitamin and mineral therapies in the treatment of deficiency disorders.

5. Identify several drug–vitamin and drug–mineral interactions.

6. Compare and contrast the functions of major minerals and trace minerals.

7. Compare and contrast enteral and parenteral methods of providing nutrition.

enteral nutrition 537

hemoglobin (HEE-moh-glow-bin) 534

hypervitaminosis 530

intrinsic factor 532

major mineral (macromineral) 532

pernicious (megaloblastic) anemia (pur-NISH-us ah-NEE-mee-ah) 531

provitamin 529

recommended dietary allowance (RDA) 530

total parenteral nutrition (TPN) 538

trace mineral 532

undernutrition 537

vitamins 529

The vitamin, mineral, and nutritional supplement business is a multibillion dollar industry. Although aggressive marketing often leads patients to believe that dietary supplements are essential to maintain health, most people obtain all necessary nutrients through a balanced diet. Once the body has obtained the amounts of vitamins or minerals it needs to carry on metabolism, the excess is simply excreted or stored. There are some conditions, however, in which dietary supplementation is necessary and will benefit the patient's health. This chapter focuses on these conditions and explores the role of vitamins, minerals, and nutritional supplements in pharmacology.

Vitamins are needed to promote growth and maintain health.

CORE CONCEPT 30.1

Vitamins are organic compounds required by the body in small amounts for growth and for the maintenance of normal metabolic processes. Since the discovery of thiamine in 1911, over a dozen vitamins have been identified. Because scientists did not know the chemical structures of the vitamins when they were discovered, they were assigned letters and numbers such as A, B_{12}, and C. These names are still widely used today.

An important characteristic of vitamins is that, with the exception of vitamin D, human cells cannot synthesize them. They or their precursors—known as **provitamins**—must be supplied in the diet. A second important characteristic is that if the vitamin is not present in adequate amounts, the body's metabolism will be disrupted and disease will result. Furthermore, the symptoms of the deficiency can be reversed by the administration of the missing vitamin.

pro = *before*
vitamin = *essential substance*

Vitamins serve diverse and important roles in human physiology. For example, the B complex vitamins are coenzymes essential to many metabolic pathways. Vitamin A is a precursor of retinal, a pigment needed for normal vision. Calcium metabolism is regulated by a hormone that is derived from vitamin D. Without vitamin K, abnormal prothrombin is produced, and blood

Fast Facts Vitamins, Minerals, and Dietary Supplements

■ About 40% of Americans take vitamin supplements daily.

■ There is no difference between the chemical structure of a natural vitamin and a synthetic vitamin, yet consumers pay much more for the natural type.

■ Vitamin B_{12} is present in animal products only. Vegetarians may find adequate amounts in fortified cereals, nutritional supplements, or yeast.

■ Administration of folic acid during pregnancy has been found to reduce birth defects in the nervous system of the baby.

■ Patients who never receive sun exposure may need vitamin D supplements.

■ Heavy menstrual periods may result in considerable iron loss.

■ Technically, vitamins and minerals cannot increase a patient's energy levels. Energy can be provided only by adding calories in carbohydrates, proteins, and fats.

■ "Organic" foods do not necessarily contain a higher concentration of vitamins or minerals than nonorganic foods.

clotting is affected. Patients having a low or unbalanced dietary intake, those who are pregnant, and those experiencing a chronic disease may benefit from vitamin therapy.

CORE CONCEPT 30.2

Vitamins are classified as fat soluble or water soluble.

A simple way to classify vitamins is by their ability to mix with water. Those that dissolve easily in water are called water-soluble vitamins. Examples include vitamin C and the B vitamins. Those that dissolve in lipids are called fat soluble or lipid soluble and include vitamins A, D, E, and K.

The difference in solubility affects the way the vitamins are absorbed by the gastrointestinal (GI) tract and stored in the body. The water-soluble vitamins are absorbed along with water in the digestive tract and readily dissolve in blood and body fluids. When excess water-soluble vitamins are ingested, they cannot be stored for later use and are simply excreted in the urine. Because they are not stored to any significant degree, they must be ingested daily; otherwise deficiencies will quickly develop.

Fat-soluble vitamins, however, cannot be absorbed in sufficient quantity in the small intestine unless they are ingested with other fats. These vitamins can be stored in large quantities in the liver and fat. Should the patient not ingest sufficient quantities, fat-soluble vitamins are removed from storage depots in the body as needed. Unfortunately, this storage can lead to dangerously high levels of the fat-soluble vitamins if they are taken in excessive amounts.

CORE CONCEPT 30.3

Recommended dietary allowances (RDAs) for vitamins have been established for the average healthy adult.

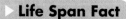

NATIONAL COUNCIL AGAINST HEALTH FRAUD

Based on scientific research on humans and animals, the Food and Nutrition Board of the National Academy of Sciences has established levels for the intake of vitamins and minerals, called **recommended dietary allowances (RDAs)**. Canada publishes similar data called the recommended nutrient intake (RNI). The RDA values represent the *minimum* amount of a vitamin or mineral needed to prevent a deficiency in a healthy adult. The RDAs are revised periodically to reflect the latest scientific research. Current RDAs for vitamins are listed in Table 30.1. A newer standard, the Dietary Reference Index (DRI), is sometimes used to represent the *optimum* level of nutrient needed to ensure wellness.

Vitamin, mineral, or nutritional supplements should never substitute for a balanced diet. Sufficient intake of proteins, carbohydrates, and fats is needed for proper health. Furthermore, although the label on a vitamin supplement may indicate that it contains 100% of the RDA for a particular vitamin, the body may absorb as little as 10% to 15% of the amount ingested. With the exception of vitamins A and D, it is not harmful for most patients to consume two to three times the recommended levels of vitamins.

CORE CONCEPT 30.4

Vitamin therapy is indicated for specific conditions.

hyper = *above*
vitamin = *vitamin*
osis = *condition*

▶ **Life Span Fact**

Infancy and childhood are times of potential vitamin deficiency due to the high growth demands placed on the body.

Most people who eat a normal, balanced diet obtain all the necessary nutrients without vitamin supplementation. Indeed, megavitamin therapy is not only expensive but may be harmful to health if taken for long periods. **Hypervitaminosis**, or toxic levels of vitamins, has been reported for vitamins A, C, D, E, B_6, niacin, and folic acid. In the United States, it is actually more common to observe syndromes of vitamin *excess* than those of vitamin *deficiency*. Most patients are unaware that taking too much of a vitamin or mineral can cause serious adverse effects.

Vitamin deficiencies may have a number of causes. Table 30.1 lists the functions of the vitamins and some common causes of deficiencies. In the United States deficiencies are most often the result of poverty, fad diets, chronic alcoholism, or prolonged parenteral feeding. Infants, pregnant women, nursing mothers, older adults, and those eating a vegan or vegetarian diet often require larger amounts of vitamins and minerals to maintain optimal health. Men and women can have different vitamin and mineral needs, as do persons who participate in vigorous exercise. Vitamin deficiencies in patients with chronic liver and kidney disease are well documented. Patients with alcohol or serious drug dependency are often deficient in the quality and quantity of their nutritional intake. In cases in which dietary needs are increased, the RDAs will need adjustment, and supplements are indicated to achieve optimum wellness.

Certain drugs affect vitamin metabolism. Alcohol is well known for its ability to inhibit the absorption of thiamine and folic acid; alcohol abuse is the most common cause of thiamine defi-

TABLE 30.1	Vitamins				
		RDA		
VITAMIN	**FUNCTION(S)**	**MEN**	**WOMEN**	**COMMON CAUSE(S) OF DEFICIENCY**
A	Visual pigments, epithelial cells	1000 RE*	800 RE	Prolonged dietary deprivation, particularly when rice is the main food source; pancreatic disease; cirrhosis
B complex: Biotin (B₇)	Coenzyme in metabolic reactions	30 mcg	30 mcg	Deficiencies are rare
Pr Cyanocobalamin (B₁₂) (Crystamine, others)	Coenzyme in nucleic acid metabolism	2.4 mcg	2.4 mcg	Lack of intrinsic factor, inadequate intake of foods from animal origin
Folic acid/folate (B₉)	Coenzyme in amino acid and nucleic acid metabolism	400 mcg	400 mcg	Pregnancy, alcoholism, cancer, oral contraceptive use
Niacin (B₃)	Coenzyme in metabolic reactions	16 mg	14 mg	Prolonged dietary deprivation, particularly when Indian corn (maize) or millet is the main food source; chronic diarrhea; liver disease; alcoholism
Pantothenic acid (B₅)	Coenzyme in metabolic reactions	5 mg	5 mg	Deficiencies are rare
Pyridoxine (B₆)	Coenzyme in amino acid metabolism	1.3 mg	1.3 mg	Alcoholism; oral contraceptive use; malabsorption diseases
Riboflavin (B₂)	Coenzyme in metabolic reactions	1.3 mg	1.1 mg	Inadequate consumption of milk or animal products; chronic diarrhea; liver disease; alcoholism
Thiamine (B₁)	Coenzyme in metabolic reactions	1.2 mg	1.1 mg	Prolonged dietary deprivation, particularly when rice is the main food source; hyperthyroidism, pregnancy, liver disease; alcoholism
C	Coenzyme and antioxidant	60 mg	60 mg	Inadequate intake of fruits and vegetables; pregnancy; chronic inflammatory disease; burns; diarrhea; alcoholism
D	Calcium and phosphate metabolism	5 mcg	5 mcg	Low dietary intake; inadequate exposure to sunlight
E	Antioxidant	10 TE**	8 TE	Premature infants; malabsorption diseases
K	Cofactor in blood clotting	70 mcg	65 mcg	Newborns; liver disease; long-term parenteral nutrition; certain drugs such as cephalosporins and salicylates

*RE = retinoid equivalents
**TE = alpha-tocopherol equivalents

ciency in the United States. Folic acid levels may be reduced in patients taking phenothiazines, oral contraceptives, phenytoin (Dilantin), or barbiturates. Vitamin D deficiency can be caused by therapy with certain anticonvulsants. Inhibition of vitamin B_{12} absorption has been reported with a number of drugs, including trifluoperazine, alcohol, and oral contraceptives.

One of the most common and clinically important vitamin syndromes is deficiency of vitamin B_{12}. The most obvious consequence of B_{12} deficiency is a type of anemia called **pernicious** or **megaloblastic anemia**. Insufficient vitamin B_{12} creates a lack of activated folic acid, which is essential for DNA synthesis and cell division. Lack of vitamin B_{12} also affects the nervous system, causing tingling or numbness in the limbs, mood disturbances, and even hallucinations in severe deficiencies.

Treatment of vitamin B_{12} deficiency is most often accomplished by weekly or biweekly IM or subcutaneous injections. Although oral supplements are available, they are effective only in patients who have sufficient intrinsic factor and normal absorption in the small intestine (see Drug

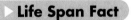

▶ **Life Span Fact**

The absorption of food diminishes with age, and often the quantity of ingested food is reduced, leading to vitamin deficiencies in elderly patients.

megalo = *large*
blastic = *embryonic state*

an = *lack of*
emia = *blood condition*

DRUG PROFILE: 🅟 *Cyanocobalamin (Crystamine, Others)*

Therapeutic Class: Agent for anemia
Pharmacologic Class: Vitamin supplement

Actions and Uses:

Cyanocobalamin is a purified form of vitamin B_{12} that is administered in deficiency states. Vitamin B_{12} is not synthesized by either plants or animals; only bacteria perform this function. Because only miniscule amounts of vitamin B_{12} are required, deficiency of this vitamin is not usually caused by insufficient dietary intake. The most common cause of vitamin B_{12} deficiency is lack of a chemical called **intrinsic factor**, which is secreted by stomach cells. Intrinsic factor is required for vitamin B_{12} to be absorbed from the intestine. Figure 30.1 ■ illustrates the metabolism of vitamin B_{12}/cyanocobalamin. Inflammatory diseases of the stomach or surgical removal of the stomach (gastrectomy) may result in deficiency of intrinsic factor. Inflammatory diseases of the small intestine that affect food and nutrient absorption may also cause vitamin B_{12} deficiency.

Intranasal spray and gel formulations (Nascobal) are available that provide for once-weekly dosage. Because these intranasal formulations exhibit variable absorption and bioavailability, they are used for *maintenance therapy* after normal vitamin B_{12} levels have been restored by parenteral preparations.

Adverse Effects and Interactions:

Adverse effects from cyanocobalamin are uncommon. Hypokalemia is possible; thus, serum potassium levels are monitored periodically.

Alcohol, aminosalicylic acid, neomycin, and colchicine may decrease absorption of oral cyanocobalamin. Chloramphenicol may interfere with therapeutic response to cyanocobalamin.

Refer to MyNursingKit for a Nursing Process Focus specific to this drug.

Life Span Fact

Elderly patients who have less exposure to direct sunlight may need vitamin D supplements.

Life Span Fact

Infants fed only breast milk receive insufficient amounts of vitamin D, which can result in rickets.

Profile for cyanocobalamin). Parenteral administration rapidly reverses most signs and symptoms of B_{12} deficiency. If the disease has been prolonged, symptoms may take longer to resolve, and some neurologic damage may be permanent. Treatment may need to continue for the remainder of the patient's life.

Vitamins are indicated for several additional conditions. Vitamin K is administered to patients with certain clotting disorders and as an antidote to warfarin (Coumadin) overdose. B complex vitamins such as folic acid, thiamine, and riboflavin are commonly administered to patients with chronic alcoholism. The role of vitamin D therapy in the pharmacotherapy of bone disorders is discussed in Chapter 33 ⃠.

Concept Review   30.1

■ What are some conditions in which the RDA for a vitamin may not be sufficient?

CORE CONCEPT 30.5

Minerals are inorganic substances needed in very small amounts to maintain normal body metabolism.

Minerals are inorganic substances that constitute about 4% of body weight. The most common minerals are the bone salts, calcium and phosphorus, which make up about 75% of the total mineral content in the body. Minerals are classified as **major minerals (macrominerals)** or **trace minerals**, depending on how much is needed in the diet. The seven major minerals must be obtained daily from dietary sources in amounts of 100 mg or higher. Required daily amounts of the nine trace minerals are 20 mg or less. These minerals are listed in Table 30.2.

FIGURE 30.1

Metabolism of vitamin B₁₂

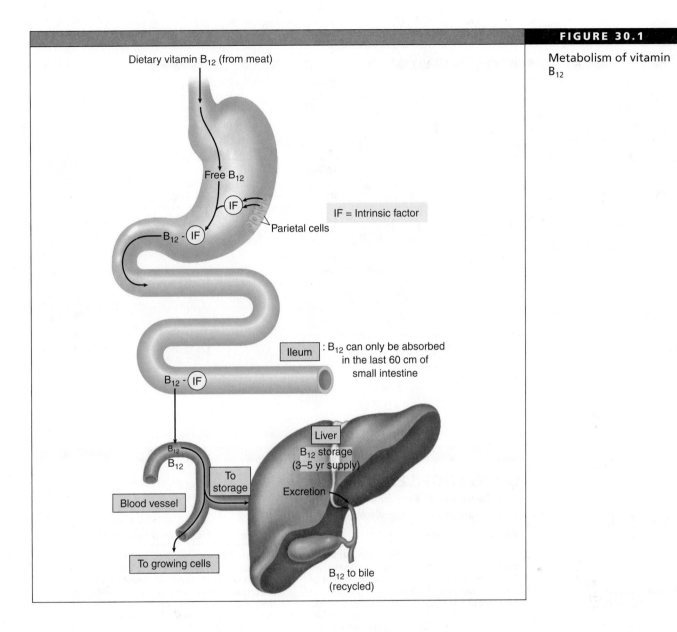

Minerals serve many important and diverse functions in the body. Some minerals, such as sodium and magnesium, appear primarily as ions in body fluids. Others, such as iron and cobalt, are usually bound to organic molecules. The functions of many of the minerals in human physiology, such as calcium, sodium, and potassium, are well known. The functions of some of the trace minerals, such as aluminum, silicon, arsenic, and nickel, are less understood.

Because minerals are needed in very small amounts for human metabolism, a balanced diet will supply the necessary quantities for most patients. Like vitamins, excess amounts of minerals can lead to toxicity, and patients should be advised not to exceed recommended doses. For example, arsenic, chromium, and nickel have been implicated as human carcinogens, and excess sodium intake can lead to water retention and hypertension.

Mineral therapy is indicated for certain disorders. Iron-deficiency anemia is the most common nutritional deficiency in the world and is a primary indication for iron supplements. Women at high risk for osteoporosis are advised to consume extra calcium, either in their diet or as a supplement (see Chapter 33 ⚭). Magnesium deficiencies are promptly treated with oral or IV magnesium salts because lack of sufficient amounts of this electrolyte can lead to weakness, dysrhythmias, and hypertension. Iodine-based drugs serve a number of functions, including use as topical antiseptics, as contrast agents in radiologic procedures of the urinary and cardiovascular systems, and the treatment of thyroid abnormalities (see Chapter 31 ⚭). Selected minerals used in pharmacotherapy are shown in Table 30.3.

▶ **Life Span Fact**

For each decade after age 40, bone mass decreases approximately 3–5%. To avoid bone fractures, older adults must ensure a substantial dietary intake of calcium or take calcium supplements.

osteo = *bone*
por = *passage*
osis = *condition*

TABLE 30.2	Minerals		
MAJOR MINERALS	**RECOMMENDED DAILY INTAKE**	**TRACE MINERALS**	**RECOMMENDED DAILY INTAKE**
Calcium	800–1200 mg	Chromium	0.05–20 mg
Chloride	750 mg	Cobalt	0.1 mcg
Magnesium	Men: 420 mg Women: 320 mg	Copper	1.5–3 mg
Phosphorus	700 mg	Fluoride	1.5–4 mg
Potassium	2 g	Iodide	150 mcg
Sodium	500 mg	Iron	Men: 10 mg Women: 15 mg
Sulfur	Not established	Manganese	2–5 mg
		Molybdenum	75–250 mg
		Selenium	Men: 70 mcg Women: 55 mcg
		Zinc	12–15 mg

DRUG PROFILE: ℗ *Ferrous Sulfate (Feosol, Feostat, Others)*

Therapeutic Class: Agent for anemia
Pharmacologic Class: Iron supplement

Actions and Uses:

Ferrous sulfate is an iron supplement. Iron is a mineral essential to the function of several biological molecules, the most significant of which is **hemoglobin**. Each molecule of hemoglobin in a red blood cell contains four iron atoms, each of which can bind reversibly to an oxygen atom. Sixty to eighty percent of all iron in the body is associated with hemoglobin.

Because free iron is toxic, the body binds the mineral to protein complexes called ferritin, hemosiderin, and transferrin. After red blood cells die, nearly all of the iron in their hemoglobin is recycled for later use. Because of this recycling, very little iron is excreted; thus, dietary iron requirements in most individuals are small.

Iron deficiency is a common cause of anemia. The usual cause of iron-deficiency anemia is blood loss, such as may occur during menstruation or from peptic ulcers. Certain patients have an increased demand for iron, including those who are pregnant and those undergoing intensive athletic training. Ferrous sulfate is available in a wide variety of dosage forms to prevent or rapidly reverse symptoms of iron-deficiency anemia.

Adverse Effects and Interactions:

The most common adverse effect of iron sulfate is GI upset. Although taking iron with meals will lessen GI upset, food can decrease the absorption of iron by as much as 70%. It is recommended that iron preparations be administered 1 hour before or 2 hours after a meal. However, if major gastric irritation is experienced, the iron may be taken with meals. Patients should be advised that iron preparations may darken stools and that this is a harmless adverse effect. Excessive doses of iron are very toxic, and patients should be advised to take their medication exactly as directed.

Antacids and food decrease the absorption of iron. Vitamin C increases the absorption of iron, whereas calcium (including dairy products) and bran block its absorption. Ferrous sulfate may decrease the absorption of penicillamine. Vitamin C may increase the absorption of ferrous sulfate.

hemo = *blood*
globin = *protein*

 Refer to MyNursingKit for a Nursing Process Focus specific to this drug.

TABLE 30.3	Selected Minerals Used for Pharmacotherapy	

DRUG	ROUTE AND ADULT DOSE	REMARKS
potassium chloride (KCl) (see page 379 for the Drug Profile box)	PO; 10–100 mEq/hr in divided doses	
	IV; 10–40 mEq/hr diluted to at least 10–20 mEq/100 ml of solution (max: 200–400 mEq/day)	Electrolyte levels should be frequently assessed and the drug discontinued immediately if hyperkalemia is suspected
sodium bicarbonate (NaHCO$_3$) (see page 380 for the Drug Profile box)	PO; 0.3–2 g once or twice daily or 1 tsp of powder in a glass of water	For treatment of metabolic acidosis, to enhance renal excretion of certain drugs, and as an antacid
CALCIUM		
calcium acetate (PhosLo)	PO; two to four tablets with each meal (each tablet contains 169 mg)	To prevent high blood phosphate levels in patients who are on dialysis
calcium carbonate (Rolaids, Tums, Os-Cal, others)	PO; 1–2 g bid–tid	For calcium supplementation and as an antacid
calcium citrate (Citracal)	PO; 1–2 g bid–tid	For calcium supplementation
calcium gluconate (Kalcinate) (see page 599 for the Drug Profile box)	PO; 1–2 g bid–qid	For calcium supplementation and to reverse cardiac signs of hyperkalemia
calcium lactate (Cal-Lac)	PO; 325 mg–1.3 g tid with meals	To correct mild hypokalemia
IRON		
ferrous fumarate (Feostat, others)	200 mg tid–qid	For iron supplementation
ferrous gluconate (Fergon, others)	325–600 mg qid; may be gradually increased to 650 mg qid as needed and tolerated	For iron supplementation
(Pr) ferrous sulfate (Feosol, Feostat, others)	750–1500 mg/day in one to three divided doses	For iron supplementation
iron dextran (Dexferrum, others)	IM/IV; dose is individualized and determined from a table of correlations between the patient's weight and hemoglobin, as per package insert (max: 100 mg [2 ml] of iron dextran within 24 hours)	For iron supplementation when oral administration is not indicated
MAGNESIUM		
magnesium chloride (Chloromag, Slo-Mag)	PO; 270–400 mg/day	For magnesium supplementation
magnesium hydroxide (Milk of Magnesia)	PO; 5–15 mL or two to four tablets up to 4 times/day	For constipation, hyperacidity, or magnesium supplementation
magnesium oxide (Mag-Ox, Maox, others)	PO; 400–1200 mg/day in divided doses	For constipation, hyperacidity, or magnesium supplementation
magnesium sulfate (Epsom salt)	IV/IM; 0.5–3 g/day	For constipation, to control seizures, or for magnesium supplementation
PHOSPHORUS		
potassium/sodium phosphates (K-Phos original, K-Phos MF, K-Phos neutral, Neutra-Phos-K, Uro-KP neutral)	PO; 250–1000 mg /day	For correction of phosphate deficiency and to lower urinary calcium concentration
ZINC		
zinc gluconate	PO; 20–100 mg (20-mg lozenges may be taken to a max of six/day)	For correction of zinc deficiency
zinc sulfate (Orazinc, Zincate, others)	PO; 15–220 mg/day	For correction of zinc deficiency

NURSING PROCESS FOCUS

Patients Receiving Iron Supplements

ASSESSMENT

Prior to administration:
- Obtain a complete health history (physical/mental), including allergies, drug history, and possible drug reactions
- Assess reason for drug administration, such as presence/history of anemia or prophylaxis during infancy, childhood, and pregnancy
- Assess complete blood count, specifically hematocrit and hemoglobin levels, to establish baseline values
- Assess vital signs

POTENTIAL NURSING DIAGNOSES

- Risk for Imbalanced Nutrition related to inadequate iron intake.
- Risk for Injury (weakness, dizziness, syncope) related to anemia.
- Deficient Knowledge related to information about drug therapy.

PLANNING: PATIENT GOALS AND EXPECTED OUTCOMES

The patient will:
- Exhibit an increase in hematocrit level and experience improvement in anemia-related symptoms
- Demonstrate an understanding of the drug's action by accurately describing drug adverse effects and precautions
- Immediately report significant adverse effects such as GI distress

IMPLEMENTATION

Interventions and (Rationales)	Patient Education/Discharge Planning
Monitor vital signs, especially pulse. (Increased pulse is an indicator of decreased oxygen content in the blood.)	Instruct the patient to monitor pulse rate and report irregularities and changes in rhythm.
Monitor complete blood count to evaluate effectiveness of treatment. (Increases in hematocrit and hemoglobin values indicate increased red blood cell [RBC] production.)	Instruct the patient: • On the need for initial and continuing laboratory blood monitoring • To keep all laboratory appointments
Monitor changes in stool. (May cause constipation, change stool color, and cause false positives when stool tested for occult blood.)	Instruct the patient: • That stool color may change, and that this is no cause for alarm • On measures to relieve constipation, such as including fruits and fruit juices in the diet and increasing fluid intake and exercise
Plan activities and allow for periods of rest to help the patient conserve energy. (Diminished iron levels result in decreased formation of hemoglobin, leading to weakness.)	Instruct the patient to: • Rest when he or she is feeling tired and not to overexert • Plan activities to avoid fatigue
Administer oral forms of ferrous sulfate (iron) 1 hour before or 2 hours after meals with a full glass of water or juice for better absorption.	Instruct the patient: • Not to crush or chew sustained-release preparations; take with a full glass of water or juice • That medication may cause GI upset and may be taken with food if this becomes a problem
Administer liquid iron preparations through a straw or place on the back of the tongue (to avoid staining the teeth).	Instruct the patient to: • Dilute liquid medication before using and to use a straw to take the medication • Rinse the mouth after swallowing to decrease the chance of staining the teeth
Monitor dietary intake to ensure adequate intake of foods high in iron.	Instruct the patient to increase intake of iron-rich foods such as liver, egg yolks, brewer's yeast, wheat germ, and muscle meats.
Monitor for potential for child access to the medication. (Iron poisoning can be fatal to young children.)	Advise the parent to store iron-containing vitamins out of reach of children and in childproof containers.

EVALUATION OF OUTCOME CRITERIA

Evaluate the effectiveness of drug therapy by confirming that patient goals and expected outcomes have been met (see "Planning").

NATURAL THERAPIES

Sea Vegetables

Sea vegetables, or seaweeds, are a form of marine algae that grow in the upper levels of the ocean, where sunlight can penetrate. Examples of these edible seaweeds include spirulina, kelp, chlorella, arame, and nori, many of which are used in Asian cooking. Sea vegetables are found in coastal locations throughout the world. Kelp, or *Laminaria*, is found in the cold waters of the North Atlantic and Pacific oceans.

Sea vegetables contain a multitude of vitamins as well as protein. Their most notable nutritional aspect, however, is their mineral content. Plants from the sea contain more minerals than most other food sources, including calcium, magnesium, phosphorus, iron, potassium, and all essential trace elements. Because they are so rich in minerals, seaweeds act as alkalizers for the blood, helping to rid the body of acid conditions (acidosis). Spirulina, kelp, and chlorella are available in capsule or tablet form.

Certain drugs affect mineral metabolism. For example, loop or thiazide diuretics can cause significant urinary potassium loss. Corticosteroids, oral contraceptives, and a number of other drugs can cause sodium retention. The uptake of iodine by the thyroid gland can be impaired by certain oral hypoglycemics and lithium (Eskalith). Oral contraceptives have been reported to lower the plasma levels of zinc and increase those of copper.

Concept Review 30.2

■ What is the difference between a vitamin and a mineral?

Enteral and total parenteral nutrition are therapies that deliver essential nutrients to patients with deficiencies.

CORE CONCEPT 30.6

When a patient is eating or drinking fewer nutrients than required for normal body growth and maintenance, **undernutrition** occurs. Undernutrition can also occur in certain malabsorption disorders of the intestinal tract. The two primary goals in treating undernutrition are to *identify* the specific type of deficiency and *supply* the missing nutrients. Nutritional supplements may be needed for short-term therapy or for the remainder of the patient's life.

Causes of undernutrition range from simple to complex. Common causes of undernutrition include the following:

- Advanced age
- HIV-AIDS
- Alcoholism
- Severe burns
- Cancer
- Chronic inflammatory bowel disease
- Eating disorders

The most obvious cause for undernutrition is low dietary intake. Reasons for the inadequate intake must be carefully assessed. Patients may have no resources to purchase food and may be suffering from starvation. Clinical depression leads many patients to shun food. Elderly patients may have poorly fitting dentures or difficulty chewing or swallowing after a stroke. In terminal disease, patients may be comatose or otherwise unable to take food orally. Although the causes differ, patients with insufficient intake exhibit a similar pattern of general weakness, muscle wasting, and loss of subcutaneous fat.

Many different types of nutritional supplements are available to assist patients suffering from undernutrition. Products administered via the GI tract, either orally or through a feeding tube, are called **enteral nutrition**. Oral feeding allows natural digestive processes to occur and requires less nursing care. Tube feeding is necessary when the patient has difficulty swallowing or is otherwise unable to take meals orally. An advantage of tube feeding is that the amount of enteral nutrition the patient is receiving can be precisely measured and recorded.

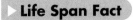

▶ **Life Span Fact**

Elderly patients may have poor-fitting dentures or difficulty chewing or swallowing following a stroke.

The particular enteral product is chosen to address the specific nutritional needs of the patient. For example, some contain mixtures of amino acids and protein, whereas others contain primarily carbohydrates or fats. There are many different formulations of enteral products available, each designed to meet a specific nutrient need. Examples of enteral products include Vivonex T.E.N. Peptamen Liquid, Sustacal Powder, Ensure-Plus, Casec, Polycose, Microlipid, and MCT Oil.

Patients sometimes exhibit vomiting, nausea, or diarrhea when first receiving enteral nutrition. Therapy is often started slowly, with small quantities so that adverse effects can be assessed.

When the metabolic needs of the patient cannot be met through enteral nutrition, **total parenteral nutrition (TPN)** is indicated. For short-term therapy, peripheral vein TPN may be used. Because of the risk of phlebitis, however, long-term therapy often requires central vein TPN. Because the GI tract is not being used, patients with severe malabsorption disease may be successfully treated with TPN.

TPN is able to provide all the patient's nutritional needs with solutions containing amino acids, fats, carbohydrate (as dextrose), electrolytes, vitamins, and minerals. The particular formulation may be specific to the disease state, such as products for renal failure or hepatic failure. TPN is administered through an infusion pump so that nutrition can be precisely monitored. Patients in various settings such as acute care, long-term care, and home health care often benefit from TPN therapy.

PATIENTS NEED TO KNOW

Patients treated with vitamins, minerals, or herbs need to know the following:

In General

1. If receiving regular monthly injections of vitamin B_{12}, do not take additional oral supplements of vitamin B_{12} or folic acid without the advice of a health care provider.
2. Do not take more than the recommended doses of any vitamin or mineral without first checking with a health care provider. Although small amounts of these substances are beneficial, large amounts may be dangerous.
3. Ensure that diet is nutritionally adequate, adding foods that naturally supply the needed vitamins and minerals before taking supplements. See a dietician for advice, particularly for special needs such as pregnancy or diabetes.
4. Avoid foods with high zinc or oxalate content if a calcium supplement is being taken because these may interfere with absorption. These foods include nuts, peas, beans, spinach, and soy products.
5. Know that niacin, or vitamin B_3, is also effective at lowering lipid levels. The dose for lowering cholesterol, however, is 2 to 3 grams per day, whereas the vitamin dose is only 25 mg per day.
6. When providing a medical or drug history to the physician or dentist, always report vitamins, minerals, herbs, or dietary supplements being taken. If allergies to any dietary supplements are known, be sure to report these also.

Regarding Iron Preparations

7. Because liquid iron preparations can stain teeth, dilute these solutions with juice or water and rinse the mouth after taking the medication to reduce staining.
8. Take oral forms of ferrous sulfate (iron) 1 hour before or 2 hours after meals for better absorption. Take with a full glass of water or juice.

SAFETY ALERT

Overuse of Vitamin and Mineral Supplements

While talking with the nurse in her son's pediatrician office, a young mother remarks to the nurse, "I insist that my children take iron-fortified vitamins every day. My children really enjoy taking the cute little cartoon vitamins. They call the vitamins their morning candy." Adults are often unaware that accidental iron poisoning is now the leading cause of deaths by poisoning in children under 5 years old. In 1997 the Food and Drug Administration (FDA) enforced labeling of all iron-containing drugs to include the warning for young children. The number of accidental iron poisonings has doubled since the mid-1980s. To avoid this tragedy, the nurse should teach patients to store all iron medicines out of the reach of children. In addition, to help combat iron-deficiency anemia, the nurse should teach patients to increase the intake of iron-rich foods such as lean red meats, blackstrap molasses, leafy green and yellow vegetables, and selected seafood.

CORE CONCEPTS SUMMARY

30.1 Vitamins are needed to promote growth and maintain health.

With the exception of vitamin D, vitamins cannot be synthesized by the body and must be provided in the diet. Although only very small amounts of vitamins are needed, lack of sufficient quantity will result in disease.

30.2 Vitamins are classified as fat soluble or water soluble.

Water-soluble vitamins include vitamins C and B. Fat-soluble vitamins include vitamins A, D, E, and K. Water-soluble vitamins cannot be stored and must be ingested daily, whereas excess fat-soluble vitamins can be stored for later use.

30.3 Recommended dietary allowances (RDAs) for vitamins have been established for the average healthy adult.

RDA values represent the minimum amount of vitamin or mineral needed to prevent a deficiency in a healthy adult. These values must be adjusted for changes in health status, such as athletic training, pregnancy, or chronic disease.

30.4 Vitamin therapy is indicated for specific conditions.

Most people do not need vitamin supplementation, and excess intake may lead to hypervitaminosis. Indications for vitamin therapy include alcoholism, pregnancy or breast-feeding, chronic kidney or liver disease, therapy with certain drugs that affect vitamin metabolism, and reduced food intake in elderly patients.

30.5 Minerals are inorganic substances needed in very small amounts to maintain normal body metabolism.

Like vitamins, most people receive all the minerals they need through a balanced diet. Certain conditions, such as osteoporosis or iron-deficiency anemia, do warrant mineral therapy.

30.6 Enteral and total parenteral nutrition are therapies that deliver essential nutrients to patients with deficiencies.

Enteral nutrition supplies patients all the essential nutrients via the oral route or through feeding tube. For patients who cannot take oral supplements, nutrients are supplied parenterally by way of total parenteral nutrition.

REVIEW QUESTIONS

The following questions are written in NCLEX-PN® style. Answer these questions to assess your knowledge of the chapter material, and go back and review any material that is not clear to you.

1. Vitamin B_{12} is indicated for which of the following conditions?

1. Liver disease
2. Chronic inflammatory disease
3. Pernicious anemia
4. Inadequate exposure to sunlight

2. This vitamin is indicated for the patient who is experiencing warfarin (Coumadin) overdose.

1. Vitamin A
2. Vitamin D
3. Vitamin E
4. Vitamin K

3. If the patient is taking ferrous sulfate, what instructions should be given?

1. Do not take antacids with this medication.
2. This medication can cause severe diarrhea.
3. This medication should never be taken on an empty stomach.
4. Blood pressure must be monitored closely.

4. Patients with a history of alcohol abuse should be especially monitored for a _____ deficiency.

1. Biotin
2. Thiamine
3. Niacin
4. Riboflavin

5. The patient on a thiazide or loop diuretic, such as Lasix, should have which electrolyte monitored?

1. Sodium
2. Calcium
3. Potassium
4. Magnesium

6. The patient taking liquid iron should be instructed to:

1. Swish medication in his mouth for 1 minute
2. Take medication with food
3. Avoid foods with high iron content
4. Rinse his mouth with water afterward

7. The patient is exhibiting weakness, hypertension, and dysrhythmias. Which of the following should be checked?

1. Sodium
2. Magnesium
3. Aluminum
4. Chromium

8. Vitamins A, D, E, and K are:

1. Trace minerals
2. Minerals
3. Water-soluble vitamins
4. Fat-soluble vitamins

9. The patient's GI tract is not functioning. Which type of feeding is the patient receiving?

1. Oral
2. Enteral
3. TPN
4. GI

10. The patient asks the nurse if it would be okay to increase her vitamin intake. The nurse's best response would be:

1. "While you can safely take additional vitamins, there is no need."
2. "You probably need to take more vitamins every day."
3. "You will need to speak with your physician."
4. "You may safely increase your intake of water-soluble vitamins only."

CASE STUDY QUESTIONS

For questions 1–4, please refer to the following case study, and choose the correct answer from choices 1–4.

Ms. Davis has been taking a multivitamin for several years. Lately, she has been taking four times the label dose because she heard that this can prevent colds.

1. In Ms. Davis's multivitamin, which of the following is a water-soluble vitamin?

1. A
2. B complex
3. D
4. E

2. Ms. Davis asks you the meaning of RDA. What would be the best response?

1. "It is the amount of nutrient required by all people."
2. "It is the maximum amount of nutrient required by all people."

3. "It is the amount of nutrient needed by an average person."
4. "It is the minimum amount of nutrient required by all people."

3. What would be your advice to Ms. Davis?

1. Stop taking multivitamins.
2. Continue taking four times the label dose because this is considered safe.
3. Take only the dose stated on the label.
4. Continue taking four times the label dose until she develops abnormal symptoms.

4. Which of the following is a common indication for vitamin or mineral pharmacotherapy?

1. Chronic alcoholism
2. Liver failure
3. Iron-deficiency anemia
4. All of the above

FURTHER STUDY

- The role of vitamin D and calcium therapy in the pharmacotherapy of bone disorders is discussed in Chapter 33 ⊕ .

- Iodine-based drugs serve a number of functions, including the treatment of thyroid abnormalities, which is discussed in Chapter 31 ⊕ .

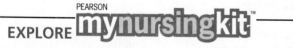

EXPLORE PEARSON **mynursingkit**™

MyNursingKit is your one stop for online chapter review materials and resources. Prepare for success with additional NCLEX®-style practice questions, interactive assignments and activities, web links, animations and videos, and more!

Register your access code from the front of your book at
www.mynursingkit.com

31 Drugs for Endocrine Disorders

CORE CONCEPTS

31.1 The endocrine system maintains homeostasis by using hormones as chemical messengers.

31.2 Hormones are used as replacement therapy, as antineoplastics, and for their natural therapeutic effects.

31.3 The hypothalamus and the pituitary gland secrete hormones that control other endocrine organs.

31.4 Insulin and glucagon are secreted by the pancreas.

31.5 Type 1 diabetes is treated by dietary restrictions and insulin injections.

31.6 Type 2 diabetes is controlled through lifestyle changes and oral hypoglycemic agents.

31.7 The thyroid gland controls the basal metabolic rate and affects virtually every cell in the body.

31.8 Thyroid disorders may be treated by administering thyroid hormone or by decreasing the activity of the thyroid gland.

31.9 Glucocorticoids are released during periods of stress and influence carbohydrate, lipid, and protein metabolism in most cells.

31.10 Glucocorticoids are prescribed for adrenocortical insufficiency and a wide variety of other conditions.

31.11 Of the many pituitary and hypothalamic hormones, only a few have clinical applications as drugs.

DRUG SNAPSHOT

The following drugs are discussed in this chapter:

DRUG CLASSES	DRUG PROFILES
Insulins	**Pr** regular insulin (Humulin R, Novolin R, Pork Regular Iletin II, Regular Purified Pork Insulin)
Oral hypoglycemics	**Pr** glipizide (Glucotrol)

DRUG CLASSES	DRUG PROFILES
Thyroid Drugs	
Thyroid agents	**Pr** levothyroxine (Synthroid)
Antithyroid agents	**Pr** propylthiouracil (PTU)
Adrenal Drugs	
Glucocorticoids	**Pr** hydrocortisone (Cortef, Hydrocortone, Solu-Cortef, others)

LEARNING OUTCOMES

After reading this chapter, the student should be able to:

1. Describe the general structure and functions of the endocrine system.

2. Compare and contrast the functions of the pancreatic hormones.

3. Compare and contrast the causes, signs, symptoms, and treatment of type 1 and type 2 diabetes mellitus.

4. Identify the five types of insulin.

5. Describe the signs and symptoms of insulin overdose and underdose.

6. Explain the primary functions of the thyroid gland.

7. Identify the signs and symptoms of hypothyroidism and hyperthyroidism.

8. Explain the primary functions of the adrenal cortex.

9. Describe the signs and symptoms of Addison's disease and Cushing's syndrome.

10. For each of the drug classes listed in the Drug Snapshot, identify representative drugs and explain the mechanisms of drug action, primary actions, and important adverse effects:

11. Categorize drugs used in the treatment of endocrine disorders based on their classifications and mechanisms of action.

KEY TERMS

Addison's disease (ADD-iss-uns) 560

adrenocorticotropic hormone (ACTH) (uh-dreen-oh-kor-tik-o-TRO-pik) 558

atrophy (AT-troh-fee) 561

cretinism (KREE-ten-izm) 555

Cushing's syndrome (KUSH-ings) 561

diabetes insipidus (die-uh-BEE-tees in-SIP-uh-dus) 564

diabetes mellitus, type 1 (die-uh-BEE-tees MEL-uh-tiss) 547

diabetes mellitus, type 2 549

dwarfism 564

follicular cells (fo-LIK-yu-lur) 555

glucocorticoid (glu-ko-KORT-ik-oyd) 558

Graves' disease 556

hormones 543

hyperglycemia (hi-pur-gli-SEEM-ee-uh) 545

hypoglycemia (hi-po-gli-SEEM-ee-uh) 545

hypothalamus (hi-po-THAL-ih-mus) 545

incretin (in-KREE-ten) **enhancers** 553

islets of Langerhans (EYE-lits of LANG-gur-hans) 545

ketoacids (KEY-to-ass-ids) 548

mineralocorticoid (min-ur-al-oh-KORT-ik-oyd) 558

myxedema (mix-uh-DEEM-uh) 556

parafollicular cells (par-uh-fo-LIK-u-lur) 555

pituitary gland (pit-TOO-it-air-ee) 545

releasing factors 545

somatotropin (so-mat-oh-TROH-pin) 564

vasopressin (vaz-oh-PRESS-in) 564

Like the nervous system, the endocrine system is a major controller of homeostasis. Although a nerve may exert instantaneous control over a single muscle or gland, a hormone from the endocrine system may affect all body cells and take as long as several days to produce a measurable response. Small amounts of hormones may produce very serious effects on the body. Conversely, deficiencies of small quantities may produce equally serious physiologic changes. This chapter examines common endocrine disorders and their pharmacotherapy. The reproductive hormones are covered in Chapter 32 ⬭ .

endo = *within*
crine = *to secrete*

The endocrine system maintains homeostasis by using hormones as chemical messengers.

CORE CONCEPT 31.1

The endocrine system consists of various glands that secrete chemical messengers called **hormones**. Hormones are released in response to a change in the body's internal environment. For example, when the level of glucose in the blood rises, the pancreas secretes insulin. When blood levels of calcium fall, parathyroid hormone (PTH) is released from the parathyroid gland. The various endocrine glands are illustrated in Figure 31.1 ■.

After they are secreted, hormones enter the blood and are transported throughout the body. Some hormones, such as insulin and thyroid hormone, have receptors on nearly every cell in the body and thus produce widespread physiologic changes. Others, such as parathyroid hormone and oxytocin, have receptors on only a few specific types of cells.

In the endocrine system, it is common for one hormone to control the secretion of another hormone. In addition, it is common for the last hormone or action in the pathway to provide feedback to turn off the action of the first hormone. For example, as serum calcium level falls, PTH is released. PTH causes an increase in serum calcium level, which provides feedback to the parathyroid glands to shut off PTH secretion. This is a common feature of endocrine homeostasis known as *negative feedback*.

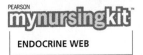

PEARSON
mynursingkit

ENDOCRINE WEB

FIGURE 31.1

The endocrine system *Source: Pearson Education/PH College*

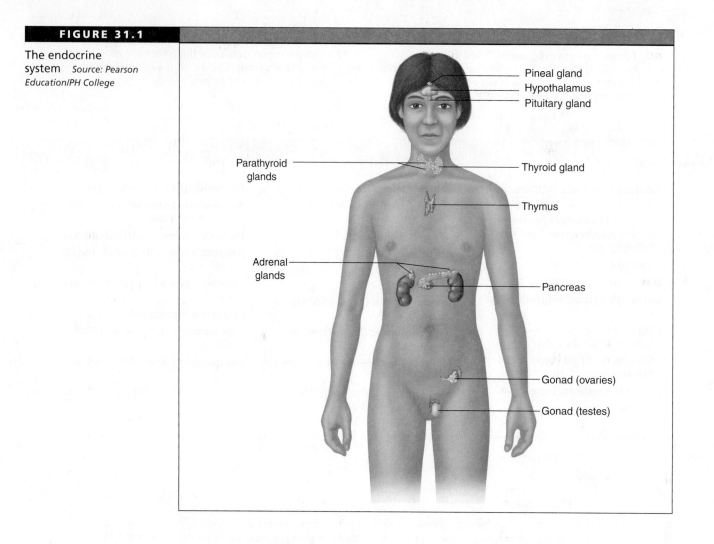

Pineal gland
Hypothalamus
Pituitary gland

Parathyroid glands

Thyroid gland

Thymus

Adrenal glands

Pancreas

Gonad (ovaries)

Gonad (testes)

CORE CONCEPT 31.2

Hormones are used as replacement therapy, as antineoplastics, and for their natural therapeutic effects.

The goals of hormone pharmacotherapy vary widely. In many cases, the hormone is administered simply as replacement therapy for patients who are unable to secrete sufficient quantities of their own endogenous hormones. Examples of replacement therapy include the administration of thyroid hormone after the thyroid gland has been surgically removed or supplying insulin to a patient whose pancreas is not functioning. Replacement therapy usually supplies the same low-level amounts of the hormone that would normally be present in the body. A summary of selected endocrine disorders and their drug therapy is given in Table 31.1.

Some hormones are used in cancer chemotherapy. Examples include testosterone for breast cancer and estrogen for testicular cancer. The antineoplastic mechanism of action of these hormones is not known. When used as antineoplastics, the doses of the hormones far exceed those levels normally present in the body (see Chapter 27 ⊂⊃).

Another goal of hormone therapy may be to produce an exaggerated response that is part of the normal action of the drug to achieve some therapeutic advantage. Supplying hydrocortisone to suppress inflammation is an example of taking advantage of the normal action of the glucocorticoids but at higher amounts than would normally be present in the body. Supplying small amounts of estrogen or progesterone at specific times during the menstrual cycle can prevent ovulation and pregnancy. In this example, the patient is supplied natural hormones; however, they are given at a time when levels in the body are normally low.

TABLE 31.1	Endocrine Disorders and Their Drug Treatment		
GLAND	**HORMONE(S)**	**DISORDER**	**DRUGS**
Adrenal Cortex	Glucocorticoids	Hypersecretion: Cushing's syndrome	None
		Hyposecretion	Glucocorticoids
Pancreas (Islets of Langerhans)	Insulin	Hyposecretion: diabetes mellitus	Insulin
Pituitary	Growth hormone	Hyposecretion: dwarfism	somatrem (Protropin) and somatropin (Humatrope and others)
	Antidiuretic hormone	Hyposecretion: diabetes insipidus	vasopressin desmopressin (DDAVP, Stimate)
Thyroid	Thyroid hormone (T_3 and T_4)	Hypersecretion: Graves' disease	propylthiouracil (PTU)
		Hyposecretion: myxedema (adults) and cretinism (children)	thyroid hormone (Synthroid)

The hypothalamus and the pituitary gland secrete hormones that control other endocrine organs.

CORE CONCEPT 31.3

Two endocrine structures in the brain deserve special recognition because they control many other endocrine glands. The **hypothalamus** secretes chemicals called **releasing factors** or *releasing hormones* that travel via blood vessels a short distance to an area immediately below, called the anterior **pituitary gland**. These releasing factors tell the pituitary which hormone to release. After the pituitary releases the appropriate hormone, it travels to its target organ to cause its effect. For example, the hypothalamus secretes thyrotropin-releasing hormone, which travels to the pituitary gland with the message to secrete thyroid-stimulating hormone (TSH). TSH then travels to its target organ—the thyroid gland—to stimulate the release of thyroid hormone. Hormones associated with the pituitary gland are illustrated in Figure 31.2 ■.

Insulin and glucagon are secreted by the pancreas.

CORE CONCEPT 31.4

Located behind the stomach and between the duodenum and spleen, the pancreas is a gland that is essential to both the digestive and endocrine systems. It is responsible for the secretion of several enzymes into the pancreatic duct that then flow into the duodenum to assist in the chemical digestion of nutrients. This is its *exocrine* function. Certain cells in the pancreas, called **islets of Langerhans**, control its *endocrine* function: the secretion of glucagon and insulin. As with other endocrine organs, the pancreas secretes these hormones directly into blood capillaries, where they are available for transport to body tissues.

exo = *out/away from*
crine = *to secrete*

Insulin secretion is regulated by various chemical, hormonal, and neural regulators. One of the most important regulators is the level of glucose in the blood stream. After a meal, when glucose levels levels fall (**hyperglycemia**), the pancreas is stimulated to secrete insulin. The islet cells sends the pancreas a message to stop secreting the hormone when blood glucose levels fall (**hypoglycemia**) or when high levels of insulin counter the need for more glucose in the bloodstream.

hyper = *elevated*
hypo = *lowered*
glyc = *sugar*
emia = *blood*

Insulin affects carbohydrate, fat, and protein metabolism in most cells of the body. One of its most important actions is to assist in glucose transport. Without insulin, glucose cannot enter a cell. Cells may be swimming in glucose, but it cannot enter and be used for fuel by the cell without insulin. The brain is an important exception, not requiring insulin for glucose transport. Insulin is said to have a hypoglycemic effect because its presence causes glucose to leave the bloodstream and enter cells.

Islet cells in the pancreas also produce glucagon. Glucagon is best thought of as a blocker of insulin because its actions are opposite to those of insulin. When levels of glucose are low,

FIGURE 31.2

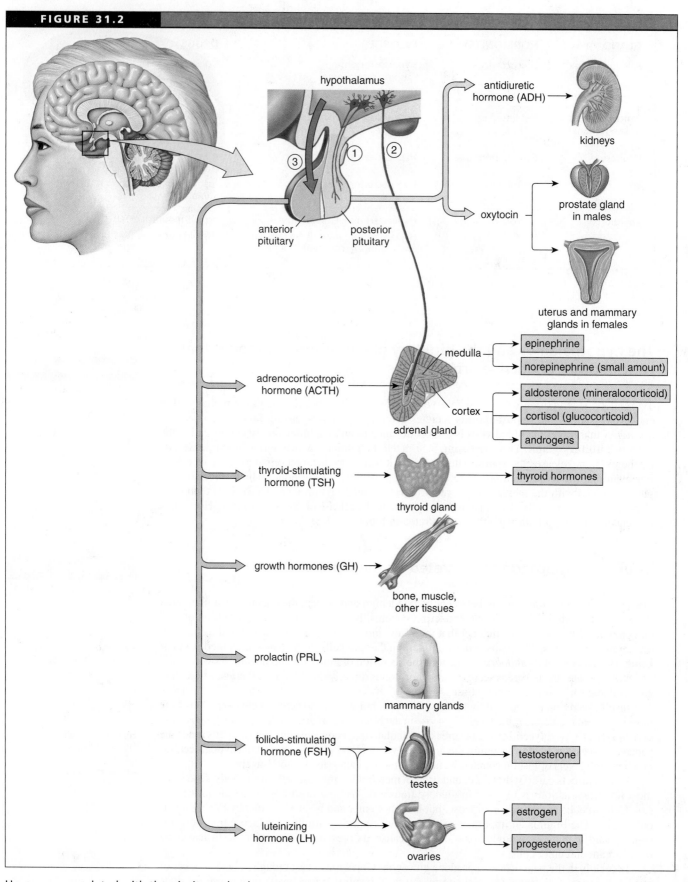

Hormones associated with the pituitary gland   *Source: Adapted by permission of Pearson Education, Inc., Upper Saddle River, NJ*

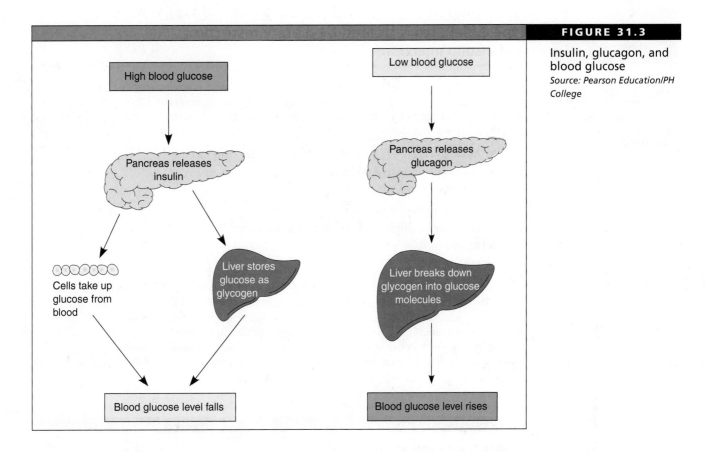

FIGURE 31.3

Insulin, glucagon, and blood glucose
Source: Pearson Education/PH College

Fast Facts Diabetes Mellitus

- Of the 16 million Americans who have diabetes, 5 million probably do not know that they have the disease.
- Each day, 2,200 people are diagnosed with diabetes.
- Diabetes causes more than 198,000 deaths each year; it is the sixth leading cause of death.
- Diabetes is the leading cause of blindness in adults; each year 12,000–24,000 people lose their sight because of diabetes.
- Diabetes is responsible for 50% of nontraumatic lower limb amputations; 56,000 amputations are performed each year in diabetics.
- Costs for diabetes treatment exceed $100 billion annually—one in every seven health care dollars.
- Diabetes is the leading cause of end-stage renal disease, accounting for about 40% of new cases.

glucagon is secreted. Its primary function is to maintain adequate levels of glucose in the blood between meals. It has a hyperglycemic effect: its presence moves glucose from cells, primarily in the liver, to the bloodstream. Figure 31.3 ■ illustrates the relationships between blood glucose, insulin, and glucagon.

TYPE 1 DIABETES MELLITUS

Type 1 diabetes mellitus is one of the most common diseases of childhood. Sometimes called *juvenile-onset diabetes* because it is often diagnosed between the ages of 11 to 13, the disease results from a lack of insulin secretion by the pancreas. There is a genetic component to type 1 diabetes, and children and siblings of people with the disease have a higher risk of acquiring the disorder.

dia = *through*
betes = *to go*
mellitus = *sweet*

CORE CONCEPT 31.5

Type 1 diabetes is treated by dietary restrictions and insulin injections.

AMERICAN DIABETES ASSOCIATION AND HEALTHY LIVING

The signs and symptoms of type 1 diabetes are consistent from patient to patient. The most diagnostic sign is sustained hyperglycemia. Fasting plasma glucose levels of 126 mg/dl or greater on at least two separate occasions is diagnostic for diabetes. Following are the typical signs and symptoms of type 1 diabetes:

- *Hyperglycemia*—fasting blood glucose greater than 126 mg/dl
- *Polyuria*—excessive urination
- *Polyphagia*—increase in hunger
- *Polydipsia*—increased thirst
- *Glucosuria*—high levels of glucose in the urine
- *Weight loss*
- *Fatigue*

Untreated diabetes produces serious long-term damage to arteries that leads to heart disease, stroke, kidney disease, and blindness. Lack of adequate circulation to the feet often causes gangrene of the toes, which may require amputation. Nerve degeneration is common and may produce symptoms ranging from tingling in the fingers or toes to complete loss of sensation. Because glucose cannot enter cells, lipids are used as an energy source, and **ketoacids** are produced as waste products. These ketoacids can give the patient's breath an acetone-like, fruity odor. More

---

DRUG PROFILE: Ⓡ *Regular Insulin (Humulin R, Novolin R, Pork Regular Iletin II, Regular Purified Pork Insulin)*

Therapeutic Class: Antidiabetic
Pharmacologic Class: Natural (biologic) hormone, hypoglycemic agent

Actions and Uses:

Regular insulin is prepared from pork pancreas or as human insulin through recombinant DNA technology. It is classified as short-acting insulin, with an onset of action of 30 to 60 minutes, a peak effect at 2 to 3 hours, and a duration of 5 to 7 hours. Its primary action is to promote the entry of glucose into cells. For the emergency treatment of acute ketoacidosis, it may be given subcutaneously or IV. Regular insulin is also available as Humulin 70/30 (a mixture of 30% regular insulin and 70% isophane insulin) or as Humulin 50/50 (a mixture of 50% of both regular and isophane insulin).

Adverse Effects and Interactions:

The most serious adverse effect from insulin therapy is hypoglycemia. Hypoglycemia may result from taking too much insulin, not properly timing the insulin injection with food intake, or skipping a meal. Dietary carbohydrates must be in the blood when insulin is injected; otherwise the drug will remove too much glucose, and signs of hypoglycemia—tachycardia, confusion, sweating, and drowsiness—will ensue. If severe hypoglycemia is not quickly treated with glucose, convulsions, coma, and death may follow.

Regular insulin interacts with many drugs. For example, the following substances may increase hypoglycemic effects: alcohol, salicylates, monoamine oxidase inhibitors (MAOIs), anabolic steroids, and guanethidine. The following substances may decrease hypoglycemic effects: corticosteroids, thyroid hormones, and epinephrine. Serum glucose levels may be increased with furosemide or thiazide diuretics. Symptoms of hypoglycemic reaction may be hidden if beta blockers are used at the same time.

Use cautiously with herbal supplements such as garlic and ginseng, which may increase the hypoglycemic effects of insulin.

 Refer to MyNursingKit for a Nursing Process Focus specific to this drug.

important, high levels of ketoacids change the pH of the blood, producing acidosis and possibly coma (see Chapter 23 ⬭).

Type 1 diabetes requires drug therapy with insulin or hypoglycemics. Insulin is reserved for the more severe deficiency states, whereas the oral hypoglycemics are given for milder forms of diabetes. Type 1 diabetes is treated with a combination of proper meal planning, exercise, and insulin. Food must be eaten regularly, every 4 to 5 hours, because skipping meals can have serious effects on blood glucose. Regular, moderate exercise helps the cellular responsiveness to insulin.

The treatment goal with insulin therapy is to maintain blood glucose levels within strict, normal limits. Several types of insulin are available, differing in their onset and duration of action. Until the 1980s, the source of all insulin was beef or pork pancreas. Most insulin today, however, is human insulin obtained through recombinant DNA technology. The most common route of administration for insulin is subcutaneous, although research is being conducted to discover more convenient routes of drug administration, including nasal spray. In 2006, an inhaled form of insulin (Exubera) was approved by the Food and Drug Administration (FDA). This product was withdrawn from the U.S. market in 2007 due to lack of consumer demand. The insulin was packaged as a dry powder in a device for inhalation through the mouth. Insulin pumps are used to dispense regular doses of insulin.

All insulin preparations produce the same actions and adverse effects. Doses of insulin are highly individualized for each patient; some patients may need two or more injections daily. Occasionally, two different types of insulin are mixed to obtain the desired therapeutic effect. Common insulin preparations are given in Table 31.2.

TYPE 2 DIABETES MELLITUS

There are a number of differences between type 1 and type 2 diabetes. Unlike type 1, which begins in the early teens, **type 2 diabetes mellitus** begins in the middle-age group and is sometimes referred to as *adult-onset diabetes*. It is more common in patients who are overweight and those with low HDL-cholesterol and high triglyceride levels. Approximately 90% of all patients with diabetes are type 2.

Type 2 diabetes is controlled through lifestyle changes and oral hypoglycemic agents.

CORE CONCEPT 31.6

Unlike those with type 1 diabetics, patients with type 2 are capable of secreting insulin, although in amounts that are too small. The fundamental problem in type 2, however, is that insulin receptors in the target tissues have become insensitive or resistant to the hormone. Thus the small amount of insulin present does not bind effectively to its receptors, and no effect is achieved. Whereas patients with type 1 diabetes must take insulin, those with type 2 diabetes are usually controlled with oral hypoglycemic agents. In severe, unresponsive cases, insulin may also be necessary for patients with type 2 diabetes. The long-term consequences of type 1 and type 2 diabetes are the same.

Another important difference is that proper diet and exercise can sometimes increase the sensitivity of insulin receptors to the point that drug therapy is unnecessary in type 2 diabetes. Many patients with type 2 diabetes are obese and need a medically supervised plan to help them reduce weight gradually and exercise safely. This is an important lifestyle change for such patients; they will need to maintain these changes for the remainder of their lives.

Oral hypoglycemic medications are prescribed after diet and exercise have failed to bring blood glucose levels to within normal values. The six general classes of oral hypoglycemic medications used for type 2 diabetes are sulfonylureas, biguanides, thiazolidinediones, alpha-glucosidase inhibitors, meglitinides, and dipeptidyl-peptase 4 inhibitors. Classification of oral hypoglycemic drugs is based on their chemical structures and mechanisms of action.

Therapy with oral hypoglycemics is usually initiated with a single agent. If therapeutic goals are not achieved, two agents may be administered together. Failure to achieve normal blood glucose levels with two oral hypoglycemics usually indicates a need for insulin. The general oral hypoglycemic classes are listed in Table 31.3.

TABLE 31.2	Insulin Preparations	
DRUG	**ROUTE AND ADULT DOSE**	**REMARKS**
INSULIN ANALOGS (RAPID ACTING)		
insulin aspart (NovoLog)	Subcutaneous; 0.25–0.7 unit/kg/day given 5–10 min before each meal For type 2 diabetes: if already taking oral hypoglycemic drugs, start with 10 units subcutaneous at bedtime daily, and adjust according to patient's needs	Must give 5–10 min before meal. Initial hypoglycemic response begins within 15 min and peaks 45–120 min after injection.
insulin glulisine (Apidra)	Subcutaneous; 0.5–1 unit/kg/day	Must give 5–10 min before meal. Initial hypoglycemic response begins within 15 min and peaks 45–90 min after injection.
insulin lispro (Humalog)	Subcutaneous; 5–10 units given 0–15 min ac	Give 0–15 min before meals. Assess for hypoglycemia from 60–180 min after injection.
INSULIN ANALOGS (LONGER ACTING)		
insulin glargine (Lantus)	For type 1 diabetes: subcutaneous; if not taking insulin, 10 units at bedtime each day; if taking NPH* or ultralente insulin daily, give same dose at bedtime; if taking NPH insulin bid, give 80% of total daily dose at bedtime	Do not give this product IV. Give at same time each day (usually at bedtime) and do not mix with any other insulin product.
INSULIN MIXTURES (SHORT TO INTERMEDIATE ACTING)		
NPH 70% Regular 30% (Humulin 70/30, Novolin 70/30)	IM/subcutaneous; individualized doses	The insulin substance must be uniformly mixed with the contents of the insulin reservoir before a dose is given. The insulin mixture should appear cloudy or milky.
NPH 50% Regular 50%	IM/subcutaneous; individualized doses	The insulin mixture should appear cloudy or milky.
SHORT-ACTING INSULIN (PEAK ACTIVITY IS USUALLY BETWEEN 2 AND 4 HOURS)		
Ⓟ regular insulin (Humulin R, Novolin R, Pork Regular Iletin II, Regular Purified Pork Insulin)	Subcutaneous; 5–10 units given 15–30 min ac and at bedtime	Give regular insulin 30 min before a meal. Frequency of blood glucose monitoring is determined by the type of insulin regimen and health status of the patient.
INTERMEDIATE-ACTING INSULIN (PEAK ACTIVITY IS USUALLY BETWEEN 4 AND 12 HOURS)		
isophane insulin suspension (NPH, NPH Iletin II, Humulin N, Novolin N)	IM/subcutaneous; individualized doses	Give 30 min before the first meal of the day. If necessary, a second smaller dose may be prescribed 30 min before supper or at bedtime.
insulin zinc suspension (Lente Iletin II, Lente L, Humulin L, Novolin L)	IM/subcutaneous; individualized doses	Give 30 min before breakfast. Some patients require another injection 30 min before supper or at bedtime.
LONGER-ACTING INSULIN (PEAK ACTIVITY IS USUALLY 6–20 HOURS)		
extended insulin zinc suspension (Humulin U, Ultralente)	IM/subcutaneous; individualized doses	Give 30 min before breakfast by deep subcutaneous injection. Ultralente may be mixed with Semilente but not with other modified insulin preparations.

NPH* = Neutral Protamine Hagedorn

NURSING PROCESS FOCUS

Patients Receiving Insulin Therapy

ASSESSMENT

Prior to administration:
- Obtain a complete health history (physical/mental), including allergies, drug history, and possible drug interactions
- Assess vital signs. If the patient has a fever or elevated pulse, assess further to determine the cause, because infection can alter the amount of insulin required
- Assess blood glucose level
- Assess appetite and presence of symptoms that indicate the patient may not be able to consume or retain the next meal
- Assess subcutaneous areas for potential insulin injection sites
- Assess knowledge of insulin and ability to self-administer insulin

POTENTIAL NURSING DIAGNOSES

- Risk for Injury (hypoglycemia) related to adverse effects of drug therapy.
- Deficient Knowledge related to information about disease process and self-care regimen.
- Risk for Imbalanced Nutrition related to adverse effects of drug therapy.
- Risk for Infection related to blood glucose elevations and impaired circulation.

PLANNING: PATIENT GOALS AND EXPECTED OUTCOMES

The patient will:
- Immediately report irritability, dizziness, diaphoresis, hunger, behavior changes, and changes in level of consciousness (LOC)
- Demonstrate ability to self-administer insulin
- Demonstrate an understanding of lifestyle modifications necessary for successful maintenance of drug therapy

IMPLEMENTATION

Interventions and (Rationales)	Patient Education/Discharge Planning
■ Monitor blood glucose at least several times a day. Check urine for ketones if blood glucose is over 300. (Ketones will spill into the urine at this glucose level and provide an early sign of diabetic ketoacidosis.)	■ Teach the patient how to monitor blood glucose and test urine for ketones.
■ Increase frequency of blood glucose monitoring if the patient is experiencing fever, nausea, vomiting, or diarrhea. (Illness usually requires adjustments in insulin doses.)	■ Instruct the patient to increase blood glucose monitoring when experiencing fever, nausea, vomiting, or diarrhea.
■ Monitor weight on a routine basis. (Changes in weight will alter insulin needs.)	■ Instruct the patient to weigh self on a routine basis at the same time each day and to report significant changes (e.g., plus or minus 10 lb).
■ Monitor vital signs. (Increased pulse and blood pressure are early signs of hypoglycemia. Patients with diabetes may have circulatory problems and/or impaired kidney function that can increase blood pressure.)	■ Teach the patient how to take blood pressure and pulse and to report significant changes.
■ Monitor potassium level. (Insulin causes potassium to move into the cell and may cause hypokalemia.)	■ Instruct the patient to report the first sign of heart irregularity.
■ Check blood glucose and feed patient some form of simple sugar at the first sign of hypoglycemia. (Using a simple sugar will raise blood sugar immediately.)	Advise the patient: ■ That exercise may increase insulin needs ■ To check blood glucose before and after exercise and to keep a simple sugar on his or her person while exercising ■ To eat some form of simple sugar or complex carbohydrate before strenuous exercise as prophylaxis against hypoglycemia

EVALUATION OF OUTCOME CRITERIA

Evaluate the effectiveness of drug therapy by confirming that patient goals and expected outcomes have been met (see "Planning").

See Table 31.2 for a list of drugs to which these nursing actions apply.

TABLE 31.3   Oral Hypoglycemics

DRUG	ROUTE AND ADULT DOSE	REMARKS
ALPHA-GLUCOSIDASE INHIBITORS		
acarbose (Precose)	PO; 25–100 mg tid (max: 300 mg/day)	Avoid use in patients with chronic intestinal diseases associated with marked disorders of digestion or absorption
miglitol (Glyset)	PO; 25–100 mg tid (max: 300 mg/day)	Use cautiously in patients with renal impairment.
BIGUANIDES		
metformin HCl (Glucophage)	PO; 500 mg one to three times/day (max: 3 g/day)	Extended-release form available. Lactic acidosis may be a complication.
MEGLITINIDES		
nateglinide (Starlix)	PO; 60–120 mg tid	Similar to second-generation sulfonylureas. Use cautiously in patients with hepatic or renal impairment.
repaglinide (Prandin)	PO; 0.5–4 mg bid–qid	Glitazone type. Use cautiously in patients with hepatic or renal impairment.
SULFONYLUREAS, FIRST GENERATION		
chlorpropamide (Diabinese, Novopropamide)	PO; 100–250 mg/day (max: 750 mg/day)	Known sensitivity to sulfonylureas and to sulfonamides.
tolazamide (Tolamide, Tolinase)	PO; 100–500 mg one or two times/day (max: 1 g/day)	Short-acting, older drug used when other drugs fail to control blood glucose levels.
tolbutamide (Orinase)	PO; 250–1500 mg one or two times/day (max: 3 g/day)	Very similar to tolazamide; used when other drugs fail to control blood glucose levels.
SULFONYLUREAS, SECOND GENERATION		
glimepiride (Amaryl)	PO; 1–4 mg/day (max: 8 mg/day)	Not recommended during pregnancy.
Pr glipizide (Glucotrol)	PO; 2.5–20 mg one or two times/day (max: 40 mg/day)	Glucotrol XL is an extended-release form. Serious reactions may occur with overdose.
glyburide (DiaBeta, Micronase, Glynase)	PO; 1.25–10 mg one or two times/day (max: 20 mg/day)	Glucovance is a combination drug containing glyburide and metformin. Serious reactions may occur with overdose.
THIAZOLIDINEDIONES		
pioglitazone (Actos)	PO; 15–30 mg/day (max: 45 mg/day)	Glitazone type. Give without regard to meals.
rosiglitazone (Avandia)	PO; 2–4 mg one or two times/day (max: 8 mg/day)	Often used in combination with metformin or insulin to control blood glucose levels.
DIPEPTIDYL-PEPTIDASE 4 INHIBITORS		
saxaglipton (Onglyza)	PO; 2.5–5 mg once daily	Approved in 2009; may be used in combination with other antidiabetics.
sitagliptin (Januvia)	PO; 100 mg once daily	Actions occur only in the presence of rising serum glucose levels; type of incretin enhancement therapy.
COMBINATION DRUGS		
glipizide/metformin (Metaglip)	PO; 2.5/250 mg/day (max: 10 mg glipizide and 2000 mg metformin/day)	Lactic acidosis is a complication in many cases if these medications are not taken properly.
glyburide/metformin (Glucovance)	PO; 1.25 mg/250 mg one or two times/day (max: 20 mg glyburide and 2000 mg metformin/day)	
rosiglitazone/metformin (Avandamet)	PO; variable dose (max: 8 mg rosiglitazone and 1000 mg metformin/day)	

NATURAL THERAPIES

The Hypoglycemic Effects of Bitter Melon

Bitter melon (*Momordica charantia*) is a climbing vine that bears a knobby, cucumber-shaped fruit. It is grown in many parts of the world, including Asia, Africa, India, and Central and South America. Preparations include fresh juice and capsules. Although the fresh juice is said to have more activity, its taste is extremely bitter and unpalatable.

Extracts of bitter melon were used to lower blood sugar hundreds, and perhaps thousands, of years before the availability of injectible insulin. Two chemicals isolated from this plant—charantin and mormordin—have been found to have hypoglycemic activity. The fruit may also contain substances that have antimicrobial, antiviral, and antitumor properties. Patients with diabetes should use bitter melon only under medical supervision because the combined use of this botanical with insulin or other antidiabetic drugs could lead to hypoglycemia.

In 2005, the FDA approved two new injectable drugs for diabetes: pramlintide (Symlin) and exenatide (Byetta). Symlin is used to enhance the effects of insulin in patients with type 1 or type 2 diabetes mellitus. This drug suppresses glucagon secretion. Byetta stimulates glucose-dependent release of insulin from beta cells in the pancreas and is used to improve control of blood glucose levels in patients taking metformin or sulfonylurea medication.

In 2006, a relatively new class of oral medications was approved and brought to the market called dipeptidylpeptidase 4 (DDP-4) inhibitors. Examples of DDP-4 inhibitors, in clinical trial testing are vildagliptin (Galvus), denagliptin (Redona), and alogliptin (Takeda). Sitagliptin (Januvia) and saxagliptin (Onglyza) are currently used to help lower blood glucose in patients with type 2 diabetes who are unable to achieve normal glucose levels with diet and exercise. DDP-4 inhibitors suppress enzymes responsible for breaking down gastric hormones called *incretins*. In response to the presence of food in the small intestine, incretins normally inhibit the release of glucagon, stimulating the release of insulin from the pancreas; they also delay gastric emptying and convey impulses to the brain about satiety (feeling of being full). When incretin action is enhanced, the result is decreased glucagon secretion, increased insulin secretion, and stablization of hormone fluctuations after a meal. Thus, when taken within proper parameters, DDP-4 inhibitors or **incretin enhancers** are effective at lowering blood glucose without causing extreme hypoglycemia.

DRUG PROFILE: 🅟 *Glipizide (Glucotrol)*

Therapeutic Class: Antidiabetic
Pharmacologic Class: Oral hypoglycemic, sulfonylurea (second generation)

Actions and Uses:

Glipizide belongs to the sulfonylurea group of hypoglycemics. It is a second-generation sulfonylurea that offers the advantages of higher potency, once-a-day dosing, fewer adverse effects, and fewer drug–drug interactions than the first-generation medications in this class. Glipizide stimulates the pancreas to secrete more insulin and also increases the sensitivity of insulin receptors in target tissues. Some degree of pancreatic function is required for glipizide to lower blood glucose. Maximum effects are achieved if the drug is taken 30 minutes prior to the primary meal of the day.

Adverse Effects and Interactions:

Hypoglycemia is less frequent with glipizide than with first-generation sulfonylureas. Patients should stay out of the sun because rashes and photosensitivity are possible. Some patients experience mild, gastrointestinal (GI)-related effects such as nausea, vomiting, or loss of appetite. Glipizide and other sulfonylureas have the potential to interact with a number of drugs; thus, the patient should always consult with a health care provider before adding a new medication or herbal supplement. Ingestion of alcohol will result in distressing symptoms that include headache, flushing, nausea, and abdominal cramping.

Mechanism in Action:

Glipizide, an oral hypoglycemic agent, lowers blood glucose levels by stimulating insulin release from pancreatic cells. This drug is used for the treatment of type 2 diabetes mellitus. Because it is a sulfonylurea drug, sensitivity reactions are possible.

Refer to MyNursingKit for a Nursing Process Focus specific to this drug.

NURSING PROCESS FOCUS

Patients Receiving Oral Hypoglycemic Therapy

ASSESSMENT

Prior to administration:
- Obtain a complete health history (physical/mental), including allergies, drug history, and possible drug interactions
- Assess for pain location and level
- Assess knowledge of drug
- Assess ability to conduct blood glucose testing

POTENTIAL NURSING DIAGNOSES

- Risk for Injury (hypoglycemia) related to adverse effects of drug therapy.
- Pain (abdominal) related to adverse effects of drug.
- Deficient Knowledge related to information about drug therapy.
- Deficient Knowledge related to information about blood glucose testing.

PLANNING: PATIENT GOALS AND EXPECTED OUTCOMES

The patient will:
- Describe signs and symptoms that should be reported immediately, including nausea, diarrhea, jaundice, rash, headache, anorexia, abdominal pain, tachycardia, seizures, and confusion
- Demonstrate an ability to accurately self-monitor blood glucose; maintain blood glucose within a normal range

IMPLEMENTATION

Interventions and (Rationales)	Patient Education/Discharge Planning
■ Monitor blood glucose at least daily and monitor urinary ketones if blood glucose is over 300. (Ketones will spill into the urine at high blood glucose levels and provide an early sign of diabetic ketoacidosis.)	■ Teach the patient how to monitor blood glucose and test urine for ketones, especially when ill.
■ Monitor for signs of lactic acidosis if the patient is receiving a biguanide. (Mitochondrial oxidation of lactic acid is inhibited, and lactic acidosis may result.)	■ Instruct the patient to report signs of lactic acidosis such as hyperventilation, muscle pain, fatigue, and increased sleeping.
■ Review laboratory tests for any abnormalities in liver function. (These drugs are metabolized in the liver and may cause elevations in AST and LDH. Metformin decreases absorption of vitamin B_{12} and folic acid, which may result in deficiencies of these substances.)	■ Instruct the patient to report the first sign of yellow skin, pale stools, or dark urine.
■ Obtain accurate history of alcohol use, especially if the patient is receiving a sulfonylurea or biguanide. (These drugs may cause an Antabuse-like reaction.)	■ Advise the patient to abstain from alcohol and to avoid liquid over-the-counter (OTC) medications, which may contain alcohol.
■ Monitor for signs and symptoms of illness or infection. (Illness may increase blood glucose levels.)	■ Instruct the patient to report the first signs of fatigue, muscle weakness, and nausea. ■ Discuss importance of adequate rest and healthy routines.
■ Monitor blood glucose frequently, especially at the beginning of therapy and in elderly patients. ■ Monitor carefully patients who also take a beta blocker, because early signs of hypoglycemia may not be apparent.	Teach the patient: ■ Signs and symptoms of hypoglycemia, such as hunger, irritability, sweating ■ At first sign of hypoglycemia, to check blood glucose and eat a simple sugar; if symptoms do not improve, call 911 ■ To monitor blood glucose before breakfast and supper ■ Not to skip meals and to follow a diet specified by the health care provider
■ Monitor weight, weighing at the same time of day each time. (Changes in weight will affect the amount of drug needed to control blood glucose.)	■ Instruct the patient to weigh each week, at the same time of day, and report any significant loss or gain.

continued . . .

NURSING PROCESS FOCUS *(continued)*

Interventions and (Rationales)	Patient Education/Discharge Planning
■ Monitor vital signs. (Increased pulse and blood pressure are early signs of hypoglycemia.)	■ Teach the patient how to take accurate blood pressure, temperature, and pulse.
■ Monitor the skin for rashes and itching. (These are signs of an allergic reaction to the drug.)	■ Advise the patient of the importance of immediately reporting skin rashes and itching that are not due to dry skin.
■ Monitor activity level. (Dose may require adjustment with change in physical activity.)	■ Advise the patient to increase activity level, which will help lower blood glucose. ■ Advise the patient to closely monitor blood glucose when involved in vigorous physical activity.

EVALUATION OF OUTCOME CRITERIA

Evaluate the effectiveness of drug therapy by confirming that patient goals and expected outcomes have been met (see "Planning").

See Table 31.3 for a list of drugs to which these nursing actions apply.

Concept Review 31.1

■ Why are oral hypoglycemic drugs ineffective for treating type 1 diabetes?

THYROID DISORDERS

The thyroid gland controls the basal metabolic rate and affects virtually every cell in the body.

CORE CONCEPT **31.7**

The thyroid gland lies in the neck, just below the larynx and in front of the trachea. **Follicular cells** in the gland secrete thyroid hormone, which is actually a combination of two different hormones: thyroxine (tetraiodothyronine or T_4) and triiodothyronine (T_3). Iodine is essential for the synthesis of these hormones and is provided through the dietary intake of common iodized salt. **Parafollicular cells** in the thyroid gland secrete calcitonin, a hormone that is involved with calcium homeostasis (see Chapter 33 ⬭).

Thyroid function is regulated through multiple levels of hormonal control. Thyroid-releasing hormone (TRH) from the hypothalamus stimulates the pituitary gland to secrete TSH. TSH then stimulates the thyroid gland to release thyroid hormone. After thyroid hormone has reached a certain level in the blood, it operates in a negative feedback loop to shut off secretion of TRH and TSH. The negative feedback mechanism for the thyroid gland is depicted in Figure 31.4 ■.

Thyroid hormone affects nearly every cell in the body by regulating *basal metabolic rate,* the baseline speed at which cells perform their functions. By increasing cellular metabolism, thyroid hormone increases body temperature. Thyroid hormone is critical to the growth of the nervous system. Deficiency during infancy may result in a combination of dwarfism and severe mental retardation known as **cretinism**.

Thyroid disorders may be treated by administering thyroid hormone or by decreasing the activity of the thyroid gland.

CORE CONCEPT **31.8**

Thyroid disorders are quite common, and drug therapy is often indicated. The correct dose of thyroid or antithyroid drug is highly individualized and may require periodic adjustment.

FIGURE 31.4

Feedback mechanisms
of the thyroid gland

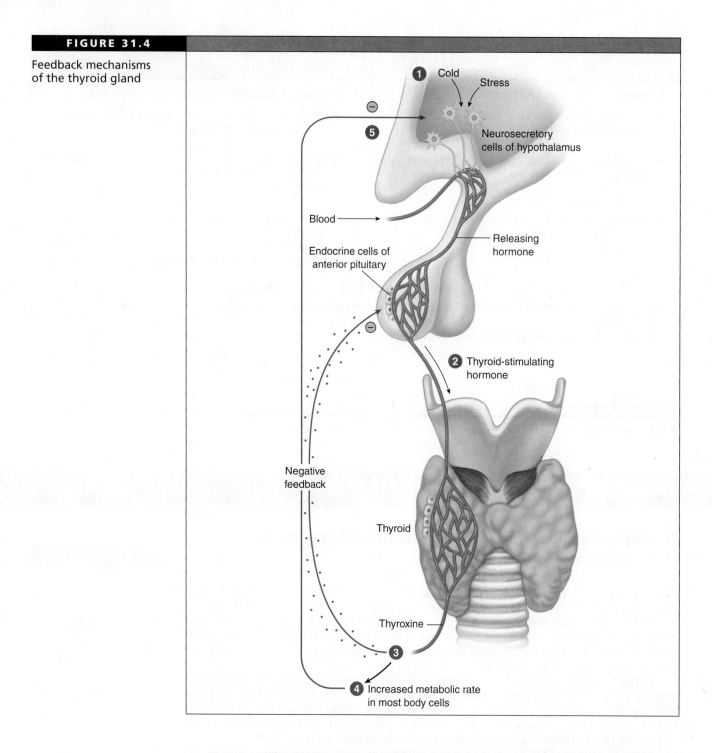

Hypothyroidism is a common disease caused by insufficient secretion of either TSH or thy-roid hormone. Symptoms of hypothyroidism in adults, also known as **myxedema**, include slowed body metabolism, slurred speech, bradycardia, weight gain, low body temperature, and intoler-ance to cold environments. Low or absent thyroid function may be a consequence of autoimmune disease, surgical removal of the gland, or aggressive treatment with antithyroid drugs. Hypothy-roidism is treated with natural or synthetic thyroid hormone.

Hypersecretion of thyroid hormone results in symptoms that are the opposite of hypothy-roidism, such as increased body metabolism, tachycardia, weight loss, high body temperature, and anxiety. A particularly severe form of hyperthyroidism is called **Graves' disease**. If the cause of the hypersecretion is found to be a tumor, the disease is corrected through surgical re-moval of the thyroid gland, or thyroidectomy. In less severe conditions, the patient may receive antithyroid medications or ionizing radiation to kill or inactivate some of the hyperactive thy-

Fast Facts Thyroid Disorders

- Hypothyroidism is 10 times more common in women than men; hyperthyroidism is 5–10 times more common in women.
- The two most common thyroid disorders, Graves' disease and Hashimoto's thyroiditis, are autoimmune diseases and may run in families.
- One of every 4,000 babies is born without a working thyroid gland.
- About 15,000 new cases of thyroid cancer are diagnosed each year.
- One of every five women older than age 75 has Hashimoto's thyroiditis.
- Postpartum thyroiditis occurs in 5–9% of women after giving birth and may recur in future pregnancies.
- Both hyperthyroidism and hypothyroidism can affect a woman's ability to become pregnant; both also can cause miscarriages.

roid cells. Antithyroid agents are sometimes given 10 to 14 days prior to thyroidectomy to decrease bleeding during surgery.

The thyroid is the organ most susceptible to nuclear and radiation exposure. (See Chapter 1 for a discussion of bioterrorism.) Symptoms of radiation exposure remain some of the most difficult to treat pharmacologically. Apart from the symptomatic treatment of *acute radiation syndrome*, taking potassium iodide (KI) tablets after an incident or an attack is the only recognized therapy.

Following a nuclear explosion, one of the resultant radioisotopes is iodine-131. Because iodine is naturally concentrated in the thyroid gland, I-131 will immediately enter the thyroid and damage thyroid cells. If taken prior to, or immediately following, a nuclear incident, KI can prevent up to 100% of the radioactive iodine from entering thyroid tissue. Unfortunately, KI only protects the thyroid gland from I-131. It has no protective effects on other body tissues, and it offers no protection against the dozens of other harmful radioisotopes generated by a nuclear blast. Interestingly, I-131 is also a medication used to shrink the size of overactive thyroid glands. The thyroid and antithyroid medications are listed in Table 31.4.

Concept Review   31.2

- If thyroid hormone is secreted by the thyroid gland, how can a deficiency in this hormone be caused by disease in the hypothalamus or pituitary gland?

TABLE 31.4   Thyroid and Antithyroid Medications

DRUG	ROUTE AND ADULT DOSE	REMARKS
THYROID PREPARATIONS		
levothyroxine (Synthroid)	PO; 100–400 mcg/day	Synthetic T_4; IV form available
liothyronine (Cytomel)	PO; 25–75 mcg/day	Synthetic T_3
liotrix (Euthroid, Thyrolar)	PO; 12.5–30 mcg/day	Mixture of synthetic T_3 and synthetic T_4 in a 1:4 ratio
thyroid (S-P-T, Thyrar, Thyroid USP)	PO; 60–100 mg/day	Animal thyroid glands
ANTITHYROID PREPARATIONS		
methimazole (Tapazole)	PO; 5–15 mg tid	10 times more potent than propylthiouracil
potassium iodide and iodine (Lugol's solution, Thyro-block)	PO; 0.1–1.0 ml tid	IV form available; Lugol's is a mixture of 5% elemental iodine and 10% potassium iodide
propylthiouracil (PTU)	PO; 100–150 mg tid	May take 6-12 months for full therapeutic effect
radioactive iodide (^{131}I, Iodotope)	PO; 0.8–150 mCi (based on radiation quantity)	May take 2–3 months for full therapeutic effect

DRUG PROFILE: (Pr) *Levothyroxine (Synthroid)*

Therapeutic Class: Thyroid replacement agent
Pharmacologic Class: Natural (biologic) hormone, metabolic enhancing drug

Actions and Uses:

Levothyroxine is a synthetic form of thyroxine (T_4) used for replacement therapy in patients with low thyroid function. Actions are those of thyroid hormone and include loss of weight, improved tolerance to environmental temperature, increased activity, and increased pulse rate. Blood levels of thyroid hormone are monitored carefully until the patient's symptoms stabilize. To achieve the proper level of thyroid function, doses may require periodic adjustments for several months or longer.

Adverse Effects and Interactions:

The difference between a therapeutic dose of levothyroxine and one that produces adverse effects is quite narrow. Adverse effects of levothyroxine resemble symptoms of hyperthyroidism and include tachycardia, anxiety, insomnia, weight loss, and heat intolerance. Menstrual irregularities may occur in women. Long-term use of levothyroxine has been associated with osteoporosis in women.

Levothyroxine interacts with many other drugs; for example, cholestyramine and colestipol decrease the absorption of levothyroxine. Using it with epinephrine and norepinephrine increases the risk of cardiac insufficiency. Oral anticoagulants may increase hypoprothrombinemia.

Herbal supplements such as lemon balm should be used cautiously. Lemon balm may interfere with thyroid hormone function.

Refer to MyNursingKit for a Nursing Process Focus specific to this drug.

CORE CONCEPT 31.9

Glucocorticoids are released during periods of stress and influence carbohydrate, lipid, and protein metabolism in most cells.

An adrenal glands lie on top of each kidney. Structurally the adrenal glands are made up of two general regions—the cortex and the medulla. The outer cortex releases three important classes of hormones, called *mineralocorticoids, glucocorticoids,* and *androgens.* Collectively, these hormones are referred to as *corticosteroids* or *adrenocortical hormones.*

The **mineralocorticoid** aldosterone is responsible for increasing the renal absorption of sodium in exchange for potassium. Discussion of aldosterone is more relevant to the subject of diuretics because drugs or conditions may disrupt aldosterone release and alter the levels of fluids and electrolytes and important minerals in the bloodstream (see Chapter 23 ⬯). Aldosterone release is also affected by **adrenocorticotropic hormone (ACTH)**, although the main action of this hormone is the direct release of the important glucocorticoid hormone cortisol.

gluco = sugar
corti = cortex
oid = resemble

Cortisol is one of about 30 **glucocorticoids** secreted from the outer portion, or cortex, of the adrenal gland. Glucocorticoids affect the metabolism of nearly every cell in the body. During long-term stress, these hormones mobilize the formation of glucose and increase the breakdown and use of proteins and lipids. They have a potent anti-inflammatory effect that was discussed in Chapters 24 and 28 ⬯. They also serve to promote homeostasis of the cardiovascular, nervous, and musculoskeletal systems.

Control of glucocorticoid levels begins with corticotropin-releasing factor (CRF), secreted by the hypothalamus. CRF travels to the pituitary, where it causes the release of ACTH. ACTH travels through the blood and reaches the adrenal cortex, causing it to release cortisol and other corticosteroids. When the level of cortisol in the blood rises, it provides negative feedback to the hypothalamus and pituitary to shut off further release of glucocorticoids from the adrenal gland. This negative feedback mechanism is depicted in Figure 31.5 ■.

FIGURE 31.5

Feedback control of the adrenal cortex

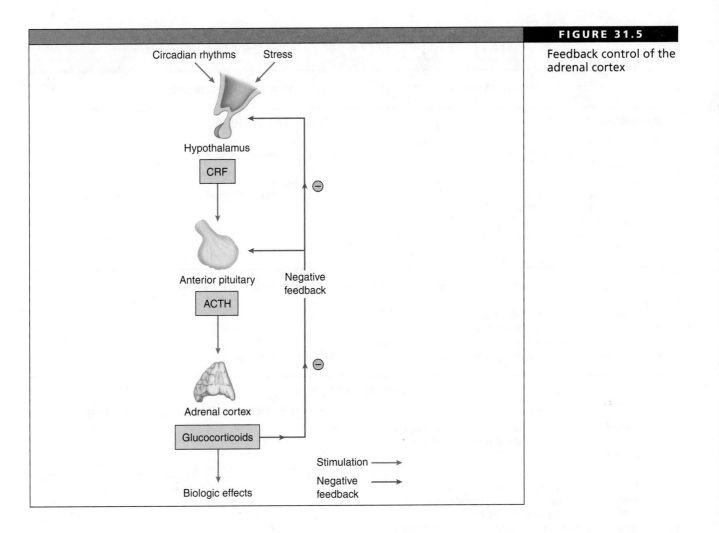

Circadian rhythms   Stress

Hypothalamus

CRF

⊖

Anterior pituitary

ACTH

⊖

Negative feedback

Adrenal cortex

Glucocorticoids

Biologic effects

Stimulation ⟶
Negative feedback ⟶

DRUG PROFILE: ℞ *Propylthiouracil (PTU)*

Therapeutic Class: Hyperthyroidism drug
Pharmacologic Class: Thyroid hormone synthesis inhibitor, antithyroid agent

Actions and Uses:

Propylthiouracil is administered to patients with hyperthyroidism, sometimes prior to surgery. It acts by interfering with the synthesis of T_3 and T_4. Because it does not affect thyroid hormone that has already been secreted, its action may be delayed from several days to as long as 6 to 12 weeks. Effects include a return to normal thyroid function: weight gain, reduction in anxiety, less insomnia, and slower pulse rate.

Adverse Effects and Interactions:

Overtreatment with propylthiouracil produces symptoms of hypothyroidism. In addition, a small percentage of patients display blood changes such as decreased platelet and white blood cell counts. Periodic laboratory blood counts and thyroid hormone values are necessary to establish the proper dosage.

Antithyroid medications interact with many other drugs. For example, propylthiouracil can reverse the effectiveness of drugs such as aminophylline, anticoagulants, and cardiac glycosides.

 Refer to MyNursingKit for a Nursing Process Focus specific to this drug.

NURSING PROCESS FOCUS

Patients Receiving Thyroid Hormone Replacement

ASSESSMENT

Prior to administration:
- Obtain a complete health history (physical/mental), including allergies, drug history, and possible drug interactions
- Obtain a complete physical examination
- Assess for the presence/history of symptoms of hypothyroidism
- Obtain an ECG and laboratory studies including T_4, T_3, and serum TSH levels

POTENTIAL NURSING DIAGNOSES

- Activity Intolerance related to disease process.
- Fatigue related to impaired metabolic status.
- Deficient Knowledge related to information drug therapy.
- Infective Health Maintenance related to adverse effects of drug.

PLANNING: PATIENT GOALS AND EXPECTED OUTCOMES

The patient will:
- Exhibit normal thyroid hormone levels
- Report a decrease in hypothyroid symptoms
- Experience no significant adverse effects from drug therapy
- Demonstrate an understanding of hypothyroidism and the need for life-long therapy

IMPLEMENTATION

Interventions and (Rationales)	Patient Education/Discharge Planning
Monitor vital signs. (Changes in metabolic rate will be manifested as changes in blood pressure, pulse, and body temperature.)	Instruct the patient to report dizziness, palpitations, and intolerance to temperature changes.
Monitor for decreasing symptoms related to hypothyroidism, such as fatigue, constipation, cold intolerance, lethargy, depression, and menstrual irregularities. (Decreasing symptoms will determine that the drug is achieving therapeutic effect.)	Instruct the patient about the signs of hyperthyroidism and to report symptoms.
Monitor for symptoms related to hyperthyroidism, such as nervousness, insomnia, tachycardia, dysrhythmias, heat intolerance, chest pain, and diarrhea. (Symptoms of hyperthyroidism indicate the drug is at a toxic level.)	Instruct the patient about the signs of hyperthyroidism and to report symptoms.
Monitor T_3, T_4, and TSH levels. (This helps to determine the effectiveness of pharmacotherapy.)	Instruct the patient about the importance of ongoing monitoring of thyroid hormone levels and to keep all laboratory appointments.
Monitor blood glucose levels, especially in individuals with diabetes mellitus. (Thyroid hormones increase metabolic rate and may alter glucose utilization.)	Instruct the patient with diabetes to monitor blood glucose levels and adjust insulin doses as directed by the health care provider.
Provide supportive nursing care to cope with symptoms of hypothyroidism, such as constipation, cold intolerance, and fatigue until the drug has achieved therapeutic effect.	Instruct the patient to: - Increase fluid and fiber intake, as well as activity, to reduce constipation - Wear additional clothing and maintain a comfortable room environment for cold intolerance - Plan activities and include rest periods to avoid fatigue
Monitor weight at least weekly. (Weight loss is expected due to increased metabolic rate. Weight changes help to determine the effectiveness of drug therapy.)	Instruct the patient to weigh weekly and to report significant changes.

continued . . .

NURSING PROCESS FOCUS (continued)

Interventions and (Rationales)	**Patient Education/Discharge Planning**
■ Monitor the patient for signs of decreased compliance with therapeutic regimen.	■ Instruct the patient about the disease, the importance of life-long therapy, and the importance of follow-up care.

EVALUATION OF OUTCOME CRITERIA

Evaluate the effectiveness of drug therapy by confirming that patient goals and expected outcomes have been met (see "Planning").

See Table 31.4 for a list of drugs to which these nursing actions apply.

Glucocorticoids are prescribed for adrenocortical insufficiency and a wide variety of other conditions.

CORE CONCEPT 31.10

Lack of adequate corticosteroid production, known as *adrenocortical insufficiency*, may be caused by hyposecretion by the adrenal cortex or by inadequate secretion of ACTH from the pituitary. Symptoms include hypoglycemia, fatigue, hypotension, and GI disturbances such as anorexia, vomiting, and diarrhea. Primary adrenocortical insufficiency, known as **Addison's disease**, is quite rare and includes a deficiency of both glucocorticoids and mineralocorticoids.

Secondary adrenocortical insufficiency is relatively common and may result from long-term therapy with glucocorticoids. When glucocorticoids are taken as medications for long periods, the pituitary receives a message through the negative feedback mechanism to stop secreting ACTH. Without stimulation from ACTH, the adrenal cortex shrinks in size and stops secreting endogenous glucocorticoids, a condition known as adrenal **atrophy**. If a patient abruptly discontinues the glucocorticoid medication, the shrunken adrenal glands will not be able to secrete enough glucocorticoids, and symptoms of adrenocortical insufficiency will appear.

a = *without*
trophy = *nourishment*

The goal of replacement therapy is to achieve the same physiologic level of glucocorticoids in the blood that would be present if the adrenal glands were functioning properly. Patients requiring replacement therapy may need to take glucocorticoids their entire lives.

Many glucocorticoid preparations are available via the topical, oral, IM, IV, and other routes to treat a variety of disorders. The role of corticosteroids in the treatment of inflammation and allergic rhinitis is presented in Chapters 24 and 28 ⚭ , respectively. Following is a list of the various disorders that may be treated with corticosteroids:

- Allergies
- Asthma
- Seasonal rhinitis
- Skin disorders such as contact dermatitis and rashes
- Neoplastic disease such as Hodgkin's disease, leukemias, and lymphomas
- Shock
- Rheumatic disorders such as rheumatoid arthritis, ankylosing spondylitis, and bursitis
- Post-transplant surgery to suppress the immune system
- Chronic inflammatory bowel disease such as ulcerative colitis and Crohn's disease
- Adrenal insufficiency
- Hepatic, neurologic, and renal disorders characterized by edema

Significant adverse effects can occur during long-term therapy with corticosteroids. An array of signs and symptoms known as **Cushing's syndrome** includes adrenal atrophy, osteoporosis, increased risk of infections, delayed wound healing, peptic ulcers, and a redistribution of fat around the shoulders and neck. Mood and personality changes may occur, with the patient becoming psychologically dependent on the therapeutic effects of the drug. Some of the glucocorticoids, such as hydrocortisone, also have mineralocorticoid activity and thus can cause retention of sodium and water. Alternate-day dosing, whereby the drug is administered every other day, is sometimes used to limit adrenal atrophy. Patients taking inhaled or topical corticosteroids, or who receive the drugs for 2 weeks or less, exhibit few adverse effects. Some of the glucocorticoids used in replacement therapy are listed in Table 31.5.

TABLE 31.5   Selected Glucocorticoids

DRUG	ROUTE AND ADULT DOSE	REMARKS
betamethasone (Celestone, others)	PO; 0.6–7.2 mg/day	Long acting; IV, topical, and IM forms available; has little mineralocorticoid activity
cortisone (Cortistan, Cortone)	PO; 20–300 mg/day	Short acting; IM form available; also has mineralocorticoid activity
dexamethasone	PO; 0.25–4 mg bid–qid	Long acting; IV, ophthalmic, topical, intranasal, inhalation, and IM forms available; has little mineralocorticoid activity
fludrocortisone (Florinef)	PO; 0.1–0.2 mg/day	Long acting; also has strong mineralocorticoid activity
Pr hydrocortisone (Cortef, Hydrocortone, Solu-Cortef, others)	PO; 2–80 mg tid–qid	Short acting; IV, topical, and IM forms available; also has mineralocorticoid activity
methylprednisolone (Solu-Medrol, Medrol)	PO; 2–60 mg one to four times/day	Intermediate acting; IV and IM forms available; has little mineralocorticoid activity
prednisolone (Delta-Cortef)	PO; 5–60 mg one to four times/day	Intermediate acting; IV and IM forms available; has little mineralocorticoid activity
prednisone (see page 394 for the Drug Profile box)	PO; 5–60 mg one to four times/day	Intermediate acting; has little mineralocorticoid activity
triamcinolone (Aristocort, Atolone, Kenacort, Kenalog-E)	PO; 4–48 mg one to four times/day	Intermediate acting; IV, intra-articular, subcutaneous, topical, inhalation, and IM forms available; has little mineralocorticoid activity

DRUG PROFILE: Pr *Hydrocortisone (Cortef, Hydrocortone, Solu-Cortef, Others)*

Therapeutic Class: Drug for moderate to severe asthma and allergies, antineoplastic, and adrenal hormone replacement therapy

Pharmacologic Class: Systemic glucocorticoid

Actions and Uses:

Structurally identical to the natural hormone cortisol, hydrocortisone is a synthetic corticosteroid that is the drug of choice for treating adrenocortical insufficiency. When used for replacement therapy, it is given at physiologic doses. Once proper dosing is achieved, its therapeutic effects should mimic those of natural corticosteroids. Hydrocortisone is also available for the treatment of inflammation, allergic disorders, and many other conditions. Intra-articular injections may be given to decrease severe inflammation in affected joints.

Adverse Effects and Interactions:

When used at physiologic doses for replacement therapy, adverse effects of hydrocortisone should not be evident. The patient and the health care professional must be vigilant, however, in observing for signs of Cushing's syndrome, which can develop with high doses. If taken for longer than 2 weeks, hydrocortisone should be discontinued gradually.

Hydrocortisone interacts with many drugs. For example, barbiturates, phenytoin, and rifampin may increase liver metabolism, thus decreasing hydrocortisone levels. Estrogens increase the effects of hydrocortisone. Nonsteroidal anti-inflammatory drugs (NSAIDs) increase the risk of ulcers. Cholestyramine and colestipol decrease hydrocortisone absorption. Diuretics and amphotericin B increase hypokalemia. Anticholinesterase agents may produce severe weakness. Hydrocortisone may cause a decrease in immune response to vaccines and toxoids.

Herbal supplements, such as aloe and buckthorn (a laxative), may cause potassium deficiency.

Refer to MyNursingKit for a Nursing Process Focus specific to this drug.

Concept Review **31.3**

■ Why does administration of glucocorticoids for extended periods result in adrenal atrophy?

NURSING PROCESS FOCUS

Patients Receiving Systemic Glucocorticoid Therapy

ASSESSMENT

Prior to administration:
- Obtain a complete health history (physical/mental), including allergies, drug history, and possible drug interactions
- Obtain a complete physical examination, focusing on presenting symptoms
- Determine the reason the medication is being administered
- Obtain laboratory studies (long-term therapy), including serum sodium and potassium levels, hematocrit and hemoglobin levels, blood glucose level, and blood urea nitrogen (BUN)

POTENTIAL NURSING DIAGNOSES

- Risk for Infection related to immunosuppression.
- Risk for Injury related to adverse effects of drug therapy.
- Deficient Knowledge related to information about drug therapy.

PLANNING: PATIENT GOALS AND EXPECTED OUTCOMES

The patient will:
- Exhibit a decrease in the symptoms for which the drug is being given
- Exhibit no symptoms of infection
- Demonstrate an understanding of the drug's action, drug administration, and adverse effects

IMPLEMENTATION

Interventions and (Rationales)	Patient Education/Discharge Planning
■ Monitor vital signs. (Blood pressure may increase because of increased blood volume and potential vasoconstriction effect.)	■ Instruct the patient to report dizziness, palpitations, or headaches.
■ Monitor for infection. Protect the patient from potential infections. (Glucocorticoids increase susceptibility to infections by suppressing the immune response.)	Instruct the patient to: ■ Avoid people with infections ■ Report fever, cough, sore throat, joint pain, increased weakness, and malaise ■ Consult with the health care provider before taking any immunizations
■ Monitor the patient's compliance with drug regimen. (Sudden discontinuation of these agents can precipitate an adrenal crisis.)	Instruct the patient: ■ To never suddenly stop taking the medication ■ In proper use of self-administering tapering dose pack ■ To take oral medications with food
■ Monitor for symptoms of Cushing's syndrome, such as moon face, "buffalo hump" contour of shoulders, weight gain, muscle wasting, and increased deposits of fat in the trunk. (Symptoms may indicate excessive use of glucocorticoids.)	Instruct the patient: ■ To weigh self daily ■ That initial weight gain is expected; provide the patient with weight gain parameters that warrant reporting ■ That there are multiple adverse effects to therapy and that changes in health status should be reported
■ Monitor blood glucose levels. (Glucocorticoids cause an increase in gluconeogenesis and reduce glucose utilization.)	Instruct the patient to: ■ Report symptoms of hyperglycemia, such as excessive thirst, copious urination, and insatiable appetite ■ Adjust insulin dose based on blood glucose level, as directed by the health care provider

continued . . .

NURSING PROCESS FOCUS *(continued)*

Interventions and (Rationales)	Patient Education/Discharge Planning
■ Monitor skin and mucous membranes for lacerations, abrasions, or breaks in integrity. (Glucocorticoids impair wound healing.)	Instruct the patient to: ■ Examine skin daily for cuts and scrapes and to cover any injuries with sterile bandage ■ Watch for symptoms of skin infection such as redness, swelling, and drainage ■ Notify the health care provider of any nonhealing wound or symptoms of infection
■ Monitor GI status for peptic ulcer development. (Glucocorticoids decrease gastric mucus production and predispose patients to peptic ulcers.)	■ Instruct the patient to report GI adverse effects such as heartburn, abdominal pain, or tarry stools.
■ Monitor serum electrolytes. (Glucocorticoids cause hypernatremia and hypokalemia.)	Instruct the patient to: ■ Consume a diet high in protein, calcium, and potassium but low in fat and concentrated simple carbohydrates ■ Keep all laboratory appointments
■ Monitor changes in the musculoskeletal system. (Glucocorticoids decrease bone density and strength and cause muscle atrophy and weakness.)	Instruct the patient: ■ To participate in exercise or physical activity to help maintain bone and muscle strength ■ That the drug may cause weakness in bones and muscles; avoid strenuous activity that may cause injury
■ Monitor emotional stability. (Glucocorticoids may produce mood and behavior changes such as depression or feeling of invulnerability.)	■ Instruct the patient that mood changes may be expected and to report mental status changes to the health care provider.

EVALUATION OF OUTCOME CRITERIA

Evaluate the effectiveness of drug therapy by confirming that patient goals and expected outcomes have been met (see "Planning").

See Table 31.5 for a list of drugs to which these nursing actions apply.

CORE CONCEPT 31.11

Of the many pituitary and hypothalamic hormones, only a few have clinical applications as drugs.

Of the 15 different hormones secreted by the pituitary gland and hypothalamus, only a few are used for drug therapy. This is because some of these hormones can only be obtained from natural sources rather than from the pituitary or hypothalamus, and it is usually easier to give drugs affecting the target organs. Two pituitary hormones, prolactin and oxytocin, affect the reproductive system and are discussed in Chapter 32. Of those remaining, growth hormone and antidiuretic hormone have some clinical use.

Growth hormone, known as **somatotropin**, stimulates the growth of nearly every cell in the body. Deficiency of this hormone in children results in **dwarfism**. Unlike a deficiency of thyroid hormone, however, growth hormone deficiency usually does not cause mental impairment. Two preparations of human growth hormone, somatrem (Protropin) and somatropin (Humatrope and others), are available as replacement therapy in children. If therapy is begun early in life, as much as 6 inches of growth may be achieved.

As its name implies, antidiuretic hormone (ADH) conserves water in the body. ADH is secreted from the posterior pituitary gland and acts on the collecting ducts in the kidney to increase water reabsorption. A deficiency of ADH, known as **diabetes insipidus**, causes the patient to lose large volumes of water. ADH is also called **vasopressin** because it has the capability to raise blood pressure when secreted in large amounts. Two preparations of ADH are available for the treatment of diabetes insipidus: vasopressin and desmopressin (DDAVP, Stimate). Desmopressin is occasionally used by the intranasal route to treat enuresis (bedwetting).

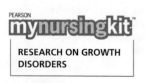

PATIENTS NEED TO KNOW

Patients treated for endocrine disorders need to know the following:

Regarding Corticosteroids

1. When taking oral corticosteroids for more than 2 weeks, do not miss doses or discontinue the drug without consulting a health care provider.
2. See a physician if any infections, cuts, or injuries appear to be healing abnormally slowly while on corticosteroids.
3. If taking hydrocortisone for replacement therapy, take the medication between 6:00 a.m. and 9:00 a.m. because this is the time when natural corticosteroids are released.

Regarding Diabetic Medications

4. When taking insulin or oral hypoglycemics, report any signs of hypoglycemia, such as weakness, sweating, dizziness, tremor, anxiety, or tachycardia, to a health care provider immediately. Mild symptoms may be treated with small amounts of sugar in the form of candy or fruit juice.
5. Always take insulin or oral hypoglycemics at the same time each day.
6. When self-monitoring blood glucose, recall that normal values are 80 to 120 mg/dl before meals, and 100 to 140 mg/dl before bedtime.
7. Store unopened vials of insulin in the refrigerator. Do not use after the expiration date.
8. If taking insulin or oral hypoglycemics, read the directions for all medications very carefully because many drug–drug interactions are possible. Medications such as corticosteroids, thiazide diuretics, and sympathomimetics can raise blood glucose levels and inhibit the effects of insulin.
9. If diagnosed with diabetes mellitus, check with a health care provider before beginning a vigorous exercise program. Often, insulin doses should be reduced or extra food should be ingested just prior to intense exercise.
10. If self-injecting insulin is used, follow all instructions provided by the health care provider carefully to avoid injury or infection.

Regarding Thyroid Medications

11. Because pulse rate is a good indicator of the effectiveness of thyroid medications, take it regularly. If the pulse rate consistently exceeds 100 or any other significant change is noted, contact the health care provider.
12. Because finding the correct dosage of thyroid hormone often takes several months, do not change the prescribed dose without being advised to do so by a health care provider.

SAFETY ALERT

Problems with Insulin Pens–OptiClik Injector Pen

A potential problem that can result in medication errors has been reported by the Institute for Safe Medication Practices (ISMP) involving the use of the OptiClik injector pen for administering insulin glargine or insulin glulisine. Patients who are left-handed could administer the wrong dose by using the pen with the dosing window viewed upside down and the needle facing to the right. Because an estimated 20% of people are left-handed, there are many opportunities for this error to occur. For example, when the needle is facing to the right (upside down), a dose of 52 units would look like 25 units, 12 units would look like 21 units, and 1 unit will appear to be 10 units. Nurses should be alert to this problem and emphasize to patients using this device that when dialing in a dose, they should make sure they are holding the pen so that the "OptiClik" printing on the pen can be read right-side-up.

Source: Institute for Safe Medication Practices. (2007).

CORE CONCEPTS SUMMARY

31.1 The endocrine system maintains homeostasis by using hormones as chemical messengers.

Hormones are secreted by endocrine glands in response to changes in the internal environment. The hormones act on their target cells to return the body to homeostasis. Negative feedback prevents the body from overresponding to internal changes.

31.2 Hormones are used as replacement therapy, as antineoplastics, and for their natural therapeutic effects.

Hormones are often given as replacement therapy to patients who are not able to secrete sufficient quantities of endogenous hormones. In high doses, several hormones may be used as antineoplastics. Hormones may also be used therapeutically to take advantage of their natural physiologic effects.

31.3 The hypothalamus and the pituitary gland secrete hormones that control other endocrine organs.

The hypothalamus secretes releasing hormones that signal the anterior pituitary gland to release its hormones. Pituitary hormones travel throughout the body to affect many other organs.

31.4 Insulin and glucagon are secreted by the pancreas.

The pancreas secretes insulin after a meal, when blood glucose levels are high. Insulin permits glucose to leave the blood and enter cells. Glucagon has effects opposite to those of insulin, causing glucose to leave tissues and enter the blood.

31.5 Type 1 diabetes is treated by dietary restrictions and insulin injections.

Type 1 diabetes is diagnosed in late childhood and is caused by a lack of insulin secretion by the pancreas. Parenteral insulin is provided and must be carefully timed to coincide with meals. Taking too much insulin or skipping meals may result in acute hypoglycemia. Untreated diabetes leads to serious long-term consequences.

31.6 Type 2 diabetes is controlled through lifestyle changes and oral hypoglycemic agents.

Type 2 diabetes is more common than type 1, occurs in older patients, and is primarily due to a lack of sensitivity of insulin receptors. Drug therapy starts with oral hypoglycemics and may proceed to insulin injections if the disease is not controlled appropriately.

31.7 The thyroid gland controls the basal metabolic rate and affects virtually every cell in the body.

The thyroid gland secretes thyroid hormone, which is essential for the growth and metabolism of cells in the body. Thyroid hormone is a combination of two different hormones, thyroxine and triiodothyronine, both of which require iodine for their synthesis.

31.8 Thyroid disorders may be treated by administering thyroid hormone or by decreasing the activity of the thyroid gland.

Hypothyroidism produces symptoms such as slowed body metabolism, slurred speech, bradycardia, weight gain, low body temperature, and intolerance to cold environments. Administration of thyroid hormone reverses these effects. Hyperthyroid patients exhibit the opposite symptoms. Hyperthyroidism may be treated with drugs that kill or inactivate thyroid cells.

31.9 Glucocorticoids are released during periods of stress and influence carbohydrate, lipid, and protein metabolism in most cells.

The adrenal cortex secretes glucocorticoids in response to stimulation by ACTH from the pituitary. Glucocorticoids affect the metabolism of nearly every cell in the body and have a potent anti-inflammatory effect.

31.10 Glucocorticoids are prescribed for adrenocortical insufficiency and a wide variety of other conditions.

Glucocorticoids are given to patients whose adrenal glands are unable to produce adequate amounts of these hormones and for a wide variety of other conditions. When used at high doses, oral therapy is often limited to 2 weeks because of the potential for producing Cushing's syndrome and adrenal atrophy.

31.11 Of the many pituitary and hypothalamic hormones, only a few have clinical applications as drugs.

Growth hormone, or somatotropin, is used to increase the height of children with growth hormone deficiencies. ADH, or vasopressin, increases water reabsorption in the kidney and is used to treat diabetes insipidus.

REVIEW QUESTIONS

The following questions are written in NCLEX-PN® style. Answer these questions to assess your knowledge of the chapter material, and go back and review any material that is not clear to you.

1. The patient is exhibiting hypoglycemia, fatigue, hypotension, anorexia, vomiting, and diarrhea. The nurse suspects:

1. Cushing's syndrome
2. Graves' disease
3. Adrenal insufficiency
4. Diabetes mellitus

2. Which of the following is not a symptom of diabetes?

1. Polyphagia
2. Polyuria
3. Polydipsia
4. Weight gain

3. The mechanism of action of oral hypoglycemic agents includes:

1. Decreased uptake and utilization of glucose by body cells
2. Stimulated insulin release from the pancreas
3. Increased insulin production by the pancreas
4. Decreased amount of insulin produced by the pancreas

4. The patient has a history of hypothyroidism and has been on levothyroxine (Synthroid) 250 mcg/day. The nurse recognizes the medication is being effective when:

1. The patient sleeps more hours per day
2. The patient's weight increases
3. The patient's pulse rate increases
4. The patient states she feels tired

5. The patient has been on methylprednisolone (Medrol) for an exacerbation of asthma. Which of the following instructions to the patient is of the highest priority?

1. "This medication may cause weight gain."
2. "Do not stop taking this medication abruptly."
3. "This medication can cause sleeplessness."
4. "This medication may cause restlessness."

6. Patients should be instructed to take oral glucocorticoids?

1. In the early morning hours
2. With lunch
3. With dinner
4. At bedtime

7. The patient with diabetes has decided to start an exercise program. What effect does exercise have on the body?

1. It increases the need for insulin.
2. It decreases the need for insulin.
3. The need for insulin is not affected.
4. Oral hypoglycemics may be required.

8. The patient has been started on desmopressin (DDAVP). The nurse understands the medication is effective when:

1. The patient's urinary output increases
2. The patient's blood pressure is within normal limits
3. The patient's blood sugar level is between 80 and 120 mg/dl
4. The patient's urinary output decreases

9. Glipizide (Glucotrol) should be administered:

1. Subcutaneously only
2. After meals
3. At bedtime
4. Just before breakfast

10. Insulin glargine (Lantus) should be administered:

1. Before meals
2. After meals
3. At bedtime
4. Before and after meals

CASE STUDY QUESTIONS

For questions 1–4, please refer to the following case study, and choose the correct answer from choices 1–4.

*M*r. Jones is a 35-year-old firefighter who smokes and is somewhat overweight. Over the last 5 years, he has begun to develop slightly elevated blood pressure as determined by annual physical exams. He feels like he should lose weight and is concerned about his energy level. He has always felt "fit" despite the fact that he smokes, but recently he has begun to feel sluggish and is wondering whether his physical condition is changing. He thinks to himself, "Maybe I'm just getting older." At his last visit to the doctor, laboratory results revealed fasting blood glucose levels above 126

mg/dl. His blood pressure was 150/90 mmHg. Mr. Jones has not been taking medications for any reported disorder.

1. The most likely reason for the slightly elevated blood pressure in this instance is:

1. Hypertension, a common condition associated with smokers
2. Vascular damage brought on by hypertension, a common problem with the onset of diabetes
3. High stress levels associated with the profession of firefighting
4. Hypertension caused by being overweight

2. Noninsulin-dependent diabetes mellitus (NIDDM) or type 2 diabetes is a condition treated by a group of oral hypoglycemic agents that stimulate the pancreas to produce or release insulin. These agents are called:

1. Sulfonylureas
2. Biguanides
3. Alpha-glucosidase inhibitors
4. Thiazolidinediones

3. As a health care provider, which of the following words of advice would you give to Mr. Jones when considering the adverse effects of oral hypoglycemic agents?

1. "Be sure to take your medication after the last meal of the day."

2. "Ingestion of alcohol will not matter, so go ahead . . . a few beers won't hurt you."
3. "Although rare, lactic acidosis may occur with some medications if you don't take them properly."
4. "You are relatively safe if you start taking antihypertensive medication at the same time . . . don't worry."

4. Type 2 diabetes can be controlled by:

1. Lifestyle changes
2. Both hypoglycemic agents and insulin
3. Choice 1 or choice 2
4. Choice 1 and hypoglycemic agents only

FURTHER STUDY

- High levels of ketoacids seen in diabetics change the pH of the blood, producing acidosis, as discussed in Chapter 23 ⦾.

- Chapter 32 ⦾ discusses reproductive hormones.

- Hormones used as antineoplastics are detailed in Chapter 27 ⦾.

- Aldosterone release affects the balance of fluids, electrolytes, and minerals in the bloodstream, as discussed in Chapter 23 ⦾.

- The anti-inflammatory effects of glucocorticoids are discussed in more depth in Chapters 24 and 28 ⦾.

- Prolactin and oxytocin are presented in Chapter 32 ⦾.

- Drugs that block the renin-angiotensin pathway also inhibit aldosterone secretion and are used to treat hypertension (see Chapter 17 ⦾) and heart failure (see Chapter 18 ⦾).

PEARSON
EXPLORE **mynursingkit**™

MyNursingKit is your one stop for online chapter review materials and resources. Prepare for success with additional NCLEX®-style practice questions, interactive assignments and activities, web links, animations and videos, and more!

Register your access code from the front of your book at
www.mynursingkit.com

32

Drugs for Disorders and Conditions of the Reproductive System

CORE CONCEPTS

32.1 Testosterone, estrogen, and progesterone are the primary hormones contributing to the growth, health, and maintenance of the reproductive system.

32.2 Low doses of estrogens and progestins are used for contraception.

32.3 Estrogens have been used for replacement therapy and in the treatment of prostate cancer.

32.4 Progestins are prescribed for dysfunctional uterine bleeding.

32.5 Oxytocin and tocolytics are drugs used to influence uterine contractions.

32.6 Androgens are used to treat hypogonadism or delayed puberty in men and breast cancer in women.

32.7 Erectile dysfunction is a common disorder successfully treated with drug therapy.

32.8 In its early stages, benign prostatic hyperphasia may be treated successfully with drug therapy.

DRUG SNAPSHOT

The following drugs are discussed in this chapter:

DRUG CLASSES	DRUG PROFILES
Oral Contraceptives	
Estrogen-progestin combinations	**Pr** ethinyl estradiol with norethindrone (Ortho-Novum 1/35)
Progestin-only drugs	
Emergency contraceptives	
Hormone Replacement Therapy	**Pr** conjugated estrogens (Premarin) and conjugated estrogens with medroxyprogesterone (Prempro)
Drugs for Dysfunctional Uterine Bleeding	**Pr** medroxyprogesterone (Prempro)
Uterine Stimulants and Relaxants	**Pr** oxytocin (Pitocin)
Drugs for Male Hypogonadism	**Pr** Androgens testosterone base (Andro)
Drugs for Erectile Dysfunction	**Pr** sildenafil (Viagra)
Drugs for Benign Prostatic Hyperplasia	**Pr** finasteride (Proscar)

After reading this chapter, the student should be able to:

1. Identify and describe the primary functions of the steroid sex hormones.
2. Explain the mechanisms by which estrogen and progestins prevent conception.
3. Describe the role of drug therapy in the treatment of menopausal and postmenopausal symptoms.
4. Identify the role of the steroid sex hormones in the chemotherapy of cancer.
5. Describe the uses of progestins in the therapy of dysfunctional uterine bleeding.
6. Compare and contrast oxytocin and tocolytics in antepartum and postpartum treatment.

7. Explain the role of androgens in the treatment of hypogonadism.
8. Describe the role of drug therapy in the treatment of erectile dysfunction and benign prostatic hyperplasia (BPH).
9. For each of the classes in the Drug Snapshot, identify representative drugs and explain their mechanisms of action, primary actions, and important adverse effects.
10. Categorize drugs used in the treatment of reproductive disorders and conditions based on their classifications and mechanisms of action.

KEY TERMS

amenorrhea (ah-men-oh-REE-ah) *578*

androgens (AN-droh-jens) *571*

antepartum (an-teh-PART-um) *583*

benign prostatic hypertrophy (BPH) (bee-NINE pros-TAT-ik hy-PURR-tro-fee) *586*

breakthrough bleeding *578*

corpus cavernosum (KORP-us kav-ver-NOH-sum) *586*

dysfunctional uterine bleeding *578*

endometrium (en-doh-MEE-tree-um) *571*

estrogen (ES-troh-jen) *570*

follicle-stimulating hormone (FSH) *571*

hypogonadism (hy-poh-GO-nad-izm) *583*

hysterectomy (hiss-ter-EK-toh-mee) *578*

impotence (IM-poh-tense) *585*

libido (lih-BEE-do) *584*

luteinizing hormones (LH) (LEW-ten-iz-ing) *571*

menopause (MEN-oh-paws) *576*

menorrhea (men-oh-REE-uh) *578*

oligomenorrhea (ol-ego-men-oh-REE-uh) *578*

ovulation (ov-you-LAY-shun) *571*

oxytocin (ox-ee-TOH-sin) *582*

postpartum (post-PART-um) *583*

progesterone (pro-JESS-ter-own) *570*

prolactin (pro-LAK-tin) *582*

tocolytic (toh-koh-LIT-ik) *583*

virilization (veer-you-lih-ZAY-shun) *584*

The male and female reproductive systems are regulated by a small number of hormones that are responsible for the growth and maintenance of the reproductive organs. These hormones can be supplemented with natural or synthetic hormones to achieve a variety of therapeutic goals, ranging from replacement therapy to prevention of pregnancy to milk production. This chapter examines drugs used to treat disorders and conditions of the reproductive system.

CORE CONCEPT 32.1

Testosterone, estrogen, and progesterone are the primary hormones contributing to the growth, health, and maintenance of the reproductive system.

estro = *desire*
gen = *producing/forming*

The sex hormones are steroids synthesized from cholesterol. Although the male and female gonads produce the vast majority of sex hormones, the adrenal cortex also secretes small amounts. Male and female hormones are present in both sexes.

The ovaries synthesize the female sex hormones **estrogen** and **progesterone**. *Estrogen* is actually a generic term for three different female sex hormones: estradiol, estrone, and estriol. Es-

Fast Facts Reproductive Conditions and Disorders

- Erectile dysfunction affects 10 to 15 million Americans—about one man in four older than age 65.
- BPH affects 50% of men older than age 60, and 90% of men older than age 80.
- There is a wide range of ages when women reach menopause: 8% women will stop menstruating before age 40, and 5% will continue beyond age 60.
- About half the cases of dysfunctional uterine bleeding are diagnosed in women older than 45; however, 20% of cases occur in those younger than 20.
- Compared to just 10 years ago, oral contraceptives now contain two to four times less estrogen.
- The primary reason why a woman may become pregnant while on oral contraceptives is skipping a dose.
- A nonsmoking woman aged 25 to 29 has a 2 in 100,000 chance of dying from complications due to oral contraceptives. By comparison, the risk of a woman in this age group dying in an automobile accident is 74 in 100,000.
- Oral contraceptives have more benefits than simply contraception. It is estimated that each year they prevent:

  51,000 cases of pelvic inflammatory disease
  9,900 hospitalizations for ectopic pregnancy
  27,000 cases of iron-deficiency anemia
  20,000 hospitalizations for certain types of nonmalignant breast disease

trogen is responsible for the maturation of the reproductive organs and for the appearance of the secondary sex characteristics in women. Estrogen also has numerous metabolic effects on nonreproductive tissues, including the brain, kidneys, blood vessels, and skin. For example, estrogen helps to maintain low blood cholesterol levels and facilitates calcium uptake by bones to help maintain proper bone density (see Chapter 33 ⊂⊃). At about age 50 to 55, the ovaries stop secreting estrogen as women enter menopause.

The ovaries also secrete a class of hormones called *progestins,* the most common of which is progesterone. Progesterone, in combination with estrogen, promotes breast development and the monthly changes in the ovaries and uterus known as the menstrual cycle. When progesterone levels fall sharply at the end of the cycle, a portion of the inner lining of the uterus, the **endometrium**, is shed, and menstrual bleeding occurs. During pregnancy, progesterone secreted by the placenta maintains a healthy endometrium for the fetus and prevents premature labor contractions.

Androgens are male sex hormones. The testes secrete testosterone, the primary androgen responsible for maturation of the male sex organs and the secondary sex characteristics of men. Unlike the cyclic secretion of estrogen and progesterone in women, the secretion of testosterone is relatively constant in adult men. Like estrogen, testosterone has metabolic effects in tissues outside the reproductive system. Of particular note is its ability to build muscle mass, which contributes to the difference in muscle strength and body composition between men and women.

andro = *male*
gen = *producing/forming*

The ovaries and testes are regulated by the pituitary hormones **follicle-stimulating hormone (FSH)** and **luteinizing hormone (LH)**. FSH regulates sperm or egg production. LH in the female triggers the release of the egg, a process known as **ovulation**, and promotes the secretion of estrogen and progesterone by the ovary. In males, LH—sometimes called *interstitial cell-binding hormone*—regulates the production of testosterone. The relationships between the hypothalamus, pituitary, and the reproductive hormones are illustrated in Figure 32.1 ■.

CONTRACEPTION

Low doses of estrogens and progestins are used for contraception.

CORE CONCEPT 32.2

The most widespread pharmacologic use of the female sex hormones is for the prevention of pregnancy. When used appropriately, they are nearly 100% effective. Most oral contraceptives contain a combination of estrogen and progestin, although a few contain only progestin. The most common estrogen used in these preparations is ethinyl estradiol, and the most common progestin is norethindrone.

FIGURE 32.1

Control of the
reproductive hormones

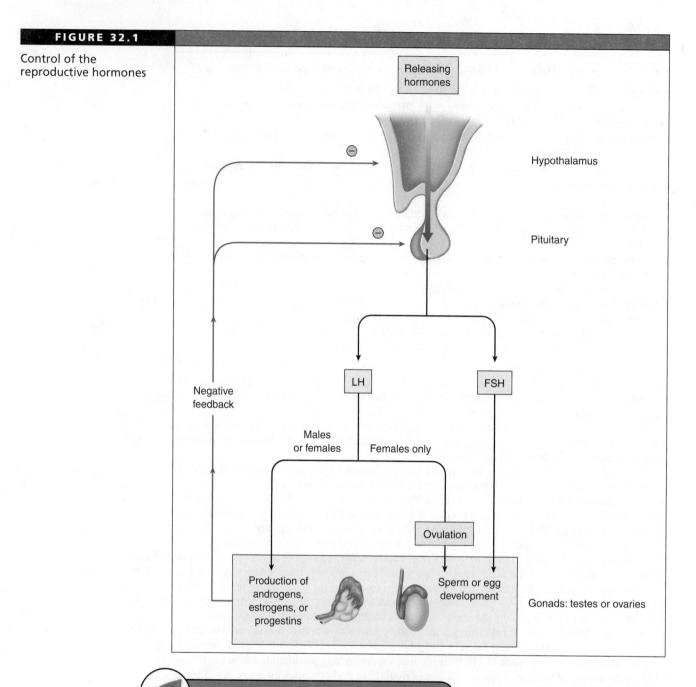

NATURAL THERAPIES

Dong Quai for Premenstrual Syndrome

Since antiquity, dong quai has been recognized as an important herb for women's health in Chinese medicine. Obtained from *Angelica sinensis,* a small plant that grows in China, dong quai contains a number of active substances that are said to exert analgesic, antipyretic, anti-inflammatory, and antispasmodic activity. The dried root is available as capsules, tablets, teas, and tinctures.

The reproductive effects of dong quai may be due to active substances that have estrogenic activity. These estrogenic ingredients act as a "uterine tonic" to improve the overall hormonal balance of the female reproductive system. dong quai is used to treat the symptoms of premenstrual syndrome, as well as other disorders such as irregular menstrual periods or painful menstruation.

Dong quai has also been used for its cardiovascular effects. It is claimed to increase circulation by dilating blood vessels. Because some of the active ingredients of Dong quai may have anticoagulant activity, patients taking warfarin (Coumadin) or high doses of aspirin should not take the herb without notifying their health care practitioner.

A wide variety of oral contraceptive preparations is available, they differ in dose and type of estrogen and progestin. Selection of a specific formulation is individualized to each patient and determined by which drug gives the best contraceptive protection with the fewest adverse effects. Table 32.1 lists some of the oral contraceptives and their compositions. As shown in Figure 32.2 ■, special packaging assists the patient in taking this medication on a daily basis.

TABLE 32.1   Selected Oral Contraceptives

TRADE NAME	ESTROGEN	PROGESTIN
MONOPHASIC		
Alesse	ethinyl estradiol; 20 mcg	levonorgestrel; 0.1 mg
Desogen	ethinyl estradiol; 30 mcg	desogestrel; 0.15 mg
Loestrin Fe 1.5/30	ethinyl estradiol; 30 mcg	norethindrone; 1.5 mg
Lo-Ovral	ethinyl estradiol; 30 mcg	norgestrel; 0.3 mg
Ortho-Cept	ethinyl estradiol; 30 mcg	desogestrel; 0.15 mg
Ortho-Cyclen	ethinyl estradiol; 35 mcg	norgestimate; 0.25 mg
Pr Ortho-Novum 1/35	ethinyl estradiol; 35 mcg	norethindrone; 1 mg
Yasmin 28	ethinyl estradiol; 30 mcg	drospirenone; 3.0 mg
Zovia 1/50-21 and 28	ethinyl estradiol; 50 mcg	ethynodiol diacetate; 1 mg
BIPHASIC		
Mircette	ethinyl estradiol; 20 mcg for 21 days; 10 mcg for 5 days	desogestrel, 0.15 mg for 21 days
Ortho-Novum 10/11	ethinyl estradiol; 35 mcg ethinyl estradiol; 35 mcg	norethindrone; 0.5 mg (Phase 1) norethindrone; 1.0 mg (Phase 2)
TRIPHASIC		
Ortho-Novum 7/7/7	ethinyl estradiol; 35 mcg ethinyl estradiol; 35 mcg ethinyl estradiol; 35 mcg	norethindrone; 0.5 mg (Phase 1) norethindrone; 0.75 mg (Phase 2) norethindrone; 1.0 mg (Phase 3)
Ortho-Tri-Cyclen	ethinyl estradiol; 35 mcg ethinyl estradiol; 35 mcg ethinyl estradiol; 35 mcg	norgestimate; 0.5 mg (Phase 1) norgestimate; 0.75 mg (Phase 2) norgestimate; 1.0 mg (Phase 3)
Tri-Levlen	ethinyl estradiol; 30 mcg ethinyl estradiol; 40 mcg ethinyl estradiol; 30 mcg	levonorgestrel; 0.05 mg (Phase 1) levonorgestrel; 0.075 mg (Phase 2) levonorgestrel; 0.125 mg (Phase 3)
Tri-Nessa	ethinyl estradiol; 35 mcg ethinyl estradiol; 35 mcg ethinyl estradiol; 35 mcg	norgestimate; 0.180 mg (Phase 1) norgestimate; 0.215 mg (Phase 2) norgestimate; 0.250 mg (Phase 3)
Triphasil	ethinyl estradiol; 30 mcg ethinyl estradiol; 40 mcg ethinyl estradiol; 30 mcg	norgestrel; 0.05 mg (Phase 1) norgestrel; 0.075 mg (Phase 2) norgestrel; 1.25 mg (Phase 3)
PROGESTIN ONLY		
Micronor	None	norethindrone; 0.35 mg
Nor-Q.D	None	norethindrone; 0.35 mg
Ovrette	None	norgestrel; 0.075 mg
EMERGENCY CONTRACEPTIVE		
Plan B (two tablets)	None	levonorgestrel; 0.75 mcg

Photograph of an oral contraceptive showing the daily doses and the different formulation taken in the last 7 days of the 28-day cycle

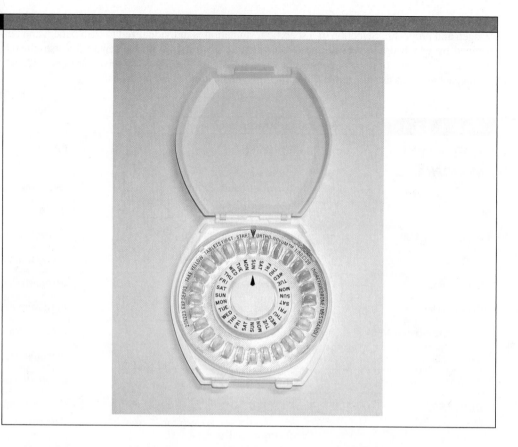

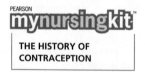

THE HISTORY OF CONTRACEPTION

The estrogen-progestin oral contraceptives prevent ovulation, which is required for conception to occur. These hormones act by providing negative feedback to the pituitary gland that shuts down secretion of LH and FSH. Without these pituitary hormones, the egg cannot mature, and ovulation is prevented. The estrogen-progestin agents also make the lining of the uterus less favorable to receiving an embryo.

There are three basic estrogen-progestin formulations: monophasic, biphasic, and triphasic. The most common is the monophasic, which delivers a constant amount of estrogen and progestin throughout the menstrual cycle. In biphasic agents, the amount of estrogen in each pill remains constant, but the amount of progestin is increased toward the end of the menstrual cycle to better nourish the uterine lining. In triphasic formulations, the amounts of both estrogen and progestin vary in three distinct phases during the 28-day cycle.

The progestin-only oral contraceptives prevent pregnancy primarily by producing a thick, viscous mucus at the entrance to the uterus that prevents penetration by sperm. Progestin-only agents are less effective than estrogen-progestin combinations and produce a higher incidence of menstrual irregularities. Because of this, they are generally reserved for women who are at high risk for adverse effects from estrogen.

Several long-term formulations of oral contraceptives are available. A deep intramuscular injection of medroxyprogesterone acetate (Depo-Provera) provides 3 months of contraceptive protection. Ortho-Evra is a transdermal patch containing ethinyl estradiol and norelgestromin that is worn on the skin. The patch is changed every 7 days for the first 3 weeks, followed by no patch during week 4. NuvaRing is a 2-inch-diameter ring containing estrogen and progestin that is inserted into the vagina to provide 3 weeks of contraceptive protection. The ring is removed during week 4, and a new ring is inserted during the first week of the next menstrual cycle. Mirena consists of a polyethylene cylinder placed in the uterus to release levonorgestrel. This drug acts locally to prevent conception over 5 years. The effectiveness of these long-term formulations is similar to the oral contraceptives. They offer a major advantage for women who are likely to forget their daily pill or who prefer a greater ease of use.

NURSING PROCESS FOCUS

Patients Receiving Oral Contraceptive Therapy

ASSESSMENT

Prior to administration:
- Obtain a health history (physical/mental), including cigarette smoking
- Obtain a drug history to determine possible drug interactions and allergies
- Assess cardiovascular status, including hypertension, history of myocardial infarction (MI), cerebrovascular accident (CVA), and thromboembolic disease
- Determine if the patient is pregnant or lactating

POTENTIAL NURSING DIAGNOSES

- Deficient Knowledge related to drug therapy.
- Nausea related to adverse effects of drug therapy.
- Noncompliance related to medication regimen.

PLANNING: PATIENT GOALS AND EXPECTED OUTCOMES

The patient will:
- Report effective birth control
- Demonstrate an understanding of the drug's action by accurately describing drug adverse effects and precautions
- Take the medication exactly as ordered to prevent pregnancy
- Immediately report effects such as symptoms of thrombophlebitis, difficulty breathing, visual disturbances, and severe headache

IMPLEMENTATION

Interventions and (Rationales)	Patient Education/Discharge Planning
■ Monitor for the development of breast or other estrogen-dependent tumors. (Estrogen may cause tumor growth or proliferation.)	■ Instruct the patient to immediately report if a first-degree relative is diagnosed with any estrogen-dependent tumor.
■ Monitor for thrombophlebitis or other thromboembolic disease. (Estrogen predisposes to thromboembolic disorders by increasing levels of clotting factors.)	■ Instruct the patient to immediately report pain in the calves, limited movement in the legs, dyspnea, sudden severe chest pain, headache, seizures, anxiety, or fear.
■ Monitor for cardiac disorders and hypertension. (These drugs increase blood levels of angiotensin and aldosterone, which increase blood pressure.)	Instruct the patient to: ■ Report immediately signs of possible cardiac problems such as chest pain, dyspnea, edema, tachycardia or bradycardia, and palpitations ■ Monitor blood pressure regularly ■ Report symptoms of hypertension such as headache, flushing, fatigue, dizziness, palpitations, tachycardia, and nosebleeds
■ Encourage the patient not to smoke. (Smoking increases risk of thromboembolic disease.)	Instruct the patient to: ■ Be aware that the combination of oral contraceptives and smoking greatly increases risk of cardiovascular disease, especially MI ■ Be aware that the risk increases with age (>35) and with number of cigarettes smoked (15 or more/day)
■ Monitor blood and urine glucose levels. (These drugs increase serum glucose levels.)	■ Instruct the patient to monitor urine and blood glucose regularly and contact the health care provider if hyperglycemia or hypoglycemia occurs.

continued . . .

NURSING PROCESS FOCUS *(continued)*

Interventions and (Rationales)

- Monitor the patient's knowledge level of proper administration. (Incorrect use may lead to pregnancy.)

- Encourage compliance with follow-up treatment. (Follow-up is necessary to avoid serious adverse effects.)

Patient Education/Discharge Planning

Instruct the patient to:
- Discontinue the medication and notify the health care provider if significant bleeding occurs at midcycle
- Take the missed dose as soon as remembered or take two tablets the next day; if three consecutive tablets are missed, begin a new compact of tablets, starting 7 days after the last tablet was taken
- Contact the health care provider if two consecutive periods are missed because pregnancy may have occurred

Instruct the patient to:
- Schedule annual Pap smears
- Perform breast self-exams (BSEs) monthly and obtain routine mammograms as recommended by the health care provider

EVALUATION OF OUTCOME CRITERIA

Evaluate the effectiveness of drug therapy by confirming that patient goals and expected outcomes have been met (see "Planning").

See Table 32.1 for a list of drugs to which these nursing actions apply.

MENOPAUSE

meno = *month*
pause = *cessation*

Menopause is the permanent cessation of menses, resulting in a lack of estrogen secretion by the ovaries. Menopause is neither a disease nor a disorder but a natural consequence of aging that is often accompanied by a number of unpleasant symptoms. The potential consequences of estrogen loss related to menopause are listed in Table 32.2.

Over the past 20 years, health care providers have commonly prescribed hormone replacement therapy (HRT) to treat unpleasant symptoms of menopause and related osteoporotic bone fractures. However, studies have raised questions regarding the safety of HRT for these conditions. Data suggest that patients may have an increased risk of coronary artery disease, stroke, and venous thromboembolism. Women are now encouraged to discuss alternatives with their health care provider, as discussed in Chapter 33 . Undoubtedly, research will continue to provide

TABLE 32.2	Potential Consequences of Estrogen Loss Related to Menopause
Early menopausal symptoms	Mood disturbances, depression, irritability
	Insomnia
	Hot flashes
	Irregular menstrual cycles
	Headaches
Mid-menopausal symptoms	Vaginal atrophy, increased infections, painful intercourse
	Skin atrophy
	Stress urinary incontinence
	Sexual disinterest
Postmenopausal conditions	Cardiovascular disease
	Osteoporosis
	Alzheimer's-like dementia
	Colon cancer

valuable information on the long-term effects of HRT. Until then, the choice of HRT to treat menopausal symptoms will remain a highly individualized one between the patient and her health care provider.

In addition to their use as oral contraceptives, estrogens are used to reduce unpleasant symptoms associated with menopause and to treat certain cancers. Higher doses are used for these conditions; thus, more adverse effects are observed.

Estrogens have been used for replacement therapy and in the treatment of prostate cancer.

CORE CONCEPT 32.3

When estrogen secretion becomes deficient, as with menopause or with irregular or painful menstrual cycles, replacement drug therapy may be indicated. In addition, surgical removal of the ovaries usually requires estrogen supplementation because the adrenal glands cannot supply sufficient quantities of estrogen. Some of the estrogen and estrogen-progesterone combinations used for replacement therapy are listed in Table 32.3.

DRUG PROFILE: ℗ *Ethinyl Estradiol with Norethindrone (Ortho-Novum 1/35)*

Therapeutic Class: Ovulation inhibitor, luteinizing hormone (LH) inhibitor
Pharmacologic Class: Oral contraceptive

Actions and Uses:

Ortho-Novum is typical of the monophasic oral contraceptives, containing fixed amounts of estrogen and progesterone for 21 days followed by placebo tablets for 7 days. It is nearly 100% effective at preventing conception. If a dose is missed, the patient should take the dose as soon as possible, or take two tablets the next day. If two consecutive doses are missed, conception is possible, and the patient should use other birth control methods until the regular dosing schedule is reestablished. Ortho-Novum should not be continued if two consecutive menstrual periods are missed or the woman otherwise suspects she is pregnant. Ortho-Novum is also available as a biphasic and triphasic preparation.

Adverse Effects and Interactions:

Like most oral contraceptives, Ortho-Novum can increase the risks of thromboembolic disease: the potential for blood clots, hemorrhage, pulmonary embolism, or stroke. This is particularly true in smokers, who carry a five times greater risk of a fatal MI than nonsmokers. Because of this risk, Ortho-Novum is contraindicated in women with a history of stroke, MI, or other serious vascular disease. It should be used with caution in women with hypertension because it has the potential to raise blood pressure. Bleeding in the early or mid-menstrual cycle, known as *breakthrough bleeding,* is relatively common and may be severe enough to require a medication change in some women. Any unusual breast lumps should be reported immediately to the health care practitioner; estrogen stimulates certain types of pre-existing breast cancer.

Ethinyl estradiol interacts with many drugs. For example, rifampin, some antibiotics, barbiturates, anticonvulsants, and antifungals decrease efficacy of oral contraceptives, so the risks of breakthrough bleeding and pregnancy are higher. Ortho-Novum may also decrease the effects of oral anticoagulants.

Use cautiously with herbal supplements. For example, breakthrough bleeding has been reported in women taking St. John's wort at the same time.

Mechanism in Action:

Ethinyl estradiol with norethindrone is a monophasic oral contraceptive. This preparation prevents ovulation by negative feedback control targeted at the hypothalamic-pituitary axis. When the right combination of estrogens and progestins are present in the bloodstream, the release of FSH and LH is inhibited. LH is the hormone responsible for ovulation.

Refer to MyNursingKit for a Nursing Process Focus specific to this drug.

TABLE 32.3	Selected Estrogens and Progestins Used for Hormone Replacement Therapy	
DRUG	**ROUTE AND ADULT DOSE**	**REMARKS**
ESTROGENS		
estradiol (Estrace, Estraderm)	PO; 1–2 mg/day Transdermal patch, 50–100 mcg applied twice weekly	Available as vaginal cream and as a transdermal patch; also for breast and prostate cancer and to relieve postpartum breast engorgement
estradiol cypionate (depGynogen, Depogen)	IM; 1–5 mg every 3–4 weeks	Menopausal and postmenopausal symptoms
estradiol valerate (Delestrogen, Duragen-10, Valergen)	IM; 10–20 mg every 4 weeks	Also for breast cancer and to relieve postpartum breast engorgement
Pr estrogen, conjugated (Premarin)	PO; 0.3–1.25 mg/day for 21 days each month	Also for postcoital contraception and breast cancer
estropipate (Ogen)	PO; 0.75–6 mg/day for 21 days each month	Also for female hypogonadism and palliative treatment of prostate cancer; available as a vaginal cream
PROGESTINS		
Pr medroxyprogesterone (Prempo)	PO; 5–10 mg/day on days 1–12 of menstrual cycle	Also for endometrial and renal carcinoma; IM form available
norethindrone (Micronor, Nor-Q.D)	PO; 0.35 mg/day beginning on day 1 of menstrual cycle	Also for endometriosis
norethindrone acetate	PO; 5 mg/day for 2 weeks; increase by 2.5 mg/day every 2 weeks (max: 15 mg/day)	Also for endometriosis
progesterone micronized (Prometrium)	PO; 400 mg at bedtime for 10 days	IM and rectal forms available; intrauterine insert available for contraception

High doses of estrogens have also been used to treat prostate and breast cancer. Prostate cancer is usually dependent on androgens for growth, and administration of estrogens will suppress androgen secretion. As an antineoplastic hormone, estrogen is rarely used alone: it is one of many agents used in combination for the chemotherapy of cancer, as discussed in Chapter 27 ⚭ .

UTERINE ABNORMALITIES

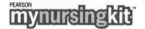

PSYCHOLOGICAL AND PHARMACOLOGICAL ASPECTS OF MENOPAUSE

Dysfunctional uterine bleeding is a condition in which hemorrhage occurs on a noncyclic basis or in abnormal amounts. It is the health problem most frequently reported by women and a common reason for **hysterectomy** or surgical removal of the uterus. Types of dysfunctional uterine bleeding include the following conditions:

- **Amenorrhea**—absence of menstruation
- **Oligomenorrhea**—infrequent menstruation
- **Menorrhea**—prolonged or excessive menstruation
- **Breakthrough bleeding**—hemorrhage between menstrual periods
- **Postmenopausal bleeding**—uterine hemorrhage after menopause

DRUG PROFILE: Ⓟ Conjugated Estrogens (Premarin)
and Conjugated Estrogens with Medroxyprogesterone (Prempro)

Therapeutic Class: Menopausal hormone therapy

Pharmacologic Class: Hormone replacement therapy, estrogen, and estrogen–progestin combination

Actions and Uses:

Premarin contains a mixture of different estrogens. It exerts several positive metabolic effects, including an increase in bone mass and a reduction in low-density lipoprotein (LDL) cholesterol. It may also increase the risk of coronary artery disease and colon cancer. When used as postmenopausal replacement therapy, it is typically combined with a progestin, as in Prempro.

Adverse Effects and Interactions:

Adverse effects from Prempro or Premarin include nausea, fluid retention, breast tenderness, and weight gain. As with oral contraceptives, estrogens are contraindicated in women with a history of thromboembolic disease.

The risks and benefits of replacement therapy have been discussed for a number of years. It is believed that the long-term use of estrogen increases uterine and ovarian cancers. Whether or not estrogen causes breast cancer is being investigated. Adding a progestin exerts a protective effect by countering the effects of estrogen on the growth and proliferation of the endometrial lining. Unfortunately, studies have suggested that although progestins protect against uterine cancer, they may increase the risk of breast cancer following long-term use. The risks of adverse effects increase in women older than age 35. Conjugated estrogens are a category X drug and should not be taken during a known or suspected pregnancy.

Drug interactions include decreased effect of tamoxifen, enhanced corticosteroid effects, and decreased effects of anticoagulants, especially warfarin. The effects of estrogen may be decreased if taken with barbiturates or rifampin, and there is a possible increased effect of tricyclic antidepressants if taken with estrogens.

Use cautiously with herbal supplements. Red clover and black cohosh may interfere with estrogen therapy. Effects of estrogen may be enhanced if combined with ginseng.

Refer to MyNursingKit for a Nursing Process Focus specific to this drug.

NURSING PROCESS FOCUS

Patients Receiving Hormone Replacement Therapy

ASSESSMENT

Prior to administration:
- Obtain a complete health history (physical/mental), including personal or familial history of breast cancer, gallbladder disease, diabetes mellitus, and liver or kidney disease
- Obtain a drug history to determine possible drug interactions and allergies
- Assess cardiovascular status, including hypertension, and history of MI, CVA, and thromboembolic disease
- Determine if the patient is pregnant or lactating

POTENTIAL NURSING DIAGNOSES

- Excess Fluid Volume related to edema secondary to adverse effect of drug.
- Ineffective Tissue Perfusion related to development of thrombophlebitis, pulmonary embolism, or cerebral embolism.

continued . . .

NURSING PROCESS FOCUS *(continued)*

PLANNING: PATIENT GOALS AND EXPECTED OUTCOMES

The patient will:
- Report relief from symptoms of menopause
- Demonstrate an understanding of the drug's action by accurately describing drug adverse effects and precautions
- Immediately report such effects as symptoms of thrombophlebitis, difficulty breathing, visual disturbances, severe headache, and seizure activity

IMPLEMENTATION

Interventions and (Rationales)	Patient Education/Discharge Planning
■ Monitor for thromboembolic disease. (Estrogen increases risk for thromboembolism.)	■ Instruct the patient to report shortness of breath, feeling of heaviness, chest pain, severe headache, warmth, or swelling in the affected part, usually the legs or pelvis.
■ Monitor for abnormal uterine bleeding. (If an undiagnosed tumor is present, these drugs can increase its size and cause uterine bleeding.)	■ Instruct the patient to report excessive uterine bleeding or that which occurs between menstruations.
■ Monitor breast health. (Estrogens promote the growth of certain breast cancers.)	■ Instruct the patient to have regular breast exams, perform monthly BSE, and obtain routine mammograms, as recommended by the health care provider.
■ Monitor for vision changes. (These drugs may worsen myopia or astigmatism and cause intolerance of contact lenses.)	Instruct the patient to: ■ Obtain regular eye exams during HRT ■ Report changes in vision ■ Report any difficulty in wearing contact lenses
■ Encourage the patient not to smoke. (Smoking increases risk of cardiovascular disease.)	■ Instruct the patient to avoid smoking and participate in smoking cessation programs, if necessary.
■ Encourage the patient to avoid caffeine. (Estrogens and caffeine may lead to increased central nervous system [CNS] stimulation.)	Instruct the patient to: ■ Restrict caffeine consumption ■ Recognize common foods that contain caffeine: coffee, tea, carbonated beverages, chocolate, certain over-the-counter (OTC) medications ■ Report unusual nervousness, anxiety, and insomnia
■ Monitor glucose levels. (Estrogens may increase blood glucose levels.)	Instruct the patient to: ■ Monitor blood and urine glucose frequently, if diabetic ■ Report any consistent changes in blood glucose
■ Monitor for seizure activity. (Estrogen-induced fluid retention may increase risk of seizures.)	■ Instruct the patient to be alert for possibility of seizures, even at night, and report any seizure-type symptoms.
■ Monitor the patient's understanding and proper self-administration. (Improper administration may increase incidence of adverse effects.)	Instruct the patient to: ■ Administer proper dose, form, and frequency of medication ■ Take with food to decrease gastrointestinal (GI) irritation ■ Take daily dose at bedtime to decrease occurrence of adverse effects ■ Document menstruation and any problems that occur

EVALUATION OF OUTCOME CRITERIA

Evaluate the effectiveness of drug therapy by confirming that patient goals and expected outcomes have been met (see "Planning").

See Table 32.3 for a list of drugs to which these nursing actions apply.

Progestins are prescribed for dysfunctional uterine bleeding.

Besides being used in oral contraceptives, progestins are prescribed for various uterine abnormalities. They are occasionally used for specific cancers in combination with other antineoplastics.

The function of natural progesterone is to prepare the uterus for implantation of the embryo and pregnancy. If implantation does not occur, levels of progesterone fall dramatically and menses begins. If pregnancy occurs, the ovaries continue to secrete progesterone until the placenta develops sufficiently to begin producing the hormone.

The noncontraceptive indications for progesterone include the treatment of various uterine disorders. Dysfunctional uterine bleeding is often caused by a hormonal imbalance between estrogen and progesterone. While estrogen increases the thickness of the endometrium, bleeding occurs sporadically unless balanced by an adequate amount of progesterone secretion. Administration of a progestin in a pattern starting 5 days after the onset of menses and continuing for the next 20 days can sometimes help to establish a normal, monthly cyclic pattern. Oral contraceptives may also be prescribed for this disorder.

Progestins are occasionally prescribed for the treatment of metastatic endometrial carcinoma. In these cases, they are used for palliation, usually in combination with other antineoplastics. Selected progestins and their dosages are listed in Table 32.3.

hyster = *womb or uterus*
ectomy = *excision*
a = *lack of*
dys = *abnormal*
oligo = *scanty*
meno = *month*
rhagia = *excessive*
rhea = *flow*

Concept Review   32.1

■ Why is a progestin usually prescribed along with estrogen in oral contraceptives and when treating postmenopausal symptoms?

DRUG PROFILE: ℗ *Medroxyprogesterone (Prempro)*

Therapeutic Class: Drug for the treatment of endometriosis and abnormal uterine bleeding, antineoplastic
Pharmacologic Class: Inhibitor of endometrial proliferation, progestin

Actions and Uses:

Medroxyprogesterone is a synthetic progestin with a long duration of action. Like its natural counterpart, the primary target tissue for medroxyprogesterone is the endometrium of the uterus. It inhibits the negative effect of estrogen on the uterus, thus restoring normal hormonal balance. When used for dysfunctional uterine bleeding, it is typically administered for 5 to 10 days. Three to seven days after discontinuation of the drug, withdrawal bleeding occurs. The medication is often timed so that the withdrawal bleeding occurs during the estimated normal menses time. Several cycles of drug administration may be required to restore normal cyclic function. Medroxyprogesterone may also be given IM for the palliation of metastatic uterine or renal carcinoma.

Adverse Effects and Interactions:

Medroxyprogesterone is a category X drug and should be discontinued if pregnancy is suspected or confirmed. The most common adverse effects are breakthrough bleeding and breast tenderness. The most serious adverse effects relate to thromboembolic disease.

Serum levels of medroxyprogesterone are decreased by aminoglutethimide, barbiturates, primidone, rifampin, rifabutin, and topiramate.

Use cautiously with herbal supplements. For example, St. John's wort may cause intermenstrual bleeding and loss of effectiveness.

 Refer to MyNursingKit for a Nursing Process Focus specific to this drug.

LABOR AND BREASTFEEDING

Oxytocin and tocolytics are drugs used to influence uterine contractions.

Oxytocin is a natural hormone that has two primary functions: to stimulate uterine contractions during childbirth and to eject milk from the mammary glands following delivery. Other drugs, known as *tocolytics,* are used to inhibit uterine contractions during premature labor.

Oxytocin is a hormone secreted by the posterior portion of the pituitary gland, whose target organs are the uterus and the breast. It is secreted in larger and larger amounts as the growing fetus distends the uterus. This is an example of positive feedback: As distention increases, oxytocin secretion increases. As blood levels of oxytocin rise, the uterus is stimulated to contract, thus assisting in labor and the delivery of the fetus and the placenta. In postpartum patients, oxytocin is also released in response to suckling, whereby it causes milk to be ejected from the mammary glands following delivery. Oxytocin does not increase the volume of milk production. This function is provided by the pituitary hormone **prolactin**, which increases the synthesis of milk. The actions of oxytocin during breastfeeding are illustrated in Figure 32.3 ■.

FIGURE 32.3

Oxytocin and breastfeeding

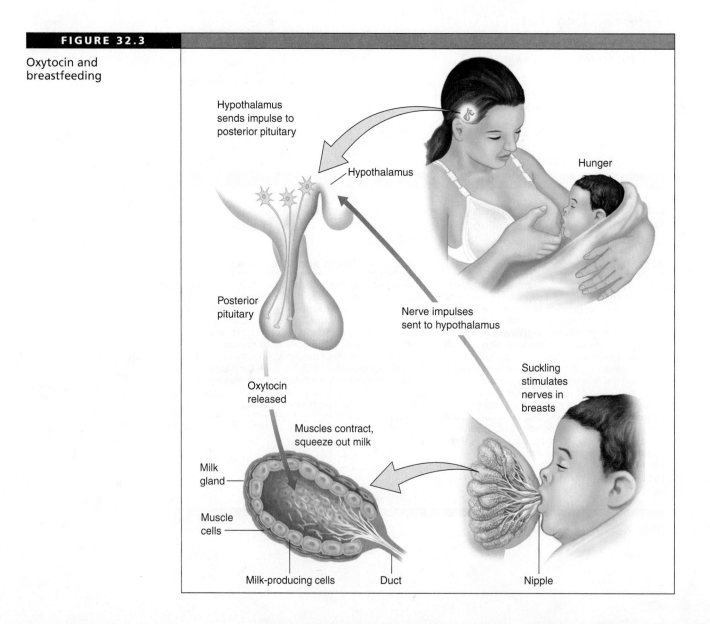

Hypothalamus sends impulse to posterior pituitary

Hypothalamus

Hunger

Posterior pituitary

Nerve impulses sent to hypothalamus

Oxytocin released

Suckling stimulates nerves in breasts

Muscles contract, squeeze out milk

Milk gland

Muscle cells

Milk-producing cells   Duct   Nipple

DRUG PROFILE: Ⓟ *Oxytocin (Pitocin)*

Therapeutic Class: Labor induction drug
Pharmacologic Class: Uterine stimulant, hormonal agent

Actions and Uses:

Oxytocin is given by several different routes depending on its intended action. Given IV immediately prior to birth, or **antepartum**, oxytocin causes labor by stimulating contractions of the smooth muscle in the uterus. It is timed to the final stage of pregnancy, after the cervix is dilated and presentation of the fetus has occurred. Oxytocin may also be infused after delivery, or **postpartum**, to reduce hemorrhage after expulsion of the placenta and to aid in returning normal muscular tone to the uterus.

Adverse Effects and Interactions:

Adverse effects of oxytocin are uncommon in the mother or fetus. When given IV, vital signs of the fetus and mother are monitored continuously to avoid fetal complications such as dysrhythmias or intracranial hemorrhage. Serious complications in the mother may include uterine rupture, seizures, or coma.

Oxytocin interacts with several drugs. For example, vasoconstrictors used with oxytocin cause severe hypertension.

Use cautiously with herbal supplements. For example, ephedra or ma-huang used with oxytocin may lead to hypertension.

Refer to MyNursingKit for a Nursing Process Focus specific to this drug.

Several other drugs may be used to promote uterine contractions. Dinoprostone (Cervidil and others) is used to initiate labor or to expel a fetus that has died. Mifepristone (Mifeprex, RU 486) is used for the emergency prevention of pregnancy and is nearly 100% effective if taken within 3 days following unprotected intercourse. Given from weeks 3 to 7 following conception, the combination of mifepristone with misoprostol (Cytotec) is 80–90% effective at terminating pregnancy.

There are certain clinical situations in which it is desirable to slow uterine contractions. **Tocolytics** are drugs used to inhibit the uterine contractions experienced in premature labor. Terminating premature labor allows additional time for the fetus to develop and may permit the pregnancy to reach normal term. Typically, the mother is given a monitor with a sensor that records uterine contractions. This information is used to determine the doses and timing of tocolytic medications. The drugs used as uterine stimulants and tocolytics are listed in Table 32.4.

toco = *childbirth*
lytic = *destructive*

Concept Review 32.2

■ What is the difference between the effects of prolactin and oxytocin on the breast?

HYPOGONADISM

Androgens are used to treat hypogonadism or delayed puberty in men and breast cancer in women.

CORE CONCEPT 32.6

Androgens are male sex hormones that affect male sex characteristics and promote the maturation of the sex organs. Therapeutically they are used to treat hypogonadism and certain cancers.

Deficiency of testosterone in prepubertal men can result in a lack of maturation of the sex organs, a condition called **hypogonadism**. In adult males, lack of testosterone can lead to impotence and low sperm counts. Failure of the testes to produce adequate amounts of testosterone may be the result of pituitary disease, hereditary disorders, or unknown causes. Drug therapy with

TABLE 32.4	Uterine Stimulants and Relaxants	
DRUG	**ROUTE AND ADULT DOSE**	**REMARKS**
STIMULANTS (OXYTOCICS)		
dinoprostone (Cervidil, Prepidil, Prostin E₂)	Intravaginal; 10 mg	For terminating pregnancy through second trimester or following fetal death; or for cervical ripening prior to induction of labor
ergonovine (Ergotrate maleate)	PO; 1 tablet (0.2 mg) tid–qid after childbirth	Ergot alkaloid
methylergonovine maleate (Methergine)	PO; 0.2–0.4 mg bid–qid	IV and IM forms available; usually for postpartum delivery of the placenta
mifepristone (RU 486)	PO; 600 mg as a single dose	For termination of early pregnancy in combination with misoprostol
misoprostol (Cytotec)	PO; 400 mcg as a single dose	For termination of early pregnancy in combination with mifepristone; also for peptic ulcers
Pr oxytocin (Pitocin)	IV (antepartum); 1 m unit/min starting dose to a maximum of 20 m unit/min	
RELAXANTS (TOCOLYTICS)		
magnesium sulfate	IV; 1–4 g in 5% dextrose by slow infusion	Also used as an anticonvulsant in pre-eclampsia; IM form available
nifedipine (Adalat, Procardia) (see page 277 for the Drug Profile box)	PO; 10 mg as a single dose (max: 40 mg in 1 hr)	Calcium channel blocker also used for cardiovascular disorders
ritodrine hydrochloride (Yutopar)	IV; 50–100 mcg/min starting dose, increased by 50 mcg/min every 10 min	Selective for beta₂-adrenergic receptors; oral form available
terbutaline sulfate (Brethine)	IV; 10 mcg/min (max: 80 mcg/min)	Selective for beta₂-adrenergic receptors; also available in oral and inhalation form for bronchodilation

DRUG PROFILE: **Pr** *Androgens Testosterone Base (Andro)*

Therapeutic Class: Male hypogonadism drug, female breast cancer agent

Pharmacologic Class: Androgen, hormonal agent

Actions and Uses:

The primary therapeutic use of testosterone is for the treatment of hypogonadism in men. Less frequent applications are breast cancer and replacement therapy in menopausal women. The administration of testosterone to young men who have an abnormally delayed puberty will stimulate normal secondary sex characteristics to appear, including enlargement of the sexual organs, facial hair, and a deepening of the voice. In adult men, testosterone administration will increase interest in sexual activity, or **libido**, and restore masculine characteristics that may be deficient. Long-duration IM injections are available that last up to 2 weeks. Transdermal patches are also available.

Adverse Effects and Interactions:

An obvious adverse effect of testosterone therapy is **virilization** or appearance of masculine characteristics, which is usually only of concern when the drug is taken by women. Salt and water are often retained, causing edema. Liver damage is a rare, although potentially serious, adverse effect. Acne and skin irritation is common during therapy. Testosterone is a category X drug and thus should not be taken if pregnancy is confirmed or suspected.

Testosterone base interacts with many drugs. For example, when taken with oral anticoagulants, testosterone base may increase hypoprothrombinemia. Insulin requirements may decrease, and the risk of liver toxicity may increase when used with echinacea. Use cautiously with herbal supplements.

 Refer to MyNursingKit for a Nursing Process Focus specific to this drug.

TABLE 32.5	Selected Androgens	
DRUG	**ROUTE AND ADULT DOSE**	**REMARKS**
danazol (Danocrine)	PO; 200–400 mg bid × 3–6 months	For endometriosis, fibrocystic breast disease, and hereditary angioedema
fluoxymesterone (Halotestin)	PO; 2.5–20 mg/day for replacement therapy	For hypogonadism, breast cancer, and postpartum breast engorgement
methyltestosterone (Android, Testred)	PO; 10–50 mg/day	For hypogonadism, breast cancer, and postpartum breast engorgement
nandrolone phenpropionate (Durabolin, Hybolin)	IM; 50–100 mg every week	For breast cancer only
testolactone (Teslac)	PO; 250 mg qid	For breast cancer only
ⓟ testosterone (Andro 100, Histerone, Testoderm)	PO; 10–25 mg every 2–3 days	IM, topical, and buccal forms available; for hypogonadism and breast cancer; also for postpartum breast engorgement
testosterone cypionate (Depotest, Andro-Cyp, Depo-testosterone)	IM; 50–400 mg every 2–4 weeks	For hypogonadism, breast cancer, and postpartum breast engorgement
testosterone enanthate (Andro LA, Delatest, Delatestryl)	IM; 50–400 mg every 2–4 weeks	For hypogonadism and breast cancer

testosterone or other androgens promotes normal gonadal development and may restore normal reproductive function. Some of the androgens used therapeutically are listed in Table 32.5.

High doses of androgens are occasionally used to treat certain types of breast cancer. Androgens are normally used as a palliative measure in combination with other antineoplastics.

Anabolic steroids are testosterone-like compounds with hormonal activity. They are frequently taken inappropriately by athletes who hope to build muscle mass and strength, thereby obtaining a competitive edge. When taken in large doses for long periods, anabolic steroids can produce significant adverse effects, some of which may persist for many months after discontinuation of the drugs. These drugs tend to raise cholesterol levels and may cause low sperm counts and impotence in men. In women, menstrual irregularities are likely, with an obvious increase in masculine characteristics. Permanent liver damage may result. Behavioral changes include aggression and psychological dependence. The use of anabolic steroids is strongly discouraged by physicians and athletic associations.

ERECTILE DYSFUNCTION

Erectile dysfunction, or **impotence**, is a common disorder in men. The defining characteristic of this condition is the inability to either obtain an erection or to sustain an erection long enough to achieve successful intercourse.

Erectile dysfunction is a common disorder successfully treated with drug therapy.

CORE CONCEPT 32.7

The incidence of erectile dysfunction increases with advancing age, although it may occur in adult men of any age. Certain diseases, most notably atherosclerosis, diabetes, stroke, and hypertension, are associated with a higher incidence of the condition. Psychogenic causes may include depression, fatigue, guilt, or fear of sexual failure. A number of common drugs cause impotence as an adverse effect, including the thiazide diuretics, phenothiazines, serotonin-reuptake inhibitors, tricyclic antidepressants, propranolol (Inderal, InnoPran XL), and diazepam (Valium).

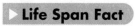

▶ **Life Span Fact**

Erectile dysfunction affects about 1 in 4 men older than age 65.

DRUG PROFILE: ℗ *Sildenafil (Viagra)*

Therapeutic Class: Erectile dysfunction drug

Pharmacologic Class: Phosphodiesterase 5 inhibitor

Actions and Uses:

When sildenafil was approved as the first pharmacologic treatment for erectile dysfunction in 1998, it set a record for pharmaceutical sales for any new drug in U.S. history. Sildenafil acts by relaxing the erectile tissues in the penis, called the **corpus cavernosum**, which allows increased blood flow into the organ. The increased blood flow results in a firmer and longer-lasting erection in about 70% of men taking the drug. The onset of action is relatively rapid, usually less than 1 hour, and its effects last 2 to 4 hours. Despite considerable research interest, no effects of sildenafil have been shown on female sexual function, and this drug is not approved for use by women.

Adverse Effects and Interactions:

The most serious adverse effects with sildenafil occur in men who are concurrently taking organic nitrates, common drugs used in the therapy of angina (see Chapter 20 ⊙⊙). Because life-threatening hypotension has been reported, sildenafil is contraindicated for patients taking organic nitrates. Minor adverse effects include headache, flushing, and nasal congestion. Sildenafil should not be taken more than once per day.

Sildenafil interacts with many drugs. Cimetidine, erythromycin, and ketoconazole increase serum levels of sildenafil and require lower drug doses. Protease inhibitors (ritonavir, amprenavir, and others) will cause increased sildenafil levels, which may lead to toxicity. Rifampin may decrease sildenafil levels, leading to decreased effectiveness.

Mechanism in Action:

Through a series of complex biomolecular interactions, sildenafil (Viagra) causes dilation of blood vessels that empty blood directly into the corpora cavernosa of the penis. This results in engorgement of the corpora cavernosa, leading to an erection and improved sexual performance. Sexual performance is prolonged by occlusion of penile blood vessels.

See the Mechanism in Action feature specific to this drug.
Refer to MyNursingKit for a Nursing Process Focus specific to this drug.

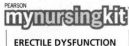

ERECTILE DYSFUNCTION RESOURCES

The marketing of sildenafil (Viagra) has revolutionized the medical therapy of erectile dysfunction. The drug is the most effective treatment for this disorder. Two other similar drugs, vardenafil (Levitra) and tadalafil (Cialis), have been approved by the Food and Drug Administration (FDA) for this disorder. Levitra and Cialis may be effective in treating long-term impotence in men who have not reacted favorably to Viagra. In many instances, Cialis produces a longer lasting effect, up to 12 hours. In comparison, other drug products may last up to 4 hours.

Concept Review **32.3**

■ Why do you think that sildenafil is used to treat erectile dysfunction instead of testosterone?

BENIGN PROSTATIC HYPERPLASIA (BPH)

hyper = *above*
plasia = *growth*

Benign prostatic hyperplasia (BPH) is an enlargement of the prostate gland that occurs in most men of advanced age. It is a nonmalignant disorder that progressively decreases the outflow of urine by obstructing the urethra, causing difficult urination. Common symptoms include increased urinary frequency (usually with small amounts of urine), increased urgency to urinate, excessive nighttime urination, decreased force of the urinary stream, and a sensation that the bladder did not empty completely. In severe cases, surgery is needed to restore the patency of the urethra. In milder cases, drug therapy may be of benefit. BPH is illustrated in Figure 32.4 ■.

CORE CONCEPT 32.8

In its early stages, benign prostatic hyperplasia may be treated successfully with drug therapy.

A few drugs are available to treat benign enlargement of the prostate. Although the drugs have limited efficacy, they have some value in treating mild disease. Because drug therapy alleviates

FIGURE 32.4

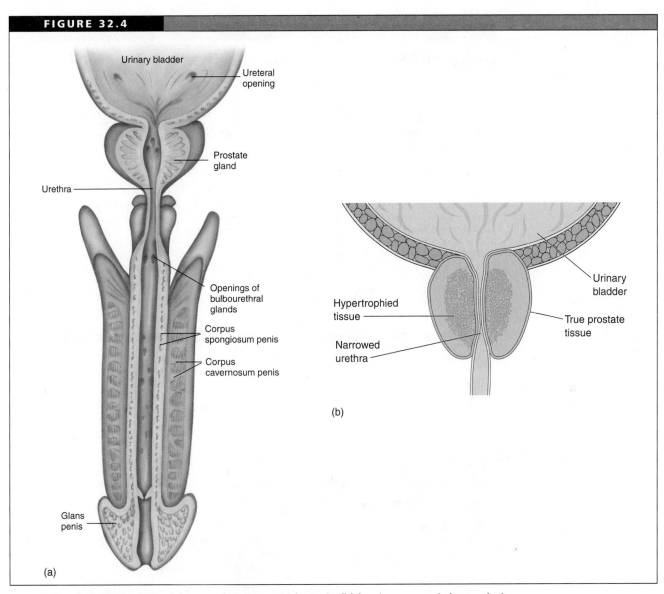

Benign prostatic hyperplasia: (a) normal prostate with penis; (b) benign prostatic hyperplasia   *Source: Pearson Education/PH College*

the symptoms but does not cure the disease, these medications must be taken the remainder of the patient's life, or until surgery is indicated.

Although primarily used for hypertension, several alpha$_1$-adrenergic blockers have been approved for BPH. Alpha blockers relax smooth muscle in the prostate gland, thus easing the urinary obstruction. Doxazocin (Cardura) and terazocin (Hytrin) are of particular value to patients who have both hypertension and BPH. A third alpha$_1$-blocker, tamsulosin (Flomax), has no effect on blood pressure, and its only indication is BPH. Additional information on the alpha blockers is presented in Chapter 17 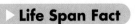 .

Finasteride (Proscar) is also used to promote shrinkage of enlarged prostates and to help restore urinary function in men with BPH. Finasteride acts by inhibiting an enzyme responsible for converting testosterone to one of its metabolites, 5-alpha-dihydrotestosterone. This drug is also marketed as Propecia, which is prescribed to promote hair regrowth in patients with male-pattern baldness. Doses of finasteride are five times higher when prescribed for BPH than when prescribed for baldness. Finasteride is a category X drug, and women who are pregnant or who may become pregnant should avoid the semen of men taking the drug.

▶ **Life Span Fact**

BPH affects 50% of men older than age 60, and 90% of men older than age 80.

DRUG PROFILE: ℗ *Finasteride (Proscar)*

Therapeutic Class: Drug for benign prostatic hyperplasia drug

Pharmacologic Class: 5-alpha reductase enzyme inhibitor

Actions and Uses:

Finasteride acts by inhibiting 5-alpha reductase, the enzyme responsible for converting testosterone to one of its metabolites. This metabolite causes growth of prostate cells and promotes enlargement of the gland. Because it inhibits the metabolism of testosterone, finasteride is sometimes called an antiandrogen. Finasteride shrinks enlarged prostates and helps to restore urinary function. It is most effective in patients with larger prostates. This drug is also marketed as Propecia, which is prescribed to promote hair regrowth in patients with male-pattern baldness. Doses of finasteride are five times higher when prescribed for BPH than when prescribed for baldness.

Adverse Effects and Interactions:

Finasteride causes various types of sexual dysfunction in up to 16% of patients, including impotence, diminished libido, and ejaculatory dysfunction.

No clinically significant drug interactions have been established.

Use with caution with herbal supplements. For example, saw palmetto may increase the effects of finasteride.

Refer to MyNursingKit for a Nursing Process Focus specific to this drug.

PATIENTS NEED TO KNOW

Patients treated for reproductive disorders need to know the following:

Regarding Oral Contraceptives

1. If taking oral contraceptives, schedule frequent medical checkups. Take blood pressure periodically and report any persistent changes to a health care provider.
2. Discontinue oral contraceptives, estrogen, or progestins immediately if pregnancy is suspected. Continued use may injure the fetus.
3. Be certain to inform the health care provider if oral contraceptives are being taken. Some drugs decrease the effectiveness of oral contraceptives and could result in pregnancy. These drugs include several common antibiotics and anticonvulsants.
4. A balanced diet is important when taking oral contraceptives, because these drugs may lower levels of folic acid and vitamin B_6.

Regarding Hormone Replacement Therapy

5. Before beginning HRT, a baseline mammogram should be performed. Monthly BSEs should be conducted in addition to an annual exam by a health care provider.

Regarding Erectile Dysfunction Medications

6. If taking antihypertensive drugs, monitor blood pressure carefully when taking sildenafil. An increased risk of hypotension is possible.

Regarding Androgens

7. When taking androgens, expect virilization to occur. Prolonged erections, known as *priapism*, should be reported to a health care provider immediately. This is a sign of overdose, and permanent damage to the penis may result.

SAFETY ALERT

Missing Information

It has been a very busy morning on the nursing unit, with multiple patient discharges and several new admissions. One patient is a 35-year-old woman who is being released from the hospital with a discharge order that reads, *Prempro one tablet daily at bedtime.* The nurse should clarify the order before the patient leaves. Prempro (conjugated estrogens/medroxyprogesterone acetate) is one of the drugs frequently ordered without specifying the dose. However, the drug is now marketed in two strengths (0.625 mg/2.5 mg and 0.625 mg/5 mg). With the advent of new drugs, and with new strengths being developed daily, there is no way to keep current with all the changes. This is why it is imperative to accept only complete orders that specify the strength.

CHAPTER REVIEW

CORE CONCEPTS SUMMARY

32.1 Testosterone, estrogen, and progesterone are the primary hormones contributing to the growth, health, and maintenance of the reproductive system.

Estrogen and progesterone are secreted by the ovary and are responsible for reproductive health in women. Testosterone is secreted by the testes and is responsible for the growth and maintenance of the male reproductive system. The sex hormones are controlled by FSH and LH from the pituitary.

32.2 Low doses of estrogens and progestins are used for contraception.

The most common oral contraceptives contain low doses of an estrogen combined with a progestin. Nearly 100% effective, these drugs act by preventing ovulation. Thromboembolic disease is a potentially serious adverse effect in some patients.

32.3 Estrogens have been used for replacement therapy and in the treatment of prostate cancer.

Estrogens have been used to reduce the symptoms and consequences of estrogen loss in menopausal and postmenopausal women. Thromboembolic disease is a contraindication for estrogen therapy.

32.4 Progestins are prescribed for dysfunctional uterine bleeding.

Abnormal uterine bleeding may be the result of an imbalance between progesterone and estrogen secretion. Administration of progestins can often reestablish a normal cyclic menstrual pattern. High doses of progestins are also used as antineoplastics.

32.5 Oxytocin and tocolytics are drugs used to influence uterine contractions.

Oxytocin is administered to stimulate uterine contractions to aid in labor and delivery. Intranasally, it assists in milk letdown. Mifepristone is a uterine stimulant that is used to prevent and terminate pregnancy. Tocolytics are used to relax uterine smooth muscle so that pregnancy may reach term.

32.6 Androgens are used to treat hypogonadism or delayed puberty in men and breast cancer in women.

Administration of testosterone promotes the appearance of masculine characteristics, a desirable action in men with hypogonadism. Anabolic steroids are testosterone-like drugs taken illegally to increase athletic performance, which may produce serious, permanent adverse effects in both men and women.

32.7 Erectile dysfunction is a common disorder successfully treated with drug therapy.

Erectile dysfunction is a common disorder with many possible physiologic and psychogenic causes. Sildenafil is effective at promoting more rigid and longer-lasting erections. It is contraindicated in patients taking organic nitrates.

32.8 In its early stages, benign prostatic hyperplasia may be treated successfully with drug therapy.

BPH results in urinary difficulties that may be treated by drug therapy or surgery. Alpha$_1$-blockers relax smooth muscle in the prostate to promote urine flow. Finasteride shrinks the prostate to improve urinary function. Drugs are effective only in mild cases of BPH.

REVIEW QUESTIONS

The following questions are written in NCLEX-PN® style. Answer these questions to assess your knowledge of the chapter material, and go back and review any material that is not clear to you.

1. With which type of birth control does estrogen level remain constant throughout the cycle, although progestin level increases toward the end of the menstrual cycle?

1. Monophasic
2. Biphasic
3. Triphasic
4. Quadriphasic

2. High doses of estrogen:

1. Increase androgen levels
2. Decrease androgen levels
3. Increase progestin levels
4. Decrease progestin levels

3. Which of the following patients should not be placed on medroxyprogesterone (Prempro)?

1. A 37-year-old woman with dysfunctional uterine bleeding
2. A 65-year-old woman diagnosed with metastatic uterine cancer
3. A 40-year-old woman with a history of deep vein thrombosis
4. A healthy 21-year-old who needs birth control

4. The patient states she had sexual intercourse yesterday and is concerned she may be pregnant. She is requesting emergency prevention. Which of the following drugs may be ordered?

1. Oxytocin (Pitocin)
2. Dinoprostone (Prepidil)
3. Medroxyprogesterone (Prempro)
4. Magnesium sulfate

5. Complications of oxytocin (Pitocin) include all of the following except:

1. Uterine rupture
2. Seizures
3. Fetal dysrhythmias
4. Hypotension

6. Complications of testosterone therapy may include:

1. Renal failure
2. Hepatic failure
3. Decreased cholesterol levels
4. Maturation of male sex organs

7. Your patient states that she has forgotten to take her birth control pills for the last 2 days. You should instruct her to:

1. Take her missed pills immediately
2. Get back on schedule as soon as possible
3. Use additional birth control until a regular schedule is established
4. Get a home pregnancy kit

8. At her yearly exam, your 37-year-old patient states that she has discovered a lump in her left breast. She has been taking monophasic oral contraceptives for 5 years. You suspect that the physician will:

1. Change the patient's monophasic oral contraceptive to a triphasic oral contraceptive
2. Order a mammogram
3. Closely observe the patient
4. Take her off oral contraceptives

9. Your patient states that she is experiencing menopausal symptoms and asks for your advice regarding hormone replacement therapy (HRT). Your best response is:

1. "HRT is dangerous and should never be prescribed."
2. "HRT is perfectly safe, with no risks."
3. "You are not a candidate for HRT."
4. "You need to discuss risks versus benefits of HRT with your physician."

10. Your patient with BPH is complaining of feeling like he "cannot empty his bladder." You suspect that the physician will order which of the following?

1. Propecia
2. Sildenafil (Viagra)
3. Estrogen
4. Finasteride (Proscar)

CASE STUDY QUESTIONS

For questions 1–4, please refer to the following case study, and choose the correct answer from choices 1–4.

*M*s. Marge, a 29-year-old female, enters the clinic with complaints of lower abdominal pain and irregular menstrual bleeding with prolonged menstruation. Blood *pressure and pulse are slightly elevated due. . She states that she has had problems with frequently being tired. Ms. Marge's last physical exam was 1 year ago.*

1. Based on the information obtained from Ms. Marge, her symptoms would probably be related to:

1. Thyroid disorder
2. Pelvic neoplasms
3. Pregnancy
4. Dysfunctional uterine bleeding

2. The best course of treatment for Ms. Marge would include:

1. Progestins
2. Antibiotics and examination for reproductive scarring
3. Nonsteroidal anti-inflammatory drugs
4. High doses of conjugated estrogens

3. Methods used to treat dysfunctional uterine bleeding include:

1. Use of condoms
2. Visiting the doctor only when the pain gets really bad
3. Possible use of oral contraceptives
4. Screening of sexual partner

4. If Ms. Marge begins oral contraceptives, she will need to know:

1. It doesn't matter if she smokes
2. That it is OK to miss taking the medication for several days in a row
3. To notify her healthcare provider if two or more consecutive periods are missed
4. That caffeine will actually be beneficial

FURTHER STUDY

- Maintenance of bone density and alternatives to estrogen-replacement therapy are discussed in Chapter 33 ⬥.

- Chapter 27 ⬥ presents information on the use of reproductive hormones as antineoplastic agents.

- Chapter 17 ⬥ discusses alpha blockers for use in treating hypertension.

- Nitrates used for the treatment of angina pectoris are covered in Chapter 21 ⬥.

UNIT 7

The Skeletal System, Integumentary System, and Eyes and Ears

UNIT CONTENTS

33 Drugs for Bone and Joint Disorders

CORE CONCEPTS

33.1 Adequate levels of calcium, vitamin D, parathyroid hormone, and calcitonin are necessary for normal body processes.

33.2 Hypocalcemia is a serious condition that requires immediate therapy.

33.3 Treatment for osteomalacia consists of calcium and vitamin D supplements.

33.4 Treatment for osteoporosis includes calcitonin, estrogen-receptor modulator drugs, and bisphosphonates.

33.5 Treatment for Paget's disease includes bisphosphonates and calcitonin.

33.6 Analgesics and anti-inflammatory drugs are important components of pharmacotherapy for osteoarthritis.

33.7 Glucocorticoids, immunosuppressants, and disease-modifying drugs are additional therapies used to treat rheumatoid arthritis.

33.8 Drug therapy for gout requires agents that inhibit uric acid buildup.

DRUG SNAPSHOT

The following drugs are discussed in this chapter:

DRUG CLASSES	DRUG PROFILES
Calcium Supplements and Vitamin D Therapy	**Pr** calcium gluconate (Kalcinate)
	Pr calcitriol (Calcijex, Rocaltrol)
Bone Resorption Inhibitors	
Estrogen receptor modulators	**Pr** raloxifene (Evista)
Bisphosphonates	**Pr** alendronate (Fosamax)

DRUG CLASSES	DRUG PROFILES
Disease-Modifying Antirheumatic Drugs (DMARDs)	**Pr** hydroxychloroquine (Plaquenil)
Uric Acid Inhibitors for Gout	**Pr** colchicine (Colcrys)

LEARNING OUTCOMES

After reading this chapter, the student should be able to:

1. Identify the different body systems contributing to body movement.

2. Discuss nonpharmacologic therapies used to treat bone and joint disorders.

3. Identify important symptoms or disorders associated with an imbalance of calcium, vitamin D, parathyroid hormone, and calcitonin.

4. Describe the pharmacologic management of disorders caused by calcium and vitamin D deficiency and disorders related directly to bones and joints.

5. Discuss drug treatments for hypocalcemia, osteomalacia, and rickets.

6. Identify important disorders characterized by weak, fragile bones and abnormal joints.

7. For each of the drug classes, identify representative drugs and explain their mechanisms of action, primary actions, and important adverse effects.

Disorders associated with movement are some of the most difficult conditions to treat. Their underlying causes relate to at least four important systems in the body: the nervous, muscle, endocrine, and skeletal systems. Appropriate body movement depends on intact neural pathways and properly functioning muscles. For muscles to function well, the body needs adequate levels of minerals such as sodium, potassium, and calcium. The skeletal system and joints are at the core of movement and must be free from any defect that would destabilize the other body systems. Disorders associated with bones and joints affect a patient's ability to fulfill daily activities and lead to immobility.

This chapter focuses on the pharmacotherapy of skeletal disorders such as osteomalacia, osteporosis, arthritis, and gout. The importance of calcium balance and the action of vitamin D are both stressed because both relate to the proper functioning of bones and joint tissue. Drugs used to treat important bone and joint disorders are important because of the major mobility problems that would occur without medical intervention.

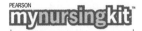

PEARSON
mynursingkit™

THE NATIONAL INSTITUTE OF ARTHRITIS AND MUSCULOSKELETAL AND SKIN DISEASES

Adequate levels of calcium, vitamin D, parathyroid hormone, and calcitonin are necessary for normal body processes.

CORE CONCEPT 33.1

One of the most important minerals in the body responsible for nerve conduction, muscle contraction, and formation of bone is calcium. Levels of calcium in the blood are controlled by two endocrine glands: the parathyroid glands, which secrete parathyroid hormone (PTH), and the thyroid gland, which secretes calcitonin, as depicted in Figure 33.1 ■. PTH stimulates bone cells called *osteoclasts*. These cells accelerate the process of **bone resorption**, the demineralization process that breaks down bone into its mineral components. Once bone is resorbed or broken down, calcium becomes available for transport and is used elsewhere in the body. The opposite of this process is **bone deposition**, or bone building. This process, which removes calcium from the blood, is stimulated by the hormone calcitonin.

PTH and calcitonin control calcium homeostasis in the body by influencing three major target organs: the bones, kidneys, and gastrointestinal (GI) tract. The GI tract is mainly influenced by PTH. Calcium homeostasis and vitamin D metabolism are interrelated: Calcium disorders are often associated with vitamin D disorders.

Vitamin D is unique among vitamins in that the body is able to synthesize it from precursor molecules. In the skin, the inactive form of vitamin D, called **cholecalciferol**, is synthesized from cholesterol. Exposure of the skin to sunlight or ultraviolet light increases the level of cholecalciferol in the bloodstream. Cholecalciferol can also be obtained from dietary products such as milk or other foods fortified with vitamin D. Figure 33.2 ■ illustrates the metabolism of vitamin D.

Once cholecalciferol is absorbed or formed in the body, it is converted to an intermediate vitamin form called **calcifediol**. Enzymes in the kidneys metabolize calcifediol to **calcitriol**, the active form of vitamin D. PTH stimulates the formation of calcitriol in the kidneys. Patients with extensive kidney disease are unable to synthesize adequate levels of calcitriol.

FIGURE 33.1

(a) Parathyroid hormone (PTH); (b) calcitonin action

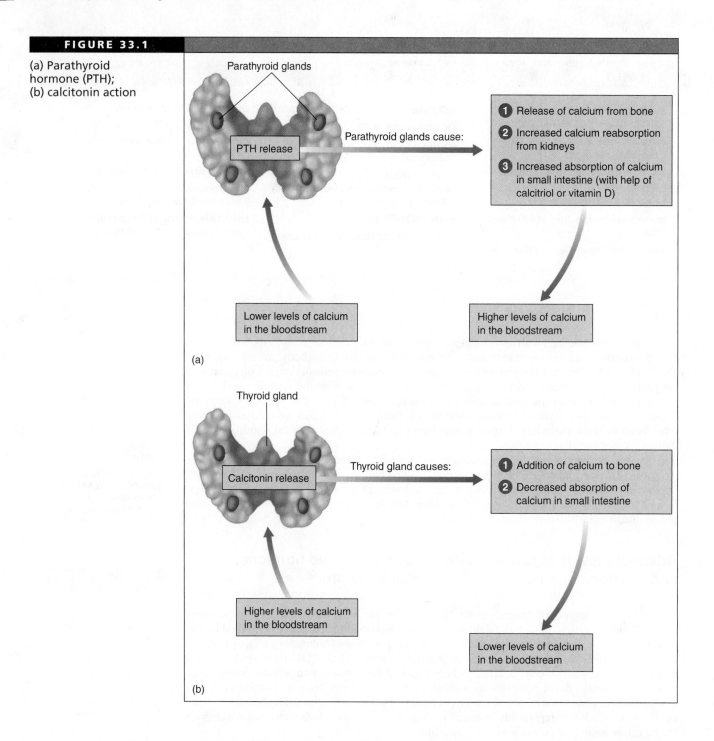

Parathyroid glands

PTH release

Parathyroid glands cause:

1 Release of calcium from bone
2 Increased calcium reabsorption from kidneys
3 Increased absorption of calcium in small intestine (with help of calcitriol or vitamin D)

Lower levels of calcium in the bloodstream

Higher levels of calcium in the bloodstream

(a)

Thyroid gland

Calcitonin release

Thyroid gland causes:

1 Addition of calcium to bone
2 Decreased absorption of calcium in small intestine

Higher levels of calcium in the bloodstream

Lower levels of calcium in the bloodstream

(b)

The primary function of calcitriol is to increase calcium absorption from the GI tract. Dietary calcium is absorbed better in the presence of PTH and active vitamin D to produce higher levels of calcium in the bloodstream.

The importance of proper calcium balance in the body cannot be overstated. Calcium ions influence the excitability of all neurons. When calcium concentrations are too high (*hypercalcemia*), sodium permeability decreases across cell membranes. This is dangerous because nerve conduction depends on the proper influx of sodium into cells. When calcium levels in the bloodstream are too low (*hypocalcemia*), cell membranes become hyperexcitable. If hypocalcemia becomes severe, seizures or muscle spasms may result. Calcium is also important for the normal functioning of other body processes such as blood coagulation, neurotransmitter release, and stability of the entire skeletal system.

hyper = *elevated*
hypo = *lowered*
calc = *calcium*
emia = *blood level*

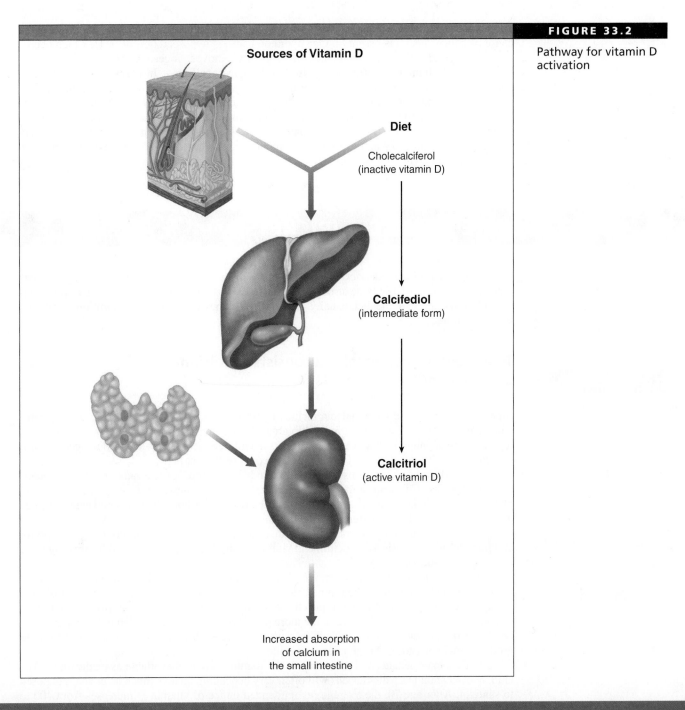

FIGURE 33.2

Pathway for vitamin D activation

HYPOCALCEMIA

Hypocalcemia, or lowered levels of calcium in the blood, is associated with a range of conditions, including poor nutrition, seizures, muscle spasms, and endocrine and bone disorders.

Hypocalcemia is a serious condition that requires immediate therapy.

CORE CONCEPT 33.2

Therapies for calcium disorders may involve calcium supplements, vitamin D supplements, bisphosphonates, and/or several miscellaneous agents. Conditions of calcium and vitamin D metabolism are hypocalcemia, osteomalacia, osteoporosis, and Paget's disease.

Hypocalcemia is not a disease, but a sign of underlying pathology; therefore, diagnosis of the cause of hypocalcemia is essential. One common cause is hyposecretion of PTH, which occurs when the thyroid and parathyroid glands are surgically removed. Digestive-related malabsorption disorders and vitamin D deficiencies also result in hypocalcemia. In cases of hypocalcemia, health care practitioners should assess for the adequate intake of calcium-containing foods.

With hypocalcemia, numbness and tingling of the extremities may occur, and convulsions are possible. Symptoms of hypocalcemia are nerve and muscle excitability. Muscle twitching, tremor, or cramping may be evident. A patient may be confused or behave abnormally. Severe hypocalcemia requires IV administration of calcium salts, whereas less severe hypocalcemia can often be reversed with oral supplements.

OSTEOMALACIA (RICKETS)

Osteomalacia, referred to as *rickets* in children, is a disorder characterized by softening of bones without alteration of basic bone structure. The cause of osteomalacia and rickets is a lack of vitamin D and calcium in the diet, usually as a result of kidney failure or malabsorption of calcium from the GI tract.

CORE CONCEPT 33.3

Treatment for osteomalacia consists of calcium and vitamin D supplements.

Signs and symptoms of osteomalacia include hypocalcemia, muscle weakness, muscle spasms, and diffuse bone pain, especially in the hip area. Patients may also experience pain in the arms, legs, and spinal column. Classic signs of rickets in children include bowlegs and a pigeon breast. Children may also develop a slight fever and become restless at night.

Tests performed to verify osteomalacia include bone biopsy; bone radiographs; computerized tomography (CT) scan of the vertebral column; and determination of serum calcium, phosphate, and vitamin D levels. Many of these tests are routine for bone disorders and are performed as needed to determine the extent of bone health.

In extreme cases, surgical correction of disfigured limbs may be required. Drug therapy for children and adults consists of calcium and vitamin D supplements. Drugs used for treating these conditions are shown in Table 33.1.

The two major forms of calcium are complexed and elemental. Most calcium supplements are in the form of complexed calcium. These products are often compared on the basis of their ability to release elemental calcium into the bloodstream. The greater the ability of complexed calcium to release elemental calcium, the more potent is the supplement. Elemental calcium may be obtained from dietary sources such as dark green vegetables, canned salmon, and fortified products, including tofu, orange juice, and milk.

Inactive, intermediate, and active forms of vitamin D are also available as medications. The amount of vitamin D a patient needs will often vary depending on how much he or she is exposed to sunlight. After age 70, the average recommended intake of vitamin D increases from 400 to 600 units/day. Because vitamin D is needed to absorb calcium from the GI tract, many supplements combine vitamin D and calcium into a single tablet.

Concept Review **33.1**

■ Identify the major drug therapies used for hypocalcemia, osteomalacia, and rickets.

WEAK AND FRAGILE BONES

Two important disorders characterized by weak and fragile bones are osteoporosis and Paget's disease. Although these disorders are not the same, they share many of the same symptoms.

TABLE 33.1	Calcium Supplements and Vitamin D Therapy	
DRUG	**ROUTE AND ADULT DOSE**	**REMARKS**
CALCIUM SUPPLEMENTS (ALL DOSES ARE IN TERMS OF ELEMENTAL CALCIUM)		
calcium acetate (Phos-Ex, PhosLo)	PO; 1–2 g bid–tid	1 gram calcium acetate equals 250 mg (12.6 mEq) elemental calcium; phosphate binder used to treat hypophosphatemia in dialysis patients
calcium carbonate (BioCal, Calcite-500, others)	PO; 1–2 g bid–tid	1 gram calcium carbonate equals 400 mg (20 mEq) elemental calcium
calcium chloride	IV; 0.5–1 g daily every 3 days	1 gram calcium chloride equals 272 mg (13.6 mEq) elemental calcium; may be irritating to body tissues
calcium citrate (Citracal)	PO; 1–2 g bid–tid	1 gram calcium citrate equals 210 mg (12 mEq) elemental calcium
calcium gluceptate	IV; 1.1–4.4 g daily IM; 0.5–1.1 g daily	1 gram calcium gluceptate equals 82 mg (4.1 mEq) elemental calcium; not availabe in the U.S.
ⓟ calcium gluconate (Kalcinate)	PO; 1–2 g bid–qid	1 gram calcium gluconate equals 90 mg (4.5 mEq) elemental calcium
calcium lactate	PO; 325 mg–1.3 g tid with meals	1 gram calcium lactate equals 130 mg (6.5 mEq) elemental calcium
calcium phosphate tribasic (Posture)	PO; 1–2 g bid–tid	1 gram calcium phosphate equals 390 mg (19.3 mEq) elemental calcium
VITAMIN D SUPPLEMENTS		
calcifediol	PO; 50–100 mcg daily or every other day	For metabolic bone disease and hypocalcemia associated with chronic kidney failure
ⓟ calcitriol (Calcijex, Rocaltrol)	PO; 0.25 mcg daily	For hypocalcemia in chronic renal failure and with hypoparathyroidism
ergocalciferol (Deltalin, Calciferol)	PO/IM; 25–125 mcg daily for 6–12 weeks	For osteomalacia; also used for vitamin D-dependent rickets and hypoparathyroidism

DRUG PROFILE: ⓟ *Calcium Gluconate (Kalcinate)*

Therapeutic Class: Drug for treatment of hypocalcemia, hypoparathyroidism, osteoporosis, and Paget's disease

Pharmacologic Class: Calcium supplement

Actions and Uses:

Calcium gluconate and other calcium compounds are used to correct hypocalcemia and to treat osteoporosis and Paget's disease. The objective of calcium therapy is to return serum levels of calcium to normal. People at high risk for developing these conditions include postmenopausal women; those with little physical activity over a prolonged period; and patients taking certain medications such as corticosteroids, immunosuppressive drugs, and some antiseizure medications. Calcium gluconate is available in tablets or as a 10% solution for IV injection. Calcium gluconate is pregnancy category B.

Adverse Effects and Interactions:

The most common adverse effect of calcium gluconate is hypercalcemia, which is brought on by taking too much of this supplement. Symptoms include drowsiness, lethargy, weakness, headache, anorexia, nausea and vomiting, increased urination, and thirst. IV administration of calcium may cause hypotension, bradycardia, dysrhythmia, and cardiac arrest.

Using this drug with cardiac glycosides increases the risk of dysrhythmias. Magnesium may compete for GI absorption. Calcium decreases the absorption of tetracyclines.

Refer to MyNursingKit for a Nursing Process Focus specific to this drug.

DRUG PROFILE: ℗ Calcitriol (Calcijex, Rocaltrol)

Therapeutic Class: Drug for treatment of hypocalcemia, osteoporosis, osteomalacia, and rickets
Pharmacologic Class: Vitamin D agent

Actions and Uses:

Calcitriol is the active form of vitamin D and is available in both oral and IV formulations. It promotes the intestinal absorption of calcium and elevates serum levels of calcium. This medication is used when patients have impaired kidney function or have hypoparathyroidism. Calcitriol reduces bone resorption and is useful in treating rickets. The effectiveness of calcitriol depends on the patient receiving an adequate amount of calcium; therefore, it is usually prescribed in combination with calcium supplements.

Adverse Effects and Interactions:

Common adverse effects include hypercalcemia, headache, weakness, dry mouth, thirst, increased urination, and muscle or bone pain. Thiazide diuretics may increase the effects of vitamin D, causing hypercalcemia. Too much vitamin D may cause dysrhythmias in patients who are receiving cardiac glycosides. Magnesium supplements should not be given together with calcitriol because of the increased risk of hypermagnesemia.

Mechanism in Action:

Calcitriol is an active form of vitamin D responsible for increasing calcium absorption. Calcium is important for the proper functioning of the muscular, skeletal, and nervous systems. All three systems, as well as organs of the endocrine and renal systems, play a critical role in maintaining a proper balance of calcium in the bloodstream.

Refer to MyNursingKit for a Nursing Process Focus specific to this drug.

OSTEOPOROSIS

Osteoporosis, the most common metabolic bone disease, is responsible for as many as 1.5 million fractures annually. This disorder is usually asymptomatic until the bones become brittle enough to fracture or a vertebra collapses. In some cases, a lack of dietary calcium and vitamin D contribute to bone deterioration. In other cases, osteoporosis is due to disrupted bone homeostasis.

CORE CONCEPT 33.4

Treatment for osteoporosis includes calcitonin, estrogen-receptor modulator drugs, and bisphosphonates.

Simply stated, bone resorption outpaces bone deposition, and patients develop weak bones. Following are risk factors for osteoporosis:

- Postmenopauseal status
- High alcohol or caffeine consumption
- Anorexia nervosa
- Tobacco use
- Physical inactivity
- Testosterone deficiency, particularly in elderly men
- Lack of adequate vitamin D or calcium in the diet
- Drugs such as corticosteroids, some anticonvulsants, and immunosuppressants that lower calcium levels in the bloodstream

The most common risk factor associated with the development of osteoporosis is the onset of menopause. When women reach menopause, estrogen secretion declines and bones become weak and fragile. One theory to explain this occurrence is that normal levels of estrogen may limit the life span of osteoclasts, the bone cells that resorb bone. When estrogen levels become low, osteoclast activity is no longer controlled, and bone demineralization accelerates, resulting in loss of bone density. In women with osteoporosis, fractures often occur in the hips, wrists, forearms, or spine. The metabolism of calcium in osteoporosis is illustrated in Figure 33.3 ∎.

PEARSON
mynursingkit™

OSTEOPOROSIS AND
RELATED BONE DISEASES
NATIONAL RESOURCE
CENTER

FIGURE 33.3

Calcium metabolism in osteoporosis: (a) normal calcium intake; (b) low calcium intake

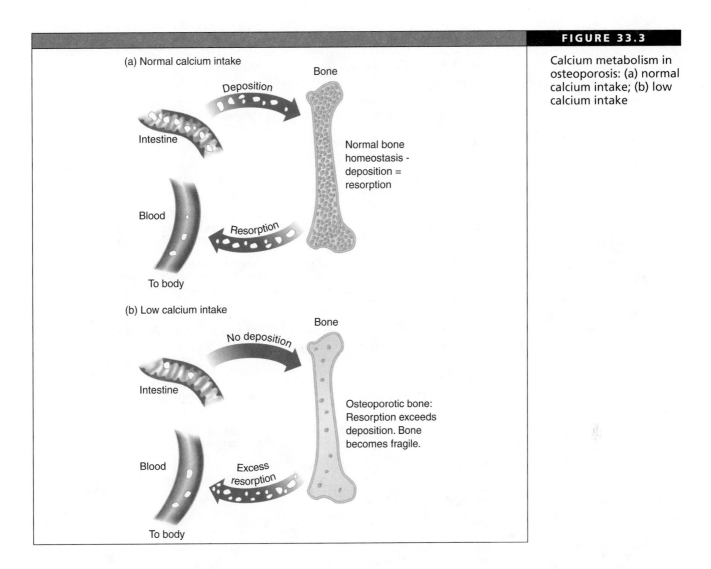

Many drug therapies are available for osteoporosis. These include calcium and vitamin D therapy, hormone therapy with estrogen, estrogen-receptor modulators, calcitonin, statins, slow-release sodium fluoride, and bisphosphonates. Many of these drug classes are also used for other bone disorders or conditions unrelated to the skeletal system. Selected drugs for osteoporosis and related bone disorders are listed in Table 33.2.

PEARSON
mynursingkit

NATIONAL
OSTEOPOROSIS
FOUNDATION

Hormone Therapy with Estrogen

Until recently, hormone therapy (HT) with estrogen was one of the most common treatments for osteoporosis in postmenopausal women. Because of increased risks of cardiovascular events, thromboembolic disease, uterine cancer, breast cancer, urinary incontinence, and other chronic disorders, the use of HT in treating osteoporosis has been carefully monitored. Accordingly, black box warnings advise health care providers and patients to be extremely careful. Additional information about HT and estrogen may be found in Chapter 32 ⬭ .

Selective Estrogen-Receptor Modulators

Selective estrogen-receptor modulators (SERMs) bind to estrogen receptors and comprise a relatively new class of drugs used in the prevention and treatment of osteoporosis. SERMs may be estrogen agonists or antagonists, depending on the specific drug and the tissue involved. For example, raloxifene (Evista) blocks estrogen receptors in the uterus and breast; thus, it has no estrogen-like proliferative effects on these tissues that might promote cancer. Evista decreases bone resorption, thus increasing bone density and making fractures less likely. Like estrogen, it has a cholesterol-lowering effect.

TABLE 33.2	Bone Resorption Inhibitors and Selected Drugs	
DRUG	**ROUTE AND ADULT DOSE**	**REMARKS**
HORMONAL (BIOLOGIC) AND SELECTED DRUGS		
calcitonin–salmon (Fortical; Miacalcin)	Paget's disease: subcutaneous human, 0.5 mg daily; subcutaneous/IM salmon, 100 units daily Hypercalcemia: subcutaneous/IM salmon, 4 units/kg bid	Calcium regulating hormone; used commonly for hypercalcemia and Paget's disease
cinacalcet (Sensipar)	PO; start with 30 mg once daily; may increase every 2–4 weeks until target PTH of 150–300 mg/mL (max: 300/day)	For secondary hyperparathyroidism
Pr raloxifene (Evista)	PO; 60 mg daily	Selective estrogen-receptor modulator; mimics the effects of estrogen on bone
teriparatide (Forteo)	SC; 20 mcg/day	Parathyroid hormone (rDNA origin); for osteoporosis in postmenopausal women; for male patients with high risk of fractures
BISPHOSPHONATES		
Pr alendronate (Fosamax)	Osteoporosis treatment: PO 10 mg daily Osteoporosis prevention: PO 5 mg daily Paget's disease: PO 40 mg daily for 6 months	For osteoporosis in men and women; for Paget's disease
etidronate (Didronel)	PO; 5–10 mg/kg daily for 6 months or 11–20 mg/kg daily for 3 months	For Paget's disease
ibandronate (Boniva)	PO; 2.5 mg daily or 150 mg once monthly	For treatment and prevention of postmenopausal osteoporosis
pamidronate (Aredia)	IV; 15–90 mg in 1000 ml NS or D_5W over 4–24 hours	For Paget's disease and moderate hypercalcemia of malignancy
risedronate (Actonel)	PO; 30 mg daily at least 30 minutes before the first drink or meal of the day for 2 months	For Paget's disease
tiludronate (Skelid)	PO; 400 mg daily taken with 6–8 ounces of water 2 hours before or after food for 3 months	For Paget's disease
zoledronate (Reclast)	IV; 4 mg, may be repeated in 7 days	For hypercalcemia of malignancy; treatment of steroid-induced osteoporosis, postmenopausal osteoporosis, and bone density medication

Calcitonin

Calcitonin, a natural product obtained from salmon, is approved for the treatment of osteoporosis in women who are more than 5 years postmenopausal. It is available by nasal spray or subcutaneous injection. Calcitonin increases bone density and reduces the risk of vertebral fractures. Adverse effects are generally minor; the nasal formulation may irritate the nasal mucosa, and allergies are possible. Parenteral forms may produce nausea and vomiting. In addition to treating osteoporosis, calcitonin is indicated for Paget's disease and hypercalcemia.

Bisphosphonates

The most common drug class used to treat osteoporosis is the **bisphosphonates**. These drugs are structural analogs of pyrophosphate, a natural inhibitor of bone resorption. Bisphosphonates inhibit bone resorption by suppressing osteoclast activity, thereby increasing bone density and reducing the incidence of fractures. Examples include etidronate (Didronel), alendronate (Fosamax), risedronate (Actonel), tiludronate (Skelid), pamidronate (Aredia), and zoledronate (Zometa); several forms are available as injectable drugs. Adverse effects include GI problems such as nausea, vomiting, abdominal pain, and esophageal irritation. Because these drugs are

DRUG PROFILE: ⓟ *Raloxifene (Evista)*

Therapeutic Class: Treatment of postmenopausal osteoporosis in women
Pharmacologic Class: Bone resorption inhibitor, selective estrogen-receptor modulator

Actions and Uses:

Raloxifene is a SERM. It decreases bone resorption and increases bone mass and density by acting through the estrogen receptor. Raloxifene is primarily used for the prevention of osteoporosis in postmenopausal women. This drug also reduces serum total cholesterol and low-density lipoprotein (LDL) without lowering high-density lipoprotein (HDL) or triglycerides.

Adverse Effects and Interactions:

Common adverse effects are hot flashes, migraine headache, flulike symptoms, endometrial disorder, breast pain, and vaginal bleeding. Patients should not take cholesterol-lowering drugs or estrogen replacement therapy concurrently with this medication.
    Use with estrogen is not recommended. Absorption is reduced by cholestyramine.

 Refer to MyNursingKit for a Nursing Process Focus specific to this drug.

poorly absorbed, they should be taken on an empty stomach, as tolerated by the patient. Recent studies suggest that once-weekly dosing may give the same bone-density benefits as daily dosing because of these drugs' extended duration of action.

Concept Review 33.2

■ What are the major drug therapies used for the treatment of osteoporosis and related bone disorders?

DRUG PROFILE: ⓟ *Alendronate (Fosamax)*

Therapeutic Class: Drug for osteoporosis
Pharmacologic Class: Bone resorption inhibitor, bisphosphonate

Actions and Uses:

Alendronate is approved for the following indications: prevention of osteoporosis in postmenopausal women, treatment of glucocorticoid-induced osteoporosis in both women and men, to increase bone mass in men with osteoporosis, and treatment of symptomatic Paget's disease in both women and men. Alendronate is also used off-label for treating hypercalcemia due to malignancy. Therapeutic effects may take from 1 to 3 months to appear and may continue for several months after therapy is discontinued. All doses must be taken on an empty stomach, preferably in a fasting state 2 hours before breakfast.

Adverse Effects and Interactions:

Common adverse effects of alendronate are diarrhea, nausea, vomiting, esophageal irritation, and a metallic or altered taste perception. Pathologic fractures may occur if the drug is taken longer than 3 months. Calcium supplements may decrease absorption of alendronate; therefore, use of these drugs together should be avoided. Food–drug interactions are common. Milk and other dairy products and medications, such as calcium, iron, antacids, and other mineral supplements, must be reviewed before beginning bisphosphonate therapy because they have the potential to decrease the effectiveness of bisphosphonates. Blood levels of the enzyme alkaline phosphatase are lowered with this drug.

Refer to MyNursingKit for a Nursing Process Focus specific to this drug.

PAGET'S DISEASE

Paget's disease, or *osteitis deformans*, is a chronic, progressive condition characterized by enlarged and abnormal bones. With this disorder, the processes of bone resorption and bone formation occur at a high rate. Excessive bone turnover causes the new bone to be weak and brittle, which may result in deformity and fractures. The patient may be asymptomatic or have only vague, nonspecific complaints for many years. Symptoms include pain of the hips and femurs, joint inflammation, headaches, facial pain, and hearing loss if bones around the ear cavity are affected. Nerves along the spinal column may be pinched in the compressed vertebrae.

CORE CONCEPT 33.5

PEARSON
mynursingkit
THE PAGET FOUNDATION

Treatment for Paget's disease includes bisphosphonates and calcitonin.

Paget's disease is sometimes confused with osteoporosis because some of the symptoms are similar. In fact, medical treatments for osteoporosis are similar to those for Paget's disease. The cause of Paget's disease, however, is quite different. Blood levels of the enzyme alkaline phosphatase are elevated because of the extensive bone turnover. Detection of this enzyme in the blood often provides early confirmation of the disease. Calcium blood levels are also increased. The symptoms of Paget's disease can be treated successfully when diagnosis is made early. If the diagnosis is made late in the disease's progression, permanent skeletal abnormalities may develop, and other disorders may appear, including arthritis, kidney stones, and heart disease.

Bisphosphonates are drugs of choice for the pharmacotherapy of Paget's disease. Therapy is usually cyclic: Bisphosphonates are administered until serum alkaline phosphatase levels return to normal; then a drug-free period of several months follows. When serum alkaline phosphatase levels become elevated, therapy is begun again. The pharmacologic goals are to slow the rate of bone reabsorption and encourage the deposition of strong bone. Calcitonin nasal spray is used as an option for patients who cannot tolerate bisphosphonates. Surgery may be indicated in cases of severe bone deformity, degenerative arthritis, or fracture. Patients with Paget's disease should receive adequate daily dietary intake of calcium and vitamin D. Sufficient exposure to sunlight is also important.

Concept Review 33.3

■ Identify two important disorders characterized by weak and fragile bones. What are the major drug therapies used in their treatments?

ARTHRITIC AND JOINT DISORDERS

Arthritis is a general term meaning inflammation of a joint. There are several types of arthritis, each having somewhat different characteristics based on the etiology. Because joint pain is common to both arthritic and joint disorders, analgesics and/or anti-inflammatory drugs are important components of pharmacotherapy. A few additional drugs are specific to the particular pathologies.

OSTEOARTHRITIS

Osteoarthritis is a degenerative, age-onset disease in which the cartilage at articular joint surfaces wears away. It is not accompanied by the degree of inflammation associated with other forms of arthritis.

Analgesics and anti-inflammatory drugs are important components of pharmacotherapy for osteoarthritis.

Osteoarthritis (OA) is the most common type of arthritis and produces localized pain and stiffness, joint and bone enlargement, and limitations in movement. The cause of OA is thought to be excessive wear and tear of weight-bearing joints; the knee, spine, and hip are particularly affected. Many consider this disorder to be a normal part of the aging process.

The goals of pharmacotherapy for OA include reduction of pain and inflammation. The COX-2 inhibitors (see Chapter 24 ⚭) were once the preferred therapy for OA, but in 2004 their safety and effectiveness came under review by the Food and Drug Administration (FDA), and several drugs of the class were removed from the market.

Topical medications (capsaicin cream and balms), nonsteroidal anti-inflammatory drugs (NSAIDs) (including aspirin), acetaminophen, and tramadol (Ultram) are valuable for treatment of pain associated with OA. In acute cases, intra-articular glucocorticoids may be used on a temporary basis.

A new type of drug therapy for patients with moderate OA who do not respond adequately to analgesics has been sodium hyaluronate (Hyalgan). This chemical is normally found in high amounts within synovial fluid. Administered by injection directly into the knee joint, this drug replaces or supplements the body's natural hyaluronic acid that deteriorates due to the condition of OA. Treatment consists of three to five injections at the rate of one per week. By coating the articulating cartilage surface, Hyalgan helps to provide a barrier, thus preventing friction and further injury to the joint. Patients should be told that adverse effects can include pain and/or swelling at the injection site, and they must avoid strenuous activities for approximately 48 hours after an injection.

osteo = *bone*
rheuma = *watery discharge*
toid = *associated*
arthr = *joint*
itis = *associated disease, often linked with inflammation*

RHEUMATOID ARTHRITIS

Rheumatoid arthritis is a systemic autoimmune disorder that causes disfigurement and inflammation of multiple joints and usually occurs at an earlier age than OA.

Glucocorticoids, immunosuppressants, and disease-modifying drugs are additional therapies used to treat rheumatoid arthritis.

Rheumatoid arthritis (RA) is the second most common form of arthritis and has an autoimmune etiology. In RA, **autoantibodies**, called *rheumatoid factors*, activate other inflammatory substances called *complement proteins* and draw leukocytes into an area where they attack normal cells. This results in ongoing injury and formation of inflammatory fluid within the joints. Joint capsules, tendons, ligaments, and skeletal muscles may also be affected. Unlike OA, which causes local pain in affected joints, patients with RA may develop systemic manifestations that include infections, pulmonary disease, pericarditis, abnormal numbers of blood cells, and symptoms of metabolic dysfunction such as fatigue, anorexia, and weakness.

Pharmacotherapy for RA includes the same classes of analgesics and anti-inflammatory drugs used to treat OA. Additional drugs are sometimes prescribed to control the severe inflammation and the immune aspects of the disease. Additional therapies, usually prescribed as a second course of treatment after analgesics and anti-inflammatories, include the following:

auto = *self-directed*
anti = *against*
bodies = *things*

- Glucocorticoids
- **Disease-modifying antirheumatic drugs (DMARDs):** hydroxychloroquine (Plaquenil), gold salts, sulfasalazine (Azulfidine), D-penicillamine (Cuprimine)
- Immunosuppressants: methotrexate (Rheumatrex), leflunomide (Arava), azathioprine (Imuran), cyclosporine (Neoral, Sandimmune), cyclophosphamide (Cytoxan)
- Biologic agents; tumor necrosis factor blockers and interleukin-1 blockers: etanercept (Enbrel), infliximab (Remicade), adalimumab (Humira), anakinra (Kineret)

DMARDs not only treat arthritis symptoms, but they are remittive and can slow down progressive joint destruction. They are often used as a second form of treatment, after other anti-inflammatory drugs have failed. These and additional therapies may require several months of

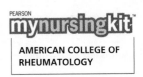

treatment before maximum therapeutic effects are achieved. Because many of these drugs can be toxic, patients should be closely monitored. Adverse effects vary depending on the type of drug. These agents are listed in Table 33.3.

Nonpharmacologic therapies for the pain of arthritis are common. The use of nonimpact and passive range-of-motion (ROM) exercises to maintain flexibility along with rest is encouraged. Splinting may help keep joints positioned correctly and relieve pain. Other therapies commonly used to relieve pain and discomfort include thermal therapies, meditation, visualization, distraction techniques, and massage therapy. Knowledge of proper body mechanics and posturing, provided by physical and occupational therapists, offers some benefit. Surgical techniques such as joint replacement and reconstructive surgery may be necessary when other methods are ineffective.

Concept Review 33.4

■ Identify the major types of arthritis. What are the general differences between these disorders?

TABLE 33.3	**Disease-Modifying and Related Drugs for Rheumatoid Arthritis**	
DRUG	**ROUTE AND ADULT DOSE**	**REMARKS**
adalimumab (Humira)	SC; 40 mg every other week; without methotrexate, dose can be increased up to 40 mg every week	Tumor necrosis factor blocker
anakinra (Kineret)	SC; 100 mg per day	Interleukin-1 blocker
auranofin (Ridaura)	PO; 3–6 mg daily; may increase up to 3 mg tid after 6 months	Gold salt
aurothioglucose (Gold thioglucose, Solganal)	IM; 10 mg week 1, 25 mg week 2; then 50 mg/week to a cumulative dose of 1 g	Gold salt
azathioprine (Imuran)	PO; 0.5–1.0 mg/kg/day (max: 2.5 mg/kg/day)	Immunosuppressant and anti-inflammatory; may cause bone marrow depression
etanercept (Enbrel)	SC; 50 mg once weekly	Tumor necrosis factor blocker
gold sodium thiomalate (Myochrysine)	IM; 10 mg week 1, 25 mg week 2; then 25–50 mg/week to a cumulative dose of 1 g	Gold salt; expected adverse effects with administration: flushing, dizziness, fainting
(Pr) hydroxychloroquine (Plaquenil)	PO; 400–600 mg daily	Has been used for acute malaria and malaria suppression
infliximab (Remicade)	IV; 3 mg/kg followed by 3 mg/kg 2 weeks and 6 weeks after initial dose and then every 8 weeks	Tumor necrosis factor-alpha blocker, used in combination with methotrexate
leflunomide (Arava)	PO; loading dose 100 mg/day for 3 days; maintenance dose 10–20 mg daily	Immunomodulator with anti-inflammatory effects; may cause Stevens-Johnson syndrome
methotrexate (Rheumatrex, Trexall) (see page 466 for the Drug Profile box)	PO; 2.5–5 mg every 12 hours for three doses each week	Folic acid blocker; antineoplastic and immunosuppressant; may cause liver toxicity, sudden death, and pulmonary fibrosis
penicillamine (Cuprimine, Depen)	PO; 125–250 mg daily (max: 1–1.5 g/day)	Also used to promote increased excretion of excess copper; used to limit urinary excretion of cystine
rituximab (Rituxan)	IV; 1,000 mg every 2 weeks for a total of two doses (give a corticosteroid 30 min prior to treatment)	Also indicated for the treatment of non-Hodgkin's lymphoma (NHL)
sulfasalazine (Azulfidine)	PO; 250–500 mg daily (max: 8 g/day)	Also for ulcerative colitis

DRUG PROFILE: Ⓟ *Hydroxychloroquine (Plaquenil)*

Therapeutic Class: Disease-modifying antirheumatic drug (DMARD)

Pharmacologic Class: Protein synthesis inhibitor, inhibitor of DNA and RNA polymerase, rheumatoid agent

Actions and Uses:

Hydroxychloroquine is prescribed for RA and lupus erythematosus in patients who have not responded well to other anti-inflammatory drugs. This agent relieves the severe inflammation characteristic of these disorders. For full effectiveness, hydroxychloroquine is most often prescribed with salicylates and glucocorticoids. This drug has also been used for prophylaxis and treatment of malaria.

Adverse Effects and Interactions:

Adverse symptoms include blurred vision, GI disturbances, loss of hair, headache, and mood and mental changes. Hydroxychloroquine has possible ocular effects that include blurred vision, photophobia, diminished ability to read, and blacked out areas in the visual field.

Antacids with aluminum and magnesium may prevent absorption. This drug interferes with the patient's response to the rabies vaccine. Hydroxychloroquine may increase the risk of liver toxicity when administered with drugs that are toxic to the liver. Alcohol use should be eliminated during therapy. It also may lead to increased digoxin levels.

Refer to MyNursingKit for a Nursing Process Focus specific to this drug.

Fast Facts Arthritis and Joint Disorders

- Between 20 million and 40 million patients in the United States are affected by OA.

- After age 40, more than 90% of the population has symptoms of OA in major weight-bearing joints. After 70 years of age, almost all patients have symptoms of OA.

- Of the world's population, 1% has RA, which most often affects patients between 30 and 50 years of age. Women are three to five times more likely to develop RA than men.

- Between 1% and 3% of the U.S. population is affected by gout. Most of the patients are men between the ages of 30 and 60. Most women are affected after menopause.

GOUT

Gout, a form of acute arthritis, is a metabolic disorder caused by the accumulation of uric acid in the bloodstream or joint cavities; this disorder is extremely painful.

Drug therapy for gout requires agents that inhibit uric acid buildup.

CORE CONCEPT **33.8**

Gout is a disorder characterized by an accumulation of uric acid crystals that occurs when excretion of uric acid by the kidneys is reduced. One metabolic step important to the pharmacotherapy of this disease is the conversion of hypoxanthine to uric acid by the enzyme xanthine oxidase. Uric acid is the final breakdown product of DNA and RNA metabolism. An elevated blood level of uric acid is called *hyperuricemia.*

Gout may be classified as primary or secondary. *Primary gout,* caused by genetic errors in uric acid metabolism, is most commonly observed in Pacific Islanders. *Secondary gout* is caused by diseases or drugs that increase the metabolic turnover of nucleic acids or that interfere with uric acid excretion. Examples of drugs that may cause gout include thiazide diuretics, aspirin, cyclosporine, and alcohol (when ingested on a chronic basis). Conditions that can cause secondary gout include diabetic ketoacidosis, kidney failure, and diseases associated with a rapid cell turnover, such as leukemia, hemolytic anemia, and polycythemia.

hyper = *elevated*
uric = *uric acid*
emia = *blood level*

TABLE 33.4	Uric Acid-Inhibiting Drugs for Gout and Gouty Arthritis	
DRUG	**ROUTE AND ADULT DOSE**	**REMARKS**
allopurinol (Lopurin, Zyloprim)	PO (primary); 100 mg daily; may increase by 100 mg/week (max: 800 mg/day) PO (secondary); 200–800 mg daily for 2–3 days or longer	For primary hyperuricemia, secondary hyperuricemia, and prevention of gout flare-up
colchicine (Colcrys)	PO; 0.5–1.2 mg followed by 0.5–0.6 mg every 1–2 hours until pain relief (max: 1.2 mg/day)	For acute gouty attack; may cause gastric upset at higher doses; IV form available
febuxostat (Uloric)	PO; 40–80 mg once daily	For chronic management of hyperuricemia in patients with gout
probenecid (Benemid, Probalan)	PO; 250 mg bid for 1 week; then 500 mg bid (max: 3 g/day)	For gout; also used as an adjunct for penicillin or cephalosporin therapy
sulfinpyrazone (Anturane)	PO; 100–200 mg bid for 1 week; then increase to 200–400 mg bid	For gout; also used for inhibition of platelet aggregation

Acute gouty arthritis occurs when needle-shaped uric acid crystals accumulate in joints, resulting in red, swollen, and inflamed tissue. Attacks have a sudden onset; often occur at night; and may be triggered by diet, injury, or other stresses. Gouty arthritis most often occurs in the big toes, heels, ankles, wrists, fingers, knees, and elbows. About 90% of patients with gout are men.

Uric acid-inhibiting drugs block the accumulation of uric acid within the blood, or uric acid crystals within the joints. The goals of gout pharmacotherapy are twofold: termination of acute attacks and prevention of future attacks. NSAIDs are the drugs of choice for treating the pain and inflammation of acute attacks. Indomethacin (Indocin) is an NSAID that has been widely used for acute gout.

The uric acid inhibitors (Table 33.4) such as colchicine (Colcrys), probenecid (Benemid), sulfinpyrazone (Anturane), and allopurinol (Lopurin) are also used for acute gout. In 2009, the first new antigout drug in over 40 years was approved by the FDA. Febuxostat (Uloric) acts by the same mechanism as allopurinol but is safer for patients with renal impairment because it is not excreted by the kidneys. Uric acid inhibitors block the accumulation of uric acid within the blood or of uric acid crystals within the joints. When uric acid accumulation is blocked, symptoms associated with gout diminish. About 80% of the patients using uric acid inhibitors experience GI complaints such as abdominal cramping, nausea, vomiting, and/or diarrhea. Glucocorticoids are useful for the short-term therapy of acute gout, particularly when the symptoms are in a single joint and the medication is delivered intra-articularly.

Prophylaxis of gout includes dietary management, avoidance of drugs that worsen gout, and treatment with antigout medications. Patients should avoid high-purine foods such as meat, legumes, alcoholic beverages, mushrooms, and oatmeal because nucleic acids will be formed when they are metabolized. Prophylactic therapy with drugs that lower serum uric acid is used for patients who suffer frequent and acute gout attacks. Probenecid and sulfinpyrazone are *uricosuric* drugs that increase the excretion of uric acid by blocking its reabsorption in the kidney. Allopurinol blocks xanthine oxidase, thus inhibiting the formation of uric acid. Prophylactic therapy is used for patients who suffer frequent and acute gout attacks.

Concept Review **33.5**

■ Identify drug therapies used to treat the major arthritic and joint disorders.

NATURAL THERAPIES

Glucosamine and Chondroitin for Osteoarthritis

Glucosamine sulfate is a natural substance that is an important building block of cartilage. With aging, glucosamine is lost with the natural thinning of cartilage. As cartilage wears down, joints lose their normal cushioning ability, resulting in the pain and inflammation of OA. Glucosamine sulfate is available as an over-the-counter (OTC) dietary supplement. Some studies have shown it to be more effective than a placebo in reducing mild arthritis and joint pain. It is claimed to promote cartilage repair in the joints. Although reliable long-term studies are not available, glucosamine is marketed as a safe and inexpensive alternative to prescription anti-inflammatory drugs.

Chondroitin sulfate is another dietary supplement claimed to promote cartilage repair. It is a natural substance that forms part of the matrix between cartilage cells. Chondroitin is usually combined with glucosamine in specific arthritis formulas.

DRUG PROFILE: Ⓡ *Colchicine (Colcrys)*

Therapeutic Class: Antigout agent
Pharmacologic Class: Inhibitor of uric acid accumulation

Actions and Uses:

Colchicine inhibits inflammation and reduces pain associated with gouty arthritis. It may be taken prophylactically for acute gout or in combination with other uric acid-inhibiting agents. Colchicine works by inhibiting the synthesis of subcellular microtubules, decreasing the movement of white blood cells into the inflamed area. It disrupts the accumulation of uric acid deposits and inhibits formation of a glycoprotein that is produced when white blood cells phagocytize the uric acid crystals. In 2009, colchicine became the first drug approved by the FDA to treat familial Mediterranean fever (FMF), a hereditary disorder characterized by acute inflammation and arthritis.

Adverse Effects and Interactions:

Adverse effects such as nausea, vomiting, diarrhea, and GI upset are more likely to occur at the beginning of therapy. These adverse effects are related to disruption of microtubules responsible for cell proliferation. Colchicine may also directly interfere with the absorption of vitamin B_{12}.

Colchicine interacts with many drugs. For example, NSAIDs may increase GI symptoms, and cyclosporine may increase bone marrow suppression. Erythromycin may increase colchicine levels. Phenylbutazone may increase the risk for blood disorders. Loop diuretics may decrease colchicine effects. Alcohol or products that contain alcohol may cause skin rashes and increased liver damage.

Refer to MyNursingKit for a Nursing Process Focus specific to this drug.

PATIENTS NEED TO KNOW

Patients taking drugs for bone or joint disorders need to know the following:

In General

1. When receiving treatment for problems with mobility, it often takes several weeks for effectiveness to begin. Follow the advice of a health care provider in order to achieve full therapeutic effect.

Regarding Calcium and Bone-Regulating Medications

2. When taking calcium or vitamin D supplements, be aware of the signs and symptoms of hypercalcemia. Check with the health care provider or pharmacist before taking supplements of any kind. In some cases, only proper diet and sunshine are needed for successful therapy.
3. Zinc-rich food products (nuts, seeds, tofu, and legumes) may interfere with calcium absorption. Calcium may react with some foods or interfere with the absorption of iron and bisphosphonates.
4. Be familiar with the risks and long-term effects of vitamin D therapy, corticosteroids, hormone therapy involving estrogen, and estrogen receptor modulators. Major undesirable adverse effects could occur in some cases.
5. Know how to use a nasal pump if taking calcitonin by this method. Be aware that some vitamins may interfere with the pharmacologic effects of calcitonin.
6. Some medications cause GI discomfort. Drugs like these can be taken after meals or with milk to minimize discomfort.

Regarding Arthritic and Joint-Related Medications

7. Report any unfavorable symptoms such as bone pain, restricted mobility, inflammation, or fracture to a health care provider. Report any muscle pain because muscles that have not been moved for a while may feel stiff and tender.
8. When taking some antigout medications, drink plenty of fluids to avoid kidney stones. To ensure proper fluid balance, monitor intake and output of fluids.
9. When taking probenecid, avoid taking aspirin for pain because it interferes with the drug's action. Take acetaminophen instead.
10. Be careful when taking sulfa drugs because they may produce unfavorable reactions.

SAFETY ALERT

Soundalike Drug Names – Celecoxib (Celebrex) and Celexa

Mary Clark will be discharged today from the hospital. Earlier this week she slipped on the icy pavement and injured her back. She has been given a prescription for celecoxib (Celebrex). While she is preparing to leave the hospital she mentions to the nurse that the new medication written on the prescription sounded a lot like the medication she routinely takes for depression (Celexa). Confusing drugs with similar names accounts for about 10% of all medication errors, according to the FDA. The nurse needs to counsel the patient about ways to avoid a self-medication error. One way to avoid the error is to instruct the patient to talk with the pharmacist who will be filling the prescription about the "soundalike" drugs. The drug may need to be packaged in a distinctly different type of container that will help prevent confusion that could occur with similar bottles. The patient can also label the bottles with large letters using the words ANTIDEPRESSION and PAIN PILLS. Storing the medication in two different locations may also be helpful. While the patient is taking both drugs, it might be best to have someone else double-check the medication with the patient to be certain that the appropriate medication is being taken.

CHAPTER REVIEW

CORE CONCEPTS SUMMARY

33.1 Adequate levels of calcium, vitamin D, parathyroid hormone, and calcitonin are necessary for normal body processes.

One of the most important minerals in the body responsible for proper nerve conduction, muscle contractions, and bone formation is calcium. Calcium homeostasis is controlled by two important hormones, PTH and calcitonin. These hormones influence major body targets: the bones, kidneys, and GI tract. They direct the processes of bone resorption and bone deposition. Active vitamin D increases calcium absorption from the GI tract and helps to keep proper calcium balance in the body.

33.2 Hypocalcemia is a serious condition that requires immediate therapy.

Hypocalcemia, or lowered calcium levels in the bloodstream, is a sign of an underlying disorder; therefore, identifying its cause is essential. Signs of hypocalcemia are nerve and muscle excitability, muscle twitching, tremor, or cramping. These conditions are often reversed with calcium supplements. Calcium supplements consist of complexed and elemental calcium. Elemental calcium may be obtained from dietary sources.

33.3 Treatment for osteomalacia consists of calcium and vitamin D supplements.

Osteomalacia, called rickets in children, is a disorder characterized by softening of bones without alteration of basic bone structure. Drug therapy for children and adults consists of calcium supplements and vitamin D.

33.4 Treatment for osteoporosis includes calcitonin, estrogen-receptor modulator drugs, and bisphosphonates.

Osteoporosis, or weak bones caused by disrupted bone homeostasis, is the most common metabolic bone disease. The onset of menopause is the most frequent risk factor. Many drug therapies are available for this disorder, including calcium and vitamin D therapy, estrogen therapy, estrogen receptor modulators, statins, slow-release sodium fluoride, bisphosphonates, and calcitonin.

33.5 Treatment for Paget's disease includes bisphosphonates and calcitonin.

Paget's disease is a chronic progressive condition characterized by enlarged and abnormal bones. Although the cause of Paget's disease is different from that of osteoporosis, medical treatments are similar. Bisphosphonates are drugs of choice for the pharmacotherapy of Paget's disease.

33.6 Analgesics and anti-inflammatory drugs are important components of pharmacotherapy for osteoarthritis.

Arthritis is a general term meaning inflammation of the joints. The goals of pharmacotherapy for osteoarthritis include reduction of pain and inflammation.

33.7 **Glucocorticoids, immunosuppressants, and disease-modifying drugs are additional therapies used to treat rheumatoid arthritis.**

Rheumatoid arthritis (RA) is the second most common form of arthritis and has an autoimmune etiology. Pharmacotherapy for RA includes these same classes of analgesics and anti-inflammatory drugs, plus additional therapies of glucocorticoids, disease-modifying drugs, immunosuppressants, and biologic agents.

33.8 **Drug therapy for gout requires agents that inhibit uric acid buildup.**

Gout is caused by an accumulation of uric acid in the bloodstream. Gout may be classified as primary or secondary gout. Acute gouty arthritis occurs when needle-shaped uric acid crystals accumulate in the joints. The goals of gout pharmacotherapy include termination of acute attacks and prevention of future attacks with the use of uric acid inhibitors.

REVIEW QUESTIONS

The following questions are written in NCLEX-PN® style. Answer these questions to assess your knowledge of the chapter material, and go back and review any material that is not clear to you.

1. This medication lowers serum alkaline phosphatase.

1. Sulfasalazine (Azulfidine)
2. Etidoronate (Didronel)
3. Colchicine
4. Baclofen (Lioresal)

2. The patient on raloxifene (Evista) has had warfarin (Coumadin) ordered. The nurse understands the patient may experience:

1. Decreased effectiveness of raloxifene
2. Increased effectiveness of raloxifene
3. Increased clotting times
4. Decreased clotting times

3. The patient taking calcitriol should be assessed for:

1. Dysrhythmias
2. Hypercalcemia
3. Fluid overload
4. Flulike symptoms

4. Which of the following statements demonstrates that the patient with gout needs additional instructions?

1. "I will take my allopurinol as prescribed by my physician."
2. "I will stop having alcoholic beverages."
3. "I will avoid high purine foods."
4. "I will continue my aspirin therapy."

5. Because esophageal irritation can occur, this medication should not be used if the patient cannot remain in an upright position for 30 minutes after taking it.

1. HT with estrogen
2. Calcitonin

3. Alendronate (Fosamax)
4. Raloxifene (Evista)

6. This medication, when used intranasally, may cause irritation of the nasal mucosa.

1. Calcitonin
2. Vitamin D
3. Calcium
4. Raloxifene (Evista)

7. The patient has had a total thyroidectomy. The nurse will assess for all of the following except:

1. Cramping
2. Confusion
3. Tingling of extremities
4. Bone pain

8. Calcium levels in the blood are lowered by the action of:

1. Calcitriol
2. Parathyroid hormone
3. Thyroid hormone
4. Vitamin D

9. Calcitonin is not indicated for which of the following?

1. Paget's disease
2. Hypercalcemia
3. Hypocalcemia
4. Osteoporosis

10. The patient taking calcium channel blockers should not take:

1. Dantrolene sodium (Dantrium)
2. Calcifediol
3. Ergocalciferol (Deltalin)
4. Calcium gluconate (Kalcinate)

CASE STUDY QUESTIONS

For questions 1–4, please refer to the following case study, and choose the correct answer from choices 1–4.

*M*r. Hurtt is a 60–year-old white male. In an office visit, Mr. Hurtt complains of joint pain in the knees, ankles, and shoulders. Over the last several years, he has taken aspirin for overall pain, but he generally has not been compliant with regular office visits to the clinic. Thus, there is little historical information about this patient on file. Laboratory and physical examination yield the following information: persistent cough, small nodules found sporadically under the skin, complaint of intense pain in one of the metatarsophalangeal joints, acute swelling of the knees, and elevated blood urea nitrogen, serum creatinine, white blood cell (WBC) count, and serum lipids.

1. Mr. Hurtt most likely has which of the following disorders?

1. Paget's disease
2. Gouty arthritis
3. Osteoarthritis
4. Rheumatoid arthritis

2. Which of the following medications will most effectively treat Mr. Hurtt's symptoms?

1. Calcitriol (Calcijex, Rocaltrol)
2. Azathioprine (Imuran)
3. Allopurinol (Lopurin, Zyloprim)
4. Raloxifene (Evista)

3. The small nodules found underneath the surface of the skin are most likely linked to:

1. An unexplained allergic reaction
2. Infection, as supported by the persistent cough
3. Monosodium urate crystals
4. Vasodilation of skin tissue due to NSAID use

4. In order for successful pharmacotherapy in Mr. Hurtt's case, which of the following medications would probably NOT INVOLVE suspension of aspirin therapy?

1. Colchicine
2. Probenecid (Benemid, Probalan)
3. Sulfinpyrazone (Anturane)
4. Indomethacin (Indocin)

FURTHER STUDY

- Physiologic processes involving calcium are mentioned throughout the text in Chapters 8, 12, 13, 17, 19, 20, 23, 30, and 31 ∞ .

- Causes of muscle and joint stiffness can include overmedication with antipsychotic drugs, which are discussed in Chapter 11 ∞ .

- Additional information on HT and the effects of estrogen may be found in Chapter 32 ∞ .

- Drugs for relieving pain are discussed in Chapter 14 ∞ .

- Anti-inflammatory agents are presented in Chapter 24 ∞ .

34 Drugs for Skin Disorders

CORE CONCEPTS

34.1 Layers of skin provide protection to the body.

34.2 The major causes of skin disorders are injury, aging, inherited factors, and other medical conditions.

34.3 Scabicides and pediculicides treat parasitic mite and lice infestations.

34.4 The goal of drug therapy for sunburn is to eliminate discomfort until healing occurs.

34.5 Problems of acne and rosacea are treated by a combination of OTC and prescription drugs.

34.6 Topical glucocorticoids are used mainly to treat dermatitis and related symptoms.

34.7 Several topical and systemic medications are used to treat psoriatic symptoms.

DRUG SNAPSHOT

The following drugs are discussed in this chapter:

DRUG CLASSES	DRUG PROFILES
Scabicides and Pediculicides	**Pr** permethrin (Acticin, Elimite, Nix)
Drugs for Sunburn and Minor Irritations	**Pr** benzocaine (Americaine, Anbesol, others)
Drugs for Acne and Rosacea	
OTC agent	
Retinoids	**Pr** tretinoin (Avita, Retin-A, Trentin-X)
Hormones	
Antibiotics	

DRUG CLASSES	DRUG PROFILES
Drugs for Dermatitis and Eczema	
Topical glucocorticoids	
Drugs for Psoriasis	
Topical glucocorticoids	
Topical immunomodulators	
Retinoids	
Systemic agents	

LEARNING OUTCOMES

After reading this chapter, the student should be able to:

1. Identify important skin layers and explain how superficial skin cells must be replaced after they become damaged or lost.

2. Describe major symptoms associated with stress and injury to the skin versus those associated with a patient's changing age or health.

3. For each of the classes in the Drug Snapshot, identify representative drugs and explain their mechanisms of action, primary actions, and important adverse effects.

4. Identify the major actions of the following types of drugs as they pertain to treatment of skin disorders: scabicides, pediculicides, topical anesthetics, antibiotics, retinoids, keratolytic agents, glucocorticoids, emollients, and psoralens.

5. Describe popular treatments used in conjunction with available drug therapies for skin disorders.

closed comedones (KOME-eh-dones) *622*

dermatitis (dur-mah-TIE-tiss) *623*

eczema (ECK-zih-mah) *623*

emollients (ee-MOLE-ee-ents) *625*

erythema (ear-ih-THEE-mah) *616*

keratinization (keh-RAT-en-eye-zay-shun) *621*

keratolytic agents (keh-RAT-oh-lih-tik) *623*

open comedones *622*

papules (PAP-yools) *622*

pediculicides (puh-DIK-you-lih-sides) *619*

pruritus (proo-RYE-tus) *615*

psoralen (SOR-uh-len) *625*

pustules (PUSS-chools) *622*

retinoids (RETT-ih-noydz) *623*

retinol (RETT-in-nall) *624*

rosacea (roh-ZAY-shee-uh) *622*

scabicides (SKAY-bih-sides) *619*

scabies (SKAY-beez) *619*

seborrhea (seb-oh-REE-ah) *621*

The integumentary system consists of the skin, hair, nails, sweat glands, and oil glands. The largest of all organs is the skin. Because of its large surface area, it normally provides an effective barrier between extreme conditions in the outside environment and the body's internal organs. At times, however, external conditions become too extreme or conditions within the body change, resulting in unhealthy skin. When this happens, either the body's natural defense system must try to correct the problem, or therapy must be provided to improve the skin's condition. The relationship between the integumentary system and other systems in the body is depicted in Figure 34.1 ■.

The purpose of this chapter is to examine the broad scope of skin disorders and the medications used for skin therapy. Particular attention is given to drugs that are of direct benefit to lice and mite infestations; sunburn; acne; inflammation; and dry, scaly skin. Pharmacotherapy of these conditions provides the basis for a more complete understanding of the many drugs applied to the skin's surface.

CORE CONCEPT 34.1   Layers of skin provide protection to the body.

The skin has three major layers: the epidermis, dermis, and a subcutaneous layer called the hypodermis. Each layer is distinct in form and function and provides the basis for how drugs are injected or applied to the surface of the skin (see Chapter 3 ⚭). The most superficial skin layer is the epidermis. Depending on its thickness, the epidermis has either four or five sublayers. The strongest and outermost sublayer is the stratum corneum, or horny layer. It is called this because of the abundance of the protein keratin, also found in the hair, hooves, and horns of many vertebrate mammals. Not every part of the skin has a large amount of keratin—only those areas that are subject to mechanical stress–for example, the soles of the feet and the palms of the hands.

The deepest sublayer of the epidermis is the stratum germanitivum. It supplies the epidermis with new cells after older, superficial cells have been damaged or lost by normal wear. Cells must migrate over their lifetime to the outermost layers of the skin, where they eventually fall off. As these cells are pushed to the surface, they are flattened and covered with a water-insoluble material, forming a protective seal. The average time it takes for a cell to move from the germanitivum layer to the outer body surface is about 3 weeks. Specialized cells within the deeper layers of the epidermis called *melanocytes* secrete the dark pigment melanin, which offers a degree of protection from the sun's ultraviolet rays.

The next major layer of skin, the dermis, is made up of dense, irregular connective tissue, named this way because of its irregular arrangement of thick protein fibers. The dermis provides a foundation for the epidermis and appendages such as hair and nails. Most receptor nerve endings, sweat glands, oil glands, and blood vessels are found within the dermis.

Below the dermis is the subcutaneous layer, or hypodermis. This layer is composed mainly of adipose tissue or fat that cushions, insulates, and provides a source of energy for the body. The hypodermis is involved with the maintenance of body homeostasis, temperature regulation, and metabolism.

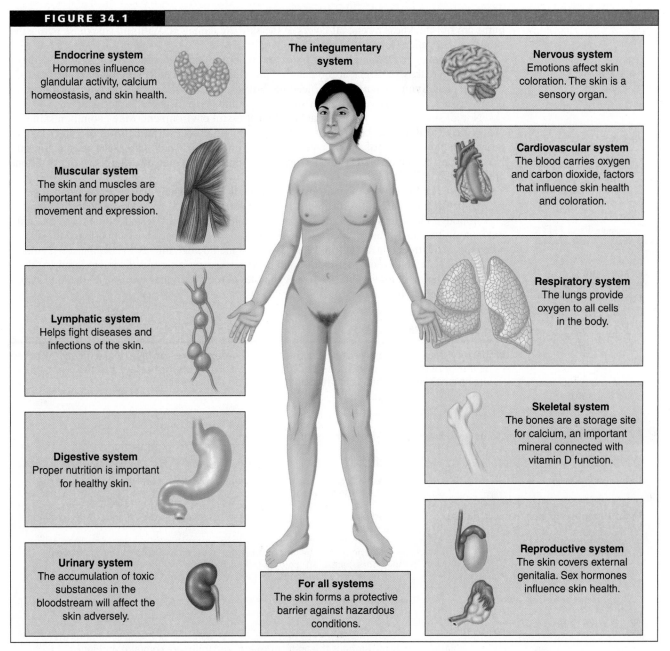

FIGURE 34.1

Endocrine system
Hormones influence glandular activity, calcium homeostasis, and skin health.

Muscular system
The skin and muscles are important for proper body movement and expression.

Lymphatic system
Helps fight diseases and infections of the skin.

Digestive system
Proper nutrition is important for healthy skin.

Urinary system
The accumulation of toxic substances in the bloodstream will affect the skin adversely.

The integumentary system

For all systems
The skin forms a protective barrier against hazardous conditions.

Nervous system
Emotions affect skin coloration. The skin is a sensory organ.

Cardiovascular system
The blood carries oxygen and carbon dioxide, factors that influence skin health and coloration.

Respiratory system
The lungs provide oxygen to all cells in the body.

Skeletal system
The bones are a storage site for calcium, an important mineral connected with vitamin D function.

Reproductive system
The skin covers external genitalia. Sex hormones influence skin health.

The integumentary system (skin) and how the other body systems affect it

The major causes of skin disorders are injury, aging, inherited factors, and other medical conditions.

CORE CONCEPT 34.2

Skin that is dry, cracked, scaly, or worn represents a disturbance in the outermost skin layer. **Pruritus**, or itching, is a symptom often associated with dry, scaly skin, or it may be a symptom of infestation with mites and lice. The thick, horny layer is designed to protect the skin and keep it from drying out.

prur = *itching*
itus = *condition*

Some forceful or noxious stresses may damage deeper layers of the epidermis. When this happens, the role of the germanitivum layer is to replace any skin that might be lost or damaged due to special stresses.

Burns are a unique type of stress that may affect all layers of the skin. They are classified according to the degree of skin damage. First-degree burns affect only the outer layers of the epidermis, are characterized by redness, and are analogous to sunburn. Second-degree burns affect most of the epidermis and part of the dermis, resulting in inflammation and blisters. Third-degree burns are full-thickness burns; all layers of the skin are damaged. With full-thickness burns, the skin cannot regenerate, and skin grafting is required.

eryth = *red*
ema = *appears*

Inflammation, a characteristic of burns and other traumatic disorders, occurs when damage to the skin is extensive. Signs accompanying inflammation include **erythema** or redness, irritation, and pain. Symptoms including bleeding, bruises, and infections may accompany trauma to deeper tissues. Common symptoms of stress or skin injury are listed in Table 34.1.

Not all skin disorders are associated with a stressful environment. Many common skin disorders are related to inherited factors or the normal aging process. Sometimes the skin may appear unhealthy because of another medical condition, or, in some cases, the reason for skin irritation may be unclear and indirect. Common symptoms associated with a range of conditions are presented in Table 34.2.

As listed in Table 34.3, the reasons for skin conditions are many. They can be grouped based on whether they are infectious disorders, inflammatory disorders, or cancer-related disorders.

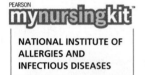

NATIONAL INSTITUTE OF
ALLERGIES AND
INFECTIOUS DISEASES

Although there are many skin disorders, a limited number are less debilitating and require only intermittent drug therapy. A few irritating disorders are of particular importance to patients who require treatment on a walk-in basis. Examples include lice infestation, sunburn with minor irritation, and acne. Eczema, dermatitis, and psoriasis are more serious disorders requiring therapy for a longer time. Figure 34.2 ■ shows examples of regions of the body where irritating symptoms most likely appear.

Concept Review 34.1

■ Identify the skin layers protecting the body. Give examples of layers specifically affected by minor or major external stresses. What skin disorders are not related to the external environment? How would you categorize most skin disorders?

TABLE 34.1	Symptoms Associated with Stress or Injury to the Skin
SYMPTOM	**DESCRIPTION**
Blisters and calluses	Improperly fitting shoes or clothing may cause mechanical stress and abrasion, leading to these lesions.
Bruises, scrapes, and small-impact injuries	Increased physical activity sometimes wears away at the skin and results in minor skin damage.
Crusty and cracked areas	These may be caused by lack of moisture, extremely dry conditions, or severe temperatures; areas affected by lack of moisture include the lips, corners of the mouth, nose, between the fingers and toes, and joint areas.
Cuts, abrasions, and larger wounds	These signs may accompany more dramatic stress, such as sudden trauma or serious accidental injury.
Infections and infestations	There are many types of bacterial, fungal, parasitic, and viral conditions that occur throughout the body; ticks, lice, and mites are common problems associated with hairy skin.
Inflammation and redness	Tissue damage almost always results in inflammation; other signs may also accompany inflammation, as with some allergies, drugs, insect bites, stings, and plant toxins.
Irritated areas	Burning and itching are common symptoms of irritated skin; many chemical agents (for example, household or industrial detergents, greases, and volatile organic agents) may cause skin irritation.
Rash	Exposure to wet conditions for long periods may cause rash; examples are an infant's wet diaper or someone staying in a wet bathing suit for too long.
Sores and lesions	Lack of attention to an area of the body for a long time may cause unhealthy skin, as occurs in elderly, bedridden patients or those who are wheelchair-bound.
Sunburn	The sun's hazardous rays may damage the skin; also, prolonged sun exposure may cause some types of skin cancer.

TABLE 34.2	**Signs and Symptoms of Skin Conditions Associated with a Patient's Changing Health, Age, or Weakened Immune System**
SYMPTOM	**DESCRIPTION**
Delicate skin, wrinkles, and hair loss	Many degenerative changes occur in the skin; some are found in elderly patients; others are genetically related (fragile epidermis, wrinkles, reduced activity of oil and sweat glands, male pattern baldness, poor blood circulation); hair loss may also be linked to some medical procedures; such as radiation and chemotherapy.
Discoloration of the skin	Discoloration is often a useful sign of another medical disorder (for example, anemia, cyanosis, fever, jaundice, or Addison's disease); some medications have photosensitive properties, making a patient's skin sensitive to the sun and causing erythema.
Scales, patches, and itchy areas	Some symptoms may be related to a combination of genetics, stress, and immunity; other symptoms may be related to a fast turnover of skin cells; some symptoms develop for unknown reasons.
Seborrhea/oily skin and bumps	This condition is usually associated with a younger age group; examples include cradle cap in infants and an oily face, chest, arms, and back in teenagers and young adults; pustules, cysts, papules, and nodules represent lesions connected with oily skin.
Tumors	Tumors may be genetic or may occur because of exposure to harmful agents or conditions.
Warts, skin marks, and moles	Some skin marks are congenital; others are acquired or may be linked to environmental factors.

TABLE 34.3	**Classification of Skin Disorders**
DISORDER	**EXAMPLE**
Infectious disorders	Bacterial infections such as boils, impetigo, infected hair follicles; fungal infections such as ringworm, athlete's foot, jock itch, nail infection; parasitic infections such as mosquito bites, ticks, mites, lice; viral infections such as cold sores, fever blisters (herpes simplex), chickenpox, warts, shingles (herpes zoster), measles (rubeola), and German measles (rubella). (See Chapter 25 ⊙⊙ for information on anti-infectives.)
Inflammatory disorders	Injury and exposure to the sun such as sunburn and other environmental stresses; disorders marked by a combination of overactive glands, increased hormone production, or infection such as acne, blackheads, whiteheads, rosacea; disorders marked by itching, cracking, and discomfort, such as eczema (atopic dermatitis), other forms of dermatitis (contact dermatitis, seborrheic dermatitis, stasis dermatitis), and psoriasis.
Skin cancers	There are several types of malignant skin cancers: squamous cell carcinoma, basal cell carcinoma, and malignant melanoma. Malignant melanoma is the most dangerous. Other types of cancer (benign type) include keratosis and keratoacanthoma.

Fast Facts Skin Disorders

- An estimated 3 million people with new cases of lice infestation are treated each year in the United States.
- Nearly 17 million people in the United States have acne, making it the most common skin disease.
- More than 15 million people in the United States have symptoms of dermatitis.
- Ten percent of infants and young children experience symptoms of dermatitis. Roughly 60% of these infants continue to have symptoms into adulthood.
- Psoriasis affects 1–2% of the U.S. population. This disorder occurs in all age groups—adults mainly—affecting about the same number of men as women.

FIGURE 34.2

Anatomical distribution of common skin disorders: (a) contact dermatitis due to footwear; (b) cosmetics; (c) seborrheic dermatitis; (d) acne; (e) scabies; (f) sunburn

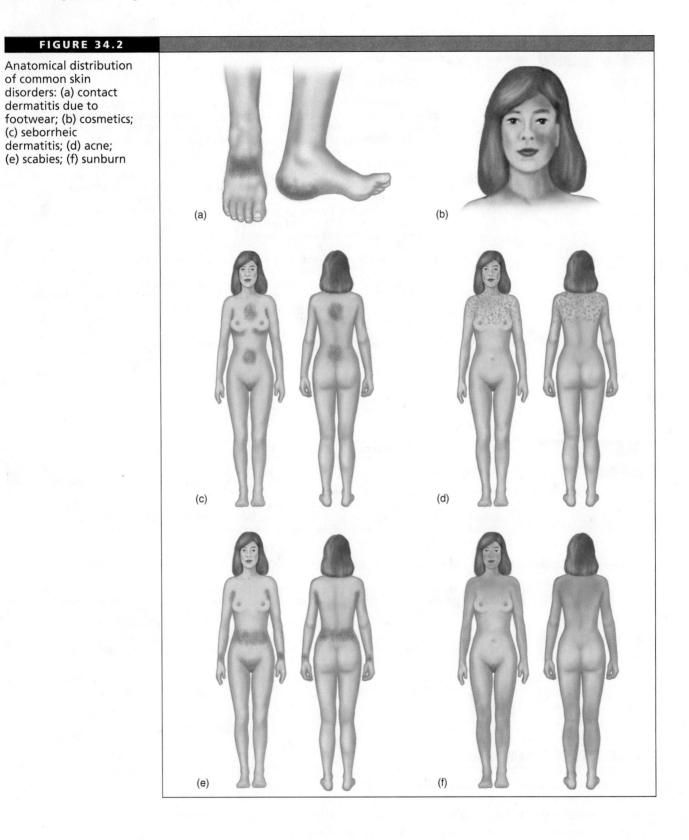

SKIN PARASITES

Common skin parasites include mites and lice. Mites cause a skin disorder called **scabies**, based on their scientific name, *Sarcoptes scabiei*. Scabies is an eruption of the skin caused by the female mite burrowing into the skin and laying eggs. This causes intense itching, most commonly between the fingers, extremities, and around the trunk and pubic area. Scabies is readily spread among family members and sexual partners.

Lice, scientific name *Pediculus,* are another type of skin parasite readily passed on by infected clothing or close personal contact. Lice often infest the pubic area or the scalp and lay eggs that attach to body hairs.

Scabicides and pediculicides treat parasitic mite and lice infestations.

CORE CONCEPT 34.3

Scabicides are pharmacologic agents that kill mites; **pediculicides** kill lice. Either treatment may be effective for both types of parasites. The choice of drug often depends on where the infestation has occurred.

Several important drugs kill lice and mites. These are lindane, sometimes referred to by its chemical name, gamma benzene hexachloride; crotamiton (Eurax); malathion (Ovide); pyrethrin (Rid); and permethrin (Nix). Unlike lindane or crotamiton, permethrin is an insecticide and should be rinsed from the body within 10 minutes after being applied. Malathion and pyrethrin are also insecticides that kill lice by affecting the nervous system of the parasite. Antiparasitic drugs are most often applied to the pubic or scalp area. Patients should be cautioned against applying any lice or mite medication to the mouth, open skin lesions, or eyes.

Lice lay eggs called *nits.* Fine-toothed nit combs are useful in removing nits after the lice have been killed. Patients should comb the infested area after the hair has been dried. To ensure that drug therapy is effective, patients should inspect hair shafts daily for at least 1 week after treatment. Because nits may be present in bedding and other upholstery material, all material coming in close contact with the patient should be washed or treated with the medication.

Concept Review 34.2

■ Name examples of medications used to treat mite and lice infestations. What precautions should be taken when using these medications?

DRUG PROFILE: ℗ *Permethrin (Acticin, Elimite, Nix)*

Therapeutic Class: Antiparasitic drug
Pharmacologic Class: Scabicide, pediculicide

Actions and Uses:

Nix is marketed as a cream or shampoo to kill head and crab lice. It will also kill mites and eradicate their ova. A 1% lotion is approved for lice, and 5% lotion for mites. The medication should be allowed to remain on the hair and scalp 10 minutes before removal. Patients should be aware that itching may last up to 2 or 3 weeks even after parasites have been killed. Successful elimination of parasitic infestations should include removing the nits with a comb, washing bedding, and cleaning or removing objects that have been in contact with the head or hair.

Adverse Effects and Interactions:

Permethrin causes few systemic effects. Local reactions may occur and include pruritus, rash, transient tingling, burning, stinging, erythema, and edema of the infested area.

Contraindications include hypersensitivity to pyrethrins, chrysanthemums, sulfites, or other preservatives. Permethrin should be used cautiously on inflamed skin, in those with asthma, or in lactating women. No significant clinical drug interactions have been documented.

 Refer to MyNursingKit for a Nursing Process Focus specific to this drug.

NURSING PROCESS FOCUS

Patients Receiving Treatment for Lice

ASSESSMENT

Prior to administration:
- Obtain a complete health history, including allergies, drug history, and possible drug interactions
- Assess vital signs
- Assess the skin for presence of lice and/or mite infestation, skin lesions, raw or inflamed skin, and open cuts
- Assess history of seizure disorders
- Obtain the patient's age
- Assess pregnancy and lactation status
- Obtain social history of close contacts, including household members and sexual partners

POTENTIAL NURSING DIAGNOSES

- Deficient Knowledge related to condition and information about drug therapy.
- Noncompliance related to treatment regimen.
- Risk for Impaired Skin Integrity related to drug therapy.

PLANNING: PATIENT GOALS AND EXPECTED OUTCOMES

- Patient and significant others will be free of lice or mites and experience no reinfestation.
- Patient will express an understanding of how lice and mites are spread; proper administration of lindane; necessary household hygiene; and the need to notify household members, sexual partners, and other close contacts (such as classmates) about infestation.
- Skin will be intact and free of secondary infection and/or irritation.

IMPLEMENTATION

Interventions and (Rationales)	Patient Education/Discharge Planning
■ Examine for presence of lice or mites. (This determines the effectiveness of drug therapy.)	Instruct the patient to: ■ Monitor for nits on hair shafts; lice on skin or clothes, inner thigh areas, and seams of clothes that come in contact with axilla, neckline, or beltline ■ Monitor for mites between the fingers, on the extremities, in the axillary and gluteal folds, around the trunk, and in the pubic area
■ Apply prescribed medication properly. (Proper application is critical to elimination of infestation.)	Instruct the patient: ■ To wear gloves during application, especially if applying lindane to more than one person, or if pregnant ■ That all skin lotions, creams, and oil-based hair products should be removed completely by scrubbing the whole body well with soap and water, and drying the skin prior to application ■ To apply permethrin to clean and dry affected body area as directed, using no more than 2 oz per application ■ That eyelashes can be treated with the application of petroleum jelly twice a day for 8 days followed by combing to remove nits ■ To use fine-toothed comb to comb affected hair following lindane application to the hair and scalp; to treat all household members and sexual contacts simultaneously ■ To recheck affected hair or skin daily for at least 1–2 weeks after treatment
■ Inform the patient and others living in the home about proper care of clothing and equipment. (Contaminated articles can cause reinfestation.)	Instruct the patient: ■ To wash all bedding and clothing in hot water, and to dry-clean all nonwashable items that came in close contact with the patient ■ To clean combs and brushes and rinse thoroughly

EVALUATION OF OUTCOME CRITERIA

Evaluate the effectiveness of drug therapy by confirming that patient goals and expected outcomes have been met (see "Planning").

DRUG PROFILE: ℞ *Benzocaine (Americaine, Anbesol, Others)*

Therapeutic Class: Agent for sunburn pain and minor skin irritations

Pharmacologic Class: Local anesthetic, sodium channel blocker

Actions and Uses:

Benzocaine provides temporary relief for pain and discomfort in cases of sunburn, pruritus, minor wounds, and insect bites. Its pharmacologic action is caused by local anesthesia of skin receptor nerve endings. Preparations are also available to treat the skin and other areas such as the ear, mouth, throat, rectal, and genital areas.

Adverse Effects and Interactions:

Benzocaine should not be used for treatment of patients with open lesions, traumatized mucosal areas, or a history of drug sensitivity. Benzocaine may interfere with the activity of some antibacterial sulfonamides. Patients should use preparations only in areas of the body for which the medication is intended.

Refer to MyNursingKit for a Nursing Process Focus specific to this drug.

SUNBURN AND MINOR IRRITATION

Sunburn, a common problem among the general public, is associated with factors such as light skin complexion and lack of proper sun protection. Nonpharmacologic approaches to sun protection include the appropriate use of sunscreens, sunglasses, and sufficient clothing. Limiting the amount of time spent directly in the sun is essential to avoiding sunburn. Many dangers result from sun exposure, including eye injury and skin cancer. Some of these disorders may not appear until years after the exposure.

PEARSON
mynursingkit

THE AMERICAN ACADEMY OF DERMATOLOGY

The goal of drug therapy for sunburn is to eliminate discomfort until healing occurs.

CORE CONCEPT 34.4

Drugs for sunburn and minor irritation include mild lotions and topical anesthetic medications. These are meant to provide temporary relief of painful symptoms.

Pharmacologic treatments for sunburn may not be necessary. Remaining calm until the minor irritation passes is one common approach to mild sunburn. In cases in which pharmacologic intervention is necessary, topical anesthetics such as benzocaine (Solarcaine, others), dibucaine (Nupercainal), and tetracaine (Pontocaine) may be applied. Some of these medications may also provide minor relief from insect bites and pruritus. In cases of more lengthy sun exposure, more potent pain medications may be administered (see Chapters 14 and 24 ⚭), or tetanus toxoid might be administered to prevent infection (see Chapter 25 ⚭).

Concept Review   34.3

■ What is the major purpose of drugs used to treat sunburn, insect bites, and related injuries? What major class of drugs would be used for this purpose?

ACNE AND ACNE-RELATED DISORDERS

Acne is a common condition found most often in adolescents and young adults. The disorder usually begins 1 or 2 years before puberty and is caused by overproductive oil glands or **seborrhea**. Acne is also caused by abnormal **keratinization** or development of the horny layer

sebor = *oil*
rhea = *flow*

of the epithelial tissue of skin. This activity results in blocked oil glands. Administration of androgens or testosterone-like hormones may cause extensive acne by increasing keratinization and the production of sebum (oil). Following this, the bacterium *Propionibacterium acnes* grows within gland openings and modifies the sebum into an acidic and irritating substance. As a result, small inflamed bumps appear on the surface of the skin.

Blackheads, or **open comedones**, are a type of acne in which sebum has plugged the oil gland, causing it to become black because of the presence of melanin granules. Whiteheads, or **closed comedones**, are a type of acne that develops just beneath the surface of the skin and appears white rather than black. In more severe cases of acne, deeper bumps called *nodules* may appear and become very painful because of the intense inflammation and pus found within pore pockets.

Another related skin disorder characterized by inflammation but without pus is **rosacea**. Unlike pimples or **pustules**—the technical name given to pus-filled bumps—rosacea is characterized by small **papules** or inflammatory bumps that swell, thicken, and become very painful. Characteristic of rosacea is its swelling just beneath the surface of the skin. The face of a patient with rosacea may take on a flushed appearance, particularly around the nose and cheek area. Rosacea is exacerbated by many factors, including sunlight, stress, increased temperature, and agents that dilate facial blood vessels such as alcohol, spicy foods, and warm beverages.

Problems of acne and rosacea are treated by a combination of OTC and prescription drugs.

CORE CONCEPT 34.5

Most acne drugs slow down the turnover of skin cells, especially those surrounding pore openings. Some inhibit bacterial growth because they are combined with antibiotics such as doxycycline and tetracycline (see Chapter 25 ⟳). Some drugs must be used carefully because of their ability to dramatically reduce oil gland activity and skin cell turnover.

Important medications for acne-related disorders are summarized in Table 34.4. Benzoyl peroxide (Benzaclin, Benzamycin, and others) is one of the primary over-the-counter (OTC) medications used to treat acne-related disorders. This medication may be dispensed as a lotion, cream, or gel and is available in various concentrations. Benzoyl peroxide decreases symptoms of acne by

TABLE 34.4	Drugs for Acne and Acne-Related Disorders
DRUG	**REMARKS**
OTC Medication—Topical Preparation	
benzoyl peroxide (Benzaclin, Fostex, others)	Often combined with erythromycin or clindamycin to fight bacterial infection; refer to Chapter 25 ⟳
Prescription Medications—Topical	
adapalene (Differin)	Retinoid-like compound used to treat acne formation
azelaic acid (Azelex, Finacea, others)	For mild to moderate inflammatory acne
sulfacetamide sodium (Cetamide, Klaron, others)	For sensitive skin; sometimes combined with sulfur to promote peeling, as in rosacea; also used for conjunctivitis
tazarotene (Tazorac)	A retinoid drug that may also be used for plaque psoriasis; has antiproliferative and anti-inflammatory effects
(Pr) tretinoin (Avita, Retin-A, Trentin-X)	Used to prevent clogging of pore follicles; the oral form (Versanoid) is used for the treatment of acute promyelocytic leukemia and wrinkles
Prescription Medications—Oral	
doxycycline (Adoxa Doryx, Periostat Vibramycin)	Antibiotic; refer to Chapter 25 ⟳
ethinyl estradiol (Estinyl)	Oral contraceptives are sometimes used for acne treatment; combination drugs may be helpful, for example, ethinyl estradiol plus norgestimate (Ortho Tri-Cyclen-28); refer to Chapter 32 ⟳
minocycline (Minocin)	Antibiotic; refer to Chapter 25 ⟳
tetracycline (Sumycin, others) (see page 417 for the Drug Profile box)	Antibiotic; refer to Chapter 25 ⟳

inhibiting bacterial growth and suppressing the turnover of skin cells at the pore's opening. Sometimes benzoyl peroxide is combined with antibiotics to directly fight bacterial infections.

Retinoids are vitamin A-like compounds. Vitamin A provides improved resistance to bacterial infection by reducing oil production and the occurrence of clogged pores. Retinoids are not recommended during pregnancy because of possible harmful effects to the fetus. A common reaction to retinoids is sensitivity to sunlight.

Prescription medications for acne include adapalene (Differin), a retinoid-like compound, and related compounds such as azelaic acid (Alzelex), sulfacetamide (Cetamide), and tretinoin (Retin-A). Tretinoin is sometimes used for wrinkle removal. When acne is particularly severe, resorcinol, salicylic acid, or sulfur may be used as additional treatments to promote shedding of old skin. These are called **keratolytic agents**.

kerato = *horny layer*
lytic = *loosening*

Some drugs may be taken in combination with or in lieu of other acne medications, including doxycycline (Vibramycin and others), tetracycline (Samycin, others), and ethinyl estradiol (Estinyl, Feminone). Doxycycline and tetracycline are antibiotics (see Chapter 25 ⬤). Ethinyl estradiol is an estrogen commonly found in birth control medications (see Chapter 32 ⬤).

Concept Review	34.4

- What is the major purpose of drugs used to treat acne and related skin conditions? Give examples of both topical and systemic medications. Which medications are OTC, and which are prescription medications?

DERMATITIS AND ECZEMA

Eczema, also called *atopic dermatitis,* is a skin disorder with symptoms resembling an allergic reaction, including inflammation, itching, and rash. Long-term itching and scaling may cause the skin to appear thickened and leathery. Exposure to environmental irritants may make these symptoms worse. Other conditions, including stress, too little or too much moisture, and extreme temperature fluctuations, may worsen symptoms. Blisters and other lesions may also develop. In infants and small children, lesions usually begin on the face and progress to other parts of the body. The skin may become raw and infected from scratching.

atopic = *out of place*

Contact dermatitis is a delayed type of allergic reaction resulting from exposure to specific allergens—for example, perfume, cosmetics, detergents, latex, or jewelry. Accompanying the allergic reaction may be various degrees of cracking, bleeding, or small blisters.

Seborrheic dermatitis is a disorder caused by overactive oil glands. This condition is sometimes seen in newborns and in teenagers after puberty. Oily and scaly patches of skin appear in areas of the face, scalp, chest, back, or pubic area. Bacterial infection or dandruff may accompany these symptoms.

Stasis dermatitis is seen more commonly in older women. It is found primarily in the lower extremities. Redness and scaling may be observed in areas where venous circulation is impaired or where deep venous blood clots have formed.

Topical glucocorticoids are used mainly to treat dermatitis and related symptoms.

CORE CONCEPT 34.6

Topical glucocorticoids or corticosteroids are used in cases of **dermatitis** and eczema to treat symptoms of inflammation, burning, and pruritus. In conjunction with other medical therapies, topical corticosteroids are also used for the treatment of psoriasis.

dermat = *skin*
itis = *inflammation*

Topical glucocorticoids are the most effective treatment for dermatitis. As seen in Table 34.5, there are many varieties of glucocorticoids supplied at different levels of potency. Creams, lotions, solutions, gels, and pads are specially formulated to cross skin membranes. These medications are especially intended for the relief of local inflammation and itching. In cases of long-term use, however, adverse affects such as irritation, redness, and thinning of the skin membranes may occur. If absorption occurs, topical glucocorticoids may produce undesirable systemic effects, including adrenal insufficiency, mood changes, serum imbalances, and bone defects, as discussed in Chapter 24 ⬤.

DRUG PROFILE: Pr *Tretinoin (Avita, Retin-A, Trentin-X)*
Therapeutic Class: Antiacne drug
Pharmacologic Class: Retinoid receptor drug, vitamin derivative

Actions and Uses:

This drug is indicated for the early treatment and control of mild to moderate acne vulgaris. Symptoms take 4 to 8 weeks to improve, and maximum therapeutic benefit may take up to 5 or 6 months. This drug is most often reserved for cystic acne or severe keratinization disorders.

The principal action of tretinoin is regulation of skin growth and cell turnover. As cells from the germanitivum grow toward the skin's surface, skin cells are lost from the pore openings, and their replacement is slowed down. Tretinoin also decreases oil production by reducing the size and number of oil glands.

Adverse Effects and Interactions:

Tretinoin is a natural derivative of **retinol** or vitamin A. Thus, vitamin A supplements, which increase toxicity, should be avoided.

Common adverse effects are conjunctivitis (visual disturbance), dry mouth, inflammation of the lip, dry nose, increased serum concentrations of triglycerides, bone and joint pain, and photosensitivity. Additive phototoxicity can occur if tretinoin is used concurrently with other phototoxic drugs such as tetracyclines, fluoroquinolones, or sulfonamides.

Liver function, serum glucose, and serum triglyceride tests should be performed when taking tretinoin. Using tretinoin together with hypoglycemic agents may lead to loss of glycemic control as well as increased risk of cardiovascular disease due to elevated triglyceride levels.

Patients should not take this drug while pregnant. Topical preparations are category C; PO preparations are category D.

Refer to MyNursingKit for a Nursing Process Focus specific to this drug.

TABLE 34.5	Selected Topical Glucocorticoids for Dermatitis and Related Symptoms
GENERIC NAME	**TRADE NAMES**
HIGHEST POTENCY	
betamethasone	Diprolene
clobetasol	Temovate
diflorasone	Maxiflor
HIGH POTENCY	
amcinonide	Cyclocort
desoximetasone	Topicort
fluocinonide	Lidex
halcinonide	Halog
mometasone	Elocon
triamcinolone	Aristocort, Kenalog
MEDIUM POTENCY	
clocortolone	Cloderm
fluocinolone	Synalar
flurandrenolide	Cordran
fluticasone	Flonase
hydrocortisone	Cutivate
LOWER POTENCY	
alclometasone	Aclovate
desonide	Desonate, DesOwen, Verdeso
dexamethasone	Decaspray

PSORIASIS

Psoriasis is a chronic disorder characterized by red patches of skin covered with flaky, silver-colored scales. The silver-colored scales are called *plaques.* The reason for the appearance of plaques is an extremely fast skin turnover rate. The skin reacts as if it has been injured, but skin cells reach the surface much more quickly than usual, in about 4 days, which is six to seven times faster than usual. The reason for this kind of reaction is not known, although scientists believe that it may be a genetic immune reaction. Plaques are ultimately shed from the skin's surface, while the underlying skin becomes inflamed and irritated.

Several topical and systemic medications are used to treat psoriatic symptoms.

CORE CONCEPT 34.7

Because psoriatic symptoms may be extreme, numerous drugs are employed to soothe the patient's symptoms, including **emollients**, topical glucocorticoids, and immunosuppressant medications.

emolli = *to soften*
ent = *causing*

Drugs used for the treatment of psoriasis include topical and systemic medications. Examples are provided in Table 34.6. One of the main treatments for psoriasis is topical glucocorticoids, which reduce the inflammation associated with fast skin turnover. Other agents applied topically are retinoid-like compounds such as calcipotriene (Dovonex) and tazarotene (Tazorac). These drugs provide the same benefits as topical glucocorticoids, but they are much less toxic. Calcipotriene produces elevated levels of calcium in the bloodstream, so this medication is not used on an extended basis.

Systemic medications for psoriasis include acitretin (Soriatane) and etretinate (Tegison). These drugs are taken orally to inhibit skin cell growth. Methotrexate (Rheumatrex, Texall) produces similar effects in the body (see Chapter 27 ⚭). Other medications that are used for different disorders but provide relief of severe psoriatic symptoms are hydroxyurea (Hydrea) and cyclosporine (Sandimmune, Neoral). Hydroxyurea is a sickle cell anemia medication. Cyclosporine is an immunosuppressive agent, discussed in Chapter 24 ⚭ .

Skin therapy techniques may be used with or without other psoriasis medications. These include various forms of tar treatment (coal tar) and a material called *anthralin.* Both substances are applied to the skin's surface. Tar and anthralin inhibit DNA synthesis and arrest abnormal cell growth.

Ultraviolet B (UVB) and ultraviolet A (UVA) phototherapy are techniques used in cases of severe psoriasis. UVB therapy is less hazardous than UVA therapy. UVB light has a wavelength similar to sunlight; it reduces widespread lesions that normally resist topical treatments. With close supervision, this type of phototherapy can be administered at home. Keratolytic pastes are often applied between treatments. The second type of phototherapy is often referred to as PUVA therapy because **psoralens** are often administered in conjunction with phototherapy. Psoralens are oral or topical agents that, when exposed to UV light, produce a photosensitive reaction. This reaction seems to provide benefit to the patient by reducing the number of lesions, but unpleasant adverse effects such as headache, nausea, and skin sensitivity still occur, limiting the effectiveness of this therapy. Immunosuppressant drugs such as cyclosporine are not used in conjunction with PUVA therapy because they increase the risk of skin cancer.

TABLE 34.6	Drugs for Psoriasis and Related Disorders	
DRUG	**ROUTE AND ADULT DOSE**	**REMARKS**
TOPICAL MEDICATIONS		
anthralin (Dritho-Scalp, Psoriatec)	Topically to lesions daily or as directed	Second-line therapy after tolerance to corticosteroids has developed
calcipotriene (Dovonex)	Topically to lesions once or twice daily up to 8 weeks	Synthetic form of vitamin D_3; may raise the level of calcium in the body to unhealthy levels
coal tar (Balnetar, Cutar, others)	Topically to lesions daily or as directed	Second-line therapy after tolerance to corticosteroids has developed
salicylic acid (Salax, Neutrogena, others)	Topically to lesions (concentrations ranging from 2–10%) as directed	Wide range of delivery: creams, foams, gels, lotions, ointments, pads, plasters, shampoos, soaps, and skin solutions
tacrolimus (Protopic)	Topically as directed; apply a thin layer to affected area	Immunosuppressant drug; for moderate to severe eczema
tazarotene (Tazorac)	Acne: Apply thin film to clean, dry area daily; plaque psoriasis: apply a thin film daily in the evening	Topical retinoid; less toxic than corticosteroids
SYSTEMIC MEDICATIONS		
acitretin (Soriatane)	PO; 10–50 mg/day with the main meal	Retinoid; category X drug
cyclosporine (Neoral, Gengraf) (see page 401 for Drug Profile box)	PO; 1.25 mg/kg bid (max: 4 mg/kg/day)	Immunosuppressant drug
etanercept (Enbrel)	Subcutaneous; 50 mg twice weekly (given 3–4 days apart); maintenance dose 50 mg/week	For rheumatoid arthritis
hydroxyurea (Hydrea)	PO; 80 mg/kg every 3 days or 20–30 mg/kg daily	Off label use for psoriasis; also used for sickle cell anemia
methotrexate (Rheumatrx, Trexall) (see page 466 for the Drug Profile box)	PO; 2.5–5 mg bid × 3 doses each week (max: 25–30 mg/week)	For rheumatoid arthritis and neoplasia

PATIENTS NEED TO KNOW

Patients taking medications for skin disorders need to know the following:

1. Inform family members, sexual partners, school personnel, and any other persons with whom close contact has occurred about skin infestations. Treat clothes, bed linens, and personal items properly to avoid reinfestation.
2. Be informed and understand the proper way to apply medication or to remove nits if necessary. Scabicides and pediculicides should not be applied to the face, mouth, open skin lesions, or the eyes.
3. For acne and related disorders, apply medication only to areas where it is supposed to be applied. Follow instructions in package inserts, and do not deviate from the precautions communicated by the health care provider.
4. Do not share skin medications with family or friends. Be familiar with medication adverse effects, especially those of retinoids, retinoid-like products, or medications used to treat severe skin disorders.
5. Use medications only during the time for which they are intended. With extended use, some medications (for example, corticosteroids) may cause adverse effects. Take a medication suitable for the disorder; avoid those that are too potent or not potent enough.
6. Give medications a chance to work. Some systemic medications must be taken exactly as prescribed without skipping or stopping early.
7. Avoid contact with agents that are known to cause allergy or dermatitis. Try to avoid scratching, if possible. For severe skin disorders, see a dermatologist.

■ In most cases, which drug category is used to treat symptoms of dermatitis and psoriasis? What other drug therapies and techniques are used to provide a measure of relief for these symptoms?

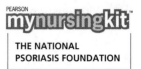

CHAPTER REVIEW

CORE CONCEPTS SUMMARY

34.1 **Layers of skin provide protection to the body.**

Two layers of skin and one underlying layer protect the body: the epidermis, dermis, and hypodermis. The most superficial layer is the epidermis, in which skin cells are replenished every 3 weeks. New cells arise from the bottom layer, called the germanitivum, and are pushed to the outermost layer.

34.2 **The major causes of skin disorders are injury, aging, inherited factors, and other medical conditions.**

Many symptoms are associated with skin stress and injury. Others are associated with a patient's changing age or health. Skin disorders fit into three main categories: infectious, inflammatory, and cancerous disorders.

34.3 **Scabicides and pediculicides treat parasitic mite and lice infestations.**

Mites affect the skin and hair, whereas lice remain localized in hairy regions of the body. Both conditions are treatable with medications. Scabicides kill mites; pediculicides kill lice.

34.4 **The goal of drug therapy for sunburn is to eliminate discomfort until healing occurs.**

Local anesthetics are the primary medication used to treat mild sunburn and irritation. Often drugs are used for temporary relief of minor discomfort; in some cases, drugs may not be needed at all.

34.5 **Problems of acne and rosacea are treated by a combination of OTC and prescription drugs.**

Blackheads, whiteheads, and rosacea are disorders in which pores become blocked, inflamed, or infected because of accelerated skin processes. Topical drugs for acne are those that inhibit bacterial growth (antibiotics) or promote shedding of old skin (keratolytic agents). Vitamin A-like compounds (retinoids) provide an improved resistance to bacterial infections by reducing oil production and the occurrence of clogged pores.

34.6 **Topical glucocorticoids are used mainly to treat dermatitis and related symptoms.**

Dermatitis is treated by agents that reduce symptoms of inflammation, itchiness, flaking, cracking, bleeding, and lesions. Topical corticosteroids are the primary drug treatment for dermatitis. Potency depends on the type of drug formulation and whether it is packaged as a cream, lotion, solution, gel, or pad.

34.7 **Several topical and systemic medications are used to treat psoriatic symptoms.**

Psoriasis is a chronic disorder characterized by extreme discomfort and flaky areas called plaques. The treatments for psoriasis include topical glucocorticoids, retinoid-like compounds, drugs that arrest skin cell growth, and immunosuppressants. Skin therapy techniques are also used, including keratolytic agents, coal tar, anthralin, psoralens, and phototherapy.

REVIEW QUESTIONS

The following questions are written in NCLEX-PN® style. Answer these questions to assess your knowledge of the chapter material, and go back and review any material that is not clear to you.

1. This skin disorder may be caused by lack of moisture and extremely dry conditions.

1. Sunburn
2. Crusty and cracked areas
3. Blisters and calluses
4. Sores and lesions

2. With this type of burn, there is inflammation and blisters.

1. Full thickness
2. First degree
3. Second degree
4. Third degree

3. This medication must be rinsed from the body within 10 minutes after being applied.

1. Lindane
2. Crotamiton (Eurax)
3. Hexachloride
4. Permethrin (Nix)

4. The patient is complaining of discomfort related to minor sunburn. Which of the following would be recommended?

1. Benzocaine (Americaine)
2. Hexachloride
3. Benzoyl peroxide
4. Doxycycline

5. Patients that are pregnant should not take this medication.

1. Hydrocortisone
2. Trentinoin (Retin-A)
3. Benzoyl peroxide
4. Benzocaine

6. The patient is using topical glucocorticoids. The nurse will assess for all the following systemic effects of the medication except:

1. Mood changes
2. Osteoporosis
3. Liver toxicity
4. Adrenal insufficiency

7. Which of the following drugs would be used to treat severe psoriasis?

1. Calcipotriene (Dovonex)
2. Tarzarotene (Tazorac)
3. Acitreten (Soriatane)
4. Cyclosporine (Neoral, Gengraf)

8. This group of medications promotes shedding of old skin.

1. Pediculicides
2. Keratolytic agents
3. Retinoids
4. Glucocorticoids

9. Patients with this skin disorder exhibit bumps without pus that are swollen, thick, and painful.

1. Pustules
2. Erythema
3. Rosacea
4. Papules

10. When teaching the patient about the long-term use of topical glucocorticoids for dermatitis, the nurse should inform the patient about the possibilities of the following adverse effects:

1. Irritation
2. Reddness
3. Thinning of the skin membranes
4. all of the above

CASE STUDY QUESTIONS

For questions 1–4, please refer to the following case study, and choose the correct answer from choices 1–4.

*B*urt is a 16-year-old white male with a family history of various allergy disorders. He is complaining of itching (pruritus), dryness, and general irritation around the face, neck, and forearm. On examination, the nurse pays close attention to the scalp, forehead, behind the ears, and eyes. Nothing unusual is observed–only a slight case of acne in the face, no excessive oil, no erythema, no lesions, no burrows, no nits. Although areas around the neck and forearm are inflamed, these do not appear to be infected.

1. The condition described is probably:

1. Seborrheic dermatitis
2. Scabies
3. Sunburn
4. Atopic dermatitis

2. Effective treatment of the neck and arms would include:

1. Cleansing of the skin with antibacterial soap
2. Application of topical benzocaine (Americaine)
3. Short-term application of topical glucocorticoids
4. Application of a Retinoid (Retin-A)

3. Undesirable systemic effects from the medication used to treat Burt's condition would include:

1. Cardiac arrest
2. Adrenal insufficiency
3. Irritation to the eyes and mucous membranes
4. Adverse central nervous system (CNS) effects, including restlessness, dizziness, and tremors

4. Which of the following interventions would not be helpful in a plan to care for the appearance of acne?

1. Establish rapport with the patient
2. Tell the patient to avoid products that will irritate the skin, such as cologne, perfumes, and other alcohol-based products
3. Encourage use of nonoily face creams
4. Tell the patient to avoid foods that make the acne worse

FURTHER STUDY

- A discussion of topical drug administration is detailed in Chapter 3 ⚭ .

- Chapters 14 and 24 ⚭ cover pain medications that may be of use in severe sunburn.

- Detailed information on the systemic effects of glucocorticoids are discussed in Chapters 24 and 31 ⚭ .

- Systemic medications that are used for psoriasis, such as methotrexate and cyclosporine, are also presented in Chapters 27 and 24 ⚭ , respectively.

- Anti-infective agents used for skin infections are covered in Chapter 25 ⚭ .

- Local anesthetics such as benzocaine are presented in Chapter 14 ⚭ .

EXPLORE PEARSON **mynursingkit**™

MyNursingKit is your one stop for online chapter review materials and resources. Prepare for success with additional NCLEX®-style practice questions, interactive assignments and activities, web links, animations and videos, and more!

Register your access code from the front of your book at www.mynursingkit.com

35 Drugs for Eye and Ear Disorders

CORE CONCEPTS

35.1 Knowledge of basic eye anatomy is required for an understanding of eye disorders and drug therapy.

35.2 Glaucoma is one of the leading causes of blindness.

35.3 Glaucoma therapy centers on adjusting the circulation of aqueous humor.

35.4 Some antiglaucoma medications increase the outflow of aqueous humor.

35.5 Other antiglaucoma medications decrease the formation of aqueous humor.

35.6 Drugs provide relief for minor eye conditions and are used for eye exams.

35.7 Otic preparations treat infections, inflammation, and earwax buildup.

DRUG SNAPSHOT

The following drugs are discussed in this chapter:

DRUG CLASSES	DRUG PROFILES
Drugs for Glaucoma that Increase the Outflow of Aqueous Humor	
Direct-acting miotics (Cholinergic agents)	
Indirect-acting miotics (Cholinesterase inhibitors)	
Sympathomimetics	
Prostaglandins and prostamides	(Pr) latanoprost (Xalatan)
Drugs for Glaucoma that Decrease the Formation of Aqueous Humor	
Beta-adrenergic blockers	(Pr) timolol (Timoptic, Timoptic XE)
Alpha$_2$-adrenergic agents	

DRUG CLASSES	DRUG PROFILES
Carbonic anhydrase inhibitors	
Osmotic diuretics	
Drugs for Eye Examinations and Minor Eye Conditions	
Mydriatics—sympathomimetics	
Cycloplegics—anticholinergics	
Lubricants	
Drugs for Ear Conditions	
Antibiotics	
Earwax (cerumen) softeners	

LEARNING OUTCOMES

After reading this chapter, the student should be able to:

1. Describe important eye anatomy relevant to glaucoma development.

2. Identify the major risk factors associated with glaucoma.

3. Explain how intraocular pressure is related to nerve damage in the eye.

4. Compare and contrast the two principal types of glaucoma, and explain their reasons for development.

5. Explain two major mechanisms by which drugs reduce intraocular pressure.

6. Identify examples of important drugs for treating glaucoma, and explain their basic actions and adverse effects.

7. Identify examples of drugs that dilate or constrict pupils, relax ciliary muscles, constrict ocular blood vessels, or moisten eye membranes.

8. Identify examples of drugs for treating ear infections, earaches, or a buildup of earwax.

KEY TERMS

closed-angle glaucoma (glaw-KOH-mah) *633*

cycloplegia (sy-kloh-PLEE-jee-ah) *635*

cycloplegic drug (sy-kloh-PLEE-jik) *639*

external otitis (oh-TYE-tiss) *639*

mastoiditis (mass-toy-DYE-tuss) *639*

miosis (my-OH-sis) *634*

miotics (my-AH-tiks) *633*

mydriasis (mih-DRY-uh-siss) *634*

mydriatic drugs (my-DRY-at-tik) *639*

open-angle glaucoma (glaw-KOH-mah) *633*

otitis media (oh-TYE-tuss MEE-dee-ah) *639*

tonometry (toh-NAHM-uh-tree) *633*

The eye is one of the most precious sensory organs. A simple scratch can cause the patient almost unbearable discomfort. Other eye disorders may be more bearable but are extremely dangerous, including glaucoma, one of the leading causes of blindness. The first part of this chapter covers various drugs used for the treatment of glaucoma. Drugs used routinely by ophthalmic practitioners are also discussed. The remaining part of the chapter covers examples of drugs used for treatment of ear disorders, including infections, inflammation, and the buildup of earwax (cerumen).

Knowledge of basic eye anatomy is required for an understanding of eye disorders and drug therapy.

CORE CONCEPT 35.1

To understand eye disorders and drug action, one must be familiar with basic eye anatomy. As shown in Figure 35.1 ■, a watery fluid called *aqueous humor* is found in the anterior cavity of the eye. The anterior cavity has two major subcavities: the anterior chamber and the posterior chamber. In the posterior chamber (Figure 35.2 ■), aqueous humor originates from an important muscle structure called the *ciliary body*. From there, aqueous humor flows through the pupil and into the anterior chamber. Within the anterior chamber and around the periphery is a network of spongy connective tissue called *trabecular meshwork*. Connected with trabecular meshwork is an opening called the canal of Schlemm, the location where aqueous humor drains from the anterior cavity.

trabecular = *strut-like*

GLAUCOMA

Glaucoma is one of the most dreaded eye disorders. In some cases, glaucoma is genetic; in other cases, glaucoma may be caused by nongenetic factors, including eye injury and disease. Some medications may contribute to the development of glaucoma, including long-term use of topical glucocorticoids, some antihypertensives, antihistamines, and antidepressants. The major risk factors associated with glaucoma include high blood pressure, migraine headaches, refractive disorders such as nearsightedness or farsightedness, and older age.

FIGURE 35.1

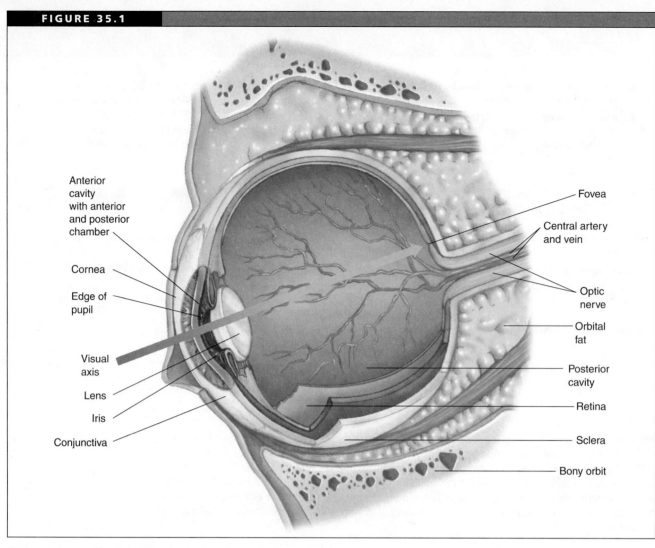

Internal structures of the eye   *Source: Pearson Education/PH College*

FIGURE 35.2

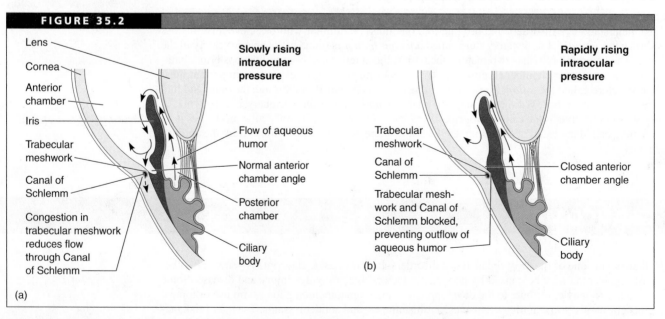

Forms of primary adult glaucoma: (a) in chronic, open-angle glaucoma, the anterior chamber angle remains open, but drainage of aqueous humor through the canal of Schlemm is impaired; (b) in acute, narrow angle-closure glaucoma, the angle of the iris and anterior chamber is smaller, obstructing the outflow of aqueous humor   *Source: Pearson Education/PH College*

Fast Facts Glaucoma

- Worldwide, more than 5 million people have lost their vision as a result of glaucoma. More than 50,000 are in the United States.
- Individuals of African heritage are affected more by glaucoma than any other ethnic group.
- Glaucoma is most common in patients older than 60 years of age.
- Acute glaucoma is often caused by head trauma, cataracts, tumors, or hemorrhage.
- Chronic simple glaucoma accounts for 90% of all glaucoma cases.

Glaucoma is one of the leading causes of blindness.

CORE CONCEPT 35.2

Tests such as tonometry may confirm the presence of glaucoma. **Tonometry** is an ophthalmic technique for measuring increased pressure inside the eye. Other routine refractory and visual field tests may uncover glaucoma signs. One problem with testing is that patients with glaucoma typically do not experience symptoms and, therefore, do not seek medical attention. In some cases, glaucoma occurs so gradually that patients do not notice a problem until later in the disease process.

tono = *pressure*
metry = *measurement*

Glaucoma is characterized by increased pressure inside the eyeball, termed *intraocular pressure* (IOP). The reason why IOP develops is because the flow of aqueous humor becomes blocked. Over time, pressure around the optic nerve can build, leading to blindness. In some cases, eye injury may be sudden, but in most cases it is gradual.

intra = *inside*
ocular = *eye*

As shown in Figure 35.2 ■, the two principal types of glaucoma are **closed-angle glaucoma** and **open-angle glaucoma**. Both disorders result from the same problem: pressure inside the anterior cavity puts pressure on the posterior cavity, leading to progressive damage of the optic nerve. The difference between these two disorders includes how quickly the IOP develops.

Open-angle, or *chronic simple glaucoma,* is the most common type of glaucoma. With this disorder, IOP develops more slowly. It is called "open angle" because the iris does not cover the trabecular meshwork (Figure 35.2a ■).

Closed-angle glaucoma, sometimes referred to as *acute glaucoma,* is usually caused by stress, impact injury, or medications. Pressure inside the anterior chamber increases suddenly because the iris is pushed over the area where the aqueous fluid normally drains (Figure 35.2b ■). Symptoms include intense headaches, difficulty concentrating, bloodshot eyes, and blurred vision.

Glaucoma therapy centers on adjusting the circulation of aqueous humor.

CORE CONCEPT 35.3

There are several approaches to glaucoma therapy. In cases of acute gluacoma, conventional or laser surgery might be performed to return the iris to its original position. Most therapies focus on reducing the amount of aqueous humor formed or unblocking its drainage. Generally, drug therapy for glaucoma functions by either increasing the outflow of aqueous humor (canal of Schlemm location) or by decreasing the formation of aqueous humor (ciliary body location).

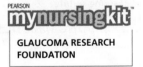

GLAUCOMA RESEARCH FOUNDATION

Concept Review   35.1

- Which components of the eye are specifically affected by glaucoma? Why is glaucoma such a dreaded eye disease? Drug therapy for glaucoma centers around which major approach?

Some antiglaucoma medications increase the outflow of aqueous humor.

CORE CONCEPT 35.4

Drugs increasing the outflow of aqueous humor include miotics, sympathomimetics, prostaglandins, and prostamides. **Miotics** are drugs that cause the pupils to constrict. Sympathomimetics are drugs that mimic activation of the sympathetic nervous system (see Chapter 8 ⚭). Prostaglandins and

mio = *constricting*
sis = *condition*

mydria = *dilating*
sis = *condition*

prostamides are chemical agents that change vascular permeability in selected body tissues. Drugs that increase the outflow of aqueous humor are summarized in Table 35.1.

Miotic drugs produce an effect like acetylcholine; sympathomimetic drugs produce an effect like norepinephrine. Acetylcholine normally causes constriction of pupils or **miosis**. Norepinephrine causes dilation of pupils or **mydriasis**. (Review Chapter 8 ⬭.) Although no antiglaucoma agents are intended to directly alter pupil diameter, they often produce this effect because of their physiologic properties. Prostaglandins do not affect pupil diameter at all, but instead directly dilate trabecular meshwork within the anterior chamber. One of the drawbacks of prostaglandins is that they change pigmentation of the eyes. A related class of drugs called *prostamides* also directly affects trabecular meshwork but with less dramatic effects on iris pigmentation. Although their long-term effectiveness remains to be established, prostamides represent a promising class of drugs for the treatment of open-angle glaucoma.

Direct-Acting Miotics (Cholinergic Agents)

uveo = *uvea, vascular*
    (blood vessel) layer
scler = *sclera*
al = *related to*

Acetylcholine chloride (Miochol), carbachol (Isopto Carbachol, Miostat), and pilocarpine (Adsorbocarpine, Isopto Carptine, and others) are cholinergic agents. These agents directly activate the cholinergic receptors, producing various responses in the eye, including dilation of trabecular meshwork, so that the canal of Schlemm can absorb more aqueous humor. When more aqueous humor is absorbed, IOP is reduced. Thus, uveoscleral draining of the aqueous humor has an

TABLE 35.1	Antiglaucoma Drugs That Increase the Outflow of Aqueous Humor	
DRUG	**ROUTE AND ADULT DOSE**	**REMARKS**
MIOTICS, DIRECT-ACTING CHOLINERGIC AGENTS		
acetylcholine chloride (Miochol)	0.5–2 ml 1% intraocular solution instilled into the eye	Intraocular treatment before surgery; cholinergic agent
carbachol (Isopto Carbachol, Miostat)	One or two drops 0.75–3% solution in the lower conjunctival sac every 4 hours three times a day	Ophthalmic solution; cholinergic agent; less useful in glaucoma than other drugs; causes stinging of the eyes
pilocarpine hydrochloride (Adsorbocarpine, Isopto Carptine, Pilopine, others)	Acute glaucoma: one drop 1–2% solution every 5–10 minutes for 3–6 doses; chronic glaucoma: one drop 0.5–4% solution every 4–12 hours	Ophthalmic solution; cholinergic agent; may be prescribed as an ocular therapeutic system, a slow release delivery method (Ocusert); Ocusert effects can last up to 7 days
MIOTICS, CHOLINESTERASE INHIBITORS		
demecarium bromide (Humorsol)	One or two drops 0.125–0.25% solution 2 × per week	Ophthalmic solution; longer-acting medication (2–3 days)
echothiophate iodide (Phospholine iodide)	One drop 0.03–0.25% solution once or twice daily	Ophthalmic solution; must be prepared immediately before use because of instability
physostigmine salicylate (Eserine sulfate)	One drop 0.25–0.5% solution one to four times/day	Ophthalmic solution; also constricts ciliary muscle, decreasing intraocular pressure
SYMPATHOMIMETICS		
dipivefrin HCl (Propine)	One drop 0.1% solution bid	Ophthalmic solution; converted to epinephrine in the eye
epinephrine borate (Epinal, Eppy/N)	One or two drops 0.25–2% solution once or twice daily	Ophthalmic solution; causes mydriasis
PROSTAGLANDINS AND PROSTAMIDES		
bimatoprost (Lumigan)	One drop 0.03% solution daily in the evening	Ophthalmic solution; prostamide; approved by the Food and Drug Administration (FDA), March 2001
(Pr) latanoprost (Xalatan)	One drop (1.5 mg) solution daily in the evening	Ophthalmic solution; prostaglandin
travoprost (Travatan)	One drop 0.004% solution daily in the evening	Ophthalmic solution; prostamide; maximum effect after about 12 hours
unoprostone isopropyl (Rescula)	One drop 0.15% solution bid	Ophthalmic solution; prostaglandin

DRUG PROFILE: ℞ *Latanoprost (Xalatan)*

Therapeutic Class: Antiglaucoma agent
Pharmacologic Class: Prostaglandin, reducer of IOP

Actions and Uses:

Latanoprost is a prostaglandin analog believed to reduce IOP by increasing the outflow of aqueous humor. The recommended dose is one drop in the affected eye(s) in the evening. It is metabolized to its active form in the cornea, reaching its peak effect in about 12 hours. It is used to treat open-angle glaucoma and elevated IOP.

Adverse Effects and Interactions:

Adverse effects include ocular symptoms such as conjunctival edema, tearing, dryness, burning, pain, irritation, itching, sensation of a foreign body in the eye, photophobia, and visual disturbances. The eyelashes on the treated eye may grow, thicken, and darken. Changes may occur in pigmentation of the iris of the treated eye and in the periocular skin. The most common systemic adverse effect is a flulike upper respiratory infection. Rash, asthenia, or headache may occur.

Latanoprost interacts with thimerosal: If mixed with eyedrops containing thimerosal, precipitation may occur.

Refer to MyNursingKit for a Nursing Process Focus specific to this drug.

---

impact on building eye pressure. Adverse effects, however, include temporary **cycloplegia**, or blurred vision, and accommodation defects.

cyclop = *round eye*
plegia = *paralysis*

Indirect-Acting Miotics (Cholinesterase Inhibitors)

Demecarium bromide (Humorsol), echothiophate iodide (Phosphaline iodide), and physostigmine salicylate (Eserine sulfate) are indirect-acting cholinergic agents. They produce about the same effects as direct-acting drugs, except that they block cholinesterase, the enzyme responsible for breaking down the natural neurotransmitter acetylcholine.

Sympathomimetics

Dipivefrin (Propine) and epinephrine borate (Ipinal and others) are sympathomimetic drugs. Dipiverdin is converted to epinephrine; epinephrine produces mydriasis, increased outflow of aqueous humor, and the subsequent fall of IOP. As discussed in Chapter 22 ⚭ , when epinephrine is released into the general circulation, it increases blood pressure and heart rate.

hypo = *reduced*
tensive = *tension*

Prostaglandins and Prostamides

Bimatoprost (Lumigan), latanoprost (Xalatan), travoprost (Travatan), and unoprostone isopropyl (Rescula) also increase aqueous humor outflow by reducing congestion in trabecular meshwork. Their main adverse effect is heightened pigmentation, usually brown color of the iris in patients with lighter colored eyes. These medications cause cycloplegia, local irritation, and stinging of the eyes. Because of these effects, prostaglandins are normally administered just before the patient goes to bed. Although prostaglandins can be irritating to the eyes, they usually do not prevent the patient from falling asleep.

Other antiglaucoma medications decrease the formation of aqueous humor.

CORE CONCEPT 35.5

Beta-adrenergic blockers, alpha₂-adrenergic agents, carbonic-anhydride inhibitors, and osmotic diuretics are drug classes that decrease the formation of aqueous humor. These are summarized in Table 35.2. Beta blockers do not alter pupil diameter or produce cycloplegic effects. Similarly, alpha₂ agents produce fewer ocular symptoms. For patients who cannot use beta-blocking agents, carbonic-anhydrase inhibitors and osmotic diuretics are other alternatives.

Beta-blocking agents are used more often than the other antiglaucoma medications. These include betaxolol (Betaoptic), carteolol (Ocupress), levobunolol (Betagan), metipranolol

TABLE 35.2	Antiglaucoma Drugs That Decrease the Formation of Aqueous Humor	
DRUG	**ROUTE AND ADULT DOSE**	**REMARKS**
BETA-ADRENERGIC BLOCKERS		
betaxolol (Beoptic)	One drop 0.5% solution bid	Ophthalmic solution; available as ophthalmic suspension; beta$_1$-blocker; reduces blood pressure, heart rate
carteolol (Ocupress)	One drop 1% solution bid	Ophthalmic solution; nonspecific beta blocker; causes bronchoconstriction
levobunolol (Betagan)	One or two drops 0.25–0.5% solution one or twice daily	Ophthalmic solution; nonspecific beta blocker
metipranolol (OptiPranolol)	One drop 0.3% solution bid	Ophthalmic solution; nonspecific beta blocker
(Pr) timolol (Timoptic, Timoptic XE)	Drops: one or two drops of 0.25–0.5% solution once or twice daily; gel (salve): apply daily	Ophthalmic solution; nonspecific beta blocker
ALPHA$_2$-ADRENERGIC AGENTS		
apraclonidine (Iopidine)	One drop 0.5% solution bid	Ophthalmic solution
brimonidine tartrate (Alphagan)	One drop 0.2% solution tid	Ophthalmic solution
CARBONIC ANHYDRASE INHIBITORS		
acetazolamide (Diamox)	PO; 250 mg one to four times/day	Oral diuretic; sulfonamide; also for seizures, high altitude sickness, and renal impairment
brinzolamide (Azopt)	One drop 1% solution tid	Ophthalmic solution; sulfonamide
dorzolamide hydrochloride (Trusopt)	One drop 2% solution tid	Ophthalmic solution; sulfonamide
methazolamide (Neptazane)	PO; 50–100 mg bid or tid	Oral sulfonamide; less diuretic activity than acetazolamide
OSMOTIC DIURETICS		
isosorbide (Ismotic)	PO; 1–3 g/kg bid–qid	Used before and after eye surgery
mannitol (Osmitrol)	IV; 1.5–2 mg/kg as a 15–25% solution over 30–60 minutes	Raises osmotic pressure, causing diuresis; IV medication

(OptiPranolol), and timolol (Timoptic, Timoptic XE). The exact mechanism by which these drugs produce their effects is not fully understood. However, they all reduce IOP effectively without the ocular adverse effects of miotic and sympathomimetic drugs. Systemic beta-blocker effects can be problematic; however, the doses of beta blockers used for glaucoma treatment are generally not high enough to enter the general circulation. Systemic adverse effects, if they occur, include bronchoconstriction, bradycardia, and hypotension.

Alpha$_2$-adrenergic agents are less frequently prescribed than the other antiglaucoma medications. These medications include apraclonidine (Iopidine) and brimonidine (Alphagan). They produce minimal cardiovascular and pulmonary adverse effects. The most significant adverse effects are headache, drowsiness, dry mucosal membranes, blurred vision, and irritated eyelids.

Carbonic-anhydrase inhibitors may be administered topically or systemically to reduce IOP. Usually these medications are used as a second choice if beta blockers are not effective. Examples include acetazolamide (Diamox), brinzolamide (Azopt), dichlorphenamide (Daranide, Oratrol), dorzolamide (Trusopt), and methazolamide (Neptazane). These medications are more effective in cases of open-angle glaucoma. Patients must be cautioned when taking these medications because they are *sulfonamides*—agents that may cause an allergic reaction. All of these drugs are diuretics, which means they can reduce IOP rather quickly and dramatically, altering serum electrolytes with continuous treatment.

Osmotic diuretics are most often used in cases of eye surgery or acute closed-angle glaucoma. Examples include isosorbide (Ismotic) and mannitol (Osmitrol). Because they have an ability to reduce plasma volume very quickly (see Chapter 23 ⚭), they may produce unpleasant adverse effects, including headache, tremors, dizziness, dry mouth, fluid and electrolyte imbalance, and *thrombophlebitis* (venous clot formation) near the site of IV administration.

thrombo = *clot*
phleb = *vein*
itis = *inflammation*

Concept Review   35.2

■ Describe two major approaches for controlling IOP in patients with glaucoma. What major drug classes are used in each case?

EYE EXAMINATIONS AND MINOR EYE CONDITIONS

Drugs for minor irritation and injury come from a broad range of classes, including antimicrobials, local anesthetics, glucocorticoids, and nonsteroidal anti-inflammatory drugs (NSAIDs).

Drugs provide relief for minor eye conditions and are used for eye exams.

CORE CONCEPT 35.6

A range of drug preparations may be used, including drops, salves, optical inserts, and injectable formulations. Some agents only provide moisture to the eye's surface. For example, approved in

---

DRUG PROFILE: ℞ *Timolol (Timoptic, Timoptic XE)*

Therapeutic Class: Antiglaucoma agent
Pharmacologic Class: Beta-adrenergic blocker, reducer of IOP, ocular hypotensive agent

Actions and Uses:

Timolol is a nonselective beta-adrenergic blocker available as a 0.25% or 0.5% ophthalmic solution. Timolol reduces elevated IOP in chronic open-angle glaucoma by reducing the formation of aqueous humor. The usual dose is one drop in the affected eye(s) twice a day. Timoptic XE allows for once-a-day dosing. Treatment may require 2 to 4 weeks for maximum therapeutic effect. It is also available in tablets, which are prescribed to treat mild hypertension.

Adverse Effects and Interactions:

The most common adverse effects are local burning and stinging on instillation. In most patients there is no significant systemic absorption to cause adverse effects as long as timolol is applied correctly. If significant systemic absorption occurs, however, drug interactions could occur. Anticholinergics, nitrates, reserpine, methyldopa, and/or verapamil use could lead to increased hypotension and bradycardia. Indomethacin and thyroid hormone use could lead to decreased antihypertensive effects of timolol. Epinephrine use could lead to hypertension followed by severe bradycardia. Theophylline use could lead to decreased bronchodilation.

 Refer to MyNursingKit for a Nursing Process Focus specific to this drug.

NURSING PROCESS FOCUS

Patients Receiving Ophthalmic Solutions for Glaucoma

ASSESSMENT

Prior to drug administration:
- Obtain a complete health history (physical/mental), including allergies, drug history, and possible drug interactions
- Obtain a complete physical examination focusing on visual acuity and visual field assessments
- Assess for the presence/history of ocular pain

POTENTIAL NURSING DIAGNOSES

- Risk for Injury related to visual acuity deficits.
- Self-Care Deficit related to impaired vision.
- Pain related to disease process.

PLANNING: PATIENT GOALS AND EXPECTED OUTCOMES

The patient will:
- Exhibit no progression of visual impairment
- Demonstrate an understanding of the disease process
- Safely function within own environment without injury
- Report absence of pain

IMPLEMENTATION

Interventions and (Rationales)	Patient Education/Discharge Planning
Monitor visual acuity, blurred vision, papillary reactions, extraocular movements, and ocular pain.	Instruct the patient to report changes in vision and headache.
Monitor the patient for specific contraindications for the prescribed drug. (There are many physiologic conditions for which ophthalmic solutions may be contraindicated.)	Instruct the patient to inform the health care provider of all health-related problems and prescribed medications.
Remove contact lenses before administration of ophthalmic solutions.	Instruct the patient to remove contact lenses prior to administering eyedrops and wait 15 minutes before reinsertion.
Administer ophthalmic solutions using proper technique.	Instruct the patient in the proper administration of eyedrops: - Wash hands prior to eye drop administration - Avoid touching the tip of the container to the eye, which may contaminate the solution - Administer the eyedrop in the conjunctival sac - Apply pressure over the lacrimal sac for 1 minute - Wait 5 minutes before administering other ophthalmic solutions - Schedule glaucoma medications around daily routines such as waking, mealtimes, and bedtime to lessen the chance of missed doses
Monitor for ocular reaction to the drug such as conjunctivitis and lid reactions.	Instruct the patient to report itching, drainage, ocular pain, or other ocular abnormalities.
Assess intraocular pressure readings. (These are used to determine effectiveness of drug therapy.)	Instruct the patient that IOP readings will be done prior to beginning treatment and periodically during treatment.
Monitor the color of the iris and periorbital tissue of the treated eye.	Instruct the patient that: - More brown color may appear in the iris and in the periorbital tissue of the treated eye only - Any pigmentation changes develop over months to years

continued . . .

NURSING PROCESS FOCUS *(continued)*

Interventions and (Rationales)	Patient Education/Discharge Planning
■ Monitor for systemic absorption of ophthalmic preparations. (Ophthalmic drugs for glaucoma can cause serious cardiovascular and respiratory complications if the drug is systemically absorbed.)	■ Instruct the patient to immediately report palpitations, chest pain, shortness of breath, and irregularities in pulse.
■ Monitor and adjust environmental lighting to aid in patient's comfort. (People who have glaucoma are sensitive to excessive light, especially extreme sunlight.)	Instruct the patient to: ■ Adjust environmental lighting as needed to enhance vision or reduce ocular pain ■ Wear darkened glasses as needed
■ Encourage compliance with the treatment regimen.	Instruct the patient: ■ To adhere to medication schedule for eyedrop administration ■ About the importance of regular follow-up care with the ophthalmologist

EVALUATION OF OUTCOME CRITERIA

Evaluate the effectiveness of drug therapy by confirming that patient goals and expected outcomes have been met (see "Planning").

See Tables 35.1 and 35.2 for lists of drugs to which these nursing actions apply.

2009, bepotastine (Bepreve) is an antihistamine approved for twice daily dosing for itching associated with allergic conjunctivitis. Others penetrate and affect a specific area of the eye.

Some drugs are specifically designed for ophthalmic examinations. These include **cycloplegic drugs** to relax ciliary muscles and **mydriatic drugs** to dilate the pupils. One has to be especially careful with anticholinergic mydriatics because these drugs can increase IOP and worsen the condition of patients with glaucoma. In addition, anti-cholinergic agents have the potential for producing unfavorable central adverse effects such as confusion, unsteadiness, or drowsiness in adults. Children generally become restless and spastic. Examples of cycloplegic, mydriatic, lubricant, and corneal edema drugs are listed in Table 35.3.

Concept Review 35.3

■ List examples of commonly used drugs for minor eye irritation and injury. What are the major actions of cycloplegic and mydriatic drugs?

EAR CONDITIONS

The ear has two major sensory functions: hearing and maintenance of equilibrium and balance. Three important structural areas—the outer ear, middle ear, and inner ear—carry out these functions (Figure 35.3 ■).

Otitis, inflammation of the ear, most often occurs in the outer and middle ear compartments. **External otitis** or *otitis externa,* commonly referred to as *swimmer's ear,* is inflammation of the outer ear; **otitis media** is inflammation of the middle ear. Outer ear infections most often occur with water exposure. Middle ear infections most often occur with upper respiratory infections, allergies, or auditory tube irritation. Of all ear infections, the most difficult ones to treat are infections of the inner ear (*otitis interna*). **Mastoiditis,** or inflammation of the mastoid sinus, can be a serious problem because if left untreated, it can result in hearing loss.

externa = *outside*
ot = *ear*
itis = *inflammation*
media = *middle*

interna = *inside*

TABLE 35.3	Drugs for Eye Examinations and Moistening Eye Membranes	
DRUG	**ROUTE AND ADULT DOSE**	**REMARKS**
MYDRIATICS: SYMPATHOMIMETICS		
phenylephrine hydrochloride (Mydfrin, Neo-Synephrine)	One drop 2.5% or 10% solution before eye exam	Decongestant and vasoconstriction properties; smaller doses provide temporary relief of eye redness; also for pupil dilation in closed-angle glaucoma
CYCLOPLEGICS: ANTICHOLINERGICS		
atropine sulfate (Isopto Atropine, others)	One drop 0.5% solution daily	Also provided as ointment; should not be administered to patients with glaucoma; effects may be prolonged
cyclopentolate (Cyclogyl, Pentalair)	One drop 0.5–2% solution 40–50 minutes before procedure	Not for patients with glaucoma; causes burning and irritation; possible central adverse effects with higher doses
homatropine (Isopto Homatropine, others)	One or two drops 2% or 5% solution before eye exam	Not for patients with glaucoma; effects may be prolonged after treatment
scopolamine hydrobromide (Isopto Hyoscine)	One or two drops 0.25% solution 1 hour before eye exam	Not for patients with glaucoma; effects may be prolonged after treatment; possible central adverse effects with higher doses
tropicamide (Mydriacyl, Tropicacyl)	One or two drops 0.5–1% solution before eye exam	Not for patients with glaucoma; central adverse effects with higher doses
LUBRICANTS CAUSING OCULAR VASOCONSTRICTION		
naphazoline hydrochloride (Albalon, Allerest, ClearEyes, others)	One to three drops 0.1% solution every 3–4 hours prn	Over-the-counter (OTC) and prescription medications available
oxymetazoline hydrochloride (OcuClear, Visine LR)	One or two drops 0.025% solution qid	OTC and prescription medications available
tetrahydrozoline hydrochloride (Collyrium, Murine Plus, Visine, others)	One or two drops 0.05% solution bid–tid	Primarily OTC medication
GENERAL PURPOSE LUBRICANTS		
lanolin alcohol (Lacri-lube)	Apply a thin film to the inside of the eyelid	Mixed with mineral oil and petroleum jelly as a salve
methylcellulose (Methulose, Visculose, others)	One or two drops prn	Artificial tear solution
polyvinyl alcohol (Liquifilm, others)	One or two drops prn	Artificial tear solution
CORNEAL EDEMA AGENTS AND ITCHING		
sodium chloride hypertonicity ointment (Muro 128 5% Ointment)	Apply a thin film to the inside of the eyelid; instill one drop into the affected eye(s) twice a day (bid)	Ophthalmic ointment for corneal edema; mixed with lanolin, mineral oil, purified water, and white petrolatum as a salve; for itching associated with allergic conjunctivitis

Otic preparations treat infections, inflammation, and earwax buildup.

CORE CONCEPT 35.7

Combination drugs effectively treat many different types of ear conditions, including infections, earaches, edema, and earwax.

FIGURE 35.3

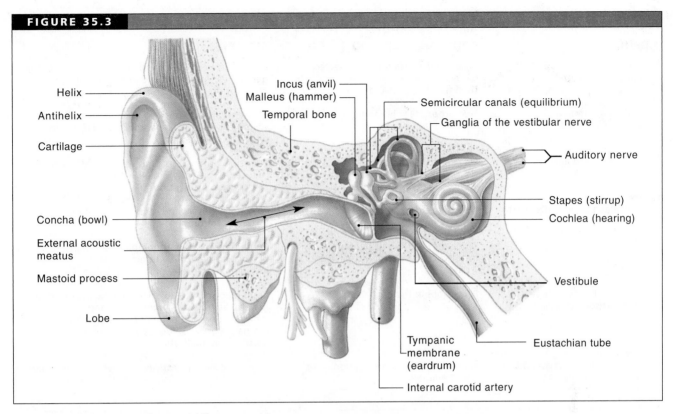

Structures of the external ear, middle ear, and inner ear   *Source: Pearson Education/PH College*

The basic treatment for ear infection is essentially the same as in all places of the body: antibiotics. Topical antibiotics in the form of eardrops may be administered for external ear infections. Systemic antibiotics (see Chapter 25 ⊙) may be needed in cases in which outer ear infections are extensive or in cases of middle or inner ear infections. Medications for pain, edema, and itching may also be necessary. Glucocorticoids are often combined with antibiotics or with other drugs when inflammation is present. Examples of these drugs are listed in Table 35.4.

Mineral oil, earwax softeners, and commercial products are also used for proper ear health. When earwax accumulates, it narrows the ear canal and may interfere with hearing. This is especially true for older patients who are not able to properly groom themselves. Health care providers working with elderly patients are trained to take appropriate measures when removing impacted earwax.

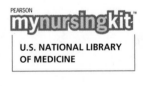

PEARSON
mynursingkit™

U.S. NATIONAL LIBRARY OF MEDICINE

NATURAL THERAPIES

Aloe Vera for Improving Eye and Ear Health

For centuries, *Aloe vera* has been hailed as the "medicine plant" because of its ability to treat burns, cuts, scrapes, rashes, and abrasions. It has a reputation for treating inflammation and acid indigestion, and even lowering blood cholesterol. *Aloe* may be able to treat eye irritation and conjunctivitis in addition to many other disorders.

One does not have to put *Aloe* directly into the eyes to obtain its therapeutic effect. The benefit comes from treating areas around the eyes, including the bridge of the nose and the outside of the eyelids and cheeks. The skin around the ears may also be treated. The antiseptic properties of *Aloe* probably come from the many agents found within its sap and leaves. Other agents have a reputation for killing microorganisms, including salicylic acid, urea nitrogen, cinnamonic acid, phenols, sulphur, and lupeol. Other groups of agents that qualify as substances with healing properties include plant sterols, immune modulating peptides, anti-inflammatory fatty acids, and viscous-like polysaccharides.

TABLE 35.4	Otic Preparations	
DRUG	**ROUTE AND ADULT DOSE**	**REMARKS**
acetic acid and hydrocortisone (Vosol HC)	Three to five drops in the affected ear every 4 hours–qid × 24 hours, then five drops tid–qid	Combination of acetic acid and glucocorticoid; for general ear infections and inflammation; prescription medication
aluminum sulfate and calcium acetate (Domeboro)	Two drops 2% solution tid–qid	For general ear infections and the prevention of swimmer's ear; may be administered using an ear wick; OTC medication
benzocaine and antipyrine (Auralgan)	Fill the ear canal with solution tid × 2 for 3 days	For acute otitis media and the removal of earwax; reduces earache associated with the infection; prescription medication
carbamide peroxide (Debrox)	One to five drops 6.5% solution bid × 4 days	To soften, loosen, and remove excessive earwax; OTC medication
ciprofloxacin (Cipro)	Three drops of the suspension instilled into the affected ear bid × 7 days	Combination of fluoroquinolone antibiotic and glucocorticoid; for ear infections and inflammation; prescription medication
polymyxin B, neomycin, and hydrocortisone (Cortisporin)	Four drops in the ear tid–qid	Combination of antibiotics and glucocorticoid; for general ear or mastoid infections and inflammation; some patients may develop dermatitis as a result of sensitivity to neomycin; prescription medication
triethanolamine polypeptide oleate 10% condensate (Cerumenex)	Fill the ear canal with solution; wait 10–20 minutes	Drug dissolved in propylene glycol; breaks apart earwax; small risk of sensitivity; OTC medication

Concept Review 35.4

■ Identify areas of the ear where microbial infections are most likely. What kind of otic preparations treat infections, inflammation, and earwax buildup?

PATIENTS NEED TO KNOW

Patients taking medications for eye and ear disorders need to know the following:

Regarding Eye Medications
1. Have regular eye exams after the age of 40.
2. Do not strain or lift heavy objects if risk for glaucoma is present. Any effort that might produce eyestrain should be avoided.
3. Make sure that all allergies or sensitivities, including those to sulfa drugs, are known to the health care providers.
4. Do not take OTC medications that "get the red out" for longer than 24 hours. Use eye lubricants instead. Persistent irritation should be reported immediately.
5. Keep eye solutions clear and sterile; do not actually touch the eye when instilling drops.

Regarding Ear Medications
6. Take precautions to keep the ear canal dry when in or around water for an extensive time. Use appropriate earplugs or a bathing cap.
7. Apply 2% acetic acid to the ear canal after swimming. Acetic acid acts as a drying agent and restores the ear canal to its normal acidic condition.
8. Avoid using glucocorticoids for long periods. They could cause eye or ear damage.
9. Rather than placing objects like cotton swabs in the ear canal, use a bulb syringe approved for removing debris and warm water. Use any cerumen dissolving agent responsibly.

CHAPTER REVIEW

CORE CONCEPTS SUMMARY

35.1 Knowledge of basic eye anatomy is required for an understanding of eye disorders and drug therapy.

The anterior cavity of the eye is the place where aqueous humor is circulated. Aqueous humor originates from the ciliary body located in the posterior chamber and drains into the canal of Schlemm found in the anterior chamber.

35.2 Glaucoma is one of the leading causes of blindness.

Glaucoma develops because the flow of aqueous humor in the anterior eye cavity becomes disrupted, leading to increasing intraocular pressure (IOP). Two principal types of glaucoma are closed-angle glaucoma and open-angle glaucoma.

35.3 Glaucoma therapy centers on adjusting the circulation of aqueous humor.

Glaucoma therapy generally works by increasing the outflow of aqueous humor or decreasing aqueous humor formation.

35.4 Some antiglaucoma medications increase the outflow of aqueous humor.

Drugs that increase the outflow of aqueous humor include miotics, sympathomimetics, prostaglandins, and prostamides.

35.5 Other antiglaucoma medications decrease the formation of aqueous humor.

Medications that decrease the formation of aqueous humor include beta blockers, alpha$_2$-adrenergic agents, carbonic-anhydrase inhibitors, and osmotic diuretics. The beta-adrenergic blockers are the most commonly prescribed drug class.

35.6 Drugs provide relief for minor eye conditions and are used for eye exams.

Mydriatic or pupil-dilating drugs and cyclopegic or ciliary-muscle relaxing drugs are routinely used for eye examinations. Some drugs constrict local blood vessels. Others lubricate the eyes.

35.7 Otic preparations treat infections, inflammation, and earwax buildup.

Combination drugs provide relief of conditions associated with the outer, middle, and inner ear. Drugs include antibiotics, corticosteroids, and earwax dissolving agents.

REVIEW QUESTIONS

The following questions are written in NCLEX-PN® style. Answer these questions to assess your knowledge of the chapter material, and go back and review any material that is not clear to you.

1. This class of drugs causes the pupils to constrict.

1. Miotics
2. Mydriatics
3. Constrictors
4. Glucocorticoids

2. This medication relieves pressure in the eye by increasing the outflow of aqueous humor.

1. Timolol (Timoptic)
2. Betaxolol (Betaoptic)
3. Pilocarpine (Ocusert)
4. Ciprofloxacin (Cipro)

3. This medication relieves pressure by decreasing production of aqueous humor.

1. Timolol (Timoptic)
2. Atropine sulfate
3. Pilocarpine (Ocusert)
4. Ciprofloxacin (Cipro)

4. Patients with glaucoma should not take which of the following classes of medications?

1. Osmotic diuretics
2. Beta-adrenergic blockers
3. Anticholinergics
4. Alpha$_2$-adrenergic blockers

5. If the patient has an ear infection with inflammation, which of the following medications may be added?

1. Glucocorticoids
2. Aluminum sulfate and calcium acetate (Domeboro)
3. Osmotic diuretics
4. Carbonic-anhydrase inhibitors

6. Prior to administering eardrops, the nurse should instruct the patient that:

1. The solution should stay in the ear for 1 hour
2. The solution will be removed within 1 hour
3. There may be a decrease in hearing for a few minutes
4. The medication will take effect immediately

7. If the patient has closed-angle glaucoma, the nurse will assess for:

1. Blindness
2. Blurred vision
3. Loss of consciousness
4. Hyperactivity

8. The goal of treatment in glaucoma patients is to:

1. Decrease aqueous humor production and increase outflow of aqueous humor
2. Increase aqueous humor production and decrease outflow of aqueous humor
3. Decrease aqueous humor production and decrease outflow of aqueous humor
4. Increase aqueous humor production and increase outflow of aqueous humor

9. The patient started on travoprost (Travatan) should be instructed that:

1. This medication is administered in the morning only
2. Due to pupil constriction, visual acuity may be affected
3. This medication may change the pigmentation of the eyes
4. Due to dilation of the pupils, visual acuity may be affected

10. If the patient is allergic to sulfonamides, he should not take:

1. Methazolamide (Neptazane)
2. Betaxolol (Betaoptic)
3. Carteolol (Ocupress)
4. Beta blockers

CASE STUDY QUESTIONS

For questions 1–4, please refer to the following case study, and choose the correct answer from choices 1–4.

Ms. Saunders is a 45-year-old African American female presenting with severe pain in the right eye, headache, and blurred vision. She has a history of primary hypertension. Her blood pressure is 140/90 mmHg. No other obvious signs are noted. In the course of the examination, she mentions that she and her family have recently relocated. It has been a particularly stressful time because she has not had much help from her family. She has not been taking her medication. At a recent hospital visit, she was prescribed the beta blocker, timolol (Timoptic).

1. The primary diagnosis of Ms. Saunders is:

1. Diabetes
2. Myopia
3. Glaucoma
4. Fibroplasia

2. The nurse examining the eye of Ms. Saunders should be cautious of the potential adverse reactions to which of the following drugs?

1. Cholinergic-blocking drugs
2. Miotic medications
3. Prostaglandins
4. Antibiotic drops

3. Which of the following could be a potential contraindication to the use of timolol (Timoptic)?

1. Hyperthyroidism
2. Liver disease
3. Organic nitrates for angina
4. Theophylline for asthma

4. In counseling Ms. Saunders, the nurse explains that if left untreated pharmacologically, the condition could lead to:

1. Mydriasis
2. Cycloplegia
3. Blindness
4. Vertigo

FURTHER STUDY

- Sympathomimetics, cholinergic agents, and cholinesterase inhibitors are autonomic agents that are discussed in Chapter 8 ⊗ .

- Chapters 8, 17, and 22 ⊗ present details of epinephrine's effect on blood pressure and heart rate.

- Osmotic diuretics are discussed in Chapter 23 ⊗ .

- Chapter 25 ⊗ discusses the use of systemic antibiotics that may be utilized for eye or ear infections.

- Use of the beta blocker timolol in the treatment of hypertension is presented in Chapter 17 ⊗ .

EXPLORE **PEARSON mynursingkit™**

MyNursingKit is your one stop for online chapter review materials and resources. Prepare for success with additional NCLEX®-style practice questions, interactive assignments and activities, web links, animations and videos, and more!

Register your access code from the front of your book at
www.mynursingkit.com

APPENDIX A: References

General References

Adams, M. P., & Koch, R. W. (2010). Pharmacology: Connections to nursing practice. Upper Saddle River, NJ: Prentice Hall.

Audesirk, T., Audesirk, G., & Beyers, B. E. (2008). *Biology: Life on earth* (8th ed.). Upper Saddle River, NJ: Pearson.

Beers, M. H., & Berkow, R. (Eds.). (2001). *Merck manual: Diagnosis and therapy* (17th ed.). Whitehouse Station, NJ: Merck & Co., Inc.

Brunton, L. L., Lazo, J. S., & Parker, K. L. (Eds.). (2006). *The pharmacological basis of therapeutics* (11th ed.). New York: McGraw-Hill.

Krogh, D. (2009). *Biology: A guide to the natural world* (4th ed.). Upper Saddle River, NJ: Prentice Hall.

LeMone, P., & Burke, K. M. (2008). *Medical-surgical nursing: Critical thinking in client care* (4th ed.). Upper Saddle River, NJ: Prentice Hall.

Martini, F. H. (2001). *Fundamentals of human anatomy and physiology* (5th ed.). Upper Saddle River, NJ: Prentice Hall.

Medical Economics Staff (Ed.). (2001). *Physicians' desk reference for non-prescription drugs and dietary supplements.* Montvale, NJ: Medical Economics.

Medical Economics Staff (Ed.). (2006). *Physicians' desk reference* (60th ed.). Montvale, NJ: Medical Economics.

Mulvihill, M. L., Zelman, P., Holdaway, P., Tompary, E., & Turchany, J. (2010). *Human diseases: A systemic approach* (7th ed.). Upper Saddle River, NJ: Prentice Hall.

Osborn, K. S., Wraa, C. E. & Watson, A. (2009). Medical Surgical Nursing: Preparation for Practice, Upper Saddle River, NJ: Prentice Hall.

Silverthorn, D. U. (2010). *Human physiology: An integrated approach* (5th ed.). Upper Saddle River, NJ: Benjamin-Cummings.

Wilson, B. A., Shannon, M. T., & Shields, K. M., C. L. (2010). *Nurse's drug guide 2010.* Upper Saddle River, NJ: Prentice Hall.

CHAPTER 1
Introduction to Pharmacology: Drug Regulation and Approval

Bond, C. A., Raehl, C. L., & Franke, T. (2001). Medication errors in United States hospitals. *Pharmacotherapy, 21*(9), 1023–1036.

Brown, S. D., & Landry, F. J. (2001). Recognizing, reporting, and reducing adverse drug reactions. *Southern Medical Journal, 94*(4), 370–373.

Carrico, J. M. (2000). Human Genome Project and pharmacogenomics: Implications for pharmacy. *Journal of American Pharmacology Association, 40*(1), 115–116.

Gaither, C. A., Kirking, D. M., Ascione, F. J., & Welage, L. S. (2001). Consumers' views on generic medications. *Journal of the American Pharmaceutical Association, 41*(5), 729–736.

Kacew, S. (1999). Effects of over-the-counter drugs on the unborn child: What is known and how should this influence prescribing? *Pediatric Drugs, 1*(2), 75–80.

Lazarou, J., Pomeranz, B. H., & Corey, P. N. (1998). Incidence of adverse drug reactions in hospitalized patients. *Journal of the American Medical Association, 279*(15), 1200–1205.

Moore, T. J., Cohen, M. R., Furberg, C. D. QuarterWatch 2008 quarter 2. Retrieved from Institute for Safe Medication Practices website: http://www.ismp.org/QuarterWatch/200901.pdf.

Newton, G. D., Pray, W. S., & Popovich, N. G. (2001). New OTC drugs and devices 2000: A selective review. *Journal of the American Pharmaceutical Association, 41*(2), 273–282.

Oates, J. A. (2006). The science of drug therapy. In L. L. Brunton, J. S. Lazo, & K. L. Parker (Eds.), *Goodman & Gilman's The pharmacological basis of therapeutics* (11th ed., pp. 117–136). New York, NY:McGraw-Hill.

Phillips, K. A., Veenstra, D. L., Oren, E., Lee, J. K., & Sardee, W. (2001). Potential role of pharmacogenomics in reducing adverse drug reactions: A systematic review. *Journal of the American Medical Association, 286,* 2270–2279.

CHAPTER 2
Drug Classes, Schedules, and Categories

Brass, E. P. (2001). Drug therapy: Changing the status of drugs from prescription to over-the-counter availability. *New England Journal of Medicine, 345,* 810–816.

Drug Enforcement Agency. (2005). *Drugs of abuse.* Retrieved May 27, 2005, from http://www.usdoj.gov/dea/pubs/abuse/doa-p.pdf

Force, M. V., Deering, L., Hubbe, J., Andersen, M., Hagemann, B., Cooper-Hahn, M., & Peters,W. (2006). Effective strategies to increase reporting of medication errors in hospitals. *Journal of Nursing Administration, 36*(1) 34–41.

Smith, S. F., Duell, D. J., & Martin, B. C. (2004). *Clinical nursing skills* (6th ed.). Upper Saddle River, NJ: Prentice Hall.

CHAPTER 3
Methods of Drug Administration

Berman, A. J., Snyder, S., Kozier, B., & Erb, G. (2008). *Kozier & Erb's Fundamentals of Nursing Concepts, Process, and Practice* (8th ed.). Upper Saddle River, NJ: Prentice Hall.

Institute for Safe Medical Practices. (2003). List of error-prone abbreviations, symbols, and dose designations. *ISMP MedicationSafetyAlert!, 8.*

Joint Commission on Accreditation of Healthcare Organizations. (2002). *The official "do not use" list.* Retrieved June 2, 2005, from http://www.jcaho.org/accredited+organizations/patient+safety/dnu.htm

Olsen, J. L., Giangrasso, A. P., & Shrimpton, D. M. (2008). *Medical dosage calculations* (9th ed.). Upper Saddle River, NJ: Prentice Hall.

Rosenthal, K. (2003). Keeping I.V. therapy safe with needleless systems. *Nursing Management, 34,* 16–20.

Smith, S. F., Duell, D. J., & Martin, B. C. (2002). *PhotoGuide of nursing skills.* Upper Saddle River, NJ: Prentice Hall.

CHAPTER 4
What Happens After a Drug Has Been Administered

Bateman, D. N. (2001). Introduction to pharmacokinetics and pharmacodynamics. *Journal of Toxicology—Clinical Toxicology, 39*(3), 207.

Buxton, I. L. (2006). Pharmacokinetics and pharmacodynamics: The dynamics of drug absorption, distribution, action and elimination. In L. L. Brunton, J. S. Lazo, & K. L. Parker (Eds.), *The pharmacological basis of therapeutics* (11th ed., pp. 1–39). New York: McGraw-Hill.

Consider racial, ethnic, and cultural differences in cardiovascular drug effectiveness. (2001). *Progress in Cardiovascular Nursing, 16*(4), 152–160+.

Levy, R. H., Thummel, K. E., Trager, W. F., Hansten, P. D., & Eichelbaum, M. (Eds.). (2000). *Metabolic drug interactions.* Philadelphia: Lippincott Williams & Wilkins.

CHAPTER 5
The Nursing Process

American Nurses Association (ANA). (2007). *Scope of nursing informatics practice.* Retrieved May 7, 2007, from http://nursingworld.org/practice/niworkgroup/ANA.

Berman, A., Snyder, S., Kozier, B., & Erb, G. (2008). *Kozier & Erb's fundamentals of nursing* (8th ed.). Upper Saddle River, NJ: Prentice Hall.

LeMone, P., & Burke, K. (2008). *Medical-surgical nursing: Critical thinking in patient care* (4th ed.). Upper Saddle River, NJ: Prentice Hall.

North American Nursing Diagnosis Association. (2001). *NANDA: Nursing diagnoses: Definitions & classification 2001–2002.* Philadelphia: Author.

Potter, P., Wolf, L., Boxerman, S., Grayson, D., Sledge, J., Dunagan, C., et al. (2005). Understanding the cognitive work of nursing in the acute care environment. *Journal of Nursing Administration, 35*(7–8), 327–335.

Wilkinson, J. M. (2005). *Nursing diagnosis handbook: NIC interventions and NOC outcomes* (8th ed.). Upper Saddle River, NJ: Prentice Hall.

Wilkinson, J. M. (2007). *Nursing process and critical thinking* (4th ed.). Upper Saddle River, NJ: Prentice Hall.

CHAPTER 6
Herbs and Dietary Supplements

Atwater, J., Montgomery-Salguero, J., & Roll, D. B. (2005). The USP dietary supplement verification program: Helping pharmacists and consumers select dietary supplements. *U.S. Pharmacist, 30*(6), 61–64.

Barnes, P., Powell-Griner, E., McFann, K., & Nahin, R. (2004). Complementary and alternative medicine use among adults: United States, 2002 (CDC Advance Data Report No. 343). Hyattsville, MD: National Center for Health Statistics.

Blumenthal, M. (Ed.). (2000). Herbal medicine: Expanded Commission E monographs. Austin, TX: American Botanical Council.

Blumenthal, M. (Ed.). (1988). The complete German Commission E monographs: Therapeutic guide to herbal medicines. Austin, TX: American Botanical Council.

Chavez, M. L. (2005). Herbal-drug interactions. *InetCE, 9*(10), 2–30.

Facts and ComparisonsTM. (n.d.). The review of natural products (4th ed.). St. Louis: Wolters Kluwer Health.

Fontaine, K. L. (2009). Complementary and alternative therapies for nursing practice (3rd ed.). Upper Saddle River, NJ: Prentice Hall.

Gagnier, J. J., van Tulder, M., Berman, B., & Bombardier, C. (2007). Herbal medicine for low back pain: A Cochrane review. *Spine, 32*(1), 82–92.

Gardiner, P., Graham, R., Legedza, A. T., Ahn, A. C., Eisenberg, D. M., & Phillips, R. S. (2007). Factors associated with herbal therapy use by adults in the United States. *Alternative Therapies Health Medicine, 13*(2), 22–29.

Marcus, D. M., & Snodgrass, W. R. (2005). Do no harm: Avoidance of herbal medicines during pregnancy. *Obstetrics & Gynecology, 105,* 1119–1122.

Medical Economics Staff (Ed.). (2007). PDR for herbal medicines (4th ed.). Montvale, NJ: Thomson Healthcare.

Snyder, M., & Lundquist, R. (2006). Complementary/alternative therapies in nursing. New York: Springer. U.S. Department of Health and Human Services, U.S. Food and Drug Administration. (1994). Dietary Supplement Health and Education Act of 1994, Pub. L. No. 103-417. Retrieved May 8, 2008, at http://www.fda.gov/opacom/laws/dshea.html#sec3

White House commission on complementary and alternative medicine policy, final report. (2002, March). Retrieved May 8, 2008, at http://govinfo.library.unt.edu/whccamp.

CHAPTER 7
Substance Abuse

Haseltine, E. (2001). The unsatisfied mind: Are reward centers in your brain wired for substance abuse? *Discover, 22*(11), 88.

Jason, L. A., Davis, M. I., Ferrari, J. R., & Bishop, P. D. (2001). A review of research and implications for substance abuse recovery and community research. *Journal of Drug Education, 31*(1), 1–28.

Manoguerra, A. S. (2001). Methamphetamine abuse. *Journal of Toxicology. Clinical Toxicology, 38*(2), 187.

Naegle, M. A., & D'Avanzo, C. E. (2001). *Addictions and substance abuse: Strategies for advanced practice nursing.* Upper Saddle River, NJ: Prentice Hall.

O'Brien, C. P. (2006). Drug addiction and drug abuse. In L. L. Brunton, J. S. Lazo, and K. L. Parker (Eds.), *The pharmacological basis of therapeutics* (11th ed., pp. 607–627). New York: McGraw-Hill.

Sindelar, J. L., & Fiellin, D. A. (2001). Innovations in treatment for drug abuse: Solutions to a public health problem. *Annual Review of Public Health, 22,* 249.

Wasilow-Mueller, S., & Erickson, C. K. (2001). Drug abuse and dependency: Understanding gender differences in etiology and management. *Journal of American Pharmacology Association, 41*(1), 78–90.

CHAPTER 8
Drugs Affecting Functions of the Autonomic Nervous System

Westfall, T. C., & Westfall, D. P. (2006). Neurotransmission: The autonomic and somatic nervous systems. In L. L. Brunton, J. S. Lazo, and K. L. Parker (Eds.), *The pharmacological basis of therapeutics* (11th ed., pp. 137–181). New York: McGraw-Hill.

CHAPTER 9
Drugs for Anxiety and Insomnia

Baldessarini, R. J. (2006). Drug therapy of depression and anxiety disorders. In L. L. Brunton, J. S. Lazo, and K. L. Parker (Eds.), *The pharmacological basis of therapeutics* (11th ed., pp. 429–460). New York: McGraw-Hill.

Charney, D. S., Mihic, J., & Harris, A. (2006). Hypnotics and sedatives. In L. L. Brunton, J. S. Lazo, and K. L. Parker (Eds.), *The pharmacological basis of therapeutics* (11th ed., pp. 401–438). New York: McGraw-Hill.

Fontaine, K. L., & Fletcher, J. S. (2003). *Mental health nursing* (5th ed.). Upper Saddle River, NJ: Prentice Hall.

Gorman, J. N. (2001). Generalized anxiety disorder. *Clinical Corner, 3*(3), 37–46.

Lippmann, S., Mazour, I., & Shahab, H. (2001). Insomnia: Therapeutic approach. *Southern Medical Journal, 94*(9), 866–873.

Smock, T. K. (2001). *Physiological psychology: A neuroscience approach.* Upper Saddle River, NJ: Prentice Hall.

Stahl, S. M. (1999). Antidepressants: The blue chip psychotropic for the modern treatment of anxiety disorders. *Journal of Clinical Psychiatry, 60,* 6.

Vitiello, M. V. (2000). Effective treatment of sleep disturbances in older adults. *Clinical Corner, 2*(5), 16–27.

CHAPTER 10
Drugs for Emotional and Mood Disorders

American Academy of Pediatrics. (2000). Diagnosis and evaluation of the child with attention deficit-hyperactivity disorder. *Pediatrics, 105*(5), 1158–1170.

Baldessarini, R. J., & Tarazi, F. I. (2006). Pharmacotherapy of psychosis and mania. In L. L. Brunton, J. S. Lazo, and K. L. Parker (Eds.), *The pharmacological basis of therapeutics* (11th ed., pp. 461–500). New York: McGraw-Hill.

Desai, H. D., & Jann, M. W. (2000). Major depression in women: A review of the literature. *Journal of American Pharmacology Association, 40*(4), 525–537.

Emslie, G. J., & Mayes, T. L. (1999). Depression in children and adolescents: A guide to diagnosis and treatment. *CNS Drugs, 11*(3), 181–189.

Janicak, P. G., Dowd, S. M., Martis, B., Alam, D., Beedle, D., Krasuski, J., et al. (2002, April 15). Repetitive transcranial magnetic stimulation versus electroconvulsive therapy for major depression: Preliminary results of a randomized trial. *Biological Psychiatry, 51*(8), 659–667.

Nelson, J. C. (2000). Augmentation strategies in depression. *Journal of Clinical Psychiatry, 61,* 13–19.

Rosenburg, P. B., Mehndiratta, R. B., Mehndiratta, Y. B., Wamer, A., Rosse, R. B., & Balish, M. (2002). Repetitive transcranial magnetic stimulation treatment of comorbid posttraumatic stress disorder and major depression. *Journal of Neuropsychiatry and Clinical Neurosciences, 14*(3), 270–276.

CHAPTER 11
Drugs for Psychoses

Bailey, K. (2003). Aripiprazole: The newest antipsychotic agent for the treatment of schizophrenia. *Pyschological Nursing and Mental Health Services, 41*(2), 14–18.

Baldessarini, R. J., & Tarazi, F. I. (2006). Pharmacotherapy of psychosis and mania. In L. L. Brunton, J. S. Lazo, and K. L. Parker (Eds.), *The pharmacological basis of therapeutics* (11th ed., pp. 461–500). New York: McGraw-Hill.

Brown, C. S., Markowitz, J. S., Moore, T. R., & Parker, N. G. (1999). Atypical antipsychotics: Part II. Adverse effects, drug interactions, and costs. *Annals of Pharmacotherapy, 33,* 210–217.

Burns, M. J. (2001). The pharmacology and toxicology of atypical antipsychotic agents. *Journal of Toxicology—Clinical Toxicology, 39*(1), 1.

Canales, P. L., Olsen, J., Miller, A. L., & Crismon, M. L. (1999). Role of antipsychotic polypharmacotherapy in the treatment of schizophrenia. *CNS Drugs, 12,* 179–188.

Markowitz, J. S., Brown, C. S., & Moore, T. R. (1999). Atypical antipsychotics: Part I. Pharmacology, pharmacokinetics, and efficacy. *Annals of Pharmacotherapy, 33,* 73–85.

Owen, W., & Castle, D. J. (1999). Late-onset schizophrenia: Epidemiology, diagnosis, management, and outcomes. *Drugs and Aging, 15*(2), 81–89.

Tandon, R., Milner, K., & Jibson, M. D. (1999). Antipsychotics from theory to practice: Integrating clinical and basic data. *Journal of Clinical Psychiatry, 8,* 21–28.

Vitiello, B. (2001). Psychopharmacology for young children: Clinical needs and research opportunities. *Pediatrics, 108*(4), 983.

CHAPTER 12
Drugs for Degenerative Diseases and Muscles

About Alzheimer's. Retrieved from http://www.alzfdn.org *Alzheimer's disease; Unraveling the mystery: The search for new treatments.* (2003, April 11). Retrieved from http://www.alzheimers.org.

Birks, J., & Grimley, Evans J. Ginkgo Biloba for Cognitive Impairment and Dementia. *Cochrane Database of Systematic Reviews* 2009, Issue 1.

Capozza, K. (2003, April 2). Drug slows progression of Alzheimer's. *Medline Plus.* Retrieved from http://www.nlm.nih.gov/medlineplus.

DeKosky, S. T.,Williamson, J. D., Fitzpatrick, A. L., Kronmal, R. A., Ives, D. G., Saxton, J.A., . . . & Furberg,C. D. (2008). Ginkgo biloba for prevention of dementia: A randomized controlled trial. *Journal of the American Medical Association, 300*(19), 2253–2262.

Disorders and Stroke. (2003). *NINDS spasticity information page.* Retrieved from http://nindsupdate.ninds.nih.gov/health_and_medical/disorders/spasticity_doc.htm.

Dystonia Medical Research Foundation. (2003a). *Botulism toxin injections.* Retrieved from http://www.dystonia-foundation.org/pages/botulinum_toxin_injections/124.php.

Dystonia Medical Research Foundation. (2003b). *Complementary therapy.* Retrieved from http://www.dystonia-foundation.org/pages/complementary_therapy/156.php.

Dystonia Medical Research Foundation. (2003c). *Dystonia defined.* Retrieved from http://www.dystonia-foundation.org/defined/

Gruetzner, H. (2001). Alzheimer's: *A caregiver's guide and sourcebook* (3rd ed.). Indianapolis, IN:Wiley.

National Institutes of Health. (2003). *Spasticity.* Retrieved from http://www.nlm.nih.gov/medlineplus/ency/article/003297.htm National Institutes of Health, National Institute of Neurological.

Richter, R. (Ed.). (2003). *Alzheimer's disease: The physician's guide to practical management.* Totowa, NJ: Human Press. Sierpina,V. S.,Wollschlaeger, B., & Blumenthal M. (2003). Ginkgo biloba. American Family Physician, 68(5), 923–926.

Standaert, D. G., & Young, A. B. (2006). Treatment of central nervous system degenerative disorders. In L. L. Brunton, J. S. Lazo, & K. L. Parker (Eds.), *Goodman & Gilman's The pharmacological basis of therapeutics* (11th ed., pp. 527–546). New York, NY: McGraw-Hill.

CHAPTER 13
Drugs for Seizures

Bourdet, S. V., Gidal, B. E., & Alldredge, B. K. (2001). Pharmacologic management of epilepsy in the elderly. *Journal of the American Pharmaceutical Association, 41*(3), 421–436.

Landover, M. D. (1999). *Epilepsy: A report to the nation* [on-line]. Retrieved 2005, from http://www.efa.org/epusa/nation/nation/html.

McNamara, J. O. (2006). Pharmacotherapy of the epilepsies. In L. L. Brunton, J. S. Lazo, and K. L. Parker (Eds.), *The pharmacological basis of therapeutics* (11th ed., pp. 501–526). New York: McGraw-Hill.

Schachter, S. C. (2000). The next wave of anticonvulsants: Focus on levetiracetam, oxcarbazepine, and zonisamide. *CNS Drugs, 14*(3), 229–249.

Stahl, S. M. (1999). Antidepressants: The blue chip psychotropic for the modern treatment of anxiety disorders. *Journal of Clinical Psychiatry, 60,* 6.

Tatum, W. O., Galvez, R., Benbadis, S., & Carrazana, E. (2000). New antiepileptic drugs: Into the new millennium. *Archives of Family Medicine, 9,* 1135–1141.

Winkelman, C. (1999). Pharmacology update: A review of pharmacodynamics and pharmacokinetics in seizure management. *Journal of Neuroscience Nursing, 31*(1), 50–53.

CHAPTER 14
Drugs for Pain Control

Bannwarth, B. (1999). Risk-benefit assessment of opioids in chronic noncancer pain. *Drug Safety, 21*(4), 283–296.

Barkin, R. L., & Barkin, D. (2001). Pharmacologic management of acute and chronic pain: Focus on drug interactions and patient-specific pharmacotherapeutic selection. *Southern Medical Journal, 94*(8), 756–812.

Broadbent, C. (2000). The pharmacology of acute pain—Part 3. *Nursing Times, 96*(26), 39.

elt-Hansen, P., DeVries, P., & Saxena, P. R. (2000). Triptans in migraine: A comparative review of pharmacology, pharmacokinetics, and efficacy. *Drugs, 60*(6), 1259–1287.

FDA News. (2004, September 30). *FDA issues Public Health Advisory on Vioxx as its manufacturer voluntarily recalls the product.* Retrieved June 8, 2005, from http://www.fda.gov/bbs/topics/news/2004/NEW01122.html.

Glajchen, M. (2001). Chronic pain: Treatment barriers and strategies for clinical practice. *Journal of the American Board of Family Practice, 14*(3), 178–183.

Guay, D. R. P. (2001). Adjunctive agents in the management of chronic pain. *Pharmacotherapy, 21*(9), 1070–1081.

Gunstein, H. B., & Akil, H. (2006). Opioid analgesics. In L. L. Brunton, J. S. Lazo, and K. L. Parker (Eds.), *The pharmacological basis of therapeutics* (11th ed., pp. 547–590). New York: McGraw-Hill.

Khouzam, H. R. (2000). Chronic pain and its management in primary care. *Southern Medical Journal, 93*(10), 946–952.

Tepper, S. J., & Rapoport, A. M. (1999). The triptans: A summary. *CNS Drugs, 12*(5), 403–417.

CHAPTER 15
Drugs for Anesthesia

Catterall, W. A., & Mackie, K. (2006). Local anesthetics. In L. L. Brunton, J. S. Lazo, and K. L. Parker (Eds.), *The pharmacological basis of therapeutics* (11th ed., pp. 369–386). New York: McGraw-Hill.

Colbert, B. J., & Mason, B. J. (2002). *Integrated cardiopulmonary pharmacology.* Upper Saddle River, NJ: Prentice Hall.

Cross, J. H. (2009). The ketogenic diet. *Advances in Clinical Neurosciences & Rehabilitation, 8*(6), 8–10.

Evers, A. S., Crowder, C. M., & Balser, J. R. (2006). General anesthetics. In L. L. Brunton, J. S. Lazo, and K. L. Parker (Eds.), *The pharmacological basis of therapeutics* (11th ed., pp. 341–368). New York: McGraw-Hill.

Nagelhout, J. J., Nagelhout, K., & Zaglaniczny, V. H. (2001). *Handbook of nurse anesthesia* (2nd ed.). Philadelphia: W. B. Saunders.

Omoigui, S. (2001). *Sota Omogui's anesthesia drugs handbook* (4th ed.). Hawthorne, CA: State of the Art Technologies.

Stoelting, R. K. (2006). *Pharmacology and physiology in anesthetic practice* (4th ed.). Philadelphia: Lippincott Williams & Wilkins.

Waugaman, W. R., Foster, S. D., & Rigor, B. M. (1999). *Principles and practice of nurse anesthesia* (3rd ed.). Upper Saddle River, NJ: Prentice Hall.

CHAPTER 16
Drugs for Lipid Disorders

Ballantyne, C. M., O'Keefe, J. H., Jr., & Gotto, A. M., Jr. (2005). Dyslipidemia essentials. Royal Oak, MI: Physician's Press.

Florentin, M., Liberopoulos, E. N., Mikhailidis, D. P., & Elisaf, M. S. (2008). Fibrate-associated adverse effects beyond muscle and liver toxicity. *Current Pharmaceutical Design, 14*(6), 574–587.

Insull, W., Jr. (2006). Clinical utility of bile acid sequestrants in the treatment of dyslipidemia: A scientific review. *Southern Medical Journal, 99*(3), 257–273.

Law, M., & Rudnicka, A. (2006). Statin safety: A systematic review. *American Journal of Cardiology, 97*(8), S52–S60.

Mahley, R. W., & Bersot, T. P. (2006). Drug therapy for hypercholesterolemia and dyslipidemia. In L. L. Brunton, J. S. Lazo, & K. L. Parker (Eds.), The pharmacological basis of therapeutics (pp. 933–964). New York: McGraw-Hill.

Marcoff, L., & Thompson, P. (2007). The role of coenzyme Q10 in statin-associated myopathy: A systematic review. *Journal of the American College of Cardiology, 49*(23), 2231–2237.

McLoughlin, C. (2004). Statins. *Professional Nurse, 19*(11), 51–52.

Nichols, N. (2004). Clinical practice guidelines for the management of dyslipidemia. *Canadian Journal of Cardiovascular Nursing, 14*(2), 7–10.

Rundek, T., Naini, A., Sacco, R., Coates, K., & DiMauro, S. (2004). Atorvastatin decreases the coenzyme Q10 level in the blood of patients at risk for cardiovascular disease and stroke. *Archives of Neurolology, 61,* 889–892.

CHAPTER 17
Drugs for Hypertension

American Heart Association. (2008). Heart disease and stroke statistics. Retrieved December 11, 2009, from http://www.americanheart.org/downloadable/heart/1240250946756LS-1982%20Heart%20and%20Stroke%20Update.042009.pdf

Burnier, M. (2006). Medication adherence and persistence as the cornerstone of effective antihypertensive therapy. *American Journal of Hypertension, 19*(11), 1190–1196.

Colbert, B. J., & Mason, B. J. (2008). Integrated cardiopulmonary pharmacology (2nd ed.). Upper Saddle River, NJ: Prentice Hall.

Feldman, P. H., & McDonald, M. V. (2006). Clinical guidelines and recent research on hypertension and heart failure. *Home Healthcare Nurse, 24*(1), 50–53.

Grossman, E., & Messerli, F. (2006). Long-term safety of antihypertensive therapy. *Progress in Cardiovascular Diseases, 49*(1), 16–25.

Gu, Q., Paulose-Ram, R., Dillon, C., & Burt, V. (2006). Antihypertensive medication use among U.S. adults with hypertension. *Circulation, 113*(1), 213–221.

Hoffman, B. B. (2006). Therapy of hypertension. In L. Brunton, J. Lazo, & K. Parker (Eds.), The pharmacological basis of therapeutics (pp. 845–968). New York: McGraw-Hill.

Israili, Z. H., Hernandez-Hernandez, R., & Valasco, M. (2007). The future of antihypertensive treatment. *American Journal of Therapeutics, 14*(2), 121–134.

Kaplan, N., & Opie, L. (2006). Controversies in hypertension. *The Lancet, 367*(9505), 168–176.

Manach, C., Mazur, A., & Scalbert, A. (2005). Polyphenols and prevention of cardiovascular diseases. *Current Opinion in Lipidology, 16*(1), 77–84.

McLean, D. L. (2007). Nurses managing high blood pressure in patients with diabetes in community pharmacies. *Canadian Journal of Cardiovascular Nursing, 17*(2), 17–21.

Ong, K. L., Cheung, B. M. Y., Man, Y. B., Lau, C. P., & Lam, K. S. L. (2007). Prevalence, awareness, treatment, and control of hypertension among United States adults 1999–2004. *Hypertension, 49*(12), 69–75.

CHAPTER 18
Drugs for Heart Failure

Albert, N. M. (2006). Evidence-based nursing care for patients with heart failure. *AACN Advanced Critical Care, 17*(2), 170–185.

Amabile, C. M., & Spencer, A. P. (2004). Keeping your patient with heart failure safe: A review of potentially dangerous medications. *Archives of Internal Medicine, 164*(7), 709–720.

American College of Cardiology/American Heart Association Task Force on Practice Guidelines. (2005). ACC/AHA 2005 guideline update for the diagnosis and management of chronic heart failure in the adult. A Report of the (Writing Committee to Update the 2001 Guidelines for the Evaluation and Management of Heart Failure). *Circulation, 112,* e154-e235.

Bell, J., Kimber, J.,Mattick, R., Ali, R., Lintzers, N.,Monhert, B., . . . & White, J. (2003). *Interim clinical guidelines: Use of naltrexone in relapse prevention for opioid dependence* (abbreviated version).

Evans, R.W., & Taylor, F. R. (2006)."Natural" or alternative medications for migraine prevention. *Headache: The Journal of Head and Face Pain, 46*(6), 1012–1018.

Gislason, G. H., Rasmussen, J. N., Abildstrom, S. Z., Schramm, T. K., Hansen, M. L., Buch, P., et al. (2007). Persistent use of evidence-based pharmacotherapy in heart failure is associated with improved outcomes. *Circulation, 116*(10), 734–744.

Kendler, B. S. (2006). Supplemental conditionally essential nutrients in cardiovascular disease therapy. *Journal of Cardiovascular Nursing, 21*(1), 9–16.

Lovlien, M., Schei, B., & Hole, T. (2006). Women with myocardial infarction are less likely than men to experience chest symptoms. *Scandinavian Cardiovascular Journal, 40*(6), 342–347.

McCarthy, P. M., & Young, J. B. (Eds.). (2007). Heart failure: A combined medical and surgical approach. Malden, MA: Blackwell.

National Coalition for Women with Heart Disease. (2008). Women and heart disease fact sheet. Retrieved December 11, 2009, from http://womenheart.org/resources/cvdfactsheet.cfm.

Pauly, D. F. (2005). Cardiac function and heart failure. *Journal of the American College of Cardiology, 45*(11 Suppl B), 24B–29B.

Rocco, T. P., & Fang, J. C. (2006). Pharmacotherapy of congestive heart failure. In L. L. Brunton, J. S. Lazo, & K. L. Parker (Eds.), The pharmacological basis of therapeutics (11th ed., pp. 869–898). New York: McGraw-Hill.

Torpy, J. M., Lynm, C., & Glass, R. M. (2007). Heart failure. *Journal of the American Medical Association, 297*(22), 2548.

Tweed, V. (2006). Heart-warming nutrients. *Better Nutrition, 68*(9), 24–25.

Wagner, J. A. (2006). Top ten challenges in heart failure management. *Journal for Nurse Practitioners, 2*(8), 528–532.

CHAPTER 19
Drugs for Dysrhythmias

American College of Cardiology, American Heart Association Task Force, European Society of Cardiology. (2006). ACC/AHA/ESC 2006 guidelines for management of patients with ventricular arrhythmias and the prevention of sudden cardiac death—Executive Summary. *Journal of the American College of Cardiology, 48,* 1064–1108.

Ball, J. W., & Bindler, R. C. (2006). Child health nursing: Partnering with children and families. Upper Saddle River, NJ: Pearson Education.

Berry, C., Rankin, A. C., & Brady, A. (2004). Bradycardia and tachycardia occurring in older people: An introduction. *British Journal of Cardiology, 11*(1), 61–64.

De Bruin, M. L., Langendijk, P. N. J., Koopmans, R. P., Wilde, A. A. M., Leufkens, H. G. M., & Hoes, A. M. (2007). In-hospital cardiac arrest is associated with use of non-antiarrhythmic QTc-prolonging drugs. *British Journal of Clinical Pharmacy, 63*(2), 216–223.

Laidlaw, D. W., Homoud, M. K., Weinstock, J., Mark Estes III, N. A., & Link, M. S. (2007). Prognosis and treatment of ventricular arrhythmias following myocardial infarction. *Current Cardiology Reviews, 3*(1), 23–33.

Roden, D. M. (2006). Antiarrhythmic drugs. In L. L. Brunton, J. S. Lazo, and K. L. Parker (Eds.), The pharmacological basis of therapeutics (11th ed., pp. 899–932). New York: McGraw-Hill.

Tong, G. M., & Rude, R. K. (2005). Magnesium deficiency in critical illness. *Journal of Intensive Care Medicine, 20*(1), 3–17.

CHAPTER 20
Drugs for Coagulation Disorders

Cooney, M. F. (2006). Heparin-induced thrombocytopenia: Advances in diagnosis and treatment. *Critical Care Nurse, 26*(6), 30–36.

Eriksson, B. I., & Quinlan, D. J. (2006). Oral anticoagulants in development: Focus on thromboprophylaxis in patients undergoing orthopaedic surgery. *Drugs, 66*(11), 1411–1429.

Franchini, M., Zaffanello, M., & Veneri, D. (2005). Recombinant factor VIIa: An update on its clinical use. *Thrombosis and Haemostasis, 93*(6), 1027–1035.

Gallagher, D., & Rix, E. (2006). Understanding the implications of oral anticoagulants. *Nursing Times, 102*(25), 30–32.

Hairon, N. (2007). Prevention of venous thromboembolism in patients. *Nursing Times, 103*(18), 24–25.

Heit, J.A. (2008). The epidemiology of venous thromboembolism in the community. *Arteriosclerosis, Thrombosis and Vascular Biology, 28*(3), 370–372.

Hirsh, J., Guyatt, G., Albers, G. W., Harrington, R., & Shünemann, H. J. (2008). Antithrombotic and thrombolytic therapy: American College of Chest Physicians Guidelines (8th ed.). *Chest, 133,* 110S–112S.

Lambing, A. (2005). Clearing the way: Treating venous thromboembolism and deep vein thrombosis. *Advance for Nurse Practitioners, 13*(6), 24–30.

Lins, S., Guffey, D., VanRiper, S., & Kline-Rogers, E. (2006). Decreasing vascular complications after percutaneous coronary interventions: Partnering to improve outcomes. *Critical Care Nurse, 26*(6), 38–45.

Rahman, K., & Lowe, G. M. (2006). Garlic and cardiovascular disease: A critical review. *Journal of Nutrition, 136*(3 Suppl), 736S–740S.

Segal, J. B., Streiff, M. B., Hofmann, L. V., Thornton, K., & Bass, E. B. (2007). Management of venous thromboembolism: A systematic review for a practice guideline. *Annals of Internal Medicine, 146*(3), 211–222.

Spader, C. (2006). Keeping a grip on anticoagulant therapy. *Nursing Spectrum, 18A*(12), 46–49.

CHAPTER 21
Drugs for Angina Pectoris, Myocardial Infarction, and Cerebrovascular Accident

Aronow, W. S., Frishman, W. H., & Cheng-Lai, A. (2007). Cardiovascular drug therapy in the elderly. *Cardiology in Review, 15*(4), 195–215.

Decker, C., Garavalia, L., Chen, C., Buchanan, D. M., Nugent, K., Shipman, A., et al. (2007). Acute myocardial infarction: Patients' information needs over the course of treatment and recovery. *Journal of Cardiovascular Nursing, 22*(6), 459–465.

Demaerschalk, B. M. (2003). Diagnosis and management of stroke (brain attack). *Seminars in Neurology, 23*(3), 241–252.

Gehi, A. K., Ali, S., Na, B., & Whooley, M. A. (2007). Self-reported medication adherence and cardiovascular events in patients with stable coronary heart disease: The heart and soul study. *Archives of Internal Medicine, 167*(16), 1798–1803.

Harvey, S. (2004). The nursing assessment and management of patients with angina. *British Journal of Nursing, 13*(10), 598–601.

Jackevicius, C. A., Li, P., & Tu, J. V. (2008). Prevalence, predictors, and outcomes of primary nonadherence after acute myocardial infarction. *Circulation, 117*(2), 1028–1036.

Manfredini, R., Salmi, R., & Manfredini, F. (2008). Survival patterns with in-hospital cardiac arrest. *Journal of the American Medical Association, 299*(22), 2625–2626.

McGovern, R., & Rudd, A. (2003). Management of stroke. *Postgraduate Medical Journal, 79*(928), 87–92.

Michel, T. (2006). Treatment of myocardial ischemia. In L.L. Brunton, J. S. Lazo, & K. L. Parker (Eds.), The pharmacological basis of therapeutics (11th ed.) (pp. 823–844). New York: McGraw-Hill.

Quinn, T. (2004). Managing acute myocardial infarction. *Emerging Nurse, 12*(3), 17–19.

Rasmussen, J. N., Chong, A., & Alter, D. A. (2007). Relationship between adherence to evdence-based pharmacotherapy and long-term mortality after acute myocardial infarction. *Journal of the American Medical Association, 297*(2), 177–186.

CHAPTER 22
Drugs for Shock and Anaphylaxis

Bench, S. (2004). Clinical skills: Assessing and treating shock: a nursing perspective. *British Journal of Nursing, 13*(12), 715–721.

Brown, S. G. (2005). Cardiovascular aspects of anaphylaxis: Implications for treatment and diagnosis. *Current Opinion in Allergy and Clinical Immunology, 5*(4), 359–364.

Crusher, R. (2004). Anaphylaxis. *Emerging Nurse, 12*(3), 24–31.

Dellinger, R. P. (2003). Cardiovascular management of septic shock. *Critical Care Medicine, 31*(3), 946–955.

Leone, M., & Martin, C. (2008). Vasopressor use in septic shock: An update. *Current Opinion in Anaesthesiology, 21*(2), 141–147.

Liolios, A. (2004). Volume resuscitation: The crystalloid vs. colloid debate revisited paper given at the 24th International Symposium on Intensive Care and Emergency Medicine. *Medscape Today.* Retrieved December 13, 2009, from http://www.medscape.com/viewarticle/480288.

Menon, V., & Fincke, R. (2003, January–February). Cardiogenic shock: A summary of the randomized SHOCK trial. *Congestive Heart Failure, 9*(1), 35–39.

Tang, A. W. (2003). A practical guide to anaphylaxis. *American Family Physician, 68*(7), 1325–1332.

CHAPTER 23
Diuretics and Drugs for Electrolyte and Acid-Base Disorders

Bard, R. L., Bleske, B. E., & Nicklas, J. M. (2004). Food: An unrecognized source of loop diuretic resistance. *Pharmacotherapy, 24*(5), 630–637.

Bunn, F., Alderson, P., & Hawkins, V. (2004). Colloid solutions for fluid resuscitation. *Cochrane Reviews Abstract.*

Charlesworth, J. A., Gracey, D. M., & Pussell, B. A. (2008). Adult nephrotic syndrome: Non-specific strategies for treatment. *Nephrology, 13*(1), 45–50.

Gallagher, M., Perkovic, V., & Chalmers, J. (2006). Diuretics: A modern day treatment option? *Nephrology, 11*(5), 419–427.

Jackson, E. K. (2006). Diuretics. In L. L. Brunton, J. S. Lazo, & K. L. Parker (Eds.), The pharmacological basis of therapeutics (11th ed., pp. 737–770). New York: McGraw-Hill.

National Kidney Foundation. (2009). End stage renal disease in the United States. Retrieved December 13, 2009, from http://www.kidney.org/news/newsroom/fs_new/esrdinUS.cfm.

Schiffrin, E. L., Lipman, M. L., & Mann, J. F. E. (2007). Chronic kidney disease: Effects on the cardiovascular system. *Circulation, 116*(1), 85–97.

Sica, D., Gehr, T., & Frishman, W. (2006). Use of diuretics in the treatment of heart failure in the elderly. *Heart Failure Clinics, 3*(4), 455–464.

CHAPTER 24
Drugs for Inflammation and Immune Modulation

Advisory Committee on Immunization Practices, Centers for Disease Control. Prevention of varicella: Recommendations of the Advisory Committee on Immunization Practices. (2007). *Morbidity and Mortality Weekly Report, 56*(RR-4), 1–40.

Braunstahl, G., & Hellings, P. W. (2003). Allergic rhinitis and asthma: The link further unraveled. *Current Opinion in Pulmonary Medicine, 9*(1), 46–51.

Centers for Disease Control and Prevention. (2009). *Vaccines and Immunizations.* Retrieved December 14, 200, from http://www.cdc.gov/vaccines/default.htm.

Krensky, A. M., Vincenti, F., & Bennett, W. M. (2006). Immunosuppressants, tolerogens, and immunostimulants. In L. L. Brunton, J. S. Lazo, & K. L. Parker (Eds.), *The pharmacological basis of therapeutics* (11th ed., pp. 1405–1431). New York: McGraw-Hill.

Moonan, M., Fowler, K., Cook, C., Shermont, H., Powers, D., & O'Sullivan, J. (2007). The gift of life: A nursing grand rounds presentation on organ and tissue donations. *Pediatric Nursing, 33*(5), 458–461.

Santamaria, P. (2003). *Cytokines and autoimmune disease.* New York: Plenum.

Stillman, M. J., & Stillman, M. T. (2007). Choosing nonselective NSAIDs and selective COX-2 inhibitors in the elderly. A clinical use pathway. *Geriatrics, 62*(2), 26–34.

CHAPTER 25
Drugs for Bacterial Infections

Centers for Disease Control and Prevention. (2007). Get smart: Know when antibiotics work. Retrieved December 15, 2009, from http://www.cdc.gov/getsmart/.

Chambers, H. F. (2006). General considerations of antimicrobial therapy. In L. L. Brunton, J. S. Lazo, & K. L. Parker (Eds.), *The pharmacological basis of therapeutics* (11th ed., pp. 1095–1110). New York: McGraw-Hill.

Cisneros-Farrar, F., & Parsons, L. (2007). Antimicrobials: Classifications and uses in critical care. *Critical Care Nursing Clinics of North America, 19*(1), 43–51.

Gleckman, R. A. (2004). Selected issues in antibiotic resistance. *Infections in Medicine, 21*(3), 114–122.

Kenyon, N. J., & Albertson, T. E. (2004). Current issues in treatment of respiratory infections. *Infections in Medicine, 21*(4), 167–173.

Owens, R. C., & Ambrose, P. G. (2005). Antimicrobial safety: Focus on fluoroquinolones. *Clinical Infectious Diseases, 41*(2), S144–S157.

Petri, W. A. (2006). Chemotherapy of tuberculosis, *Mycobacterium avium* complex disease, and leprosy. In L. L. Brunton, J. S. Lazo, & K. L. Parker (Eds.), *The pharmacological basis of therapeutics* (11th ed., pp. 1203–1224). New York: McGraw-Hill.

Petri, W. A. (2006). Penicillins, cephalosporins, and other beta-lactam antibiotics. In L. L. Brunton, J. S. Lazo, & K. L. Parker (Eds.), *The pharmocological basis of therapeutics* (11th ed., pp. 1127–1154). New York: McGraw-Hill.

Petri, W. A. (2006). Sulfonamides, trimethoprim-sulfamethoxazole, quinolones, and agents for urinary tract infections. In L. L. Brunton, J. S. Lazo, & K. L. Parker (Eds.), *The pharmacological basis of therapeutics* (11th ed., pp. 1111–1126). New York: McGraw-Hill.

Turkoski, B. B. (2005). Fighting infection: An ongoing challenge—antibacterials. *Orthopaedic Nursing, 24*(3), 210–223.

CHAPTER 26
Drugs for Fungal, Viral, and Parasitic Diseases

Baird, J. K. (2005). Effectiveness of antimalarial drugs. *New England Journal of Medicine, 352*(15), 1565–1577.

Bennet, J. E. (2006). Antifungal agents. In L. L. Brunton, J. S. Lazo, & K. L. Parker (Eds.), *The pharmacological basis of therapeutics* (11th ed., pp. 1225–1242). New York: McGraw-Hill.

Brown, T., & Chin, T. (2006). Superficial fungal infections. In J. T. De Piro (Ed.), Pharmcotherapy: A pathophysiologic approach (6th ed., pp. 2145–2160). New York: McGraw-Hill

Burkhart, C. G. (2005). Herpes acquisition and transmission. *Journal of Drugs in Dermatology, 3,* 378–383.

Dickson, R., Awasthi, S., Dimellweek, C., & Williamson, P. (2003). Antihelmintic drugs for treating worms in children: Effects on growth and cognitive performance. *Cochrane Review.* Retrieved from http://www.medscape.com.

Gupta, A. (2006). Therapies for onychomycosis: A review. *Dermatologic Clinics, 24*(3), 375–379.

Panel on Antiretroviral Guidelines for Adults and Adolescents, Department of Health and Human Services. (2008, January 29). Guidelines for the use of antiretroviral agents in HIV-1-infected adults and adolescents.

Shapiro, T. A., & Goldberg, D. E. (2006). Chemotherapy of protozoal infections: Malaria. In L. L. Brunton, J. S. Lazo, & K. L. Parker (Eds.), *The pharmacological basis of therapeutics* (11th ed., pp. 869–898). New York: McGraw-Hill.

van Voorhis, W. C., & Weller, P. F. (2004, November 19). Protozoan infections. *ACP Medicine.*

Wilson, T. R. (2005). The ABCs of hepatitis. *Nurse Practitioner, 30*(6), 12–21.

CHAPTER 27
Drugs for Neoplasia

Birner, A. (2003). Safe administration of oral chemotherapy. *Clinical Journal of Oncological Nursing, 7*(2), 158–162.

Chabner, B. A., Amrein, P. C., Druker, B., Michaelson, M. D., Mitsiades, C. S., Goss, P. E., et al. (2006). Chemotherapy of neoplastic diseases. In L. L. Brunton, J. S. Lazo, & K. L. Parker (Eds.), *The pharmacological basis of therapeutics* (11th ed., pp. 1315–1403). New York: McGraw-Hill.

Fitzgerald, M. (2007). Herbal facts, herbal fallacies. *American Nurse Today, 2*(12), 27–33.

Fortenbaugh, C., & Rummel, M. (2004). Chemotherapy safety. *Clinical Journal of Oncologcal Nursing, 8*(4), 424–425.

Fortenbaugh, C., & Rummel, M. (2004). Chemotherapy safety. *Clinical Journal of Oncological Nursing, 8*(4), 424–425.

Hood, L. E. (2003). Chemotherapy in the elderly: Supportive measures for chemotherapy-induced myelotoxicity. *Clinical Journal of Oncological Nursing, 2*(7), 185–190.

Marek, C. (2003). Antiemetic therapy in patients receiving cancer chemotherapy. *Oncological Nursing Forum, 30*(2), 259–271.

Szetala, A., & Gibson, D. (2007). How the new oral antineoplastics affect nursing practice. *American Journal of Nursing, 107*(12), 40–49.

CHAPTER 28
Drugs for Respiratory Disorders

Altman, E. E. (2004). Update on COPD. Today's strategies improve quality of life. *Advanced Nursing Practices, 12*(3), 49–54.

Banasiak, N. (2007). Childhood asthma part one: Initial assessment, diagnosis, and education. *Journal of Pediatric Health Care, 21*(1), 44–48.

Colbert, B. J., & Mason, B. J. (2008). *Integrated cardiopulmonary pharmacology 2e.* Upper Saddle River, NJ: Pearson Education, Inc.

Dahlin, C. (2006). It takes my breath away end-stage COPD: Part 1: A case study and an overview of COPD. *Home Healthcare Nurse, 24*(3), 148–155.

Luggen, A. S. (2004). Pharmacology tips: Medications that complicate asthma control in older people. *Geriatric Nursing, 25*(3), 184.

Ratner, P. H., Stoloff, S., Metzer, E. O., & Hadley, J. A. (2007). Intranasal corticosteroids in the treatment of allergic rhinitis. *Allergy and Asthma Proceedings, 28*(Suppl. 1), s25–s32.

Smith, S. M., Schroeder, K., & Fahey, T. (2008). Over-the-counter medications for acute cough in children and adults in ambulatory settings. Cochrane Database of Systematic Reviews 2007, 3. Art. No.: CD001831. DOI: 10.1002/14651858.CD001831.pub3.

Stevens, N. (2003). Inhaler devices for asthma and COPD: Choice and technique. *Professional Nurse, 18*(11), 641–645.

Undem, B. J. (2006). Pharmacotherapy of asthma. In L. L. Brunton, J. S. Lazo, & K. L. Parker (Eds.), *The pharmacological basis of therapeutics* (11th ed., pp. 717–735). New York: McGraw-Hill.

Vega, C. (2005). Budesonide/formoterol may be effective for maintenance and acute relief of asthma. *American Journal of Respiratory Critical Care Medicine, 171,* 129–136.

Weir, P. (2004). Quick asthma assessment. A stepwise approach to treatment. *Advanced Nurse Practitioner, 12*(1), 53–56.

CHAPTER 29
Drugs for Gastrointestinal Disorders

Blair, K., & Beltz, J. (2006, March). Dyspepsia: Is it gastroesophageal reflux disease, or peptic ulcer disease? *The American Journal for Nurse Practitioners,* 157–163.

Comar, K., & Kirby, D. F. (2005). Herbal remedies in gastroenterology. *Journal of Clinical Gastroenterology, 39*(6), 457–468.

Feldman, M., & Le, M. (2007). Gastroenterology II: Peptic ulcer diseases, May 2007 update. Philadelphia: APC Medicine.

Herrstedt, J. (2008). Antiemetics: An update and the MASCC guidelines applied to clinical practice. *Nature Clinical Practice Oncology, 5*(1), 32–43.

Hoogerwerf, W. A., & Pasricha, P. J. (2006). Pharmacotherapy of gastric acidity, peptic ulcers and gastroesophageal reflux disease. In L. L. Brunton, J. S. Lazo, & K. L. Parker (Eds.), *The pharmacological basis of therapeutics* (11th ed., pp. 967–982). New York: McGraw-Hill.

Huggins, R. M., Scates, A. C., & Latour, J. K. (2003). Intravenous proton-pump inhibitors versus H$_2$-antagonists for treatment of GI bleeding. *Annals of Pharmacotherapy, 37*(3), 433–437.

Petersen, A. M. (2003). *Helicobacter pylori:* An invading microorganism? A review. *FEMS Immunology and Medical Microbiology, 36*(3), 117–126.

Sharma, P., & Vakil, N. (2003). *Helicobacter pylori* and reflux disease. *Alimentary Pharmacology and Therapeutics, 17*(3), 297–305.

Spiller, R. (2008). Review article: Probiotics and prebiotics in irritable bowel syndrome. *Alimentary Pharmacology and Therapeutics, 28*(4), 385–396.

Stanghellini, V. (2003). Management of gastroesophageal reflux disease. *Drugs Today, 39* (Suppl. A), 15–20.

CHAPTER 30
Vitamins, Minerals, and Nutritional Supplements

Jean-Marie, S. (2007). Vitamin supplements: Ensuring a healthy start in life. *Nursing in Practice: The Journal for Today's Primary Care Nurse, 18*(33), 43–44, 46.

Kaushansky, K., & Kipps, T. J. (2006). Hematopoietic agents: Growth factors, minerals and vitamins. In L. L. Brunton, J. S. Lazo, & K. L. Parker (Eds.), *The pharmacological basis of therapeutics* (11th ed., pp. 1433–1466). New York: McGraw-Hill.

Methany, N. A. (2006). Preventing respiratory complications of tube feedings: Evidence-based practice. *American Journal of Critical Care, 15*(4), 360–369.

More, J. (2007). Who needs vitamin supplements? *Journal of Family Health Care, 17*(2), 57–60.

Prentice, R. L. (2007). Clinical trials and observational studies to assess the chronic disease benefits and risks of multivitamin-multimineral supplements. *American Journal of Clinical Nutrition, 85*(Suppl. 1), 308S–313S.

Rosenberg, I. H. (2007). Challenges and opportunities in the translation of the science of vitamins. *American Journal of Clinical Nutrition, 85*(Suppl. 1), 325S–327S.

Sinatra, S. T. (2007). Cutting edge: Refuel your heart—Four nutritional supplements play critical roles in new approach to heart disease. *Alternative Medicine Magazine, 14*(52), 67–70.

Sudakin, T. (2006). Supporting nutrition with T.E.N or T.P.N. *Nursing 2006, 36*(12), 52–55.

CHAPTER 31
Drugs for Endocrine Disorders

American Diabetes Association. (2000). Clinical practice recommendations. *Diabetes Care, 23*(Suppl. 1), S1–S16.

American Diabetes Association. (2001). Standards of care. *Diabetes Care, 24*(Suppl. 1), S33–S43.

Bell, D. S. H., & Ovalle, F. (2000, Spring). Management of type 2 diabetes. *Clinical Reviews,* 93–96.

Chehade, J. M., & Mooradian, A. D. (2000). A rational approach to drug therapy of type 2 diabetes mellitus. *Drugs, 60*(1), 95–113.

Davis, S. N. (2006). Insulin, oral hypoglycemic agents, and the pharmacology of the endocrine pancreas. In L. L. Brunton, J. S. Lazo, & K. L. Parker (Eds.), *The pharmacological basis of therapeutics* (11th ed., pp. 1613–1646). New York: McGraw-Hill.

Demester, N. (2001). Diseases of the thyroid: A broad spectrum. *Clinical Reviews, 11*(7), 58–64.

Farwell, A. P., & Braverman, L. E. (2006). Thyroids and antithyroid drugs. In L. L. Brunton, J. S. Lazo, & K. L. Parker (Eds.), *The pharmacological basis of therapeutics* (11th ed., pp. 1511–1540). New York: McGraw-Hill.

Harrigan, R. A., Nathan, M. S., & Beattie, P. (2001). Oral agents for the treatment of type 2 diabetes mellitus: Pharmacology, toxicity, and treatment. *Annals of Emergency Medicine, 38*(1), 68.

Hovens, M. M., Tamsma, J. T., Beishuizen, E. D., & Huisman, M.V. (2005). Pharmacological strategies to reduce cardiovascular risk in type 2 diabetes mellitus: An update. *Drugs, 65*(4), 433–445.

Margioris, A. N., & Chrousos, G. P. (Eds.). (2001). *Adrenal disorders.* Totowa, NJ: Humana Press.

Mokdad, A. H., Bowman, B. A., Ford, E. S., Vinicor, F., Marks, J. S., & Koplan, J. P. (2001). The continuing epidemics of obesity and diabetes in the United States. *Journal of the American Medical Association, 286,* 1195–1200.

Parker, K. L., & Schimmer, B. P. (2006). Pituitary hormones and their hypothalamic releasing factors. In L. L. Brunton, J. S. Lazo, & K. L. Parker (Eds.), *The pharmacological basis of therapeutics* (11th ed., pp. 1489–1510). New York: McGraw-Hill.

Winqvist, O., Rorsman, F., & Kampe, O. (2000). Autoimmune adrenal insufficiency: Recognition and management. *BioDrugs, 13*(2), 107–114.

CHAPTER 32
Drugs for Disorders and Conditions of the Reproductive System

Basaria, S., & Dobs, A. S. (1999). Risk versus benefits of testosterone therapy in elderly men. *Drugs and Aging, 15*(2), 131–142.

Frackiewicz, E. J., & Shiovitz, T. M. (2001). Evaluation and management of premenstrual syndrome and premenstrual dysphoric disorder. *Journal of the American Pharmaceutical Association, 41*(3), 437–447.

Loose, D. S., & Stancel, G. M. (2006). Estrogens. In L. L. Brunton, J. S. Lazo, & K. L. Parker (Eds.), *The pharmacological basis of therapeutics* (11th ed., pp. 1541–1572). New York: McGraw-Hill.

Nelson, A. (2000). Contraceptive update Y2K: Need for contraception and new contraceptive options. *Clinic Corner, 3*(1), 48–62.

Rozenberg, S., Vasquez, J. B., Vandromme, J., & Kroll, M. (1998). Educating patients about the benefits and drawbacks of hormone replacement therapy. *Drugs and Aging, 13*(1), 33–41.

Shepherd, J. E. (2001). Effects of estrogen on cognition, mood, and degenerative brain diseases. *Journal of the American Pharmaceutical Association, 41*(2), 221–228.

Snyder, P. J. (2006). Androgens. In L. L. Brunton, J. S. Lazo, & K. L. Parker (Eds.), *The pharmacological basis of therapeutics* (11th ed., pp. 1573–1586). New York: McGraw-Hill.

CHAPTER 33
Drugs for Bone and Joint Disorders

Burke, A., Smyth, E. M., & Fitzgerald, G. A. (2006). Analgesic-antipyretic agents; pharmacotherapy of gout. In L. L. Brunton, J. S. Lazo, & K. L. Parker (Eds.), *The pharmacological basis of therapeutics* (11th ed., pp. 671–716). New York: McGraw-Hill.

Cashman, J. N. (2000). Current pharmacotherapeutic strategies in rheumatic diseases and other pain states. *Clinical Drug Investigation, 19*(Suppl. 2), 9–20.

Clemett, D., & Goa, K. L. (2000). Celecoxib: A review of its use in osteoarthritis, rheumatoid arthritis, and acute pain. *Drugs, 59*(4), 957–980.

Friedman, P. A. (2006). Agents affecting mineral ion homeostasis and bone turnover. In L. L. Brunton, J. S. Lazo, & K. L. Parker (Eds.), *The pharmacological basis of therapeutics* (11th ed., pp. 1647–1677). New York: McGraw-Hill.

Jelley, M. J., & Wortmann, R. (2000). Practical steps in the diagnosis and management of gout. *Biodrugs, 14*(2), 99–107.

Lacki, J. K. (2000). Management of the patient with severe refractory rheumatoid arthritis: Are the newer treatment options worth considering? *BioDrugs, 13*(6), 425–435.

Orwoll, E. S. (1999). Osteoporosis in men. *New Dimensions in Osteoporosis, 1*(5), 2–8, 12.

Prestwood, K. M. (2000). Prevention and treatment of osteoporosis. *Clinic Corner, 2*(6), 34–44.

Watts, N. B. (1999). Treatment of postmenopausal osteoporosis. *New Dimensions in Osteoporosis, 1*(4), 2–6.

CHAPTER 34
Drugs for Skin Disorders

Fox, L. P., Merk, H. F., & Bickers, D. R. (2006). Dermatological pharmacology. In L. L. Brunton, J. S. Lazo, & K. L. Parker (Eds.), *The pharmacological basis of therapeutics* (11th ed., pp. 1679–1706). New York: McGraw-Hill.

Feldman, S. (2000). Advances in psoriasis treatment. *Dermatology Online, 6*(1), 4.

Roos, T. C., & Merk, H. F. (2000). Important drug interactions in dermatology. *Drugs, 59*(2), 181–192.

CHAPTER 35
Drugs for Eye and Ear Disorders

APhA drug treatment protocols: Management of pediatric acute otitis media. *Journal of the American Pharmaceutical Association, 40*(5), 599–608.

Beers, S. L., & Abramo, T. J. (2004). Otitis externa review. *Pediatric Emergency Care, 20*(4), 250–256.

Brook, I. (1999). Treatment of otitis externa in children. *Paediatric Drugs, 1*(4), 283–289.

Camras, C. B., & Tamesis, R. R. (1999). Efficacy and adverse effects of medications used in the treatment of glaucoma. *Drugs and Aging, 15*(5), 377–388.

Henderer, J. D., & Rapuano, C. J. (2006). Ocular pharmacology. In L. L. Brunton, J. S. Lazo, & K. L. Parker (Eds.), *The pharmacological basis of therapeutics* (11th ed., pp. 1707–1737). New York: McGraw-Hill.

Hoyng, P. F. J., & van Beek, L. M. (2000). Pharmacological therapy for glaucoma: A review. *Drugs, 59*(3), 411–434.

Leibovitz, E., & Dagan, R. (2001a). Otitis media therapy and drug resistance: Current concepts and new directions. *Infections in Medicine, 18*(5), 263–270.

Leibovitz, E., & Dagan, R. (2001b). Otitis media therapy and drug resistance: Management principles. *Infections in Medicine, 18*(4), 212–216.

Pray, S. (2001). Swimmer's ear: An ear canal infection. *U.S. Pharmacist, 26*(8).

Schwartz, K. A., & Budenz, D. B. (2004). Current management of glaucoma. *Current Opinion in Ophthalmology, 15*(2), 119–126. Tripathi, R. C., Tripathi, B. J., & Haggerty, C. (2003). Drug-induced glaucomas: Mechanism and management. *Drug Safety, 26*(11), 749–767.

Chapter 1

Answers to NCLEX-PN® Questions
1. 4
2. 3
3. 4
4. 4
5. 2
6. 4
7. 2
8. 4
9. 3
10. 4

Chapter 2

Answers to NCLEX-PN® Questions
1. 1
2. 2
3. 4
4. 4
5. 4
6. 2
7. 2
8. 3
9. 2
10. 3

Chapter 3

Answers to NCLEX-PN® Questions
1. 3
2. 2
3. 1
4. 3
5. 1
6. 1
7. 4
8. 4
9. 2
10. 3
11. 4
12. 1

Chapter 4

Answers to NCLEX-PN® Questions
1. 3
2. 2
3. 4
4. 3
5. 1
6. 4
7. 2
8. 3
9. 2
10. 1

Chapter 5

Answers to NCLEX-PN® Questions
1. 1
2. 3
3. 2

4. 1, 3, and 4
5. 4
6. 3
7. 4
8. 3

Chapter 6

Answers to NCLEX-PN® Questions
1. 1, 2, 3
2. 2
3. 2
4. 1
5. 3
6. 2
7. 2
8. 4
9. 3
10. 4

Chapter 7

Answers to NCLEX-PN® Questions
1. 3
2. 2
3. 4
4. 1
5. 2
6. 2
7. 3
8. 1
9. 3
10. 2

Chapter 8

Answers to NCLEX-PN® Questions
1. 4
2. 2
3. 4
4. 3
5. 2
6. 2
7. 3
8. 2
9. 4
10. 3

Answers to Case Study Questions
1. 3
2. 2, 3, and 4
3. 3
4. 4

Chapter 9

Answers to NCLEX-PN® Questions
1. 4
2. 2
3. 3
4. 3
5. 2
6. 4
7. 3
8. 2

9. 2
10. 1

Answers to Case Study Questions
1. 4
2. 1

Chapter 10

Answers to NCLEX-PN® Questions
1. 3
2. 3
3. 4
4. 1
5. 1
6. 2
7. 2
8. 3
9. 2
10. 3

Answers to Case Study Questions
1. 4
2. 3
3. 2
4. 4

Chapter 11

Answers to NCLEX-PN® Questions
1. 2
2. 2
3. 3
4. 3
5. 4
6. 1
7. 2
8. 3
9. 4
10. 2

Answers to Case Study Questions
1. 1
2. 1, 2, and 3
3. 2
4. 2

Chapter 12

Answers to NCLEX-PN® Questions
1. 4
2. 2
3. 3
4. 3
5. 2
6. 2
7. 3
8. 1

Answers to Case Study Questions
1. 4
2. 3
3. 2
4. 3

Chapter 13

Answers to NCLEX-PN® Questions
1. 4
2. 3
3. 4
4. 1
5. 2
6. 3
7. 4
8. 4
9. 3
10. 1

Answers to Case Study Questions
1. 3
2. 3
3. 3
4. 4

Chapter 14

Answers to NCLEX-PN® Questions
1. 4
2. 1
3. 1
4. 4
5. 3
6. 2
7. 3
8. 1
9. 2
10. 2

Answers to Case Study Questions
1. 4
2. 1
3. 2
4. 2

Chapter 15

Answers to NCLEX-PN® Questions
1. 4
2. 2
3. 1
4. 2
5. 3
6. 2
7. 1
8. 2
9. 3
10. 3

Answers to Case Study Questions
1. 2
2. 3
3. 4
4. 4

Chapter 16

Answers to NCLEX-PN® Questions

1. 3
2. 3
3. 2
4. 4
5. 1
6. 3
7. 1
8. 1
9. 3
10. 1

Answers to Case Study Questions

1. 2
2. 1
3. 3
4. 4

Chapter 17

Answers to NCLEX-PN® Questions

1. 4
2. 1
3. 2
4. 2
5. 4
6. 3
7. 2
8. 3
9. 4
10. 2

Answers to Case Study Questions

1. 3
2. 2
3. 1
4. 4

Chapter 18

Answers to NCLEX-PN® Questions

1. 2
2. 4
3. 2
4. 1
5. 2
6. 3
7. 1
8. 1
9. 1
10. 3

Answers to Case Study Questions

1. 2
2. 2
3. 1
4. 3

Chapter 19

Answers to NCLEX-PN® Questions

1. 3
2. 2

3. 4
4. 3
5. 1
6. 2
7. 1
8. 2
9. 2
10. 1

Answers to Case Study Questions

1. 4
2. 2
3. 3
4. 1

Chapter 20

Answers to NCLEX-PN® Questions

1. 4
2. 2
3. 3
4. 2
5. 4
6. 2
7. 3
8. 1
9. 4
10. 2

Answers to Case Study Questions

1. 4
2. 3
3. 2
4. 1

Chapter 21

Answers to NCLEX-PN® Questions

1. 2
2. 1
3. 2
4. 2
5. 3
6. 3
7. 4
8. 1
9. 3
10. 3

Answers to Case Study Questions

1. 2
2. 2
3. 1
4. 1

Chapter 22

Answers to NCLEX-PN® Questions

1. 2
2. 4
3. 2
4. 4
5. 1
6. 4
7. 2

8. 3
9. 2
10. 2

Answers to Case Study Questions

1. 4
2. 1
3. 4
4. 4

Chapter 23

Answers to NCLEX-PN® Questions

1. 3
2. 4
3. 2
4. 2
5. 2
6. 2
7. 1
8. 2
9. 4
10. 2

Answers to Case Study Questions

1. 3
2. 1
3. 4
4. 2

Chapter 24

Answers to NCLEX-PN® Questions

1. 3
2. 3
3. 3
4. 4
5. 2
6. 4
7. 2
8. 3
9. 4
10. 1

Answers to Case Study Questions

1. 2
2. 1
3. 3
4. 2

Chapter 25

Answers to NCLEX-PN® Questions

1. 4
2. 2
3. 3
4. 1
5. 2
6. 3
7. 4
8. 3
9. 4
10. 2

Answers to Case Study Questions

1. 1
2. 3
3. 1
4. 1

Chapter 26

Answers to NCLEX-PN® Questions

1. 3
2. 4
3. 3
4. 1
5. 3
6. 4
7. 4
8. 2
9. 4
10. 1

Answers to Case Study Questions

1. 3
2. 2
3. 1
4. 2

Chapter 27

Answers to NCLEX-PN® Questions

1. 3
2. 2
3. 4
4. 2
5. 1
6. 4
7. 2
8. 3
9. 3
10. 2

Answers to Case Study Questions

1. 3
2. 2
3. 2
4. 1

Chapter 28

Answers to NCLEX-PN® Questions

1. 1
2. 3 or 4
3. 4
4. 2
5. 2
6. 4
7. 1
8. 4
9. 2
10. 1

Answers to Case Study Questions

1. 4
2. 3
3. 1
4. 2

Chapter 29

**Answers to NCLEX-PN®
Questions**
1. 3
2. 1
3. 1
4. 2
5. 1
6. 2
7. 2
8. 1
9. 3
10. 1

**Answers to Case Study
Questions**
1. 1
2. 4
3. 1
4. 1

Chapter 30

**Answers to NCLEX-PN®
Questions**
1. 3
2. 4
3. 1
4. 2
5. 3
6. 4
7. 2
8. 4
9. 3
10. 4

**Answers to Case Study
Questions**
1. 2
2. 3
3. 3
4. 4

Chapter 31

**Answers to NCLEX-PN®
Questions**
1. 3
2. 4
3. 2
4. 3
5. 2
6. 1
7. 2
8. 4
9. 4
10. 3

**Answers to Case Study
Questions**
1. 2
2. 1
3. 3
4. 2

Chapter 32

**Answers to NCLEX-PN®
Questions**
1. 2
2. 2
3. 3
4. 2
5. 4
6. 2
7. 3
8. 2
9. 4
10. 4

**Answers to Case Study
Questions**
1. 4
2. 1
3. 3
4. 3

Chapter 33

**Answers to NCLEX-PN®
Questions**
1. 2
2. 4
3. 1
4. 4
5. 3
6. 1
7. 4
8. 2
9. 3
10. 1

**Answers to Case Study
Questions**
1. 2
2. 3
3. 3
4. 4

Chapter 34

**Answers to NCLEX-PN®
Questions**
1. 2
2. 3
3. 4
4. 1
5. 2
6. 3
7. 4
8. 2
9. 4
10. 4

**Answers to Case Study
Questions**
1. 4
2. 3
3. 2
4. 3

Chapter 35

**Answers to NCLEX-PN®
Questions**
1. 1
2. 3
3. 1
4. 3
5. 1
6. 3
7. 2
8. 1
9. 3
10. 1

**Answers to Case Study
Questions**
1. 3
2. 1
3. 1
4. 3

Rank	Top 100 Generic Drugs	Top 100 Brand Name Drugs	Rank	Top 100 Generic Drugs	Top 100 Brand Name Drugs
1.	Hydrocodone w/APAP	Lipitor	52.	Carisoprodol	Chantix
2.	Lisinopril	Nexium	53.	Allopurinol	Avapro
3.	Simvastatin	Lexapro	54.	Methylprednisolone Tabs	Proventil HFA
4.	Levothyroxine	Singulair	55.	Meloxicam	Abilify
5.	Amoxicillin	Plavix	56.	Amlodipine/benazepril	Yasmin 28
6.	Azithromycin	Synthroid	57.	Potassium chloride	Budeprion XL
7.	Hydrochlorothiazide	Prevacid	58.	Clonidine	Niaspan
8.	Alprazolam	Advair Diskus	59.	Promethazine Tabs	Combivent
9.	Atenolol	Effexor XR	60.	Isosorbide mononitrate	Januvia
10.	Metformin	Diovan	61.	Folic Acid	Boniva
11.	Metoprolol succinate	Crestor	62.	Spironolactone	TriNessa
12.	Furosemide Oral	Vytorin	63.	Glimepiride	NuvaRing
13.	Metoprolol tartrate	Cymbalta	64.	Pantoprazole	Risperdal
14.	Sertraline	Pro-Air HFA	65.	Glyburide	Polymagma Plain
15.	Omeprazole	Klor-Con	66.	Verapamil SR	Flovent HFA
16.	Zolpidem tartrate	Diovan HCT	67.	Albuterol Nebulizer Solution	Imitrex oral
17.	Oxycodone w/APAP	Levaquin	68.	Cefdidnir	Evista
18.	Ibuprofen	Actos	69.	Temazepam	Avelox
19.	Prednisone Oral	Flomax	70.	Triamcinolone acetonide Topical	Depakote ER
20.	Fluoxetine	Seroquel	71.	Penicillin VK	Protonix
21.	Warfarin	Zetia	72.	Oxycodone	Avalide
22.	Cephalexin	Tricor	73.	Metformin HCl ER	Lioderm
23.	Lorazepam	Celebrex	74.	Benazepril	Zyprexa
24.	Clonazepam	Nasonex	75.	Glipizide	Namenda
25.	Citalopram	Premarin-Tabs	76.	Clindamycin Systemic	Tussionex
26.	Tramadol	Lantus	77.	Ramipril	Thyroid, Armour
27.	Gabapentin	Viagra	78.	Metronidazole Tabs	Humalog
28.	Ciprofloxacin	Yaz	79.	Digoxin	Vigamox
29.	Propoxyphene w/APAP	Lyrica	80.	Metoclopramide	Tamiflu
30.	Lisinopril/HCTZ	Adderall XR	81.	Estradiol Oral	Budeprion SR
31.	Triamterene/HCTZ	Valtrex	82.	Hydroxyzine	Suboxone
32.	Amoxicillin/clavulanate	Cozaar	83.	Amphetamine salt combination	Lanoxin
33.	Cyclobenzaprine	Topamax	84.	Diclofenac	Loestrin 24 Fe
34.	Trazodone	Concerta	85.	Gemfibrozil	Avodart
35.	Fexofenadine	Levoxyl	86.	Propranolol HCl	Coumadin tabs
36.	Fluticasone Nasal	Actonel	87.	Vitamin D	Wellbutrin XL
37.	Paroxetine	Ambien CR	88.	Quinapril	Endocet
38.	Lovastatin	Spiriva	89.	Promethazine/Codeine	Skelaxin
39.	Trimethoprim/Sulfa	Benicar	90.	Doxazosin	Nasacort AQ
40.	Albuterol Aerosol	Xalatan	91.	Mirtazapine	Keppra
41.	Diazepam	Benicar HCT	92.	Glipizide ER	Allegra D 12 hr
42.	Pravastatin	Aricept	93.	Phentermine	Strattera
43.	Acetaminophen/Codeine	Ortho Tri-Cyclen Lo	94.	Acyclovir	Lovaza
44.	Alendronate	Hyzaar	95.	Meclizine	Avandia
45.	Amitriptyline	Tri-Sprintec	96.	Potassium chloride	Ocella
46.	Naproxen	Cialis	97.	Nitrofurantoin	Vyvanse
47.	Fluconazole	OxyContin	98.	Sulfamethoxazole/trimethoprim	Toprol XL
48.	Enalapril	AcipHex	99.	Fentanyl Transdermal	Levitra
49.	Carvedilol	Lunesta	100.	Buspirone	Astelin
50.	Ranitidine	Lamictal			
51.	Doxycycline	Detrol LA			

Data retrieved September 24, 2009, from http://drugtopics.modernmedicine.com/drugtopics/data/articlestandard//drugtopics/222009/599844/article.pdf
http://drugtopics.modernmedicine.com/drugtopics/data/articlestandard//drugtopics/222009/599845/article.pdf

High-alert medications are drugs that bear a heightened risk of causing significant patient harm when they are used in error. Although mistakes may or may not be more common with these drugs, the consequences of an error are clearly more devastating to patients. We hope you will use this list to determine which medications require special safeguards to reduce the risk of errors. This may include strategies such as improving access to information about these drugs; limiting access to high-alert medications; using auxiliary labels and automated alerts; standardizing the ordering, storage, preparation, and administration of these products; and employing redundancies such as automated or independent double-checks when necessary. (Note: Manual independent double-checks are not always the optimal error-reduction strategy and may not be practical for all of the medications on the list.)

Classes/Categories of Medications

adrenergic agonists, IV (e.g., epinephrine, phenylephrine, norepinephrine)

adrenergic antagonists, IV (e.g., propranolol, metoprolol, labetalol)

anesthetic agents, general, inhaled and IV (e.g., propofol, ketamine)

antiarrhythmics, IV (e.g., lidocaine, amiodarone)

antithrombotic agents (anticoagulants), including warfarin, low-molecular-weight heparin, IV unfractionated heparin, Factor Xa inhibitors (fondaparinux), direct thrombin inhibitors (e.g., argatroban, lepirudin, bivalirudin), thrombolytics (e.g., alteplase, reteplase, tenecteplase), and glycoprotein IIb/IIIa inhibitors (e.g., eptifibatide)

cardioplegic solutions

chemotherapeutic agents, parenteral and oral

dextrose, hypertonic, 20% or greater

dialysis solutions, peritoneal and hemodialysis

epidural or intrathecal medications

hypoglycemics, oral

inotropic medications, IV (e.g., digoxin, milrinone)

liposomal forms of drugs (e.g., liposomal amphotericin B)

moderate sedation agents, IV (e.g., midazolam)

moderate sedation agents, oral, for children (e.g., chloral hydrate)

narcotics/opiates, IV, transdermal, and oral (including liquid concentrates, immediate and sustained-release formulations)

neuromuscular blocking agents (e.g., succinylcholine, rocuronium, vecuronium)

radiocontrast agents, IV

total parenteral nutrition solutions

© ISMP 2008

Specific Medications

epoprostenol (Flolan), IV
insulin, subcutaneous and IV
magnesium sulfate injection
methotrexate, oral, nononcologic use
opium tincture
oxytocin, IV
nitroprusside sodium for injection
potassium chloride for injection concentrate
potassium phosphates injection
promethazine, IV
sodium chloride for injection, hypertonic (greater than 0.9% concentration)
sterile water for injection, inhalation, and irrigation (excluding pour bottles) in containers of 100 mL or more

Background

Based on error reports submitted to the USP-ISMP Medication Errors Reporting Program, reports of harmful errors in the literature, and input from practitioners and safety experts, ISMP created and periodically updates a list of potential high-alert medications. During February–April 2007, 770 practitioners responded to an ISMP survey designed to identify which medications were most frequently considered high-alert drugs by individuals and organizations. Further, to ensure relevance and completeness, the clinical staff at ISMP, members of our advisory board, and safety experts throughout the United States were asked to review the potential list. This list of drugs and drug categories reflects the collective thinking of all who provided input.

APPENDIX E: Calculating Dosages

I. Calculating Dosage Using Ratios and Proportions

A. *ratio* is used to express a relationship between two or more quantities. Ratios may be written using the following notations.

1:10 means 1 part of drug A to 10 parts of solution/solvent.

In drug calculations, ratios are usually expressed as a fraction:

$$\frac{1 \text{ part drug A}}{10 \text{ parts solution}} = \frac{1}{10}$$

A *proportion* shows the relationship between two ratios. It is a simple and effective means for calculating certain types of doses.

$$\frac{\text{Dose on hand}}{\text{Quantity on hand}} = \frac{\text{Desired dose}}{\text{Quantity desired } (X)}$$

Using cross-multiplication, we can write the same formula as follows:

$$\text{Quantity desired } (X) = \frac{\text{Desired dose} \times \text{Quantity on hand}}{\text{Dose on hand}}$$

Example 1: The health care provider orders erythromycin 500 mg. It is supplied in a liquid form containing 250 mg in 5 ml. How much drug should the nurse administer?

To calculate the dosage, use the formula:

$$\frac{\text{Dose on hand (250 mg)}}{\text{Quantity on hand (5 ml)}} = \frac{\text{Desired dose (500 mg)}}{\text{Quantity desired } (X)}$$

Then, cross-multiply:

$$250 \text{ mg} \times X = 5 \text{ ml} \times 500 \text{ mg}$$

Therefore, the dose to be administered is 10 ml.

B. The same proportion method can be used to solve solid dosage calculations.

Example 2: The health care provider orders methotrexate 20 mg/day. The methotrexate is available in 2.5-mg tablets. How many tablets should the nurse administer each day?

$$\frac{\text{Dose on hand (2.5 mg)}}{1 \text{ tablet}} = \frac{\text{Desired dose (20 mg)}}{\text{Quantity desired } (X \text{ tablets})}$$

Cross-multiplication gives:

$$2.5 \text{ mg } X = 20 \text{ mg} \times 1 \text{ tablet}$$

Therefore, the nurse should administer 8 tablets daily.

II. Calculating Dosage by Weight

Doses for pediatric patients are often calculated by using body weight. The nurse must use caution to convert between pounds and kilograms, as necessary (see Table 3.2 in Chapter 3, page 29). Use the formula:

Body weight (kg) × amount mg/kg = X mg of drug

Example 3: The health care provider orders 10 mg/kg of methsuximide for a client who weighs 90 kg. How much should be administered?

The patient should receive 900 mg of methsuximide.

Example 4: The health care provider orders 5 mg/kg/day of amiodarone. The patient weighs 110 pounds. How much of the drug should be administered daily?

Step 1: Convert pounds to kilograms.

110 lb × 1 kg/2.2 lb = 50 kg

Step 2: Perform the drug calculation.

50 kg (body weight) × 5 mg/ kg = 250 mg

The patient should receive 250 mg of amiodarone per day.

III. Calculating Dosage by Body Surface Area

Many antineoplastic drugs and most pediatric doses are calculated using body surface area (BSA).

The formula for BSA in metric units is:

$$\text{BSA} = \sqrt{\frac{\text{weight (kg)} \times \text{height (cm)}}{3600}}$$

The formula for BSA in household units is

$$\text{BSA} = \sqrt{\frac{\text{weight (lb)} \times \text{height (inches)}}{3131}}$$

Example 5: The health care provider orders 10 mg/m^2 of an antibiotic for a child who is 2 feet tall and weighs 30 lb. How many milligrams should be administered?

Step 1: Calculate the BSA of the child.

$$\text{BSA} = \sqrt{\frac{30 \times 24}{3131}}$$

$$\text{BSA} = \sqrt{\frac{720}{3131}}$$

$$\text{BSA} = \sqrt{0.230} = 0.48 \text{ m}^2$$

Step 2: Calculate the drug amount.

$$10 \text{ mg/m}^2 \times 0.48 \text{ m}^2$$

The nurse should administer 4.8 mg of the antibiotic to the child.

IV. Calculating IV Infusion Rates

Intravenous fluids are administered over time in units of ml/min or gtt/min (gtt = drops). The basic equation for IV drug calculations is as follows:

$$\frac{\text{ml of solution} \times \text{gtt/ml}}{\text{h of administration} \times 60 \text{ min/h}} = \frac{\text{gtt}}{\text{min}}$$

Example 6: The health care provider orders 1,000 ml of 5% normal saline to infuse over 6 hours. What is the flow rate?

$$\frac{1,000 \text{ ml} \times 10 \text{ gtt/ml}}{6 \text{ h} \times 60 \text{ min/h}} = \frac{28 \text{ gtt}}{\text{min}}$$

Other IV conversion formulas you may use include the following:

$$\text{mcg/kg/h} \rightarrow \text{ml/h}$$

$$\text{kg} \times \frac{\text{mcg/kg}}{\text{h}} \times \frac{\text{mg}}{1,000 \text{ mcg}} \times \frac{\text{ml}}{\text{mg}} = \frac{\text{ml}}{\text{h}}$$

$$\text{mcg/m}^2\text{/h} \rightarrow \text{ml/h}$$

$$\text{m}^2 \times \frac{\text{mcg/m}^2}{\text{h}} \times \frac{\text{mg}}{1,000 \text{ mcg}} \times \frac{\text{ml}}{\text{mg}} = \frac{\text{ml}}{\text{h}}$$

$$\text{mcg/kg/min} \rightarrow \text{gtt/min}$$

$$\text{kg} \times \frac{\text{mcg/kg}}{\text{min}} \times \frac{\text{mg}}{1,000 \text{ mcg}} \times \frac{\text{ml}}{\text{mg}} \times \frac{10 \text{ gtt}}{\text{ml}} = \frac{\text{gtt}}{\text{min}}$$

Name of Drug	Therapeutic Class	Pharmacologic Class	Page
Acetaminophen (Tylenol)	Antipyretic, nonopioid analgesic	Central noninflammatory-type prostaglandin inhibitor	222
Acyclovir (Zovirax)	Antiviral for herpesviruses	Nucleoside analog	447
Alendronate (Fosamax)	Drug for osteoporosis	Bone resorption inhibitor, bisphosphonate	603
Alteplase (Activase)	Drug for dissolving clots	Thrombolytic	331
Aminocaproic Acid (Amicar)	Clot stabilizer	Hemostatic/Antifibrinolytic	333
Amiodarone (Cardarone)	Antidysrhythmic (Class III)	Potassium channel blocker	315
Amphotericin B (AmBisome, Fungizone, Others)	Antifungal (systemic type)	Polyene	437
Androgens Testosterone Base (Andro)	Male hypogonadism drug, female breast cancer agent	Androgen, hormonal agent	584
Aspirin (Acetylsalicylic Acid, ASA)	Nonopioid analgesic, nonsteriodal anti-inflammatory drug (NSAID), antipyretic; drug for myocardial infarction prophylaxis and transient ischemia	Salicylate, cyclooxygenase (COX) inhibitor, prostaglandin synthesis inhibitor platelet aggregation inhibitor	222
Atenolol (Tenormin)	Drug for angina, hypertension or MI	Beta-adrenergic blocker	345
Atorvastatin (Lipitor)	Antilipemic drug	HMG-CoA reductase inhibitor (statin)	258
Atropine (Atro-Pen, Atropair, Atropisol)	Antidote for anticholinerase poisoning, antidysrhythmic, mydriatic (pupil dilating drug)	Anticholinergic, cholinergic receptor blocker	102
Benzocaine (Americaine, Anbesol, Others)	Agent for sunburn pain and minor skin irritations	Local anesthetic, sodium channel blocker	621
Benztropine (Cogentin)	Antiparkinson agent	Centrally acting cholinergic receptor blocker	175
Bethanechol (Urecholine)	Urinary retention (incomplete bladder emptying) treatment	Parasympathomimetic, cholinergic receptor drug	99
Calcitriol (Calcijex, Rocaltrol)	Drug for treatment of hypocalcemia, osteoporosis, osteomalacia, and rickets	Vitamin D agent	600
Calcium Gluconate (Kalcinate)	Drug for treatment of hypocalcemia, hypoparathyroidism, osteoporosis, and Paget's disease	Calcium supplement	599
Carvedilol (Coreg)	Drug for heart failure and HTN	Beta-adrenergic blocker	300
Cefotaxime (Claforan)	Antibacterial	Cell wall inhibitor; third-generation cephalosporin	416
Chlorothiazide (Diuril)	Antihypertensive, agent for reducing edema	Thiazide diuretic	374
Chlorpromazine (Thorazine)	Conventional antipsychotic, schizophrenia agent	Phenothiazine, D_2 dopamine receptor blocker	158
Cholestyramine (Questran)	Antilipemic drug	Bile acid resin	258
Ciprofloxacin (Cipro)	Antibacterial	Fluoroquinolone, bacterial DNA synthesis inhibitor	421
Clopidogrel (Plavix)	Antiplatelet agent	ADP receptor blocker	330
Colchicine (Colcrys)	Antigout agent	Inhibitor of uric acid accumulation	609
Conjugated Estrogens (Premarin) and Conjugated Estrogens with Medroxyprogesterone (Prempro)	Menopausal hormone therapy	Hormone replacement therapy, estrogen, and estrogen-progestin combination	579
Cyanocobalamin (Crystamine, Others)	Agent for anemia	Vitamin supplement	532
Cyclobenzaprine (Cycloflex, Flexeril)	Skeletal muscle relaxant, central-acting	Catecholamine reuptake inhibitor	182

Name of Drug	Therapeutic Class	Pharmacologic Class	Page
Cyclophosphamide (Cytoxan)	Antineoplastic	Alkylating agent	464
Cyclosporine (Neoral, Sandimmune)	Immunosuppressant	Calcineurin inhibitor	401
Dantrolene Sodium (Dantrium)	Skeletal muscle relaxant, peripheral-acting	Skeletal muscle calcium release blocker	186
Diazepam (Valium)	Antiseizure drug, sedative-hypnotic, anxiolytic, anesthetic adjunct, skeletal muscle relaxant (centrally acting)	Benzodiazepine, GABA$_A$ receptor drug	199
Digoxin (Lanoxin)	Drug for heart failure	Cardiac glycoside	299
Diltiazem (Cardizem, Cartia XT, Dilacor XR, Taztia XT, Tiazac)	Drug for angina and hypertension	Calcium channel blocker	346
Diphenhydramine (Benadryl, Others)	Drug to treat allergies	H$_1$-receptor blocker, antihistamine	487
Diphenoxylate with Atropine (Lomotil)	Antidiarrheal	Opioid	519
Donepezil (Aricept, Aricept ODT)	Alzheimer's disease agent	Acetylcholinerase inhibitor	178
Dopamine (Dopastat, Intropin)	Drug for shock	Nonselective adrenergic agonist, inotropic agent	361
Doxazosin (Cardura)	Drug for hypertension and BPH	Alpha$_1$-adrenergic blocker	283
Doxorubicin (Adriamycin)	Antineoplastic	Antitumor antibiotic	467
Enalapril (Vasotec)	Drug for hypertension and heart failure	ACE inhibitor	282
Epinephrine (Adrenalin)	Drug for anaphylaxis and shock	Sympathomimetic, vasoconstrictor	362
Epoetin Alfa (Epogen, Procrit)	Drug for anemia	Hematopoietic growth factor, erythropoietin	472
Erythromycin (E-Mycin, Erythrocin)	Antibacterial	Macrolide protein synthesis inhibitor	418
Ethinyl Estradiol with Norethindrone (Ortho-Novum 1/35)	Ovulation inhibitor, luteinizing hormone (LH) inhibitor	Oral contraceptive	577
Ethosuximide (Zarontin)	Antiseizure drug	Succinimide, low-threshold calcium channel blocking drug	203
Ferrous Sulfate (Feosol, Feostat, Others)	Agent for anemia	Iron supplement	534
Finasteride (Proscar)	Drug for benign prostatic hyperplasia drug	5-alpha reductase enzyme inhibitor	588
Fluoxetine (Prozac)	Antidepressant	Selective serotonin reuptake inhibitor (SSRI)	141
Fluticasone (Flonase, Veramyst)	Drug for allergic rhinitis	Intranasal corticosteroid	490
Furosemide (Lasix)	Drug for heart failure and HTN	Diuretic (loop type)	298
Gemfibrozil (Lopid)	Antihyperlipidemic drug	Fibric acid agent	262
Gentamicin	Antibacterial	Aminoglycoside, protein synthesis inhibitor	419
Glipizide (Glucotrol)	Antidiabetic	Oral hypoglycemic, sulfonylurea (second generation)	553
Haloperidol (Haldol)	Conventional antipsychotic, schizophrenia agent	Nonphenothiazine, D$_2$ dopamine receptor blocker	159
Halothane (Fluothane)	General anesthetic	Inhalation volatile liquid	241
Heparin	Anticoagulant	Indirect thrombin inhibitor	327
Hepatitis B Vaccine (Energix-B, Recombivax HB)	Vaccine	Vaccine	398
Hydralazine (Apresoline)	Drug for hypertension and heart failure	Direct-acting vasodilator	285
Hydrochlorothiazide (Microzide)	Drug for hypertension and edema	Thiazide diuretic	276
Hydrocortisone (Cortef, Hydrocortone, Solu-Cortef, Others)	Drug for moderate to severe asthma and allergies, antineoplastic, and adrenal hormone replacement therapy	Systemic glucocorticoid	562

Name of Drug	Therapeutic Class	Pharmacologic Class	Page
Hydroxychloroquine (Plaquenil)	Disease-modifying antirheumatic drug (DMARD)	Protein synthesis inhibitor, inhibitor of DNA and RNA polymerase, rheumatoid agent	607
Imipramine (Tofranil)	Antidepressant, treatment of nocturnal enuresis (bed-wetting) in children	Tricyclic antidepressant (TCA), serotonin and norepinephrine reuptake inhibitor (SNRI)	137
Interferon alfa-2b (Intron A)	Immunostimulant	Interferon, biologic response modifier	472
Isoniazid (INH, Nydrazid)	Antituberculosis agent	Mycolic acid inhibitor	426
Latanoprost (Xalatan)	Antiglaucoma agent	Prostaglandin, reducer of IOP	635
Levodopa (Larodopa)	Antiparkinson agent	Dopamine precursor	174
Levothyroxine (Synthroid)	Thyroid replacement agent	Natural (biologic) hormone, metabolic enhancing drug	558
Lidocaine (Xylocaine)	Anesthetic (local/regional/topical), antidysrhythmic (class IB)	Sodium channel blocker; amide	237
Lisinopril (Prinivil, Zestril)	Drug for heart failure and HTN	ACE inhibitor	295
Lithium (Eskalith)	Bipolar affective disorder drug, antimanic, antidepressant	Serotonin receptor blocker, glutamate inhibiting agent, inhibitor of glycogen synthase kinase-3 beta	144
Lorazepam (Ativan)	Sedative-hypnotic, anxiolytic, anesthetic adjunct	Benzodiazepines, GABA receptor agent	122
Medroxyprogesterone (Prempro)	Drug for the treatment of endometriosis and abnormal uterine bleeding, antineoplastic	Inhibitor of endometrial proliferation, progestin	581
Methotrexate (Rheumatrex, Trexall)	Antineoplastic	Antimetabolite, folic acid analog	466
Methylphenidate (Ritalin)	Drug for attention-deficit-hyperactivity disorder, narcolepsy drug	Central nervous system stimulant, norepinephrine and dopamine releasing agent	146
Metronidazole (Flagyl)	Anti-infective, antiprotozoan	Agent that disrupts nucleic acid synthesis	450
Milrinone (Primacor)	Drug for heart failure	Phosphodiesterase inhibitor	301
Morphine (Astramorph PF, Duramorph, Others)	Opioid analgesic	Opioid receptor drug	216
Naloxone (Narcan)	Drug for treatment of acute opioid overdose and misuse	Opioid receptor blocker	217
Naproxen (Naprosyn) and Naproxen Sodium (Aleve, Anaprox)	Analgesic, anti-inflammatory drug, antipyretic	Nonsteroidal anti-inflammatory drug (NSAID)	391
Nifedipine (Adalat, Procardia)	Drug for hypertension and angina	Calcium channel blocker	277
Nitroglycerin (Nitrostat, Nitro-Bid, Nitro-Dur, Others)	Antianginal drug	Organic nitrate, vasodilator	342
Nitrous Oxide	General anesthetic	Inhalation gaseous agent	240
Norepinephrine (Levophed)	Drug for shock	Sympathomimetic, vasoconstrictor	361
Normal Serum Albumin (Albuminar, Plasbumin, Others)	Fluid replacement agent	Blood product, colloid	358
Nystatin (Mycostatin, Nystop, Others)	Topical antifungal	Polyene	438
Omeprazole (Prilosec)	Antiulcer drug	Proton-pump inhibitor	513
Oxymetazoline (Afrin, Others)	Decongestant	Sympathomimetic	492
Oxytocin (Pitocin)	Labor induction drug	Uterine stimulant, hormonal agent	583
Penicillin G Sodium/Potassium	Antibacterial	Cell wall inhibitor, natural penicillin	414
Permethrin (Acticin, Elimite, Nix)	Antiparasitic drug	Scabicide, pediculicide	619
Phenelzine (Nardil)	Antidepressant	Monoamine oxidase inhibitor (MAOI)	142
Phenobarbital (Luminal)	Antiseizure drug, sedative, hypnotic	Barbiturate, $GABA_A$ receptor drug	199

Name of Drug	Therapeutic Class	Pharmacologic Class	Page
Phenylephrine (Neo-Synephrine)	Nasal decongestant, mydriatic agent, antihypotensive	Sympathomimetic, alpha$_1$-adrenergic drug	104
Phenytoin (Dilantin)	Antiseizure drug, antidysrhythmic	Hydantoin, sodium influx suppressing drug	202
Potassium Chloride (KCl)	Potassium supplement	Electrolyte	379
Prazosin (Minipress)	Antihypertensive	Sympatholytic, alpha$_1$-adrenergic blocker	107
Prednisone	Anti-inflammatory agent	Glucocorticoid	394
Procainamide (Procanbid)	Antidysrhythmic (Class 1A)	Sodium channel blocker	313
Prochlorperazine (Compazine)	Antiemetic antipsychotic	Phenothiazine	522
Propranolol (Inderal, InnoPran XL)	Antidysrhythmic (Class II)	Beta-adrenergic blocker	314
Propylthiouracil (PTU)	Hyperthyroidism drug	Thyroid hormone synthesis inhibitor, antithyroid agent	559
Psyllium Mucilloid (Metamucil, Others)	Agent for constipation	Bulk-type laxative	517
Raloxifene (Evista)	Treatment of postmenopausal osteoporosis in women	Bone resorption inhibitor, selective estrogen-receptor modulator	603
Ranitidine (Zantac)	Antiulcer drug	H$_2$-receptor blocker	513
Regular Insulin (Humulin R, Novolin R, Pork Regular Iletin II, Regular Purified Pork Insulin)	Antidiabetic	Natural (biologic) hormone, hypoglycemic agent	548
Reteplase (Retavase)	Drug for dissolving clots	Thrombolytic	348
Risperidone (Risperdal, Risperdal Consta)	Atypical antipsychotic, schizophrenia agent, psychotic depression agent	Serotonin (5-HT) receptor antagonist, D$_2$ dopamine receptor antagonist (weaker affinity)	162
Salmeterol (Serevent)	Bronchodilator	Beta-adrenergic agent	497
Sibutramine (Meridia)	Antiobesity agent, appetite suppressant	Anorexiant, SSRI	523
Sildenafil (Viagra)	Erectile dysfunction drug	Phosphodiesterase 5 inhibitor	586
Sodium Bicarbonate (NaHCO$_3$)	Agent to treat acidosis or bicarbonate deficiency	Electrolyte	380
Spironolactone (Aldactone)	Antihypertensive, drug for reducing edema	Potassium-sparing diuretic, aldosterone antagonist	375
Succinylcholine (Anectine)	Skeletal muscle paralytic agent, neuromuscular blocker	Depolarizing blocker, acetylcholine receptor blocking agent	244
Sumatriptan (Imitrex)	Antimigraine drug	Triptan, 5-HT (serotonin) receptor drug, vasoconstrictor of intracranial arteries	227
Tamoxifen	Antineoplastic	Hormonal agent, estrogen receptor blocker	470
Tetracycline (Sumycin, Others)	Antibacterial	Tetracycline, protein synthesis Inhibitor	417
Thiopental (Pentothal)	General anesthetic	Intravenous induction agent; short-acting barbiturate	243
Timolol (Timoptic, Timoptic XE)	Antiglaucoma agent	Beta-adrenergic blocker, reducer of IOP, ocular hypotensive agent	637
Tretinoin (Avita, Retin-A, Trentin-X)	Antiacne drug	Retinoid receptor drug, vitamin derivative	624
Trimethoprim-sulfamethoxazole (Bactrim, Septra)	Antibacterial	Sulfonamide, folic acid inhibitor	422
Valproic Acid (Depakene)	Antiseizure drug, bipolar disorder drug, migraine prophylaxis	Valproate, sodium influx suppressing drug, calcium influx suppressing drug, GABA potentiating drug	203
Vancomycin (Vancocin)	Antibiotic	Bacterial cell wall synthesis inhibitor	424
Verapamil (Calan, Isoptin, Others)	Antidysrhythmic (Class IV)	Calcium channel blocker	316

Name of Drug	Therapeutic Class	Pharmacologic Class	Page
Vincristine (Oncovin)	Antineoplastic	Vinca alkaloid, plant extract	468
Warfarin (Coumadin)	Anticoagulant	Vitamin K antagonist	329
Zidovudine (AZT, Retrovir)	Antiretroviral	Nucleoside reverse transcriptase inhibitor (NRTI)	444
Zolpidem (Ambien)	Sedative-hypnotic	Nonbenzodiazepine, nonbarbiturate CNS depressant, GABA receptor agent	125

Aδ fibers nerves that transmit sensations of sharp pain / *page 212*

absorption (ab-SORP-shun) the process of moving a drug across body membranes / *page 49*

acetylcholine (Ach) (ah-SEET-ul-KOH-leen) primary neurotransmitter of the parasympathetic nervous system; also present at somatic neuromuscular junctions and at parasympathetic and sympathetic preganglionic nerves / *page 96*

acetylcholinesterase (AchE) (AS-ee-til-KOH-lin-ES-ter-ays) an enzyme that degrades acetylcholine within the synapse, enhancing the effects of the neurotransmitter / *page 176*

acidosis (ah-sid-OH-sis) condition of having too much acid; plasma pH below 7.35 / *page 379*

acquired resistance when a microbe is no longer affected by a drug following treatment with anti-infectives / *page 410*

action potential (poh-TEN-shial) an electrical signal of a single cell (muscle or nerve) generated by the opening and closing of special ion channels located on the cell's membrane / *page 200*

activated partial thromboplastin time (aPTT): (thrombow-PLAS-tin) blood test used to determine how long it takes clots to form to regulate heparin dosage / *page 325*

active immunity stimulating the body to produce antibodies through the administration of a vaccine / *page 396*

acute gouty arthritis (ah-CUTE GOW-ty are-THRYE-tis) condition where uric acid crystals quickly accumulate in the joints of the big toes, heels, ankles, wrists, fingers, knees, or elbows, resulting in red, swollen, or inflamed tissue / *page 608*

addiction (ah-DIK-shun) the continued use of a substance despite its negative health and social consequences / *page 78*

Addison's disease (ADD-iss-uns) hyposecretion of glucocorticoids and aldosterone by the adrenal cortex / *page 561*

adenoma (AH-den-OH-mah) benign tumor of glandular tissue / *page 456*

adjuvant chemotherapy (AD-ju-vent) technique in which antineoplastics are administered *after* surgery or radiation to effect a cure / *page 458*

adrenergic (add-rah-NUR-jik) a term relating to nerves that release norepinephrine or epinephrine / *page 96*

adrenergic agent (add-rah-NUR-jik drug) another name for a sympathomimetic drug / *page 97*

adrenergic blocker a drug that blocks the actions of the sympathetic nervous system / *page 97*

adrenocorticotropic hormone (ACTH) (uh-dreen-oh-kor-tik-o-TRO-pik) hormone secreted by the pituitary that stimulates the release of glucocorticoids by the adrenal cortex / *page 558*

aerosol (AIR-oh-sol) suspension of small liquid droplets of drug, usually to cause bronchodilation / *page 483*

afterload pressure that must be overcome for the ventricles to eject blood from the heart / *page 292*

agonists (AG-on-ists) drugs that are capable of binding with receptors in order to cause a cellular response / *page 53*

akathisia (ACK-ah-THEE-shea) uncontrolled limb and body movements / *page 157*

alcohol intoxication (AL-ku-hol in-tak-su-KA-shun) a condition of altered mental and physical function resulting from drinking more alcoholic beverages within a time frame than the body can tolerate / *page 82*

aldosterone (al-DOH-stair-own) hormone secreted by the adrenal cortex that increases sodium reabsorption in the distal tubule of the kidney / *pages 280, 375*

alimentary canal (AL-uh-MEN-tare-ee) the hollow tube in the digestive system that starts in the mouth and includes the esophagus, stomach, small intestine, and large intestine / *page 507*

alkalosis (al-kah-LOH-sis) condition of having too much base; plasma pH above 7.45 / *page 379*

alkylation (AL-kill-AYE-shun) process by which certain chemicals attach to DNA and change its structure and function / *page 461*

allergic reaction a hyperresponse of body tissues to a foreign substance (allergen), in which patients experience uncomfortable and potentially serious symptoms, including difficulty breathing, pain, swelling, skin rash, and other unfavorable signs / *page 26*

allergic rhinitis (rye-NYE-tis) syndrome of sneezing, itchy throat, watery eyes, and nasal congestion resulting from exposure to antigens; also known as *hay fever* / *page 484*

alopecia (AL-oh-PEESH-ee-uh) hair loss / *page 461*

alpha receptor type of subreceptor found in the sympathetic nervous system / *page 96*

alternate-day therapy taking a drug every other day in order to minimize adverse effects / *page 394*

alveoli (al-VEE-oh-lie) dilated sacs at the end of the bronchial tree where gas exchange occurs / *page 481*

Alzheimer's disease (AD) (ALLZ-heye-mers) most common dementia, characterized by loss of memory, confusion, disorientation, and loss of judgment; hallucinations and delusions may also occur / *page 174*

amenorrhea (ah-men-oh-REE-ah) lack of normal menstrual periods / *page 578*

amides (AM-ides) type of chemical linkage found in some local anesthetics involving carbon, nitrogen, and oxygen (—NH—CO—) / *page 236*

analgesic (an-ul-JEE-zik) drug used to reduce or eliminate pain / *page 212*

anaphylaxis (ANN-a-fah-LAX-iss) an acute allergic response to an antigen that results in severe hypotension and may cause death if untreated / *pages 26, 355, 388*

androgens (AN-droh-jens) steroid sex hormones that promote the appearance of masculine characteristics / *page 571*

anemia (ah-NEE-mee-ah) shortage of functional red blood cells / *page 471*

anesthesia (ANN-ess-THEE-zee-uh) medical procedure involving drugs that block the transmission of nerve impulses and cause loss of sensation and/or consciousness / *page 233*

angina pectoris (an-JEYE-nuh PEK-tore-us) acute pain in the chest on physical or emotional exertion due to inadequate oxygen supply to the myocardium / *page 328*

angiotensin II (AN-geo-TEN-sin) chemical released in response to falling blood pressure that causes vasoconstriction and release of aldosterone / *page 279*

angiotensin-converting enzyme (ACE) (angeo-TEN-sin) enzyme responsible for converting angiotensin I to angiotensin II / *page 279*

anorexia (AN-oh-REX-ee-uh) loss of appetite / *page 509*

anorexiant (AN-oh-REX-ee-ant) drug used to suppress appetite / *page 522*

antacid (an-TASS-id) drug that neutralizes stomach acid / *page 515*

antagonism type of drug interaction in which one drug inhibits the effectiveness of another / *page 412*

antagonists (an-TAG-oh-nists) drugs that block the response of another drug / *page 53*

antepartum (an-teh-PART-um) prior to the onset of labor / *page 583*

antibiotic (ann-tie-bye-OT-ik) substance produced by a microorganism that inhibits or kills other microorganisms / *page 409*

antibody (ANN-tee-BOD-ee) protein produced by the body in response to an antigen; used interchangeably with the term *immunoglobulin* / *page 395*

anticholinergic a drug that inhibits the action of acetylcholine at its receptor / *page 97*

anticoagulant (ANT-eye-co-AG-you-lent) an agent that inhibits the formation of blood clots / *page 323*

antidepressants (AN-tee-dee-PRESS-ahnts) drugs used for the treatment of depression and a range of anxiety disorders, including panic, obsessive-compulsive, social phobia, and post-traumatic stress disorders / *pages 117, 132*

antidiuretic hormone (ADH) (ANT-eye-deye-your-ET-ik) hormone produced by the hypothalamus that stimulates the kidneys to conserve water / *page 272*

antiemetic (AN-tie-ee-MET-ik) drug that prevents vomiting / *page 520*

antiflatulent (an-tie-FLAT-u-lent) drug that reduces gas formation in the GI tract / *page 515*

antigen (ANN-tih-jen) a foreign organism or substance that induces the formation of antibodies / *pages 362, 394*

anti-infective (ann-tie-in-FEK-tive) general term for any medication effective against pathogens / *page 409*

antiretroviral (an-tie-RET-roh-veye-ral) type of drug effective against retroviruses / *page 442*

antitussive (anti-TUSS-ive) drug used to suppress cough / *page 492*

anxiety state of apprehension and autonomic nervous system activation resulting from exposure to a nonspecific or unknown cause / *page 113*

anxiolytics (ANG-zee-oh-LIT-iks) drugs that relieve anxiety / *page 115*

apothecary system (ah-POTH-eh-kare-ee) former system of weights and measures used by health care providers and pharmacists; replaced by the metric system / *page 29*

ASAP order means "as soon as possible"; a physician's order referring to the time frame that is often defined as less than 30 minutes / *page 28*

assessment appraisal of a patient's condition that involves gathering and interpreting data / *page 58*

asthma (AZ-muh) chronic inflammatory disease of the airways / *page 493*

astringent effect (ah-STRIN-jent) the shrinkage of swollen membranes or binding together of body surface material / *page 33*

atherosclerosis (ath-ur-oh-skler-OH-sis) a buildup of fatty substances and loss of elasticity of the arterial walls / *pages 251, 339*

atrioventricular (AV) node (ay-tree-oh-ven-TRIK-you-lur noad) mass of cardiac tissue that receives electrical impulses from the SA node and conveys them to the ventricles / *page 308*

atrioventricular bundle (ay-tree-oh-ven-TRIK-you-lur BUN-dul) specialized cardiac tissue that receives electrical impulses from the AV node and sends them to the bundle branches also known as the *bundle of His* / *page 308*

atrophy (AT-troh-fee) shrinkage or wasting away of a tissue / *page 561*

attention deficit disorder (ADD) consistent difficulty in focusing attention on a task for a sufficient length of time / *page 85*

attention deficit–hyperactivity disorder (ADHD) a disorder typically diagnosed in childhood and adolescence characterized by hyperactivity as well as attention, organization, and behavior control issues / *page 145*

aura (AUR-uh) sensory cue such as bright lights, smells, or tastes that precede a migraine / *page 225*

autoantibodies (AW-tow-ANN-tee-BAH-dees) proteins called rheumatoid factors released by B lymphocytes; these tear down the body's own tissue / *page 605*

automaticity (aw-toh-muh-TISS-uh-tee) ability of certain myocardial cells to spontaneously generate an action potential / *page 308*

B cell type of lymphocyte that is essential for the humoral immune response / *page 394*

bacteriocidal (bak-teer-ee-oh-SY-dall) substance that has ability to kill bacteria / *page 409*

bacteriostatic (bak-teer-ee-oh-STAT-ik) substance that can inhibit the growth of bacteria / *page 409*

barbiturates (bar-bi-CHUR-ates) class of drugs derived from barbituric acid; they act as CNS depressants and are used for their sedative and antiseizure effects / *page 122*

baroreceptors (BARE-oh-ree-sep-tours) nerves located in the walls of the atria, aortic arch, vena cava, and carotid sinus that sense changes in blood pressure / *page 271*

benign prostatic hypertrophy (BPH) (bee-NINE pros-TAT-ik hy-PURR-tro-fee) nonmalignant enlargement of the prostate gland / *page 586*

benign (bee-NINE) neither life-threatening nor fatal / *page 456*

benzodiazepines (ben-zo-di-AZ-eh-peenz) class of drugs used to treat anxiety and insomnia / *page 120*

beta-lactamase/penicillinase (bay-tuh-LAK-tam-ace/pen-uh-SILL-in-ace) enzyme present in certain bacteria that is able to inactivate many penicillins and some cephalosporins / *page 412*

beta-lactam ring (bay-tuh LAK-tam) chemical structure found in most penicillins and some cephalosporins / *page 412*

beta receptor type of subreceptor found in the sympathetic nervous system / *page 96*

bile acid (BEYE-ul) chemicals secreted in bile that aid in the digestion of fats / *page 257*

bioavailability (BEYE-oh-ah-VALE-ah-BILL-ih-TEE) the ability of a drug to reach its target cells and produce its effect / *page 18*

biologic response modifiers natural substances that are able to enhance or stimulate the immune system / *pages 399, 470*

biologics (beye-oh-LOJ-iks) chemical agents that produce biological responses within the body; they are synthesized by cells of the human body, animal cells, or microorganisms / *page 4*

biotransformation (BEYE-oh-trans-for-MAY-shun) the chemical conversion of drugs from one form to another that may result in increased or decreased activity / *page 49*

bipolar disorder (bi-PO-ler) a disorder characterized by extreme and opposite feelings, such as euphoria and depression or calmness and rage; also called *manic depression* / *page 142*

bisphosphonates (bis-FOSS-foh-nayts) family of drugs that block bone resorption by inhibiting osteoclast activity / *page 602*

black box warning warning label surrounded by a black border and issued by the FDA to emphasize the important and serious life-threatening risks associated with use of the drug / *page 118*

bone deposition the opposite of bone resorption; the process of depositing mineral components into bone / *page 595*

bone resorption (ree-SORP-shun) process of bone demineralization or the breaking down of bone into mineral components / *page 595*

booster an additional dose of a vaccine given months or years after the initial dose to increase the effectiveness of the vaccine / *page 396*

botanicals (boh-TAN-ik-uls) a plant extract used to treat or prevent illness / *page 67*

bradycardia (bray-dee-KAR-DEE-ah) a condition of slow heartbeat / *page 285*

bradykinin (bray-dee-KYE-nin) chemical mediator of pain released following tissue damage / *page 223*

breakthrough bleeding bleeding at abnormal times during the menstrual cycle / *page 578*

broad-spectrum antibiotic anti-infective that is effective against many different gram-positive and gram-negative organisms / *page 412*

bronchi (BRON-ky) primary passageway of the bronchial tree that contains smooth muscle / *page 481*

bronchioles (BRON-key-oles) very small bronchi / *page 481*

bronchoconstriction (BRON-koh-kun-STRIK-shun) decrease in diameter of the airway due to contraction of bronchial smooth muscle / *page 493*

bronchodilation (BRON-koh-dye-LAY-shun) increase in diameter of the airway due to relaxation of bronchial smooth muscle / *page 495*

bronchospasm (bron-koh-SPAZ-um) rapid constriction of the airways / *page 493*

buccal route (BUCK-ahl) the administration of medications by the cheek or mouth / *page 32*

bundle branches (BUN-dul BRAN-chez) electrical conduction pathway in the heart leading from the AV bundle and through the wall between the ventricles / *page 308*

calcifediol (kal-SIF-eh-DYE-ol) intermediate form of vitamin D / *page 595*

calcitonin (kal-sih-TOH-nin) treatment typically administered to women who cannot take estrogen or bisphosphonate therapy or for clients with Paget's disease / *page 602*

calcitriol (kal-si-TRY-ol) substance that is transformed in the kidneys during the second step of the conversion of vitamin D to its active form / *page 595*

calcium channel blocker (CCB) a drug that blocks the flow of calcium ions into myocardial cells / *page 275*

calcium ion channel (KAL-see-um) pathway in a plasma membrane through which calcium ions enter and leave / *page 309*

cancer (KAN-sir) malignant disease characterized by rapidly growing, invasive cells that spread to other regions of the body and eventually kill the host / *page 455*

capsid (CAP-sid) protein coat that surrounds a virus / *page 438*

carbonic anhydrase (kar-BON-ik an-HY-drase) enzyme that forms carbonic acid by combining carbon dioxide and water / *page 375*

carcinogen (kar-SIN-oh-jen) any physical, chemical, or biological factor that causes or promotes cancer / *page 456*

cardiac output amount of blood pumped by each ventricle in 1 minute / *page 270*

cardiogenic shock (kar-dee-oh-JEN-ik) type of shock caused when the heart is diseased such that it cannot maintain circulation to the tissues / *page 355*

cardioversion/defibrillation (kar-dee-oh-VER-shun/dee-fib-ree-LAY-shun) conversion of fibrillation to a normal heart rhythm / *page 310*

cathartic (kah-THAR-tik) drug that causes complete evacuation of the bowel / *page 516*

cerebrovascular accident/stroke (sir-ree-bro-VASK-u-lur) an acute condition of a blood clot or bleeding in a vessel in the brain / *page 349*

C fibers nerves that transmit dull, poorly localized pain / *page 212*

chemical name strict chemical nomenclature used for naming drugs established by the International Union of Pure and Applied Chemistry (IUPAC) / *page 16*

chemoprophylaxis (kee-moh-pro-fill-AX-is) use of a drug to prevent an infection / *page 411*

chemotherapy drug treatment of cancer / *page 457*

cholecalciferol (KOH-lee-kal-SIF-er-ol) inactive form of vitamin D / *page 595*

cholinergic (kol-in-UR-jik) a term relating to nerves that release acetylcholine / *page 96*

cholinergic drug another name for a parasympathomimetic drug / *page 97*

cholinergic blocker a drug that blocks the actions of the parasympathetic nervous system / *page 97*

chronic bronchitis (KRON-ik bron-KEYE-tis) chronic disease of the lungs characterized by excess mucus production and inflammation / *page 500*

clinical pharmacology an area of medicine devoted to the evaluation of drugs used for human therapeutic benefit / *page 8*

closed-angle glaucoma (glaw-KOH-mah) called acute glaucoma, this type of glaucoma is caused by the iris blocking trabecular meshwork, hindering outflow of aqueous fluid / *page 633*

closed comedones (KOME-eh-dones) commonly called whiteheads, this type of acne develops just beneath the surface of the skin / *page 622*

clotting factors substances contributing to the process of blood clotting / *page 321*

CNS depressants (dee-PRESS-ahnts) drugs that lower neuronal activity within the CNS / *page 117*

coagulation (co-ag-you-LAY-shun) the process of blood clotting / *page 321*

coagulation cascade (cass-KADE) a complex series of steps by which blood flow stops / *page 321*

colloids (KO-loyds) type of IV fluid replacement solution consisting of large protein molecules that are unable to cross membranes / *page 359*

combination drugs drug product with more than one active generic ingredient / *page 17*

complementary and alternative medicine (CAM) general term for treatments that consider the health of the whole person and promote disease prevention / *page 66*

compliance (kom-PLY-ans) taking a medication in the way it was prescribed by the practitioner; in the case of OTC drugs, following the instructions found on the label / *page 26*

constipation (kon-stah-PAY-shun) infrequent passage of abnormally hard and dry stools / *page 516*

contractility (kon-trak-TILL-eh-tee) the strength by which the myocardial fibers contract / *page 292*

controlled substance in the United States, a drug restricted by the Comprehensive Drug Abuse Prevention and Control Act. In Canada, a drug subject to guidelines outlined in Part III, Schedule G, of the Canadian Food and Drugs Act / *page 18*

convulsions (kon-VULL-shuns) uncontrolled muscle contractions or spasms that occur in the face, torso, arms, or legs / *page 192*

coronary arterial bypass graft (CABG) surgery surgical procedure performed to restore blood flow to the myocardium by using a section of the saphenous vein or internal mammary artery to go around the obstructed coronary artery / *page 340*

coronary arteries (KOR-un-air-ee AR-tur-ees) vessels that bring oxygen and nutrients to the myocardium / *page 338*

corpus cavernosum (KORP-us kav-ver-NOH-sum) tissue in the penis that fills with blood during an erection / *page 586*

cretinism (KREE-ten-izm) dwarfism and mental retardation caused by lack of thyroid hormone during infancy / *page 555*

Crohn's disease (KROHNS) chronic inflammatory bowel disease affecting the ileum and sometimes the colon / *page 510*

cross-tolerance (krause TOL-er-ans) the process of adapting to a new drug as a result of having already been exposed to a related drug / *page 80*

crystalloids (KRIS-tuh-loyds) type of IV fluid replacement solution that resembles blood plasma and is capable of crossing membranes / *page 359*

culture and sensitivity testing laboratory test used to identify bacteria and to determine which antibiotic is most effective / *page 412*

Cushing's syndrome (KUSH-ings) condition caused by excessive corticosteroid secretion by the adrenal glands or by overdosage with corticosteroid medication / *pages 394, 561*

cyclooxygenase (COX) (sye-klo-OK-sah-jen-ays) key enzyme in the prostaglandin metabolic pathway that is blocked by aspirin and other NSAIDs / *pages 220, 390*

cycloplegia (sy-kloh-PLEE-jee-ah) blurred vision / *page 635*

cycloplegic drug (sy-kloh-PLEE-jik) drugs that relax or temporarily paralyze ciliary muscles / *page 639*

cytokines (SYE-toh-kines) chemicals produced by white blood cells, such as interleukins, leukotrienes, interferon, and tumor necrosis factor, that guide the immune response / *page 395*

cytotoxic T cell type of lymphocyte that directly attacks and destroys antigens / *page 395*

defecation (def-ah-KAY-shun) evacuation of the colon; bowel movement / *page 516*

dementia (dee-MEN-she-ah) degenerative disorder characterized by progressive memory loss, confusion, and the inability to think or communicate effectively / *page 175*

depolarization (dee-po-lur-eye-ZAY-shun) condition in which the plasma membrane charge is changed such that the inside is made less negative / *page 309*

dermatitis (dur-mah-TIE-tiss) inflammatory condition of the skin characterized by itching and scaling / *page 623*

dermatophytic (der-MAT-oh-FIT-ik) superficial fungal infection / *page 435*

designer drugs (de-ZEYE-ner drugs) drugs that are produced in a laboratory and are intended to mimic the effects of other psychoactive controlled substances / *page 77*

diabetes insipidus (die-uh-BEE-tees in-SIP-uh-dus) excessive urination due to lack of secretion of antidiuretic hormone / *page 564*

diabetes mellitus, type 1 (die-uh-BEE-tees MEL-uh-tiss) disease characterized by lack of secretion of insulin by the pancreas that usually begins in the early teens / *page 547*

diabetes mellitus, type 2 disease characterized by insufficient secretion of insulin by the pancreas or by lack of sensitivity of insulin receptors that usually begins in middle age / *page 549*

diarrhea abnormal frequency and liquidity of bowel movements / *page 518*

diastolic pressure (DEYE-ah-stall-ik) blood pressure during the relaxation phase of heart activity / *page 269*

dietary fiber substance neither digested nor absorbed that contributes to the fecal mass / *page 516*

dietary supplement a nondrug substance regulated by the DSHEA / *page 67*

Dietary Supplement and Nonprescription Drug Consumer Protection Act law that requires companies that market herbal and dietary supplements to include their address and phone number on the product labels so consumers can report adverse events / *page 73*

Dietary Supplement Health and Education Act (DSHEA) of 1994 primary law in the United States regulating herb and dietary supplements / *page 72*

digestion (dye-JES-chun) process by which the body breaks down ingested food into small molecules that can be absorbed / *page 507*

disease-modifying antirheumatic (ANTY-roo-MATIK) drugs (DMARDs) agents that reduce destruction of the joints and progression of rheumatoid arthritis / *page 605*

distribution (dis-tree-BU-shun) the process of transporting drugs through the body / *page 49*

diuretic (deye-your-ET-ik) drug that increases urine flow / *pages 271, 371*

dry powder inhaler (DPI) device used to convert a solid drug to a fine powder for the purpose of inhalation / *page 483*

dwarfism below normal height caused by a deficiency in thyroid hormone or growth hormone / *page 564*

dysentery (DISS-en-tare-ee) severe diarrhea that may include bleeding / *page 448*

dysfunctional uterine bleeding hemorrhage that occurs at abnormal times or in abnormal quantity during the menstrual cycle / *page 578*

dyspnea (DISP-nee-uh) shortness of breath / *page 493*

dysrhythmia (diss-RITH-mee-uh) abnormality in cardiac rhythm / *page 306*

dysthymic disorder (dis-THEYE-mick) less severe type of mood disorder that may prevent a person from feeling well or functioning normally / *page 131*

dystonia (diss-TONE-ee-ah) muscle spasm characterized by rigidity and abnormal, occasionally painful, movements or postures / *page 184*

eclampsia (ee-KLAMP-see-uh) condition in which seizures and/or a coma develop in a patient with preeclampsia / *page 194*

ectopic foci/pacemakers (ek-TOP-ik FO-si) cardiac tissue outside the normal cardiac conduction pathway that generates action potentials / *page 308*

eczema (ECK-zih-mah) also called *atopic* dermatitis, a skin disorder with unexplained symptoms of inflammation, itching, and scaling / *page 623*

efficacy (EFF-ik-ah-see) the effectiveness of a drug in producing a more intense response as its concentration is increased / *page 53*

electrocardiogram (ECG) (e-lek-tro-KAR-dee-oh-gram) device that records the electrical activity of the heart / *page 308*

electrolytes (ee-LEK-troh-lites) charged substances in the blood, such as sodium, potassium, calcium, chloride, and phosphate / *pages 274, 377*

embolus (EM-boh-luss) a blood clot carried in the bloodstream / *page 324*

emesis (EM-eh-sis) vomiting / *page 520*

emetic (ee-MET-ik) drug used to induce vomiting / *page 520*

emollients (ee-MOLE-ee-ents) agents used to soothe and soften the skin / *page 625*

emphysema (em-fuss-EE-muh) terminal lung disease characterized by dilation of the alveoli / *page 501*

endogenous opioids (en-DAHJ-en-nuss O-pee-oyds) chemicals produced naturally within the body that decrease or eliminate pain; they closely resemble the actions of morphine / *page 212*

endometrium (en-doh-MEE-tree-um) inner lining of the uterus / *page 571*

enteral nutrition treatment of undernutrition by the oral route or through a feeding tube / *page 537*

enteral route (EN-tur-ul) the major route by which drugs enter the body through the digestive tract / *page 30*

enteric coated (in-TARE-ik) hard, waxy coating that enables drugs to resist the acidity of the stomach; enables drugs to dissolve in the small intestine / *page 30*

enterohepatic recirculation (EN-ter-oh-HEE-pah-tik) recycling of drugs and other substances by the circulation of bile through the intestine and liver / *page 51*

epilepsy (EPP-ih-lepp-see) disorder of the CNS characterized by seizures and/or convulsions / *page 192*

erythema (ear-ih-THEE-mah) redness associated with skin irritation / *page 616*

erythropoietin (ee-rith-ro-po-EE-tin) hormone secreted by the kidney that stimulates red blood cell production / *page 371*

esters (ES-turs) type of chemical linkage found in some local anesthetics involving carbon and oxygen (—CO—O—) / *page 236*

estrogen (ES-troh-jen) class of steroid sex hormones produced by the ovary / *page 570*

etiologies (e-tee-OL-o-gees) causes of the patient's disease or condition / *page 59*

evaluation criteria objective assessment of the effectiveness and impact of interventions / *page 60*

evaluation phase part of the nursing process that provides an objective assessment of the effectiveness of the interventions/ *page 62*

excretion (eks-KREE-shun) the process of removing substances from the body / *page 51*

expectorant (eks-PEK-tor-ent) drug used to increase bronchial secretions / *page 493*

external otitis (oh-TYE-tiss) commonly called swimmer's ear, this is inflammation of the outer ear / *page 639*

extrapyramidal symptoms (EPS) (peh-RAM-ed-el) symptoms where muscles become very rigid because of overmedication with antipsychotics or by lack of dopamine function in the corpus striatum / *page 157*

false neurotransmitter (NYUR-oh-TRANS-mitt-ur) chemical that simulates a natural neurotransmitter but does not produce the same physiologic effect / *page 285*

febrile seizures abnormal state of neuronal discharge resulting from high fever / *page 193*

fibrillation (fi-bruh-LAY-shun) type of dysrhythmia in which the chambers beat in a highly disorganized manner / *page 307*

fibrin (FEYE-brin) an insoluble protein formed from fibrinogen by the action of thrombin in the blood-clotting process / *page 321*

fibrinogen (feye-BRIN-oh-jen) blood protein converted to fibrin by the action of thrombin in the blood-clotting process / *page 321*

fibrinolysis (feye-brin-OL-oh-sis) removal of a blood clot / *page 323*

filtrate (FIL-trate) fluid in the nephron that is filtered at Bowman's capsule / *page 368*

first-pass effect a mechanism whereby drugs are absorbed across the intestinal wall and enter into blood vessels, known as the hepatic portal circulation, which carries blood directly to the liver / *page 50*

folic acid (FOH-lik) B vitamin that is a coenzyme in protein and nucleic acid metabolism; also known as *folate* / *page 466*

follicle-stimulating hormone (FSH) hormone secreted by the pituitary gland that regulates sperm or egg production / *page 571*

follicular cells (fo-LIK-yu-lur) cells in the thyroid gland that secrete thyroid hormone / *page 555*

formularies (FOR-mew-LEH-reez) lists of drugs and drug recipes commonly used by pharmacists / *page 5*

fungi (FUN-jeye) kingdom of organisms that includes mushrooms, yeasts, and molds / *page 434*

ganglia (GANG-lee-ah) collections of neuron cell bodies located outside the CNS / *page 96*

gastroesophageal reflux disease (GERD) (GAS-troh-ee-SOF-ah-JEEL REE-flux) the regurgitation of stomach contents into the esophagus / *page 510*

general anesthesia medical procedure that produces loss of sensation throughout the entire body and unconsciousness / *page 233*

generalized anxiety disorder (GAD) difficult-to-control, excessive anxiety that lasts 6 months or more / *page 113*

generalized seizures seizures that travel throughout the entire brain on both sides / *page 194*

generic name (je-NARE-ik) nonproprietary name of a drug assigned by the government / *page 17*

glioma (glee-OH-muh) malignant tumor of the brain / *page 456*

glucocorticoid (glu-ko-KORT-ik-oyd) type of hormone secreted by the outer portion of the adrenal gland that includes cortisol / *page 558*

glycoprotein IIb/IIIa (GLEYE-koh-proh-teen) enzyme responsible for platelet aggregation / *page 328*

goal an objective that the patient or nurse seeks to attain or achieve / *page 60*

gout (GOWT) metabolic disorder characterized by the accumulation of uric acid in the bloodstream or joint cavities / *page 607*

Graves' disease syndrome caused by hypersecretion of thyroid hormone / *page 556*

H^+, K^+-ATPase enzyme responsible for pumping acid onto the mucosal surface of the stomach / *page 510*

H_1-receptor blocker drug that blocks the effects of histamine in smooth muscle in the bronchial tree / *page 486*

H_2-receptor blocker drug that inhibits the effects of histamine at its receptors in the GI tract / *page 511*

half-life ($t_{1/2}$) the length of time required for a drug to decrease its concentration in the plasma by one half of the original amount / *page 52*

heart failure (HF) disease in which the heart muscle cannot contract with sufficient force to meet the body's metabolic needs / *page 291*

***Helicobacter pylori* (hee-lick-oh-BAK-tur py-LOR-eye)** bacterium associated with a large percentage of peptic ulcer disease / *page 509*

helminth (HELL-minth) type of flat, round, or segmented worm / *page 448*

helper T cell type of lymphocyte that coordinates both the humoral and cell-mediated immune responses and that is the target of the human immunodeficiency virus / *page 395*

hemoglobin (HEE-moh-glow-bin) substance in a red blood cell that contains iron and transports oxygen and CO_2 / *page 534*

hemorrhagic stroke (hee-moh-RAJ-ik) type of stroke caused by bleeding from a blood vessel in the brain / *page 350*

hemostasis (hee-moh-STAY-sis) the slowing or stopping of blood flow / *page 321*

hemostatics (hee-moh-STAT-iks) drugs used to prevent and treat excessive bleeding from surgical sites / *page 324*

herbs plants with a soft stem that is used in healing or as a seasoning / *page 67*

high-density lipoprotein (HDL) lipid-carrying particle in the blood that contains high amounts of protein and lower amounts of cholesterol; considered to be "good" cholesterol / *page 253*

highly active antiretroviral therapy (HAART) type of drug therapy for HIV infection that includes high doses of multiple medications that are given together / *page 442*

histamine (HISS-tuh-meen) chemical released by mast cells in response to an antigen; causes dilation of blood vessels, smooth muscle constriction, tissue swelling, and itching / *page 388*

HMG-CoA reductase (ree-DUCK-tase) primary enzyme in the biochemical pathway for the synthesis of cholesterol / *page 256*

hormones chemicals secreted by endocrine glands that act as chemical messengers to affect homeostasis / *page 543*

host an organism that is being infected by a microbe / *pages 441, 543*

host flora (host FLOR-uh) normal microorganisms found in or on a patient / *page 412*

household system older system of measurement involving teaspoons, tablespoons, cups, drops, pounds, etc. / *page 29*

humoral immunity (HYOU-mor-ul eh-MEWN-uh-tee) a specific body defense mechanism involving the production and release of antibodies / *page 394*

hypercholesterolemia (HEYE-purr-koh-LESS-tur-ol-EEM-ee-uh) high levels of cholesterol in the blood / *page 253*

hyperglycemia (heye-pur-gli-SEEM-ee-uh) abnormally high level of glucose in the blood / *page 545*

hyperkalemia (heye-purr-kah-LEE-mee-ah) high potassium levels in the blood / *pages 275, 374*

hyperlipidemia (HEYE-purr-LIP-id-EEM-ee-uh) excess amounts of lipids in the blood / *page 253*

hypernatremia high sodium level in the blood / *page 378*

hypertension (heye-purr-TEN-shun) high blood pressure / *page 267*

hypervitaminosis excess intake of vitamins / *page 530*

hypoglycemia (heye-po-gli-SEEM-ee-uh) abnormally low level of glucose in the blood / *page 545*

hypogonadism (hy-poh-GO-nad-izm) below normal secretion of the steroid sex hormones / *page 583*

hypokalemia (heye-poh-kah-LEE-mee-ah) low potassium levels in the blood / *pages 275, 372*

hyponatremia (hy-po-nay-TREE-mee-uh) low levels of sodium in the blood / *page 378*

hypothalamus (hi-po-THAL-ih-mus) region of the brain that affects emotions and drives and that secretes releasing factors that affect the pituitary gland / *page 545*

hypovolemic shock (high-poh-voh-LEEM-ik) type of shock caused by loss of fluids such as occurs during hemorrhaging, extensive burns, or severe vomiting or diarrhea / *page 355*

hysterectomy (hiss-ter-EK-toh-mee) surgical removal of the uterus / *page 578*

immunoglobulin (Ig) (ih-MEW-noh-GLOB-you-lin) protein produced by the body in response to an antigen; used interchangeably with the term *antibody* / *page 395*

immunosuppressant (ih-MEW-noh-suh-PRESS-ent) any drug, chemical, or physical agent that lowers the natural immune defense mechanisms of the body / *page 400*

implementation phase part of the nursing process during which the nurse carries out activities that assist in accomplishing established goals / *page 61*

impotence (IM-poh-tense) inability to obtain or sustain an erection; also called erectile dysfunction / *page 585*

incretin (in-KREE-ten) enhancers a group of drugs that boost the action of gastrointestinal hormones, which stimulate the pancreas to release insulin after a meal before blood glucose levels can become too elevated / *page 553*

inflammation (IN-flah-MAY-shun) nonspecific body defense that occurs in response to an injury or antigen / *page 388*

influenza (in-flew-EN-zah) common viral infection of the respiratory system; often called *flu* / *page 447*

inotropic drug (eye-noh-TROW-pik) medication that changes the force of contraction of the heart / *page 360*

inotropic effect (in-oh-TRO-pik) change in the strength or contractility of the heart / *page 292*

insomnia (in-SOM-nee-uh) the inability to fall asleep or stay asleep / *page 116*

international normalized ratio (INR) laboratory value used to monitor the degree of blood anticoagulation during warfarin therapy / *page 327*

intervention action that produces an effect or that is intended to alter the course of a disease or condition / *page 59*

intracellular parasite an infectious microbe that lives inside host cells / *page 441*

intradermal (ID) route (IN-trah-DERM-ul) method of parenteral drug delivery in which drugs are injected into the dermis of the skin / *page 37*

intramuscular (IM) route (IN-trah-musk-u-lar) method of parenteral drug delivery in which drugs are injected into layers of muscle beneath the skin / *page 41*

intravenous (IV) route (IN-trah-VEE-nus) method of parenteral drug delivery in which drugs are injected into the venous circulation / *page 41*

intrinsic factor chemical secreted by the stomach that is required for absorption of vitamin B_{12} / *page 532*

islets of Langerhans (EYE-lits of LANG-gur-hans) clusters of cells in the pancreas responsible for the secretion of insulin and glucagon; also called the *pancreatic islets* / *page 545*

keratinization (keh-RAT-en-eye-zay-shun) development of the stratum corneum or horny layer of epithelial tissue / *page 621*

keratolytic agents (keh-RAT-oh-lih-tik) drugs used to promote shedding of old skin / *page 623*

ketoacids (KEY-to-ass-ids) waste products of fat metabolism that lower the pH of the blood / *page 548*

lecithin (LESS-ih-thin) phospholipid that is an important part of cell membranes / *page 252*

leukemia (lew-KEE-mee-ah) cancer of the blood characterized by overproduction of white blood cells / *page 456*

libido (lih-BEE-do) interest in sexual activity / *page 584*

limbic system (LIM-bik) area in the brain responsible for emotion, learning, memory, motivation, and mood / *page 114*

lipoma (lip-OH-mah) benign tumor of fat tissue / *page 456*

lipoprotein (LIP-oh-PROH-teen) substance carrying lipids in the bloodstream / *page 253*

liposomes (LIP-oh-sohms) small sacs of lipids designed to carry drugs inside them / *page 456*

local anesthesia loss of sensation to a relatively small part of the body without loss of consciousness / *page 233*

low molecular weight heparins (LMWHs) heparin-like drugs that inhibit blood clotting / *page 325*

low-density lipoprotein (LDL) lipid-carrying particle that contains lower amounts of protein and high amounts of cholesterol; considered to be "bad" cholesterol / *page 253*

lumen (LOO-men) the cavity or channel of a hollow tube such as a blood vessel / *page 271*

lutinizing hormone (LH) (LEW-ten-iz-ing) hormone secreted by the pituitary gland that triggers ovulation in the female and stimulates sperm production in the male / *page 571*

lymphocyte (LIM-foh-site) type of white blood cell formed in lymphoid tissue / *page 394*

lymphoma (lim-FOH-mah) cancer of lymphatic tissue / *page 456*

major depressive disorder a disorder characterized by at least five symptoms of depression / *page 131*

major mineral (macromineral) inorganic compound needed by the body in amounts of 100 mg or more daily / *page 532*

malaria (mah-LARE-ee-ah) tropical disease characterized by severe fever and chills; caused by the protozoan *Plasmodium* / *page 448*

malignant (mah-LIG-nent) life threatening or fatal / *page 456*

mast cell connective tissue cell located in tissue spaces that releases histamine following injury / *page 388*

mastoiditis (mass-toy-DYE-tuss) inflammation of the mastoid sinus / *page 639*

mechanism of action how a drug exerts its effects / *page 15*

menopause (MEN-oh-paws) time when females stop secreting estrogen and menstrual cycles cease / *page 576*

menorrhea (men-oh-REE-uh) prolonged or excessive menstruation / *page 578*

metabolism (meh-TAHB-oh-liz-ehm) the sum total of all chemical reactions in the body or an organ (for example, the liver) / *page 49*

metastasis (mah-TAS-tah-sis) travel of cancer cells from their original site to a distant tissue / *page 456*

metered-dose inhaler (MDIs) device used to deliver a precise amount of drug to the respiratory system / *page 483*

metric system the most common system of measurement; involves kilograms (kg), grams (g), milligrams (mg), or micrograms (mcg), etc. / *page 29*

migraine (MYE-grayne) severe headache preceded by auras that may include nausea and vomiting / *page 225*

mineralocorticoid (min-ur-al-oh-KORT-ik-oyd) hormone involved in the regulation of fluid and electrolytes by its effects in the kidney / *page 558*

miosis (my-OH-sis) constriction of the pupil / *page 634*

miotics (my-AH-tiks) drugs that cause pupil constriction / *page 633*

monoamine oxidase inhibitors (MAOIs) (mon-oh-AHM-een OK-se-daze) drugs inhibiting monoamine oxidase, an enzyme that terminates the actions of neurotransmitters such as dopamine, norepinephrine, epinephrine, and serotonin / *page 140*

mood disorder a disorder involving a change in behavior, such as major depressive disorder or bipolar disorder / *page 130*

mood stabilizers drugs that level mood to treat bipolar disorder and mania / *page 143*

mucolytic drug used to loosen thick mucus / *page 483*

multiple sclerosis (MS) (skle-ROH-sis) autoimmune disorder of the central nervous system; a condition in which antibodies slowly destroy tissues in the brain and spinal cord / *page 178*

muscarinic (MUS-kah-RIN-ik) type of cholinergic receptor found in smooth muscle, cardiac muscle, and glands / *page 96*

mutations (myou-TAY-shuns) permanent, inheritable changes to DNA / *page 409*

mycoses (my-KOH-sees) diseases caused by fungi/ *page 434*

mydriasis (mih-DRY-uh-siss) dilation of the pupil / *page 634*

mydriatic drugs (my-DRY-at-tik) drugs that cause pupil dilation / *page 639*

myocardial infarction (MI) (meye-oh-KAR-dee-ul in-FARK-shun) medical emergency in which a blood clot blocks a portion of a coronary artery / *page 346*

myocardial ischemia (meye-oh-KAR-dee-ul ik-SKEE-mee-uh) condition in which there is a lack of blood supply to the myocardium due to a constriction or obstruction of a blood vessel / *page 339*

myxedema (mix-uh-DEEM-uh) condition caused by insufficient secretion of thyroid hormone / *page 556*

narcolepsy (NAR-koh-lep-see) condition characterized by uncontrolled daytime sleepiness / *page 85*

narcotic (nar-KOT-ik) natural or synthetic drug related to morphine; may be used as a broader legal term referring to hallucinogens (LSD), CNS stimulants, marijuana, and other illegal drugs / *page 212*

narrow-spectrum antibiotic anti-infective that is effective against only one or a small number of organisms / *page 412*

natriuretic peptide (hBNP) (na-tree-ur-ET-ik) hormone that increases the urinary excretion of sodium and dilates blood vessels / *page 302*

natural alternative therapies herbs, natural extracts, vitamins, minerals, or dietary supplements / *page 4*

nebulizer (NEB-you-lyes-ur) device used to convert liquid drugs into a fine mist for the purpose of inhalation / *page 483*

negative symptoms symptoms that *subtract from* normal behavior; signs that are used to assist with the diagnosis of schizophrenia / *page 154*

neoplasm (NEE-oh-PLAZ-um) same as *tumor;* an abnormal swelling or mass / *page 456*

nephron (NEF-ron) functional unit of the kidney / *page 368*

nephrotoxicity (NEF-row-toks-ISS-ih-tee) an adverse effect on the kidneys / *page 420*

neurogenic shock (nyoor-oh-JEN-ik) type of shock resulting from brain or spinal cord injury / *page 355*

neuroleptic malignant syndrome (NMS) (noo-roh-LEP-tik) a potentially fatal condition caused by some antipsychotic medications; symptoms include an extremely high body temperature, drowsiness, changing blood pressure, irregular heartbeat, and muscle rigidity / *page 158*

neuroleptics (noo-roh-LEP-ticks) drugs used to treat "nervous-type" conditions such as psychoses / *page 156*

neuromuscular blocking agents (NEWR-oh-musc-you-lahr) drugs that bind to acetylcholine receptors, preventing contraction of skeletal muscle / *page 186*

nicotinic (NIK-oh-TIN-ik) type of cholinergic receptor found in ganglia of both the sympathetic and parasympathetic nervous systems / *page 96*

nitrogen mustards class of chemicals that are alkylating agents / *page 461*

nociceptor (no-si-SEPP-ter) receptor connected with nerves that receive and transmit pain signals to the spinal cord and brain / *page 210*

norepinephrine (nor-EH-pin-NEF-rin) primary neurotransmitter in the sympathetic nervous system / *page 96*

nosocomial infections (noh-soh-KOH-mee-ul) infections acquired in a health care setting such as a hospital, physician's office, or nursing home / *page 410*

nursing diagnosis clinically based judgment about the patient and his or her response to health and illness / *page 59*

nursing process five-part decision-making system that includes assessment, nursing diagnosis, planning, implementation, and evaluation / *page 58*

obsessive-compulsive disorder (OCD) anxiety characterized by recurrent, intrusive thoughts or repetitive behaviors that interfere with normal activities or relationships / *page 114*

oligomenorrhea (ol-ego-men-oh-REE-uh) infrequent menstruation / *page 578*

open-angle glaucoma (glaw-KOH-mah) also called chronic simple glaucoma, this type of glaucoma is caused by congestion in trabecular meshwork, hindering outflow of aqueous fluid / *page 633*

open comedones type of acne in which sebum has plugged the oil gland; commonly called blackheads / *page 622*

opiate (OH-pee-aht) natural substance extracted from the poppy plant / *page 212*

opioid (OH-pee-oyd) natural or synthetic morphine-like substance obtained from the unripe seeds of the poppy plant / *pages 77, 212*

orthostatic hypotension (or-tho-STAT-ik) fall in blood pressure that occurs when someone changes position from recumbent to upright / *page 285*

osteoarthritis (OA) (OSS-tee-oh-are-THRYE-tis) disorder characterized by degeneration of joints such as the fingers, spine, hips, and knees / *page 605*

osteomalacia (OSS-tee-oh-muh-LAY-shee-uh) rickets in children; disease characterized by softening of the bones without alteration of basic bone structure / *page 598*

osteoporosis (OSS-tee-oh-poh-ROH-sis) condition in which bones become brittle and susceptible to fracture / *page 600*

otitis media (oh-TYE-tuss MEE-dee-ah) inflammation of the middle ear / *page 639*

ototoxicity (OH-toh-toks-ISS-ih-tee) an adverse effect on hearing / *page 420*

outcome objective measures of goals / *page 60*

ovulation (ov-you-LAY-shun) release of an egg by the ovary / *page 571*

oxytocin (ox-ee-TOH-sin) hormone secreted by the pituitary gland that stimulates uterine contractions and milk ejection / *page 582*

Paget's disease (PAH-jets) disorder characterized by weak, enlarged, and abnormal bones / *page 604*

palliation (PAL-ee-AYE-shun) form of chemotherapy intended to alleviate symptoms rather than cure the disease / *page 458*

pancreatic insufficiency condition in which the pancreas is not secreting sufficient amounts of digestive enzymes, resulting in malabsorption syndromes / *page 523*

panic disorder anxiety characterized by intense feelings of immediate apprehension, fearfulness, terror, or impending doom / *page 113*

papules (PAP-yools) inflammatory bumps without pus that swell, thicken, and become painful / *page 622*

parafollicular cells (par-uh-fo-LIK-u-lur) cells in the thyroid gland that secrete calcitonin / *page 555*

parasympathetic nervous system (PAIR-ah-SIM-pah-THET-ik) portion of the autonomic system that is active during periods of rest and digestion / *page 93*

parasympathomimetics (PAIR-ah-SIM-path-oh-mah-MET-iks) drugs that mimic the actions of the parasympathetic nervous system / *page 97*

parenteral route (pah-REN-tur-ul) the major route by which drugs enter the body other than the enteral or topical route / *page 36*

parkinsonism degenerative disorder of the nervous system caused by a deficiency of the brain neurotransmitter dopamine; this deficiency results in disturbances of muscle movement / *pages 157, 171*

partial (focal) seizures seizures that start on one side of the brain and travel a short distance before stopping / *page 194*

passive immunity administration of antibodies; provides short-term immunity / *page 396*

pathogen (PATH-oh-jen) organism that is capable of causing disease / *page 407*

pathogenicity (path-oh-jen-ISS-ih-tee) ability of an organism to cause disease in humans / *page 407*

pathophysiology (PATH-oh-fiz-ee-OL-oh-jee) the study of diseases and the functional changes occurring in the body as a result of diseases / *page 3*

patient-controlled analgesia (PCA) (patient-controlled an-ul-JEE-ziah) use of an infusion pump to deliver a prescribed amount of pain relief medication over a designated time / *page 216*

pediculicides (puh-DIK-you-lih-sides) medications that kill lice / *page 619*

peptic ulcer erosion of the mucosa in the alimentary canal, most commonly in the stomach and duodenum / *page 508*

percutaneous transluminal coronary angioplasty (PTCA) (per-cue-TAIN-ee-us trans-LOO-min-ul KOR-un-air-ee ANN-gee-oh-plas-tee) procedure by which a balloon-shaped catheter is used to compress fatty plaque against an arterial wall for the purpose of restoring normal blood flow / *page 340*

perfusion (purr-FEW-shun) blood flow through a tissue or organ / *page 482*

peripheral edema (purr-IF-ur-ul eh-DEE-mah) swelling in the limbs, particularly the feet and ankles, due to an accumulation of interstitial fluid / *page 292*

peripheral resistance (per-IF-ur-ul) the amount of friction encountered by blood as it travels through the vessels / *page 271*

peristalsis (pair-ih-STAL-sis) involuntary wave-like contraction that occurs in the alimentary canal / *page 507*

pernicious (megaloblastic) anemia (pur-NISH-us ah-NEE-mee-ah) type of anemia usually caused by lack of secretion of intrinsic factor / *page 531*

pH a measure of the acidity or alkalinity of a solution / *page 379*

pharmaceutics (far-mah-SOO-tiks) the science of preparing and dispensing drugs / *page 5*

pharmacodynamics (FAR-mah-koh-deye-NAM-iks) the study of how the body responds to drugs and natural substances / *page 52*

pharmacokinetics (FAR-mah-koh-kee-NET) the study of what the body does to drugs / *page 48*

pharmacologic classification (FAR-mah-koh-LOJ-ik) method for organizing drugs on the basis of their mechanism of action (how they work pharmacologically) / *page 15*

pharmacology (far-mah-KOL-oh-jee) the study of medicines; the discipline pertaining to how drugs improve the health of the human body / *page 3*

pharmacopoeia (far-mah-KOH-pee-ah) medical reference summary indicating standards of drug purity, strength, and directions for synthesis / *page 5*

pharmacotherapeutics (far-mah-koh-THER-ah-PEW-tiks) treatment of diseases by the use of drugs / *page 4*

phobias (FO-bee-ahs) fearful feelings attached to situations or objects / *page 114*

phosphodiesterase (fos-fo-die-ES-tur-ase) enzyme in muscle cells that cleaves phosphodiester bonds; its inhibition increases myocardial contractility / *page 302*

phospholipid (FOS-foh-LIP-id) type of lipid that contains two fatty acids, a phosphate group, and a chemical backbone of glycerol / *page 252*

photosensitivity condition that occurs when the skin is very sensitive to sunlight / *page 417*

physical dependence (FI-zi-kul dee-PEN-dens) the condition of experiencing unpleasant withdrawal symptoms when a substance is discontinued / *page 79*

pituitary gland (pit-TOO-it-air-ee) endocrine gland in the brain responsible for controlling many other endocrine glands / *page 545*

planning phase stage of the nursing process that links strategies or interventions to established goals and outcomes / *page 60*

plaque (PLAK) fatty material that builds up in the lining of blood vessels and may lead to hypertension, stroke, myocardial infarction, or angina / *pages 252, 339*

plasma cell type of cell derived from B cells that produces antibodies / *page 395*

plasmid (PLAZ-mid) small piece of circular DNA found in some bacteria that is able to transfer resistance from one bacterium to another / *page 410*

plasmin (PLAZ-min) enzyme formed from plasminogen that dissolves blood clots / *page 323*

plasminogen (plaz-MIN-oh-jen) protein that prevents fibrin clot formation / *page 323*

polarized (POLE-uh-rized) condition in which the inside of a cell is more negatively charged than the outside of the cell / *page 309*

positive symptoms symptoms that *add on to* normal behavior; signs that are used to assist with the diagnosis of schizophrenia / *page 154*

postpartum (post-PART-um) occurring after childbirth / *page 583*

post-traumatic stress disorder (PTSD) anxiety characterized by a sense of helplessness and the reexperiencing of a traumatic event, for example, war, physical or sexual abuse, natural disasters, or murder / *page 114*

potassium ion channel (po-TASS-ee-um) pathway in a plasma membrane through which potassium ions enter and leave / *page 309*

potency (POH-ten-see) the power or strength of a drug at a specified concentration or dose / *page 53*

pre-eclampsia (pree-ee-KLAMP-see-uh) condition in which hypertension develops because of pregnancy or recent pregnancy. Hypertension is accompanied by proteinuria and/or edema / *page 194*

preload degree of stretch of the cardiac muscle fibers just before they contract / *page 292*

prn order Latin: *pro re nata;* physician's order; means "to administer as required by the patient's condition" / *page 28*

prodrugs drugs that become more active after they are metabolized / *page 49*

progesterone (pro-JESS-ter-own) hormone responsible for building up the uterine lining in the second half of the menstrual cycle and during pregnancy / *page 570*

prolactin (pro-LAK-tin) hormone secreted by the pituitary gland that stimulates milk production in the mammary glands / *page 582*

prostaglandins (pros-tah-GLAN-dins) chemicals released after tissue damage, leading to pain, inflammation, and other body reactions / *page 223*

prothrombin (PRO-throm-bin) blood protein converted to thrombin in the blood-clotting process / *page 321*

prothrombin time (PT) blood test used to determine the time needed for plasma to clot, used to regulate warfarin dosage / *page 325*

proton-pump inhibitor (PPI) drug that inhibits the enzyme H^+, K^+-ATPase / *page 510*

prototype drug (PRO-toh-type) an original, well-understood drug model from which other drugs in a pharmacologic class have been developed / *page 16*

protozoan (PRO-toh-ZOH-en) single-celled microorganism / *page 448*

provitamin an inactive chemical that is converted to a vitamin in the body / *page 529*

pruritus (proo-RYE-tus) itching associated with dry, scaly skin / *page 615*

psoralen (SOR-uh-len) drug used along with phototherapy for the treatment of psoriasis and other severe skin disorders / *page 625*

psychedelics (seye-keh-DEL-iks) substances that alter perception and reality / *page 83*

psychological dependence (seye-koh-LOJ-i-kul dee-PEN-dens) an unpleasant, intense craving for a drug after it has been withdrawn / *page 79*

purine (PYUR-een) building block of DNA and RNA, either adenine or guanine / *page 462*

Purkinje fibers (purr-KEN-gee FI-burrs) electrical conduction pathway leading from the bundle branches to all portions of the ventricles / *page 308*

pustules (PUSS-chools) inflammatory bumps with pus / *page 622*

pyrimidine (peer-IM-uh-deen) building block of DNA and RNA, either thymine or cytosine in DNA, and cytosine and uracil in RNA / *page 462*

reabsorption movement of substances from the kidney tubule back into the blood / *page 369*

rebound congestion a condition of hypersecretion of mucus following use of intranasal sympathomimetics / *page 491*

rebound insomnia increased sleeplessness that occurs when long-term antianxiety or hypnotic medication is discontinued / *page 117*

receptor (ree-SEP-tor) the structural component of a cell to which a drug binds in a dose-related manner to produce a response / *page 52*

receptor theory a cellular mechanism by which most drugs produce their effects / *page 52*

recommended dietary allowance (RDA) amount of vitamin or mineral needed daily to avoid a deficiency in a healthy adult / *page 530*

red-man syndrome rash on the upper body caused by certain anti-infectives / *page 424*

reflex tachycardia (ta-kee-CAR-dee-ah) temporary speeding up of heart rate that occurs when blood pressure falls / *page 272*

refractory period (ree-FRAK-tor-ee) time during which the myocardial cells rest and are not able to contract / *page 310*

releasing factors hormones secreted by the hypothalamus that affect secretions in the pituitary gland / *page 545*

renal failure decrease in the kidneys' ability to maintain electrolyte and fluid balance and excrete waste products / *page 370*

renin-angiotensin-aldosterone system (REN-in–an-geo-TEN-sin-al-DOS-ter-own) series of enzymatic steps by which the body raises blood pressure / *page 272*

respiration (res-purr-AY-shun) exchange of oxygen and carbon dioxide / *page 481*

restricted drug in Canada, a drug not intended for human use, covered in Part IV, Schedule H, of the Canadian Food and Drugs Act / *page 19*

reticular activating system (RAS) the brain structure that projects from the brainstem and thalamus to the cerebral cortex; responsible for sleeping and wakefulness and performs an alerting function / *page 115*

reticular formation (re-TIK-u-lurr) a network of neurons found along the entire length of the brainstem connected with the reticular activating system / *page 115*

retinoids (RETT-ih-noydz) vitamin A-like compounds used in the treatment of severe acne and psoriasis / *page 623*

retinol (RETT-in-nall) chemical name for vitamin A / *page 624*

reverse transcriptase (ree-VERS trans-CRIP-tace) viral enzyme that converts RNA to DNA / *page 442*

rheumatoid arthritis (RA) (ROO-mah-toyd are-THRYE-tis) systemic autoimmune disorder characterized by inflammation of multiple joints / *page 605*

rosacea (roh-ZAY-shee-uh) skin disorder characterized by clusters of papules / *page 622*

routine orders standard order usually carried out within 2 hours of the time it was written by the physician / *page 28*

salicylism (sal-IH-sill-izm) poisoning due to aspirin and aspirin-like drugs / *page 391*

scabicides (SKAY-bih-sides) drugs that kill scabies and mites / *page 619*

scabies (SKAY-beez) skin disorder caused by the female mite burrowing into the skin and laying eggs / *page 619*

scheduled drugs in the United States, a term describing a drug placed into one of five categories (I through V) based on its potential for misuse or abuse / *page 18*

schizoaffective disorder (SKIT-soh-ah-FEK-tiv) disorder with symptoms similar to schizophrenia and mood disorders / *page 154*

schizophrenia (SKIT-soh-FREN-ee-uh) type of psychosis characterized by abnormal thoughts and thought processes, withdrawal from other people and the outside environment, and apparent preoccupation with one's own mental state / *page 154*

seborrhea (seb-oh-REE-ah) condition characterized by overactivity of oil glands / *page 621*

secondary hypertension high blood pressure caused as a result of another disorder / *page 268*

secretion movement of substances from the blood into the kidney tubule after filtration has occurred / *page 369*

sedative-hypnotic (SED-ah-tiv hip-NOT-ik) drug that produces a calming effect when given in lower doses, and produces sleep when given in higher doses / *page 117*

sedatives (SED-ah-tivs) drugs that relax or calm the patient / *page 117*

seizure (SEE-zhurr) symptom of epilepsy characterized by abnormal neuronal discharges within the brain / *page 192*

selective estrogen-receptor modulators (SERMS) drugs that directly produce an action similar to estrogen in body tissues; used for the treatment of osteoporosis in postmenopausal women / *page 601*

selective serotonin-reuptake inhibitors (SSRIs) (sir-eh-TO-nin) drugs that selectively inhibit the reuptake of serotonin into nerve terminals / *page 135*

septic shock (SEP-tik) type of shock caused by severe infection in the bloodstream / *page 355*

serotonin-norepinephrine reuptake inhibitors (SNRIs) drugs that block the recycling of two neurotransmitters, serotonin and norepinephrine / *page 136*

serotonin syndrome (SES) a set of signs and symptoms associated with overmedication with antidepressants / *page 136*

shock condition in which there is inadequate blood flow to meet the body's needs / *page 355*

single order a physician's order for a drug that is to be given only once and at a specific time; an example is a preoperative order / *page 28*

sinoatrial (SA) node (si-no-AYE-tree-ul noad) pacemaker of the heart located in the wall of the right atrium / *page 308*

sinus rhythm (SI-nuss) number of beats per minute normally generated by the SA node / *page 308*

six rights of drug administration practical guidelines for nurses to use during drug preparation, delivery, and administration of drugs / *page 26*

sodium ion channel (SO-dee-um) pathway in a plasma membrane through which sodium ions enter and leave / *page 309*

somatotropin (so-mat-oh-TROH-pin) another name for growth hormone / *page 564*

spasticity (spas-TISS-ih-tee) condition in which certain muscle groups remain in a continuous contracted state / *page 182*

specialty supplement a nonherbal dietary supplement used to enhance body functions / *page 67*

stable angina type of angina that occurs in a predictable pattern, usually relieved by rest / *page 339*

standing order a physician's order written in advance of a situation, which is to be carried out under specific circumstances / *page 28*

STAT order comes from *statim,* the Latin word meaning "immediately"; the time frame between writing the STAT order and administering the drug may be 5 minutes or less, depending on facility rules / *page 27*

status asthmaticus (STAT-us az-MAT-ik-us) acute form of asthma requiring immediate medical attention / *page 493*

status epilepticus (ep-ih-LEP-tih-kus) condition characterized by repeated seizures / *page 195*

stepped care a systematic approach to treatment of hypertension / *page 273*

steroid (STAIR-oyd) type of lipid that consists of four rings and comprises certain hormones and drugs / *page 251*

steroid nucleus (STAIR-od NUK-lee-us) ring structure common to all steroids / *page 251*

subcutaneous (SC or SQ) route (sub-kew-TAY-nee-us) method of parenteral drug delivery in which drugs are injected into the hypodermis of the skin / *page 38*

sublingual (SL) route (sub-LIN-gwal) method of enteral drug delivery in which drugs are placed under the tongue / *page 31*

substance P neurotransmitter within the spinal cord involved in the neural transmission of pain / *page 212*

superficial mycoses fungal diseases of the hair, skin, nails, and mucous membranes / *page 435*

superinfection condition caused when a microorganism grows rapidly as a result of having less competition in its environment / *page 412*

supraventricular (sue-prah-ven-TRIK-you-lur) lying above the ventricles or in the atria / *page 307*

sustained-release tablets or capsules that are designed to dissolve very slowly / *page 30*

sympathetic nervous system (SIM-pah-THET-ik) portion of the autonomic system that is active during periods of stress and which produces the fight-or-flight response / *page 93*

sympatholytic (SIM-path-oh-LIT-ik) a drug that blocks the actions of the sympathetic nervous system / *page 97*

sympathomimetic (SIM-path-oh-mih-MET-ik) a drug that mimics the actions of the sympathetic nervous system / *page 97*

systemic mycoses fungal diseases affecting internal organs / *page 435*

systolic pressure (SIS-tol-ik) blood pressure during the contraction phase of heart activity / *page 269*

T cell type of lymphocyte that is essential for the cell-mediated immune response / *page 395*

tardive dyskinesia (TAR-div dis-ki-NEE-zee-uh) involuntary movements of facial muscles and the tongue that occur due to long-term antipsychotic therapy / *page 157*

taxanel a type of drug that blocks cell growth by stopping mitosis / *page 464*

tension headache common type of head pain caused by stress and relieved by nonnarcotic analgesics / *page 225*

tetrahydrocannabinol (THC) (TEH-trah-HEYE-droh-cah-NAB-in-ol) the active chemical in marijuana / *page 83*

therapeutic classification (ther-ah-PEW-tik) method for organizing drugs on the basis of their *therapeutic usefulness* / *page 15*

therapeutic lifestyle changes nondrug changes which, when implemented, can reduce blood cholesterol levels / *page 254*

therapeutics (ther-ah-PEW-tiks) the branch of medicine concerned with the treatment of disease and suffering / *page 4*

three checks of drug administration checks used by nurses together with the six rights to help ensure patient safety and drug effectiveness / *page 26*

thrombin (THROM-bin) enzyme formed in coagulating blood from prothrombin; it converts fibrinogen to fibrin, which forms the basis of a blood clot / *page 321*

thromboembolic disorders (THROM-bow-EM-bow-lik) diseases associated with the formation of blood clots / *page 323*

thrombolytics (throm-bow-LIT-iks) drugs used to dissolve existing blood clots / *page 324*

thrombotic stroke (throm-BOT-ik) type of stroke caused by a blood clot blocking an artery in the brain / *page 349*

thrombus (THROM-bus) blood clot / *page 324*

tissue plasminogen activator (tPA) natural enzyme and a drug that dissolves blood clots / *page 323*

titer (TIE-ter) measurement of the amount of a substance in the blood / *page 396*

tocolytic (toh-koh-LIT-ik) drug used to inhibit uterine contractions / *page 583*

tolerance (TOL-er-ans) the process of adapting to a drug over time and requiring higher doses to achieve the same effect / *page 80*

tonometry (toh-NAHM-uh-tree) technique for measuring eye tension and pressure / *page 633*

topical route (TOP-ik-ul) the route by which drugs are placed directly onto the skin and associated membranes / *page 32*

topoisomerase (TOH-poh-eye-SOM-er-ase) enzyme that assists in the repair of DNA damage / *page 464*

total parenteral nutrition (TPN) treatment of undernutrition through the parenteral infusion of dextrose, amino acids, emulsified fats, vitamins, and minerals / *page 538*

toxin (TOX-in) chemical produced by a microorganism that is able to cause injury to its host / *page 408*

toxoid (TOX-oid) toxin that has been chemically modified to remove its harmful nature but is still able to cause an immune response in the body / *page 396*

trace mineral inorganic compound needed by the body in amounts of 20 mg or less daily / *page 532*

trade name proprietary name of a drug assigned by the manufacturer; also called the *brand name* or *product name* / *page 17*

transdermal (trans-DER-mul) method of drug delivery, usually by a patch, in which drugs are absorbed across the layers of the skin for the purpose of entering the bloodstream / *page 33*

transmucosal (trans-mew-KOH-sul) method of topical drug delivery in which drugs are applied directly to mucosal membranes, including the nasal and respiratory pathways and vagina / *page 33*

transplant rejection when the immune system recognizes a transplanted tissue as being foreign and attacks it / *page 400*

tricyclic antidepressants (TCAs) (treye-SICK-lick) drugs with a three-ring chemical structure that inhibit the reuptake of norepinephrine and serotonin into nerve terminals / *page 132*

triglyceride (tri-GLISS-ur-ide) type of lipid that contains three fatty acids and a chemical backbone of glycerol / *page 251*

tubercles (TOO-burr-kyouls) cavity-like lesions in the lung characteristic of infection by *Mycobacterium tuberculosis* / *page 426*

tumor (TOO-more) abnormal swelling or mass / *page 456*

tumor suppressor genes genes that inhibit the transformation of normal cells into cancer cells / *page 457*

ulcerative colitis (UL-sir-ah-tiv koh-LIE-tuss) inflammatory bowel disease of the colon / *page 510*

undernutrition taking in or absorbing fewer nutrients than required for normal body growth and maintenance / *page 537*

unstable angina type of angina that occurs frequently with severe symptoms and which is not relieved by rest / *page 339*

vaccine (vaks-EEN) preparation of microorganism particles that is injected into a patient to stimulate the immune system with the intention of preventing disease / *page 396*

vaccination/immunization (VAK-sin-AYE-shun/IH-mewn-ize-AYE-shun) receiving a vaccine or toxoid to prevent disease / *page 396*

vasomotor center (VAZO-mo-tor) area of the medulla that controls baseline blood pressure / *page 271*

vasopressin (vaz-oh-PRESS-in) another name for antidiuretic hormone / *page 564*

vasospastic (Prinzmetal's) angina type of angina in which decreased myocardial blood flow is caused by *spasms* of the coronary arteries / *page 339*

ventilation (ven-tah-LAY-shun) process by which air is moved into and out of the lungs / *page 482*

very low-density lipoprotein (VLDL) lipid-carrying particle that is converted to LDL in the liver / *page 253*

vinca alkaloids (VIN-ka AL-kah-loids) chemicals obtained from the periwinkle plant / *page 464*

virulence (VEER-you-lens) the severity of disease that an organism in able to cause / *page 407*

virulization (veer-you-lih-ZAY-shun) appearance of masculine secondary sex characteristics / *page 584*

virus nonliving particle containing RNA or DNA that is able to cause disease / *page 438*

vitamins organic compounds required by the body in small amounts / *page 529*

withdrawal syndrome (with-DRAW-ul SIN-drom) unpleasant symptoms experienced when a physically dependent client discontinues the use of an abused drug / *page 79*

yeast (YEEST) type of fungus that is unicellular and divides by budding / *page 434*

Zollinger-Ellison syndrome (ZOLL-in-jer ELL-ih-sun) disorder of having excess acid secretion in the stomach / *page 513*

INDEX

Page numbers followed by *f* indicate figures and those followed by *t* indicate tables, boxes, or special features. The titles of special features (e.g., Life Span Facts, Nursing Process Focus) are also capitalized.

Profile drugs appear in **boldface**, drug classifications are in SMALL CAPS, and trade names are capitalized and cross-referenced to their generic name. Disease, disorders, and conditions are in purple type.

5-FU. *See* fluorouracil
5-HT (serotonin), 135
6-MP. *See* mercaptopurine
6-TG. *See* thioguanine

A

abacavir, 440*t*
abbreviations, drug administration, 27*t*
abciximab, 324*f*, 328*t*
Abilify. *See* aripiprazole
Abreva. *See* docosanol
absence seizures, 195, 196*t*, 200, 205. *See also* seizure(s)
absorption, 48*f*, 49
acamprosate calcium, 82
acarbose, 552*t*
Accolate. *See* zafirlukast
Accupril. *See* quinapril
ACE (angiotensin-converting enzyme), 279
ACE (angiotensin-converting enzyme) inhibitors. *See* ANGIOTENSIN-CONVERTING ENZYME (ACE) INHIBITORS
acebutolol:
    actions, 106*t*
    clinical uses, 106*t*
        angina and myocardial infarction, 343*t*
        dysrhythmias, 313*t*
        hypertension, 284*t*
    route and adult dose, 284*t*
Aceon. *See* perindopril
acetaminophen:
    clinical uses, 221*t*, 223
    Drug Profile, 222*t*
    Nursing Process Focus, 224*t*
    route and adult dose, 221*t*
acetazolamide, 375, 375*t*, 636*t*
acetic acid and hydrocortisone, 642*t*
acetohexamide, 552*t*
acetylcholine (Ach), 96, 97*t*, 177*f*
acetylcholine chloride, 634, 634*t*
acetylcholinesterase (AchE), 176, 177*f*
ACETYLCHOLINESTERASE INHIBITORS:
    adverse effects, 176
    for Alzheimer's disease, 176–77, 176*t*, 177*f*
    drugs classified as, 98*t*, 176*t*
acetylcysteine, 493
Acetylsalicylic acid. *See* **aspirin**
Achromycin. *See* **tetracycline**
acid-base imbalances, 379–80, 380*t*, 381*f*
acidosis, 379–80, 380*t*, 381*f*
AcipHex. *See* rabeprazole sodium
acitretin, 625, 626*t*
Aclovate. *See* alclometasone
acne, 621–23, 622*t*, 625*t*
Acova. *See* argatroban
acquired resistance, 410, 411*f*
ACTH (adrenocorticotropic hormone), 558
ActHIB. *See* *Haemophilus influenza* type B conjugate vaccine

Acticin. *See* **permethrin**
Actifed. *See* pseudoephedrine
Actifed Cold and Allergy, 487*t*
action potential, 200, 308
Actiq. *See* fentanyl citrate
Activase. *See* **alteplase**
activated partial thromboplastin time (aPTT), 325
active immunity, 396, 398*f*
Actonel. *See* risedronate sodium
Actos. *See* pioglitazone
Actron. *See* ketoprofen
Acuprin. *See* **aspirin**
acute glaucoma, 632*f*, 633
acute gouty arthritis, 608
acute radiation syndrome, 557
acyclovir:
    Drug Profile, 447*t*
    pregnancy category, 20*t*
    route and adult dose, 441*t*
Adalat. *See* nifedipine
adalimumab, 606*t*
adapalene, 622*t*, 623
(ADD) attention deficit disorder, 85
Adderall. *See* d- and l-amphetamine racemic mixture
addiction, 18, 78–79. *See also* substance abuse
Addison's disease, 560
adefovir, 448
Aδ fibers, 212
Adenocard. *See* adenosine
adenoma(s), 456
Adenoscan. *See* adenosine
adenosine, 316*t*, 317
adenosine diphosphate (ADP) receptor blockers, 328, 328*t*
ADH (antidiuretic hormone; vasopressin), 272, 545*t*, 564
ADHD. *See* attention deficit hyperactivity disorder
adjuvant chemotherapy, 458
adrenal disorders, 545*t*
adrenal gland(s), 272*f*, 544*f*, 546*f*, 559*f*, 561
Adrenalin. *See* **epinephrine**
adrenergic, 96
ADRENERGIC BLOCKERS (sympatholytics):
    actions, 97, 97*t*, 106, 294*f*
    clinical uses, 106, 106*t*
        angina and myocardial infarction, 343*t*
        anxiety, 123, 124*t*
        heart failure, 296*t*
        hypertension, 283–85, 284*t*
    drugs classified as, 106*t*, 284*t*, 343*t*
    Nursing Process Focus, 107–8*t*
    Patients Need to Know, 109*t*
adrenergic drugs. *See* SYMPATHOMIMETICS
adrenocorticotropic hormone (ACTH), 558
Adriamycin. *See* **doxorubicin**
Adsorbocarpine. *See* pilocarpine

Advicor, 261
Advil. *See* ibuprofen
AEB (as evidenced by), 60
AeroBid. *See* flunisolide
Aeroseb-HC. *See* **hydrocortisone**
aerosol, 483
Afluria. *See* influenza, vaccine
African Americans, antihypertension therapy in, 273
Afrin. *See* **oxymetazoline**
Aftate. *See* tolnaftate
afterload, 292, 341
age-onset diabetes, 549. *See also* diabetes mellitus
Aggrastat. *See* tirofiban
agonist(s), 53, 53*f*
agoraphobia, 114
akathisia, 157, 157*t*
Akineton. *See* biperiden
Albalon. *See* naphazoline
albendazole, 449*t*, 451
Albenza. *See* albendazole
Albuminar. *See* **normal serum albumin**
Albutein. *See* **normal serum albumin**
albuterol:
    actions, 104*t*
    clinical uses, 101, 104*t*
        asthma, 496*t*
        shock, 363
alclometasone, 624*t*
alcohol:
    abuse of, 77*t*, 82
    cross-tolerance, 80
    metabolism, 82
    Patients Need to Know, 87*t*
    withdrawal syndrome, 80*t*, 82
alcohol intoxication, 82
Aldactone. *See* **spironolactone**
aldesleukin, 399, 470
Aldomet. *See* methyldopa
aldosterone, 280, 375*t*
alemtuzumab, 471*t*
alendronate:
    Drug Profile, 603*t*
    route and adult dose, 602*t*
Alesse, 573*t*
Aleve. *See* **naproxen sodium**
Alfenta. *See* alfentanil hydrochloride
alfentanil hydrochloride, 242*t*, 243*t*
alimentary canal, 507
Alimta. *See* pemetrexed
alkalosis, 379–80, 380*t*, 381*f*
Alka-Seltzer, 512*t*
Alkeran. *See* melphalan
ALKYLATING AGENTS, 461, 462*t*, 463*f*
alkylation, 461
Allegra. *See* fexofenadine
Allerdryl. *See* **diphenhydramine**
Allerest. *See* naphazoline

adjunct to anesthesia, 243*t*
intravenous anesthetic, 242*t*
sedation and insomnia, 122–23, 123*t*
seizures, 198–200, 198*t*
drugs classified as, 123*t*, 198*t*, 242*t*, 243*t*
interactions
with clopidogrel, 330*t*
with herbal products, 71*t*
with hydrocortisone, 562*t*
with lidocaine, 237*t*
with prednisone, 394*t*
tolerance, 122
withdrawal syndrome, 80*t*
baroreceptors, 271, 272*f*
basal metabolic rate, 555
baseline data, 58
basiliximab, 400*t*
Bayer aspirin. *See* **aspirin**
BCG (bacille Calmette-Guérin) vaccine, 399
beclomethasone:
inhaled, 499*t*
intranasal, 490*t*
Beconase AQ. *See* beclomethasone
behavioral insomnia, 116
Benadryl. *See* **diphenhydramine**
Benadryl Allergy/Cold, 487*t*
Benahist. *See* **diphenhydramine**
benazepril, 279*t*
bendamustine, 462*t*
bendroflumethiazide and nadolol, 373*t*
Bendylate. *See* **diphenhydramine**
Benemid. *See* probenecid
Benicar. *See* olmesartan
benign prostatic hyperplasia (BPH), 571*t*,
586–87, 587*f*
benign tumors, 456
Bentyl. *See* dicyclomine
Benzaclin. *See* benzoyl peroxide
Benzamycin. *See* benzoyl peroxide
benzocaine:
Drug Profile, 621*t*
as local anesthetic, 236, 236*t*
for sunburn and minor skin irritation, 621
benzocaine and antipyrine, 642*t*
BENZODIAZEPINES, 120
abuse of, 81
actions, 120
adverse effects, 120
chemical structure, 120
clinical uses, 122
anxiety and insomnia, 120*t*, 122
bipolar disorder, 144
intravenous anesthetic, 242*t*
muscle relaxation, 181*t*, 182
seizures, 196*t*, 198*t*, 200
drugs classified as, 120*t*, 198*t*, 242*t*
interactions
with fluoxetine, 141*t*
with herbal products, 71*t*
parenteral administration, 120
Patients Need to Know, 126*t*
withdrawal syndrome, 80*t*
benzonatate, 493
benzoyl peroxide, 622, 622*t*
benztropine:
clinical uses, 101*t*, 157, 173*t*, 175*t*

Drug Profile, 175*t*
route and adult dose, 173*t*
bepridil, 343*t*
BETA (β) BLOCKERS, 106, 106*t*. *See also*
ADRENERGIC BLOCKERS
actions, 274*f*, 341*f*
adverse effects, 345
clinical uses
angina and myocardial infarction, 341,
343*t*, 345, 349
anxiety, 124, 124*t*
dysrhythmias, 313, 313*t*
glaucoma, 635–36, 636*t*
heart failure, 296*t*, 299–300
hypertension, 284*t*
migraine prophylaxis, 226*t*
drugs classified as, 106*t*, 284*t*, 313*t*, 343*t*
interactions, 159*t*
with amiodarone, 315*t*
with aspirin, 222*t*
with digoxin, 299*t*
with diltiazem, 346*t*
with dopamine, 361*t*
with epinephrine, 362*t*
with fluoxetine, 141*t*
with haloperidol, 159*t*
with insulin, 548*t*
with lidocaine, 237*t*
with norepinephrine, 361*t*
Patients Need to Know, 317*t*
beta (β) receptors, 96, 97*t*
BETA-ADRENERGIC AGENTS, 484*f*, 495–97, 496*t*
Betagan. *See* levobunolol
beta-lactam ring, 412
beta-lactamase, 412
betamethasone, 393*t*, 562*t*, 624*t*
Betapace. *See* sotalol
Betapace AF. *See* sotalol
Betaseron. *See* interferon beta-1b
betaxolol, 284*t*, 636*t*
bethanechol:
clinical uses, 99*t*, 243*t*, 245
Drug Profile, 99*t*
Betimol. *See* timolol
Betoptic. *See* betaxolol
bevacizumab, 471*t*
Bextra. *See* valdecoxib
BGTD (Biologic and Genetic Therapies
Directorate), 10
Biaxin. *See* clarithromycin
bicalutamide, 469*t*
Bicillin. *See* penicillin G benzathine
BiCNU. *See* carmustine
BiDil, 273, 276*t*, 300
BIGUANIDES, 552*t*
bilberry, 68*t*
BILE ACID-BINDING AGENTS:
actions, 261*f*, 267
adverse effects, 257
drugs classified as, 257*t*
Patients Need to Know, 262*t*
bile acids, 257
Biltricide. *See* praziquantel
bimatoprost, 634*t*, 635
binding, 49
bioavailability, 18, 49

BioCal. *See* calcium carbonate
Biologic and Genetic Therapies Directorate
(BGTD), 10
BIOLOGIC RESPONSE MODIFIERS, 396, 399,
470–71, 471*t*
biologic therapies, 66*t*. *See also* herbal
products; Natural Therapies
biologics, 4, 4*t*
Biologics Control Act, 5, 6*t*
bioterrorism, 10–11
anthrax, 397, 399, 420
nerve agents, 98
biotin (vitamin B₇), 531*t*
biotransformation, 49
biperiden, 173*t*
bipolar disorder, 142
pharmacotherapy, 143–45, 144*t*
symptoms, 143
bisacodyl, 517*t*
bismuth salts, 515, 519*t*, 520
bisoprolol, 284*t*
BISPHOSPHONATES:
drugs classified as, 602*t*
for osteoporosis, 602–3
for Paget's disease, 602–3
bitter melon, 553*t*
bivalirudin, 325, 325*t*
black box warning, 118, 140
black cohosh:
interactions, 579*t*
labeling, 72*f*
primary uses, 68*t*
standardization, 69*t*
blackheads, 622
Blastomyces dermatitidis, 435*t*
Blenoxane. *See* bleomycin
bleomycin, 466*t*
Blocadren. *See* timolol
blockers (antagonists), 53, 53*f*. *See also*
ADRENERGIC BLOCKERS
alpha (α), 106, 106*t*
beta. *See* beta (β) blockers
blood-brain barrier, 49
blood-placental barrier, 49
blood pressure. *See also* hypertension
control of, 271–72, 271*f*, 272*f*
diastolic, 269
factors affecting, 270–71, 270*f*
physiology, 269–70, 269*f*
systolic, 269, 270*f*
variations through the life span, 268*t*
BLOOD PRODUCTS, 358–59, 358*t*
blood-testicular barrier, 49
blood volume, 271
bone deposition, 585
bone resorption, 585
Bonine. *See* meclizine
Boniva. *See* ibandronate sodium
boosters, 396
Borrelia burgdorferi, 408*t*
botanical, 67. *See also* herbal products
Botox. *See* botulinum toxin A
botulinum toxin, 184, 185*f*
botulinum toxin A, 185*t*
botulinum toxin B, 185*t*
Bowman's capsule, 368

multiple sclerosis. *See* multiple sclerosis
Parkinson's disease. *See* Parkinson's disease
neurofibrillary tangles, 175
neurogenic shock, 355, 355t. *See also* shock
neurolept anesthesia, 241
neuroleptic(s), 156. *See also* ANTIPSYCHOTICS
neuroleptic malignant syndrome, 157t, 158t
NEUROMUSCULAR BLOCKING AGENTS:
    actions, 185f, 186, 245
    classification, 186
    clinical uses, 186–87
        as adjunct to anesthetics, 243t, 245
    drugs classified as, 187t, 243t
    Patients Need to Know, 187t
neuron, 94, 95f
Neurontin. *See* gabapentin
neuropathic pain, 210–11
neurotransmitter(s), 94
    false, 285
    in pain transmission, 212, 213f
    receptors, 53f
Neutra-Phos-K. *See* potassium/sodium phosphates
Neutrogena. *See* salicylic acid
Neuvil. *See* ibuprofen
nevirapine, 440t
new drug application (NDA), 8–9, 8f
Nexium. *See* esomeprazole
NF (National Formulary), 5, 6t
Niac. *See* niacin
niacin (vitamin B₃), 531t
    as lipid-lowering agent, 257t, 259–60, 261f, 262t
nicardipine, 276t, 343t
Nicobid. *See* niacin
nicotinamide, 260
nicotine:
    dependence, 87
    effects, 87
    Patients Need to Know, 87t
    withdrawal syndrome, 80t
nicotinic, 96
nicotinic acid. *See* niacin
nicotinic blocking agents, 186
nicotinic receptors, 96, 97t
nifedipine:
    actions, 274f, 277t
    clinical uses, 277t
        angina and myocardial infarction, 343t
        hypertension, 276t
        migraine prophylaxis, 226t
        as tocolytic, 584t
    Drug Profile, 277t
    interactions, 277t
        with calcium supplements, 63t
nifurtimox, 449t
Nilandron. *See* nilutamide
nilutamide, 469t
Nimbex. *See* cisatracurium
nimodipine, 226t
Nimotop. *See* nimodipine
Nipent. *See* pentostatin
Nisocor. *See* nisoldipine
nisoldipine, 276t
Nitro-Bid. *See* **nitroglycerin**
Nitro-Dur. *See* **nitroglycerin**

nitrofurantoin, 423t, 517t
nitrogen mustards, 461, 462t
nitroglycerin:
    actions and uses, 341f, 342, 342t
    Drug Profile, 342t
    Nursing Process Focus, 344t
    Patients Need to Know, 351t
Nitropress. *See* nitroprusside
nitroprusside, 286, 286t
nitrosoureas, 462t
Nitrostat. *See* **nitroglycerin**
nitrous oxide:
    clinical uses, 240, 240t
    contraindications, 241
    Drug Profile, 240t
    interaction with succinylcholine, 244t
nits, 619
Nix. *See* **permethrin**
nizatidine, 512t
Nizoral. *See* ketoconazole
NMDA (*N*-methyl-D-aspartate) receptors, 177
N-methyl-D-aspartate (NMDA) receptors, 177
NNRTIs (NONNUCLEOSIDE REVERSE TRANSCRIPTASE INHIBITORS), 440t, 443
nociceptor pain, 210, 223, 223f
NoDoz, 86t
NONBENZODIAZEPINE, NONBARBITURATE CNS AGENTS:
    for anxiety and insomnia, 123, 124t, 125
    drugs classified as, 124t
noncompliance, 26, 27t, 63t
nondepolarizing blockers, 186, 187t. *See also* NEUROMUSCULAR BLOCKING AGENTS
NONNUCLEOSIDE REVERSE TRANSCRIPTASE INHIBITORS (NNRTIs), 440t, 443
NONOPIOID ANALGESICS:
    acetaminophen. *See* **acetaminophen**
    centrally acting, 221t, 223
    nonsteroidal anti-inflammatory drugs. *See* NONSTEROIDAL ANTI-INFLAMMATORY DRUGS
NONPHENOTHIAZINES:
    actions, 157–59
    adverse effects, 157t, 158
    drugs classified as, 158t
    Nursing Process Focus, 160–61t
NONSTEROIDAL ANTI-INFLAMMATORY DRUGS (NSAIDs):
    actions, 220, 223
    adverse effects, 220
    drugs classified as
        ibuprofen and ibuprofen-like drugs, 221t, 390t, 391
        salicylates, 221t, 390, 390t
        selective COX-2 inhibitors, 221t, 223, 223f, 390t, 391
    interactions
        with alteplase, 331t
        with aspirin, 222t
        with cefotaxime, 416t
        with enalapril, 282t
        with herbal products, 71t
        with hydralazine, 285t
        with hydrocortisone, 562t
        with methotrexate, 466t
        with warfarin, 329t
    Nursing Process Focus, 224t, 392–93t

Patients Need to Know, 402t
    usage statistics, 387t
Norcuron. *See* vecuronium
Nordryl. *See* **diphenhydramine**
norepinephrine (NE), 96
    actions, 104t
    clinical uses, 104t
    Drug Profile, 361t
norethindrone, 20t, 578t
norethindrone acetate, 578t
Norflex. *See* orphenadrine citrate
norfloxacin, 420t
Norgesic. *See* aspirin
Norlutin. *See* norethindrone
normal serum albumin, Drug Profile, 358t
Noroxin. *See* norfloxacin
Norpace. *See* disopyramide
Norplant, 574
Norpramin. *See* desipramine
Nor-Q.D., 573t
North American Nursing Diagnosis Association (NANDA), 59
nortriptyline, 119t, 133t
Norvasc. *See* amlodipine
Norvir. *See* ritonavir
nosocomial infections, 410
Notice of Compliance (NOC), 10
Novantrone. *See* mitoxantrone
Novastan. *See* argatroban
Novocaine. *See* procaine
Novolin L. *See* insulin zinc suspension
Novolin N. *See* isophane insulin suspension
Novolin R. *See* **regular insulin**
Novoprofen. *See* ibuprofen
Novopropamide. *See* chlorpropamide
NPH. *See* isophane insulin suspension
NPH Iletin II. *See* isophane insulin suspension
NSAIDs. *See* NONSTEROIDAL ANTI-INFLAMMATORY DRUGS
Nubain. *See* nalbuphine hydrochloride
NUCLEOSIDE REVERSE TRANSCRIPTASE INHIBITORS (NRTIs), 440t, 442
NUCLEOTIDE REVERSE TRANSCRIPTASE INHIBITORS (NtRTIs), 440t, 442
Numorphan. *See* oxymorphone hydrochloride
Nupercainal. *See* dibucaine
Nupercaine. *See* dibucaine
Nuprin. *See* ibuprofen
Nuromax. *See* doxacurium
nurse(s), substance abuse in, 88
nursing diagnosis, 59–60, 59t
nursing process, 58, 58f
    assessment, 58–59
    diagnosis, 59–60, 59t
    evaluation phase, 62–63
    implementation, 61–62, 62f
    planning, 60–61
Nursing Process Focus:
    ACE inhibitor therapy, 280–82t
    acetaminophen, 224t
    adrenergic blocker therapy, 107–8t
    antianxiety therapy, 121t
    antibacterial therapy, 424–25t
    anticholinergic therapy, 102–3t
    anticoagulant therapy, 326–27t
    antidepressant therapy, 137–39t
    antidysrhythmic drugs, 311t

SPECIAL FEATURES

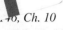

SPECIAL FEATURES

711

SPECIAL FEATURES

711

SPECIAL FEATURES

711

.0, *Ch. 10*

Allergies, *p. 486, Ch. 28*

Alternative Therapies in America, *p. 67, Ch. 6*

Anesthesia and Anesthetics, *p. 233, Ch. 15*

Angina Pectoris and Coronary Heart Disease, *p. 340, Ch. 21*

Anxiety Disorders, *p. 114, Ch. 9*

Arthritis and Joint Disorders, *p. 607, Ch. 33*

Asthma, *p. 495, Ch. 28*

Bacterial Infections, *p. 406, Ch. 25*

Cancer, *p. 455, Ch. 27*

Cerebrovascular Accident, *p. 350, Ch. 21*

Clotting Disorders, *p. 323, Ch. 20*

Diabetes Mellitus, *p. 547, Ch. 31*

Dysrhythmias, *p. 306, Ch. 19*

Epilepsy, *p. 193, Ch. 13*

Fungal, Viral, and Parasitic Diseases, *p. 434, Ch. 26*

Gastrointestinal Tract Disorders, *p. 506, Ch. 29*

Glaucoma, *p. 633, Ch. 35*

Grapefruit Juice and Drug Interactions, *p. 27, Ch. 3*

Heart Failure, *p. 291, Ch. 18*

High Blood Cholesterol, *p. 251, Ch. 16*

Hypertension, *p. 269, Ch. 17*

Inflammatory and Allergic Disorders, *p. 387, Ch. 24*

Insomnia, *p. 116, Ch. 9*

Muscle Spasms, *p. 180, Ch. 12*

Myocardial Infarction, *p. 348, Ch. 21*

Neurodegenerative Diseases, *p. 170, Ch. 12*

Pain, *p. 211, Ch. 14*

Potentially Fatal Drug Reactions, *p. 27, Ch. 3*

Psychosis, *p. 153, Ch. 11*

Renal Disorders, *p. 368, Ch. 23*

Reproductive Conditions and Disorders, *p. 571, Ch. 32*

Shock, *p. 356, Ch. 22*

Skin Disorders, *p. 617, Ch. 34*

Substance Abuse in the United States, *p. 77, Ch. 7*

Thyroid Disorders, *p. 557, Ch. 31*

Vaccines and Organ Transplants, *p. 399, Ch. 24*

Vitamins, Minerals, and Dietary Supplements, *p. 529, Ch. 30*

► Life Span Fact

Absorption of Food Diminishes with Age, *p. 531, Ch. 30*

ADHD in Children, *p. 145, Ch. 10*

Administering Ophthalmic Drugs to Children, *p. 33, Ch. 3*

Administering Otic Drugs to Children, *p. 33, Ch. 3*

Anticholinergic Side Effects in Older Adults, *p. 313, Ch. 19*

Benign Prostatic Hypertrophy in Older Men, *p. 587, Ch. 32*

Bleeding Complications in Elderly Patients, *p. 325, Ch. 20*

Bone Mass Decreases About 3–5% per Decade After Age 40, *p. 533, Ch. 30*

Breastfeeding May Contribute to Vitamin D Deficiency, *p. 532, Ch. 30*

Childhood Vaccine Act, *p. 6, Ch. 1*

Constipation in Older Adults, *p. 516, Ch. 29*

Control of Blood Pressure in Elderly Patients, *p. 273, Ch. 17*

Crushing Medications for Children and Elderly Patients, *p. 30, Ch. 3*

Depression in Elderly Patients, *p. 130, Ch. 10*

Drug Compliance Among Elderly Patients, *p. 27, Ch. 3*

Elderly Patients May Need Vitamin D Supplements, *p. 532, Ch. 30*

Elderly Patients with Poor-fitting Dentures May Require Nutritional Supplements, *p. 537, Ch. 30*

Epilepsy in Youth and Elderly, *p. 194, Ch. 13*

Erectile Dysfunction in Older Adults, *p. 585, Ch. 32*

Herbs and Dietary Supplements for Elderly Patients, *p. 68, Ch. 6*

High Fever in Children, *p. 195, Ch. 13*

IM Injections in Pediatric Patients, *p. 41, Ch. 3*

Laxative Misuse in Older Adults, *p. 517, Ch. 29*

Medication-related Sleeping Problems in Elderly Patients, *p. 116, Ch. 9*

Nonadherence, *p. 63, Ch. 5*

Older Adults at Particular Risk for Dehydration, *p. 274, Ch. 17*

Potassium Channel Blocker Side Effects in Older Adults, *p. 315, Ch. 19*

Potential Vitamin Deficiency in Infancy and Childhood, *p. 530, Ch. 30*

Reduced Metabolic Enzyme Activity in Very Young and Elderly Patients, *p. 51, Ch. 4*

TCA Use in Elderly Patients, *p. 134, Ch. 10*

Ventrogluteal Site for IM Injections in Children, *p. 41, Ch. 3*

NATURAL THERAPIES

NURSING PROCESS FOCUS

PATIENTS NEED TO KNOW

SAFETY ALERT